Principles of Nutritional Assessment

PRINCIPLES OF NUTRITIONAL ASSESSMENT

Second Edition

Rosalind S. Gibson

Professor of Human Nutrition
University of Otago
Dunedin, New Zealand

OXFORD
UNIVERSITY PRESS
2005

OXFORD
UNIVERSITY PRESS

Oxford University Press, Inc., publishes works that further
Oxford University's objective of excellence
in research, scholarship, and education.

Oxford   New York
Auckland   Cape Town   Dar es Salaam   Hong Kong   Karachi
Kuala Lumpur   Madrid   Melbourne   Mexico City   Nairobi
New Delhi   Shanghai   Taipei   Toronto

With offices in
Argentina   Austria   Brazil   Chile   Czech Republic   France   Greece
Guatemala   Hungary   Italy   Japan   Poland   Portugal   Singapore
South Korea   Switzerland   Thailand   Turkey   Ukraine   Vietnam

Published by Oxford University Press, Inc.
198 Madison Avenue, New York, New York 10016
http://www.oup.com

Library of Congress Cataloging-in-Publication Data
Gibson, Rosalind S.
Principles of nutritional assessment / Rosalind S. Gibson. – 2nd ed.
p. cm.
Includes bibliographical references and index.
ISBN-13 978-0-19-517169-3

1. Nutrition–Evaluation. I. Title
RC621.G52 2005
613.2–dc22   2004054778

Typeset in Adobe Times Roman 11/12, with headings in Optima; figures are annotated in
Adobe Helvetica. The text was prepared using Professor Donald E. Knuth's program TEX
and Dr Leslie Lamport's package LATEX. Most diagrams and figures were generated using
Harvard Graphics, Adobe Illustrator, and CorelDraw. Book design by Philip Taylor and
Ian L. Gibson with the assistance of Oxford University Press.

9 8 7 6 5

Printed in the United States of America
on acid-free paper

This book is dedicated to our son Simon (1968 – 1990) and daughter Isobel who instigated the first edition, and to my former and present graduate students who continue to be a source of inspiration.

Preface

The larger size and two-column format of this new edition of *Principles of Nutritional Assessment* reflect the growth in the importance of assessment since the publication of the first edition in 1990. This has led to a complete rewriting of the volume, but its aim remains unchanged: to provide an up-to-date, authoritative reference source and working textbook for the four major nutritional assessment methods — dietary, anthropometric, laboratory, and clinical — currently being used. The international perspective of this second edition has been enhanced in the hope that the book will continue to have widespread use among health professionals involved in nutritional assessment in hospital and community settings in both industrialized and low income countries. Senior undergraduate and graduate students studying dietetics, nutritional sciences, home economics, sports nutrition, nursing, medicine, and public health will also find the revised book a valuable resource.

The last decade has been marked by numerous studies highlighting the role of diet in health and chronic disease. These studies have often involved large multicenter collaborative trials such as the European Prospective Investigation into Cancer and Nutrition (EPIC), in which the use of standardized and validated methods are critical to ensure comparability among measurements of foods, nutrients, and biomarkers collected from diverse populations. This has led to some significant technical advances in the measurement and evaluation of usual food and nutrient intakes of individuals. Efforts have also increased to standardize all the methods used, improve their accuracy, and reduce respondent burden. Attention has focused on ways to harmonize food composition databases, and to correct for systematic errors that may mask associations between diet and disease. Widespread underreporting in food consumption studies is now recognized. This has led to the increasing use of independent biomarkers of dietary intake to validate dietary intake methods in large-scale epidemiological studies and national nutrition surveys.

These new advances are described in detail in Chapters 2–7 of this revised edition. Chapter 8 presents more reliable ways to evaluate the adequacy of nutrient intakes at both the individual and population levels using the newly defined multiple nutrient-based levels. The latter now focus on optimizing health and reducing the risk of chronic disease, and not solely on the prevention of nutritional deficiencies as they did in the past. Indeed, tolerable upper intake levels have been set in some countries to help people avoid adverse health effects from taking too much of a nutrient in view of the dramatic rise in the use of nutritional supplements and fortified foods in many countries. Newly revised tables of these nutrient reference levels are now available for the United Kingdom, Europe, the United States and Canada, and from a joint FAO/WHO expert consultation; details are given in Chapter 8. More emphasis is now given to qualitative methods for evaluating the adequacy of a healthy diet through guidelines for healthy food choices, a topic that is also now addressed in Chapter 8.

Since the publication of the first edition of *Principles of Nutritional Assessment*, several large-scale national nutrition surveys have been undertaken in the United States, United Kingdom, Continental Europe, and Australasia. In some countries, anthropometric data from these surveys have been used to generate revised growth charts designed to overcome some of the limitations and technical defects of the earlier growth reference data; details of all these new growth charts and their interpretation are given in the anthropometric section of this revised edition (i.e., Chapters 9–13). A new international growth reference for infants and children up to 5 y old is also being developed by the World Health Organization, together with new reference data for mid-upper-arm circumference (MUAC) by age and MUAC-for-height.

National nutrition surveys have highlighted that overweight and obesity are now the major nutritional problems in many industrialized and emerging countries. This has led to increased emphasis on the use of body mass index (BMI) as an indirect indicator of overweight and obesity across all age groups, not just for adults as was the practice at the time of the first edition of this book. Further, because of the importance of intra-abdominal fat as a critical factor for obesity-related illnesses and metabolic disorders, waist-hip circumference ratio and waist circumference alone are now being used as anthropometric surrogates of intra-abdominal fat. Use of all these new indicators is outlined in the anthropometric section of this revised edition, and where possible, national survey results have been integrated into the relevant chapters.

I have continued to emphasize the scientific principles, advantages, limitations, and applicability of the various assessment methods, and the use of appropriate reference data. The inclusion of biochemical markers in many of the latest epidemiological studies and national nutrition surveys has highlighted the critical importance of confounding factors, such as infection and the use of hormonal agents, in the evaluation of nutritional assessment data and interrelationships with diseases. Therefore, in this revised publication, I have included new sections that address confounding factors affecting biomarkers, where relevant, and separate details of their interpretive criteria and measurement in each of the laboratory assessment chapters. Reference to these new sections will allow the reader to take into account important confounders during the design of a study and the statistical analysis of the results.

Another important development since the publication of the first edition has been the growing awareness that micronutrient deficiencies rarely occur in isolation. Indeed, in most developing countries, where diets are predominantly plant-based, multiple micronutrient deficiencies coexist. This and interactions among micronutrients can lead to multiple clinical signs and symptoms that are difficult to interpret. To identify such multiple micronutrient deficits and their adverse health outcomes, a combination of sensitive and specific biochemical and functional laboratory tests are required, whereas to confirm their etiology, careful investigations of food and nutrient intakes must be conducted. I hope that having one volume that encompasses comprehensive information on anthropometric, laboratory, and dietary assessment methods will facilitate investigations of these complex multi-micronutrient interactions.

Remarkable progress has been made over the last decade for the micronutrients iron, iodine, vitamin A, and more recently zinc, encouraged and facilitated by the recognition by the United Nations Agencies of the global importance of these micronutrient deficiencies. This has spurred the refinement of new laboratory indices for these micronutrients, especially the development of new simple, noninvasive approaches to measure the risk of deficiency, and in some cases, excess of these micronutrients, as well as to monitor and evaluate the effects of nutrition interventions. These new approaches include the measurement of nutrients in dried blood spots prepared from a fingerprick or heelprick blood sample, thus avoiding the necessity for venous blood collection and refrigerated storage. For some nutrients, on-site analysis is now possible, enabling researchers and subjects to obtain results immediately. I have attempted to summarize these new and important developments by significantly expanding the chapters dealing with these four micronutrients in the revised edition.

Research on the micronutrient folate has been precipitated by the recognition of its importance in neural tube defects. However, an additional factor here has been the discovery that the risk of neural tube defects may be associated with a folate status that would not conventionally be classed as deficient. This finding has led to the recognition that adverse health outcomes might be associated with subclinical deficiency states of other micronutrients such as iron, iodine, zinc, vitamin A, and vitamin D. Such discoveries have prompted the development of multiple cutoffs for some of these micronutrients, which have each been discussed in the appropriate chapter, although there is often limited agreement among investigators.

This volume continues to be based on the research and reports of many investigators, but I am particularly grateful to the private individuals, editors, and publishers who granted permission to reproduce figures and tables containing numerical data. In most cases these tables have been reset and the figures redrawn; the sources have been acknowledged in the caption. I am also indebted to my colleagues — Dr. I. Brouwer, Dr. K.R. Cavan, Dr. S. DePee, Dr. N. DeJong, Dr. J. Elmslie, Dr. D. O'Connor, Dr. E.L. Ferguson, Ms. S. Fitzgerald, Dr. T. Green, Dr. R. Hanning, Dr. A.-L. Heath, Dr. L. Hodson, Dr. L. Hoffman-Goetz, Dr. C. Hotz, Dr. C.M. Mac-Donald, Mrs. W. Parnell, Dr. M. Skeaff, Dr. S. Skeaff, Dr. C. Thomson, Ms. P. Vandekooy, Dr. H. Weiler, and Dr F. Yeudall, who kindly read drafts of one or more of the individual chapters and suggested improvements; I would also like to thank Amy Dick, Marleen Overtoom, Kylie Smith, and Lara Temple, for their assistance in checking proofs and dealing with permissions, although I continue to be responsible for defects of fact, treatment, judgment, or style.

To speed publication, the book has been printed directly from computer-typeset files prepared by myself and my husband, Ian L. Gibson. I am particularly grateful to Mr. Philip Taylor, Royal Holloway College, University of London, for assistance with the design and typesetting of this second edition. Mr. Jeffrey House, Ms. Nancy Wolitzer, and the staff at Oxford University Press, New York, not only agreed to our typesetting the book, but kindly provided advice and guidance on this process, and allowed us to depart in some measure from the Oxford house style; I am grateful to the publisher for their forbearance and help in this matter.

Dunedin, New Zealand   R.S.G.

Contents

Introduction

Nutritional assessment procedures were first used in surveys designed to describe the nutritional status of populations on a national basis. The methods used were initially described following a conference held in 1932 by the Health Organization of the League of Nations.

In 1955, the Interdepartmental Committee on Nutrition for National Defense (ICNND) was organized to assist low-income countries in assessing the nutritional status of their populations and to identify problems of malnutrition and the ways in which they could be solved. The ICNND teams conducted medical nutrition surveys in 24 countries. A comprehensive manual was then produced (ICNND, 1963), with the intention of standardizing both the methods used for the collection of nutrition survey data and the interpretation of the results.

On the recommendation of a World Health Organization (WHO) Expert Committee on Medical Assessment of Nutritional Status, a second publication was prepared by Jelliffe (1966) in consultation with 25 specialists from various countries. This monograph was directed specifically at the assessment of the nutritional status of vulnerable groups in low-income countries of the world. Many of the methods described in this monograph are still applicable today.

Many industrialized countries now collect data on the nutritional status of the population. The data can be used to identify public health nutrition problems so that effective intervention programs can be designed. In some countries, data are collected on an ongoing basis using nutrition surveillance systems. In the past, these systems have targeted high-risk populations, especially low-income mothers, children under five, and pregnant women. Now with the growing awareness of the role of nutrition as a risk factor for chronic diseases, surveillance systems often encompass all age groups.

Today, nutritional assessment in many low-income countries emphasizes new simple, noninvasive approaches that can be used to measure the risk of both nutrient deficits and excesses, as well as to monitor and evaluate the effects of nutrition interventions (Section 1.1.4) (Solomons, 2002). These new approaches include the measurement of nutrients in dried blood spots prepared from a finger-prick blood sample, avoiding the necessity for venous blood collection and refrigerated storage (Mei et al., 2001). In addition, for some nutrients, on-site analysis is now possible, enabling researchers and subjects to obtain results immediately. For example, in recent years methods have been developed for the

- Assessment of hemoglobin from a finger-prick blood sample with a portable battery-operated hemocue
- Analysis of retinol-binding protein using a reliable, easily calibrated, and transported fluorometer (Craft, 2001)
- Measurement of an individual's dark adaptation threshold to assess vitamin A deficiency (Congdon et al., 1995).

1

Many of these new approaches can also be applied to biomarkers for monitoring risk of chronic diseases. These may include markers of antioxidant protection, soft-tissue oxidation, and free-radical formation, all of which have numerous clinical applications.

Nutritional assessment is also an essential component of the nutritional care of the hospitalized patient. The important relationship between nutritional status and health, and particularly the critical role of nutrition in recovery from acute illness or injury, is well documented. Although it is now many years since the prevalence of malnutrition among hospitalized patients was first reported (Bistrian et al., 1974, 1976), such malnutrition still persists (Corish and Kennedy, 2000). The failure to identify and treat malnourished patients in hospitals appears to be associated with a lack of physician awareness (Roubenoff et al., 1987; Anonymous, 1988). Consequently, it is essential that physicians appreciate the most effective means of diagnosing, evaluating, and monitoring the nutritional status of high-risk hospital patients.

Health-care administrators and the community in general, continue to demand demonstrable benefits from the investment of public funds in nutrition intervention programs. This requires improved techniques in both nutritional assessment and the evaluation of nutrition interventions. The aim of this book is to provide guidance on some of these new, improved techniques, as well as a comprehensive and critical appraisal of many of the older, established methods in nutritional assessment.

1.1 Nutritional assessment systems

Nutritional assessment can be defined as

> The interpretation of information from dietary, laboratory, anthropometric and clinical studies.

The information is used to determine the nutritional status of individuals or population groups as influenced by the intake and utilization of nutrients.

Nutritional assessment systems can take one of four forms: surveys, surveillance, screening, or interventions. These are described briefly below.

1.1.1 Nutrition surveys

The nutritional status of a selected population group is often assessed by means of a cross-sectional survey. The survey may either establish baseline nutritional data or ascertain the overall nutritional status of the population. Cross-sectional nutrition surveys can also identify and describe population subgroups "at risk" for chronic malnutrition. They are unlikely to identify acute malnutrition or provide information on the possible causes of malnutrition, although they are often a necessary first step in an investigation into the causes.

National nutrition surveys generate valuable information on the extent of existing nutritional problems which can be used both to allocate resources to those population subgroups in need and to formulate policies to improve the overall nutrition of the population. They can also be used to evaluate nutrition interventions by collecting baseline data before and at the end of a nutrition intervention program.

Several large-scale national nutrition surveys have been conducted in industrialized countries during the last decade. They include surveys in the United States (NCHS, 1994), the United Kingdom (Gregory et al., 1990, 1995, 2000; Finch et al., 1998), Ireland (SLAN, 1999), New Zealand (Russell et al., 1999; Parnell et al., 2003), and Australia (McLennan and Podger, 1995), as well as in some low-income countries, including Thailand and the Philippines (MOPH, 1999; Kuizon et al., 1997).

1.1.2 Nutrition surveillance

The characteristic feature of surveillance is the continuous monitoring of the nutritional status of selected population groups. Surveillance studies therefore differ from nutrition surveys because the data are collected, analyzed, and utilized over an extended period of time. Sometimes, the surveillance only involves specific at-risk subgroups, identified in earlier nutrition surveys.

Surveillance studies, unlike cross-sectional nutrition surveys, identify the possible causes of both chronic and acute malnutrition and, hence, can be used to formulate and initiate intervention measures at either the population or the subpopulation level. Additional objectives of nutrition surveillance may include monitoring the effect of government nutrition policies and evaluating the efficacy and effectiveness of nutrition intervention programs (WHO, 1976).

In the United States, a program of national nutrition surveillance, known as the National Health and Nutrition Examination Survey (NHANES), was conducted in 1971. Since then, NHANES II (1976–1980) and NHANES III (1988–1994) have been completed (Gunter and McQuillan, 1990) and further surveys are planned. Presently, these surveys are coordinated by the Centers for Disease Control (CDC). The United Kingdom has conducted an annual national nutrition surveillance system — termed the National Food Survey — since 1950. In 1996, this was extended to cover Northern Ireland, as well as England, Wales, and Scotland (Section 2.3).

Note that the term "nutrition monitoring," rather than nutrition surveillance, is often used when the subjects are selected high-risk individuals (e.g., pregnant women).

1.1.3 Nutrition screening

The identification of malnourished individuals requiring intervention can be accomplished by nutrition screening. This involves a comparison of measurements on individuals with predetermined risk levels or "cutoff" points (Section 1.5.3), using measurements that are simple and cheap, and that can be applied rapidly on a large scale.

Nutrition screening can be carried out on the whole population, targeted to a specific subpopulation considered to be at risk, or on selected individuals. In the United States, for

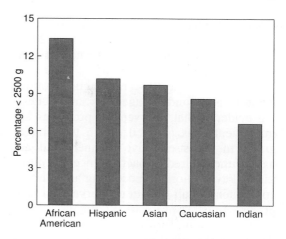

Figure 1.1: The prevalence of low birth weight in 1988 as recorded by the Pediatric Nutrition Surveillance System. From Trowbridge et al., Journal of Nutrition 120: 1512–1518, 1990, American Society for Nutritional Sciences.

example, screening is used to identify individuals who might benefit from the Food Stamp Program, the Women Infants and Children Special Supplemental Food Program (WIC), and the Pediatric Nutrition Surveillance System (PedNSS) (Trowbridge et al., 1990; IOM, 1996). Screening programs are usually less comprehensive than surveys or surveillance studies.

The measurements used in the WIC program and the PedNSS include height, weight, hemoglobin or hematocrit, birth weight, and infant feeding practices by self-report from the mother. Indicators for short stature, underweight or overweight, anemia, low birth weight, and breastfeeding prevalence are then derived from these simple measures (Trowbridge et al., 1990). Figure 1.1 depicts the prevalence of low birth weight by ethnic group for children who participated in the PedNSS in 1988. The highest prevalence of low birth weight was among African American infants.

1.1.4 Nutrition interventions

Nutrition interventions often target population subgroups identified as "at-risk" during nutrition surveys or by nutrition screening. There are three types of nutrition interventions: supplementation, fortification, and dietary approaches (Ruel and Levin, 2001; Shrimpton and Schultink, 2002; and Darnton-Hill and Nalubola, 2002).

Increasingly, health-care program administrators and funding agencies are requesting evidence that intervention programs are implemented as planned, reach their target group in a cost-effective manner, and are having the desired impact. Hence, monitoring and evaluation are becoming an essential component of all nutrition intervention programs.

Several publications are available on the design and evaluation of nutrition interventions. The reader is advised to consult these sources for further details (Habicht et al., 1999; Rossi et al., 1999; Altman et al., 2001). Only a brief summary is given below.

Monitoring oversees the implementation of an intervention, and is discussed in detail by Levinson et al. (1999). Hence, monitoring is used to assess service provision, utilization, coverage, and sometimes the cost of the program. Effective monitoring is essential to demonstrate that the expected result is probably from the intervention.

The evaluation of any nutrition intervention program requires the choice of an appropriate design to assess the performance or effect of the intervention. The choice of the design depends on the purpose of the evaluation and the level of precision required; these aspects are discussed in detail by Habicht et al. (1999). The indicators used to address the evaluation objectives must also be carefully considered (Habicht and Pelletier, 1990; Habicht and Stoltzfus, 1997).

The simplest intervention design involves a within-group distribution of the intervention to all the target group. This design can be evaluated by assessing whether the expected changes have occurred. This can be achieved by comparing the outcome in the target group with either a previously defined goal, or with the change observed in the target group following the intervention program. This type of evaluation is termed an "adequacy evaluation." An example might be distributing iron supplements to *all* the target

group (e.g., all preschool children with iron-deficiency anemia) and assessing whether the goal of $< 10\%$ prevalence of iron-deficiency anemia in the intervention area after two years, has been met. Obviously, when evaluating the outcome by assessing the adequacy of change over time, at least baseline and final measurements are needed. Note that because there is no control group in this design, any reported improvement in the group, even if it is statistically significant, cannot be causally linked to the intervention.

The second type of design for evaluating an intervention employs a between-group quasi-experimental design in which the experimental group receives the intervention, but the control group does not. The design should preferably allow blinding (e.g., use an identical placebo). Because of the quasi-experimental design, the subjects are not randomized into the two groups, and multivariate analysis is used to control for potential confounding factors and biases, although it may not be possible to fully remove these statistically. A between-group quasi-experimental design requires more resources and is therefore more expensive than the within-group design. It is selected when decision makers require a greater degree of certainty that the outcomes that are observed are related to the nutrition intervention. Evaluation of a between-group design is termed a "plausibility evaluation."

The third and most expensive design for evaluating an intervention is a randomized, controlled, double-blind experimental trial. In this design, the subjects are randomly assigned to either the intervention or the control group. Randomization is conducted to ensure that, within the limits of chance, the treatment and control groups will be comparable at the start of the study. An intervention with such a design, when properly executed, provides the highest level of confidence that the intervention was responsible for the outcome; evaluation of such a design is called a "probability evaluation." In some randomized trials, the treatment groups are communities and not individuals, in which case they are known as "community trials."

1.1.5 Assessment systems in the clinical setting

The types of nutritional assessment systems used in the community have been adopted in clinical medicine to assess the nutritional status of hospitalized patients. This practice has arisen because of reports of the high prevalence of protein-energy malnutrition among surgical patients in North America and elsewhere (Corish and Kennedy, 2000). Today, nutritional assessment is often performed on patients with acute traumatic injury, on those undergoing surgery, on chronically ill medical patients, and on elderly patients.

Initially, screening can be carried out to identify those patients requiring nutritional management. A more detailed and comprehensive baseline nutritional assessment of the individual may then follow. This assessment will clarify and expand the nutritional diagnosis, and establish the severity of the malnutrition. Further details of protocols that have been developed to assess the nutritional status of hospital patients are given in Sections 27.1 and 27.2. Finally, a nutrition intervention may be implemented, often incorporating nutritional monitoring and an evaluation system, to follow both the response of the patient to the nutritional therapy and its impact.

1.2 Nutritional assessment methods

In the past, nutritional assessment systems have focused on methods to characterize each stage in the development of a nutritional deficiency state. These methods are based on a series of dietary, laboratory, anthropometric, and clinical observations as shown in Table 1.1, used either alone or, more effectively, in combination.

Increasingly, nutritional assessment systems are now applied to define multiple levels of nutrient status and not just the level associated with a nutrient deficiency. Such levels may be associated with the maintenance of health, or with reduction in the risk of chronic disease; sometimes, levels leading to specific health hazards or toxic effects are also defined

Depletion stage	Method(s) used
1 Dietary inadequacy	Dietary
2 Decreased level in reserve tissue store	Biochemical
3 Decreased level in body fluids	Biochemical
4 Decreased functional level in tissues	Anthropometric / Biochemical
5 Decreased activity of nutrient-dependent enzyme or mRNA for some proteins	Biochemical / Molecular techniques
6 Functional change	Behavioral /Physiological
7 Clinical symptoms	Clinical
8 Anatomical sign	Clinical

Table 1.1: Generalized scheme for the development of a nutritional deficiency. From Martorell (1984) © by the United Nations University.

(Combs, 1996) (Section 8.1.1). The methods listed in Table 1.1 are still used, but there is now increasing emphasis on the use of new functional tests to determine these multiple levels of nutrient status. Examples include functional tests that measure immune function, muscle strength, glucose metabolism, nerve function, work capacity, and oxidative stress (Lukaski and Penland, 1996; Mayne, 2003). Correct interpretation of the results of nutritional assessment methods often requires consideration of other factors, such as socioeconomic status, cultural practices, and health and vital statistics. Collectively, these factors are sometimes termed "ecological factors" and are discussed in Section 1.2.5.

1.2.1 Dietary methods

The first stage of any nutritional deficiency is identified by dietary assessment methods. During this stage, the dietary intake of one or more nutrients is inadequate, either because of a primary deficiency (low levels in the diet) or because of a secondary deficiency. In the latter case, dietary intakes may appear to meet nutritional needs, but conditioning factors (such as certain drugs, dietary components, or disease states) interfere with the ingestion, absorption, transport, utilization, or excretion of the nutrient(s).

Several dietary methods are available, the choice depending primarily on the objectives of the study and the characteristics of the study group (Section 3.3). Often, information on the proportion of the population "at risk" of inadequate intakes of nutrients is required. Such information can be used to ascertain whether assessment using more invasive laboratory methods is warranted in a specific population or subgroup.

Sometimes, knowledge, attitudes and practices, and reported food-related behaviors are also investigated. This often involves observations, as well as in-depth interviews and focus groups— approaches based on ethnological and anthropological techniques. Such methods are particularly useful when designing and evaluating nutrition interventions.

1.2.2 Laboratory methods

The laboratory methods include both static biochemical and functional tests. Static biochemical tests measure either a nutrient in biological fluids or tissues or the urinary excretion rate of the nutrient or its metabolite. They are especially useful for identifying the second and third stages in the development of a nutritional deficiency, as shown in Table 1.1, when the tissue stores, followed by the body fluid levels, become gradually depleted of the nutrient(s).

Functional tests can be further categorized into functional biochemical tests and functional physiological or behavioral tests. They are being increasingly used, not only to detect the later stages in the development of a nutritional deficiency— when for example, a decline in the activity of certain nutrient-dependent enzymes, may occur (i.e., stage 5; Table 1.1)— but also to measure nutrient status associated with optimal health and reduction in the risk of chronic disease. For example, such tests may include the in vivo assessment of a physiological function known to be dependent on a specific nutrient (Solomons, 2002). Examples of such functional tests include papillary and visual

threshold for vitamin A and taste acuity for zinc. Functional tests provide a measure of the biological importance of a given nutrient because they assess the functional consequences of deficiency or excess of a nutrient (Solomons and Allen, 1983). They are especially useful for defining optimal nutrient status levels.

In general, functional physiological tests are not suitable for large-scale nutrition surveys: they are often too invasive, they may require elaborate equipment, and the results tend to be difficult to interpret because of the lack of cutoff points. Functional physiological tests also tend to be less responsive than biochemical tests to small changes in nutrient status. In addition, many other non-nutritional factors may influence their performance, besides a deficit in one specific nutrient, reducing their specificity. For example, even the newest test for dark adaptation— papillary and visual threshold test— is not specific for vitamin A; zinc deficiency also impairs night vision (Christian and West, 1998). As a result, functional physiological tests generally show greater variability among subjects than that reported for static biochemical tests. Details of functional physiological or behavioral tests dependent on specific nutrients are summarized in Chapters 16–25.

1.2.3 Anthropometric methods

Anthropometric methods involve measurements of the physical dimensions and gross composition of the body (WHO, 1995). The measurements vary with age (and sometimes with sex and race) and degree of nutrition, and they are particularly useful in circumstances where *chronic* imbalances of protein and energy are likely to have occurred. In some cases they can detect moderate and severe degrees of malnutrition, but the methods cannot be used to identify specific nutrient deficiency states. Anthropometric measurements have the additional advantage of providing information on past nutritional history, which cannot be obtained with equal confidence using other assessment techniques.

The measurements can be performed relatively quickly, easily, and reliably using portable equipment, provided standardized methods and calibrated equipment are used (Chapters 10 and 11). To aid in the interpretation of anthropometric data, the raw measurements are generally expressed as an index, such as height-for-age (see Section 1.3).

1.2.4 Clinical methods

A medical history and a physical examination are the clinical methods used to detect signs (i.e., observations made by a qualified examiner) and symptoms (i.e., manifestations reported by the patient) associated with malnutrition (Section 26.1). These signs and symptoms are often nonspecific and only develop during the advanced stages of nutritional depletion; for this reason, diagnosis of a nutritional deficiency should not rely exclusively on clinical methods. It is obviously desirable to detect marginal nutrient deficiencies before a clinical syndrome develops, and, as a result, laboratory methods should also be included as an adjunct to clinical assessment.

1.2.5 Ecological factors

Nutritional assessment methods often include the collection of information on a variety of other factors known to influence the nutritional status of individuals or populations, including any relevant socioeconomic and demographic data. Variables may include household composition, education, literacy, ethnicity, religion, income, employment, material resources, water supply and household sanitation, access to health and agricultural services, as well as land ownership and other information. Additional data on food prices, the adequacy of food preparation equipment, the degree of food reserves, cash-earning opportunities, and the percentage of the household income spent on certain foods such as animal foods, fruits, and vegetables can also be collected, if appropriate.

Data on health and vital statistics may also be obtained, as may information on the percentage of the population with ready access to a good source of drinking water, the proportion of children immunized against measles, the proportion of infants born with a low birth weight, the percentage of mothers breastfeeding, and age- and cause-specific mortality rates.

Some non-nutritional variables are strongly related to malnutrition and can be used to identify at-risk individuals during surveillance studies. For example, Morley (1973) identified birth order over seven, breakdown of marriage, death of either parent, and episodes of infectious diseases in early life as being important factors in the prediction of West African children who were nutritionally at risk.

1.3 Nutritional assessment indices and indicators

Raw measurements alone have no meaning unless they are related to, for example, the age or sex of an individual (WHO, 1995). Hence, raw measurements derived from each of the four methods are often (but not always) combined to form "indices." Examples of such combinations include height-for-age percentile, nutrient density (i.e., nutrient intake per megajoule), body mass index (weight /height^2), and mean cell volume (i.e., hematocrit/red blood cell count). These indices are all continuous variables. Construction of indices is a necessary step for the interpretation and grouping of measurements collected by nutritional assessment systems.

Indices are often evaluated at the population level by comparison with predetermined reference limits or cutoff points (Section 1.5). Such an approach can be used to identify, for example, the proportion of children at risk of vitamin A deficiency, based on serum retinol levels < 0.70 µmol/L, as shown in Table 1.2. When used in this way, the index and its associated reference limit or cutoff become an "indicator," a term that relates to their use in nutritional assessment, often for public health, or social/medical decision-making at the population level. Nutritional indicators are sometimes classified according to the nu-

Nutritional indicator	Application
Dietary indicators	
Proportion of children with dietary phytate:Zn molar ratios > 15	Assessment of dietary quality
Proportion of population with nutrient intakes below EAR	Risk of dietary inadequacy
Anthropometric indicators	
Proportion of children (of defined age and sex) with WHZ < -2 SD	Prevalence of wasting
Proportion of children (of defined age and sex) with HAZ < -2 SD	Prevalence of stunting
Laboratory indicators	
Prevalence of serum retinol $< 0.70\,\mu$mol/L in children 6–71 mo $\geqslant 15\%$	Vitamin A deficiency likely to be a public health problem
Median urinary iodine $< 20\,\mu$g/L based on $\geqslant 300$ casual urine samples	Risk of severe IDD in the population
Proportion of children (of defined age and sex) with two or more abnormal iron indices (serum ferritin, erythrocyte protoporphyrin, transferrin saturation) plus an abnormal hemoglobin	Prevalence of iron deficiency anemia
Clinical indicators	
Proportion of children with total goiter rate $\geqslant 30\%$	Severe risk of IDD
Prevalence of maternal night blindness $\geqslant 5\%$	Vitamin A deficiency is a severe public health problem

Table 1.2: Examples of dietary, anthropometric, laboratory, and clinical indicators and their application. EAR, estimated average requirement; WHZ, weight-for-height Z-score; HAZ, height-for-age Z-score; IDD, iodine deficiency disorders.

tritional assessment methods on which they are based; examples are given in Table 1.2.

Indicators should be chosen carefully in relation to both the study objectives and their attributes. They can be used to meet a variety of objectives, and some of these are itemized in Table 1.3. The critical attributes of the indicators required to meet these objectives are also shown. For example, if the objective of the program is to evaluate the treatment of malnutrition, then the indicator chosen must have the potential to respond to the specific intervention under study and must relate to the nature and severity of the malnutrition present. Thus the same indicators are not appropriate for evaluating the treatment of stunting versus wasting. Further, several factors will affect the magnitude of the expected response of an indicator. These may include the degree of deficiency, age, sex, and physiological state of the target group. Other influencing factors may be the type and duration of the intervention, home diet, the age-specificity of the response, and

Objective
Required informational content
Prevent malnutrition
Indicate risk of future malnutrition or its consequences.
Predict benefit from intervention
Treat malnutrition
Indicate harm from past malnutrition.
Predict benefit from intervention
Treat consequences
Indicate harm from past malnutrition
Evaluate treatment
Indicate responsiveness to intervention or determinant
Promote nutrition education
Indicate normalcy

Table 1.3: Attributes of nutritional indicators needed to meet objectives. From Habicht and Pelletier, Journal of Nutrition 120: 1519–1524, 1990, by permission of the American Society for Nutritional Sciences.

whether the indicator is homeostatically controlled. A more detailed discussion of the selection criteria for indicators can be found in Habicht et al. (1982), Habicht and Pelletier (1990), and Habicht and Stoltzfus (1997).

Indicators vary in their validity, sensitivity, specificity, and predictive value; these characteristics, as well as other important factors, are described in Section 1.4 below.

1.4 The design of nutritional assessment systems

The design of the nutritional assessment system is critical if time and resources are to be used effectively. The assessment system used, the type and number of measurements selected, and the indices and indicators derived from these measurements will depend on a variety of factors.

1.4.1 Study objectives

The general design of the assessment system, the raw measurements, and, in turn, the indices and indicators derived from these measurements should be dictated by the study objectives. Possible objectives may include:

1. Determining the overall nutritional status of a population or subpopulation
2. Identifying areas, populations, or subpopulations at risk of chronic malnutrition
3. Characterizing the extent and nature of the malnutrition within the population or subpopulation
4. Identifying the possible causes of malnutrition within the population or subpopulation
5. Designing appropriate intervention programs for high-risk populations or subpopulations
6. Monitoring the progress of changing nutritional, health, or socioeconomic influences, including intervention programs
7. Evaluating the efficacy and effectiveness of intervention programs
8. Tracking progress toward the attainment of long-range goals.

The first three objectives can be met by a cross-sectional nutrition survey, often involving all the methods of nutritional assessment. Such surveys, however, are unlikely to provide information on the possible causes of malnutrition (i.e., objective no. 4). The latter can only be achieved via nutrition surveillance, an approach also needed to achieve objective no. 6. An assessment of the possible causes of malnutrition is a necessary prerequisite when implementing nutrition intervention programs (i.e., objectives nos. 5–7).

In some circumstances, the objective may be to identify only those individuals at risk of malnutrition and who require intervention (i.e., objective no. 5). To achieve this objective, a screening system is required that uses simple and cheap measurements and reflects both past and present nutritional status.

1.4.2 Sampling protocols

Nutritional assessment systems often target a large population — perhaps that of a city, province, or country. For practical reasons, only a limited number of individuals within the target population can actually be studied. These individuals must be chosen carefully to ensure the results can be used to infer information about the target population. The technique of selecting a sample representative of the target population and of a size adequate for achieving the primary study objectives, requires the assistance of a person with training in sampling techniques; only a very brief review is provided here.

A major factor influencing the choice of the sampling protocol is the availability of a sampling frame. This consists of a list from which the sample can be selected. The list may be of individuals in the population, district, village or school or of districts or households, each of which is termed a "sampling unit." Additional factors affecting the protocol selection are time, resources, and logistical constraints. When a sampling frame is not available, nonprobability sampling methods must be used, whereas when a sampling frame is available, a probability-based sampling protocol should be used.

Three nonprobability sampling protocols are available: consecutive sampling, convenience sampling, and quota sampling, each of which is described briefly in Box 1.1. Note that use of nonprobability sampling methods produces samples that are not representative of the target population and may lead to systematic bias; for example, only those with a higher level of education may volunteer to participate. In these circumstances, it is essential to fully document the characteristics of the sample and to identify the probable direction and magnitude of the bias that arises from the sample protocol and nonresponse rate. Extrapolating the results from a nonprobability sample to the general population is risky and should be avoided.

Every attempt should be made to compile some type of sampling frame, or to use one that already exists, so that probability sampling can be used (Lemeshow et al., 1990). Probability sampling is the recommended method for obtaining a representative sample with minimum bias. Several probability sampling methods exist: simple random sampling, systematic sampling, stratified random sampling, cluster sampling, and multistage sampling. Of these, three methods are described briefly in Box 1.2, and further details can be found in Varkevisser et al. (1993).

When stratified sampling is used, the sample is not necessarily representative of the

---

Simple random sampling involves drawing a random sample from the whole target population.

Stratified random sampling divides the target population into a number of categories or strata (e.g., urban and rural populations, different ethnic groups, various geographical areas or administrative regions). A separate random sample is then drawn from each stratum.

Multistage random sampling requires defining a number of levels of sampling, from each of which is drawn a random sample.

Box 1.2: Probability sampling protocols.

---

actual population. Weighting allows the imbalance to be corrected when the results are generalized to the target population. Alternatively, a sampling strategy, termed proportional stratification, can be used to adjust the sampling before selecting the sample, provided information on the size of the sampling units is available. This approach simplifies the data analysis and also ensures that subjects from larger communities have a proportionately greater chance of being selected than do subjects from smaller communities.

As can be seen, each method involves a random selection procedure to ensure that each sampling unit (often the individual) has an equal probability of being sampled. Random selection can be achieved by using a table of random numbers, a computer program that generates random numbers, or a lottery method; each of these procedures is described in Varkisser et al. (1993).

National nutrition surveys often use multistage sampling. Four stages may be appropriate: sampling at the provincial or similar level (stage one), district level (stage two), level of communities in each selected district (stage three), and level of households in each chosen community (stage four). A random sample must be drawn at each stage. The NHANES III, the U.K. Diet and Nutrition surveys, and the New Zealand and Australian national nutrition surveys all used a combination of stratified and multistage random sampling techniques to obtain a sample representative of the civilian noninstitutionalized populations of these countries.

Consecutive sampling is the best of the nonprobability techniques. It is used, for example, in clinical research, when it is feasible to recruit all available patients who meet the selection criteria, over a time period that is long enough to avoid seasonal factors or other changes over time.

Convenience sampling involves taking individuals into the study who happen to be available at the time of data collection and who consent to participate.

Quota sampling involves dividing the target population into a number of different categories (e.g., age groups or occupations) and taking a certain number of consenting individuals from each category into the final sample.

Box 1.1: Nonprobability sampling protocols.

1.4.3 Calculating sample size

A critical feature of any sampling protocol selected for a nutritional assessment system is the size of the sample required. The latter depends on the study objective, nature and scope of the study, and the expected outcomes. Again, assistance with sample size calculations should be sought from a statistician. A practical guide to calculating the sample size is published by WHO (Lwanga and Lemeshow, 1991). To perform sample size calculations, information on the following variables is needed:

- Required level of statistical significance of the expected results
- Acceptable chance of missing the real effect
- Magnitude of the effect under investigation
- Amount of disease in the population, where relevant
- Relative sizes of the groups being compared, where applicable

The WHO guide also provides tables of minimum sample size for various study conditions (e.g., studies involving population proportion, odds ratio, relative risk, and incidence rate), but the tables are only valid when the sample is selected in a statistically random manner. For each situation in which sample size is to be determined, the information needed is specified and at least one illustrative example is given. In practice, the final sample size may be constrained by cost and logistical considerations and is often a compromise.

1.4.4 Validity

Validity is an important concept in the design of nutritional assessment systems. It describes the *adequacy* with which any measurement, index, or indicator reflects what it is intended to measure. For example, if information on the long-term nutritional status of an individual is required, the dietary measurement should provide a valid reflection of the true "usual" nutrient intake rather than the intake over a single day. Similarly, the biochemical parameter selected should be a valid measure of the total body content of a nutrient, or the size of the tissue store most sensitive to deficiency, and not reflect the recent dietary intake (Solomons, 1985). This means that measurement of urinary vitamin B_6, for example, would be an inappropriate choice because it is not a valid measure of long-term vitamin B_6 status, but, instead, reflects recent dietary intake (Section 21.4). A valid measure would be measurement of the activation coefficient of aspartate aminotransferase (AsAT) (Section 21.1).

Both random and systematic errors are often associated with a measurement and will reduce its validity (Kipnis et al., 2001). Measures of sensitivity and specificity also relate to the validity of a measure. Valid measures are ideally free from random and systematic errors and are both sensitive and specific (Section 1.4.11).

In some circumstances, assessment measures only have "internal" validity, indicating that the results are valid only for the particular group of individuals being studied. In contrast, if the results have "external" validity, or generalizability, then the results are valid when applied to individuals not only in the study but in the wider universe. For example, conclusions derived from a study on African Americans may be valid for that particular population but cannot be extrapolated to the wider American population.

Internal validity is easier to achieve. It is necessary for, but does not guarantee, external validity. External validity requires external quality control of the measurements and judgment about the degree to which the results of a study can be extrapolated to the wider universe. The design of any nutritional assessment system must include consideration of both the internal and external validities of the raw measurements, the indices based on them, and any derived indicators.

1.4.5 Reproducibility or precision

The degree to which repeated measurements of the same variable give the same value is a measure of reproducibility — also referred to as "reliability" or "precision" in biochemical assessment (Section 15.4.1). The study design should always include some replicate observations (repeated but independent measurements on the same subject or sample). In this way, the reproducibility of each measurement procedure can be calculated as the coefficient of variation (CV%):

$$CV\% = \text{standard deviation} \times 100\% \, / \, \text{mean}$$

The reproducibility of a measurement is a function of the random measurement errors and, in certain cases, true variability in the measurement that occurs over time. For example, the nutrient intakes of an individual vary over time (within-subject variation), and this results in uncertainty in the estimation of usual nutrient intake. This variation characterizes the true "usual intake" of an individual. Unfortunately, within-subject variation cannot be distinguished statistically from random measurement errors, irrespective of the design of the nutritional assessment system (Section 6.2.3).

The precision of biochemical measures is similarly a function of random errors that occur during the actual analytical process *and* within-subject biological variation in the biochemical measure. The relative importance of these two sources of uncertainty varies with the different measures. For many modern biochemical measures, the within-subject biological variation exceeds the long-term analytical variation, as shown in Table 1.4.

A variety of strategies can be used to increase the precision of nutritional assessment systems. These are discussed in detail by Hulley and Cummings (1988) and include the following:

- Compiling an operations manual that contains specific written guidelines for taking each measurement, to ensure all the techniques are standardized
- Training all the examiners to use the standardized techniques consistently; the latter is especially important in large surveys involving multiple examiners, and in longitudinal studies, where maintaining stan-

Measurement	Coefficient of variation (%)	
	Within-subject	Analytical
Serum retinol		
Daily	11.3	2.3
Weekly	22.9	2.9
Monthly	25.7	2.8
Serum ascorbic acid		
Daily	15.4	0.0
Weekly	29.1	1.9
Monthly	25.8	5.4
Serum albumin		
Daily	6.5	3.7
Weekly	11.0	1.9
Monthly	6.9	8.0

Table 1.4: Within-subject and analytical variance components for some common biochemical measures. Abstracted from Gallagher et al., Clinical Chemistry 38: 1449–1453, 1992, with permission of the AACC.

dardized measurement techniques during the survey is an ongoing problem
- Carefully selecting and standardizing the instruments used for the data collection; in some cases, variability can be reduced by the use of automated instruments
- Refining and standardizing questionnaires and interview protocols, preferably with the use of computer-administered interview protocols; the latter approach was used by the United States and New Zealand for the 24-h recall interviews in their recent national nutrition surveys (NCHS, 1994; Quigley and Watts, 1997; Parnell et al., 2003)
- Reducing the effect of random errors from any source by repeating all the measurements, when feasible, or at least on a random subsample (Section 15.4.1)

1.4.6 Accuracy

The term "accuracy" is best used in a restricted statistical sense to describe the extent to which the measurement is close to the true value. It therefore follows that a measurement can be reproducible or precise, but, at the same time, inaccurate — a situation which occurs when there is a systematic bias in the measurements (see below). The greater the

	Precision or reproducibility	Accuracy
Definition	The degree to which repeated measurements of the same variable give the same value	The degree to which a measurement is close to the true value
Assess by	Comparison among repeated measures	Comparison with certified reference materials, criterion method, or criterion anthropometrist
Value to study	Increases power to detect effects	Increases validity of conclusions
Adversely affected by	Random error contributed by the measurer, the respondent, or the instrument	Systematic error (bias) contributed by the measurer, the respondent, or the instrument

Table 1.5: Precision and accuracy of measurements.

systematic error or bias, the less accurate the measurement. Accurate measurements, however, necessitate high reproducibility. Accuracy has an important effect on both the internal and external validities of a study.

Controlling the accuracy of objective biochemical measurements is relatively easy and can be accomplished by using reference materials with certified values for the nutrient of interest (Section 15.3). The control of accuracy in other assessment methods is more difficult and is discussed in more detail in later chapters. For example, the correct value of any anthropometric measurement is never known with absolute certainty. In the absence of absolute reference standards, the accuracy of anthropometric measurements is estimated by comparing them with those made by a designated criterion anthropometrist (Ulijaszek and Kerr, 1999) (Section 9.2).

Statements such as "weight-for-height is an 'accurate' reflection of wasting" should not be used. The term "valid" is more appropriate here, and confusion with the well-accepted statistical usage of "accurate" is avoided.

Several strategies exist for enhancing accuracy in nutritional assessment systems. Because accurate measurements must also be reproducible or precise, the same strategies outlined under reproducibility (Section 1.4.5) should be adopted. Additional strategies that can also be used to enhance accuracy include (a) making unobtrusive measurements, (b) blinding, and (c) calibrating the instruments. Of these strategies, the first two should always be used to help avoid bias where feasible and appropriate, together with the third when any instruments are used.

Table 1.5 compares and contrasts the important features of reproducibility or precision with accuracy. The strategies actually adopted to maximize reproducibility and accuracy will depend on several factors. These may include feasibility and cost considerations, the importance of the variable, and the magnitude of the potential impact of the anticipated degree of inaccuracy on the study conclusions (Hulley and Cummings, 1988).

1.4.7 Random errors

Random errors generate a deviation from the correct result due to chance alone. They lead to measurements that are imprecise in an unpredictable way, resulting in less certain conclusions. They reduce the precision of a measurement by increasing the variability about the mean. They do not influence the mean or median value.

There are three main sources of random error:

- Individual biological variation
- Sampling error
- Measurement error

Individual biological variation may be the major source of random error, particularly for certain biochemical measurements, such as serum iron, which are associated with large within-subject variation (Table 17.10).

Sampling may also be a major source of random error. For example, significant sampling errors may be associated with the collection of food samples for nutrient analysis or with selection of subjects, who for practical reasons, are usually a small subset of a larger population. This error will be present even if the sampling is truly random. One way to reduce this error is to increase the sample size (i.e., the number of food samples or the number of subjects).

Random measurement errors may be produced by variations in the measuring and recording process. When recording 24-h dietary recalls, for example, the major source of random measurement error may be associated with the measurement of the actual amounts of the foods consumed (Section 5.2.5). Measurement error in skinfolds may arise from variation in the duration and level of compression by calipers during the measurement (Ward and Anderson, 1993).

Random measurement errors can be minimized by using standardized measurement techniques and trained personnel and by employing rigorous quality-control procedures during the laboratory analysis. However, such errors can never be entirely eliminated. To be sure, random measurement errors may be generated when the same examiner repeats the measurements (within- or intra-examiner error), or when several different examiners repeat the same measurement (between- or inter-examiner error). Details of the quality-control procedures that can be incorporated to minimize sources of analytical measurement errors are included in Section 15.3

1.4.8 Systematic errors or bias

Unfortunately, systematic errors may arise in any nutritional assessment method, which thus may become biased. Bias may be defined as a condition that causes a result to depart from the true value in a consistent direction. The errors arising from bias reduce the accuracy of a measurement by altering the mean or median value. They have no effect on the variance and hence do not alter the reproducibility or precision of the measurement (Himes, 1987).

Several types of bias exist, but the principal

Self-selection bias results from studying only volunteers for a study, who perhaps volunteer because they are unwell.

Referral bias will be present if cases are recruited through a district health center but controls from an adjacent village.

Nonresponse bias is caused by ignoring people who do not respond to an initial attempt to include them in the study.

Diagnostic bias arises from selecting subjects for a multicenter case-control study using different diagnostic criteria in different centers.

Drop-out bias is usually the result of ignoring possible systematic differences between those who fail to complete a study and the remaining participants.

Box 1.3: Various types of selection bias.

---

biases are selection bias and measurement (or classification) bias (Sackett et al., 1991). Selection bias can occur in all types of nutritional assessment systems. It arises when there is a systematic difference between the characteristics of the individuals selected for the study and the characteristics of those who are not, making it impossible to generalize the results to the target population. Selection bias may originate in a variety of ways. Some of these are outlined in Box 1.3.

Wherever possible, a strategy should be used to obtain information on people who refuse to participate or subsequently fail to complete the study. This information can then be used to assess whether those who did not participate or dropped out of the study are similar to the participants. If they differ, then a selection bias is present.

Measurement bias can be introduced in a variety of ways. For example:

- Biased equipment may over- or underestimate weight or height. Alternatively, skinfold calipers may systematically over- or underestimate skinfold thickness, because of differences in degree of compression.
- Analytical bias may result from the use of a biochemical method that systematically under- or overestimates the nutrient content of a food or biological specimen. For

example, vitamin C may be underestimated because only the reduced form of vitamin C, and not total vitamin C, is measured.

- Social desirability bias occurs, for example, when respondents underestimate their alcohol consumption in a 24-h food record. However, scales can be used to measure the extent of the bias (Robinson et al., 1991), including the Marlowe-Crowne Social Desirability Scale (Crowne and Marlowe, 1960).

- Interviewer bias arises when interviewers differ in the way in which they obtain, record, process, and interpret information. This is a particular problem if different interviewers are assigned different segments of the population, such as different racial or age groups.

- Recall bias is a form of measurement bias of critical importance in retrospective case-control studies. In such studies, there may be differential recall of information by cases and controls. For example, persons with heart disease will be more likely to recall past exposure to saturated fat than the controls, as saturated fat is widely known to be associated with heart disease. Such a recall bias may exaggerate the degree of effect of association with the exposure or, alternatively, may underestimate the association if the cases are more likely than controls to deny past exposure.

Bias is important as it cannot be removed by subsequent statistical analysis. Consequently, care must be taken to reduce and, if possible, eliminate all sources of bias in the nutritional assessment system by the choice of an appropriate design and careful attention to the equipment and methods selected. Strategies for controlling bias and its potential effect on the measurement of a cause–effect relationship are described in most standard epidemiological texts.

1.4.9 Confounding

Confounding is a special type of bias and therefore affects the validity of a study: it masks the true effect. A confounding variable is defined as a characteristic or variable that is distributed differently in the study and control groups and that affects the outcome being assessed (Riegelman and Hirsch, 1989). Examples of typical confounders include age, gender, and social class.

In the example shown in Figure 1.2, cigarette smoking confounds the apparent relationship between coffee consumption and coronary heart disease and is thus said to be the confounding variable. The latter arises because persons who consume coffee are more likely to smoke than people who do not drink coffee, and cigarette smoking is known to be a cause of coronary heart disease (Beaglehole et al., 1993).

Some authors have drawn a distinction between confounders and other variables that may also influence outcome. The latter include outcome modifiers and effect modifiers. Outcome modifiers have an effect on the health outcome independent of the exposure of interest. Note that neither confounders nor outcome modifiers lie on the causal pathway.

In contrast, effect modifiers modify (positively or negatively) the effect of the hypothesized causal variables. Hence, unlike confounders and outcome modifiers, effect modifiers do lie on the causal pathway relating the exposure of interest to the outcome. As an example, hypertension is more frequent among African Americans than among Caucasians, whereas the prevalence of coronary heart disease is higher among Caucasians than among African Americans. Hence, some variable possibly related to lifestyle or consti-

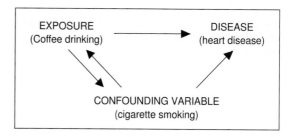

Figure 1.2: The relationship of exposure, disease, and a confounding variable. From Beaglehole et al. (1993).

tution may modify the effect of hypertension on coronary heart disease.

Several strategies exist to control for confounders and modifiers, provided they are known and measured. They can be applied at the design or, subsequently, at the analysis stage. At the design phase, strategies include randomization, stratification, restriction, and matching, each of which is discussed in detail in Hulley and Cummings (1988). At the analysis stage, the existence of confounding and outcome and effect modifiers can be controlled in large studies, either by stratification or by multivariate analysis. For guidelines on the appropriate use of each of these strategies, consult a statistician.

1.4.10 Sensitivity

The sensitivity of an index or indicator refers to the extent to which it reflects nutritional status or predicts changes in nutriture. Sensitive indices (or indicators) show large changes as a result of only small changes in nutritional status. As a result, they have the ability to identify and classify those persons within a population who are *genuinely* malnourished. An index (or indicator) with 100% sensitivity correctly identifies all those individuals who are genuinely malnourished: no malnourished persons are classified as "well" (i.e., there are no false negatives).

Numerically, sensitivity (Se) is the proportion of individuals with malnutrition who have positive tests (true positives divided by the sum of true positives and false negatives). The sensitivity of an index (or indicator) changes with prevalence, as well as with the cutoff point, as discussed in Section 1.5.3.

Unfortunately, the term "sensitivity" is also used to describe the ability of an analytical method to detect the substance of interest. The term "analytical sensitivity" should be used in this latter context (Section 15.3.3).

1.4.11 Specificity

The specificity of an index (or indicator) refers to the ability of the index (or indicator) to identify and classify those persons who are

genuinely well nourished. If an index (or indicator) has 100% specificity, all genuinely well-nourished individuals will be correctly identified: no well-nourished individuals will be classified as "ill" (i.e., there are no false positives). Numerically, specificity (Sp) is the proportion of individuals without malnutrition who have negative tests (true negatives divided by the sum of true negatives and false positives).

Table 1.6 describes the four situations that are possible when evaluating the performance of an index or indicator. These are a true-positive (TP) result: the test is positive and the subject really has, for example, anemia; a false-positive (FP) result: the test is positive but the subject does not, for example, have anemia; a false-negative (FN) result: the test is negative but the subject genuinely has anemia: and a true-negative (TN) result: the test is negative and the subject does not have anemia. Increasingly in nutritional assessment, the performance of indices, and their associated indicators is being evaluated by calculating sensitivity and specificity, as well as predictive value (Section 1.4.13).

Test result	The true situation	
	Malnutrition present	No malnutrition
Positive	True positive (TP)	False positive (FP)
Negative	False negative (FN)	True negative (TN)

Sensitivity (Se) = TP / (TP + FN)

Specificity (Sp) = TN / (FP + TN)

Predictive value (V) =
        (TP + TN) / (TP + FP + TN + FN)

Positive predictive value (V+) = TP / (TP + FP)

Negative predictive value (V−) = TN / (TN + FN)

Prevalence (P) = (TP + FN) / (TP + FP + TN + FN)

Table 1.6: Numerical definitions of sensitivity, specificity, predictive value, and prevalence for a single index used to assess malnutrition in a sample group. From Habicht, American Journal of Clinical Nutrition 33: 531–535, 1980 ⓒ Am J Clin Nutr. American Society for Clinical Nutrition.

It is important to note that sensitivity and specificity only provide information on the proportion or percentage of subjects with or without malnutrition who are correctly categorized. These measures do not predict the actual number of subjects who will be categorized as malnourished. The actual number of subjects will depend on the frequency of malnutrition in the group being studied.

The ideal test has a low number of both false positives (high specificity) and false negatives (high sensitivity), and hence the test is able to completely separate those who genuinely are malnourished from subjects who are healthy.

In practice, a balance has to be struck between specificity and sensitivity, depending on the consequences of identifying false negatives and false positives. For example, for a serious condition such as screening for neonatal phenylketonuria, it might be preferable to have high sensitivity and to accept the increased cost of a high number of false positives (reduced specificity). In such circumstances, follow-up would be required to identify the true positives and true negatives.

Factors modifying sensitivity and specificity

Cutoff points have an effect on both sensitivity and specificity. In cases where lower values of the measure are associated with malnutrition (e.g., hemoglobin), decreasing the cutoff point decreases sensitivity but increases specificity for a given test. Conversely, increasing the cutoff will increase sensitivity but decrease specificity. Table 1.7 shows that when the cutoff point for the mid-upper-arm circumference is reduced from < 14.0 cm to < 12.5 cm, the sensitivity falls from 90.4% to 55.8% and the specificity in predicting malnutrition (based on weight-for-height $< 60\%$ of median) increases from 82.7% to 98.0% (Trowbridge and Staehling, 1980). Similarly Bozzetti et al. (1985) showed that when the cutoff for total iron binding capacity was lowered from $< 310\,\mu g/dL$ to $< 270\,\mu g/dL$, the sensitivity falls from 55% to 30% but the specificity in predicting postoperative sepsis

Parameter	Cutoff	Sensitivity	Specificity
Arm circ. (cm)	< 14.0	90.4%	82.7%
	< 12.5	55.8%	98.0%

Table 1.7: Influence of change in the cutoff point on the sensitivity and specificity of mid-upper-arm circumference as a predictor of outcome. Data for arm circumference from Trowbridge and Staehling, American Journal of Clinical Nutrition 33: 687–696, 1980 © Am J Clin Nutr. American Society for Clinical Nutrition.

increases from 68% to 87% (Bozzetti et al., 1985).

Extent of the random errors associated with the raw measurements influence the specificity and sensitivity of a test. If the associated random errors are large, the test will be imprecise and the specificity (and sensitivity) will be reduced.

Non-nutritional factors such as infection, diurnal variation, and the effects of disease may reduce the specificity (Habicht et al., 1979). For example, infection is known to decrease serum zinc concentrations. As a result, the test yields a value which does not reflect true zinc status, so misclassification occurs; individuals are designated "at risk" to low serum zinc concentrations, when they are actually unaffected (false positives). In contrast, infection increases serum ferritin, so that in this case individuals may be designated "not at risk" when they are truly affected by the condition (false negatives).

Biological and behavioral processes that relate the indicator to the outcomes may influence sensitivity and specificity. For example, the sensitivity of low birth weight as an indicator of neonatal mortality will be greater in settings where it is due largely to prematurity rather than to intrauterine growth retardation.

1.4.12 Prevalence

The number of persons with malnutrition or disease during a given time period is measured by the prevalence. Numerically, the actual prevalence (P) is the proportion of individuals who really are malnourished or infected with the disease in question (the sum of true positives and false negatives) divided by the sample population (the sum of true positives, false positives, true negatives, and false negatives) (Table 1.6).

Prevalence influences the predictive value of a nutritional index more than any other factor (see below). For example, when the prevalence of malnutrition such as anemia decreases, it becomes less likely that an individual with a positive test (i.e., low hemoglobin) actually has anemia and more likely that the test represents a false positive. Therefore, the lower the prevalence of the condition, the more specific a test must be to be clinically useful (Hulley and Cummings, 1988).

1.4.13 Predictive value

The predictive value can be defined as the likelihood that a test correctly predicts the presence or absence of malnutrition or disease. Numerically, the predictive value of a test is the proportion of all tests that are true (the sum of the true positives and true negatives divided by the total number of tests) (Table 1.6). Because it incorporates information on both the test and the population being tested, predictive value is a good measure of overall clinical usefulness.

The predictive value can be further subdivided into the positive predictive value and the negative predictive value, as shown in Table 1.6. The positive predictive value of a test is the proportion of positive tests that are true (the true positives divided by the sum of the true positives and false positives). The negative predictive value of a test is the proportion of negative tests that are true (the true negatives divided by the sum of the true negatives and false negatives).

The predictive value of any test is not constant but depends on the sensitivity, specificity, and prevalence of malnutrition or disease. Table 1.8 shows the influence of prevalence on the positive predictive value of an index when the sensitivity and specificity are

constant. When the prevalence of malnutrition is low, even very sensitive and specific tests have a relatively low positive predictive value. Conversely, when the prevalence of malnutrition is high, tests with rather low sensitivity and specificity may have a relatively high positive predictive value.

The predictive value is the best indicator of the usefulness of any test of nutritional status in a particular circumstance. An acceptable predictive value for any test depends on the number of false-negative and false-positive results that are considered tolerable, taking into account the prevalence of the disease or malnutrition, its severity, the cost of the test, and, where appropriate, the availability and advantages of treatment. In general, the highest predictive value is achieved when specificity is high, irrespective of sensitivity (Habicht, 1980).

Sometimes, laboratory measurements are combined with measurements of nutrient intakes and anthropometric measurements to form a multiparameter index with an enhanced predictive value. Several examples of multiparameter indices used to identify malnourished hospital patients and predict those who are at nutritional risk are discussed in detail in Section 27.2. Of these, the Nutritional Risk Index (NRI), developed by the Veterans Affairs Total Parenteral Nutrition (TPN) Cooperative Study Group (1991) uses a formula that includes serum albumin level, present weight, and usual weight:

$$\text{NRI} = (1.519 \times \text{serum albumin})$$
$$+ 41.7 \times (\text{present weight/usual weight})$$

The NRI was found to be sensitive and spe-

Predictive Value	Prevalence					
	0.1%	1%	10%	20%	30%	40%
Positive	0.02	0.16	0.68	0.83	0.89	0.93
Negative	1.00	1.00	0.99	0.99	0.98	0.97

Table 1.8: Influence of disease prevalence on the predictive value of a test with sensitivity and specificity of 95%. From DT Dempsey and JL Mullen, Journal of Parenteral and Enteral Nutrition 11: 109S–114S, 1987 © American Society for Parenteral and Enteral Nutrition.

cific and a positive predictor for identifying patients at risk for complications in a study of 395 surgical patients (Veterans Affairs TPN Coperative Study Group, 1991). NRI > 100 indicated not malnourished; NRI 97.5–100, mild malnutrition; NRI 83.5–97.5, moderate malnutrition; NRI < 83.5, severe malnutrition.

1.4.14 Ethical issues

Formal guidelines on the general conduct of biomedical research are contained in the declaration of Helsinki and Ethics and Epidemiology, published by the Council for International Organization of Medical Sciences (CIOMS,1991). Ethical approval from the appropriate human ethics committees in the countries involved in the research study must be obtained by the principal investigators before work begins. The basic guidelines for research on human subjects must be followed. As an example, sections of the regulations of the U.S. Department of Health and Human Services (1988) are shown in Box 1.4. A more detailed discussion of ethical issues can be found in Lo et al. (1988).

Informed consent must be obtained from the participants or their principal caregivers in all studies. When securing informed consent, the investigator should also:

- Disclose details of the nature and procedures of the study
- Clearly state the associated potential risks and benefits

Risks to subjects are minimized and proportional to the anticipated benefits and knowledge.

Data are monitored to ensure safety of subjects.

Selection of subjects is equitable.

Vulnerable subjects, if included, are covered by additional safeguards.

Informed consent is obtained from the subjects.

Confidentiality is adequately protected.

Box 1.4: Some possible guidelines for research on human subjects. From DHHS (1983) Guidelines for Human Research.

- Confirm that participation in the research is voluntary
- Confirm that participants are free to withdraw from the study at any time
- Explain how the results relating to individual participants will be kept confidential
- Describe the procedures that provide answers to any questions and further information about the study

1.4.15 Additional factors

Of the many additional factors affecting the design of nutritional assessment systems, the acceptability of the method, respondent burden, equipment and personnel requirements, and field survey and data processing costs are particularly important. The methods should be acceptable to both the target population and the staff who are performing the measurements. For example, in some settings, drawing venous blood for biochemical determinations such as serum retinol may be unacceptable in infants and children, whereas the collection of breast milk samples may be more acceptable. Similarly, collecting blood specimens in populations with a high prevalence of HIV infections may be perceived to be an unacceptable risk by staff performing the tests.

To reduce the nonresponse rate and avoid bias in the sample selection, the respondent burden should be kept to a minimum. In the U.K. National Food Survey, for example, the inventory method was used initially to assess household food consumption; the method was found to have a high respondent burden and was abandoned in 1951 in favor of the food accounts method (Derry, 1984). Alternative methods for minimizing the nonresponse rate include the offering of material rewards and the provision of incentives such as regular medical checkups, feedback information, social visits, and telephone follow-up.

The requirements for equipment and personnel should also be taken into account when designing a nutritional assessment system. Measurements that require elaborate equipment and highly trained technical staff may be impractical in a field survey setting; instead, the measurements selected should be relatively noninvasive and easy to perform accurately and precisely using rugged equipment and unskilled but trained assistants. The ease with which equipment can be transported to the field, maintained, and calibrated must also be considered.

The field survey and data processing costs are also important factors. In surveillance systems, the resources available may dictate the number of malnourished individuals who can subsequently be treated in an intervention program. In such circumstances, the cutoff point for the test (Section 1.5.3) can be manipulated to select only the number of individuals who can be treated.

1.5 Evaluation of nutritional assessment indices

In population studies, nutritional assessment indices can be evaluated by comparison with a distribution of reference values (if available) using percentiles (Figure 13.2), standard deviation scores (Z-scores) (Figure 13.3), or the percent-of-median (Section 13.1). Alternatively, for classifying individuals, the values for nutritional assessment indices can be compared with either predetermined reference limits drawn from the reference distribution or cutoff points. The latter are based on data that relate the levels of the indices to low body stores of the nutrient, impaired function, clinical signs of deficiency, or mortality. Sometimes, more than one reference limit or cutoff point is used to define degrees of malnutrition (e.g., for body mass index) (Section 10.3; Table 10.7).

1.5.1 Reference distribution

Reference values are obtained from the reference sample group. The distribution of these reference values forms the reference distribution. The relationship between the terms used to define reference values is shown in Table 1.9.

Theoretically, only healthy persons are included in the reference sample group. In practice, however, this is rarely followed. Instead, the reference sample group used is drawn from the general population sampled during a nationally representative survey such as NHANES III or the U.K. National Diet and Nutrition surveys.

More rarely, a specific reference sample is compiled, consisting only of healthy individuals. For example, the reference values for hemoglobin (by age, sex, and race) compiled from NHANES III are based on a sample of healthy, nonpregnant individuals only. Data from any person with conditions known to affect iron status were excluded (Looker et al., 1997).

For comparison of the observed values of an individual with data derived from the reference sample, the person under observation should be matched as closely as possible to the reference individuals by the factors known to influence the measurement. Frequently, these factors include age, sex, race, and physiological state, and, depending on the variable, they may also include exercise, body posture, fasting status, and the procedures and time of day used for specimen collection and analysis. The latter are especially critical for comparison of serum zinc concentrations with reference data (Section 24.3.1) (Hotz et al., 2003). Only if these matching criteria are met can the observed value be correctly interpreted.

1.5.2 Reference limits

The reference distribution can also be used to derive reference limits and a reference interval. Reference limits are generally defined so that a stated fraction of the reference values would be less than or equal to the limit, with a stated probability. Two reference limits are usually defined, and the interval between and including them is termed the "reference interval." Observed values for individuals can then be classified as "unusually low," "usual," or "unusually high," according to whether they are situated below the lower reference limit, between or equal to either of the reference limits, or above the upper reference

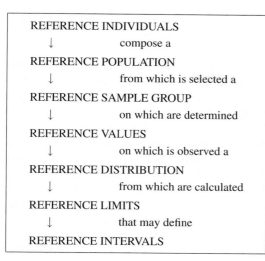

REFERENCE INDIVIDUALS
↓   compose a
REFERENCE POPULATION
↓   from which is selected a
REFERENCE SAMPLE GROUP
↓   on which are determined
REFERENCE VALUES
↓   on which is observed a
REFERENCE DISTRIBUTION
↓   from which are calculated
REFERENCE LIMITS
↓   that may define
REFERENCE INTERVALS

Table 1.9: The concept of reference values and the relationship of recommended terms. The observed value for an individual may be compared with reference values, the reference distribution, reference limits, or reference intervals. From IFCC (1987).

limit (IFCC, 1984, 1987). For anthropometric growth indices in industrialized countries, the 3rd or 5th and 95th or 97th percentiles are frequently the reference limits used to designate individuals with unusually low or unusually high anthropometric indices, whereas in low-income countries, reference limits based on standard deviation scores (Z-scores) are preferred (Section 13.2.1).

Often for biochemical indices, only a lower reference limit is defined. In NHANES III, the lower reference limit for hemoglobin corresponded to the 5th percentile (Table 17.2; Section 17.1). For serum zinc, the new lower reference limits, by age, sex, fasting status, and time of blood collection, are based on the 2.5th percentile values from a healthy reference sample derived from NHANES II (Hotz et al., 2003).

Note that these reference limits can be altered for diagnostic purposes, although it must be recognized that when the limits are changed to produce fewer false-negative results, the number of false-positive results will increase, or vice versa. The terms "abnormal," "pathological," and "normal" should not be applied when using this approach for setting the reference limits because an un-

usually high or low value for an index is not necessarily associated with any impairment in health status (Smith et al., 1985).

1.5.3 Cutoff points

Cutoff points, unlike reference limits, are based on the relationship between nutritional assessment indices and low body stores, functional impairment, or clinical signs of deficiency. Their use is less frequent than that of reference limits because information relating tests and signs of deficiency is often not available. Cutoff points may vary with the local setting because the relationship between the tests and functional outcomes is unlikely to be the same from area to area.

Sometimes more than one cutoff point is selected. For example, for body mass index (BMI), two cutoffs are often used to define overnutrition in adults (BMI > 25, overweight, BMI > 30, obesity), whereas three cutoffs are used to define degrees of underweight in adults (FAO, 1994; WHO, 1995) (Section 10.3.5). For serum 25-hydroxyvitamin D (25-OH-D) concentrations, cutoff values are sometimes used to define five stages of vitamin D status (Figure 18.12) : vitamin D deficiency, vitamin D insufficiency, hypovitaminosis D, vitamin D sufficiency, and vitamin D toxicity (Zitterman, 2003).

When selecting an index and its associated cutoff point, the relative importance of the sensitivity and specificity of the nutritional index (or indicator) must always be considered, as noted earlier (Section 1.4.11). Increasingly, receiver operator characteristic (ROC) curves are being used to select cutoff points. This is a graphical method of comparing indices and portraying the trade-offs that occur in the sensitivity and specificity of a test when the cutoffs are altered. To use this approach, a spectrum of cutoffs or thresholds over the observed range of results is used and the sensitivity and specificity for each cutoff calculated. Next, the sensitivity (or true-positive rate) is plotted against the true-negative rate (1.0–specificity), for each cutoff point. Figure 1.3 shows ROC curves for two different serum enzyme assays used to iden-

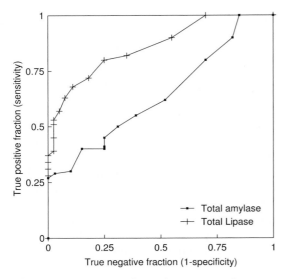

Figure 1.3: Nonparametric receiver operator characteristic (ROC) plots for two serum enzyme assays based on "binned" data. Redrawn from Zweig and Campbell, Clinical Chemistry 39: 561–577, 1993, with permission of the AACC.

tify subjects with pancreatitis. An ideal index is one that reaches the upper left corner of the graph (100% sensitivity) and 100% specificity. Neither of the two indices shown in Figure 1.3 reaches this ideal. Nevertheless, the plot does show clearly that total lipase is a better diagnostic tool in these particular circumstances, more closely approaching the ideal of perfect sensitivity and specificity. Stoltzfus et al. (1993) used this approach to compare the ability of three indicators (serum retinol, milk vitamin A concentration, and milk vitamin A per gram milk fat) to detect changes in vitamin A status of lactating women in Indonesia.

After the index to be used has been chosen on the basis of the ROC curves, the cutoff must be selected. Sometimes alternative cutoff points are selected depending on whether the consequences of a high number of subjects being classified as false positives is more, or less important than the consequences of a large number of subjects being classified as false negatives. Minimizing either misclassification may be considered more important than minimizing the total number of subjects misclassified. A detailed explana-

tion of ROC curves can be found in Zweig and Campbell (1993).

As discussed in Section 1.3, cutoff values can never separate the "deficient" and the "adequately nourished" without some misclassification occurring. In Figure 1.4, for example, the light-shaded area to the right of 110 g/L and below the left curve represents anemic persons classified as normal according to the cutoff point (110 g/L) defined by the World Health Organization (WHO, 1972). The dark-shaded area to the left of 110 g/L and below the right curve comprises persons within the normal population, classified as anemic by the WHO cutoff point but who are not found to be responsive to iron administration. Hence, the dark-shaded area represents those well-nourished persons who were incorrectly classified as "anemic" (i.e., false positives). Misclassification arises because there is always biological variation among individuals (and hence in the physiological normal levels of any indices), depending on the nutrient requirements of an individual (Beaton, 1986).

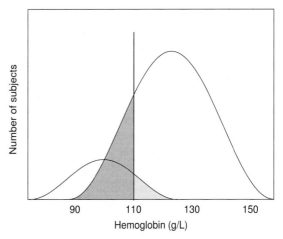

Figure 1.4: The distribution of hemoglobin values among persons with adequate intakes of iron (right curve) and those known to be responsive to an iron supplement (left curve). The two distributions overlap, showing that no single cutoff value can separate individuals with adequate iron status from those with inadequate iron status. The vertical line marks the hemoglobin value used by WHO (1972) to define anemia. From Cook et al., Blood 38: 591–603, 1971, with permission of Grune and Stratton.

Criteria	Prevalence (%)
Clinical	
Children 2–5 y	
Night blindness	> 1.0
Bitot's spots	> 0.5
Corneal xerosis	> 0.01
Corneal ulcers	> 0.01
Corneal scars	> 0.05
Women of childbearing age	
Night blindness	
during recent pregnancy	> 5.0
Biochemical	
Serum retinol < 0.70 μmol/L	> 15

Table 1.10: Various International Vitamin A Consultative Group prevalence criteria, each indicating significant vitamin A deficiency within a defined population. From Sommer and Davidson, Journal of Nutrition 132: 2845S–2850S, 2002, with permission of the American Society for Nutritional Sciences. (2002).

1.5.4 Trigger levels

In population studies, cutoff points may be combined with trigger levels to set the level of an index (or indicator) or combination of indices at which a public health problem exists of a specified level of concern. Trigger levels may highlight regions or populations, where specific nutrient deficiencies are likely to occur, or may serve to monitor and evaluate intervention programs.

Some international organizations including WHO (1995), the International Vitamin A Consultative Group (IVACG) (Sommer and Davidson, 2002), and the International Zinc Nutrition Consultative Group (IZiNCG)(Hotz and Brown, 2004) for example, have defined the prevalence criteria for selected indicators within a population that signify a public health problem in relation to specific nutrients and conditions. Table 1.10 shows some possible prevalence criteria indicating significant vitamin A deficiency in a population.

A generalized discussion of the specific procedures used for the evaluation of dietary, anthropometric, laboratory, and clinical methods of nutritional assessment are discussed more fully in Chapters 8, 13, 15, and 25, respectively.

References

Altman DG, Schulz KF, Moher D, Egger M, Davidoff F, Elbourne D, Getzsche PC, Lang T, for the CONSORT group. (2001). The revised CONSORT statement for reporting randomized trials: explanation and elaboration. Annals of Internal Medicine 134: 663–694.

Anonymous. (1988). Hospital malnutrition still abounds. Nutrition Reviews 46: 315–317.

Beaglehole R, Bonita R, Kjellström T. (1993). Basic Epidemiology. World Health Organization, Geneva.

Beaton GH. (1986). Toward harmonization of dietary, biochemical, and clinical assessments: the meanings of nutritional status and requirements. Nutrition Reviews 44: 349–358.

Bistrian BR, Blackburn GL, Hallowell E, Heddle R. (1974). Protein status of general surgical patients. Journal of the American Medical Association 230: 858–860.

Bistrian BR, Blackburn GL, Vitale J, Cochran D, Naylor J. (1976). Prevalence of malnutrition in general medical patients. Journal of the American Medical Association 235: 1567–1570.

Bozzetti F, Migliavacca S, Gallus G, Radaelli G, Scotti A, Bonalumi MG, Ammatuna M, Sequeira C, Ternø G. (1985). "Nutritional" markers, as prognostic indicators of postoperative sepsis in cancer patients. Journal of Parenteral and Enteral Nutrition 9: 464– 470.

Christian P, West KP Jr. (1998). Interactions between zinc and vitamin A: an update. American Journal of Clinical Nutrition 68: 435S–441S.

CIOMS (Council for International Organizations of Medical Sciences). (1991). International Guidelines for Ethical Review of Epidemiological Studies. Council for International Organizations of Medical Sciences, Geneva.

Combs GF. (1996). Should intakes with beneficial action, often requiring supplementation, be considered for the RDAs? Journal of Nutrition 126: 2373S–2376S.

Congdon N, Sommer A, Severns M, Humphrey J, Friedman D, Clement L, Wu LS, Natadisastra G. (1995). Pupillary and visual thresholds in young children as an index of population vitamin A status. American Journal of Clinical Nutrition 61: 1076–1082.

Cook JD, Alvarado J, Gutnisky A, Jamra M, Labardini J, Layrisse M, Linares J, Loria A, Maspes V, Restrepo A, Reynafarje C, Sanchez-Medal L, Velez H, Viteri F. (1971). Nutritional deficiency and anemia in Latin America: a collaborative study. Blood 38: 591–603.

Corish CA, Kennedy NP. (2000). Protein-energy undernutrition in hospital patients. British Journal of Nutrition 83: 575–591.

Craft NE. (2001). Innovative approaches to vitamin A assessment. Journal of Nutrition 131: 1626S–1630S.

Crowne DP, Marlowe D. (1960). A new scale of social

desirability independent of psychopathology. Journal of Consulting Psychology 24: 349–354.

Darnton-Hill I, Nalubola R. (2002). Fortification strategies to meet micronutrient needs: successes and failures. Proceedings of the Nutrition Society 61; 231–234.

Dempsey DT, Mullen JL. (1987). Prognostic value of nutritional indices. Journal of Parenteral and Enteral Nutrition 11: 109S–114S.

Derry B. (1984). Food purchases — strengths and weaknesses of the National Food Survey. In: The Dietary Assessment of Populations. Medical Research Council Scientific Report No. 4. Southampton General Hospital, Southampton, pp. 22–25.

DHHS (Department of Health and Human Services). (1983). Rules and Regulations. Title 45; Code of Federal Regulations; Part 46: Revised as of March 8, 1983. U.S. Department of Health and Human Services, Washington, DC. Services,

FAO (Food and Agriculture Organization). (1994). Body Mass Index: A Measure of Chronic Energy Deficiency in Adults. Food and Nutrition Papers No. 56. Food and Agriculture Organization, Rome.

Finch S, Doyle W, Lowe C, Bates CJ, Prentice A, Smithers G, Clarke PC. (1998). National Diet and Nutrition Survey: People Aged 65 Years and Over. Volume 1: Report of the Diet and Nutrition Survey. The Stationery Office, London.

Gallagher SK, Johnson LK, Milnes DB. (1992). Short- and long-term variability of selected indices related to nutritional status. II: Vitamins, lipids, and protein indices. Clinical Chemistry 38: 1449–1453.

Gregory J, Foster K, Tyler H, Wiseman M. (1990). The Dietary and Nutritional Survey of British Adults. Her Majesty's Stationery Office, London.

Gregory J, Collins DL, Davies PSW, Hughes JM, Clarke PC. (1995). National Diet and Nutrition Survey: Children Aged One-and-a-Half to Four-and-a-Half Years. Volume 1: Report of the Diet and Nutrition Survey. Her Majesty's Stationery Office, London.

Gregory JR, Lowe S Bates CJ, Prentice A, Jackson LV, Smithers G, Wenlock R, Farron M. (2000). National Diet and Nutrition Survey: Young People Aged 4 to 18 Years. Volume 1: Report of the Diet and Nutrition Survey. The Stationery Office, London.

Gunter EW, McQuillan G. (1990). Quality control in planning and operating the laboratory component for the Third National Health and Nutrition Examination Survey. Journal of Nutrition 120: 1451–1454.

Habicht J-P. (1980). Some characteristics of indicators of nutritional status for use in screening and surveillance. American Journal of Clinical Nutrition 33: 531–535.

Habicht J-P, Pelletier DL. (1990). The importance of context in choosing nutrition indicators. Journal of Nutrition 120: 1519–1524.

Habicht J-P, Stoltzfus RJ. (1997). What do indicators indicate? American Journal of Clinical Nutrition 66: 190–191.

Habicht J-P, Yarbrough C, Martorell R. (1979). Anthropometric field methods: criteria for selection. In: Jelliffe DB, Jelliffe EFP (eds.) Human Nutrition: A Comprehensive Treatise. Volume 2: Nutrition and Growth. Plenum Press, New York, pp. 365–387.

Habicht J-P, Meyers LD, Brownie C. (1982). Indicators for identifying and counting the improperly nourished. American Journal of Clinical Nutrition 35: 1241–1254.

Habicht J-P, Victoria CG, Vaughan JP. (1999). Evaluation designs for adequacy, plausibility and probability of public health programme performance and impact. International Journal of Epidemiology 28: 10–18.

Himes JH. (1987). Purposeful assessment of nutritional status. In: Johnston FE (ed.) Nutritional Anthropology. Alan R. Liss, New York, pp. 85–99.

Hotz C, Brown KM. (2004). Assessment of zinc deficiency in populations and options for its control. IZiNCG Technical Document No. 1. Food and Nutrition Bulletin 25(Suppl.12): S95–S204.

Hotz C, Peerson JM, Brown KH. (2003). Suggested lower cutoffs of serum zinc concentration for assessing population zinc status: a reanalysis of the second U.S. National Health and Nutrition Examination Survey data (NHANES II: 1976–1980). American Journal of Clinical Nutrition 78: 756–764.

Hulley SB, Cummings SR (eds.). (1988). Designing Clinical Research: An Epidemiological Approach. Lippincott Williams & Wilkins, Baltimore, MD.

ICNND (Interdepartmental Committee on Nutrition for National Defense). (1963). Manual for Nutrition Surveys. 2nd ed. Superintendent of Documents, U.S. Government Printing Office, Washington, DC.

IFCC (International Federation of Clinical Chemistry). (1984). The theory of reference values. Part 5: Statistical treatment of collected reference values — determination of reference limits. Clinica Chimica Acta 137: 97F–114F.

IFCC (International Federation of Clinical Chemistry). (1987). Approved recommendation (1986) on the theory of reference values. Part 1: The concept of reference values. Clinica Chimica Acta 165: 111–118.

IOM (Institute of Medicine). (1996). WIC Nutrition Risk Criteria: A Scientific Assessment. Food and Nutrition Board, Institute of Medicine, National Academy Press, Washington, DC.

Jelliffe DB. (1966). The Assessment of the Nutritional Status of the Community. WHO Monograph Series No. 53. World Health Organization, Geneva.

Kipnis V, Midthune D, Freedman LS, Bingham S, Schatzkin A, Subar A, Carroll RJ. (2001). Empirical evidence of correlated biases in dietary assessment instruments and its implications. American Journal of Epidemiology 153: 394–403.

Kuizon MD, Perlas LA, Madriaga JR, Cheong RL, Desnacido JA, Marcos JM, Fuertes RT, Valdez DH. (1997). Fourth National Nutrition Survey: Philippines, 1993. Part A, Biochemical Nutrition Survey. Philippine Journal of Nutrition 44: 66–75.

Lemeshow S, Hosmer DW, Klar J, Lwanga SK. (1990). Adequacy of Sample Size in Health Studies. John Wiley & Sons, Chichester.

Levinson FJ, Rogers BL, Hicks KM, Schaetzel T, Troy L, Young C. (1999). Monitoring and Evaluation: A Guidebook for Nutrition Project Managers in Developing Countries. Human Development Network, World Bank, Washington, DC.

Lo B, Fiegal D, Hulley SB. (1988). Addressing ethical issues. In: Hulley SB, Cummings SR (eds.) Designing Clinical Research: An Epidemiological Approach. Lippincott Williams & Wilkins, Baltimore, MD, pp. 151–158.

Looker AC, Dallman PR, Carroll MD, Gunter EW, Johnson CL. (1997). Prevalence of iron deficiency in the United States. Journal of the American Medical Association 277: 973–976.

Lukaski HC, Penland JG. (1996). Functional changes appropriate for determining mineral element requirements. Journal of Nutrition 126: 2345S–2364S.

Lwanga SK, Lemeshow S. (1991). Sample Size Determination in Health Studies: A Practical Manual. World Health Organization, Geneva.

Martorell R. (1984). Measuring the impact of nutrition intervention on physical growth. In: Sahn DE, Lockwood R, Scrimshaw NS (eds.) Methods for the Evaluation of the Impact of Food and Nutrition Programmes. United Nations University, Tokyo, Japan, pp. 65–93.

Mayne ST. (2003). Antioxidant nutrients and chronic disease: use of biomarkers of exposure and oxidative stress status in epidemiologic research. Journal of Nutrition 133: 933S–940S.

McLennan W, Podger A. (1995). National Nutrition Survey: Nutrient Intakes and Physical Measurements, Australia 1995. Australian Bureau of Statistics, Canberra.

Mei JV, Alexander JR, Adam BW, Hannon WH. (2001). Use of filter paper for the collection and analysis of human whole blood specimens. Journal of Nutrition 31: 1631S–1636S.

MOPH (Ministry of Public Health). (1999). The Fourth National Nutrition Survey 1996/97. Nutrition Division, Ministry of Public Health, Bangkok, Thailand.

Morley D. (1973). Pediatric Priorities in the Developing World. Butterworth, London.

NCHS (National Center for Health Statistics). (1994). Plan and Operation of the Third National Health and Nutrition Examination Survey, 1988–94. Vital and Health Statistics 1(32).

Parnell W, Scragg R, Wilson N, Schaaf D, Fitzgerald E. (2003). NZ Food NZ Children: Key Results of the 2002 National Children's Nutrition Survey. Ministry of Health, Wellington, New Zealand.

Quigley R, Watts C. (1997). Food Comes First: Methodologies for the National Nutrition Survey of New Zealand. Public Health Report No. 2. Public Health Group, Ministry of Health, Wellington.

Riegelman RK, Hirsch RP. (1989). Studying a Study and Testing a Test. How to Read the Medical Literature. 2nd ed. Little, Brown, Boston.

Robinson JP, Shaver PR, Wrightsman LS. (1991). Measures of Personality and Social Psychological Attitudes. Academic Press, San Diego and London.

Rossi PH, Freeman HE, Lipsey MW. (1999). Evaluation: A Systematic Approach. Sage Publications, Thousand Oaks, CA.

Roubenoff R, Roubenoff RA, Preto J, Balke CW. (1987). Malnutrition among hospitalized patients: a problem of physician awareness. Archives of Internal Medicine 147: 1462–1465.

Ruel MT, Levin CE. (2001). Food-based approaches. In: Ramakrishnan U. (ed.) Nutritional Anemias. CRC Press, Boca Raton, FL. pp. 185–214.

Russell D, Parnell W, Wilson N, Faed J, Ferguson E, Herbison P, Horwath C, Nye T, Walker R, Wilson B. (1999). New Zealand Food, New Zealand People: Key Results of the 1997 National Nutrition Survey. Ministry of Health, Wellington, New Zealand.

Sackett DL, Hayns RB, Tugwell P, Guyatt GH. (1991). Clinical Epidemiology: A Basic Science for Clinical Medicine. Lippincott Williams & Wilkins, Baltimore, MD.

Shrimpton R, Schultink W. (2002). Can supplements help meet the micronutrient needs of the developing world? Proceedings of the Nutrition Society 61: 223–229.

SLAN (Survey of Lifestyles, Attitudes and Nutrition). (1999). Dietary Habits of the Irish Population: Results from SLAN. Annual report, National Nutrition Surveillance Centre, Galway, Ireland

Smith JC, Holbrook JT, Danford DE. (1985). Analysis and evaluation of zinc and copper in human plasma and serum. Journal of the American College of Nutrition 4: 627–638.

Solomons NW. (1985). Assessment of nutritional status: functional indicators of pediatric nutriture. Pediatric Clinics of North America 32: 319–334.

Solomons NW. (2002). Methods for the measurement of nutrition impact and adaptation of laboratory methods into field settings to enhance and support community-based nutrition research. Nutrition Reviews 60: S126–S131.

Solomons NW, Allen LH. (1983). The functional assessment of nutritional status: principles, practice and potential. Nutrition Reviews 41: 33–50.

Sommer A, Davidson FR. (2002). Assessment and control of vitamin A deficiency: the Annecy Accords. Journal of Nutrition 132: 2845S–2850S.

Stoltzfus RJ, Habicht J-P, Rasmussen KM, Hakimi M. (1993). Evaluation of indicators for use in vitamin A intervention trials targeted at women. International Journal of Epidemiology 22: 1111–1118.

Trowbridge FL, Staehling N. (1980). Sensitivity and specificity of arm circumference indicators in identifying malnourished children. American Journal of Clinical Nutrition 33: 687–696.

Trowbridge FL, Wong FL, Byers TE, Serdula MK. (1990). Methodological issues in nutrition surveillance: the CDC experience. Journal of Nutrition 120: 1512–1518.

Ulijaszek SJ, Kerr DA. (1999). Anthropometric meas-

urement error and the assessment of nutritional status. British Journal of Nutrition 82: 165–177.
Erratum in 83: 95.

Varkevisser CM, Pathmanathan I, Brownlee A. (1993).
Designing and Conducting Health Systems Research
Projects. Health Systems Research Training Series,
Vol. 2, part 1. International Development Research
Centre, Ottawa.

Veterans Affairs TPN Cooperative Study Group.(1991).
Perioperative total parenteral nutrition in surgical
patients. New England Journal of Medicine 325:
525–532.

Ward R, Anderson G. (1993). Examination of the
skinfold compressibility and skinfold thickness relationship. American Journal of Human Biology 5:
541–548.

WHO (World Health Organization). (1972). Nutritional Anemia. Technical Report Series No. 3.

World Health Organization, Geneva.

WHO (World Health Organization). (1976). Report on
Methodology of Nutritional Surveillance. FAO/
UNICEF/WHO Expert Committee. Technical Re-
port Series No. 593. World Health Organization,
Geneva.

WHO (World Health Organization). (1995). Physical
Status: The Use and Interpretation of Anthropome-
try. Report of a WHO Expert Committee. Technical
Report Series No. 854. World Health Organization,
Geneva.

Zittermann A. (2003). Vitamin D in preventive medicine: are we ignoring the evidence? British Journal
of Nutrition 89: 552–572.

Zweig MH, Campbell G. (1993). Receiver operating
characteristic (ROC) plots: a fundamental evaluation tool in clinical medicine. Clinical Chemistry
39: 561–577.

2

Food consumption at the national and household levels

Food consumption can be assessed by national, household, or individual level food consumption surveys, with the resulting data expressed in terms of nutrients and/or foods. This chapter considers methods suitable for measuring the food available for consumption at the national and household levels. Chapter 3 includes a detailed discussion of methods suitable for measuring food consumption at the individual level.

2.1 Measuring food consumption at the national level

The most widely used method of assessing the food available nationally for consumption is based on food balance sheets. The data are conventionally presented on a per capita basis using population estimates, but they provide no information on the distribution of available food supplies within the country or the extent to which the food intake of individuals varies within the population. The results are frequently used both to compare the available food supply between countries, and to monitor trends over time within an individual country.

The accuracy of the estimates of available food supplies based on food balance sheets varies among countries. Systematic errors may occur, which increase as the food system becomes more sophisticated. The limitations of the data should be recognized: attempts to link trends in national food consumption data to changes in disease or mortality must

be viewed with caution; other lifestyle factors may be equally important.

2.1.1 Food balance sheets

Food balance sheets are most commonly used to assess food consumption at the national level; they provide data on the food available for consumption (i.e., the food supply within a country). National food balance sheets are published by FAO annually for 176 countries, providing data on the amounts of 95 food commodities available for human consumption. The FAO describes food balance sheets as providing

> a comprehensive picture of the pattern of a country's food supply during a specified reference period, calculated from the annual production of food, changes in stocks, imports and exports, and distribution of food over various uses within the country (FAO, 2001).

Several different terms have been used to describe food balance sheets. These include national food accounts, food moving into consumption, food consumption statistics, food disappearance data, and consumption level estimates. The various terms reflect differences in the methods of calculation, but all provide information on a country's available food supply over a specified period. The latter may be a calendar year, the agricultural year, or the crop year.

The FAO has published food balance sheets since 1949, covering the period 1934–1938, and 1947 up to the present. Fewer than 50 countries were covered in the early annual balance sheets, but the more recent three-year-average balance sheets provide coverage for at least 145 countries in a standardized format. The issue published in 1999 covers the period from 1994–1996 (FAO, 1999).

In general, the food supply is calculated from domestic food production plus imports and food taken from stocks. Exports and food added to stocks are then subtracted, to yield an estimate of total food available (the gross national food supply). Food diverted for non-human-food uses, such as animal feed, seed, and sugar in the brewing industry, together with an estimate for waste, is subtracted from the gross food supply. The result is a figure for the net food supply or the net amount of food available for human consumption in a country at the retail level (Figure 2.1) (Campbell, 1981).

The estimates for waste take into account waste on the farm and during distribution and processing. They do not include waste at the household or food service level. Waste during distribution and processing may be considerable in countries where the agricultural products reach the consumer in urban areas after passing through several marketing stages. In such cases, much food may remain unsold because of imbalances of supply and demand, especially for perishable foods such as fresh fruits and vegetables. As a result, assumptions for waste may be based on expert opinion obtained in the countries. An example of a portion of a national food balance sheet is given in Appendix A2.1. Complete balance sheet tables for other years and countries are available from www.fao.org.

The net food supply and utilization data are reported in thousand metric tons or metric tons. Once the net food supply has been calculated, it is then converted to a daily per capita basis using population estimates for that country. The FAO uses the United Nations Population Division mid-year estimates of population size for its food balance sheet data to calculate per capita food availability. In some instances, adjustments are performed to include migrants and refugees who consume the available food supply and/or to consider tourists and seasonal workers. Per capita food availability is expressed in terms of kg/y per capita of individual food commodities and major food groups.

Data in the FAO food balance sheets are also presented in terms of energy (kcal/d), protein (g/d), and fat (g/d) availability per capita. In the future, the nutrient coverage may be extended and perhaps fat broken down into saturated, monounsaturated, and polyunsaturated fatty acids.

In the FAO food balance sheets, foods are grouped into 15 food groups. These are cereals, roots and tubers, sugars and honey, pulses, nuts and oilseeds, vegetables, fruits, meat and offal, eggs, fish and seafood, milk, oils and fats, spices, stimulants, and alcoholic beverages (FAO, 2001). Processed commodities (e.g., bread) are converted back to their primary form such as wheat and added to the original commodity by FAO, producing "standardized food balance sheets." Details of this standardization procedure, and the

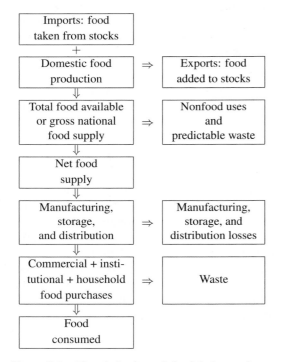

Figure 2.1: The derivation of food balance sheets. Adapted from Nelson (1984) with permission.

Region (no. of countries)	Population (millions)	Energy (kcal/d)	Zinc (mg/d)	Zinc density (mg/1000 kcal)	Phytate (mg/d)	Phytate : Zn ratio
Western Europe (20)	457	3410 ± 135	12.4 ± 1.3	3.6 ± 0.4	1596 ± 391	13.2 ± 4.8
USA and Canada (2)	305	3546 ± 164	12.2 ± 0.5	3.5 ± 0.1	1542 ± 58	12.5 ± 0.1
Eastern Europe (27)	413	2971 ± 255	10.8 ± 1.3	3.6 ± 0.3	1567 ± 211	14.5 ± 2.2
Western Pacific (13)	223	2902 ± 273	11.8 ± 1.0	4.1 ± 0.3	2123 ± 444	18.1 ± 4.7
Latin America and Caribbean (35)	498	2743 ± 313	9.9 ± 2.0	3.6 ± 0.4	2111 ± 808	21.1 ± 6.0
China including Hong Kong (1)	1262	2743 ± 33	10.9 ± 0.2	4.0 ± 0.1	2074 ± 36	18.8 ± 0.6
Southeast Asia (10)	504	2556 ± 226	9.0 ± 0.9	3.5 ± 0.1	2248 ± 586	24.5 ± 4.6
Sub-Saharan Africa (46)	581	2203 ± 379	9.3 ± 2.0	4.3 ± 0.8	2530 ± 645	26.9 ± 3.7
North Africa and E. Mediterranean (17)	342	2806 ± 450	8.7 ± 1.6	3.1 ± 0.6	2206 ± 524	25.1 ± 3.5
South Asia (6)	1297	2351 ± 99	7.6 ± 0.6	3.2 ± 0.2	2068 ± 263	26.9 ± 1.7
All regions (176)	5882	2706 ± 434	10.0 ± 2.0	3.6 ± 0.5	2045 ± 504	21.3 ± 6.0

Table 2.1: Mean (± standard deviation) daily per capita amounts of energy, zinc, and phytate in the food supply of 176 countries, by region. Reprinted with permission from Brown et al., Food and Nutrition Bulletin 22: 113–125, 2001.

accuracy of the food balance sheets, are available from http://www.fao.org/.

The validity of food supply data is affected by errors that can be introduced at each stage in the calculation of the per capita nutrient availability. For some developing countries, the coverage and quality of the statistics — especially for food diverted for nonhuman food uses, such as animal feed, seed, and manufacture — has many gaps, limiting the reliability of the food balance sheet data. Underrecording may also occur as a result of growing or catching foodstuffs for home consumption. Hence, in less-developed countries, the method is said to result in an underestimate of per capita energy availability (Poleman, 1981). Sasaki and Kesteloot (1992) have recommended that the results for nutrients are expressed per megajoule, indicating the nutrient density of the food supply rather than the per capita nutrient availability.

Food balance sheet data can be used to formulate agricultural policies concerned with the production, distribution, and consumption of foods. It can also be used to make intercountry comparisons of food supplies and to examine associations between nutrition and mortality at the national level (Gage and O'Connor, 1994). Food supply data collected over successive years can also provide useful information at the national level on trends in food consumption and, hence, changes in nutrient intakes.

Food balance sheets do not measure the food actually ingested by the population or provide information on food consumption in relation to regional, economic, demographic, seasonal, or socioeconomic differences within a country. Hence, caution should be used when food balance sheet data are used to estimate nutritional inadequacies in a particular country or region of the world (Dowler and Ok Seo, 1985; Brown et al., 2001).

Food balance sheet data have been used to compare the adequacy of the food supply among countries to meet requirements for vitamin A (West, 2000) and zinc (Brown et al., 2001). Table 2.1 presents data on the mean daily per capita availability of energy, zinc, and phytate and the zinc density and phytate-to-zinc molar ratios of the food supply in 176 countries compiled by Brown et al. (2001). Despite the sources of uncertainty emphasized by these authors, food balance sheet data clearly can provide insights into the countries and regions that are most likely to be at greatest risk for low intakes of some nutrients.

In Canada, per capita food consumption data are prepared by Statistics Canada (2002, 2003a) on an annual basis and are a measure of apparent "food disappearance." The tables indicate food available at the retail level. The data are mainly derived from farm surveys and reports from firms in the food industry that are engaged in production and marketing. These tables provide only a very gross picture of what is actually consumed in Canada. No allowance is made for processing losses and some commodities are not included; no information is provided about the intake of individual foods such as bread. Methodologies are being developed by Agriculture and Agri-foods Canada for merging the Canadian food disappearance data and the Family Food Expenditure Survey (Statistics Canada, 2003b) with the Canadian Nutrient File (CNF) (Health Canada, 1997) to yield per capita nutrient disappearance data.

In the United States, estimates of the total amount of foods consumed by the U.S. civilian population are compiled annually by the USDA Economic Research Service using food balance sheet methodologies. Thus the U.S. annual estimates can be compared with data for other countries reported in the FAO food balance sheets. Nutrient composition data from the USDA Research Service, called the "USDA Nutrient Database for Standard Reference" (USDA, 2003) (Section 4.2), are then applied to the edible portion of the foods. Results for 27 nutrients and dietary components from all foods are totaled and converted to amounts per capita per day. In addition, the percentage of total nutrients contributed by major food categories is computed (Gerrior and Bente, 2001, 2002). An example showing the sources of calcium from six major food categories is given in Figure 2.2.

One of the major strengths of U.S. food supply data is that it is compiled annually in a consistent manner. It thus provides a graphic picture of broad changes in the American diet over time (Putnam et al., 2002).

Limitations in the U.S. per capita food supply data arise from its calculation as the difference between supply and utilization. In particular, miscellaneous non-food uses for which data are not available are relegated to the food supply. For example, during the industrial processing of turkey, some parts,

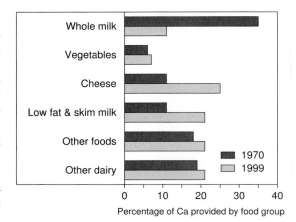

Figure 2.2: Sources of calcium in the U.S. food supply, 1970 and 1999. Data from Gerrior and Bente, Food Review 24: 39–46, 2001.

especially backs, necks, and giblets, are made into pet food; currently, this fraction is included in the food supply. Similarly, fats and oils discarded as waste during the preparation of fast foods are by default included in the food supply. Hence, the reported levels may overestimate the levels of some nutrients in the U.S. food supply (Manchester and Farrell, 1981; Kantor et al., 1997).

Some countries use food balance sheet data in place of national household food consumption surveys as a basis for estimating food consumption. This is not sound practice and should be avoided. Food balance sheets and household food consumption surveys have different objectives and yield different average per capita figures for daily energy and nutrient intakes. The size of the difference between the two methods is not necessarily constant between countries, or over time, and appears to depend in part on the gross national product (Dowler and Ok Seo, 1985).

2.1.2 Total diet studies

Total diet studies (TDSs) are defined as

studies specifically designed to establish by chemical analysis the dietary intake of food contaminants by a person consuming a typical diet (Ochuizen et al., 1991).

They involve the collection of a large number of representative foods from a particular region or country. In the United Kingdom, for example, dietary exposure to Al, As, Cr, Cu, Hg, Pb, Ni, Se, Sn, and Zn are regularly checked to see if there are any risks to health from the levels found in the U.K. diet. Total diet studies can also be used to monitor and evaluate intakes of macronutrients and vitamins in populations. They can be based on market basket studies, collection of individual food items, or duplicate portions, as discussed below.

Market basket studies

For a market basket study, food items that comprise part of the average diet of the selected age and sex group of interest are purchased from retail outlets in representative towns of the country, on one or more occasions per year. After purchase, the foods are prepared table-ready, according to normal household procedures. Next, they are combined into designated groups of similar foods, and then thoroughly homogenized and frozen until analysis.

Analysis for both toxic chemical contaminants (pesticide residues, industrial chemicals, toxic elements), and a wide range of nutrients is generally performed. From the analytical results, the average daily intake of both toxic elements and nutrients for the selected age and sex groups in the population of interest can be estimated. A limitation of this approach is that it may not provide information about the range of intakes or the risk of more extreme consumption patterns.

The U.K. total diet study has used a market basket approach every three years since 1966 to provide information on the dietary exposures of the general U.K. population to contaminants. Details of the design of the U.K. total diet study are given in Peattie et al. (1983). In the 2001 U.K. total diet study, 121 categories of foods were combined into 19 food groups for analysis. The food groups chosen were based on the amount consumed (e.g., bread, potatoes, milk) or their susceptibility to contamination (e.g., offals, fish). In the United Kingdom, both population exposure estimates and consumer exposure estimates are calculated.

Population exposure estimates are derived from the amounts of the foods consumed (based on food consumption data from the National Food Survey) and the corresponding mean concentrations of the metals and other elements detected in each food group of the market basket survey.

Consumer exposure estimates are based on consumption data for adults consuming average amounts and those who consume above-average amounts (i.e., 97.5th percentile consumers) of each food group. Ysart et al. (1999) provide data on the concentrations of 30 metals and other nutrients found in the U.K. total diet study. The results for adult consumers— mean (97.5th percentile) in mg/d — for some of the essential minerals include: Calcium 747 (1308), Copper 1.4 (3), Iron 15 (26), Selenium 0.057 (0.1), and Zinc 11 (19). The comparable nature of the mean analyzed exposure to the calculated mean intakes for British adults given by Gregory et al. (1990) suggests that the method provides valid exposure estimates. Hence, the data presented by Ysart et al. (1999) for the toxic elements may also be valid.

Total diet studies based on the market basket approach have also been conducted in many other countries in Europe (e.g., the Netherlands and Spain) (Ockhuizen et al., 1991; Urieta et al., 1996), and elsewhere, including Japan (Saito, 1991), New Zealand (Hannah et al., 1995), and Canada (Dabeka and McKenzie, 1995).

Individual food items

In this approach, a list of the most commonly consumed food items is compiled from national food consumption surveys. Samples of each of these food items are then collected, sometimes more than once a year, from major cities situated in certain geographic regions of the country. Samples of each food item are then shipped to a central laboratory where they are prepared table-ready, where necessary, after which they are homogenized and then analyzed individually. Using this approach, the food sources of specific contaminants and nutrients can then be identified. In addition, if the analyzed data are merged with data from national food surveys, then intakes of contaminants and nutrients for specific age and sex groups of the population can be estimated.

The Food and Drug Administration has used this approach for their total diet studies in the United States annually since 1961. At present, 261 foods are purchased from supermarkets or grocery stores four times a year, once from each of four regions of the country. These 261 foods are said to be representative of the over 3500 foods reported in the USDA food consumption surveys. Egan et al. (2002) have reported on the intakes of ten nutritional and four toxic elements in 1991–1996 for 14 age and sex groups in the U.S. population and have compared them with reference intakes. Contributions of specific food groups to total intakes were also determined.

Duplicate portion studies

A duplicate portion study requires the co-operation of a group of randomly selected individuals, often from a group suspected to be at risk for high levels of dietary contaminants. Hence, individuals may be living in areas where food is likely to be contaminated or may consume large amounts of food (e.g., male adolescents).

For this approach, each participant is asked to collect a duplicate portion of all foods and beverages consumed over a 24-h period in a container provided by the investigator, often for several consecutive 24-h periods. The duplicate diet composites are then homogenized and later chemically analyzed (Section 4.5). In addition, the participants are asked to make a written record of daily food intakes to ascertain the foods and quantities consumed. One of the limitations of this approach is that the participants may alter their food consumption patterns during the study.

A duplicate portion study has been used by the National Institute of Public Health and Environmental Protection in the Nether-

lands to provide data on intakes of macro- and micronutrients, as well as heavy metals, pesticides, and contaminants, for a random sample of 18–74 y old residents of the Utrecht area (Ochuizen et al. 1991).

2.1.3 Universal product codes and electronic scanning devices

Universal product codes (UPCs) in association with laser-scanning devices permit food purchases to be monitored at store checkout counters. The UPCs appear on nearly all canned and packaged foods and even some fresh items that are repackaged in food stores (Pearl, 1981). They are standard multidigit numbers with a machine-readable code that represents product, size, manufacturer, and nature of the contents. Information generated at store checkout counters can then be used to monitor food purchases and expenditure at the local, regional, and national levels.

Finnish investigators studied supermarket sales of different types of dairy products from one supermarket chain in six cities over one month. They then compared their data with reported use of dairy products derived from three health behavior surveys of adults in the same cities (Närhinen et al., 1999). The regional differences in the percentage sales of dairy products (Figure 2.3) were consis-

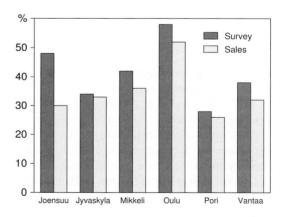

Figure 2.3: Percentage of milk-consuming subjects choosing nonfat milk as measured by survey and supermarket sales in six Finnish cities. Redrawn from Närhinen et al., Public Health Nutrition 2: 277–282, 1999.

tent with those noted in the health behavior surveys, suggesting that use of supermarket sales data may be a feasible tool for measuring regional differences in dietary habits. Den Hond et al. (1995) reached a similar conclusion when studying regional differences in consumption of 103 fat products in Belgium, based on supermarket sales from 110 branch stores.

2.2 Measuring food consumption at the household level

Household food consumption is the food and beverages available for consumption by the household, family group, or institution. It has been defined as

> the total amount of food available for consumption in the household, generally excluding that eaten away from home unless taken from the home (Klaver et al., 1982).

The household food consumption methods described in this chapter do not provide information on the consumption of food by specific individuals within the household. Instead, food consumption per capita is calculated, sometimes ignoring the age or gender distribution in the household. Alternatively, weighting may be done for the household, based on requirements by age, sex, or body size, assuming that the total household food supply is distributed according to these requirements. Generally, no record is taken of edible food waste or food obtained outside the household food supply.

Alternatively, information on the age and sex of persons in the household, their physiological state and activity level, number of meals eaten at home and away from home, income, and other socioeconomic characteristics of the household members can be collected. With this information, food consumption per capita can be calculated in terms of income level, family size, region of the country, and so on. In some cases, consumption of certain food groups, characteristic of food patterns for specific socioeconomic groups,

or rich in a specific nutrient (e.g., vitamin A or calcium), may be calculated. Estimates of nutrient intake per capita are calculated by multiplying the average food consumption data by the corresponding nutrient values for the edible portion of the food. The latter are obtained from appropriate food composition tables.

Household data are not suitable for the analysis of the quality of the diet relative to nutrient recommendations. Such comparisons necessitate adjustments for meals eaten outside of the home and assumptions about the household composition. Also, if food discarded or fed to pets is not taken into account, the food consumed will be overestimated. Only appropriately measured intakes on individuals should be compared with sex- and age-specific nutrient recommendations (Section 8.1.1).

The collection of food consumption data at both the household and individual level in the same survey can create a heavy respondent burden. In the U.S. Nationwide Food Consumption Survey 1987–1988 (USDA, 1993), this burden led to low response rates. As a result, the USDA did not include a household food consumption component in subsequent surveys.

Nationally representative Household Budget Surveys (HBSs) are undertaken in most European countries, using similar methodologies, allowing intercountry comparisons. Although HBSs are not primarily designed as nutrition surveys, they are an important source of information on food availability and on the socioeconomic factors that affect dietary choice. Greece presently coordinates the Data Food Networking (DAFNE) initiative, a collaborative European effort to examine and interpret data collected in HBSs and stored centrally (Lagiou et al., 1999; Naska et al., 2000). Note that even when consumption weightings are applied, HBSs provide only a general guide as to the adequacy of the food supply to household members.

Many of the technical problems of household surveys are similar to those of individual dietary surveys and will be discussed in later sections (Chapters 4 and 5).

2.2.1 Food account method

A food account consists of a daily record, prepared by the householder, of all food entering the household, either purchased, received as gifts, or produced for household use during a specified period — usually seven days. Quantities of each food item are recorded in retail units (where applicable) and household measures. Records may also include brand names and the retail price of the food items. The method assumes that there are no major changes in household inventories during the survey period (Burk and Pao, 1976). In the past, no account has been taken of food and beverages consumed outside the home, food discarded as plate waste or from spoilage, or food fed to pets. However, with the increasing consumption of food and drink outside the home, the food account method is now often modified accordingly.

The food account method has a low respondent burden and it is relatively inexpensive. However, it does not measure food that is actually eaten; nevertheless, the diet does not appear to be altered by the recording process. The response rate is generally high, but there is some evidence that householders agreeing to participate are of above-average socioeconomic status (Young, 1981). The food account method can be used to collect data from a large sample of the population, often several times a year to take into account seasonal variation. As a result, information on the annual mean food consumption and selection patterns of a population can be obtained (Burk and Pao, 1976). Results are often reported according to various household characteristics, including income group, geographic region, and household composition but do not provide information about intakes of food and nutrients at the individual level.

The food account method has been used since 1951 for the U.K. National Food Survey (Ministry of Agriculture, Fisheries and Food, 2000). A nationally representative sample of about 10,500 households are selected to participate in this survey each year. The person responsible for the majority of the food shopping is asked to record the weight or volume, cost, and a description of all food and drink entering the household for human consumption over a 7-d period. Since 1992, individuals aged 11 y or more in about half of the households participating in the U.K. National Food Survey have also been supplied with a separate diary to record their personal expenditure on all snacks, meals, sweets, and drinks consumed outside the home.

The food account method, with some modifications, was also used by the National Institute of Nutrition in Italy for the 1980–1984 national survey on food and nutrient intakes (Cialfa et al., 1991). Canada also used the food account method for the 2001 family expenditure survey, but asked participants to record food purchases over two successive 7-d periods (Statistics Canada, 2003b).

2.2.2 Household food record method

Food records are usually completed over at least a 1-wk period, by either the householder or a fieldworker. The record details the food actually *eaten* by the household, in contrast with the food account method in which the food *purchased or obtained* by the household is recorded. During the 1-wk survey period, the weight or volume of each food consumed at each meal is recorded separately, before subdivision into individual helpings (Burk and Pao, 1976). Detailed descriptions of all foods (including brand names) and their method of preparation are recorded. For composite dishes such as spaghetti bolognese, the amount of each raw ingredient used in the recipe and the final weight of the prepared composite dish is also recorded.

An example of a data sheet used for a weighed household food record is shown in Table 2.2. Sometimes, plate waste from each meal is collected and separated, and waste for individual food items is weighed. Generally, however, kitchen and plate waste, and food fed to pets, is not accounted for in this method. Instead, an arbitrary wastage factor of 10% of all edible portions of the foods consumed is applied, a practice sometimes also used for the food account method.

Family Name:				Date:		
Street address:				Time:		
Town/city:				Name of meal:		
Number in household:						

| Family members consuming the food (use code) | Description of food and method of cooking. One line per food. | Weight served (g/oz)[a] | Weight of waste (g/oz)[a] | LAB. USE ONLY | | Food code |
				Wt. of food (g/oz)[a]	Intake per "person"[b]	
Meals eaten outside the home: Describe foods and cooking methods. Estimate weights						

[a] Draw a circle around units in which your quantities are measured
[b] Calculate from total "man values" using the Rome Scale
Mother (M) age (...), Father (F) age (...), Son (S1) age (...), Son (S2) age (...),
Daughter (D1) age (...), Daughter (D2) age (...), Male visitor (MV1) age (...),
Female visitor (FV1) age (...)

Table 2.2: Data sheet for a weighed household food record. Modified from Weiner and Lourie (1969) with permission.

Adjustments are sometimes made in this method for food eaten outside the home and for the presence of nonhousehold members during the survey period. The number of family members and visitors eating each meal can be recorded, and a "man value" assigned to each person, weighted according to their age and sex. If the Rome scale is used, males > 14 y are assigned a value of 1.0; females > 11 y and boys 11–14 y, a value of 0.90; children 7–10 y, a value of 0.75; children 4–6 y, a value of 0.40; and children < 4 y, a value of 0.15 (Møller Jensen et al., 1984). The amount of each food consumed by the entire household can then be divided by the corresponding total "man value" to provide food intakes per "person." This adjustment produces a better estimate of the adequacy of the household food intake, particularly for families.

2.2.3 Household 24-h recall method

A technical guide for measuring household food consumption using a 24-h recall was developed by the Food and Nutrition Technical Assistance Project and its predecessors (Swindale and Ohri-Vachaspati, 1999). In this method, the household member responsible for the food preparation is interviewed to obtain information on both household composition and household food consumption over the previous 24-h period. In the first stage of the interview, information is collected on the dishes and ingredients consumed, followed by details on the quantity, focusing particularly on those foods that are important sources of energy. The amount of each food consumed by the entire household can then be divided by the number of persons in the household, to provide food intakes per "person," as described in Section 2.2.2. If information on household consumption for correlation with other household variables is required, then at least four days of recall per household are recommended.

This technical guide has been designed specifically to yield information on the number of eating occasions per day in the household, the number of different foods or food groups consumed (as an index of dietary diversity), and the percentage of households consuming the minimum daily energy requirements. Together, such data can be used to monitor changes in household food security. Detailed instructions and sample questionnaires that can be used to collect the data, quantify the portion sizes of food consumed, and analyze the results are provided.

2.3 National food consumption surveys: household methods

Several countries use household methods for their national food consumption surveys. Attention must be paid to the sampling design of these surveys to ensure that a representative national sample is obtained, as noted earlier (Section 1.4.2). The latter should account for the influence on food intake of season, holidays, weekends, socioeconomic status and region, on food consumption.

In the past, most national surveys have used an arbitrary allowance (e.g., 10%) for food waste at the domestic level (i.e., plate and kitchen wastage, spoilage, and food fed to pets) (Ministry of Agriculture, Fisheries and Food, 2000). A food waste survey established in the United Kingdom in 1976 demonstrated that 4%–6% of potential food energy was discarded, regardless of season (Wenlock et al., 1980). Kantor et al. (1997) estimated consumer and foodservice waste in the United States at about 26% of the edible food available for human consumption. The wide range in estimated waste can be attributed to the differences in the definitions of waste, the methodologies used, and the populations studied.

The U.K. National Food Survey originally used the household inventory method. At first, only urban working-class households were surveyed. In 1950, the survey was extended to cover all types of households, and in 1951, the household inventory method was replaced by the food account method (Derry, 1984), which is still used at the present time. Since 1996, the survey has been extended to cover Northern Ireland, as well as England, Wales, and Scotland.

The results from the U.K. National Food Survey are published annually. Data are collected throughout the year from a nationally representative sample of about 6000 households over a 1-wk period. Tabulated summary information on the average weight and the average amount spent on each of 23 major food categories is presented in terms of per person per week. Estimates of nutrient intake are also derived by multiplying the average consumption data by corresponding nutrient values obtained from the U.K. food composition tables (Holland et al., 1991; Food Standards Agency, 2002). The response rate for the U.K. National Food Survey in 1999 was about 65% (Ministry of Agriculture, Fisheries and Food, 2000).

In the past, allowances were made within each food category for seasonal variations in wastage, for cooking losses, and for food fed to pets or livestock. In 1998–1999, however, a separate Food Wastage Pilot Survey was undertaken in 50 households to identify a better method of recording waste food and drink. The method found to provide data of high quality and to be most acceptable to respondents was weighing waste food and drink. Therefore, this method of recording waste has now been adopted for U.K. National Food Surveys. In April 2001, the U.K. National Food Survey was merged with the Family Expenditure Survey to form the Expenditure and Food Survey (EFS).

In Canada, household food expenditure surveys were conducted in 1992, 1996, and 2001 (Statistics Canada, 2003b). They provided an estimate of food brought into the home or purchased for family use. In 2001, approximately 9000 families were asked to record the quantities and prices of all foods purchased over two consecutive 14-d periods. Snacks purchased from stores and meals bought from restaurants were recorded separately.

The European Commission have produced data on average per capita food availability for six European countries (Greece, Ireland, Luxembourg, Norway, Spain, United Kingdom) based on household budget survey data (Trichopoulou and Lagiou, 1998). Data for eight principal food items and groups (meat, fish and seafood, total added lipids, vegetables, fruits, dairy products, bread from the cereal group, and pulses) (g/person/d) are available by country and by locality and educational level. Such food availability data have the potential to provide information on nutrient intakes, provided issues such as the estimation of food portions and food waste can be taken into account. Nevertheless, caution must be used on the choice of nutrients. Inclusion of vitamin C and folate, for example, are probably not advisable in view of the known effects of food preparation on their nutrient content (Southgate, 1991).

The first U.S. nationwide household food consumption surveys (NFCS) employed the food account method. In the 1930s, this method was changed to the list-recall method because it had a lower respondent burden and hence a better response rate. The list-recall method was used at approximately 10-y intervals until 1988. In 1965–1966, 1977–1978, and 1987–1988, the U.S. NFCS included two components — household food use employing the list-recall method, and intakes by individuals, using in-person 24-h recall interviews on two nonconsecutive days.

In 1987–1988, laptop computers were used for the first time for the 24-h recall interviews. The computer was programmed to handle the extensive food list of nearly 3000 items. Nevertheless, the response rates were so low in the NFCS 1987–1988 that the USDA abandoned the list-recall method in their subsequent NFCS and now assess intakes only at the individual level, via 24-h recalls, some of which are repeated. These data permit analyses of the adequacy of nutrient intakes at the individual level by comparison with appropri-

ate nutrient recommendations. Such data are urgently needed, in view of the increasing emphasis on diet and health. Nevertheless, because food is often purchased at the household level, the elimination of the household food-use component has created a gap in tracking food in the United States from the farmer to the consumer and has made centralized food planning more difficult (Tippet, 1999).

2.4 Summary

Food consumption at the national level is most frequently determined by using food balance sheets (also termed national food accounts, food disappearance data, food consumption level estimates, etc.). These provide information on national per capita food availability, of varying quality, over a specified period but give no information on food consumption at the individual level. Furthermore, food balance sheets do not yield data on food consumption in relation to regional, economic, demographic, seasonal, or socioeconomic differences within a country. Data take into account both supply (production, imports, and existing stocks) and losses (exports, nonfood use, animal food, losses to pests, and production/manufacturing losses) prior to availability for domestic consumption, and are expressed in terms of grams per capita of individual food commodities. The latter, when multiplied by corresponding food composition values, can provide estimates of per capita energy and macronutrient availability.

Total diet studies are also carried out in industrialized countries. They involve the collection of a large number of representative foods from a particular region or country and are designed to establish, by chemical analysis, the dietary intake of food contaminants by a person consuming a typical diet. Total diet studies can also be used to monitor and evaluate intakes of macro- and micronutrients in populations. They can be based on market basket studies, collection of individual food items, or duplicate portions.

The advent of universal product codes in association with laser-scanning devices has permitted food purchases to be monitored at supermarket checkout counters. Regional differences in dietary habits, based on differences in the sales of specific food groups (e.g., dairy products) may be studied using these supermarket sales data.

Household food consumption methods attempt to measure all food and beverages available for consumption by a household, family group, or institution during a specified time period. The following methods are used: food accounts, household food records, and household 24-h recalls. These all involve collecting information on demographic and socioeconomic characteristics of the household, thereby enabling data to be presented in terms of income level, family size, region of the country, and so on. Per capita nutrient intake data are derived by multiplying the per capita food consumption data by the corresponding nutrient values obtained from appropriate food composition data. "Man values," weighted according to age and sex, are sometimes assigned to each family member and used to calculate nutrient intake per person more precisely.

The household food consumption methods vary in their complexity and respondent burden. In the past, no account has been taken of food and beverages consumed outside the home or of food wasted, spoiled, or fed to pets. Instead, in some cases, a wastage factor of all edible foods consumed is applied. However, in the U.K. National Food Surveys, respondents now weigh waste food and drink. Some households now also record their personal expenditure and snacks, meals, sweets, and drinks consumed outside the home.

Some industrialized countries are adopting household food consumption methods for national food consumption surveys, although their use in the United States has ceased.

References

Brown KH, Wuehler SE, Peerson JM. (2001). The importance of zinc in human nutrition and estimation of the global prevalence of zinc deficiency. Food and Nutrition Bulletin 22: 113–125.

Burk MC, Pao EM. (1976). Methodology for Large-Scale Surveys of Household and Individual Diets. Home Economics Research Report No. 40. U.S. Department of Agriculture, Washington, DC.

Campbell JA. (1981). An Assessment of Data Bases Relating to Nutritional Aspects of Food. Food and Nutrition Service, Marketing and Economics Branch, Agriculture Canada, Ottawa.

Cialfa E, Turrini A, Lintas C. (1991). A national food survey: food balance sheets and other methodologies — a critical overview. In: Macdonald I (ed.) Monitoring Dietary Intakes. Springer-Verlag, Berlin, pp. 23–44.

Dabeka RW, McKenzie AD. (1995). Survey of lead, cadmium, fluoride, nickel, and cobalt in food composites and estimation of dietary intakes of these elements by Canadians in 1986–1988. Journal of AOAC International 78: 897–909.

Den Hond EM, Lesaffre E, Kesteloot HE. (1995). Regional differences in consumption of 103 fat products in Belgium: a supermarket-chain sales approach. Journal of the American College of Nutrition 14: 621–627.

Derry B. (1984). Food purchases: strengths and weaknesses of the National Food Survey. In: The Dietary Assessment of Populations. Medical Research Council Environmental Epidemiology Unit. Scientific Report No. 4. Medical Research Council, Southampton, U.K.

Dowler EA, Ok Seo YI. (1985). Assessment of energy intake. Food Policy (August): 278–288.

Egan SK, Tao SS, Pennington JA, Bolger PM. (2002). U.S. Food and Drug Administration's total diet study: intake of nutritional and toxic elements, 1991–96. Food Additives and Contaminants 19: 103–125.

FAO (Food and Agriculture Organization). (1999). FAO Food Balance Sheets 1994–1996 Average. Food and Agriculture Organization of the United Nations, Rome.

FAO (Food and Agriculture Organization).(2001). Food Balance Sheets: A Handbook. Food and Agriculture Organization of the United Nations, Rome.

Food Standards Agency. (2002). McCance and Widdowson's "The Composition of Foods" 6th summary ed. Royal Society of Chemistry, Cambridge.

Gage TB, O'Connor K. (1994). Nutrition and variation in level and age patterns of mortality. Human Biology 60: 77–103.

Gerrior S, Bente L. (2001). Food supply nutrients and dietary guidance 1970–99. Food Review 24(3): 39–46.

Gerrior S, Bente L. (2002). Nutrient Content of the U.S. Food Supply, 1909–99: A Summary Report. Home Economics Research Report No. 55. Center for Nutrition Policy and Promotion, U.S. Department of Agriculture, Washington DC.

Gregory J, Foster K, Tyler H, Wiseman M. (1990). The

Dietary and Nutritional Survey of British Adults. The Stationery Office, London.

Hannah ML, Vannoort RW, Pickston L. (1995). 1990/1991 New Zealand Total Diet Survey. Part 3: Nutrients. Institute of Environmental Science and Research, Wellington, New Zealand. 65p.

Health Canada. (1997). Canadian Nutrient File. Health Canada, Ottawa.

Holland B, Welch AA, Unwin ID, Buss DH, Paul AA, Southgate DAT. (1991). McCance and Widdowsons's "The Composition of Foods" 5th ed. Royal Society of Chemistry, London.

Kantor LS, Lipton K, Manchester A, Oliveira V. (1997). Estimating and addressing America's food losses. Food Review 20(1): 2–12.

Klaver W, Knuiman JT, van Staveren WA. (1982). Proposed definitions for use in the methodology of food consumption studies. In: Hautvast JGAJ, Klaver W (eds.) The Diet Factor in Epdemiological Research. Euronut Report 1. Ponsen & Loogen, Wageningen, pp. 77–85.

Lagiou P, Trichopoulou A, Henderickx HK, Kelleher C, Leonhauser IU, Moreiras O, Nelson M, Schmitt A, Sekula W, Trygg K, Zajkas G. (1999) Household budget survey nutritional data in relation to mortality from coronary heart disease, colorectal cancer and female breast cancer in European countries. DAFNE I and II projects of the European Commission. Data Food Networking. European Journal of Clinical Nutrition 53: 328–332.

Manchester AC, Farrell KR. (1981). Measurement and forecasting of food consumption by USDA. In: Committee on Food Consumption Patterns, Food and Nutrition Board, National Research Council (ed.) Assessing Changing Food Consumption Patterns. National Academy Press, Washington, DC, pp. 51–71.

Ministry of Agriculture, Fisheries and Food. (2000). National Food Survey 1999: Annual Report on Food Expenditure, Consumption and Nutrient Intakes. The Stationery Office, London.

Møller Jensen O, Wahrendorf J, Rosenqvist A, Geser A. (1984). The reliability of questionnaire-derived historical dietary information and temporal stability of food habits in individuals. American Journal of Epidemiology 120: 281–290.

Närhinen M, Berg MA, Nissinen A, Puska P. (1999). Supermarket sales data: a tool for measuring regional differences in dietary habits. Public Health Nutrition 2: 277–282.

Naska A, Vasdekis VG, Trichopoulou A, Friel S, Leonhauser IU, Moreiras O, Nelson M, Remaut AM, Schmitt A, Sekula W, Trygg KU, Zajkas G. (2000). Fruit and vegetable availability among ten European countries: how does it compare with the "five-a-day" recommendation? DAFNE I and II projects of the European Commission. British Journal of Nutrition 84: 549–556.

Nelson M. (1984). Food production and sales. In: The Dietary Assessment of Populations. Medical Research Council Environmental Epidemiology Unit.

Scientific Report No. 4. Medical Research Council, Southampton, U.K., pp. 16–21.

Ockhuizen Th, Vaessen HAMG, de Vos RH, van Dokkum W. (1991). The validity of total diet studies for assessing nutrient intake. In: Macdonald I (ed.) Monitoring Dietary Intakes. Springer-Verlag, Berlin, pp. 9–18.

Pearl RB. (1981). Possible alternative methods for data collection on food consumption and expenditures. In: Committee on Food Consumption Patterns, Food and Nutrition Board, National Research Council (ed.) Assessing Changing Food Consumption Patterns. National Academy Press, Washington DC, pp. 198–203.

Peattie ME, Buss DH, Lindsay DG, Smart GA. (1983). Reorganization of the British total diet study for monitoring food constituents from 1981. Food and Chemical Toxicology 21: 503–507.

Poleman TT. (1981). A reappraisal of the extent of world hunger. Food Policy 6: 236–252.

Putnam J, Allshouse J, Kantor LS. (2002). U.S. per capita food supply trends: more calories, refined carbohydrates and fats. Food Review 25(3): 2–15.

Saito Y. (1991). Household food intake (market basket). In: Macdonald I (ed.) Monitoring Dietary Intakes. Springer-Verlag, Berlin, pp. 19–23.

Sasaki S, Kesteloot H. (1992). Value of Food and Agriculture Organization data on food-balance sheets as a data source for dietary fat intake in epidemiologic studies. American Journal of Clinical Nutrition 56: 716–723.

Southgate DAT. (1991). Database requirements for calculations from food balance sheet data and household budget surveys. In: Food and Health Data, Their Use in Nutrition Policy-making. WHO Regional Publications European Series 34: 85–89.

Statistics Canada. (2002). Food Consumption in Canada, Part II: 2001. Catalogue No. 32–230. Statistics Canada, Ottawa.

Statistics Canada. (2003a). Food Consumption in Canada, Part I: 2002. Catalogue No. 32–229-XIB. Statistics Canada, Ottawa.

Statistics Canada. (2003b). Food Expenditure in Canada, 2001. Catalogue No. 62–554–XIE. Statistics Canada, Ottawa.

Swindale A, Ohri-Vachaspati P. (1999). Measuring Household Food Consumption: A Technical Guide. Food and Nutrition Technical Assistance Project, Academy for Educational Development, Washington DC, pp. 1–24.

Tippett KS. (1999). Food consumption surveys in the U.S. Department of Agriculture. Nutrition Today 34: 38–44.

Trichopoulou A, Lagiou P (eds.). (1998). Methodology for the Exploitation of HBS Food Data and Results on Food Availability in Six European Countries. Office for Official Publications of the European Communities, Luxembourg.

Urieta I, Jalon M, Eguilero I. (1996). Food surveillance in the Basque Country (Spain). II: Estimation of the dietary intake of organochlorine pesticides, heavy metals, arsenic, aflatoxin M1, iron and zinc through the Total Diet Study 1990/91. Food Additives and Contaminants 13: 29–52.

USDA (U.S. Department of Agriculture, Human Nutrition Information Service). (1993). Food Consumption and Dietary Levels of Households in the United States, 1987–94. Nationwide Food Consumption Survey 1987–94, Report No. 87-H-1. U.S. Department of Agriculture, Washington DC.

USDA (U.S. Department of Agriculture, Agricultural Research Service). (2003). USDA National Nutrient Database for Standard Reference, Release 16. Nutrient Data Laboratory Home Page http://www.nal. usda.gov/fnic/foodcomp/

Weiner JS, Lourie JA. (1969). Human Biology: A Guide to Field Methods. International Biological Programme. IBP Handbook No. 9. Blackwell Scientific Publications, Oxford.

Wenlock RW, Buss DH, Derry BJ. (1980). Household food wastage in Britain. British Journal of Nutrition 43: 53–70.

West C. (2000). Meeting requirements for vitamin A. Nutrition Reviews 58: 341–345.

Young CM. (1981). Dietary methodology. In: Committee on Food Consumption Patterns, Food and Nutrition Board, National Research Council. Assessing Changing Food Consumption Patterns (eds.) National Academy Press, Washington, DC, pp. 89–118.

Ysart GE, Miller PF, Crews H, Robb P, Baxter M, De L'Argy C, Lofthouse S, Sargent C, Harrison N. (1999). Dietary exposure estimates of 30 metals and other elements from the U.K. Total Diet Study. Food Additives and Contaminants 16: 391–403.

3

Measuring food consumption of individuals

This chapter describes methods commonly used for measuring the food consumption of individuals. Subsequent chapters discuss the factors associated with the reproducibility and validity of each of these methods (Chapters 5–7) and the calculation and evaluation of nutrient intakes (Chapters 4 and 8).

3.1 Methods for measuring food consumption of individuals

Two groups of methods are used to measure the food consumption of individuals. The first group, known as quantitative daily consumption methods, consists of recalls or records designed to measure the quantity of the individual foods consumed over a 1-d period. By increasing the number of measurement days, quantitative estimates of the *usual* intakes of individuals can be obtained, using the same methods. The number, selection, and spacing of the days depend on the food intake, the nutrients of interest, the day-to-day variation in nutrient intake, and the level of precision required. Determination of the usual intake is particularly critical when relationships between diet and biological parameters or chronic disease are assessed. Estimates of usual intakes are also needed to estimate the prevalence of inadequate intakes.

The second group of methods includes the dietary history and the food frequency questionnaire. Both obtain retrospective information on the patterns of food use during a longer, less precisely defined time period.

Such methods can be used to assess the usual intake of foods or specific classes of foods. With modification, they can also provide data on usual nutrient intakes.

The measurement of food consumption at the individual level is costly and time consuming. Hence, such studies should be planned with care. Consideration should be given to the cost-effective collection of additional data from the same subjects at the same time; such additional information may significantly enhance the interpretation of the dietary data. At a minimum, socioeconomic and health-related information, simple anthropometric measures, possibly a physical activity questionnaire, and biological samples for the determination of important biomarkers (Chapter 7) should be collected when time and resources permit (Buzzard and Sievert, 1994).

The accurate assessment of the food intake of infants is a particularly difficult problem, especially when infants are receiving both breast milk and complementary foods (Piwoz et al., 1995). WHO (1998) has published guidelines that can be used to evaluate nutrient intakes of breastfed infants receiving complementary foods.

3.1.1 Twenty-four-hour recall method

In the 24-h recall method, subjects and their parents or caretakers are asked by the nutritionist, who has been trained in interviewing techniques, to recall the subject's exact food intake during the previous 24-h period or

Name:					Date:		
Street address:					Day of the week:		
Town/city:							

					LAB. USE ONLY		
Place eaten	Time	Description of food or drink. Give brand name if applicable		Amount	Day/Meal code	Food code	Amount code

Additional questions:
Was intake unusual in any way?   Yes (...) No (...)
If yes, in what way?

Do you take vitamin or mineral supplements?   Yes (...) No (...)
If yes, how many per day? (...) per week? (...)
If yes, what kind? (give brand if possible)
Multivitamin   Iron   Ascorbic acid
Other (list)

Table 3.1: Data sheet for a 24-h record. Modified from Weiner and Lourie (1969) with permission.

preceding day. Thus the method assesses the actual intake of individuals. However, a single 24-h recall is not sufficient to describe an individual's usual intake of food and nutrients; multiple 24-h recalls on the same individual over several days are required to achieve this objective (Section 3.1.2). Nevertheless, multiple single-day recalls on different individuals can give a valid measure of the intake of a group or population (Section 3.3.1).

A four stage, multiple-pass interviewing technique is often used; details are given in Gibson and Ferguson (1999). Briefly, in the first pass, a complete list of all foods and beverages consumed during the preceding day is obtained, followed, in the second pass, by a detailed description of each food and beverage consumed, including cooking methods and brand names (if possible). Standardized probe questions should be used to elicit specific details for each food item. For example, for milk products, probe questions should include the kind of dairy product, brand name (if appropriate), and percentage fat (as butterfat or milk fat). Further examples of probes that can be used to obtain detailed descrip-

tions of specified foods are outlined in Gibson and Ferguson (1999).

In the third pass, estimates of the amount of each food and beverage item consumed are obtained, generally in household measures, and entered on the data sheet (Table 3.1) or computer-based data-entry form. Photographs, a set of measuring cups, spoons, and rulers, local household utensils (calibrated for use), or food models of various types (Section 5.2.6) can be used as memory aids or to assist the respondent in assessing portion sizes of food items consumed (Gibson and Ferguson, 1999). Information on the ingredients of mixed dishes consumed by the respondents must also be collected at this time. Finally, in the fourth pass, the recall is reviewed to ensure that all items, including use of vitamin and mineral supplements, have been recorded correctly. (Methods for coding the completed 24-h recalls and potential sources of coding errors are discussed in Section 5.2.7.)

Any 24-h interview protocol must be standardized and pretested prior to use. Standardization is particularly important in large-scale national surveys and for comparisons across countries (Slimani et al., 1999). Pretesting should be undertaken in an area near the study site, using respondents similar to those who will participate in the actual study. Sometimes, the pretesting can be carried out on the field staff if they are comparable to the participants (Gibson and Ferguson, 1999).

Adherence to the interview protocol and accuracy of food coding by the interviewers should be checked periodically during the survey, and the interviewers must be retrained if necessary to minimize interviewer bias (Section 5.2.3). Detailed suggestions on how to conduct the interview can be found in Sanjur (1982) and Hughes (1986), who stressed that leading questions and judgmental comments should be avoided. An indirect approach employing open-ended questions is recommended. This enables respondents to freely express their feelings so that answers are not biased.

In general, recall interviews can be conducted on children aged $\geqslant 8$ y (Young, 1981; Livingstone and Robson, 2000) and on most adults, except for persons with poor memories (e.g., some elderly). Children aged from 4–8 y should be interviewed along with their primary caretaker, usually the mother. It may be necessary to interview several people if the children are at school or play in the homes of friends, to ensure that foods eaten away from home are reported. For this younger age group, questions should always be directed toward the child (Sobo et al., 2000).

Very often when conducting recalls, especially on children, the interviewing proceeds as a consensus recall, with family members helping the respondent to remember the amounts consumed. This consensus approach was shown to increase the accuracy of dietary recalls of U.S. children (Eck et al., 1989).

When 24-h recalls are used to characterize the average usual intake of a population group, the subjects should be representative of the population under study. In addition, the survey should be conducted in such a way that all days of the week are equally represented. In this way, any day-of-the-week effects on food or nutrient intakes will be

taken into account (Section 6.2.4). The respondent burden is small for a single 24-h recall, so that compliance is generally high. The method is quick and relatively inexpensive, and it can be used equally well with both literate and illiterate subjects.

A 24-h recall has been used in some national nutrition surveys, including the New Zealand National Nutrition Survey (MOH,1997), the U.S. National Health and Nutrition Examination Survey (NHANES) (NCHS, 1994), and the Continuing Survey of Food Intakes by Individuals (CSFII) (USDA, 1998). Since 2002, the CSFII has included a computerized multiple-pass recall with a number of built-in cues to specifically improve the recall of easily overlooked foods such as nonalcoholic and alcoholic beverages, sweets, snacks, and breads. The CSFII is now integrated with NHANES.

A modification of the 24-h recall — termed an interactive 24-h recall — has been developed to collect information on rural populations in developing countries (Ferguson et al., 1995). The modifications are listed in Box 3.1 and discussed in more detail in a manual containing practical guidelines and procedures (Gibson and Ferguson, 1999).

All recall interviews should be conducted in the respondent's home whenever possible, because the familiar environment encourages participation, improves the recall of foods consumed, and facilitates calibration of local

---

To improve the recall of food items in developing countries, investigators can:

Provide group training on portion size estimation before the actual recall.

Supply picture charts on the day before the recall for use as a checklist on the day the food is actually consumed, and for comparison with the recall to reduce memory lapses.

Provide bowls and plates for use on the recall days to help the respondents visualize the amount of food consumed.

Weigh the portion sizes of salted replicas of the actual foods consumed by the respondent.

Box 3.1: Interactive 24-h recall modifications suggested for rural populations in developing countries.

household utensils by the interviewer. In the end, the success of the 24-h recall depends on the subject's memory, the ability of the subject to convey accurate estimates of portion sizes consumed, the degree of motivation of the respondent, and the persistence of the interviewer (Acheson et al., 1980).

3.1.2 Repeated 24-h recalls

Twenty-four-hour recalls can be repeated during different seasons of the year to estimate the average food intake of individuals over a longer time period (i.e., usual food intake). The number of 24-h recalls required to estimate the usual nutrient intake of individuals depends on the day-to-day variation in food intake within one individual (i.e., within-subject variation) (Basiotis et al., 2002). In turn, this variation is affected by the nutrient under study, the study population, and seasonal variations in intake. Nonconsecutive days should be selected, when possible (Beaton et al., 1979).

Repeated 24-h recalls were recommended as part of a system for measuring food consumption patterns in the United States (NRC, 1981). For the CSFII 1994–1996 (USDA, 1998), for example, food intakes on two nonconsecutive days were recorded through an in-person 24-h recall.

If it is not feasible to carry out repeated observations on all respondents, the recalls should be repeated on a subsample of the population. In the 1988–1994 NHANES III (NCHS, 1994) and the New Zealand National Nutrition Survey (MOH, 1997), 24-h recalls were repeated on 5% and 15% of the population, respectively, across the entire age range. Section 6.1.1 provides a detailed discussion of the reproducibility of the 24-h recall method.

3.1.3 Estimated food records

For the estimated food record, the respondent is asked to record, at the time of consumption, all foods and beverages (including snacks) eaten in household measures, for a specified time period. Detailed descriptions of all foods and beverages (including brand names) and their method of preparation and cooking are also recorded. For mixed dishes such as spaghetti bolognese, the amount of each raw ingredient used in the recipe, the final weight of the mixed dish, and the amount consumed by the subject should be recorded, wherever possible. The information is recorded on a form similar to that shown in Table 3.1, except that household measures are used for food amounts. Usually, the subject, parent, or caretaker completes the food record, although in less-developed countries a local field investigator may perform this task (Dufour et al., 1999).

Food portion size can be estimated by the respondent in a variety of ways. Standard household measuring cups and spoons should be used if possible, supplemented by measurements with a ruler (for meat and cake) and counts (for eggs and bread slices). Unfortunately, errors may arise because the respondent may fail to quantify portion sizes correctly. Additional errors may also arise during the conversion of volumes to weights (Section 5.2.5). The latter step is usually completed by the investigator. Details on how to convert portion sizes to weight equivalents are given in Gibson and Ferguson (1999).

The number of days included in an estimated record varies, depending on the objective of the study. When the objective is to obtain an average intake for a group, then only one day per person is required, provided all days of the week are equally represented in the final sample. However, when estimates of usual intakes of each person are required, then the number, selection, and spacing of the days required per person depends on the factors described for the repeated 24-h recall (Section 3.1.2). Weekend days should always be proportionately included in the dietary survey period for each person, to account for potential day-of-the-week effects on food and nutrient intakes. This problem is discussed in more detail in Sections 6.1.2 and 6.2.

The European Prospective Investigation of Cancer (EPIC) study in Norfolk, U.K. collected food and nutrient intakes from 2117 men and women. EPIC is a large multicenter prospective study aimed at investigating the relationship between nutrition and various life-style factors and the etiology of cancer and other chronic diseases. The study involved 23 regional centers located in ten countries, and involved a total cohort of about 480,000 subjects. The respondents of the EPIC study in Norfolk were provided with a "diet diary" — a 45-page colored booklet in which they were asked to record the description, preparation, and amounts of foods eaten over seven consecutive days. Food portion sizes were estimated by the respondents in terms of household measures, with the help of 17 sets of color photographs of small, medium, and large portions of the different foods. A semiquantitative food frequency questionnaire (Section 3.1.6) was also used. Details are given in Bingham et al. (2001).

3.1.4 Weighed food records

Weighed food records are more frequently used in the United Kingdom and Europe because weighing scales are often used for food preparation in these areas. In the British National Diet and Nutrition Surveys of adults (Gregory et al., 1990; Finch et al., 1998; Henderson et al., 2002, 2003a, 2003b) and children (Gregory et al., 1995, 2000), 7-d weighed food records were used.

A weighed food record is the most precise method available for estimating usual food and nutrient intakes of individuals. It is the preferred method when diet counseling or correlation of intakes with biological parameters are involved.

In a weighed record, the subject, parent, or caretaker is instructed to weigh all foods and beverages consumed by the subject during a specified time period. Details of methods of food preparation, description of foods, and brand names (if known) should also be recorded. For mixed dishes such as spaghetti bolognese, the weight of the portion consumed should be recorded, along with the weights and description of all the raw ingredients, including flavors and spices used in the recipe, as well as the final total weight of the mixed dish. The method of recording is similar to that shown for a 24-h recall (Table 3.1), with the weight of the food items being recorded under "Amount."

If occasional meals are eaten away from home, respondents are generally requested to record descriptions of the amounts of food eaten. The nutritionist can then buy and weigh a duplicate portion of each recorded food item, where possible, to assess the probable weight consumed. Alternatively, if appropriate, the nutritionist can telephone a restaurant to obtain details of the portion sizes consumed.

As with the estimated record, the number, spacing, and selection of days necessary to characterize the usual nutrient intakes of an individual using the weighed record depend on the within-subject variation in food intake, which, in turn, depends on the nutrient of interest, the study population, and any seasonal variation of intake. Again, weekend days should be proportionately included to account for any weekend effect on the nutrient intake.

If a weighed food record method is to be used, respondents must be motivated, numerate, and literate. However, respondents may change their usual eating pattern to simplify the measuring or weighing process or, alternatively, to impress the investigator (Cameron and van Staveren, 1988) (Section 7.1.3). Respondent burden for food records is higher than for the 24-h recall, so individuals may be less willing to cooperate. Reproducibility is greater in the weighed record than in the estimated record method because the portion sizes are weighed. Significant underreporting (Section 5.2.2) may, however, still occur.

3.1.5 Dietary history

The dietary history method (Burke, 1947) attempts to estimate the usual food intake and meal pattern of individuals over a relatively long period of time — often a month. This interview method was originally designed to be carried out by a nutritionist trained in interviewing techniques. More recently, computerized versions have been developed (Kohlmeier et al., 1997). Such versions provide standardized methods for data collection and probing, and minimize potential interviewer bias in responses.

Initially, the dietary history had three components. The first component was an interview about the usual overall eating pattern of the subject, both at mealtimes and between meals. Such information included detailed descriptions of foods, their frequency of consumption, and usual portion sizes in common household measures. "What do you usually eat for breakfast?" is a typical question that might have been included in the interview.

The second component served as a crosscheck and consisted of a questionnaire on the frequency of consumption of specific food items. This part was used to verify and clarify the information on the kinds and amounts of foods given as the usual intake in the first component. Questions asked related to specific foods, such as: "Do you like or dislike milk." A 24-h recall of actual intake may also have been included at this stage.

In the third component, subjects recorded their food intake at home for three days. Portion sizes at this stage were estimated using a variety of techniques, including standard measuring cups and spoons, common utensils, commercial plastic food models, photographs, or real foods. Today, the original dietary history method is seldom used in this three-part format, the third component being commonly omitted.

The time periods covered by the dietary history method vary. The maximum time period that can be used has not been definitely established. When shorter time frames (i.e., $\leqslant 1$ mo) are used, reproducibility and validity are apparently higher than for longer periods (see Section 7.1.2). Measurements of food intake over 1-y periods are probably unrealistic unless seasonal variations in food intakes are taken into account.

Dutch investigators used a three-part dietary history method covering 1 mo to record usual food consumption on weekdays, Saturdays, and Sundays separately (van Staveren et al., 1985). This approach takes into account the potential effect of weekends on nutrient intake. The portion size of foods most fre-

quently consumed in this study were weighed by a dietitian in the home. A weighted daily average intake was then calculated from the data, using the following formula:

$$((5 \times \text{weekday}) + \text{Saturday} + \text{Sunday}) / 7$$

A modified version of this dietary history method was adopted in the Survey in Europe on Nutrition in the Elderly: A Concerted Action (SENECA). This multicenter survey was designed to examine cross-cultural variations in the nutrition, lifestyle, health, and performance of elderly Europeans (Euronut-SENECA, 1991). The method involved the completion of a 3-d estimated record, followed by an interview during which respondents were questioned about their usual dietary intake over the past month. Portions of the most commonly eaten foods were weighed by the interviewer (van Staveren et al., 1996).

The recording of a dietary history can be very labor intensive, with interviews taking up to 2 h per subject (Slattery et al., 2000). Several investigators have reported that the dietary history tends to overestimate nutrient intakes, when compared with results from weighed records. Nes et al. (1991), for example, used the dietary history developed for the SENECA study and showed that the history generated consistently higher intakes of energy and nutrients than the 3-d weighed records. Livingstone and Robson (2000) reported similar findings in a study of children and adolescents, but claimed that the results obtained from the dietary history were more representative of habitual intake than those obtained from 7-d weighed records. In general, because dietary histories, unlike food frequency questionnaires, do not limit the variability in the responses, they overcome many of the limitations of a food frequency questionnaire.

3.1.6 Food frequency questionnaire

The food frequency questionnaire aims to assess the frequency with which food items or food groups are consumed during a specified time period. It was originally designed to provide descriptive qualitative informa-

For each food item, indicate with a checkmark the category that best describes the frequency with which you usually eat that particular food item.

Food item	More than once per day	Once per day	3–6 times per week	Once or twice per week	Twice per month or less	Never
Beef, hamburger	☐	☐	☐	☐	☐	☐
Pork, ham	☐	☐	☐	☐	☐	☐
Liver	☐	☐	☐	☐	☐	☐
Poultry	☐	☐	☐	☐	☐	☐
Eggs	☐	☐	☐	☐	☐	☐
Dried peas/beans	☐	☐	☐	☐	☐	☐
. . .	☐	☐	☐	☐	☐	☐

Enter other foods not listed that are eaten regularly:

1	☐	☐	☐			
2	☐	☐	☐			
3	☐	☐	☐			

Table 3.2: Abbreviated food frequency questionnaire. A few foods and food categories are shown as examples. A complete questionnaire might contain more than 100 items.

tion about usual food-consumption patterns. With the addition of portion-size estimates and the introduction of improved computerized self-administered questionnaires, the method has become semi-quantitative, allowing the derivation of energy and selected nutrient intakes (Willet et al., 1985; Block et al., 1986).

In its simplest form, the questionnaire consists of a list of foods and an associated set of frequency-of-use response categories (Table 3.2). The list of foods may focus on specific groups of foods, particular foods, or foods consumed periodically in association with special events or seasons. Alternatively, the food list may be extensive to enable estimates of total food intake and dietary diversity to be made. The frequency-of-use response categories may be daily, weekly, monthly, or yearly, depending on the study objective.

Specific combinations of foods can be used as predictors for intakes of certain nutrients or non-nutrients, provided that the dietary components are concentrated in a relatively small number of foods or specific food groups. Examples include the frequency of consumption of fresh fruits and fruit juices as predictors of vitamin C intake (Tsugane et al., 1998); green leafy vegetables and carrots as predictors of carotenoid intakes (O'Neill et al., 2001); whole grain cereals, legumes, nuts, fruits, and vegetables as predictors of dietary fiber intakes (Merchant et al., 2003); and dairy products as predictors of calcium intakes (Barr et al., 2001). The method can also be used to assess the intake of fats and cholesterol (Feunekes et al., 1993), artificial sweeteners, certain contaminants present in specific foods (MacIntosh et al., 1997), alcohol (Kesse et al., 2001), and condiments (Maskarinec et al., 2000).

The food frequency questionnaires should feature simple, well-defined foods and food categories, and open-ended questions should be avoided as preformatted lists of food categories act as a memory prompt. The method may use a standardized interview, a self-administered machine-readable printed questionnaire, or a computer-administered questionnaire. Most questionnaires take from 15–30 min to complete (see abbreviated example given in Table 3.2). Hence, the food frequency questionnaire imposes less burden on respondents than most of the other dietary assessment methods. The results are easy to collect and process and are generally taken to represent usual intakes over an extended period of time. Nevertheless, the validity and feasibility of the food frequency questionnaire for estimating food intakes in the remote past has not been clearly established (van Staveren et al., 1986; Dwyer and Coleman, 1997; Ambrosini et al., 2003).

Food scores can be calculated from qualitative food frequency data and the frequency of consumption of certain food groups. The U.S. Food Guide Pyramid (USDA, 1992), or an equivalent standard, listing the optimum number of servings of the major food groups per person per day, can serve as a basis for the scores. The scores can then be examined in relation to psychosocial influences (e.g., level of education, income), as well as vital statistics, season, geographic distribution, and so on.

Figure 3.1 illustrates the use of a food scoring system—termed the Healthy Eating Index (HEI)—developed by the USDA for evaluating the quality of diets of U.S. children, using data from USDA's Continuing Survey of Food Intakes by Individuals (Basiotis et al., 2002). The HEI has ten components in total, five of which are based on the suggested number of servings of each of the five food groups recommended in the U.S. Food Guide Pyramid. The application of the HEI shown in Figure 3.1 demonstrates that, of these subjects, it is the youngest children who consume the best diets. A more detailed description of the HEI and other food scoring systems designed to evaluate the overall quality of the diet is given in Section 8.4.1.

Kant et al. (2000) used food frequency information to calculate a Recommended Food Score (RFS) in a prospective study of diet quality and mortality in women from the United States. They showed that the RFS was inversely associated with all-cause mortality.

Many recent users of food frequency questionnaires have quantified portion sizes of food items of interest, often using photographs (Nelson et al., 1994). Portion sizes can be ranked as small, medium, and large,

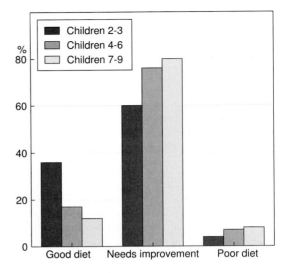

Figure 3.1: Healthy eating index rating for children aged from two to nine, 1998. From Bowman et al. (1998).

preferably based on age- and sex-specific portion size data generated from country-specific national nutrition surveys (Willett et al., 1985; Block et al., 1986). Note that inclusion of information on portion sizes produces semi-quantitative food frequency data. This can be converted to data on energy and nutrient intakes by multiplying the fractional portion size of each food consumed per day by its energy and nutrient content, obtained from appropriate food composition data. The results are then summed to obtain an estimate of an individual's total daily intake.

Block et al. (1986) derived a food list with portion sizes from the NHANES II results. Food items selected contributed significantly to the total population intake of energy and each of 17 nutrients. Serving sizes were estimated from observed portion size distributions in the NHANES II data. Medium serving sizes for each food were specified in the food frequency questionnaire, and the respondent indicated whether his or her usual serving size was small, medium, or large, as shown in Table 3.3.

A specialized food composition database was developed for use with the food frequency questionnaire developed by Block et al. (1986), based on the frequency of con-

Food	Medium serving	Serving			How Often?				
		S	M	L	D	W	M	Y	N
Apples, apple sauce, pears	(1) or 1/2 cup								
Bananas	1 medium								
Peaches, apricots (canned)	(1) or 1/2 cup								
Peaches, apricots (fresh)	1 medium								
Cantaloupe	1/4 medium								
Watermelon	1 slice								
Strawberries	1/2 cup								
Oranges	1 medium								
Orange juice	6-oz glass								
Grapefruit or grapefruit juice	1/2 or 6-oz glass								
...									

Table 3.3: An example of part of the self-administered semiquantitative food frequency questionnaire. Abbreviations: S M L = small, medium, and large relative to the medium serving; D W M Y N = daily, weekly, monthly, yearly, and never. From Block et al., American Journal of Epidemiology 124: 453–469, 1986, with permission of the Society for Epidemiologic Research.

sumption of certain specific food items observed during NHANES II. A very similar approach has been used to design semiquantitative multi-ethnic food frequency questionnaires (Dreon et al., 1993; Deurenberg-Yap et al., 2000).

The semiquantitative food frequency questionnaire has become a widely used tool in dietary assessment. Country-specific semiquantitative food frequency questionnaires containing between 130 and 300 food items were used in the EPIC study to estimate individual usual food intakes (Margetts et al., 1997). In the EPIC study in Norfolk, U.K. (Bingham et al., 2001), for example, respondents ($n = 23,003$) estimated how frequently foods were eaten over the past year, from nine possible frequency-of-use response categories from a list of 130 foods. Reduced versions containing only 60 food items that require only 17 min to administer by an interviewer are available; even the full 98-item Block questionnaire requires only 30–35 min

of interviewer time (Block et al., 1990). In some countries, a semiquantitative food frequency questionnaire has been used in national nutrition surveys (e.g., 1995 Australia National Dietary Survey) (McLennan and Podger, 1998).

Food frequency questionnaires are often used by epidemiologists studying associations between dietary habits and disease (Willett, 1994; Levi et al., 2000; Kesse et al., 2001). In such studies, the food frequency questionnaires must be semiquantitative, with the ability to rank subjects on the basis of their intakes, so that subjects with low intakes can be separated from those with high intakes. This permits the calculation of the odds ratio or relative risk of disease in relation to intake of certain foods, food groups, or nutrients (Masson et al., 2003). This approach was followed by Holick et al. (2002) in their study of the relationship between dietary carotenoids and the risk of lung cancer; results are shown in Table 3.4.

Quintile of nutrient or intake per day (n)	Median	RR	95% CI
Carotenoids (µg)			
1 (< 2770) (397)	2170	1.00	Reference
2 (2770–3786) (364)	3281	0.94	0.82, 1.08
3 (3787–4988) (320)	4344	0.80	0.69, 0.93
4 (4989–6792) (276)	5777	0.70	0.60, 0.81
5 (> 6792) (287)	8577	0.72	0.62, 0.84
	p for trend < 0.0001		
Fruits + vegetables (g)			
1 (< 116) (407)	80	1.00	Reference
2 (116–176) (362)	147	0.88	0.76, 1.02
3 (177–241) (326)	207	0.79	0.68, 0.91
4 (242–332) (293)	280	0.71	0.61, 0.83
5 (> 332) (256)	415	0.64	0.55, 0.75
	p for trend < 0.0001		

Table 3.4: Relative risk of lung cancer according to categories of baseline carotenoid and fruit + vegetable intake in a cancer-prevention prospective study 1985–1998. RR, relative risk; CI, confidence interval. Data from Holick et al., American Journal of Epidemiology 156: 536–547, 2002, with permission of the Society for Epidemiologic Research.

3.2 Technical improvements in food consumption measurements

The increasing evidence of the relationship between diet and chronic disease has led to a number of technical advances in measurements of food consumption for individuals. These aim to improve the speed and accuracy and reduce the cost of collecting and analyzing dietary intake data during large-scale epidemiological studies and nutrition surveys.

3.2.1 Telephone

A telephone survey that is well-designed and carefully-administered appears to be a promising method of obtaining dietary information. In particular, telephoned 24-h recalls are being increasingly used. The USDA has conducted several studies to examine the feasibility of using telephone follow-up surveys instead of mail follow-up for 24-h recalls. Results have been promising: response rates for telephone follow-up were much greater than those for mail follow-up. As a result, both NHANES III (1988–1994) (NCHS, 1994), and the 1994–1996 USDA Continuing Survey of Food Intake by Individuals (CSFII/DHKS, 1994–1996; USDA, 1998) included telephone follow-up surveys rather than mail follow-up.

Casey et al. (1999) carried out a validation study in which results of 24-h recalls conducted over the telephone were compared with in-person recalls collected in the 1994–1996 USDA CSFII; good correlations were reported. Based on these results, the USDA nationwide food survey conducted in 2002 also used telephone follow-up surveys.

Several other large-scale telephone dietary surveys have been used in the United States, some of which have used a food frequency instrument rather than a 24-h recall. Lyu et al. (1998) successfully showed that agreement between telephone and face-to-face interviews of a semiquantitative food frequency questionnaire made up of 115 food items was good and unaffected by age, gender, ethnicity, or education of the Hawaii respondents. These investigators did recommend mailing photographs of foods in three portion sizes in advance, to help respondents estimate amounts eaten more accurately.

Many of the smaller telephone dietary studies have been conducted on adult women (Galasso et al., 1994; Casey et al., 1999; Tran et al., 2000; Yanek et al., 2000); very few have been carried out on adolescents and adult men (Bogle et al., 2001). In college students, food intakes by telephoned recalls have been compared against actual intakes determined surreptitiously in the college cafeteria (Krantzler et al., 1982). More studies are needed, however, among certain life-stage groups, to establish the validity of 24-h recalls or food frequency questionnaires administered over the telephone. Underreporting of self-reported food intakes may still occur in telephone recalls, as they do with in-person recalls; this occurred, for example, when total energy intakes derived from telephone-administered 24-h recalls were compared with total energy expenditure measured by doubly labeled water (Tran et al., 2000) (Section 7.2.1).

Country	Reference	No. of series	Portions per series	Order of presentation	Series per page	Instructions	Table of contents
France	Hercberg et al. (1994)	245	3	Increasing size	3	Yes	Yes
Portugal	Marques et al. (1996)	110	3	Varies	2	Yes	No
Portugal	Rombo et al. (1996)	58	4	Increasing size	2	No	No
Portugal	Galeazzi et al. (1996)	71	3	Decreasing size	2	Yes	Yes
Poland	Szczyglowa et al. (1991)	135	3	Increasing size	3	No	No
Finland	Haapa et al. (1985)	126	3	Increasing size	3	Yes	No
Russia	Martintchik et al. (1995)	63	3	Increasing or varies	1	No	No
U.K.	Nelson et al. (1997)	98	8	Increasing size	1	Yes	Yes
EPIC	van Kappel et al. (1994)	140	4–6	Increasing size	1	Yes	Yes

Table 3.5: Some photographic atlases of food portion sizes. From Nelson and Haraldsdóttir, Public Health Nutrition 1: 231–237, 1998.

Telephone surveys do have several advantages. These include their ability to reach a large number of persons at perhaps less than half the cost of face-to-face surveys. As well, with the advent of computer-assisted telephone interviewing, the interviews can be readily standardized, queries can be clarified, and responses can be coded immediately, during an interviewing time that is much shorter than a face-to-face interview. As a result, the response rate is enhanced.

Potential interviewer biases can be eliminated by using computer-assisted telephone interviewing. However, other sources of bias may occur with telephone surveys; these may arise from noncoverage and nonresponse. In the United States, although over 87% of the population owns a telephone, subgroups such as the poor, certain minorities, and the elderly still have fewer telephones than the general population. Such differential coverage can introduce bias in national surveys unless alternative compensating strategies are employed. Strategies may include using supplementary face-to-face or mail interviews for persons without telephones; statistical adjustments employing weighting for sex, age, race, and income; selective over-sampling of the non-telephone users; and random-digit dialing to contact those with unlisted numbers.

Nonresponse is also a source of potential bias that influences telephone surveys. This is especially a problem among certain subgroups such as the ethnic minorities for whom language barriers may be considerable, the elderly who may have hearing difficulties, and persons with less education.

In the future, telephone dietary surveys may become a practical, economical, and valid alternative to the conventional face-to-face methods for large-scale epidemiological studies and nutrition surveys and for developing and evaluating community-based nutrition interventions in industrialized countries.

3.2.2 Photographs

Photographs can be used as memory aids or to quantify portion sizes (Section 5.2.6). Either photographs depicting a portion (i.e., amount consumed on any one occasion) or a serving size (amount served in one helping) can be used. To quantify the portion sizes, a series of graduated portion-size photographs for each food item is used, often bound together in a photographic atlas. Table 3.5 lists some of the photographic atlases currently available. Existing atlases should be used, whenever possible, provided they have been validated by using respondents with characteristics similar to those who will participate in the planned study. For assessing intakes of individuals, a range of portion-size photographs for each food is needed, but at the group level, single average portion size photographs may suffice (Robson and Livingstone, 2000).

Practical guidelines on how to develop a photographic atlas are given in Nelson and Haraldsdóttir (1998). Factors that must be considered in relation to the format of the photographs include size of the image, number and range of portion sizes depicted, and the interval between portion sizes. In the EPIC study, for example, there was a 25% difference between the portion sizes to allow a real visual perception of differences in size (van Kappel et al., 1994). Nelson et al. (1994) used portion weights from the British Adult Dietary Survey ranging from the 5th to the 95th percentile (Gregory et al., 1990), for a series of eight photographs for each food. Other important factors that should be standardized include the order of presentation of the photographs, labels used, angle at which photographs are taken, background and use of reference objects for scale, color versus black and white, and use of one versus several foods on a plate.

Photography has also been used to reduce the respondent burden imposed by completing food records. Elwood and Bird (1983) instructed subjects to photograph, at a specified distance and angle, all food items and leftovers and to record descriptions of each foodstuff, including the method of preparation. Estimates of the weights of the food items consumed were obtained by viewing the photographs alongside previously prepared standard photographs of food portions with known weights. Such an approach appears less demanding for the subject than the conventional weighed record, and is relatively easy and acceptable. Nevertheless, this approach has not been widely adopted.

3.2.3 Graduated food models

Canada was one of the first countries to use a collection of three-dimensional graduated food models in its National Nutrition Survey (Health and Welfare Canada, 1973). The models consisted of papier-maché, wooden, or hardboard shapes of various volumes and surface areas. The surface-area models were accompanied by standard thickness indicators made of hardboard squares (Figure 3.2). These were used for the 24-h recalls to assist in assessing the overall size and thickness of foods such as cheese, cold meats, cakes and

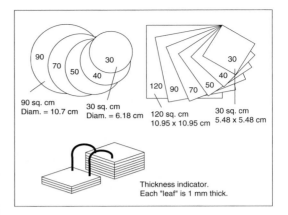

Figure 3.2: Models for use in the estimation of portion size developed by Health and Welfare Canada (1973).

cookies. Use of thickness indicators is critical for assessing portion sizes of intact cuts of meat, especially when irregular in shape. Note that the use of a range of graduated food models, like photographs depicting a range of portion sizes, prevents the tendency to generate a "direct" response. This phenomenon is observed when plastic food models representing only "average" portion sizes are used (Samuelson, 1970).

Since 1973, graduated food models have been used in many national food consumption surveys, including those in the United States (USDA, 1998; NCHS, 1994) and New Zealand (MOH, 1997; Parnell et al., 2003).

The United States has developed a new tool to measure portion sizes in the 24-h recalls conducted in their nationwide food surveys. The tool consists of a food model booklet of 32 life-size two-dimensional drawings of household vessels (glasses, mugs, bowls), abstract shapes (mounds and spreads), and geometrical models (circles, a grid, wedges, and thickness bars), together with a set of measuring cups, spoons, and rulers. This tool is now used in the dietary component of NHANES (Cleveland and Ingwersen, 2001); more details are given in Section 5.2.5.

3.2.4 Tape recorders

A portable electronic set of tape-recording scales (PETRA) has been developed in the

United Kingdom (Cherlyn Electronics, Cambridge, England). In this system, the respondent places an empty plate onto the PETRA digital recording scale, presses a switch in front of the machine, and describes the plate. The scale simultaneously records the spoken words and the weight in digitally coded form. The respondent then adds each food item separately onto the plate and, at the same time, dictates a description of the food into the microphone. At the end of the study, tapes are retrieved and read by the investigator using the PETRA Master Console. The latter plays back the description of the food and displays the decoded weight information.

The PETRA food scales are simple to operate, and the system makes it difficult for the subject to modify the digitally coded food record. Consequently, the habitual food intake is more likely to be truthfully recorded than in the conventional weighed food record (Bingham, 1987; Bingham et al., 1994). As a result, the PETRA food scales were used in the validation of the dietary assessment methods used in the U.K. EPIC study (Bingham et al., 2001).

Tape recorders have been perceived to be especially useful for populations facing memory or visual limitations such as the elderly and children. However, when Lindquist et al. (2000) compared energy intakes of children, based on both tape-recorded food records and recall interviews, with energy expenditure measured by the doubly labeled water technique, the use of a tape recorder did not result in more accurate assessments of energy intake than the recall method, especially among the older children (12–15 y).

3.2.5 Microcomputers

Stockley et al. (1986a, 1986b) were among the first investigators to develop a computerized system for recording food intake. The device consisted of a digital balance with a capacity of 1 kg interfaced to a specially developed microcomputer with a keyboard. The latter had an upper bank of color-coded control keys which registered "start," "waste," "mixed waste," "no waste," and "done," and 55 color-coded food record keys. The keyboard was fitted with a removable transparent keyboard overlay, to assist in the correct identification of the food keys. The respondent burden was reduced when using this food-recording device because the subject did not have to read the balance or keep a written diary (Stockley et al., 1986b). The device also eliminated the process of coding the food records, a task considered to be the most time-consuming part of a quantitative dietary study (Black, 1982). Details of some of the problems with coding foods are given in Section 5.2.8.

In 1990, the USDA Western Human Nutrition Research Center developed the Nutrition Evaluation Scale System (NESSy) (Fong and Kretsch, 1990) to replace the manually weighed food record. NESSy is a computerized method that uses interactive software to prompt and guide participants through the recording of food weights and descriptions. It is designed to speed up the recording of a weighed food record and can be used by participants in their own homes. Use of NESSy to record food intake saves about 80% in time and labor, and it yields accurate data at both the group and individual levels (Kretsch and Fong, 1990). The USDA Agricultural Research Service is evaluating the use of NESSy in association with internet data transfer, allowing expansion of the capabilities of the system for use by the lay person (Consumer NESSy) and for the dietetic professional (ProNeSSy).

Several large-scale national nutrition surveys, including the EPIC study, the 1988–1994 NHANES III, the USDA nationwide household food consumption survey, and the New Zealand National Nutrition Survey and Children's Nutrition Survey (Parnell et al., 2003), have adopted the use of microcomputer-based automated dietary interviews to standardize 24-h recall procedures and to automate data entry. In general, these systems allow all the recall data to be entered directly into the computer at the time of the interviews.

In the EPIC study, standardization of the 24-h recall interviews in the 23 European centers (10 countries in total) was achieved with the aid of a software program (EPIC-SOFT) (Slimani et al., 1999). EPIC-SOFT was designed specifically to prevent memory deficiency, to standardize the identification and description of foods, for quantification of portion sizes, and for handling of recipes. The specific approaches used are described in Slimani et al. (2000).

Laptop computers were used in the CS-FII for the first time in 1987–1988, to assist with interviewing (Section 2.3). The computers were programmed to handle a food list of nearly 3000 items and default codes for foods that subjects have difficulty remembering. The default codes represent the most commonly used items in a specific food category. For example meat that is not further specified may default to regular ground, pan-cooked hamburger (USDA, 1998).

In 2002, a new, automated, multiple-pass 24-h recall interview procedure was introduced by USDA in their nationwide food survey. In this revised method, there are a number of built-in cues to help jog the respondent's memory. In addition, all questions, prompts, and details about the food and how it was prepared are computerized.

In the New Zealand 1997 National Nutrition Survey (MOH, 1997), and the Children's Survey (Parnell et al., 2003), a multiple-pass 24-h recall direct data-capture program was developed to reflect the unique needs of the New Zealand surveys. The program was based on the direct data-capture program developed by the University of Minnesota (McDowell et al., 1990). Bar code scanners were also used in these New Zealand surveys to improve the accuracy of the product name information for branded items.

A different approach has been developed by Kohlmeier et al. (1997). The system is known as computer-assisted self-interviewing (CASI), and it permits the use of in-depth questionnaires using a microcomputer but without interviewers. The system also provides respondents with an evaluation of their reported nutrient intakes. A prototype CASI diet history program has been tested in several U.S. focus groups of mixed age, sex,

ethnicity, and education. The program automates data entry and ensures that responses are complete by encouraging subjects to review and correct inconsistent data.

Computerized systems have also been developed especially for use by persons with low literacy (Ammerman et al. 1994). These interactive multimedia-based dietary assessment tools will have an increasing role in improving the validity of the dietary data collected and in advancing our understanding of relationships between diet and disease.

3.3 Selecting an appropriate method

The method of choice for assessing food or nutrient intakes depends primarily on the objectives of the study. No method is devoid of random or systematic errors (Chapter 5), or prevents alterations in the food habits of the subjects. Table 3.6 summarizes the most appropriate methods for assessing food or nutrient intakes in relation to four possible levels of objectives.

Note that the number and selection of replicate 24-h recalls, or weighed or estimated 1-d food records required to obtain level two, level three, or level four data, depends on the day-to-day variation within one individual (i.e., within-subject variation) of the nutrient of interest (Section 6.2). This variation depends on the nutrient, the study population, the dietary survey method used, and the seasonal variations of intake. Nonconsecutive days should be selected when possible, to enhance the statistical power of the information: day-to-day correlations between intakes often occur when food intake data are collected over consecutive days. The length of time needed between the observation days also depends on the nutrient (IOM, 2000). Generally, for nutrients found in high concentrations in only a few foods, such as vitamins A and D and cholesterol, the number of replicates needed is greater than for those found in a wide range of foods (e.g., protein).

Additional factors that should be considered when choosing a method for assessing the food consumption of individuals are

Level	Desired information	Preferred approach
One	Mean nutrient intake of a group	A single 24-h recall, or single weighed or estimated food record, with large number of subjects and adequate representation of all days of the week
Two	Proportion of population "at risk"	Replicate observations on each individual or a subsample using 24-h recalls or weighed or estimated 1-d food records
Three	Usual intakes of nutrients in individuals for ranking within a group	Multiple replicates of 24-h recalls or food records or a semiquantitative food frequency questionnaire
Four	Usual intakes of foods or nutrients in individuals for counseling or for correlation or regression analysis	Even larger number of recalls or records for each individual. Alternatively, a semiquantitative food frequency questionnaire or a dietary history can be used.

Table 3.6: Selection of methodology to measure nutrient intakes to meet four possible levels of objectives. Modified from Gibson (2002).

the characteristics of the subjects within the study population, the respondent burden of the method, and the available resources. For instance, certain methods are unsuitable for elderly subjects with poor memories, for busy mothers with young children, or for illiterate subjects. Other methods require highly trained personnel and specialized laboratory and computing facilities, which may not be available. Generally, the more accurate methods are associated with higher costs, greater respondent burden, and lower response rates. Unfortunately, compromises often have to be made between the collection of precise data on usual nutrient intakes of individuals and a high response rate.

3.3.1 Determining the mean nutrient intake of a group: level one

Level one is the easiest objective to achieve and can be met by measuring the food intake of each subject in the group using a single 24-h recall or a 1-d food record, provided the subjects are representative of the study population and all the days of the week are equally represented in the final sample (Cole and Black, 1984). Data on average usual nutrient intakes of a group can be used for international comparisons across countries of the relationship of nutrient intakes to health and disease.

The size of the group (n) necessary to characterize the group mean usual nutrient intake depends on the degree of precision required and the day-to-day variation between subjects in the nutrient intakes (NRC, 1986; Sempos et al., 1991; IOM, 2000). The appropriate formula is

$$n = s_b^2/e^2$$

where s_b^2 is the between-subject variance of the nutrient of interest, and e is the desired standard error — a measure of precision required for the estimate of the mean intake of the nutrient of interest.

Obviously, to use this formula, an estimate of between-subject variation for the nutrient of interest is required. This is usually obtained from the literature but may be determined during a pilot study. This calculation should be repeated for each of the nutrients of interest, and the largest n (i.e., the worst case) should be used if possible.

As an example, assume the expected mean iron intake obtained from the literature is 10 mg/d, with an anticipated standard deviation (s) of 3 mg/d. Also assume that the desired margin of error in the expected mean is from 9.2 to 10.8 mg/d, or 1.6 mg/d. If a precision of 95% is required, the margin of error used is ± twice the standard error and $e = 1.6/4$ (i.e., $e = 0.4$). If a precision of 99% is required, the margin of error used is ± three times the standard error, and then $e = 1.6/6$ (i.e., $e = 0.27$. Using a precision of 95%, then

$$n = 3^2/0.4^2 = 56 \text{ subjects}$$

Alternatively, if a precision of 99% is used

then more subjects must be studied:

$$n = 3^2 / 0.27^2 = 123 \, \text{subjects}$$

If the study objective is to demonstrate a significant difference in the mean intakes of two groups, or a significant change in the mean intakes, based on unpaired or paired data, then alternative formulae must be applied; details are given in Gibson and Ferguson (1999).

3.3.2 Calculating the population percentage "at risk": level two

To determine the percentage of the population "at risk" of inadequate nutrient intakes, estimates of the usual intakes of the subjects are required. This, in turn, requires that the food consumption of subjects be measured over more than 1 day. Hence, repeated 24-h recalls, or replicate weighed or estimated 1-d food records are the methods of choice. Often, it is not feasible to carry out repeated observations on all the subjects, as in the case of a national dietary survey, and the recalls or records are repeated on a subsample of the subjects only.

To achieve a level two objective, at least two independent measurements of food intake should be obtained on at least a representative subsample of individuals in the survey. The U.S. Food and Nutrition Board (IOM, 2000) recommends that the replicate measurements should be independent and made on nonconsecutive days. However, if the data can be collected only on consecutive days, then three daily measurements should be used. The subsample should consist of 30 to 40 individuals who represent the age range of the sample. Note that it is more important to have a minimum *number* of replicate observations in the subsample than a minimum *proportion* of replicate observations.

Once a series of replicate observations on at least 30 individuals have been obtained, an adjustment can be made to the observed distribution of intakes to remove the variability introduced by day-to-day variation in nutrient intakes within an individual, i.e., to remove the within-subject variation (Section 6.2.3). Such an adjustment can be performed

using the method outlined by the National Research Council (NRC, 1986), or a more-refined NRC approach developed by Nusser et al. (1996) using SAS and PROC IML, or using the program PC-SIDE. The latter program can be downloaded from

http://www.iastate.edu/

The adjustment process provides estimates of the usual nutrient intakes for each specified age- and gender-specific subgroup. An example comparing the adjusted distributions of usual zinc intakes (using the refined NRC approach of Nusser et al., 1996) with the observed zinc intakes for New Zealand adult females aged 19–50 y is shown in Figure 3.3. The adjustment process used yields a distribution with reduced variability that preserves the shape of the original observed distribution (Gibson et al., 2003).

The adjusted distribution of "usual" nutrient intakes can then be used to predict the proportion of the population at risk of nutrient inadequacy using either the full probability approach, or the Estimated Average Requirement (EAR) cutpoint method; details are given in Sections 8.3.1 and 8.3.2. Figure 3.3 shows that, in this particular case, adjusting the distribution significantly reduces the pro-

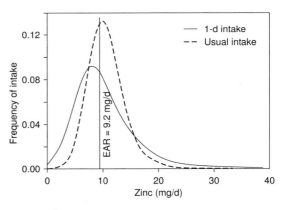

Figure 3.3: Estimates of usual intake distribution for zinc for New Zealand adults obtained from 24-h recall data and adjusted with replicate intake data using the refined NRC method. The y-axis (frequency of intake) shows the likelihood of each level of intake in the population. EAR, Estimated Average Requirement. From Gibson et al., Nutrition Today 38: 63–70, 2003 © Lippincott Williams & Wilkins.

portion of subjects considered to have intakes below the EAR.

Within-subject variation can also have a significant effect on estimates of the prevalence of abnormally high nutrient intakes. Table 3.7 shows data from NHANES II. The large differences between the observed prevalence and the calculated "true" prevalence represent the effect of removing the within-subject variation by calculation. In this case, very large numbers of repeated measurements on each subject are required to reduce the observed prevalence of abnormally high intakes of cholesterol and calcium to within 5% of the true prevalence (Sempos et al., 1991).

Data on the distribution of usual nutrient intakes of a population are essential for national food policy development and food fortification planning. Food patterns associated with inadequate nutrient intakes can also be identified using this approach, enabling food-assistance programs to be designed and improvements in nutrition education made.

3.3.3 Ranking individuals by food or nutrient intake: level three

When the study objective is at level three and involves ranking individuals within a group, often for the purpose of linking dietary intakes with risk of chronic disease, the preferred approach is to obtain multiple observations on each individual. The number of

| Variable | Prevalence (%) | | No. of repeated |
	"True"	Observed	measurements
Cholesterol > 300 mg	15	37	39
Calcium > 800 mg	12	21	9

Table 3.7: "True" and observed prevalence estimates and the number of repeated measurements needed to reduce the observed prevalence to within 5% of the "true" prevalence. Data for women aged 45–54 y from NHANES II (1976–1980). From: Sempos CT, Looker AC, Johnson CL, Woteki CE. (1991). The importance of within-person variability in estimating prevalence. In: Macdonald I (ed.), Monitoring Dietary Intakes, pp. 99–109. © Springer-Verlag, Berlin.

days required to achieve the level three objective can be calculated from the ratio of the within- to the between-subject variation in nutrient intakes (i.e., the variance ratio). Sometimes the latter can be obtained from the literature, again preferably from an earlier study on a comparable group. Alternatively, a pilot study may be necessary to obtain this information.

Several authors have developed equations for calculating the number of replicate days required to meet level three objectives (Liu et al., 1978; Black et al., 1983; Marr and Heady, 1986; Basiotis et al., 1987; Nelson et al.,1989). Black et al. (1983) suggest using the following formula for the number of days (n) of diet records needed:

$$n = (r^2/(1 - r^2)) \times (s_w^2/s_b^2)$$

In this equation, r is the unobservable correlation between the observed and true mean intakes of individuals over the period of observation, and s_w^2 and s_b^2 are the observed within- and between-subject variances, respectively. This equation should be used in association with Table 3.8 which shows the proportion of subjects correctly and incorrectly classified in the extreme fractions for different values of the correlation coefficient between the observed and true intakes (r). The value of r chosen will depend on the degree of misclassification that the investigator is prepared to accept.

As an example, assume that the investigator requires that when the subjects are divided into terciles, fewer than 5% (< 0.05) of the subjects are grossly misclassified into the opposite tercile. This will require an r value of 0.75 (Table 3.8). Assuming $s_w^2/s_b^2 = 1.7$, then

$$\text{number of days} = (r^2/(1 - r^2)) \times 1.7$$
$$= 0.75^2/(1 - 0.75^2) \times 1.7$$
$$= 3 \text{ days}$$

The number of days needed to generate a given r increases as the chosen r increases. If the size of the within-subject variation (s_w^2) in nutrient intake is small compared with the size of the between-subject (s_b^2) variation, then fewer replicate days are needed to meet level three objectives.

r		Correctly and incorrectly classified into extreme fraction		
		Thirds	Fourths	Fifths
0.75	a	0.69	0.63	0.59
	b	0.049	0.013	0.004
0.80	a	0.72	0.68	0.65
	b	0.033	0.006	0.002
0.85	a	0.76	0.72	0.69
	b	0.018	0.002	<0.001
0.90	a	0.80	0.77	0.75
	b	0.006	<0.001	<0.001
0.95	a	0.86	0.84	0.83
	b	<0.001	<0.001	<0.001

Table 3.8: Proportion of subjects correctly and incorrectly classified in the extreme fractions for different values of the correlation coefficient (r). a, correctly classified in the extreme thirds, fourths, or fifths of the distribution of intakes; b, misclassified into the opposite extreme fraction. From Nelson et al., American Journal of Clinical Nutrition 50: 155–167, 1989 © Am J Clin Nutr. American Society for Clinical Nutrition.

The U.S. subcommittee on criteria for dietary evaluation (NRC, 1986) recommended using independent days for replicating the measurements of 1-d nutrient intakes to reduce any effect of autocorrelation between intakes on adjacent days.

An alternative approach to achieving level three objectives is to use a semiquantitative food frequency questionnaire This approach is often used in epidemiological investigations to study associations between intakes and risk of disease and does not require a measurement of absolute nutrient intakes. Although this approach is much simpler, involving only a single interview with each subject, it is difficult to quantify the errors involved and to separate the effects of within- and between-subject variance.

3.3.4 Determining usual intakes of nutrients of individuals: level four

Reliable estimates of usual food or nutrient intakes of individuals that can be used with confidence to meet a level four objective, involving correlation or regression analysis with individual biochemical measures, are

the most difficult to obtain. Large numbers of measurement days for each individual are required using 24-h recalls or estimated or weighed food records.

An estimate of the within-subject variation for each nutrient of interest should be obtained from the literature, preferably from an earlier study on a comparable group or a pilot study, as noted earlier. This estimate may be expressed as the variance, s_w^2; standard deviation, s_w; or as the coefficient of variation (CV_w) expressed as a percentage:

$$CV_w = s_w/\text{mean level of intake} \times 100\%$$

This estimate can be used in the following equation to determine the number of days required per subject to estimate an individual's nutrient intake to within 20% of their true mean 95% of the time (Beaton et al., 1979):

$$n = (Z_\alpha CV_w/D_0)^2$$

where n = the number of days needed per subject, Z_α = the normal deviate for the percentage of times the measured value should be within a specified limit (i.e., 1.96 in the example below), CV_w = the within-subject coefficient of variation (as a percentage), and D_0 = the specified limit (as a percentage of long-term true intake) (i.e., 20% in the example given below).

The following example illustrates how to calculate the number of days required to estimate a Malawian woman's zinc intake using 24-h recalls to within 20% of the true mean, 95% of the time. In this example, the CV_w (i.e., 34%) for zinc intakes on Malawian women via 24-h recalls is taken from the literature (Hotz and Brown, 2004). Thus $Z_\alpha = 1.96$ and $CV_w = 34\%$. Then:

$$n = (1.96 \times 34\%/20\%)^2 = 11 \text{ days}$$

If a pilot study is undertaken in which replicate 24-h recalls are conducted, then the actual CV_w for each nutrient of interest can be calculated. In this way, the estimate of the number of days required to measure the usual intake of each of the nutrients of interest in an individual, with a required degree of precision, can be defined. In general, considerably more days are required to obtain

Method and Procedures	Uses and Limitations
24-h recall. Subject or caretaker recalls food intake of previous 24-h in an interview. Quantities estimated in household measures using food models as memory aids or to assist in quantifying portion sizes. Nutrient intakes calculated using food composition data.	Useful for assessing average *usual* intakes of a large population, provided that the sample is truly representative and that the days of the week are adequately represented. Used for international comparisons of relationship of nutrient intakes to health and susceptibility to chronic disease. Inexpensive, easy, quick, with low respondent burden so that compliance is high. Large coverage possible; can be used with illiterate individuals. Element of surprise so less likely to modify eating pattern. Single 24-h recalls likely to omit foods consumed infrequently. Relies on memory and hence unsatisfactory for the elderly and young children. Multiple replicate 24-h recalls used to estimate *usual* intakes of individuals.
Estimated food record. Record of all food and beverages "as eaten" (including snacks), over periods from one to seven days. Quantities estimated in household measures. Nutrient intakes calculated using food composition data.	Used to assess *actual* or *usual* intakes of individuals, depending on number of measurement days. Data on *usual* intakes used for diet counseling and statistical analysis involving correlation and regression. Accuracy depends on the conscientiousness of subject and ability to estimate quantities. Longer time frames result in a higher respondent burden and lower cooperation. Subjects must be literate.
Weighed food record. All food consumed over a defined period is weighed by the subject, caretaker, or assistant. Food samples may be saved individually, or as a composite, for nutrient analysis. Alternatively, nutrient intakes calculated using food composition data.	Used to assess *actual* or *usual* intakes of individuals, depending on the number of measurement days. Accurate but time consuming. Setting must permit weighing. Subjects may change their usual eating pattern to simplify weighing or to impress investigator. Requires literate, motivated, and willing participants. Expensive.
Dietary history. Interview method consisting of a 24-h recall of *actual* intake, plus information on overall *usual* eating pattern, followed by a food frequency questionnaire to verify and clarify initial data. Usual portion sizes recorded in household measures. Nutrient intakes calculated using food composition data.	Used to describe *usual* food or nutrient intakes over a relatively long time period, which can be used to estimate prevalence of inadequate intakes. Such information is used for national food policy development, for food fortification planning, and to identify food patterns associated with inadequate intakes. Labor-intensive, time-consuming, and results depend on skill of interviewer.
Food frequency questionnaire. Uses comprehensive or specific food item list to record intakes over a given period (day, week, month, year). Record is obtained by interview or self-administered questionnaire. Questionnaire can be semiquantitative when subjects asked to quantify usual portion sizes of food items, with or without the use of food models.	Designed to obtain qualitative, descriptive data on *usual* intakes of foods or classes of foods over a long time period. Useful in epidemiological studies for ranking subjects into broad categories of low, medium, and high intakes of specific foods, food components, or nutrients, for comparison with the prevalence or mortality statistics of a specific disease. Can also identify food patterns associated with inadequate intakes of specific nutrients. Method is rapid, with low respondent burden and high response rate, but accuracy is lower than for other methods.

Table 3.9: Uses and limitations of methods used to assess the food consumption of individuals.

reliable estimates of intakes of individuals to meet the level four objective, compared with level three (i.e., relative ranking of subjects into groups) (Palaniappan et al., 2003).

Sometimes, dietary histories or semiquantitative food frequency questionnaires are used to obtain this level four data on usual nutrient intakes for correlation with biomarkers (Jacques et al., 1993). Some investigators emphasize, however, that the accuracy of a semi-quantitative food frequency questionnaire is only equivalent to two to three repeat 24-h recalls (Sempos et al., 1999).

In some experimentally controlled studies such as balance studies, information on the actual nutrient intakes of an individual over a finite time period are required. For such data, weighed food records (Section 3.1.4), completed for the duration of the study period, are the recommended method. Nutrient intakes can then be calculated using food composition data. Alternatively, duplicate meals can be collected throughout the period for later analysis; details are given in Section 4.7.

3.4 Summary

Details of the available methods for assessing the food consumption of individuals, and their uses and limitations, are summarized in Table 3.9.

Technical improvements for measuring the food consumption of individuals include telephone-assisted approaches, even in national surveys; use of photographs as memory aids and to quantify portion sizes consumed; electronic devices for recording food intakes directly (e.g., tape recorders); and use of microcomputers, which can be used to automate both dietary interviews and data entry, in an effort to standardize interviews, as well as the identification and description of foods, especially in multicenter epidemiological studies. Such developments aim to reduce respondent and interviewer burden and hence increase compliance; reduce errors resulting from memory lapses and incorrect estimation of portion sizes; and, in the case of electronic devices, reduce interviewer biases and eliminate the tedious process of coding the food records.

To characterize the average usual intake of a large group (i.e., level one), a 24-h recall or record over a 1-d period is the method of choice, provided all days of the week are proportionately represented and the sample is representative of the population under study. To determine the proportion of the population "at risk" (i.e., level two) of inadequate nutrient intakes, replicate observations on each individual or a subsample of subjects are required, whereas for assessing usual nutrient intakes in individuals for ranking within a group (i.e., level three), multiple replicates of 24-h recalls or weighed or estimated 1-d food records are recommended. Alternatively, a semiquantitative food frequency questionnaire can be used. An even larger number of multiple replicates of 24-h recalls or food records for each individual are needed for individual diet counseling or correlation and regression analysis (i.e., level four). The number, spacing, and days selected for all these measurements depend on the day-to-day variation (within-subject variation) of the nutrient of interest, which, in turn, is affected by the study population, dietary survey method used, and seasonal variations in intake.

The food frequency and dietary history questionnaires yield retrospective information on patterns of food use over a relatively long time period. With certain modifications, they can also provide data on usual nutrient intakes for level three, and sometimes four objectives.

References

Acheson KJ, Campbell IT, Edholm OG, Miller DS, Stock MJ. (1980). The measurement of food and energy intake in man — an evaluation of some techniques. American Journal of Clinical Nutrition 33: 1147–1154.

Ambrosini GL, van Roosbroeck SAH, Mackerras D, Fritschi L, de Klerk NH, Musk AW. (2003). The reliability of ten-year dietary recall: implications for cancer research. Journal of Nutrition 133: 2663–2668.

Ammermann AS, Kirkley BG, Dennis B., Hohenstein C, Allison A, Strecher VJ, Bulger D. (1994). A dietary assessment for individuals with low literacy skills using interactive touch-screen computer technology. American Journal of Clinical Nutrition 59: 289 (abstr.).

Barr SI, Petit MA, Vigna YM, Prior JC. (2001). Eating attitudes and habitual calcium intake in peripubertal girls are associated with initial bone mineral content and its change over 2 years. Journal of Bone and Mineral Research 16: 940–947.

Basiotis PP, Welsh SO, Cronin FJ, Kelsay JL, Mertz W. (1987). Number of days of food intake records required to estimate individual and group nutrient intakes with defined confidence. Journal of Nutrition 117: 1638–1641.

Basiotis PP, Carlson A, Gerrior SA, Juan WY, Lino M. (2002). The Healthy Eating Index: 1999-2000, U.S. Department of Agriculture, Center for Nutrition Policy and Promotion., Washington DC. CNPP-12. www.cnpp.usda.gov

Beaton GH, Milner J, Corey P, McGuire V, Cousins M, Stewart E, de Ramos M, Hewitt D, Grambsch PV, Kassim N, Little JA. (1979). Sources of variance in 24-hour dietary recall data: implications for nutrition study, design and interpretation. American Journal of Clinical Nutrition 32: 2546–2559.

Bingham SA. (1987). The dietary assessment of individuals; methods, accuracy, new techniques and recommendations. Nutrition Abstracts and Reviews (Series A) 57: 705–742.

Bingham SA, Gill C, Welch A, Day K, Cassidy A, Khaw KT, Sneyd MJ, Key TJ, Roe L, Day NE. (1994). Comparison of dietary assessment methods in nutritional epidemiology: weighed records v. 24 h recalls, food frequency questionnaires and estimated-diet record. British Journal of Nutrition 72: 619–643.

Bingham SA, Welch AA, McTaggart A, Mulligan AA, Runswick SA, Luben R, Oakes S, Khaw KT, Wareham N, Day NE. (2001). Nutritional methods in the European Prospective Investigation of Cancer in Norfolk. Public Health Nutrition 4: 847–858.

Black AE. (1982). The logistics of dietary surveys. Human Nutrition: Applied Nutrition 36: 85–94.

Black AE, Cole TJ, Wiles SJ, White F. (1983). Daily variation in food intake of infants from 2 to 18 months. Human Nutrition: Applied Nutrition 37: 448–458.

Block G, Hartman AM, Dresser CM, Carroll MD, Gannon J, Gardner L. (1986). A data-based approach to diet questionnaire design and testing. American Journal of Epidemiology 124: 453–469.

Block G, Hartman AM, Naughton D. (1990). A reduced dietary questionnaire: development and validation. Epidemiology 1: 58–64.

Bogle M, Stuff J, Davis L, Forrester I, Strickland E, Casey PH, Ryan D, Champagne C, McGee B, Mellad K, Neal E, Zaghloul S, Yadrick K, Horton J. (2001). Validity of a telephone-administered 24-hour dietary recall in telephone and non-telephone households in the rural Lower Mississippi Delta region. Journal of the American Dietetic Association 101: 216–222.

Bowman SA, Lino M, Gerrior SA, Basiotis PP. (1998). The Healthy Eating Index: 1994–96. U.S. Department of Agriculture, Center for Nutrition Policy and Promotion, Washington, DC. CNPP-5. http://www.cnpp.usda.gov/

Burke BS. (1947). The dietary history as a tool in research. Journal of the American Dietetic Association 23: 1041–1046.

Buzzard IM, Sievert YA. (1994). Research priorities and recommendations for dietary assessment methodology: First International Conference on Dietary Assessment Methods. American Journal of Clinical Nutrition 59: 275S–280S.

Cameron ME, van Staveren WA. (eds.) (1988). Manual on Methodology for Food Consumption Studies. Oxford University Press, Oxford.

Casey PH, Goolsby SL, Lensing SY, Perloff BP, Bogle ML. (1999). The use of telephone interview methodology to obtain 24-hour dietary recalls. Journal of the American Dietetic Association 99: 1406–1411.

Cleveland LE, Ingwersen LA. (2001). Was it a slab, a slice, or a sliver? High-tech innovations take food survey to new levels. Agricultural Research, March 2001: 4–7. www.ars.usda.gov/is/AR/archive/

Cole TJ, Black AE. (1984). Statistical aspects in the design of dietary surveys. In: The Dietary Assessment of Populations. Medical Research Council Environmental Epidemiology Unit. Scientific Report No. 4. Medical Research Council, Southampton, U.K.

CSFII/DHKS. (1994–96). The Continuing Survey of Food Intakes by Individuals (CSFII) and the Diet and Health Knowledge Survey (DHKS), 1994-96. www.barc.usda.gov/bhnrc/foodsurvey/

Deurenberg-Yap M, Li T, Tan WL, van Staveren WA, Deurenberg P. (2000). Validation of a semiquantitative food frequency questionnaire for estimation of intakes of energy, fats and cholesterol among Singaporeans. Asia Pacific Journal of Clinical Nutrition 9: 282–288.

Dreon DM, John EM, DiCiccio Y, Whittemore AS. (1993). Use of NHANES data to assign nutrient densities to food groups in a multi-ethnic diet history questionnaire. Nutrition and Cancer 20: 223–230.

Dufour D, Staten LK, Waslien CI, Reina JC, Spurr GB. (1999). Estimating energy intake of urban women in Colombia: comparison of diet records and recalls. American Journal of Physical Anthropology 108: 53–63.

Dwyer JT, Coleman KA. (1997). Insights into dietary recall from a longitudinal study: accuracy over four decades. American Journal of Clinical Nutrition 65: 1153S–1158S.

Eck LH, Klesges RC, Hanson CL. (1989). Recall of a child's intake from one meal: are parents accurate? Journal of the American Dietetic Association 89: 784–789.

Elwood PC, Bird G. (1983). A photographic method of diet evaluation. Human Nutrition: Applied Nutrition 37: 474–477.

Euronut-SENECA. (1991). Nutrition and the elderly in Europe. European Journal of Clinical Nutrition 45(suppl 3): 1–196.

Ferguson EL, Gadowsky SL, Huddle J-M, Cullinan TR, Gibson RS. (1995). An interactive 24-h recall technique for assessing the adequacy of trace mineral intakes of rural Malawian women: its advantages and limitations. European Journal of Clinical Nutrition 49: 565–578.

Feunekes GIJ, van Staveren WA, De Vries JHM, Burema J, Hautvast JGAJ. (1993). Relative and biomarker based validity of a food-frequency questionnaire estimating intake of fats and cholesterol. American Journal of Clinical Nutrition 58: 489–496.

Finch S, Doyle W, Lowe C, Bates CJ, Prentice A, Smithers G, Clarke PC. (1998). National Diet and Nutrition Survey: People Aged 65 Years and Over. Vol. 1: Report of the Diet and Nutrition Survey. The Stationery Office. London.

Fong AK, Kretsch MJ. (1990). Nutrition Evaluation Scale System reduces time and labor in recording quantitative dietary intake. Journal of the American Dietetic Association 90: 664–670.

Galasso R, Panico S, Celentano E, Del Pezzo M. (1994). Relative validity of multiple telephone versus face-to-face 24-hour dietary recalls. Annals of Epidemiology 4: 332–336.

Galeazzi MAM, de Meireles AJ, de Toledo Viana RP, Zabotto CB, Domene SAM. (1966). Registro fotográfico inquéitos dietéticos. Ministry of Health, National Institute of Food and Nutrition, Goiánia, Portugal.

Gibson RS. (2002). Dietary assessment. In: Mann J, Truswell AS. (eds.) Essentials of Human Nutrition (2nd ed.). Oxford University Press, Oxford, pp. 449–466.

Gibson RS, Ferguson EL. (1999). An Interactive 24-Hour Recall for Assessing the Adequacy of Iron and Zinc Intakes in Developing Countries. International Life Sciences Institute Press, Washington, DC.

Gibson RS, McKenzie JE, Ferguson EL, Parnell WR, Wilson NC, Russell DG. (2003). The risk of inadequate zinc intake in United States and New Zealand adults. Nutrition Today 38: 63–70.

Gregory J, Foster K, Tyler H, Wiseman M. (1990). The Dietary and Nutritional Survey of British Adults. The Stationery Office, London.

Gregory J, Collins DL, Davies PSW, Hughes JM, Clarke PC. (1995). National Diet and Nutrition Survey: Children Aged 1.5–4.5 Years. Volume 1: Report of the Diet and Nutrition Survey. The Stationery Office, London.

Gregory J, Lowe S, Bates CJ, Prentice A, Jackson LV, Smithers G, Wenlock R, Farron M. (2000). National Diet and Nutrition Survey: Young People Aged 4 to 18 Years. Volume 1: Report of the Diet and Nutrition Survey. The Stationery Office, London.

Haapa E, Toponen T, Pietinen P, Rasanen L. (1985). Annoskuvakirja (Portion picture booklet). National Public Health Institute and the Department of Nutrition, University of Helsinki. (Available from authors.)

Health and Welfare Canada. (1973). Nutrition Canada National Survey. Health and Welfare, Ottawa.

Henderson L, Gregory J, Swan G. (2002). National Diet and Nutrition Survey: Adults Aged 19 to 64. Volume 1: Types and Quantities of Foods Consumed. The Stationery Office, London.

Henderson L, Gregory J, Irving K, Swan G. (2003a). Diet and Nutrition Survey: Adults Aged 19 to 64. Volume 2: Energy, Protein, Carbohydrate, Fat and Alcohol Intake. The Stationery Office, London.

Henderson L, Irving K, Gregory J, Bates CJ, Prentice A, Perks J, Swan G, Farron M. (2003b). National Diet and Nutrition Survey: Adults Aged 19 to 64. Volume 3: Vitamin and Mineral Intake and Urinary Analytes. The Stationery Office, London.

Hercberg S, Deheeger M, Preziosi P. (1994). Portions alimentaires: manuel photos pour l'estimation des quantités. Institut Scientifique et Technique de la Nutrition et de l'Alimentation, Conservatoire National des Arts et Meétiers, (CNAM) Paris Candia Polytechnica, France.

Holick CN, Michaud DS, Stolzenberg-Solomon R, Maynes ST, Pietinen P, Taylor PR, Virtamo J, Albanes D. (2002). Dietary carotenoids, serum beta-carotene, and retinol and risk of lung cancer in the alpha-tocopherol, beta-carotene cohort study. American Journal of Epidemiology 156: 536–547.

Hotz C, Brown KH (eds.). (2004). Supplement 2: International Zinc Nutrition Consultative Group (IZiNCG) Technical Document No. 1. Assessment of the risk of zinc deficiency in populations and options for its control. Food and Nutrition Bulletin 25: S96–S203.

Hughes BA. (1986). Nutrition interviewing and counselling in public health: the North Carolina experience. Topics in Clinical Nutrition 1: 43–50.

IOM (Institute of Medicine). (2000). Dietary Reference Intakes: Applications in Dietary Assessment. National Academy Press, Washington, DC.

Jacques PF, Sulsky SI, Sadowski JA, Phillips JCC, Rush D, Willett WC. (1993). Comparison of micronutrient intake measured by a dietary questionnaire and biochemical indicators of micronutrient status. American Journal of Clinical Nutrition 57: 182–189.

Kant AK, Schatzkin A, Graubard B, Schairer C. (2000). A prospective study of diet quality and mortality in women. Journal of the American Medical Association 283: 2109–2115.

Kesse E, Clavel-Chapelon F, Slimani N, van Liere M, E3N Group. (2001). Do eating habits differ according to alcohol consumption? Results of a study of the French cohort of the European Prospective Investigation into Cancer and Nutrition (E3N-EPIC). American Journal of Clinical Nutrition 74: 322–327.

Kohlmeier L, Mendez M, McDuffie J, Miller M. (1997). Computer-assisted self-interviewing: a multimedia approach to dietary assessment. American Journal of Clinical Nutrition 65: 1275S–1281S.

Krantzler NJ, Mullen BJ, Schutz HG, Grivetti LE, Holden CA, Meiselman HL. (1982). Validity of telephoned diet recalls and records for assessment of individual food intake. American Journal of Clinical Nutrition 36: 1234–1242.

Kretsch MJ, Fong AKH. (1990). Validation of a new computerized technique for quantitating individual dietary intake: the Nutrition Evaluation Scale System (NESSy) vs the weighed food record. American Journal of Clinical Nutrition 51: 477–484.

Levi F, Pasche C, Lucchini F, La Vecchia C. (2000). Selected micronutrients and colorectal cancer, a case control study from the canton in Vaud, Switzerland. European Journal of Cancer 36: 2115–2119.

Lindquist CH, Cummings T, Goran MI. (2000). Use of tape-recorded food records in assessing children's dietary intake. Obesity Research 8: 2–11.

Liu K, Stamler J, Dyer A, McKeever J, McKeever P. (1978). Statistical methods to assess and minimize the role of intra-individual variability in obscuring relationships between dietary lipids and serum cholesterol. Journal of Chronic Diseases 31: 399–418.

Livingstone MB, Robson PJ. (2000). Measurement of dietary intake in children. Proceedings of the Nutrition Society 59: 279–293.

Lyu LC, Hankin JH, Liu LQ, Wilkens LR, Lee JH, Goodman MT, Kolonel LN. (1998). Telephone vs face-to-face interviews for quantitative food frequency assessment. Journal of the American Dietetic Association 98: 44–48.

MacIntosh DL, Williams PL, Hunter DJ, Sampson LA, Morris SC, Willet WC, Rimm EB. (1997). Evaluation of a food frequency questionnaire — food composition approach for estimating dietary intake of inorganic arsenic and methylmercury. Cancer Epidemiology, Biomarkers & Prevention 6: 1043–1050.

Margetts BM, Pietinen P, Ribolo E. (1997). EPIC European prospective investigation into cancer and nutrition. Validation studies on dietary assessment methods. International Journal of Epidemiology 26 (Suppl. 1): 1–189.

Marques M, Pinho O, de Almeida MDV. (1996). Manual de quantifição de alimentos. Curso da Ciencias de Nutrição de Universidade do Porto, Porto, Portugal.

Marr JW, Heady JA. (1986). Within- and between-person variability in dietary surveys: number of days needed to classify individuals. Human Nutrition: Applied Nutrition 40A: 347–364.

Martintchik AN, Baturin AK, Baeva VS, Peskova EV, Larina TI, Zaburkhna TG. (1995). Albom portisy produktov i bljud [Album of portions of food and dishes]. Institute of Nutrition, Moscow. (Available from the authors)

Maskarinec G, Novotny R, Tasaki K. (2000). Dietary patterns are associated with body mass index in multi-ethnic women. Journal of Nutrition 130: 3068–3072.

Masson LF, McNeill G, Tomany JO, Simpson JA, Peace HS, Wei L, Grubb DA, Bolton-Smith C. (2003). Statistical approaches for assessing the relative validity of a food-frequency questionnaire: use of correlation coeffecents and the kappa statistic. Public Health Nutrition 6: 313–321.

McDowell M, Briefel RR, Warren RA Buzzard M, Seskanich D, Gardner S. (1990). The dietary data collection system: an automated interview and coding system for NHANES III. In: Proceedings of the 14th National Nutrient Databank Conference, CBORD Group Inc, Ithaca, New York, pp. 125–131.

McLennan WM, Podger A. (1998). National Nutrition Survey Nutrient Intakes and Physical Measurements, Australia 1995. Australian Bureau of Statistics, Canberra.

Merchant AT, Hu FB, Spiegelman D, Willett WC, Rimm EB, Ascherio A. (2003). Dietary fiber peripheral arterial disease risk in men. Journal of Nutrition 133: 3658–3663.

MOH (Ministry of Health). (1997). Food Comes First: Methodologies for the National Nutrition Survey of New Zealand. Ministry of Health, Wellington, New Zealand. http://www.moh.govt.nz/

NCHS (National Center for Health Statistics). (1994). Plan and operation of the Third National Health and Nutrition Examination Survey, 1988–94. Vital and Health Statistics 1(32).

Nelson M, Haraldsdóttir J. (1998). Food photographs: practical guidelines II: Development and use of photographic atlases for assessing food portion size. Public Health Nutrition 1: 231–237.

Nelson M, Black AE, Morris JA, Cole TJ. (1989). Between- and within-subject variation in nutrient intake from infancy to old age: estimating the number of days required to rank dietary intakes with desired precision. American Journal of Clinical Nutrition 50: 155–167.

Nelson M, Atkinson M, Darbyshire S. (1994). Food photography I: The perception of food portion size from photographs. British Journal of Nutrition 72: 649–663.

Nelson M, Atkinson M, Meyer J. (1997). A Photographic Atlas of Food Portion Sizes. Pub. No. PB3006. Ministry of Agriculture, Fisheries and Food, London.

Nes M, van Staveren WA, Zajkas G, Inelmen EM, Moreiras-Varela O. (1991). Validity of the dietary history method in elderly subjects. European Journal of Clinical Nutrition 45: 97–104.

NRC (National Research Council). (1981). The proposed system. In: Committee on Food Consumption Patterns, Food and Nutrition Board, National Research Council (eds.) Assessing Changing Food Consumption Patterns. National Academy Press, Washington, DC., pp. 13–18.

NRC (National Research Council). (1986). Nutrient Adequacy: Assessment using Food Consumption Surveys. National Academy Press, Washington, DC.

Nusser SM, Carriquiry AL, Dodd KW, Fuller WA. (1996). A semi-parametric transformation approach to estimating usual daily intake distributions. Journal of American Statistical Association 91: 1440–1449.

O'Neill ME, Carroll Y, Corridan B, Olmedilla B, Granado F, Blanco I, Van den Berg H, Hininger I, Roussell AM, Chopra M, Southon S, Thurnham DI. (2001). A European carotenoid database to assess carotenoid intakes and its use in a five-country comparative study. British Journal of Nutrition 85: 499–507.

Palaniappan U, Cue RI, Payette H, Gray-Donald K. (2003). Implications of day-to-day variability on measurements of usual food and nutrient intake. Journal of Nutrition 133: 232–235.

Parnell W, Scragg R, Wilson N, Schaaf D, Fitzgerald EL. (2003). NZ Food NZ Children: Key results of the 2002 National Children's Nutrition Survey. Ministry of Health, Wellington, New Zealand.

Piwoz EG, Creed de Kanashiro H, Lopez de Romana G, Black RE, Brown KH. (1995). Potential for misclassification of infants' usual feeding practices using 24-hour dietary assessment methods. Journal of Nutrition 125: 57–65.

Robson PJ, Livingtone MB. (2000). An evaluation of food photographs as a tool for quantifying food and nutrient intakes. Public Health Nutrition 3: 183–192.

Rombo M, Silveira D, Martins I, Cruz A. (1996). Modelos fotográficos para inquéritos alimentares. Centro de Estudos de Nutrição do Instituto Nacional de Saúde, Lisbon, Portugal.

Samuelson G. (1970). An epidemiological study of child health and nutrition in a northern Swedish county. 2: Methodological study of the recall technique. Nutrition and Metabolism 12: 321–340.

Sanjur D. (1982). Food consumption survey: issues concerning the process of data collection. In: Social and Cultural Perspectives in Nutrition. Prentice-Hall, Englewood Cliffs, NJ, pp. 169–194.

Sempos CT, Looker AC, Johnson CL, Woteki CE. (1991). The importance of within-person variability in estimating prevalence. In: Macdonald I (ed.), Monitoring Dietary Intakes. Springer-Verlag, Berlin, pp. 99–109.

Sempos CT, Liu K, Ernst ND. (1999). Food and nutrient exposures: what to consider when evaluating epidemiologic evidence. American Journal of Clinical Nutrition 69: 1330S–1338S.

Slattery ML, Benson J, Curtin K, Ma KN, Schaeffer D, Potter JD. (2000). Carotenoids and colon cancer. American Journal of Clinical Nutrition 71: 575–582.

Slimani N, Deharveng G, Charrondier RU, van Klappel AL, Ocke MC, Welch A, Lagiou A, van Liere M, Agudo A, Pala V, Brandstetter B, Andrea C, Stripp C, van Staveren WA, Riboli E. (1999). Structure of the standardized computerized 24-h diet recall interview used as reference method in the 22 centers participating in the EPIC project. Computer Methods and Programs in Biomedicine 58: 251–266.

Slimani N, Ferrari P, Ocke M, Welch A, Boeing H, van Liere M, Pala V, Amiano P, Lagiou A, Mattisson I, Stripp C, Engeset D, Charrondiere R, Buzzard M, van Staveren WA, Riboli E. (2000). Standardization of the 24-hour recall calibration method used in the European Prospective Investigation into Cancer and Nutrition (EPIC): general concepts and preliminary results. European Journal of Clinical Nutrition 54: 900–917.

Sobo EJ, Rock CL, Neuhouser ML, Maciel TL, Neumark-Sztainer D. (2000). Caretaker-child interaction during children's 24-hour dietary recalls: who contributes what to the recall record? Journal of the American Dietetic Association 100: 428–433.

Stockley L, Chapman RI, Holley ML, Jones FA, Prescott EHA, Broadhurst AJ. (1986a). Description of a food recording electronic device for use in dietary surveys. Human Nutrition: Applied Nutrition 40: 13–18.

Stockley L, Hurren CA, Chapman RI, Broadhurst AJ, Jones FA. (1986b). Energy, protein, and fat intake estimated using a food recording electronic device compared with a weighed diary. Human Nutrition: Applied Nutrition 40: 19–23.

Szczyglowa H, Szczepanska A, Ners A, Nowicka L. (1991). Album porcji produktow i potraw. Instytut Zywnosci i Zywienia, Warsaw, Poland. (Available from the authors)

Tran KM, Johnson RK, Soultanakis RP, Matthews DE. (2000). In-person vs telephone administered multiple-pass 24-hour recalls in women: validation with doubly labeled water. Journal of the American Dietetics Association 100: 777–783.

Tsugane S, Fahey MT, Kobayashi M, Sasaki S, Tsubono Y, Akabane M, Gey F. (1998). Four food-frequency categories of fruit intake as a predictor of plasma ascorbic acid level in middle-aged Japanese

men. Annals of Epidemiology 8: 378–383

USDA (U.S. Department of Agriculture). (1992). The Food Guide Pyramid. Home and Garden Bulletin No. 252. Washington, DC.

USDA (U.S. Department of Agriculture, Agricultural Research Service). (1998). Food and Nutrient Intakes by Individuals in the United States by Sex and Age, 1994–96. USDA Nationwide Food Surveys Report No. 96-2. Washington, DC.

van Kappel A, Amoyel J, Slimani N, Vozar B, Riboli E. (1994). EPIC-SOFT Picture Book for Estimation of Food Portion Sizes. International Agency for Research on Cancer, Lyons, France. (Available from the authors.)

van Staveren WA, de Boer JO, Burema J. (1985). Validity and reproducibility of dietary history method estimating the usual food intake during one month. American Journal of Clinical Nutrition 42: 554–559.

van Staveren WA, West CE, Hoffmans MDAF, Bos P, Kardinaal AFM, van Poppel GAFC, Schipper HJ-A, Hautvast JGAJ, Hayes RB. (1986). Comparison of contemporaneous and retrospective estimates of food consumption made by a dietary history method. American Journal of Epidemiology 123: 884–893.

van Staveren WA, Burema J, Livingstone MBE, van den Broek T, Kaaks R. (1996). Evaluation of the dietary history method used in the SENECA study. European Journal of Clinical Nutrition 50(Suppl. 2): S47–S55.

Weiner JS, Lourie JA. (1969). Human Biology: A Guide to Field Methods. International Biological Programme. Handbook No. 9. Blackwell Scientific Publications, Oxford.

WHO (World Health Organization). (1998). Complementary Feeding of Young Children in Developing Countries: A Review of Current Scientific Knowledge. World Health Organization, Geneva.

Willet WC. (1990). Nutritional Epidemiology. Oxford University Press, Oxford.

Willett WC. (1994). Future directions in the development of food frequency questionnaires. American Journal of Clinical Nutrition 59: 171S–174S.

Willett WC, Sampson L, Stampfer MJ, Rosner B, Bain C, Witschi J, Hennekens CH, Speizer FE. (1985). Reproducibility and validity of a semiquantitative food frequency questionnaire. American Journal of Epidemiology 122: 51–65.

Yanek LR, Moy TF, Raqueno JV, Becker DM. (2000). Comparison of the effectiveness of a telephone 24-h dietary recall method vs an in-person method among urban African-American women. Journal of the American Dietetic Association 100: 1172–1177.

Young CM. (1981). Dietary methodology. In: Committee on Food Consumption Patterns, Food and Nutrition Board (ed.). Assessing Changing Food Consumption Patterns. National Research Council. National Academy Press, Washington, DC., pp. 89–118.

4

Assessment of nutrient intakes from food consumption data

It is possible to calculate the nutrient intakes of individuals or population groups if quantitative or semiquantitative methods have been used to collect the relevant food consumption data. The calculations use food composition values representative of the average composition of a particular foodstuff — ideally on a year-round, nationwide basis. The values are available as food composition tables, and/or databases.

Recognition of the potential sources of error in the food composition values is important, as these errors affect the calculation of nutrient intakes. The uncertainties may result from true random variability in the nutrient content of a food or, alternatively, from systematic errors. The extent of random and systematic errors depends on the food item and the nutrient; systematic errors may produce consistent under- or overestimates of nutrient intakes, although the direction and size of the error is frequently unknown.

Food composition values indicate the total amount of the constituent in the food, rather than the amount actually absorbed. This is because the bioavailability of most nutrients in individual food items has not been quantified. As a result, intakes of most nutrients, calculated from food consumption data, represent the maximum available to the body. Consequently, when nutrient-intake data are evaluated, the potential bioavailability of the nutrients from the local diets must always be considered.

Some of the methods and uncertainties involved in the compilation of food composi-

tion data and the associated assessment of the nutrient intakes of individuals and population groups are discussed in this chapter.

4.1 Compiling or augmenting food composition data

Detailed guidelines for compiling food composition data have been published by Rand et al. (1991) and Greenfield and Southgate (1992). Murphy et al. (1991) also provide a detailed description of the development of a research food composition database for use in rural Kenya.

Five methods are used to compile food composition data; these are discussed briefly below. These same methods can also be used to augment an existing food composition database with values for local food items. Care must be taken to validate the resulting food composition database; details of this process are given in Section 4.6.

4.1.1 Direct chemical analysis

Food analysis is costly and time consuming, so a balance must be drawn between making use of existing data and augmenting a database with new chemical analyses. Priority should be given to analyzing those foods that meet all of the following criteria:

- The data for the component of interest in the food, or the food as eaten, is inadequate or nonexistent

- The food forms a significant component of the local diet
- The food contributes significantly to the intake of the dietary component of interest

Food consumption survey data on portion size and frequency of consumption should be used to identify "key foods" that contribute significantly to the overall intake of the nutrient of interest (Haytowitz et al., 2002). The average daily frequency of consumption of the key foods can then be multiplied by the average portion size consumed by the sex- and age-group of interest. Such a procedure takes into account food items that are consumed frequently but in small amounts.

Absence of data may necessitate direct chemical analysis of foods to augment a food composition database, particularly if local differences in food processing, preparation or cooking affect the concentration of the food component of interest. For example, milling, germination, fermentation, and soaking may all reduce the phytic acid content of cereals, making it essential to analyze the phytic acid values of any local cereal-based foods prepared and processed in these ways (Gibson and Hotz, 2001).

Data derived from direct chemical analyses are especially necessary for trace elements such as selenium, iodine, and zinc in plant-based staples because their content often depends on local soil trace element levels or agronomy practices (see Section 4.4.7). For example, Norwegian investigators reported major differences when Finnish instead of Norwegian selenium food composition data were used to calculate daily selenium intakes (i.e., 86 µg/d vs. 18 µg/d) (Ahola, 1991).

Once the foods have been selected for analysis, a protocol must be established to ensure that a representative sample of each food item is collected; details of the sampling protocols required are given in Section 4.4.1. After collection, food samples should be prepared and analyzed using appropriate methods.

The analytical methods chosen must be accurate, precise, and feasible. It is preferable to separately analyze each of the food samples per food type collected: this provides information on the variability within one food type. In practice, a single composite is often analyzed from the multiple samples to reduce the analytical costs (Murphy et al., 1991). In some cases, the single composite can be made up of specific proportions of different cultivars or brands to obtain a single generic value for the database. Details of each of the steps required to generate analyzed food composition values are outlined by Greenfield and Southgate (1992). The recommended AOAC International analytical methods for food analysis are documented in Horwitz (2002).

4.1.2 Using food composition data from other sources

Food composition values vary in quality. Existing values are often drawn from several sources including the food industry, published and unpublished research, contract research, and government research laboratories.

To assess the reliability of existing food composition data, a rating system has been developed, based on the following five quality criteria: (*i*) number of samples on which values are based, (*ii*) analytical method used, (*iii*) sample handling, (*iv*) sampling protocol, and (*v*) analytical quality control. Each quality criterion is further subdivided into four ratings ranging from 0 (unacceptable) to 3 (most desirable). Each of these five quality criteria should be considered when selecting food composition values from among existing data. Discrepancies often occur among existing data, sometimes arising from differences in the analytical methods used. For example, values for the selenium content of selected foods from published data were selected for the USDA nutrient database using this rating system. Details are given in Schubert et al. (1987). Further discussion on this selection process is available in Rand et al. (1991).

4.1.3 Calculating representative values

A database manager compiling new information may have analytical data for a number of different samples of the same food, or data from several sources. In such cases, a single "representative" value for each dietary component of interest must be calculated for the food and the procedure fully documented. When multiple measurements of the same food item from different samples or sources are available, the mean or median value is often weighted on the basis of sample sizes. When two or more populations appear to be represented in the data, the summary statistics should be calculated after consultation with a statistician.

A specialized food composition database may be required for the processing of food frequency questionnaire data. In these databases, different food items are combined into a single entry for a generic food (e.g., one entry for green beans based on data for several different varieties of green beans) (Block et al., 1986). The standard method for producing a single entry for a generic food from aggregated data is to calculate a weighted average. The weighting is determined from data on food consumption patterns of the population group of interest, or the market share. For normally distributed data, the arithmetic mean can be calculated, along with the standard deviation. For skewed data, the median or the geometric mean should be used. The uncertainty in the food composition data for any generic food should also be calculated; it results from both aggregating the foods and the uncertainty in the food composition values for each individual food. Calculation of the standard error can be used as a measure of this uncertainty, although it cannot differentiate between these two sources of error.

4.1.4 Estimating missing food composition values

Ideally, a food composition table or database should contain values for each nutrient for every type of food. However, values are often missing for some nutrients. It is not always clear whether these missing values arise because no analytical data are available or because the values are very small. Database compilers should clearly distinguish between these, and values that are truly zero. The term

"missing" should be assigned only when analytical data are not available and yet there is a high level of confidence that some amount of the component is present. The term "trace" should be applied when the component is present at levels below the measurement accuracy of the analytical method. "Zero" should be used when the component is not present in any detectable amount. Sometimes zero is assigned on the basis of a known biological relationship. For example, vitamin B_{12} does not occur in plant products (Rand et al., 1991).

Before using any food composition database for calculating nutrient intakes, all missing and "trace" values in the database must be replaced with calculated (Section 4.1.5) or imputed numerical nutrient values. Several procedures and sources can be used for imputing values (Box 4.1). The process is important because missing values may be

---

Cooked values from raw values. Requires data on moisture and fat loss or gain and nutrient losses during cooking.

Values for dried foods from fresh foods. Requires data on moisture loss and nutrient losses during drying.

Values for local foods from published literature. May need actual moisture content of local foods because of differences in local preparation, processing or storage conditions, etc.

Values from similar food items. Requires accurate and precise data on similar foods, matched as closely as possible to the missing food.

Generic values from specific values. Derived from aggregating data of specific foods and then applying a weighting to the mean value.

Assumed zero. Only used when the nutrient is not believed to be present in the food item in any detectable amount, based on an examination of data for similar foods.

Calculation from recipes. Requires proportions of ingredients in recipe and the nutrient values for the cooked individual ingredients (Section 4.1.5).

Box 4.1: Techniques for imputing values for missing nutrients. From Murphy et al., Development of research nutrient data bases: an example using foods consumed in rural Kenya. Journal of Food Composition and Analysis 4: 2–17, 1991 © with permission from Elsevier.

treated as zero when nutrient intakes are calculated, leading to underestimates of daily intakes. Further details are given in Murphy et al. (1991), Rand et al. (1991), and Schakel et al. (1997).

When selecting a similar food for estimating nutrient values, several factors must be considered, and the choice depends on the nutrient of interest. These factors may include color, plant maturity, processing or preparation, growing conditions, enrichment, fortification or use of other additives, or cut of meat. As an example, color of the vegetable is particularly important when imputing the carotenoid or vitamin A content of a vegetable (Schakel et al., 1997).

For these nutrient calculations, information on the refuse, yield, nutrient retention, and moisture content is often needed. Sources of such data include Matthews and Garrison (1975), and the USDA (2003a) Nutrient Retention Factors, as well as other international databases such as McCance and Widdowson's "The Composition of Foods" (Holland et al., 1991b).

Examples of how to calculate these imputed estimates can be found in Rand et al. (1991), Schakel et al. (1997), and Gibson and Ferguson (1999). All imputed food composition values should be noted in the food composition database and their source, including the citation and the calculation procedure, should be documented.

4.1.5 Calculating nutrient values of recipes from ingredient data

Recipes may be simple combinations of ingredients or may involve cooking, and require more complex adjustments that use yield or nutrient retention factors, depending on whether nutrient values for raw or cooked ingredients are used. Examples of simple combinations include preparation of raw fruit salad, and the preparation of tomato soup from condensed soup and whole milk. In these cases, nutrient values for the ingredients "as consumed" are summed and then corrected for weight or volume of the final food (Rand et al., 1991).

Calculation of the nutrient content of a cooked dish from a mixture of ingredients often involves changes in weight and nutrient content. Several stages in the calculation can be recognized. These are (*i*) selection of the recipe, (*ii*) collection of data for the nutrient content of each ingredient, (*iii*) adjustment of the nutrient content of each ingredient for the effects of preparation and where relevant cooking, (*iv*) summation of ingredient composition, (*v*) final weight (or volume) adjustment, and (*vi*) determination of the yield and final volume. An example of the procedure used to calculate the nutrient composition from a recipe is given in Section 5.2.9. Other methods have been reviewed by Powers and Hoover (1989).

It is emphasized that nutrient contents of recipes calculated in this way are estimates. Although it is preferable to use yield and retention factors based on habitual cooking methods for the region of interest, in practice the calculations often rely on yield and nutrient retention factors taken from published tables. The latter may not be a true reflection of the actual factors, as these vary with length and temperature of cooking, type of cooking, equipment used, and surface area of food contact exposure etc (Rand et al., 1991).

The recipes selected for these calculations should reflect the food as prepared by the population or subgroup of interest and should take into account any ethnic or regional variation. Sources include regional cookery books, average recipes constructed from information recorded on food record or recall forms, and recipes obtained directly from respondents. The USDA maintains a table of nutrient retention factors for calculating the retention of 25 vitamins, minerals, and alcohol during heating and food preparation (USDA, 2003a). Factors for seven additional food components are now included in this table: folic acid, food folate, β-carotene, α-carotene, β-cryptoxanthin, lycopene, and lutein/zeaxanthin. This table is available from

http://www.nal.usda.gov/fnic/foodcomp/

In some developing countries, recipes may not be available for local dishes. In such cases, recipe data can be constructed by observing and recording local cooking practices that use locally available ingredients (Gibson and Ferguson, 1999).

4.2 Food composition databases

National, and in some cases international, computer-based food composition databases are now the foundation for all calculations of nutrient intakes derived from dietary surveys: printed versions of the same information (food composition tables) are usually directly derived from the databases.

Nutrient values in food composition databases are derived from quantitative analyses of samples of each food. The data should be representative of the average composition of a particular foodstuff on a year-round, nationwide basis. In practice, however, food composition values are often of variable quality and are derived from many different sources.

Nutrient composition values are usually expressed in terms of the nutrient content of the edible portion of the food per 100 g or per common household measure. When the latter is included, the gram weight of the measure of food should also be included. In some of the early food composition tables, information on the nutrient content of the edible portion of the food "as purchased" was also given (Watt et al., 1963).

Inclusion of individual dietary components in food composition databases depends primarily on whether they affect human health: in some food composition databases, over 100 dietary components are listed. Included are components known to influence nutrient bioavailability such as dietary fiber, phytate, oxalic acid, and polyphenols, as well as more descriptive components such as water, pH, and total solids.

Most food composition databases contain a complete description of each food item and include information on the sampling and handling protocols and the quality-control procedures used for the nutrient analysis. The food composition database compiler should provide data on the number of samples used to derive the "central" nutrient value, as well as a statistical parameter to describe the observed variation (e.g., USDA, 2003b). The arithmetic mean, the number of observations, and the standard deviation or standard error should always be recorded, provided that the distribution is not skewed. The coefficient of variation ($CV\% = (SD/mean) \times 100\%$) should also be calculated. This measure expresses the variability of the nutrient content in relation to the mean and can be used for comparing errors in estimating nutrient content between several foods (NRC, 1986).

Food composition databases vary in size, comprehensiveness, the units used to express portion size and nutrient content, and the source and reliability of the values for the food components listed (Scrimshaw, 1997). Not all are updated regularly. Food items in the food composition databases are usually associated with a numerical code that varies in complexity. The INFOODS organization (Section 4.5) has developed a system for identifying foods, defining food components, and describing food component data in an effort to facilitate the global interchange of food composition data (Klensin et al., 1989). In this system, each food component is represented by a unique tagname, a name or descriptive definition of the food component (e.g., carbohydrate by difference, copper), a common or default unit of measurement (e.g., grams of protein per 100 g edible portion of food), and synonymous names for components (e.g., moisture is a synonym for water). In 1994, the INFOODS system of tagnames was adopted by the USDA and by the International Food Data Association (IFDA) (Scrimshaw, 1997).

Some food industries and food producer groups maintain their own food composition databases that contain data on their own products. These databases are used for product and recipe development, research, nutritional labeling, and quality control.

Some of the critical factors to be considered when selecting a food composition database are the geographical sources of the foods listed, the size and comprehensiveness of the database in relation to the range of

Nutrient	(n)	Nutrient	(n)	Nutrient	(n)
Protein	6661	Vitamin A (IU)	6496	Folate (DFE)	5942
Total lipids (fat)	6661	Vitamin A (RAE)	5935	Vitamin B_{12}	6133
Water	6657	Retinol	5909	Cholesterol	6548
Energy	6661	β-carotene	3676	Alcohol	3860
Carbohydrate	6661	α-carotene	3539	Caffeine	3519
Total dietary fiber	5998	β-cryptoxanthin	3524	Theobromine	3505
Total sugars	4023	Lycopene	3502	Total sat. fatty acids	6460
Ash	6655	Lutein+zeaxanthin	3495	4:0	4006
Calcium	6540	Vitamin K	3265	6:0	4032
Iron	6561	α-tocopherol	3567	8:0	4157
Magnesium	6243	Ascorbic acid	6425	10:0	4848
Phosphorus	6299	Thiamin	6272	12:0	5174
Potassium	6389	Riboflavin	6281	14:0	5620
Sodium	6656	Niacin	6274	16:0	5859
Zinc	6225	Vitamin B_6	6136	18:0	5845
Copper	6165	Folate, total	6120	Total monounsat. fat. acids	6252
Manganese	5365	Folic acid	5934	16:1 undifferentiated	5578
Selenium	5621	Food folate	5969		

Table 4.1: USDA Nutrient Database for Standard Reference (Release 16). List of the nutrients, with the number of food items (n) that contain data for that nutrient, that form the Survey Nutrient Database (SNDB) for NHANES. Data for other fatty and amino acids are also included within Release 16. IU, international units; RAE, retinol activity equivalents; DFE, dietary folate equivalents. From USDA (2003b).

foods required, the number of individual food components listed, and the methods used to indicate missing or imputed data. The competence of those involved with the database development, management, and documentation should also be considered (Hoover and Pelican, 1984). Some examples of national food composition databases are discussed briefly below.

4.2.1 United States Nutrient Databases

The USDA Agricultural Research Service maintains a large database of nutrient and non-nutrient food components. This is called the "USDA Nutrient Database for Standard Reference." This database can be searched online and downloaded for use on personal computers from

http://www.nal.usda.gov/fnic/foodcomp/

This relational database is a major source of food composition data, providing the foundation for most food composition databases in the public and private sectors in the United States. As information is updated, new versions of the database are released.

Release 16 (USDA, 2003b) contains data on 6661 food items. The release includes data for all the food groups and food components published by the USDA in the 21 volumes of Agriculture Handbook No. 8 and its four supplements. A file of food component values per 100 g constitutes the core of the information presented. The values represent the total amount of the food component present in the edible portion of the food, including any nutrients added in processing. Table 4.1 lists the number of food items that contain data for each nutrient.

The Nutrition Coordinating Center at the University of Minnesota has developed sophisticated computer software and databases for researchers collecting and analyzing dietary data, including those dealing with the 24-h recalls from NHANES III. Windows-based versions of the software are also available. The nutrient databases used have been drawn from a wide variety of sources. As a result, the number of food components in the databases is significantly larger than that in

Primary energy sources: Energy (kilocalories); Energy (kilojoules); Total Fat; Total Carbohydrate; Total Protein; Animal Protein; Vegetable Protein; Alcohol; % calories from fat; % calories from carbohydrate; % calories from protein; % calories from alcohol.

Fat and cholesterol: Cholesterol; Total Saturated Fatty acids (SFA); Total Monounsaturated Fatty acids (MFA); Total Polyunsaturated Fatty acids (PFA); Total *Trans*-Fatty acids (TRANS); Omega-3 Fatty acids % calories from SFA; % calories from MFA; % calories from PFA; Polyunsaturated to Saturated Fat Ratio; Cholesterol to Saturated Fatty Acid Index (CSI).

Carbohydrates: Total sugars; Fructose; Galactose; Glucose; Lactose; Maltose; Sucrose; Starch.

Fiber: Total Dietary Fiber; Soluble Dietary Fiber; Insoluble Dietary Fiber; Pectins.

Vitamins: Total Vitamin A Activity (Retinol Equivalents); Total Vitamin A Activity (International Units); Total Vitamin A Activity (Retinol Activity Equivalents); β-carotene Equivalents (derived from provitamin A carotenoids); Retinol; Vitamin D (calciferol); Vitamin E (International Units); Vitamin E (Total α-tocopherol); Natural α-tocopherol (RRR-α-tocopherol or d-α-tocopherol); Synthetic α-tocopherol (all rac-α-tocopherol or dl-α-tocopherol); Total α-tocopherol Equivalents; β-tocopherol; γ-tocopherol; δ-tocopherol; Vitamin K (phylloquinone); Vitamin C (ascorbic acid); Thiamin (vitamin B_1); Riboflavin (vitamin B_2); Niacin (vitamin B_3); Niacin equivalents; Pantothenic acid; Vitamin B_6 (pyridoxine, pyridoxyl, pyridoxamine); Total folate; Dietary folate equivalents; Natural folate (food folate); Synthetic folate (folic acid); Vitamin B_{12} (cobalamin).

Carotenoids: β-carotene (provitamin A carotenoid); α-carotene (provitamin A carotenoid); β-cryptoxanthin (provitamin A carotenoid); Lutein + zeaxanthin; Lycopene.

Minerals: Calcium; Phosphorus; Magnesium; Iron; Zinc; Copper; Manganese; Selenium; Sodium; Potassium.

Fatty acids: SFA 4:0, butyric acid; SFA 6:0, caproic acid; SFA 8:0, caprylic acid; SFA 10:0, capric acid; SFA 12:0, lauric acid; SFA 14:0, myristic acid; SFA 16:0, palmitic acid; SFA 17:0, margaric acid; SFA 18:0, stearic acid; SFA 20:0, arachidic acid; SFA 22:0, behenic acid; MFA 14:1, myristoleic acid; MFA 16:1, palmitoleic acid; MFA 18:1, oleic acid; MFA 20:1, gadoleic acid; MFA 22:1, erucic acid; PFA 18:2, linoleic acid; PFA 18:3, linolenic acid; PFA 18:4, parinaric acid; PFA 20:4, arachidonic acid; PFA 20:5, eicosapentaenoic acid (EPA); PFA 22:5, docosapentaenoic acid (DPA); PFA 22:6, docosahexaenoic acid (DHA); TRANS 16:1, *trans*-hexadecenoic acid; TRANS 18:1, *trans*-octadecenoic acid (elaidic acid); TRANS 18:2, *trans*-octadecadienoic acid (linolelaidic acid); incl. c-t, t-c, t-t.

Amino acids: Tryptophan; Threonine; Isoleucine; Leucine; Lysine; Methionine; Cystine; Phenylalanine; Tyrosine; Valine; Arginine; Histidine; Alanine; Aspartic acid; Glutamic acid; Glycine; Proline; Serine.

Other: Aspartame; Saccharin; Caffeine; Phytic acid; Oxalic acid; 3-Methylhistidine; Sucrose polyester; Ash; Water; User nutrients.

Table 4.2: Nutrients in the Nutrition Coordinating Center database of foods and foodstuffs, University of Minnesota. From http://www.ncc.umn.edu/

Release 16 of the USDA Nutrient Database for Standard Reference, the primary data reference. The additional food components include phytic acid and oxalic acid (Table 4.2), reflecting in part the growing awareness of the importance of components in food that affect the bioavailability of some nutrients.

4.2.2 Canadian Nutrient File

The Nutrition Research Division of Health Canada produces a large relational food composition database called the Canadian Nutrient File. The most recent release (Health Canada, 2001b) contains information on up to 112 nutrients in 4943 foods. The food composition data are derived from the USDA Nutrient Database for Standard Reference, with the addition of information based on the chemical analysis of some Canadian foods (e.g., meat) and food products. Certain adjustments have been made to some of the U.S. data to account for differences in the cuts of meat, their fat-to-lean ratio, and Canadian enrichment and fortification practices (Health Canada, 2001b).

These files are available from the Nutrition Research Division of Health Canada in a text and database format at

> http://www.hc-sc.gc.ca/food-aliment/

4.2.3 United Kingdom National Nutritional Database

Following the publication of the 6th summary edition of McCance and Widdowson's "The Composition of Foods" (Food Standards Agency, 2002), a comprehensive integrated database is in preparation. This will encompass data from all the nine supplements on specific food groups, the supplement on fatty acids, and the 6th summary edition (Section 4.3.2); only one set of food composition values per food code will be compiled.

Many of the earlier publications are available in electronic format. Inquiries relating to the material in electronic format and the comprehensive integrated database should be addressed to HMSO Licensing Division, St Clements House, 2–16 Colegate, Norwich, NR3 1BQ, England.

4.2.4 European food composition databases

In Europe, 25 countries are working collaboratively toward improving the quality and compatibility of data on food composition, in a continuation of the EUROFOODS program established in 1982. Currently there is no agreed comprehensive European nutrient database. Several countries in Europe have a national database or food composition table; details of those available in nine European countries are given in Deharveng et al. (1999). In the U.K., Denmark, France, Greece, Italy, the Netherlands, and Sweden, one national institute is responsible for the database and/or food composition table. Most nutrients in the European food composition databases (or tables) are derived from analyzed values and are expressed in a comparable way. Nevertheless, some discrepancies for certain nutrients in terms of methods of analysis, definitions, and modes of expression exist. As a result, values are not comparable for carbohydrates, dietary fiber, folate, vitamins A and E, and carotenes. Indeed, the development of a standardized European food composition database to minimize all the identified nutrient discrepancies is urgently needed to facilitate multicenter European studies.

A carotenoid database has been prepared of the most commonly consumed carotenoid-rich foods in five European countries (U.K., Republic of Ireland, Spain, France, and the Netherlands) in an effort to improve the compatibility for carotenoids. Values for five carotenoids (lycopene, β-carotene, β-cryptoxanthin, lutein, and α-carotene) are available (O'Neill et al., 2001).

4.2.5 International Minilist Nutrient Database

Readers in some developing countries may wish to use the International Minilist Nutrient Database developed at the University of California, Berkeley, in 1997. It contains data for 53 nutrients and antinutrients (including dietary fiber and phytate) in 1800 foods from six countries (Egypt, Kenya, Mexico, Senegal, India, and Indonesia), and can be modified to include food composition data for additional foods. The source of each food composition value is fully documented. The data are taken from published food composition tables or imputed where necessary; there are no missing values. The nutrient database and an associated nutrient analysis computer program — the WorldFood Dietary Assessment System — are now in the public domain and can presently be downloaded over the Internet from INFOODS at

> http://www.fao.org/infoods/

Users of the WorldFood Dietary Assessment System specify food names rather than a numerical code, and the weight consumed in grams. The nutrient analysis program is designed to also calculate intakes of available iron and zinc using the algorithms of Murphy et al. (1992) (Section 4.8.3). Note that the Office of Technology at the University of California, Berkeley, no longer provides technical support for the WorldFood Dietary Assessment System.

4.3 Food composition tables

Printed national and, in some cases, international food composition tables are usually derived directly or indirectly from the associated database. The printed tables tend to be less detailed and in some cases are not as up to date as their electronic equivalents. In some countries printed versions are specifically targeted at the general reader.

Some food composition tables contain ancillary information as separate tables or text. In the United Kingdom and New Zealand tables, for example, standardized recipes are included, whereas the German tables provide data on protein digestibility factors (Section 4.8.8). The Chinese tables include information on the effect of cooking on vitamin losses and an appendix on nutrient-based recommendations. Specialized food composition tables have also been prepared: for example, a food composition table on the carotenoid content of foods for use specifically in developing countries is available (West and Poortvliert, 1993).

A directory of food composition tables is maintained by INFOODS at

http://www.fao.org/infoods/

The directory is updated regularly and contains information on all the major national and international databases and food tables. Most of the food composition tables are not held by the INFOODS Secretariat, and many of the older printed tables are no longer available. The food composition tables for Ethiopia, West Africa, Zambia, Malaysia, and the Netherlands, are compiled predominantly from the analyses of locally grown foods — although the number of nutrients and the number of samples analyzed for any one food are sometimes small, with only the most common foods included. In some other regions, many values for local foods in the composition tables are taken from tables of other countries, with gaps in the local analytical

data being filled by using values from other food tables, as described in Section 4.1.4.

4.3.1 U.S. and Canadian food composition tables

The most recent edition of the "Nutritive Value of Foods" (USDA, 2002) contains data on 1274 foods expressed in terms of common household units. The 19 nutrients in the table are water; energy; protein; total fat; saturated, monounsaturated, and polyunsaturated fatty acids; cholesterol; total dietary fiber; calcium; iron; potassium; sodium; vitamin A in IU and RE units; thiamin; riboflavin; niacin; and ascorbic acid. This edition was developed using data from Release 13 of the USDA National Nutrient Database for Standard Reference and is available from

http://www.nal.usda.gov/fnic/foodcomp/

The Canadian Nutrient File is the basis of a more popular printed publication entitled "Nutrient Value of Some Common Foods" (Health Canada, 2001b). This contains data on 19 nutrients in 975 foods commonly consumed by Canadians. The information is for household measures of the ready-to-eat form of each food. A version of this document is presently available online from

http://www.hc-sc.gc.ca/food-aliment/

The nutrients listed are energy in kcal and kJ, protein, carbohydrate, total dietary fiber, total fat, cholesterol, calcium, iron, zinc, sodium, potassium, vitamin A, vitamin C, vitamin B_6, folate, thiamin, riboflavin, and niacin. Values for total saturated, total monounsaturated, and total polyunsaturated fatty acids are given for some foods in an appendix to the main tables.

4.3.2 U.K. food composition tables

The 6th summary edition of McCance and Widdowson's "The Composition of Foods" (Food Standards Agency, 2002) provides comprehensive nutrient data for over 1200 of the most commonly consumed foods in the United Kingdom; it lists nutrient values per 100 g portion as consumed. This edition incorporates data from the supplements published since the 4th edition and also includes some new and previously unpublished data. There are new entries for foods, such as pasta, that have become popular in more recent years. Values for a wide range of nutrients (e.g., proximates, vitamins, inorganics, non-starch polysaccharides, and fatty acid totals) are provided. Additional tables cover phytosterols, carotenoid fractions, and, for the first time, vitamin K (phylloquinone) and AOAC fiber (Section 4.4.2).

Detailed information can also be obtained from the series of supplements to the 4th and 5th editions of McCance and Widdowson's "The Composition of Foods." Supplements dealing with specific food groups include cereals and cereal products (Holland et al., 1988); milk products and eggs (Holland et al., 1989); vegetables, herbs and spices (Holland et al., 1991a); fruits and nuts (Holland et al., 1992a); vegetable dishes (Holland et al., 1992b); fish and fish products (Holland et al., 1993); miscellaneous foods (Chan et al., 1994); meat, poultry, and game (Chan et al., 1995); and meat products and dishes (Chan et al., 1996). Supplements on immigrant foods (Tan et al., 1985) and amino acids and fatty acids (per 100 g of food) (Ministry of Agriculture, Fisheries and Food, 1998) are also available.

4.3.3 European food composition tables

Details of the printed food composition tables available for the nine European countries participating in the European Prospective Investigation into Cancer and Nutrition (EPIC) are given in Deharveng et al. (1999). They are published in the national language, but most also have an English translation. Some of the tables (e.g., Greece) are based exclusively on a selected range of nutrient values taken from the 4th edition of the U.K. food composition tables (Paul and Southgate, 1978), with Greek recipes calculated using the U.K. values. Others are based on values from raw and cooked foods, all of which (e.g., the Netherlands), or most of which (e.g., Denmark, France,

Germany, Italy, Spain) have been analyzed locally but with some values compiled from other sources.

4.4 Sources of error in food composition values

The food composition values in food composition databases or food composition tables are sometimes uneven in quality. The sources of error are considered in detail below and summarized in Box 4.2.

The errors that occur in food composition values may be random or systematic. All such errors generate additional uncertainty in calculated nutrient intakes. Rules and guidelines for the identification of foods, the definition of food components, and the description of food component data have been developed by INFOODS in an effort to eliminate some of these sources of uncertainty in food composition data, and to facilitate the international exchange of such data (Klensin et al., 1989). These guidelines have been adopted by some compilers of food composition databases (e.g., New Zealand, USDA,

---

Inadequate sampling protocols result in data for unrepresentative food samples being included in the food composition databases.

Inappropriate analytical methods used for the analysis of the nutrients for the food composition data.

Errors in the analytical methods used in the analysis of the nutrients for the food composition data.

Conversion factors for calculating energy and protein content of foods included in food composition databases are not standardized.

Inconsistencies in terminology used to express certain nutrients.

Incorrect description of individual food items and/or source of nutrient values in food composition tables.

Genetic, environmental, food preparation, or processing factors result in inconsistencies in the food composition values.

Box 4.2: Sources of error in food composition tables.

Component	INFOODS tagname	Units	Analytical method
Water	WATER	g	Oven drying
Energy	ENERC	kj	Calculated
Energy	ENERC_KAL	kcal	Calculated
Protein	PROCNT	g	Calculated from total nitrogen, except where noted; FAO/WHO conversion factors
Total fat	FAT	g	Several different methods depending on food matrix
Carbohydrate	CHOAVL	g	Available carbohydrate; sum of mono-, di-, and oligosaccharides, starch and glycogen, or enzymic digestion and colorimetry
Fiber	PSCACNS	g	Non-starch polysaccharide/fiber by Englyst method
Sugar	SUGAR	g	Sum of individual mono- and disaccharides determined by GC or HPLC
Starch	STARCH	g	Enzymic digestion and colorimetry
SFA	FASAT	g	Sum of individual saturated fatty acids determined by GC of methyl esters
MUFA	FAMS	g	Sum of individual mono-unsaturated fatty acids; GC of methyl esters.
PUFA	FAPU	g	Sum of individual poly-unsaturated fatty acids; GC of methyl esters.
Cholesterol	CHOLE	g	GC
Sodium	NA	mg	Wet ashing, ICP-AES
Potassium	K	mg	Wet ashing, ICP-AES
Calcium	CA	mg	Wet ashing, ICP-AES
Iron	FE	mg	Wet ashing, ICP-AES or dry ashing, AAS
Zinc	ZN	mg	Wet ashing, ICP-AES or dry ashing, AAS
Selenium	SE	μg	Fluorometry or wet ashing ICP-AES
Vitamin A	VITA	μg	Total vitamin A equivalents/retinol equivalents; μg retinol + 1/6 μg β-carotene equivalents determined by HPLC
Carotene	CARTBEQ	μg	β-carotene equivalents; μg β-carotene + 2 μg other provitamin A carotenoids determined by HPLC
Thiamin	THIA	mg	HPLC, fluorescence detection of thiochrome
Riboflavin	RIBF	mg	HPLC, fluorescence detection
Niacin	NIAEQ	mg	Total niacin equivalents equals mg preformed niacin (HPLC, UV detection) + 1/60 mg tryptophan (HPLC)
Vitamin B_6	VITB6	mg	HPLC, fluorescence detection
Vitamin B_{12}	VITB12	μg	Microbiological
Folate	FOL	μg	Total folate by radioassay and microbiological
Vitamin C	VITC	mg	HPLC and titration

Table 4.3: The food components, INFOODS tagname, unit of measure, and methods of analyses from the Concise New Zealand Food Composition Tables. HPLC, high pressure liquid chromatography; GC, gas chromatography; ICP-AES, inductively coupled plasma – atomic emission spectrometry; AAS, atomic absorption spectrophotometry. From Athar et al. (2003).

LATINFOODS, ASEAN-FOODS). Table 4.3 presents a summary description of the food components, their designated INFOODS tagname, unit of measure, and a brief description, including methods of analyses from the Concise New Zealand Food Composition Tables (Athar et al., 2003). In the future, quality codes may also be included for all the entries in food composition databases (Scrimshaw, 1997).

4.4.1 Inadequate sampling protocols

When nutrient values for specific foods are required for a food composition database, sampling protocols must be designed which will result in the collection of representative food samples for analysis.

The sampling protocol should take into account, where appropriate, such factors as seasonal and regional differences in the composition of the food, genetic variation, stage of ripeness, handling and storage procedures, variations resulting from the effects of fertilizer application, pest control, method of food preparation, processing, and production practices (Greenfield and Southgate, 1992). In this way, random errors resulting from true variability in the nutrient composition of individual food items can be eliminated. When standardized sampling protocols are not used, nutrient composition values may not reflect the average nutrient content of a food on a year-round, nationwide basis.

Theoretically, a statistical formula should be used to estimate the number of food samples required, in order to ensure that the analyzed value is truly representative of the food item under consideration and has an acceptable level of precision. In practice, sufficient data required to perform these statistical calculations (i.e., mean, standard deviation, and level of acceptable error for the nutrient) are rarely available. Instead, 10 samples per food type are often collected. This number is thought to be large enough to reflect the variability in composition of most foods. In some cases, where variation is thought to be small, as few as five or six samples may be sufficient.

Systematic errors may occur in some food composition data, particularly with nutrient-fortified, processed, and manufactured foods. In foods such as breakfast cereals fortified with folic acid, for example, wide variations in folic acid content occur. As a result, brand-specific nutrient composition data should be used for these food items, to prevent systematic bias.

4.4.2 Inappropriate analytical methods

The methods chosen for food composition analyses must be accurate, precise, and practical. Consideration should always be given to using methods specified by AOAC International (Horwitz, 2002) at

http://www.aoac.org/

or the Codex Alimentarius Commission (especially for the analysis of pesticide residues in foods). Unfortunately, a variety of analytical procedures have been used for assaying nutrients during the compilation of most food composition data tables. Some of these methods are very unsatisfactory, resulting in erroneous estimates of the nutrient content. Greenfield and Southgate (1992) have summarized the state of development of nutrient analytical methods in foods. Earlier methodologies for nutrients such as vitamin A, carotenoids, vitamin B_{12}, folate, and vitamin C were particularly unsatisfactory, but considerable advances have now been made.

Vitamin A activity in foods should now be analyzed by high-performance liquid chromatography (HPLC). This is the preferred method for separating and quantifying both the amount of the active forms of vitamin A and the individual provitamin A carotenoids: β-carotene, α-carotene, lutein + zeaxanthin, lycopene, and β-cryptoxanthin. Improvements in HPLC methods have led to an increase in carotenoid recovery ranging from 60% to 90% (Hart and Scott, 1995).

The older colorimetric procedures used for measuring retinol and the total carotenoid content of foods often yielded an overestimate, in part because they include some carotenoids without any vitamin A activity. With the increasing use of HPLC for analyzing retinol and the individual carotenoid content of foods, the reliability of these data will improve, provided that quality-control issues are also addressed (West, 2000).

Useful guidelines on how to evaluate the published analytical data for levels of five carotenoids in foods — β-carotene, α-carotene, lutein + zeaxanthin, lycopene, and β-cryptoxanthin — are given in Mangels et al. (1993). These investigators emphasize that data on the accuracy and precision of the published methods used for carotenoid analysis are still lacking.

Vitamin E activity in foods should also be analyzed by HPLC or by gas-liquid chromatography. These are the preferred methods for analyzing α-, β-, γ-, and δ-tocopherol, as well as their corresponding tocotrienols.

Details of the HPLC method are given in Section 18.3.1

Vitamin D occurs in foods as cholecalciferol (vitamin D_3) and ergocalciferol (vitamin D_2). Small amounts of 25-hydroxy-vitamin D are also present in some animal foods and are important because of their significant vitamin D activity; 25-hydroxy-vitamin D has five times more vitamin D activity than cholecalciferol (vitamin D_3) and ergocalciferol (vitamin D_2). All forms of vitamin D in foods should be measured using HPLC (Qian and Sheng, 1998): older colorimetric or biological assays used for vitamin D are unreliable.

Thiamin, riboflavin, and niacin in food have often been assayed in the past using microbiological techniques. The latter are based on the use of a microorganism that requires a specific B vitamin for its growth. However, they are cumbersome and time consuming, and precision is often poor. HPLC methods are increasingly used for analysis of thiamin, riboflavin, and niacin, after extraction using a variety of techniques; thiamin and riboflavin can be coextracted in a single operation (Ball, 1994). Flow-injection analysis in conjunction with the AOAC fluorimetric methods for thiamin and riboflavin and the AOAC colorimetric method for niacin may replace HPLC in the future, although the preparation of sample extracts is still time-consuming (Horwitz, 2002). Similar values for thiamin and riboflavin are said to be obtained by all three methods (Deharveng et al., 1999).

Vitamin B_6 is the sum of pyridoxal, pyridoxamine, their phosphates, and pyridoxine — all of which have the same activity. In the past, vitamin B_6 has been analyzed by a microbiological assay, but this is gradually being replaced by separation of some or all of the six vitamin B_6 vitamers by HPLC, followed by measurement using fluorescence spectroscopy (Gregory et al., 1988). Care must be taken with the extraction procedure used.

Vitamin B_{12} in foods is still often analyzed using microbiological techniques. The latter, however, are not very suitable because they respond to noncobalamin corrinoids. Furthermore, they cannot be used in processed foods containing microbial growth inhibitors. To avoid these problems, competitive inhibition radioassays can be used for the analysis of vitamin B_{12}. These methods are relatively simple, and easily standardized, and they can be precise, provided that optimized extraction conditions are used (Anderson et al., 1990). Non-isotopic microtitration plate competitive protein-binding assays have also been developed, but they can be used only to determine added cyanocobalamin in fortified foods. The method is not sensitive enough to determine naturally occurring vitamin B_{12} (Alcock et al., 1990).

Folate activity in foods is usually determined by a microbiological assay, preferably using *Lactobacillus caseii* (NCIMB 10463). The bacterium *Streptococcus faecalis* is sometimes used as well but is valid for measuring only the synthetic monoglutamate form — folic acid — which is used as a fortificant or supplement.

Most naturally occurring folates in foods are conjugates with two or more γ-glutamyl residues (often called polyglutamates). As a result, prior to quantification, a thermal extraction procedure must be used to release folate from the food matrix (Gregory et al., 1990), followed by a trienzyme (α-amylase, protease, and conjugase) digestion treatment to hydrolyze the polyglutamyl folates.

The extraction and enzyme digestion procedures used in the past to release folate from the food matrix have often been incomplete for certain foods, so their actual folate content has been underestimated (Pfeiffer et al., 1997; Tamura et al., 1997). Such underestimates have sometimes been further exacerbated by the failure to use ascorbic acid to prevent oxidation of labile folate during the analysis. Work is under way, however, to improve the extraction and the quality of folate analytical data in food composition databases, by using the trienzyme extraction method followed by

HPLC (Pfeiffer et al., 1997; Konings, 1999; Konings et al., 2001).

Vitamin C analysis in foodstuffs can be carried out using methods that measure both active forms of vitamin C (i.e., L-ascorbic acid and L-dehydroascorbic acid, or only L-ascorbic acid, the reduced form of this vitamin.

Three methods are used to measure the combined activity of both of the active forms of vitamin C (total vitamin C). These are colorimetry, fluorimetry, and HPLC, each of which gives values that are broadly comparable. In Sweden, the method used for the food composition values is titrimetry, which measures only the reduced form, L-ascorbic acid (Greenfield and Southgate, 1992). Analysis of only the reduced form of vitamin C may thus underestimate the vitamin C content of a foodstuff, especially when it is cooked or processed. In fresh foods, L-ascorbic acid dominates, but the amount of the dehydroform increases with cooking and processing.

In the future, HPLC with electrochemical detection may become the preferred method for analyzing vitamin C in foods because the method can quantify both active forms of vitamin C, and it has the added advantage of distinguishing ascorbic acid from isoascorbate. The latter is a stereoisomer of ascorbic acid used increasingly by the food industry as an antioxidant, but it possesses little, if any, vitamin C activity (Kall and Andersen, 1999). Automated enzymatic assays using ascorbate peroxidase may also be used more commonly in the future.

Dietary fiber values in food depend on both the analytical method used and the chemical components included in the measurements. Dietary fiber is a complex mixture of plant materials that are often divided into two forms, based on their water solubility: insoluble and soluble dietary fiber, as shown in Table 4.4. Insoluble dietary fiber may include celluloses, some hemicelluloses, and lignin, whereas soluble dietary fiber includes β-glucans, pectins, gums, mucilages, and some hemicelluloses. Minor components of plant structures such as waxes, cutin, and

Cellulose + insoluble noncellulosic polysaccharides	Soluble noncellulosic polysaccharides	Resistant starches and lignin
Insoluble fiber[a]	Soluble fiber	
Englyst fiber (nonstarch polysaccharides)		
Southgate fiber[b] (unavailable carbohydrate)		

Table 4.4: Relationship between the dietary fiber fractions. [a] Some methods of analysis also include lignin. [b] Fiber determined by the method of Southgate (1969) may differ from the sum of the fractions shown, because it can include starch which is not necessarily the same as the resistant starch measured by the method of Englyst et al. (1982).

suberin, as well as fructans, principally inulin, may also be included in the definition of dietary fiber in some countries.

Several analytical methods are presently used to measure total dietary fiber or fractions of dietary fiber in foods. Total dietary fiber can be measured by the following methods: AOAC 985.29/AACC 32-05 or AOAC 991.43/AACC 32-07. These methods measure lignin, non-starch polysaccharides (NSP), and some resistant starch and inulin, and give similar, but not necessarily identical, results. Values for total dietary fiber in the USDA Nutrient Database for Standard Reference (Section 4.2.1), and the food composition databases of continental Europe (Section 4.2.4) have been analyzed using these AOAC methods (Deharveng et al., 1999).

Until recently, the United Kingdom has not used these AOAC methods for the analysis of dietary fiber. Instead, they used a method developed by Englyst et al. (1982) and Englyst and Cummings (1988), because until 1999 dietary fiber in the United Kingdom was defined as non-starch polysaccharides (NSP) only. Therefore, NSP values for foods were included in older editions of McCance and Widdowson's "The Composition of Foods" and in some of the published supplements. Table 4.4 shows the relationship between the total dietary fiber fractions and NSP.

Non-starch polysaccharides (Englyst fiber) are made up of insoluble and soluble forms of dietary fiber; resistant starches and lignin are excluded, as shown in Table 4.4. Hence, NSP values are generally lower than those based on the AOAC 985.29 or AOAC 991.43 methods, as shown in Table 4.5. For some processed cereal products, the differences between dietary fiber analyzed by the AOAC 985.29 and the Englyst methods could be even greater than those noted in Table 4.5 because of the presence of variable amounts of resistant starch. Three forms of resistant starch exist: protected starch molecules, unswollen granules (e.g., potato starch), and retrograded starch. For certain foods in which resistant starch is absent and which have low lignin levels, the NSP and AOAC dietary fiber values should be similar.

Some of the published supplements to McCance and Widdowson's "The Composition of Foods" — such as cereals and cereal products (Holland et al., 1988); vegetables, herbs and spices (Holland et al., 1991a); fruit and nuts (Holland et al., 1992a); and vegetable dishes (Holland et al., 1992b) — and the 1996 German food composition database also provide data for dietary fiber fractions, including soluble (hemicelluloses) and insoluble (gums, pectins, and mucilages) noncellulosic polysaccharides, lignin, cellulose, and resistant starch, as well as NSP values. These dietary fiber fractions are often measured by gas chromatography, followed by fractionation (Theander et al., 1982).

In 1999, the U.K. Joint Safety and Standards Group recommended the adoption of AOAC 991.43 as the official U.K. method

Product	AOAC	Englyst
Apples (with skin)	2.0	1.6
Bananas	1.9	1.1
Pears	2.6	2.2
Carrots (boiled)	3.1	2.5
Tomatoes (fresh)	1.7	1.0
Almonds	11.2	7.4
White bread	2.0	1.5
Brown bread	4.5	3.5
Wholemeal bread	7.4	5.8

Table 4.5: A comparison of dietary fiber (g/100 g) found in food using the AOAC 991.43 and the Englyst methods. Source: AOAC values, Spiller (1993); Englyst NSP values, Holland et al. (1991b).

for analyzing dietary fiber. They also recommended the measurement of fructans using a further method (AOAC 997.08) because fructans are also accepted as a component of dietary fiber. Hence, the method of analysis for dietary fiber used in the United Kingdom since 1999 is consistent with that used by the United States and by continental Europe (IFST, 2001). Indeed, McCance and Widdowson's "The Composition of Foods" 6th summary edition (Food Standards Agency, 2002) contains dietary fiber values analyzed by AOAC 991.43.

The U.S. definition of dietary fiber is now based on health benefits and key physiological considerations. In keeping with this new definition, dietary fiber is now recognized as a nutrient in the United States. Dietary fiber is defined as

> the edible parts of plants or analogous carbohydrates that are resistant to digestion and absorption in the human small intestine with complete or partial fermentation in the large intestine (AACC, 2001).

As such, dietary fiber includes polysaccharides, oligosaccharides, lignin, and associated plant substances.

A similar draft standard code for dietary fiber has now been adopted by the joint Food Standards Australia New Zealand (FSANZ) (Standard 1.2.8 (18)) and the U.K. Food Standards Agency (IFST, 2001). The Scandinavian countries — Denmark, Norway, and Finland — have also adopted both this definition of dietary fiber and the AOAC 985.29 and, for inulin, the AOAC 997.08 methods of analysis. However, none of the AOAC methods currently available quantifies all the unique components of dietary fiber included in the current definition (de Vries et al.,1999). Modifications to existing analytical methods are needed to ensure that, in the future, all the components that make up dietary fiber are included.

At present, food composition values for total dietary fiber are incomplete in many food composition databases. Release 16 of the USDA Nutrient Database for Standard

Reference (USDA, 2003b), for example, contains dietary fiber data for at least 80% of the foodstuffs listed. Values for some components of dietary fiber, notably the NSP fractions and lignin, are included in several of the earlier supplements to the U.K. McCance and Widdowson's "Composition of Foods," as noted earlier. Conversion of NSP fractions to total dietary fiber (TDF) values assayed using AOAC-type methods may be possible within a limited range of total dietary fiber values using a regression equation of Mongeau and Brassard (1989):

$$(TDF + 0.02) / 1.28 = NSP$$

In some older food composition tables, values for "crude fiber" measured by the classical Weende procedure are given. This fraction consists primarily of cellulose and lignin and, hence, underestimates the total dietary fiber value. No acceptable method exists for deriving total dietary fiber values from crude fiber, and the crude fiber value should not be used.

From this discussion, it is apparent that several methods exist for obtaining values for dietary fiber, some of which are incompatible, making it very difficult to make comparisons of dietary fiber intakes between — and sometimes within — countries. Therefore, details of the analytical methods used for dietary fiber must always be included when the food composition data are compiled. In this way, the user can be alerted to any potential problems and biases in the published values. The position should ease with the adoption in the United Kingdom of the same definition and analytical method for dietary fiber as is presently used in the United States and continental Europe (IFST, 2001).

4.4.3 Analytical errors

Standardized protocols must be established for the collection, handling, and storage of the food samples prior to analyses in order to avoid adventitious sources of contamination, changes in moisture during transport and storage, and losses due to oxidation; these have been discussed in Section 4.4.1. During analyses of the nutrient content of any food, further errors may occur, leading to more inaccuracies in the food composition databases (Hollman and Katan, 1988). Several rating criteria for the handling and collection of food samples, as well as the methods and quality control of the analyses, are available (Schubert et al., 1987; Lurie et al., 1989; Mangels et al., 1993). The reader is advised to consult these sources for more specific details.

Sampling errors during analysis can be minimized by analyzing homogeneous and finely ground samples. Nevertheless, sampling errors may exceed the errors that occur during the subsequent analysis. Freeze drying followed by crushing is commonly used for sample homogenization, although other techniques should be used when analyzing fatty acids and certain vitamins because freeze drying modifies these nutrients. As a check on the homogeneity of the ground sample, replicate aliquots should always be analyzed with each sample batch and the coefficient of variation for each nutrient calculated (Yuk et al. 1975) (Table 4.6).

It is important to maximize the precision of the analytical methods to allow the users of food composition data to better assess the actual variability of the nutrient in the food. To determine precision, aliquots from a homogeneous pooled sample should be repeatedly analyzed with each batch, and again the coefficient of variation of the analytical method estimated.

It is also important to control the accuracy of the analytical method (see Section 15.3).

	Mean	SE	CV
Water (g)	735	0.420	0.18
Nitrogen (g)	2.89	0.0175	1.18
Fat (g)	68.2	0.259	1.20
Iron (mg)	7.6	0.201	8.36
Energy (kJ)	5590	95.3	0.54

Table 4.6: Mean values with their standard errors (SE) and coefficients of variation (CV) for energy and selected nutrients in 10 replicate analyses of one sample of mashed potato. From Yuk et al., British Journal of Nutrition 34: 391–397, 1975.

This can be achieved by including an aliquot of a reference material, of a similar matrix to the sample and certified for the nutrient of interest, with each batch of analyses. Reference materials for method validation and quality assurance can be obtained from the National Institute of Standards and Technology (NIST), the Institute of Reference Materials and Measurement, Geel, Belgium, and Analytical Quality Control Services, Vienna. An analytical reference material with analytical values for total, insoluble, and soluble dietary fiber (Caldwell and Nelsen, 1999) can be obtained from the American Association of Cereal Chemists. Contact addresses for these agencies are given in Appendix 4.1. Food composition data should always include details on the accuracy and precision of the analytical methods used for each nutrient.

Specificity and detectability are two additional and important aspects of analytical methods that may generate errors and thus influence the quality of food composition values. Both aspects should be considered in terms of the potential uses of the food composition data. Specificity of a method refers to its ability to measure only the dietary component of interest (see Section 15.3). Examples of the impact of poor specificity on the reliability of food composition values are given in Section 4.4.2. Detectability, or limit of detection, refers to how little of the dietary component need be present before it can be measured (Section 15.4.3).

A Micronutrient Quality Assurance Program is administered by NIST with the primary goal of helping participants gain insight into the performance of their own laboratories and into the comparability of their analytical results (Duewer et al., 1999). Contact details are given in Appendix 4.1. Section 15.3 provides a more detailed discussion of factors affecting the reliability of analytical methods.

4.4.4 Uncertainties associated with energy and protein values

Despite a recommendation by INFOODS to standardize units of expression for all nutrients to facilitate the international exchange of food composition data, this has not yet been accomplished. The modes of expression differ, particularly for the two components (energy and protein) derived from other analytic measurements. Full details of the assumptions for these calculations are given in Greenfield and Southgate (1992).

Energy values in food composition tables are generally calculated indirectly from the amounts of protein, fat, carbohydrate, and alcohol in the foods, using various energy conversion factors. This approach is followed because the standard method for measuring the energy content of a food (i.e., bomb calorimetry) does not reflect the energy actually available to the body. The energy conversion factors used are all corrected to take into account the losses of energy occurring in digestion and absorption and through incomplete oxidation. Consequently, the calculated energy values represent the available, or *metabolizable*, energy content of foods.

There are no standard conversion factors for calculating the energy content of foods, leading to variations in the documented energy content of similar foods. Many countries use standard conversion factors for calculating the energy value of food items. These factors are 17 kJ/g (4 kcal/g) for protein, 37 kJ/g (9 kcal/g) for fat, 17 kJ/g (4 kcal/g) for total carbohydrate, and 29 kJ/g (7 kcal/g) for alcohol. Other areas (e.g., the United States and East Asia) use specific energy conversion factors for individual foods and food groups. These factors are based on the heat of combustion for the fat, protein, and carbohydrate in specific foods from Atwater and Bryant (1899), multiplied by the coefficient of apparent digestibility (Merrill and Watt, 1973). These specific conversion factors were recommended by FAO/WHO (1973), and a representative sample of such factors for some specific foods is shown in Table 4.7.

In the U.K. food composition tables (Food Standards Agency, 2002), the conversion factor used for available carbohydrate is 16 kJ/g (3.75 kcal/g). The latter was adopted because the free sugars (glucose, fructose, sucrose, lactose, maltose, and higher maltose homo-

Food or food group	Protein	Fat	Carbo-hydrate
Eggs, meat, milk			
Eggs	4.36	9.02	3.68
Meat	4.27	9.02	3.87
Milk and milk products	4.27	8.79	3.87
Fruits			
All (except some citrus)	3.36	8.37	3.60
Lemons and limes	3.36	8.37	2.48
Grain products			
Cornmeal (whole-ground)	2.73	8.37	4.03
Macaroni, spaghetti	3.91	8.37	4.12
Rice, white or polished	3.82	8.37	4.16
Wheat, 97%–100% extrct.	3.59	8.37	3.78
Wheat, 70%–74% extrct.	4.05	8.37	4.12
Legumes, nuts, sugars			
Peas, lima beans, cowpeas	3.47	8.37	4.07
Nuts	3.47	8.37	4.07
Cane or beet sugar	–	–	3.87
Vegetables			
Mushrooms	2.62	8.37	3.48
Potatoes and starchy roots	2.78	8.37	4.03
Most other vegetables	2.44	8.37	3.57

Table 4.7: Specific factors (kcal/g) for calculating energy values of foods or food groups. Data from Merrill and Watts (1973), Energy value of foods: basis and derivation. USDA, Agriculture Handbook No. 74, Washington, DC.

logues), dextrins, starch, and glycogen are all determined separately, by chemical analysis. Their sum represents the carbohydrate content of the food, expressed as grams of available monosaccharides. The Atwater and Bryant factors are used for protein (17 kJ/g), fat (37 kJ/g), and alcohol (27 kJ/g). Several other countries also use the factor of 16 kJ/g (3.75 kcal/g) for available carbohydrate; examples include France, Germany, and the Netherlands. These latter countries (and New Zealand) also apply specific conversion factors for the energy contribution of polyols and organic acids, but because most foods contain only very small amounts, their inclusion or exclusion does not have a major effect on the energy value (Deharveng et al. 1999).

Table 4.8 compares the energy content of

selected food items calculated using two of the methods described above. As can be seen, differences for the energy values are most marked for fruits and vegetables because in these foods much of the energy is provided by carbohydrate. An added source of confusion with the energy content of foods is that they can be expressed in kilocalories (kcal) or kilojoules (kJ).

Protein values of foods are conventionally calculated from the total nitrogen content measured using Kjeldahl-type methods. A conversion factor is then applied. In some countries, the factor of 6.25 is used indiscriminately to convert total nitrogen into protein, based on the assumption that all proteins, regardless of their source, contain 16% nitrogen. Most countries, however, apply specific nitrogen conversion factors recommended by the FAO/WHO Committee on Energy and Protein Requirements (FAO/WHO, 1973). These factors are dependent on the

Food type	(A)	(B)
Beef	273	268
Salmon, canned	143	138
Eggs	162	158
Milk	68	69
Butter	716	733
Cornmeal, degermed	363	356
Oatmeal	390	396
Rice, brown	360	356
Wheat flour, patent	364	355
Beans, snap	35	42
Peas, dry seeds	339	349
Cabbage	24	29
Carrots	42	45
Potatoes	83	85
Turnips	32	35
Apples, raw	58	64
Lemons, raw	32	44
Peaches, canned	68	75
Sugar, cane or beet	385	398

Table 4.8: A comparison of the energy values (kcal/100 g) of the edible portion of selected foods calculated using specific factors for different classes of food (Column A) and general energy conversion factors (protein × 4, fat × 9, and carbohydrate × 4) (Column B). From Périssé (1982) with permission.

Food	Factor (per g N)
Cereals	
Wheat	
Wholemeal wheat products	5.83
Other wheat products	5.70
Bran	6.31
Rice	5.95
Barley, oats, rye	5.83
Nuts	
Peanuts, Brazil nuts	5.41
Almonds	5.18
All other nuts	5.30
Milk and milk products	6.38
Gelatin	5.55
All other foods	6.25

Table 4.9: Specific factors for converting nitrogen in foods to protein. From FAO/WHO (1973).

food or food group and are derived from the data of Jones (1941). Table 4.9 presents some of these specific nitrogen conversion factors. Note that the Netherlands applies 6.38 for milk and milk products but 6.25 for all other foods in their food composition database, so the Dutch protein values for cereals, cereal products, and nuts should be higher.

Food composition tables of some countries (e.g., Ethiopia) use a conversion factor based on the amino-acid composition of the food to calculate the protein content (Ågren and Gibson, 1963). For some foods known to contain a large amount of nonprotein nitrogen in the form of urea, purine, or pyrimidine derivatives (e.g., mushrooms, beverages, cartilaginous fish, and mollusks), corrections are applied to the total nitrogen content before the protein content is calculated.

4.4.5 Inconsistencies in terminology

Confusion may arise because of inconsistencies in the terminology for nutrients such as carbohydrate, dietary fiber, vitamin A, provitamin A carotenoids, vitamin C, vitamin D, vitamin E, niacin, and folate in food composition table data. Such inconsistencies arise in part because most of these nutrients have

multiple forms, each differing in their biological activity. INFOODS provides definitions for each food component (Klensin et al., 1989).

Carbohydrate in food composition tables and databases is treated inconsistently, as noted earlier. In some, the total carbohydrate content in foods (g/100 g) is derived by difference using the following formula:

$$\text{carbohydrate (g/100 g)} =$$
$$100 - (\text{water} + \text{protein} + \text{fat} + \text{ash})\,(\text{g/100 g})$$

When this formula is used, unavailable complex carbohydrates and any noncarbohydrate residue, as well as available sugar, dextrins, and starch, are included in the total carbohydrate. Examples of food composition tables and databases that use this formula include the USDA Nutrient Data Base for Standard Reference, Ethiopia, Egypt, India, Denmark, and the Netherlands (Klensin et al., 1989). In some countries, dietary fiber is then deducted from the total carbohydrate calculated by difference (e.g., Sweden).

Elsewhere, such as the United Kingdom (Food Standards Agency, 2002), the components of available carbohydrate are analyzed separately and expressed as the sum of the free sugars, dextrins, starch, and glycogen, as noted earlier. This is the preferred approach.

Vitamin A values in nutrient databases may represent some or all of the total vitamin A activity in a foodstuff. Total vitamin A activity should include both retinol (often termed preformed vitamin A) and the carotenoids demonstrated to exhibit vitamin A activity (termed provitamin A carotenoids). Of the latter, β-carotene is the most important. The other carotenoids with significant vitamin A activity are α-carotene and α- and β-cryptoxanthins.

Unfortunately, total vitamin A activity is sometimes calculated on the basis of the contributions of only retinol and β-carotene. Most food composition tables in continental Europe, Scandinavia, and Australasia provide only limited information on the type and proportions of other provitamin A carotenoid isomers in individual foods. The U.K. food composition tables provide some data on individual carotenoids for certain food items (Food Standards Agency, 2002), whereas the USDA Nutrient Database for Standard Reference (Release 16) (USDA, 2003) includes β-carotene, α-carotene, β-cryptoxanthin, lycopene, and lutein + zeaxanthin.

Some specialized databases have been developed with detailed information on individual carotenoids in foods. West and Poortvliet (1993) have compiled a table on the carotenoid content of foods in developing countries. Values for α- and β-carotene, α- and β-cryptoxanthin, lutein, lycopene, and zeaxanthin are included. Comparable carotenoid databases exist for carotenoid-rich fruits and vegetables commonly consumed in five European countries (United Kingdom, Republic of Ireland, Spain, France, and the Netherlands) (O'Neill et al., 2001), as well as the United States (Holden et al., 1999).

The activity of vitamin A in more recent food composition tables is expressed in terms of μg retinol equivalents (RE), using the FAO/WHO interrelationships of retinol, β-carotene, and other provitamin A carotenoids, shown in Table 4.10. Recently, the correctness of the FAO/ WHO factors for the bioconversion of ingested provitamin A carotenoids to retinol has been questioned (Castenmiller and West, 1998; IOM, 2001). The U.S. Food and Nutrition Board (IOM, 2001) and the International Vitamin A Consultative Group (IVACG, 2002) now recommend new conversion factors, and these are shown

in Table 4.10 together with the FAO/WHO factors for comparison. The latter are still recommended for use by FAO/WHO (2002), until additional definitive data are available.

The amount of vitamin A activity derived from provitamin A carotenoids using the new U.S. conversion factors is half of that derived using the FAO/WHO (2002) factors. A detailed justification of these new bioconversion factors is given in IOM (2001). Note also that the U.S. has adopted the term retinol activity equivalents (RAE) rather than retinol equivalents for use when calculating the total amount of vitamin A in mixed dishes or diets, as shown in Table 4.10. If the IOM (2001) conversion factors are adopted, the vitamin A activity in a foodstuff, expressed as a retinol activity equivalency, can be calculated from the following equation:

$$\text{RAE (μg)} = \text{retinol (μg)} + (\text{β-carotene (μg)}/12.0)$$
$$+ (\text{other provitamin A carotenoids (μg)}/24.0)$$

Such inconsistencies in the values for the absorption and bioconversion of ingested provitamin A carotenoid to retinol further exacerbate existing problems when comparing vitamin A values among food composition databases and, in turn, vitamin A intakes across countries. To overcome this problem, database compilers should strive to include the content (as μg/100 g edible portion) of the individual carotenoids in foods — β-carotene, α-carotene, lutein + zeaxanthin, lycopene, and β-cryptoxanthin — so that improved estimates of intake of carotenoids can be made. Table 4.11 presents a comparison of the intakes (mg/d) of five carotenoids in adults in five European countries, calculated from a food frequency questionnaire and a European carotenoid database. The results emphasize that there are real differences in the intakes of specific carotenoids within Europe — differences that appear to be related to the consumption of different foods among the countries surveyed, and not to national differences in the food composition database used (O'Neill et al., 2001).

Some food composition databases continue to express vitamin A in terms of international units (IU). Use of these older units is

---

FAO/WHO (2002)

1 μg retinol equivalent (RE)
     = 1 μg of all-*trans*-retinol
     = 6 μg of all-*trans*-β-carotene
     = 12 μg other provitamin A carotenoids

IOM (2001), IVACG (2002)

1 μg retinol activity equivalent (RAE)
     = 1 μg of all-*trans*-retinol
     = 12 μg of all-*trans*-β-carotene
     = 24 μg other provitamin A carotenoids

Table 4.10: Interconversion of vitamin A and carotenoid units.

	β-carotene	Lutein + zeaxanthin	Lycopene	α-carotene	β-crypto-xanthin	Total carotenoids
Spain ($n = 70$)	2.96	3.25	1.64	0.29	1.36	9.54
France ($n = 76$)	5.84	2.50	4.75	0.74	0.45	16.06
U.K. ($n = 71$)	5.55	1.59	5.01	1.04	0.99	14.38
Republic of Ireland ($n = 76$)	5.16	1.56	4.43	1.23	0.78	14.53
The Netherlands ($n = 75$)	4.35	2.01	4.86	0.68	0.97	13.71

Table 4.11: Median carotenoid intake (mg/d) in adults in five European countries. Data from O'Neill et al., British Journal of Nutrition 85: 499–507, 2001, with permission of the authors.

no longer appropriate for assessing dietary adequacy of vitamin A and should be discontinued (FAO/WHO, 2002).

Vitamin C activity should be defined as the sum of L-ascorbic acid (reduced form) and the L-dehydroascorbic acid content of a food, as both forms are biologically active (Section 4.4.2). Unfortunately, some older food composition tables do not provide a definition of vitamin C activity. Swedish food composition tables provide data only for the reduced form of vitamin C, as noted earlier. To avoid confusion, these details should be checked before using any vitamin C food composition values.

Vitamin D is normally determined by measuring the sum of cholecalciferol (vitamin D_3) and ergocalciferol (vitamin D_2). Of these, vitamin D_2 occurs naturally in fungi, including yeast, but vitamin D_3 occurs only in animal products. Foods can be fortified with cholecalciferol or with synthetic ergocalciferol; both have the same vitamin D activity. Both components of vitamin D should be analyzed in fortified foods, and the total should be included in the food composition table.

In some of the earlier supplements to Mc-Cance and Widdowson's "The Composition of Foods," the values for the vitamin D activity include the sum of ergocalciferol and cholecalciferol, plus the activity arising from the small amounts of 25-hydroxy-vitamin D present in some animal foods. The activity of 25-hydroxy-vitamin D is five times greater than that of cholecalciferol (vitamin D_3) and ergocalciferol (vitamin D_2), as noted earlier (Deharveng et al., 1999).

In some older food composition data, vitamin D is expressed in terms of international units (IU). These units are no longer appropriate and should not be used.

Vitamin E activity in older food composition data is expressed in terms of international units (IU). These units are no longer appropriate and should not be used. Recent food composition databases express vitamin E activity in foods as α-tocopherol equivalents (α-TEs) where 1 α-TE is the activity of 1 mg of RRR-α-tocopherol. α-TEs include vitamin E activity from α-, β-, γ-, and δ-tocopherols and the corresponding tocotrienols, after correcting for their biological activity relative to RRR-α-tocopherol. The conversion factors used vary. In the U.K. food composition tables (Food Standards Agency, 2002), α-TEs are defined as the sum of α-tocopherol (mg × 1.0), β-tocopherol (mg × 0.4), γ tocopherol (mg × 0.1), δ-tocopherol (mg × 0.01) and α-tocotrienol (mg × 0.3), β-tocotrienol (mg × 0.05), and γ-tocotrienol (mg × 0.01) (McClaughlin and Weihrauch, 1979). These conversion factors were also used in the earlier USDA food composition database.

Some food composition databases include data for the α-tocopherol fraction only, but others (e.g., U.K. food composition tables) provide a listing of single tocopherol fractions (α-, β-, γ-, and δ-tocopherol) with some data for tocotrienols for some selected food items. The USDA Nutrient Database for Standard Reference (Release 16) (USDA, 2003) includes an expanded listing of values for α-tocopherol for all foods in the database as well as other tocopherols for some foods. Tocopherols were determined by gas-liquid chromatography (GLC) or HPLC. The USDA Release 16, however, no longer includes vitamin E reported as α-TEs. Details of how to calculate the number of milligrams of α-tocopherol in vitamin E supplements are given by IOM (2000b).

Niacin activity in foods is best expressed in terms of milligrams of niacin equivalents that include the contribution of niacin from tryptophan, as well as preformed niacin. Niacin equivalents (mg) are calculated as:

$$niacin (mg) + (tryptophan (mg)/60.0)$$

If the tryptophan intake is not known, it can be estimated by assuming that animal and vegetable proteins contain 1.4% and 1% tryptophan respectively. The most recent U.K. food composition data includes information on both preformed niacin and the potential contribution of tryptophan to the niacin content, calculated using the conversion factor shown above (Holland et al., 1991b). Large variation has been observed in the efficiency of conversion of tryptophan to niacin. When the tryptophan intake is low, less of the available tryptophan appears to be converted to niacin (Horwitt et al., 1981). In some food composition data, niacin is quoted simply as milligrams of preformed niacin (Watt et al., 1963).

Folate in foods may now include naturally occurring polyglutamates plus the synthetic monoglutamate form — folic acid — as a fortificant. Many food composition databases use the term "folic acid" as a synonym for folates and define it as the sum of the "free" and conjugated (or "bound") forms. In some databases, total folate is measured by microbiological assay, whereas in others separate values for the free and bound forms are given. In such cases, the free folate values are based on analysis before deconjugation and include the various mono-, di-, and triglutamates with a comparatively high biological activity. The bound values are derived indirectly, by calculating the difference between the amounts of total folic acid (measured after decon-

jugation) and of free folic acid. In some earlier food composition data, only values for free folate are presented; conjugated folates are excluded. Hence, free-folate values will underestimate the total folate activity in the foods (Tan et al., 1984).

In the future, in recognition of the lower bioavailability of naturally occurring dietary folates compared to synthetic folate, folate values in food composition tables will be expressed as dietary folate equivalents (see Section 4.8.8). Differentiating between the polyglutamates (naturally occurring forms in foods) and the monoglutamate form (synthetic folic acid in supplements or as a fortificant) is important because the former are often (Sauberlich et al., 1987), but not always (Brouwer et al., 1999), about half as bioavailable as the monoglutamate form (Cuskelly et al., 1996).

There is obviously an urgent need to harmonize the terminology used for carbohydrate, vitamin A, vitamin C, vitamin D, vitamin E, niacin, and folate. All published food composition databases and tables should include definitions of the terminology used and the conversion factors, where appropriate, as specified by Klensin et al. (1989).

4.4.6 Incorrect description of individual foods

Until recently, a standardized system for identifying foods, defining food components, and describing the food component data was not available. Consequently, descriptions of the foods and food components in the food composition databases have often been inadequate, making it difficult for the compiler and the user to match the food consumed with the appropriate item in the food composition database. Such difficulties can produce biases in the calculated nutrient composition of the consumed foods.

Efforts are being made by INFOODS to produce a standardized system of nomenclature and coding which will facilitate the interchange of food composition data among database compilers across countries and cultures. Details are given in Truswell et al. (1991). Food descriptions should include both the common name of the food, with local synonyms, and the scientific taxonomic name and the variety, if known. As well, details of the place and time of collection, growing conditions, number of samples collected, and preservation method (if relevant) should be recorded. Currently, two food coding systems have been developed: the Eurocode2 Food Coding System (Poortvliet et al., 1992) and the food description thesaurus Langual (Pennington and Butrum, 1991). Detailed information on these two systems can be found at

> http://www.ianunwin.demon.co.uk/eurocode/
> and   http://www.langual.org/

Development of guidelines for the definition of food components, a complete description of each food component, and their relevant methods of analysis are also essential. Such guidelines have been developed by INFOODS and are described in detail by Klensin et al. (1989). Also included in these guidelines with each food component are comments about any data manipulation arising from the use of conversion factors, or from imputing missing values, as well as a listing of selected food composition tables in which data on the specific component can be located.

4.4.7 Genetic, environmental, preparation, and processing factors

Even if all the sources of error in food composition data discussed earlier are eliminated, discrepancies in nutrient composition values for similar food items will still occur among different sets of food composition data. These variations may arise from environmental and varietal factors, or from differences in methods of preparation and processing of the food.

In some areas such as New Zealand, Finland, and certain parts of the United States, the selenium content of foods is lower than elsewhere as a result of the low selenium levels in the soil. The iodine and zinc content of foods is also very variable across countries

because of differences in the content and availability of iodine and zinc in the soil, as well as in the types and amounts of fertilizers used (Sunanda et al., 1995). In contrast, the level of carotenoids in foods is influenced by varietal differences, variable growth and harvesting, and different postharvest handling and processing methods (Mercadante and Rodriguez-Amaya, 1991).

Differences across countries may also arise from variations in the fortification or enrichment of selected foods with specific nutrients. Food-fortification programs have now been implemented in several low-income countries (Darnton-Hill and Nalubola, 2002), as well as in more affluent countries. In the United Kingdom, for example, white flour is enriched with thiamin, niacin, iron, and calcium, whereas in the United States and most of Canada it is enriched with thiamin, riboflavin, niacin, and iron.

The content of certain water-soluble and heat-labile nutrients in foods may change during food preparation and processing. For example, the content of vitamin C and thiamin in many foods varies with the cooking time and temperature used, the amount of water added, the pH in which food is prepared, and the holding time before serving (Tucker et al., 1946; Eheart and Gott, 1965). Substantial losses of folate, mainly from leaching from the food into the cooking water rather than from chemical degradation, also occur during cooking (Table 4.12) and thermal processing of certain foods; folate retention is greater

Food	Method (min)	Raw (μg/100 g)	Cooked (μg/100 g)
Spinach	Boiled (3.5)	192	94
Spinach	Steamed (3.0)	190	219
Broccoli	Boiled (10.0)	177	77
Broccoli	Steamed (10.0)	172	156
Potato	Boiled (60.0)	125	103
Beef	Grilled (11.0)	54	51

Table 4.12: Mean folate concentrations in some major folate food sources before and after typical cooking procedures. The losses are significant for boiled spinach and broccoli ($p < 0.005$, paired t-test). Data from McKillop et al., British Journal of Nutrition 88: 681–688, 2002, with permission of the authors.

with steaming rather than boiling. As well, the inherent variability of the folate content of foods also appears large.

Nutrient losses during cooking may result in large discrepancies between the actual thiamin, vitamin C, and folate content when compared with the calculated values, especially when food composition data of raw ingredients are used to compute nutrient values for cooked dishes. Data on nutrient retention during food preparation are limited, making it difficult to accurately estimate the nutrient values of a cooked composite dish (Hoover and Pelican, 1984), as noted in Section 4.1.5.

The variations in nutrient composition values arising from the factors discussed above emphasize the importance of using nutrient composition values appropriate for the country in which the food is prepared and consumed. The foods should be adequately described (Section 4.4.6) and the food components ranked by quality codes that take into account the analytical method used, sample handling, and quality control. To assess the reliability of food composition values in preexisting food composition databases, readers are advised to consult the evaluation systems devised by several authors (Holden et al., 1987; Schubert et al., 1987; Lurie et al., 1989; Mangels et al., 1993).

4.5 International Network of Food Data Systems

In an effort to eliminate some of the potential sources of error and bias in food composition data, an International Network of Food Data Systems (INFOODS) was established in 1984. This organization created a series of task forces to develop:

- Standards and guidelines for the collection of food composition data
- Standardized terminology and nomenclature so that food composition data can be understood and exchanged internationally
- Standards for data interchange
- An international directory of existing databases

- A detailed description of the needs of database users

INFOODS also created regional organizations, each of which maintains a regional database and works closely with others involved in compiling similar databases elsewhere in the world. The activities of the regional organizations also include the development of guidelines for food-sampling and analytical methods, preparation of reference materials for laboratory proficiency tests, and training support for use of appropriate software for the regional databases.

INFOODS operates a variety of electronic information and communication activities via the Internet at

http://www.fao.org/infoods/

These include the FOOD-COMP discussion list, the FOOD-TAG discussion list, and an information server. The FOOD-COMP list covers a range of topics from sampling, sample preparation, and methodological details to naming conventions and data presentation formats and expressions. Subscribers to the FOOD-TAG list are responsible for assigning food code identifiers — tagnames — according to an established formula.

4.6 Verifying nutrient values in a food composition database

After updating a food composition database using the methods outlined in Section 4.1, it is important to carry out quality-control procedures to verify that values are within expected ranges, and to check the food composition database for internal consistency. Three levels of validity checks can be recognized:

- Level 1. Between or across nutrients, but within foods
- Level 2. Between or across foods and within nutrients
- Level 3. Checks of the whole database.

An example of a check at level 1 is ensuring that the sum of the carbohydrate components (starch, sugars, fiber) does not exceed total carbohydrates. Similar checks include calculating the energy content of each food from the protein, fat, and carbohydrate values and the Atwater conversion factors, and comparing these values with the recorded energy value; comparing the sum of fatty acids with the total fat; and comparing the sum of the individual amino acids with total protein. Discrepancies between the values calculated from the algorithms and the recorded database values that fall outside acceptable ranges should be examined. Further details are provided by Buzzard et al. (1995).

Level 2 checks between or across foods can be used to verify that similar foods have comparable nutrient levels (e.g., calcium content of various milks). This task can be automated by setting edit limits which define the usual minimum and maximum nutrient values per 100 g of food within a food group. Values that fall outside the limits are flagged and subsequently investigated for possible errors.

Finally, level 3 checks of the whole database should be made. Computer programs can be used to compare all the nutrient values of the updated test nutrient database with corresponding values in the reference standard. Large discrepancies can be flagged. A diagnostic model developed by Hoover and Perloff (1981) can also be used, whereby the energy and nutrient contents of specific meals are calculated using the updated database and the results compared to known values. Results using European food composition tables have yielded discrepancies of 10% for energy and 7%–17% for macronutrients when this approach has been used (Arab, 1985), emphasizing the necessity for using a standardized model to check the quality of databases. The diagnostic model of Hoover and Perloff (1981) includes computing tasks to validate recipe calculation procedures, by calculating the nutrient content of a standard recipe.

4.7 Analysis of foods or diets

Direct chemical analysis of representative samples of the same foods is the best method for validating food composition data obtained from tables or nutrient data banks (Gibson and Scythes, 1982). Care must be taken to exclude adventitious contamination during the collection, preparation, and analysis of food samples, especially if trace elements are to be determined. Adequate storage and preliminary treatment of the sample are also essential to preserve the activity of certain vitamins (e.g., folic acid, thiamin, vitamin C, and riboflavin) (Cooke, 1983).

The individual food items must also be homogeneous, so that a representative aliquot can be removed for chemical analysis. Homogeneity can be checked by analyzing multiple aliquots of a single food, as outlined in Section 4.4.3.

Direct chemical analysis of food samples is often used for checking the reliability of the calculation procedures for mixed dishes (Section 4.1.5). It was used by the USDA Human Nutrition Information Service for their recipe calculations, and by Murphy et al. (1991) to check the composition of mixed dishes calculated using their Kenyan nutrient database (Table 4.13). Note that for the proximate nutrients shown in Table 4.13, differences between calculated and analyzed values were generally small. For vitamins and trace minerals, differences may be much larger.

Validation of the whole database is sometimes accomplished by analyzing the nutrient content of 1-d diets and comparing the results with calculated values generated using the test nutrient database. Three methods are used for collecting meals or 1-d diet composites for nutrient analysis: duplicate portions, aliquot sampling, and equivalent food composites. These methods are described below.

Duplicate portion collection involves each respondent retaining a second identical portion of all foods and beverages consumed during a 24-h period. These are preferably weighed, or sometimes estimated in household portions, by the respondent or a fieldworker. In some cases, multiple daily diet composites from each respondent may be combined into one single composite covering a multiday survey period, but this approach

Principles of Nutritional Assessment

Dish	Analyzed values			Calculated values		
	Protein	Fat	CHO	Protein	Fat	CHO
Githeri – plain (maize, beans)	6.3	1.4	31.1	5.1	1.6	29.6
Githeri – with fat and onions	4.2	1.8	24.2	4.5	1.9	25.9
Githeri – with fat and vegetables	4.5	1.9	25.9	4.3	1.8	24.3
Giwero – plain (banana, potato)	0.7	0.1	13.6	1.2	0.1	17.5
Giwero – with fat	1.0	1.7	15.8	1.2	1.4	17.1
Giwero – with fat and beans	5.0	0.6	21.2	3.0	1.1	20.5
Porridge – maize flour, water, sugar, and milk	1.1	0.4	9.2	1.1	0.7	8.9
Ugali – plain (maize flour, water)	2.1	1.3	26.2	3.3	1.7	27.6
Ugali – with beans	3.4	1.0	25.5	5.2	1.6	30.3
Ugali – with vegetables	2.3	1.2	23.3	3.3	1.3	22.3
Ugali – with beans and vegetables	3.6	1.2	24.8	4.3	1.1	25.0

Table 4.13: Analyzed and median calculated nutrient values (g/100 g) for selected Kenyan mixed dishes. The analyzed values are for a single representative sample. The calculated nutrient values are derived from nutrient values for each ingredient of the prepared dish. At least 12 examples of each dish were prepared. Data from Murphy et al., Development of research nutrient data bases: an example using foods consumed in rural Kenya. Journal of Food Composition and Analysis 4: 2–17, 1991 © with permission from Elsevier.

does not provide any data on within-subject variation in nutrient intakes (Section 6.2.3) and is not recommended. Each diet composite is then homogenized and later chemically analyzed. A comparison can then be made between analyzed values and those derived from calculations using the nutrient database.

Aliquot sampling of foods involves weighing all the foods and beverages consumed by an individual during the survey period and collecting aliquots of each food consumed, rather than the entire portion. These aliquot samples are then combined and subsequently analyzed. Care must be taken to ensure that the aliquots collected, pooled, and homogenized provide a representative sample of the total diet over the survey period.

Equivalent food composites are used less frequently than the two methods described above. In this method, weights of all foods and beverages consumed by an individual during the survey period are again recorded over a 24-h period. Subsequently, samples of raw foods, equivalent to the amount consumed by each individual are homogenized and chemically analyzed. Thus only the nutrient content of the uncooked food is determined in this method, so it is not suitable

for estimating or validating the intake of heat-labile and/or water-soluble vitamins.

Several investigators have compared energy and nutrient intakes based on direct chemical analysis of composite diets with those calculated from nutrient databases. Results suggest that for the macronutrients (e.g., protein, carbohydrate), differences between the two methods can be within 10%, especially when the nutrient intake represents a relatively long time period (e.g., 4 wks) (Bingham and Cummings, 1985). In contrast, nutrients such as fat, iron, sodium, potassium, vitamin C, and vitamin A often show poor agreement, the differences sometimes amounting to 20% or more. Some of the differences arise from the sources of variation and bias in the nutrient composition data discussed in Section 4.4. Other more specific sources of uncertainty, mainly arising during the food preparation stage, are summarized in Box 4.3. In view of these uncertainties, perfect agreement between analyzed and calculated intakes should not be expected.

It is clear that the collection of duplicate food items or composite diets followed by their direct chemical analyses is not necessarily the most accurate method available for characterizing the usual nutrient intake of in-

> **The fat content** of meat and made-up dishes varies.
> **The water content** of the analyzed and calculated diets differ.
> **Trace metal contamination** from knives and cooking utensils may be present.
> **The salt content** of processed and home prepared foods varies.
> **Heat labile and water soluble vitamins** may show a wide range in losses.

Box 4.3: Sources of discrepancies between analyzed and calculated nutrient contents.

dividuals; studies have shown that energy and nutrient intakes are consistently lower during the period of duplicate collections, compared to the other survey days. This is probably the result of subjects modifying their dietary pattern on duplicate collection days (Gibson and Scythes, 1982; Kim et al., 1984). Nevertheless, this is the most appropriate method for obtaining precise information on nutrient intakes of individuals for metabolic studies, provided that the amounts for the duplicate food items or composite diets are weighed.

4.8 Assessment of available nutrient intakes

Nutrient intakes calculated from food composition data or determined by direct chemical analysis represent the maximum amount of that nutrient available to the body. For most nutrients, however, the amount actually absorbed and used by the body is lower than the total intake and depends on the chemical form of the nutrient, the nature of the food ingested, and the composition of the total diet. The level of the body stores of the nutrient and the physiological status of the individual may also affect nutrient absorption and utilization.

The term "bioavailability" describes the degree to which a nutrient in any food is absorbed, transported, and used physiologically (O'Dell, 1983). Nutrients that are readily taken up following ingestion are termed "bioavailable." Factors that affect the nutrient bioavailability may be either extrinsic or intrinsic. Examples of these factors, some particularly affecting the bioavailability of trace elements, are summarized in Table 4.14.

At present, the dietary factors influencing the absorption or utilization of many nutrients are not well established. Hence, in many cases, algorithms have not been developed to predict nutrient bioavailability. Notable exceptions are the algorithms available for iron and zinc. These mathematical models attempt to predict bioavailability by taking into account the amount and form of iron and zinc, the presence of dietary enhancers and inhibitors, and the iron and zinc status of the individual. The models then apply certain general principles to the complex whole-diet matrix.

The accuracy of the algorithms is limited by interactions known to occur between the enhancing and inhibiting factors in the whole diet. For example, the effects of the enhancers (e.g., ascorbic acid and animal tissue) and the inhibitors (e.g., phytate and polyphenols) on nonheme iron absorption, when they are con-

Extrinsic factors

- Stability of the element species, e.g., CuS, $CuMoS_4$, and $Fe_4(P_2O_7)_3$
- Adsorption of diet components on large surfaces, e.g., fiber, silica, and $Ca_3(PO_4)_2$
- State of oxidation of element, chemical form, e.g., $Fe(II)$ vs. $Fe(III)$, $Cr(III)$ vs. $Cr(VI)$, $Mn(II)$ vs. $Mn(VII)$)
- Competitive antagonism between ions, e.g., Cu-Zn, Cd-Zn, Fe-Zn, Mn-Fe
- Chelation effects: positive or negative, depending on relative solubilities and dissociation constants

Intrinsic factors

- Species and genotype
- Age and sex
- Metabolic function: maintenance, growth, reproduction, lactation
- Nutritional status, including adaptation to dietary intake
- Physiological stress
- Intestinal microflora and infection

Table 4.14: Factors affecting the bioavailability of trace elements in the diet. From O'Dell, Federation Proceedings 42: 1714–1715, 1983, with permission of the Federation of American Societies for Experimental Biology Journal.

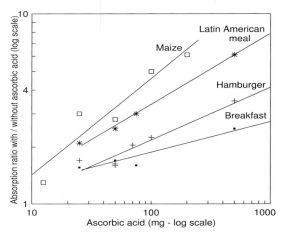

Figure 4.1: The impact of varying meal type on the enhancement of nonheme iron absorption by ascorbic acid. From Hunt JR, Journal of Nutrition 126: 2345S–2353S, 1996, with permission of the American Society for Nutritional Sciences.

tained in the same meal, are probably not additive (Reddy et al., 2000). Furthermore, most of the effects of the dietary modifiers on iron absorption have been calculated from the results of single test meals. In this regimen, the effects may be exaggerated compared to the extent of the enhancement or inhibition measured over several days (Cook et al., 1991). As well, the magnitude of the effect of the absorption modifiers may depend on the background dietary matrix. Certainly, the impact of ascorbic acid on enhancing nonheme iron absorption is greater in a maize porridge or a Latin American meal (maize or rice and beans) than with a hamburger or a breakfast of a refined wheat roll with marmalade, cheese, and coffee, as shown in Figure 4.1 (Hallberg et al., 1986). Clearly, the algorithms for iron and zinc must be revised on an ongoing basis as more quantitative information on the effect of dietary components on the absorption and utilization of these two trace elements becomes available (Hunt, 1996; Du et al., 2000).

4.8.1 Monsen's algorithms for available iron

The first algorithm for estimating available iron intakes was developed by Monsen et al.

(1978) and can be used when intakes of flesh foods, vitamin C, and total iron at *each meal* are known. In this model, 40% of the total iron found in meat, poultry, and fish is assumed to be heme iron. Nonheme iron is calculated as the difference between the total iron and heme iron.

In the initial model, absorption of heme iron was assumed to be 25%, but 23% in a later model (Monsen and Balintfy, 1982). The absorption of nonheme iron was assumed to be lower and to vary according to the amount of meat, poultry, fish, and ascorbic acid in each meal, as well as the level of iron stores of the individual. Total available iron intakes per day can be derived from the sum of available iron from each meal and snack.

The model of Monsen et al. (1978) does not take into account the amounts of any absorption inhibitors in a meal, or any possible synergistic effects of absorption enhancers that are present together in the same meal.

4.8.2 FAO/WHO algorithm

FAO/WHO (1988) has also developed a classification system for estimating iron bioavailability based on measures of iron absorption from typical meals in Asia, India, Latin America, and Western countries. In this model, diets are classified into three broad categories of low, intermediate, and high bioavailability depending on their content of flesh- vs. plant-based foods, together with their content of ascorbic acid–rich foods. The estimates of absorption are for nonanemic persons (i.e., with normal hemoglobin) with normal iron transport but no iron stores.

- Low bioavailability plant-based diets (iron absorption about 5%) are based on cereals, roots, and tubers, and contain a preponderance of foods that inhibit iron absorption (e.g., maize, beans, whole wheat flour, sorghum) along with negligible quantities of meat, fish, or ascorbic acid–rich foods. Such a dietary pattern is dominant in many developing countries.

- Intermediate bioavailability diets (iron absorption about 10%) have larger amounts of absorption enhancers such as ascorbic acid and flesh foods at the main meal, but still consist mainly of cereals, roots, and tubers.

- High bioavailability diets (iron absorption about 15%) are more diverse and contain generous amounts of meat, poultry, and/or fish, as well as foods containing high amounts of ascorbic acid. This dietary pattern is typical of most segments of the population in industrialized countries. However, a high-bioavailability diet may be reduced to the intermediate level if meals containing high amounts of inhibitors of iron absorption, such as tea or coffee, are consumed regularly.

As noted previously, the absorption values in the FAO/WHO algorithm of 5%, 10%, and 15% are for nonanemic persons with no iron stores. In cases of iron-deficiency anemia, however, each value is assumed to be increased by 50% — that is to 7.5%, 15%, and 22.5% absorption for the low, intermediate, and high bioavailability diets, respectively.

4.8.3 Algorithm of Murphy and co-workers

The algorithms of Monsen et al. (1978) and FAO/WHO (1988) were adapted by Murphy et al. (1992) to estimate iron bioavailability in diets from developing countries. Quantitative data on the intake of iron, ascorbic acid, and protein from meat, fish, and poultry are required. A tea or coffee factor can also be included to account for their inhibitory effects on nonheme iron absorption. The effect of phytate on iron absorption is not considered.

Murphy's model, like that of Monsen, also assumes that heme iron constitutes 40% of the iron in meat, poultry, and fish, and the absorption of heme iron is assumed to be 25%. Table 4.15 depicts the estimated bioavailability factors for nonheme iron for iron-deficient, nonanemic persons, taking into account the effect of two enhancers on nonheme iron absorption — meat + fish + poultry protein and ascorbic acid.

Ascorbic acid (mg / 4.18 MJ)	Meat + fish + poultry protein (g / 4.18 MJ)		
	< 9	9–27	> 27
< 35	5	10	15
35–105	10	15	15
>105	15	15	15

Table 4.15: Estimated percentage bioavailability of nonheme iron for iron-deficient, nonanemic persons with differing intakes of meat + fish + poultry protein and ascorbic acid. From Murphy et al., American Journal of Clinical Nutrition 56: 565–572, 1992 © Am J Clin Nutr. American Society for Clinical Nutrition.

The cutoffs applied for these two enhancers are those derived from Monsen but are expressed per 4.18 MJ (1000 kcal), so that the same algorithm can be used for males and females across all age groups. The percentage levels for the bioavailability of nonheme iron given for each class in Table 4.15 approximates those of the typical meals of the low, medium, and high bioavailability categories of the FAO/WHO algorithm.

For subjects with iron-deficiency anemia, the estimated absorption is increased by 50%, i.e., to 7.5%, 15%, and 22.5% absorption for low, intermediate, and high bioavailability diets, respectively, as noted previously (FAO/WHO, 1988).

The model of Murphy et al. (1992), unlike that of Monsen and Balintfy (1982), takes into account the effect of one inhibitor of nonheme iron absorption — polyphenols from tea and/or coffee. The correction factor applied depends on the average number of cups of tea or coffee per day. Tea factors range from 1 if no tea is consumed to 0.40 for at least 600 ml/d; corresponding correction factors for coffee are 1 and 0.60. The final algorithm equals:

available iron = (heme iron × 0.25) +
    (nonheme iron × availability factor × tea factor)

This model can also be used to calculate the bioavailability of iron on a daily rather than a meal basis, if the data for food intake by meal are not available. Estimates of available iron derived from day- and meal-based survey results using this model have proved comparable (Murphy et al., 1996).

The computer program supplied with the WorldFood Dietary Assessment System calculates available iron using Murphy's model (Bunch and Murphy, 1997). As noted previously, this program is available from:

http://www.fao.org/infoods/

4.8.4 Other algorithms for available iron

Several alternative algorithms have been developed for calculating available iron, each of which takes into account differing numbers of absorption modifiers. For example, Tseng et al. (1997) have refined Murphy's model so that nonheme iron absorption can be adjusted for the enhancing effect of meat, poultry, fish, and vitamin C. Separate adjustments can be made for the inhibitory effects of tea and phytates in the diet. However, this model does not account for the combined effect of enhancers and inhibitors on iron absorption and has not had extensive use.

Du et al. (2000) compared the use of the model developed by Tseng et al. (1997) with the algorithms of Monsen et al. (1978) and FAO/WHO (1988) for estimating the iron bioavailability in the diets of Chinese adults, based on 24-h recalls collected over three consecutive days. Hemoglobin as an indicator of iron status was also measured. None of the algorithms appeared to be appropriate for estimating dietary iron bioavailability in these Chinese diets. These investigators emphasized that for vegetarian diets it is important to consider the combined effect of multiple dietary factors on iron bioavailability.

Two additional algorithms are available for estimating dietary iron absorption. Reddy et al. (2000) studied the iron status (serum ferritin) and iron absorption (via extrinsic radio-iron labeling) from 25 different single meals eaten by 86 subjects. An algorithm was then developed, using multiple regression analysis, to predict the iron absorption after adjusting for each individual's iron sta-

tus and including dietary modifiers as independent variables. It is of interest that only 16.4% of the total variance in iron absorption was accounted for by the amount of animal tissue, phytic acid, and ascorbic acid in the typical Western diets studied, with the major portion being explained by the animal tissue and phytic acid contents of the meals. Nonheme iron, calcium, and polyphenols were not significant predictors of iron absorption. These results emphasize the relatively small influence of diet on the amount of iron absorbed, compared to the more important but unknown physiological factors.

Of all the algorithms available, the model of Hallberg and Hulthén (2000) is the most detailed, taking into account the affects of all the known enhancing and inhibiting factors on nonheme iron absorption, as well as interactions between the different factors. Application of this more detailed model is limited at the present time by the paucity of food composition data for the content of both phytate and iron-binding polyphenols in foods. However, this situation is changing.

4.8.5 WHO algorithm for available zinc

The bioavailability of dietary zinc, like iron, is affected by the presence of several absorption enhancers and inhibitors in the whole diet, as well as the total zinc content. Of these, only the impact of one absorption enhancer (protein from meat, fish, and poultry) and two absorption inhibitors (the proportion of phytic acid to zinc, and high levels of calcium) are taken into account in the WHO (1996) algorithm for available zinc.

Both the amount and type of protein in the diet affect zinc absorption. Increasing the level of dietary protein enhances absorption of dietary zinc; absorption is further enhanced by certain animal proteins, specifically meat, eggs, and whey protein (Lönnerdal, 2000).

Phytic acid (myo-inositol hexaphosphate) is a potent inhibitor of zinc absorption. It cannot be digested and absorbed, but instead forms insoluble complexes with zinc in the gastrointestinal tract. Only the hexa- and pentaphosphate esters of inositol significantly inhibit the bioavailability of zinc; the lower inositol phosphates have no inhibitory effect (Lönnerdal et al., 1989). This is important because household processing methods such as germination and fermentation may induce phytate hydrolysis via endogenous or microbial phytase enzymes, degrading the higher inositol phosphates. Phytic acid is present in high concentrations in unrefined cereals, legumes, and nuts, as the magnesium, calcium, or potassium salt (Gibson and Hotz, 2001).

The inhibitory effect of phytate on zinc absorption can be predicted to some degree from the phytate : zinc molar ratio in the diet. Molar ratios in excess of 15:1 progressively inhibit zinc absorption, although even molar ratios as low as 5:1 may have some negative effect. Hence, phytate : zinc molar ratios are a critical component of any algorithm used to estimate zinc bioavailability.

Calcium probably has an inhibitory effect on zinc absorption only when phytate is also present in the diet, and this inhibitory effect may arise from the formation of insoluble calcium-zinc-phytate complexes in the intestinal tract (Lönnerdal, 2000). However, the calcium content of most plant-based diets is too low to have any detrimental effect. Exceptions are diets based on tortillas prepared with lime-soaked maize, diets of lacto-vegetarians, and possibly the diets of persons who chew betel nut with lime.

In the WHO (1996) algorithm, diets are classified into low, moderate, and high bioavailability as shown below.

Low bioavailability diets are assumed to be associated with a zinc absorption of about 15%. Such diets are characterized by:

- A high content of unrefined, unfermented and ungerminated cereal grains (e.g., flat breads or sorghum), especially if fortified with inorganic calcium salts and with a negligible content of animal protein
- A phytate : zinc molar ratio >15
- High-phytate, soy-protein products constituting the primary protein source
- Approximately 50% of the energy content

accounted for either by one or a combination of the following high-phytate foods: high-extraction-rate wheat, maize grains and flours, chapatti flours and "tanok", rice, oatmeal, millet, sorghum, pigeonpeas, cowpeas, grams, blackeye beans, kidney beans, groundnut flours
- Intakes of inorganic calcium salts >1 g Ca^{2+}/d, either as supplements or as adventitious contaminants (e.g., from calcareous geophagia); low intakes of animal protein exacerbate these effects.

Moderate bioavailability diets are mostly mixed diets with a zinc bioavailability of about 30%–35%. They include:

- Mixed diets with animal or fish protein
- Lacto-ovo, ovo-vegetarian, or vegan diets not based primarily on unrefined cereal grains or high-extraction-rate flours
- Diets where the phytate : zinc molar ratio ranges from 5 to 15, or where the ratio is < 10 if more than half of the energy intake is accounted for by unfermented, unrefined cereal grains and flours and the diet is fortified with >1 g/d of inorganic calcium salts

The bioavailability of zinc in moderate availability diets improves when animal or protein sources or milk are included in the diet.

High bioavailability diets are mostly diets with an adequate protein content mainly from non-vegetable sources. They have a zinc bioavailability of about 50%–55%. They include:

- Refined diets low in cereal fiber, with a low phytic acid content and with a phytate : zinc molar ratio < 5
- Diets with adequate protein, mainly from non-vegetable sources, such as meat and fish, and including semisynthetic formula diets based on animal protein

Zinc absorption estimates for diets categorized as having high or moderate bioavailability vary according to whether the intakes

meet the basal or normative requirement estimates. When basal requirement estimates are
met, then for high and moderate bioavailability diets, zinc absorption estimates are
55% and 35%, respectively, compared to only
50% and 30% when normative requirements
are met (WHO, 1996).

These WHO (1996) zinc absorption estimates are based on data mainly from single
meals, as limited data from total diets were
available at that time. It is possible that
the effects of the dietary modifiers on zinc
absorption are exaggerated when measured
from single test meals rather than from whole
diets, as noted earlier for iron, although this
requires further investigation.

4.8.6 Algorithm of Murphy and co-workers for available zinc

The algorithm of Murphy et al. (1992) is
based on the earlier work of WHO. It takes
into account the content of animal protein
and the content of phytate and calcium in
the whole diet. For this algorithm, the phytate : zinc molar ratio of the whole diet is
calculated using the following equation:

$$[\text{phytate (mg)} / 660] / [\text{Zn (mg)} / 65.4]$$

where 660 = the molecular weight of phytate and 65.4 = the molecular weight of zinc.
Bioavailability estimates are then assigned to
the whole diets based on their phytate : zinc
molar ratios. Diets with phytate : zinc molar
ratios between 0 and 5 have an estimated
bioavailability of 55%; 5 and 15, 35%; 15 and
30, 15%; and > 30, 10%, respectively.

The bioavailability estimates are then further modified, depending on the animal protein and calcium content of the diet. If the animal protein density exceeds 16 g/1000 kcal,
the bioavailability estimate is increased by
5 percentage points (e.g., from 10% to 15%).
If the calcium density is within the range of
500–750 mg/1000 kcal, or exceeds 750 mg/
1000 kcal, then 5 and 10 percentage points,
respectively, are subtracted from the bioavailability estimate (e.g., the estimate is lowered
from 15% to 10% or from 20% to 10%).
However, the estimated bioavailability is not

allowed to fall below 10% or to rise above
55%.

In most plant-based diets in developing
countries, intakes of animal protein are generally too low to enhance zinc absorption, and
intakes of calcium are too low to reduce zinc
absorption. Even in Latin American countries where calcium intakes are often > 1g/d,
phytate intakes are so high that any further
reduction in zinc absorption is assumed to be
unlikely.

4.8.7 IZiNCG algorithm

The International Zinc Nutrition Consultative
Group (IZiNCG) have developed an algorithm for the bioavailability of zinc, based
on measurements of zinc absorption in adults
using only total diet studies; studies using
semi-purified diets, or exogenous sources of
zinc in the form of zinc salts, were excluded
(Hotz and Brown, 2004). A logit regression
model was used to describe the relationship
between four dietary factors (zinc, phytate,
protein, and calcium) and the percentage of
the zinc intake absorbed. However, in the
final model only zinc and the phytate : zinc
molar ratio were shown to be significant predictors of the percentage of zinc absorption
in adults ($r^2 = 0.41$, $p < 0.001$). Neither calcium nor protein added significant predictive
power. The IZiNCG predictive equation derived from this work is the following:

$$\text{logit (Fractional absorption of zinc)} =$$
$$1.365 - [0.6129 \times \ln{(\text{mg zinc})}]$$
$$- [0.3164 \times \ln{(\text{phytate : zinc ratio})}]$$
$$\text{and}$$
$$\text{Fractional absorption of zinc} =$$
$$\exp{[\text{logit(fractional absorption of zinc)}]}$$
$$\div \{1 + \exp{[\text{logit(fractional absorption of zinc)}]}\}$$

The applicability of this model to children is
unknown. The IZiNCG also calculated revised estimates of zinc absorption for adults
consuming diets equivalent in composition to
the moderate and low bioavailability diets
of WHO (1996). The revised bioavailability figures are 24% for men and 31% for
women consuming mixed or refined vegetarian diets (WHO moderate bioavailability)

and 16% for men and 22% for women consuming unrefined, cereal-based diets (WHO low bioavailability). Whether these bioavailability factors are appropriate for children, pregnant or lactating women, or the elderly has not been established.

4.8.8 Development of algorithms for other nutrients

Research on factors affecting the bioavailability of other nutrients in contemporary diets is urgently required. So far, steps have been taken to develop algorithms to quantify the bioavailability of protein, folate, and vitamin A in human diets; these are considered below. Niacin is discussed in Section 4.4.5.

The nutritional value of proteins in diets can be estimated from a protein digestibility-corrected amino acid score (PDCAAS), calculated using the procedures of Schaafsma (2000). This method is recommended by FAO/WHO (1990) and is based on comparison of the concentration of the first limiting amino acid in the test protein with the concentration of that amino acid in a reference pattern of essential amino acids. This reference scoring pattern is derived from the essential amino acid requirements of the preschool-age child and is given in Table 4.16. The chemical score derived in this way is then corrected for true fecal digestibility of the test protein.

Amino acid	Requirement (mg/g crude protein)
Isoleucine	28
Leucine	66
Lysine	58
Total sulfur amino acids	25
Total aromatic amino acids	63
Threonine	34
Trytophan	11
Valine	35
Total	320

Table 4.16: FAO/WHO/UNU amino acid requirement pattern based on amino acid requirements of preschool-age children. From Schaafsma, Journal of Nutrition 130: 1865S–1867S, 2000, with permission of the American Society for Nutritional Sciences.

Protein	Digestibility	AAS	PDCAAS	PER
Egg	98	121	118	3.8
Cow's milk	95	127	121	3.1
Beef	98	94	92	2.9
Soy	95	96	91	2.1
Wheat	91	47	42	1.5

Table 4.17: Measures of protein digestibility and quality in some foods. AAS, amino acid score; PDCAAS, protein digestibility-corrected amino acid score; PER, protein energy ratio. From FAO/WHO (1990). From Schaafsma, Journal of Nutrition 130: 1865S–1867S, 2000, with permission of the American Society for Nutritional Sciences, and FAO/WHO (1990).

Thus the PDCAAS (%) =

$$\frac{\text{mg of limiting amino acid in 1 g of test protein}}{\text{mg of same amino acid in 1 g of reference protein}}$$

$$\times \text{ true fecal digestibility (\%)}$$

Some values for true fecal digestibility, amino acid score, and nontruncated PDCAAS for proteins from selected foods are shown in Table 4.17. The values for proteins with a PDCAAS >100% can be truncated to 100% (FAO/WHO 1990). This approach has been adopted on the assumption that digestible essential amino acid concentrations in excess of those in the preschool-age reference pattern do not provide additional nutritional benefit. However, this assumption has been questioned because it does not take into account the ability of high-quality proteins to balance the amino acid composition of inferior proteins. This is highly relevant because, in most cases, humans consume mixed diets containing proteins from a variety of sources, rather than a single protein source (Schaafsma, 2000).

To apply this formula to habitual mixed diets, first the observed intakes of the essential amino acids are calculated from food composition data. The uncorrected amino acid score is then computed independently for each amino acid using the reference amino acid pattern for children aged 2–5 y. Lastly, the lowest amino acid score is selected and applied for the estimate of the PDCAAS (as %). Note that the digestibility of total protein intake must also be taken into account when calculating PDCAAS, because differences in digestibility affect the utilization of protein. The FAO/WHO/UNU (1985) report recommends that digestibility of total protein intake is estimated by weighted summation of the digestibility of individual protein sources. Furthermore, they provide data on the true digestibility of protein for diets based on both animal protein and on a variety of plant-based staples. An example of the use of this weighted approach is given in Table 4.18.

Alternatively, digestibility correction factors of 85% and 95% can be applied to diets based on whole grain cereals and vegetables, or refined cereals, respectively, using the following formula from FAO/WHO/UNU (1985):

digestible protein = actual dietary
    protein (Nitrogen × 6.25) × (digestibility % / 100)

Beaton et al. (1992) employed another approach for the diets of toddlers in Egypt, Kenya, and Mexico because of the absence of data on protein digestibilities of all the individual foods consumed. They imputed digestibility based on an empirical relationship between protein digestibility and dietary fiber. Large intakes of dietary fiber, especially insoluble fiber, are known to increase fecal nitrogen excretion, resulting in a reduction in apparent protein digestibility of up to approximately 10%. Beaton et al. (1992) used protein digestibility data for maize, polished rice, whole wheat, refined wheat, oatmeal, millet, mature peas, peanut butter, and soy

Food	Fraction of total dietary protein	Digestibility relative to reference protein (%)
Rice	0.40	93
Maize	0.10	89
Beans	0.35	82
Milk	0.10	100
Meat	0.05	100

Digestibility of total protein in the diet =
$(0.4 \times 93) + (0.1 \times 89) + (0.35 \times 82) +$
    $(0.1 \times 100) + (0.05 \times 100) = 90\%$

Table 4.18: Estimation of the digestibility of the protein of a mixed diet based on the protein foods it contains. From FAO/WHO/UNU (1985).

flour from FAO/WHO/UNU (1985), and that for dry beans *Phaseolus* spp. from Tobin and Carpenter (1978). Their prediction equation is:

digestibility = 1 − (0.1 × dietary fiber / dietary protein)

Such adjustments to the nutritional value of proteins are especially necessary in countries where the habitual diets are predominantly plant-based: the safe levels of protein intake, derived by FAO/WHO/UNU (1985), were calculated from studies based on animal protein.

The WorldFood Dietary Assessment system computes utilizable protein for children by adjusting intakes to account for both digestibility and amino acid score, using the FAO/WHO/UNU (1985) procedures.

Some questions have been raised regarding use of the PDCAAS method for evaluating protein quality. These questions relate to the validity of the amino acid requirement values for preschool-age children, the validity of correction for fecal instead of ileal digestibility, and the truncation of PDCAAS values to 100%, as noted earlier. For details of these concerns see Schaafsma (2000).

Folate is a naturally occurring vitamin found in foods. However, the term is also used to embrace synthetic folic acid found in fortified foods and supplements, as noted earlier (Section 4.4.5). The polyglutamate forms in foods have a lower bioavailability than does synthetic folic acid. As a result, the IOM (2000a) have introduced a new term — dietary folate equivalents (DFE) — to take into account the differences in the bioavailability of all sources of ingested folate. The dietary folate equivalent content of a food is defined as:

μg food folate + (1.7 × μg synthetic folic acid)

This equation is based on the assumption that the bioavailability of food folate is about 50%, whereas that of folic acid taken with food is 85% (i.e., folic acid is 85 / 50 = 1.7 times more available) (Sauberlich et al., 1987; Pfeiffer et al., 1997).

Many countries are now fortifying foods

such as breads and grains with the synthetic monoglutamate form, but most current food composition tables do not distinguish between folate found naturally in foods and folic acid added to foods. Work is underway in some countries to provide this information. Lewis et al. (1999) calculated folate intakes, expressed as DFEs, for the U.S population from the NHANES III data and the Continuing Survey of Food Intakes by Individuals 1994–1996. The data generated reflect intakes that account for differences in the bioavailability of all sources of ingested folate. Further research is required to improve the precision and utility of this approach for assessing the adequacy of folate intakes in diets containing foods fortified with synthetic folic acid.

Vitamin A in the diets of most industrialized countries occurs mainly as preformed vitamin A derived from animal products. In contrast, in most tropical countries the main sources of vitamin A are the provitamin A carotenoids from dark-green leafy vegetables and certain yellow- and orange-colored fruits and vegetables (West, 2000). Increasingly, synthetic sources of retinol and provitamin A compounds (mainly β-carotene) are being added to foods or used as dietary supplements in both industrialized and developing countries. Major differences exist in the bioavailability of retinol and the various provitamin A carotenoids. As a result, dietary vitamin A levels are expressed in terms of µg of retinol equivalents (RE), or as retinol activity equivalents (RAE) in the United States, as discussed in Section 4.4.5.

Currently there is uncertainty about the bioavailability of provitamin A carotenoids and the efficiency with which these absorbed carotenoids are subsequently converted to retinol (i.e., their bioconversion). Evidence suggests that the bioavailability of provitamin A carotenoids from a mixed vegetable and fruit diet is lower than was previously thought and depends primarily on the enclosing matrix.

West (2000) advocates the use of a divisor of 21.0 for β-carotene instead of the 6.0 proposed earlier by FAO/WHO (1988), when the ratio of the intake of provitamin A from dark-green leafy vegetables or carrots to that from yellow/orange fruits is ∼ 4:1. FAO/WHO (2002), however, still recommend use of their earlier factors until more definitive data are available. The U.S. Food and Nutrition Board (IOM 2001) recommends different conversion factors; these have been discussed in detail in Section 4.4.5. Consensus is urgently needed so that more reliable comparisons of the adequacy of vitamin A intakes among countries can be made.

For several other nutrients, the amount available for absorption can be only estimated. Such estimates are generally made by the expert committees formulating the nutrient recommendations, and they vary primarily according to the characteristics of the habitual diet of a country. More work is required to develop algorithms for predicting the bioavailability of nutrients in diets of differing compositions. The NRC Committee on Nutrient Adequacy (NRC, 1986), for example, emphasizes that variations in the bioavailability of iron, zinc, and folate probably have the greatest influence on the estimates of dietary intakes of these micronutrients for individuals. For estimates of the average micronutrient intakes for a group, however, the influence of such variations in bioavailability may be small in relation to other sources of measurement error.

4.9 Summary

Energy and nutrient intakes can be calculated from quantitative food consumption data by using food composition databases or tables. Food composition data are generally compiled from a variety of sources, including direct chemical analysis, the literature, sometimes imputed values, and recipe calculations. The values aim to be representative of the average composition of a particular foodstuff on a year-round, nationwide basis. They are compiled as computer-based food composition databases and/or as printed food composition tables. Both random and systematic errors may occur in food composition data, depending on the food item and the nutrient. Such errors may include inadequacies in the sampling protocols and analytical methods, use of incorrect conversion factors for calculating nutrient values, inconsistencies arising from differences in the terminology for certain nutrients, and in methods of food preparation and processing. Genetic and environmental factors and incorrect descriptions of individual food items or sources of nutrient values may be additional sources of error. Efforts to minimize these sources of error have led to the establishment of an international network of food data systems.

The validity of nutrient values in food composition databases can be checked in several ways. Consistency checks can be performed at three levels: checks between or across nutrients within foods; checks between or across foods (within nutrients), and checks of the whole database. Direct chemical analysis of individual food items or composite diets can also be used to validate food composition data. Composite diets can be prepared by three techniques: duplicate portions, aliquot sampling, and the equivalent composite method. Nutrient values derived from both food composition data and direct chemical analysis represent the maximum available to the body and not the amount actually absorbed and utilized. Algorithms have been developed for those nutrients for which the dietary factors affecting their bioavailability (e.g., iron, zinc, protein,) are well characterized. These algorithms can be used to provide more reliable assessments of the nutrient adequacy of diets. New terms have also been introduced for folate and vitamin A — dietary folate equivalent and retinol activity coefficient — to take into account the differences in the bioavailability of all sources of these micronutrients.

References

AACC (American Association of Cereal Chemists). (2001). The Definition of Dietary Fiber. Report of the Dietary Fiber Definition Committee to the Board of Directors of the American Association of Cereal Chemists, January 10, St. Paul, MN.

Ågren G, Gibson RS. (1963). Food Composition Tables for Use in Ethiopia. Children's Nutrition Unit Report No. 16. Swedish International Development Agency, Uppsala, Sweden.

Ahola M. (1991). Use of food composition data banks in nutrient intake studies. In: Macdonald I (ed.) Monitoring Dietary Intakes. Springer-Verlag, Berlin, pp. 110–116.

Alcock SC, Finglas PM, Morgan MRA. (1990). An enzyme-linked immunosorbent assay for pyridoxamine and its comparison with alternative analytical procedures. Food and Agricultural Immunology 2: 197–204.

Anderson I, Lundqvist R, Öste R. (1990). Analysis of vitamin B_{12} in milk by radioisotope dilution assay. Milchwissenschaft 45: 507–559.

Arab L. (1985). Summary of survey of food composition tables and nutrient data banks in Europe. Annals of Nutrition and Metabolism 29(suppl. 1): 39–45.

Athar N, McLaughlin J, Taylor G. (2003). The Concise New Zealand Food Composition Tables. 6th ed. Ministry of Health, Wellington, New Zealand.

Atwater WO, Bryant AP. (1899). The Availability and Fuel Value of Food Materials. Report of the Storrs Agricultural Experimental Station 1900: 73–110.

Ball GFM. (1994). Water-Soluble Vitamin Assays in Human Nutrition. Chapman & Hall, London.

Beaton GH, Calloway DH, Murphy SP. (1992). Estimated protein intakes of toddlers: predicted prevalence of inadequate intakes in village populations in Egypt, Kenya and Mexico. American Journal of Clinical Nutrition 55: 902–911.

Bingham SA, Cummings JH. (1985). Urine nitrogen as an independent validatory measure of dietary intake: a study of nitrogen balance in individuals consuming their normal diet. American Journal of Clinical Nutrition 42: 1276–1289.

Block G, Hartman AM, Dresser CM, Carroll MD, Gannon J, Gardner L. (1986). A data-based approach to diet questionnaire design and testing. American Journal of Epidemiology 124: 453–469.

Brouwer IA, van Dusseldorp M, West CE, Meyboom S, Thomas CMG, Duran M, van het Hof KH, Eskes TKAB, Hauvast JGAJ, Steegers-Theunissen RPM. (1999). Dietary folate from vegetables and citrus fruit decreases plasma homocysteine concentrations in humans in a dietary controlled trial. Journal of Nutrition 129: 1135–1139.

Bunch S, Murphy SP. (1997). User's Guide to the Operation of the WorldFood Dietary Assessment System, Version 2.0. Office of Technology Licensing, University of California, Berkeley.

Buzzard IM, Schakel SF, Ditter-Johnson J. (1995). Quality control issues in the use of food and nutrient databases for epidemiologic studies. In: Greenfield H (ed.) Quality and Accessibility of Food-

Related Data. AOAC International, Arlington, VA, pp. 241–252.

Caldwell EF, Nelsen TC. (1999). Development of an analytical reference standard for total, insoluble and soluble dietary fiber. Cereal Foods World 44: 360–362

Castenmiller JJM, West CE. (1998). Bioavailability and bioconversion of carotenoids. Annual Reviews of Nutrition 18: 19–38.

Chan W, Brown J, Buss DH. (1994). Miscellaneous Foods: Fourth Supplement to McCance and Widdowson's "The Composition of Foods" (5th ed.). The Royal Society of Chemistry, Cambridge.

Chan W, Brown J, Lee SM, Buss DH. (1995). Meat, Poultry and Game: Fifth Supplement to McCance and Widdowson's "The Composition of Foods" (5th ed.). The Royal Society of Chemistry, Cambridge.

Chan W, Brown J, Church SM, Buss DH. (1996). Meat Products and Dishes: Sixth Supplement to McCance and Widdowson's "The Composition of Foods" (5th ed.). The Royal Society of Chemistry, Cambridge.

Cook JD, Dassenko SA, Lynch SR. (1991). Assessment of the role of nonheme-iron availability in iron balance. American Journal of Clinical Nutrition 54: 717–722.

Cooke JR. (1983). Food composition tables: analytical problems in the collection of data. Human Nutrition: Applied Nutrition 37: 441–447.

Cuskelly GJ, McNutty H, Scott JM. (1996). Effect of increasing dietary folate on red-cell folate: implications for prevention of neural tube defects. Lancet 347: 657–659.

Darnton-Hill I, Nalubola R. (2002). Fortification strategies to meet micronutrient needs: successes and failures. Proceedings of the Nutrition Society 61: 231–241.

Deharveng G, Charrondière UR, Slimani N, Southgate DAT, Riboli E. (1999). Comparison of nutrients in the food composition tables available in the nine European countries participating in EPIC. European Journal of Clinical Nutrition 53: 60–79.

de Vries JW, Prosky L, Li B, Cho S. (1999). A historical perspective on defining dietary fiber. Cereal Foods World 44: 367–369.

Du S, Zhai F, Wang Y, Popkin BM. (2000). Current methods for estimating dietary iron bioavailability do not work in China. Journal of Nutrition 130: 193–198.

Duewer DL, Kline MC, Sharpless KE, Thomas JB, Gary KT, Sowell AL. (1999). Micronutrients Measurement Quality Assurance Program: helping participants use interlaboratory comparison exercise results to improve their long-term measurement performance. Analytical Chemistry 71: 1870–1878.

Eheart MS, Gott C. (1965). Chlorophyll, ascorbic acid and pH changes in green vegetables by stir fry, microwave, and conventional methods. Food Technology 19: 867–870.

Englyst HN, Cummings JH. (1988). Improved method for measurement of dietary fiber as non-starch poly-saccharides in plant foods. Journal of the Association of Official Analytical Chemists 71: 808–814.

Englyst HN, Wiggins HS, Cummings JH. (1982). Determination of the nonstarch polysaccharides in plant foods by gas-liquid chromatography of constituent sugars as alditol acetates. Analyst 107: 307–318.

FAO/WHO (Food and Agriculture Organization / World Health Organization). (1973). Energy and Protein Requirements. WHO Technical Report Series No. 522. World Health Organization, Geneva.

FAO/WHO (Food and Agriculture Organization / World Health Organization). (1988). Requirements of Vitamin A, Iron, Folate and Vitamin B_{12}. Food and Agricultural Organization, Rome.

FAO/WHO (Food and Agriculture Organization / World Health Organization). (1990). Protein Quality Evaluation. FAO Food and Nutrition Paper 51. Food and Agricultural Organization, Rome.

FAO/WHO (Food and Agriculture Organization / World Health Organization). (2002). Human Vitamin and Mineral Requirements. World Health Organization Food and Agricultural Organization, Rome.

FAO/WHO/UNU (Food and Agriculture Organization / World Health Organization / United Nations University). (1985). Energy and Protein Requirements. WHO Technical Report Series No. 724. World Health Organization, Geneva.

Food Standards Agency. (2002). McCance and Widdowson's "The Composition of Foods." 6th summary edition. The Royal Society of Chemistry, Cambridge.

Gibson RS, Ferguson EL. (1999). An Interactive 24-Hour Recall for Assessing the Adequacy of Iron and Zinc Intakes in Developing Countries. International Life Sciences Institute Press, Washington, DC.

Gibson RS, Hotz C. (2001). Dietary diversification/modification strategies to enhance micronutrient content and bioavailability of diets in developing countries. British Journal of Nutrition 85: S159–S166.

Gibson RS, Scythes CA. (1982). Trace element intakes of women. British Journal of Nutrition 48: 241–248.

Greenfield H, Southgate DAT. (1992). Food Composition Data: Production, Management, and Use. Elsevier Applied Science, London.

Gregory JF III. (1988). Methods for determination of vitamin B_6 in foods and other biological materials: a critical review. Journal of Food Composition and Analysis 1: 105–123

Gregory JF, Engelhardt R, Bhandari SD, Sartain DB, Gustafson SK. (1990). Adequacy of extraction techniques for determination of folate in foods and other biological materials. Journal of Food Composition and Analysis 3: 134–144.

Hallberg L, Hulthén L. (2000). Prediction of dietary iron absorption: an algorithm for calculating absorption and bioavailability of dietary iron. American Journal of Clinical Nutrition 71: 1147–1160.

Hallberg L, Brune M, Rossander L. (1986). Effect of ascorbic acid on iron absorption from different types of meals: studies with ascorbic-acid-rich foods and synthetic ascorbic acid given in different amounts with different meals. Human Nutrition: Applied Nutrition 40: 97–113.

Hart DJ, Scott KJ. (1995). Development and evaluation of an HPLC method for the analysis of carotenoids in foods, and the measurement of the carotenoid content of vegetables and fruits commonly consumed in the U.K. Food Chemistry 54: 101–111.

Haytowitz DB, Pehrsson PR, Holden JM. (2002). The identification of key foods for food consumption research. Journal of Food Composition and Analysis 15: 183–194.

Health Canada. (2001a). Nutrient Value of Some Common Foods. Health Services and Promotion Branch and Health Protection Branch, Health and Welfare, Ottawa. http://www.hc-sc.gc.ca/food-aliment/

Health Canada. (2001b). Canadian Nutrient File. Bureau of Nutritional Sciences, Health and Welfare, Ottawa. http://www.hc-sc.gc.ca/food-aliment/

Holden JM, Schubert A, Wolf WR, Beecher GR.(1987). A system for evaluating the quality of published nutrient data: selenium, a test case. Food Nutrition Bulletin 9(suppl.): 177–193.

Holden JM, Eldridge AL, Beecher GR, Buzzard IM, Bhagwat SA, Davis CS, Douglass Larry W, Gebhardt SE, Haytowitz DB, Schakel S. (1999). Carotenoid content of U.S. foods: an update of the database. Journal of Food Composition and Analysis 12: 169–196.

Holland B, Unwin ID, Buss DH. (1988). Cereals and Cereal Products: Third Supplement to McCance and Widdowson's "The Composition of Foods" (4th ed.). The Royal Society of Chemistry, Cambridge.

Holland B, Unwin ID, Buss DH. (1989). Milk Products and Eggs: Fourth Supplement to McCance and Widdowson's "The Composition of Foods" (4th ed.). The Royal Society of Chemistry, Cambridge.

Holland B, Unwin ID, Buss DH. (1991a). Vegetables, Herbs and Spices: Fifth Supplement to McCance and Widdowson's "The Composition of Foods" (4th ed.). The Royal Society of Chemistry, Cambridge.

Holland B, Welch AA, Unwin ID, Buss DH, Paul AA, Southgate DAT. (1991b). McCance and Widdowson's "The Composition of Foods." (5th ed.). Royal Society of Chemistry, Cambridge.

Holland B, Unwin ID, Buss DH. (1992a). Fruit and Nuts: First Supplement to McCance and Widdowson's "The Composition of Foods" (5th ed.). The Royal Society of Chemistry, Cambridge.

Holland B, Welch AA, Buss DH. (1992b). Vegetable Dishes: Second Supplement to McCance and Widdowson's "The Composition of Foods" (5th ed.). The Royal Society of Chemistry, Cambridge.

Holland B, Brown J, Buss DH. (1993). Fish and Fish Products: Third Supplement to McCance and Widdowson's The Composition of Foods (5th ed.). The Royal Society of Chemistry, Cambridge.

Hollman PCH, Katan MB. (1988). Bias and error in the determination of common macronutrients in foods: interlaboratory trial. Journal of the American Dietetic Association 88: 556–563.

Hoover LW, Pelican S. (1984). Nutrient data bases: considerations for educators. Journal of Nutrition Education 16: 58–62.

Hoover LW, Perloff BP. (1981). Model for Review of Nutrient Data Base System Capabilities. University of Missouri, Columbia.

Horwitt MK, Harper AE, Henderson LM. (1981). Niacin-tryptophan relationships for evaluating niacin equivalents. American Journal of Clinical Nutrition 34: 423–427.

Horwitz W (ed.). (2002). Official Methods of Analysis of AOAC International 17th ed., 1st rev. AOAC International, Arlington, VA.

Hotz C, Brown KH. (eds.). (2004). Supplement 2: International Zinc Nutrition Consultative Group Technical Document No.1. Assessment of the risk of zinc deficiency in populations and options for its control. Food and Nutrition Bulletin 25: S96–S203.

Hunt JR. (1996). Bioavailability algorithms in setting recommended dietary allowances: lessons from iron, applications to zinc. Journal of Nutrition 126: 2345S–2353S.

IFST (Institute of Food Science & Technology). (2001). Current Hot Topics: Dietary Fibre. http://www.ifst.org/hottop33.htm/

IVACG (International Vitamin A Consultative Group). (2002). Vitamin A Conversion to SI Units. International Life Sciences Institute Press, Washington, DC.

IOM (Institute of Medicine). (2000a). Dietary Reference Intakes for Thiamin, Riboflavin, Niacin, Vitamin B$_6$, Folate, Vitamin B$_{12}$, Pantothenic Acid, Biotin and Choline. National Academy Press, Washington, DC.

IOM (Institute of Medicine). (2000b). Dietary Reference Intakes for Vitamin C, Vitamin E, Selenium, and Carotenoids. National Academy Press, Washington, DC.

IOM (Institute of Medicine). (2001). Dietary Reference Intakes for Vitamin A, Vitamin K, Arsenic, Boron, Chromium, Copper, Iodine, Iron, Manganese, Molybdenum, Nickel, Silicon, Vanadium and Zinc. National Academy Press, Washington, DC.

Jones DB. (1941). Factors for Converting Percentages of Nitrogen in Foods and Feeds into Percentages of Protein. Circular 183. U.S. Department of Agriculture, Washington, DC.

Kall MA, Andersen C. (1999). Improved method for simultaneous determination of ascorbic acid and dehydroascorbic acid, isoascorbic acid and dehydroisoascorbic acid in food and biological samples. Journal of Chromatography. B, Biomedical Science Applications 730: 101–111.

Kim WW, Mertz W, Judd JT, Marshall MW, Kelsay JL, Prather ES. (1984). Effect of making duplicate food collections on nutrient intakes calculated from diet records. American Journal of Clinical Nutrition 40: 1333–1337.

Klensin JC, Feskanich D, Lin V, Truswell AS, Southgate DAT. (1989). Identification of Food Components for INFOOODS Data Interchange. United Nations University, Tokyo, Japan.

Konings EJM. (1999). A validated liquid chromatographic method for determining folates in vegetables, milk powder, liver and flour. Journal of AOAC International 82: 119–127.

Konings EJ, Roomans HH, Dorant E, Goldbohm RA, Saris WH, van den Brandt PA. (2001). Folate intake of the Dutch population according to newly established liquid chromatography data for foods. American Journal of Clinical Nutrition 73: 765–776.

Lewis CJ, Crane NT, Wilson DB, Yetley EA. (1999). Estimated folate intakes: data updated to reflect food fortification, increased bioavailability and dietary supplement use. American Journal of Clinical Nutrition 70: 198–207.

Lönnerdal B. (2000). Dietary factors influencing zinc absorption. Journal of Nutrition 130: 1378S–1383S.

Lönnerdal B, Sandberg A-S, Sandstrom B, Kunz C. (1989). Inhibitory effects of phytic acid and other inositol phosphates on zinc and calcium absorption in suckling rats. Journal of Nutrition 119: 211–214.

Lurie DG, Holden JM, Schubert A, Wolf WR, Miller-Ihli NJ. (1989). The copper content of foods based on a critical evaluation of published analytical data. Journal of Food Composition and Analysis 2: 298–316.

Mangels AR, Holden JM, Beecher GR, Forman MR, Lanza E. (1993). Carotenoid content of fruits and vegetables: an evaluation of analytical data. Journal of the American Dietetic Association 93: 284–296.

Matthews RH, Garrison YJ. (1975). Food Yields Summarized by Different Stages of Preparation. Agriculture Handbook No. 102. U.S. Department of Agriculture, Washington, DC.

McKillop DJ, Pentieva K, Daly D, McPartlin JM, Hughes J, Strain JJ, Scott JM, McNulty H. (2002). The effect of different cooking methods on folate retention in various foods that are amongst the major contributors to folate intake in the U.K. diet. British Journal of Nutrition 88: 681–688.

Mercadante AZ, Rodriguez-Amaya DB. (1991). Carotenoid composition of a leafy vegetable in relation to some agricultural variables. Journal of Agricultural and Food Chemistry 39: 1094–1097.

Merrill AL, Watt BK. (1973). Energy Value of Foods: Basis and Derivation. Agriculture Handbook No. 74. U.S. Department of Agriculture, Washington, DC.

Ministry of Agriculture, Fisheries and Food. (1998). Fatty Acids: Seventh Supplement to McCance and Widdowson's "The Composition of Foods" (5th ed.). The Royal Society of Chemistry, Cambridge.

Mongeau R, Brassard R. (1989). A comparison of three methods for analyzing dietary fiber in 38 foods. Journal of Food Composition and Analysis 2: 189–199.

Monsen ER, Balintfy JL. (1982). Calculating dietary iron bioavailability: refinement and computerization. Journal of the American Dietetic Association 80: 307–311.

Monsen ER, Hallberg L, Layrisse M, Hegsted DM, Cook JD, Mertz W, Finch CA. (1978). Estimation of available dietary iron. American Journal of Clinical Nutrition 31: 134–141.

Murphy SP, Weinberg-Andersson SW, Neumann C, Mulligan K, Calloway DH. (1991). Development of research nutrient data bases: an example using foods consumed in rural Kenya. Journal of Food Composition and Analysis 4: 2–17.

Murphy SP, Beaton GH, Calloway DH. (1992). Estimated mineral intakes of toddlers: predicted prevalence of inadequacy in village populations in Egypt, Kenya and Mexico. American Journal of Clinical Nutrition 56: 565–572.

Murphy SP, Allen LH, Bunch SJ. (1996). Meal-based versus day-based methods of estimating available iron in diets from rural Mexico. FASEB Journal 10: A279 (abstract).

NRC (National Research Council). (1986). Nutrient Adequacy: Assessment using Food Consumption Surveys. National Academy Press, Washington, DC.

O'Dell BL. (1983). Bioavailability of trace elements. Federation Proceedings 42: 1714–1715.

O'Neill ME, Carroll Y, Corridan B, Olmedilla B, Granado F, Blanco I, Van den Berg H, Hininger I, Rousell AM, Chopra M, Southon S, Thurnham DI. (2001). A European carotenoid database to assess carotenoid intakes and its use in a five-country comparative study. British Journal of Nutrition 85: 499–507.

Paul AA, Southgate DAT. (1978). McCance and Widdowson's "The Composition of Foods". 4th ed. Her Majesty's Stationery Office, London.

Pennington JAT, Butrum R. (1991). Food description: langual and taxonomy. Trends in Food Science and Technology 2: 285–288.

Périssé J. (1982). The heterogeneity of food composition tables. In: Hautvast JGAJ, Klaver W (eds.) The Diet Factor in Epidemiological Research. Euronut Report 1. Ponsen & Looyen, Wageningen, pp. 100–105.

Pfeiffer CM, Rogers LM, Gregory JF 3rd. (1997). Determination of folate in cereal-grain food products using trienzyme extraction and combined affinity and reversed-phase liquid chromatography. Journal of Agricultural Food Chemistry 45: 407–413.

Poortvliet EJ, Klensin JC, Kohlmeier L. (1992). Rationale document for the Eurocode food coding system. European Journal of Clinical Nutrition 46: S9–S24.

Powers PM, Hoover LW. (1989). Calculating the nutrient composition of recipes with computers. Journal of the American Dietetic Association 89: 224–233.

Qian H, Sheng M. (1998). Simultaneous determination of fat-soluble vitamins A, D and E and provitamin D2 in animal feeds by one-step extraction and high performance liquid chromatography analysis. Journal of Chromatography 825: 127–133.

Rand WM, Pennington JAT, Murphy SP, Klensin JC. (1991). Compiling Data for Food Composition Data Bases. United Nations University Press, Tokyo, Japan.

Reddy MB, Hurrell RF, Cook JD. (2000). Estimation of nonheme-iron bioavailability from meal composition. American Journal of Clinical Nutrition 71: 937–943.

Sauberlich HE, Kretsch MJ, Skala JH, Johnson HL, Taylor PC. (1987). Folate requirement and metabolism in nonpregnant women. American Journal of Clinical Nutrition 46: 1016–1028.

Schaafsma G. (2000). The protein digestibility-corrected amino acid score. Journal of Nutrition 130: 1865S–1867S.

Schakel SF, Buzzard IM, Gebhardt SE. (1997). Procedures for estimating nutrient values for food composition databases. Journal of Food Composition and Analysis 10: 102–114.

Schubert A, Holden JM, Wolf WR. (1987). Selenium content of a core group of foods based on a critical evaluation of published data. Journal of the American Dietetic Association 87: 285–299.

Scrimshaw NS. (1997). INFOODS: the international network of food data systems. American Journal of Clinical Nutrition 65: 1190S–1193S.

Sivelli LM, Bull NL, Buss DH, Wiggins R, Scuffam D, Jackson PA. (1984). Vitamin A activity in foods of animal origin. Journal of the Science of Food and Agriculture 3: 931–939.

Southgate DAT. (1969). Determination of carbohydrates in foods. II: Unavailable carbohydrates. Journal of the Science of Food and Agriculture 20: 331–335.

Spiller GA (ed.). (1993). CRC Handbook of Dietary Fiber in Human Nutrition. CRC Press, Boca Raton, FL.

Sunanda L, Sumathi S, Venkatasubbiah V. (1995). Relationship betwewn soil zinc, dietary zinc, and zinc nutritional status of humans. Plant Foods for Human Nutrition 48: 201–207.

Tamura T, Mizuno Y, Johnston KE, Jacob RA. (1997). Food folate assay with protease, α-amylase, and folate conjugase treatments. Journal of Agricultural Food Chemistry 45: 135–139.

Tan SP, Wenlock RW, Buss DH. (1984). Folic acid content of the diet in various types of British households. Human Nutrition: Applied Nutrition 38: 17–22.

Tan SP, Wenlock RW, Buss DH. (1985). Immigrant Foods: Second Supplement to McCance and Widdowson's "The Composition of Foods" (4th ed). Her Majesty's Stationery Office, London.

Theander O, Westerlund P, Åman P, Graham H. (1982). Studies on dietary fiber: a method for the chemical characterization of total dietary fiber. Journal of the

Science of Food and Agriculture 33: 340–344.

Tobin G, Carpenter KJ. (1978). The nutritional value of the dry bean (*Phaseolus vulgaris*): a literature review. Nutrition Abstracts and Reviews 48: 919–936.

Truswell AS, Bateson DJ, Madafiglio KC, Pennington JAT, Rand WM, Klensin JC. (1991). INFOODS guidelines for describing foods: a systematic approach to describing foods to facilitate international exchange of food composition data. Journal of Food Composition Analysis 4: 18–38.

Tseng M, Chakraborty H, Robinson DT, Mendez M, Kohlmeier L. (1997). Adjustment of iron intake for dietary enhancers and inhibitors in population studies: bioavailable iron in rural and urban residing Russian women and children. Journal of Nutrition 127: 1456–1468.

Tucker RE, Hinman WF, Holliday EG. (1946). The retention of thiamin and riboflavin in beef cuts during braising, frying and broiling. Journal of the American Dietetic Association 22: 877–881.

USDA (U.S. Department of Agriculture). (2002). Nutritive Value of Foods. Home and Garden Bulletin No. 72 (HG-72). U.S. Government Printing Office, Washington, DC.

USDA (U.S. Department of Agriculture). (2003a). USDA Table of Nutrient Retention Factors, Release 5. U.S. Government Printing Office, Washington, DC. http://www.nal.usda.gov/fnic/foodcomp

USDA (U.S. Department of Agriculture). (2003b). USDA National Nutrient Database for Standard Reference, Release 16. Nutrient Data Laboratory, U.S. Government Printing Office, Washington, DC. http://www.nal.usda.gov/fnic/foodcomp

Watt BK, Merrill AL, Pecot RK, Adams CF, Orr ML, Miller DF. (1963). Composition of Foods: Raw, Processed and Prepared. Agriculture Handbook No. 8. Agriculture Research Station, U.S. Department of Agriculture, Washington, DC.

West CE. (2000). Meeting requirements for vitamin A. Nutrition Reviews 58: 341–345.

West CE, Poortvliet EJ. (1993). The Carotenoid Content of Foods with Special Reference to Developing Countries: Vitamin A Field Support Project (VITAL). International Science and Technology Institute, Arlington, VA.

WHO (World Health Organization). (1996). Trace Elements in Human Nutrition and Health. World Health Organization, Geneva.

Yuk AW, Wheeler EF, Leppington IM. (1975). Variations in the apparent nutrient content of foods: a study of sampling error. British Journal of Nutrition 34: 391–398.

5

Measurement errors in dietary assessment

Random and systematic errors may occur during the measurement of food and nutrient intakes. The direction and extent of these errors vary with the method used and the population and nutrients studied. Both types of measurement error can be minimized by incorporating quality-control procedures during each stage of the measurement process.

Random measurement errors affect the reproducibility of the method (Chapter 6). They can be reduced by increasing the number of observations but cannot be entirely eliminated. In contrast, systematic measurement errors cannot be minimized by extending the number of observations. Systematic measurement errors are particularly important as they can introduce a significant bias into the results, which cannot be removed by subsequent statistical analysis unless a calibration study has been completed (Section 7.3.5).

The sources of both random and systematic errors are discussed in this chapter. Errors that can arise because of inappropriate study design and sampling of the target population are not considered. Readers are advised to consult a standard epidemiology text on these important issues. Errors associated with the compilation of nutrient composition data and the nutrient analysis of food items are discussed in Section 4.3.

5.1 Sources of measurement error

Many of the sources of error are similar in both household and individual food con-
sumption survey methods. The major errors are summarized below and then discussed in detail later in this chapter:

- **Nonresponse bias** in a dietary survey may result in an otherwise random sample of subjects not being representative of the studied population.
- **Respondent biases** result from the systematic overreporting or underreporting of foods consumed.
- **Interviewer biases** may occur if different interviewers probe for information to varying degrees, intentionally omit certain questions, or record the responses of subjects incorrectly.
- **Respondent memory lapses** may result in the unintentional omission or addition of foods in recall methods.
- **Incorrect estimation of portion size** can arise from respondents failing to quantify accurately the amount of food consumed, or from misconceptions of an "average" portion size.
- **Supplement usage** may be omitted from the dietary record or recall, causing errors in the calculated nutrient intakes.
- **Coding errors** can arise when portion size estimates are converted from household measures into grams and when food items are assigned codes (e.g., 2% milk is coded as whole milk).
- **Mistakes in the handling of mixed dishes** may result in incorrect estimates of their nutrient content per se, as well as errors in their assignment to a specific food group.

5.2 Assessment and control of measurement errors

Random and systematic measurement errors can be minimized by incorporating various quality-control procedures into each stage of the dietary assessment method. These can include training and retraining sessions for the interviewers and coders, standardization of interviewing techniques and questionnaires, pretesting of questionnaires, and administration of a pilot study prior to the survey. Each procedure in the dietary assessment method must be checked continuously to ensure compliance with standardized protocols.

Random errors, unlike systematic errors, can be minimized by increasing the number of observations. Random errors may occur across all subjects and all days. In contrast, systematic errors may be associated with only some respondents (e.g., obese or elderly subjects), specific interviewers, or certain foods (e.g., alcohol). Concerns about the effect of measurement errors on the relative risk estimates for disease have led increasingly to the use of calibration studies to quantify systematic measurement errors. The assessment of the reproducibility (Chapter 6) and validity (Chapter 7) of the dietary methods used is now essential, especially for cross-country comparisons and nutrition surveillance (Buzzard and Sievert, 1994).

5.2.1 Nonresponse bias

A lack of response or poor compliance from a specific subset of otherwise randomly selected subjects may result in a significant nonresponse bias and can occur in all types of nutritional assessment systems. This may be critical because the people who refuse to take part in the survey, or alternatively who drop out of the intervention, may have characteristics (e.g., dietary intakes or requirements) that differ from those of the responders. For example, busy working mothers may be more likely to be nonresponders in a dietary survey than those who are retired. Alternatively, in a food-for-work program, some of the participants whose nutritional status improves may

then drop out of the program resulting in an underestimate of the impact of the program (Habicht et al., 1984). In such circumstances, the results may be misleading.

Efforts should be made to minimize the nonresponse rate. Strategies include simplifying the dietary assessment methods, carrying out mailed or telephoned reminders in surveillance studies, and training interviewers to convey warmth, understanding, and trust. "Nonresponders" should be identified and examined as a group to ensure that they do not differ significantly from participants agreeing to take part, and that they are not associated with a particular interviewer. For example, in the EURONUT-SENECA project, the average participation rate was only 51%. Nevertheless, based on a study of nonparticipants, bias due to selective participation was small and insignificant for many of the variables examined (van't Hof et al., 1991).

In contrast, in the 1982–1984 Hispanic Health and Nutrition Examination Survey (HHANES), there was a 24% nonresponse rate in the examination phase which was related to socioeconomic status, sex, and age. The U.S. 1987–1988 National Food Consumption Survey had low representation from both economically poor and rich households, as well as households with working female heads, and 14–24 y old participants. Attempts should always be made to identify the reasons for nonresponse in national nutrition surveys, especially those related to age and culture, and to adjust for any nonresponse bias by reweighting, where possible (Rowland and Forthofer, 1993).

5.2.2 Respondent biases

During a survey or intervention, respondent biases may arise if the respondent misunderstands what the interviewer has requested, receives nonverbal cues to the "right answers" from the interviewer, or has a need to give "socially desirable" answers. As an example, food frequency questionnaires that focus on desirable or undesirable foods may be a source of respondent biases. These can be

The existence of underreporting can be assessed by comparing:

Total energy expenditure with the reported energy intake, using doubly labeled water techniques (Schoeller, 1990) (Section 7.3.1)

Inferred energy requirements with reported energy intake, both being expressed as multiples of basal metabolic rate (i.e., the Goldberg cutoff technique) (Goldberg et al., 1991) (Section 7.3.2)

Energy intake required to maintain body weight with self-reported intakes

Urinary cation excretion with self-reported intakes (Section 7.3.6) (Zhang et al., 2000)

Box 5.1. Methods for assessing the combined effect of all forms of underreporting of energy intake (total underreporting).

of particular concern if the data are being used to monitor the effectiveness of intervention or education programs (Buzzard and Sievert, 1994). Such biases may be systematic and associated with persons with specific characteristics (e.g., obesity) or random and observed only in some subjects on random days. For example, if the study population is stratified by weight status based on body mass index, and the overweight persons in the population tend to underreport their food intake, then there will be a systematic bias in the mean intakes of the overweight subgroup (Beaton et al., 1997).

Underreporting energy intakes

Underreporting is a common form of respondent bias and has been documented in several national surveys in North America, Europe, and the United Kingdom (Beaton et al., 1997; Briefel et al., 1997; Price et al., 1997; Heerstrass et al., 1998; Zhang et al., 2000; Johansson et al., 2001). For example, in NHANES III, 18% of men and 28% of women were classified as energy intake underreporters (Briefel et al., 1997).

Underreporting of usual energy intakes can involve both underrecording and undereating. Underrecording is a failure to record all the items consumed during the study period, or underestimating their amounts. It has been

defined as a discrepancy between reported energy intake and measured energy expenditure without any change in body mass. Undereating occurs when respondents eat less than usual or less than required to maintain body weight, and is accompanied by a decline in body mass (Goris and Westerterp, 1999). The relative importance of underrecording and undereating has been investigated by some researchers, including Goris and Westerterp (1999), Bathalon et al. (2000), Goris et al. (2000), and McCrory et al. (2002). A water balance technique based on an estimate of water loss with deuterium-labeled water has been developed to distinguish between these two errors; details are given in Goris and Westerterp (1999). In a study of obese men, total underreporting was explained by both underrecording and undereating (Goris et al., 2001), whereas when highly motivated lean women were studied, only undereating was observed (Goris and Westerterp, 1999).

The existence of total underreporting of energy intake has been confirmed using several different techniques (Box 5.1). As an example, community studies compiled by Livingstone and Black (2003) are summarized in Figure 5.1. These show the association of energy intake (EI) and energy expenditure

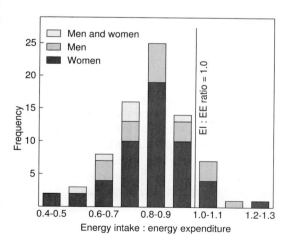

Figure 5.1: Frequency distribution of the ratio of energy intake (EI) to energy expenditure (EE) by sex in doubly labeled water studies of energy expenditure. Data from Livingstone and Black, Journal of Nutrition 133: 895S–920S, 2003, with permission of the American Society for Nutritional Sciences.

(EE) (based on doubly labeled water). The distribution of EI:EE values is not centered about the line EI:EE = 1.0 and this almost certainly indicates significant underreporting of intakes. A more detailed discussion is given in Section 7.3.1.

Three of the methods shown in Box 5.1 for assessing underreporting of energy intake depend on the assumption that energy intake must equal energy expenditure when body weight is stable (Livingstone and Black, 2003). The fourth method, urinary excretion of cations, has more limited use as a marker of energy intake because the method has a weaker relationship with dietary intake (Bingham et al., 1995).

In the future, alternative ways of measuring energy expenditure, and thus of detecting energy intake underreporting, may be employed, including heart-rate monitors, accelerometers, and/or physical activity questionnaires (Livingstone and Black, 2003).

The characteristics of energy-intake underreporters have been the subject of several studies, which have been reviewed in detail by Livingstone and Black (2003). In most of these studies, no distinction between underrecording and undereating has been made. The factors associated with low-energy reporting include weight status, age and sex effects, socioeconomic effects, health-related activities, behavioral effects, and psychological effects. These are discussed in turn below.

Weight status is the single most consistent factor related to underreporting: the probability that a subject will underreport generally increases as BMI increases (Briefel et al., 1997; Johansson et al., 1998).

Age and sex have both been associated with energy underreporting: women and older persons tend to be more at risk (Livingstone and Black, 2003), although inconsistencies have been observed (de Vries et al., 1994; Johnson et al., 1994).

Socioeconomic status does not have a consistent effect on energy underreporting (Rutishauser et al., 1994; Lafay et al., 1997). In

some cases, cultural differences may account for these inconsistencies. For example, older African Americans often have a more relaxed attitude to body image and body weight than do Caucasian Americans (Tomoyasu et al., 2000).

Health-related activities, including smoking and dieting, have often been linked with energy underreporting (Heitmann, 1993; Ballard-Barbash et al., 1996; Pryer et al., 1997; Braam et al., 1998). For example, those who practice dietary restraint, as measured by the Eating Inventory of Stunkard and Messick (1985), also typically have a lower reported energy intake for a given body weight than do unrestrained eaters (Bathalon et al., 2000).

Behavioral effects warrant more attention, including the extent to which the burden of recording the food intake may be responsible for energy underreporting associated with undereating (Goris and Westerterp, 1999). In addition, research on ways in which the behavior of the investigators and the nature of the testing environment itself may unwittingly contribute to underreporting is urgently required. In some postsurvey focus group interviews, subjects have admitted altering their eating pattern during the survey; reasons include inconvenience, embarrassment and guilt (Macdiarmid and Blundell, 1997; Mela and Aaron, 1997).

Psychological effects, including those linked to eating disorders, have been assessed with a variety of instruments to measure their impact on energy underreporting (Stunkard and Messick, 1985; van Strien et al., 1986). Again, no consistent results have been noted (Bingham et al., 1995; Bathalon et al., 2000). Associations between energy underreporting and depression (using the Beck depression inventory) (Kretsch et al., 1999), social desirability scores (Taren et al., 1999), and recent emotional problems (Price et al., 1997) have also been examined, with mixed results.

Specific foods or beverages may be selectively underreported in a way that is still not well understood. Investigators have suggested that differential underreporting can arise from some beverages or foods being perceived as "bad," such as alcohol, cakes, cookies, sugar, candies, and fats. In contrast, meat, fish, vegetables, salad, and fruit are perceived as "good" foods (Livingstone et al., 1990; Heitmann and Lissner, 1995; Pryer et al., 1997; Tonstad et al., 1999). In a U.K. study (Bingham et al., 1995), a significant difference in the reporting of cakes, sugars, fat, and breakfast cereals was observed between underreporters and the other respondents, compared to the reporting of bread, potatoes, meat, vegetables, and fruit.

In a U.S. study, those food items most often underreported were cakes and pies, savory snacks, cheese, potatoes, meat mixtures, soft drinks, fat-type spreads, and condiments (Krebs-Smith et al., 2000). Furthermore, in the U.S. National Food Consumption Survey and NHANES, intakes of alcohol for adults were underreported, compared with estimates from alcohol disappearance data (Section 2.2.1). In the NHANES III survey, however, the use of private interviews and weekend data collection reportedly improved the estimates of alcohol intake (Briefel et al., 1997).

There is also some evidence that respondents may omit certain items such as snacks from the diet (Poppitt et al., 1998), or, alternatively, items that seem too troublesome to record (Sichert-Hellert et al., 1998), although this trend has not been consistent (Goris et al., 2000). A detailed summary of those foods found to be selectively underreported is given in Livingstone and Black (2003). Data from surveys conducted in Sweden and the Netherlands (Becker and Welten, 2001) suggest that in national nutrition surveys, both general and selective underreporting of foods occur.

The selective underreporting of specific foods or alterations in food choices (or both) will affect the calculated intakes of specific macro- and micronutrients, as well as energy. This has not been extensively investigated. It appears that underreporters tend to record lower intakes of fats and higher intakes of protein and carbohydrates as a percentage of total energy (Briefel et al., 1997; Voss et al., 1998).

As expected, the reported intakes of micronutrients are usually lower for energy underreporters. However, some differences in the micronutrient density of the diets of energy underreporters relative to other subjects suggest that the reported lower intakes do not necessarily arise from underreporting of the diet as a whole. A summary of studies comparing the nutrient densities of diets of energy underreporters with those of other subjects is given in Livingstone and Black (2003).

Overreporting of energy intakes

Although generally not as prevalent as underreporting, overreporting of energy intake also occurs (Figure 5.1). In the 1990 U.K. survey of British adults, the percentage of "overreporters" was small (Gregory et al., 1990). Nevertheless, the two different types of inaccurate reporting should both be considered when identifying inaccurate energy intake reports. Currently, more emphasis is given to identifying underreporters than overreporters of energy intake.

Social desirability and approval biases

Social desirability (the tendency to respond in such a way as to avoid criticism) and social approval (the tendency to seek praise) are two prominent sources of bias that may occur in dietary assessment methods. Social desirability bias may be intentional or a form of self-deception (Roth et al., 1986).

Worsley et al. (1984) have recommended the use of a social desirability scale in dietary surveys to identify and perhaps control for social desirability variables (Table 5.1). They suggested that reported intakes of certain foods such as fresh fruits and vegetables and sweet foods are particularly susceptible to social approval needs and hence are a potential source of systematic bias. There is some evidence that gender may influence social desirability and social approval biases (Hebert et al., 1995, 1997), and their possible existence should be investigated further.

I rarely eat snacks between meals. (T)
I always brush my teeth after every meal. (T)
I hardly ever eat candies or chocolate. (T)
I often watch TV or read a newspaper
    whilst eating a meal. (F)
There have been many occasions when I
    have not washed my hands before eating. (F)
I never drink alcohol when I'm by myself. (T)
I often find myself eating food in a hurry. (F)
My table manners at home are as good as
    when I eat out in a restaurant. (T)
I try to avoid eating take-away foods. (T)
There have been few occasions when I
    have "raided the refrigerator." (F)
I usually eat everything on my plate. (T)
I have never been "really drunk" in my life. (T)

Table 5.1: Statements used to assess attitudes to food and drink. The letters (T) or (F) after each statement indicate whether the true or false answer was the socially desirable response. From Worsley et al. (1984) with permission.

5.2.3 Interviewer biases

In all dietary studies, the experimental design should allow assessment of any potential interviewer bias so that statistical methods can be applied to correct for this source of dietary measurement error (Slimani et al., 2000). Interviewer biases may include errors caused by incorrect use of probing questions, incorrect recording of responses, intentional omissions, biases associated with the interview setting, distractions, confidentiality and anonymity of the respondent, and the degree of rapport between the interviewer and the respondent (Fowler and Mangione, 1990).

Interviewer biases can be random across days and subjects, and/or systematic for a specific interviewer, or they may exist as an interaction between certain interviewers and certain respondents (Anderson, 1986). The biases are best reduced by standardizing the 24-h recall with microcomputer-based dietary interviews (Section 3.2.4).

The most common approach to assess interviewer bias has been to compare nutrient intakes calculated from multiple interviews carried out independently on the same subjects during the same 24-h eating period, using different trained interviewers. Frank et al. (1984) used this method to investigate the effect of interviewer recording practices on calculated nutrient intakes. They examined the extent of agreement of food descriptors, food quantities, codes assigned, and calculated nutrient intakes. Their results indicated difficulties in quantifying selected food items such as meat and sweets. Significant differences in calculated intakes of energy, fat, and unsaturated fat, resulting from differences in coding snack foods, were also found.

A multiple interview approach was also used successfully by the National Heart, Lung and Blood Institute for their Lipid Research Clinic Program (Beaton et al., 1979). These investigators concluded that the interviewer had no effect on the calculated energy, protein, and lipid intakes of the subjects. In contrast, despite rigorous efforts to standardize a computer-assisted 24-h recall method used in the European prospective investigation into cancer and nutrition (EPIC), an interviewer effect was observed in certain countries among the 90 interviewers involved in the collection of approximately 37,000 24-h recalls (Slimani et al., 2000), although not across centers from the same country. In this study, the interviewer effect was based on mean energy intake per interviewer, taking into account the confounding effects of age, body mass index, energy requirements, weekday, season, special diet, and physical activity.

Interviewer bias should always be considered as a potential source of error in dietary investigations (Wynder, 1994). A carefully designed and standardized interviewing protocol, preferably computer administered, may help minimize the effect. When several interviewers are employed, the assignment of interviewers-respondents-days should be randomized, and the interviewers should be trained to anticipate and recognize potential sources of distortion and bias (Wakefield, 1966). Value judgments by the interviewer should always be avoided (Hughes, 1986).

In dietary surveys involving multiple ethnic or cultural groups, it is advisable to use interviewers familiar with each language and culture. Care must also be taken to ensure that individual interviewers are not assigned just to specific ethnic or cultural groups, as interviewer and group effects can become confounded. Special attention must be given to the way the questions are asked, and how people think about and describe foods and amounts consumed in each ethnic or cultural group (Hankin and Wilkens, 1994). This will necessitate training in focused ethnographic methods (Buzzard and Sievert, 1994). In general, female interviewers are preferred because they generally have the best knowledge of foods, their ingredients, preparation and processing, and portion sizes.

5.2.4 Respondent memory lapses

Memory failure can affect recall methods in two ways: the respondent may fail to recall foods actually consumed (errors of omission) or may report foods that were not consumed during the recalled day (errors of commission). Both sources of error have been reported in several studies in which 24-h recalls were compared with unobtrusive preweighed or recorded measurements on the same day (Krantzler et al., 1982; Karvetti and Knuts, 1985; Brown et al., 1990). Certain characteristics of the subjects such as gender (Johnson et al., 1994; Briefel et al., 1997), age (Karvetti and Knuts, 1985; van Staveren et al., 1994), and level of education or ethnic group (Klesges et al., 1995), as well as the general setting of the interview (Krall et al., 1988), may also interfere with the cognitive processes of retrieving and recalling information.

The normal way to minimize errors generated by memory lapses in a 24-h recall is to use multiple-pass interviewing techniques (Section 3.1.1), "probing" questions, standardized "prompts," or memory aids such as food models. These are discussed in turn below.

Multiple-pass dietary interviews, automated by the use of a microcomputer, are now used in many national surveys. This combination minimizes the omission of possible forgotten foods and standardizes the level of detail for describing common foods and the methods used to elicit specific details

for certain food items (Briefel et al., 1997; MOH,1997; Slimani et al., 2000).

In the EPIC study, a computer-assisted 24-h diet recall method using the software program EPIC-SOFT was developed to standardize the cognitive memory aids used in the first stage (called the quick list) of the multiple-pass recall. The structure and functions of EPIC-SOFT are described in detail by Slimani et al. (1999). Similar techniques were used in the CSFII and NHANES III (NCHS, 1994; Tippett and Cypel, 1997) and New Zealand national surveys (MOH, 1997; Parnell et al., 2003).

Probing questions and standard "prompts" reduce memory lapses. For example, probing increased reported dietary intakes of hospital patients assessed by 24-h recalls by 25% compared to intakes obtained without probing (Campbell and Dodds, 1967). In a U.S. study of fourth-grade school children, the accuracy in reporting foods eaten for school lunch 90 min earlier increased to 100% after responding to prompts for additional items (Domel, 1997). In the 1994–1996 CSFII, snack foods and beverages, including alcoholic beverages, were the most common extra food items remembered after prompting. Probes are also useful for food frequency questionnaires, a method that relies mainly on generic memory.

Memory aids can also help reduce memory lapses. The aids may consist of plastic or clay simulated foods, actual foods, natural-sized colored paintings, or photographs. When these aids are available as a range of graduated portions, they have the additional advantage of reducing portion size measurement errors. In such cases, a series of graduated food models or photographs of a range of portion sizes can be used. Details are given in Section 3.2.3.

In general, food items that contribute significantly to the main part of a meal are far better remembered than condiments, salad dressings, and so on. Guthrie (1984) reported that for one in six respondents, salad dressings were forgotten.

Minimizing the time period between the actual food intake and its recall will reduce respondent memory lapses in recall methods (Smith et al., 1991). Twenty-four hours is the time period most frequently selected for memory-based recall procedures. As a check on the recall ability of the respondents, duplicate recalls, collected independently by two trained interviewers for the same 24-h period, can be obtained. Such a procedure on children demonstrated errors ranging from 9% to 21% (Frank et al., 1977).

The accurate assessment of dietary intake in children is especially challenging, and is of increasing importance with the growing concerns about childhood obesity. Children tend to have diets that are highly variable from day to day, and their food habits often change markedly. Research on the development and timing of specific cues that may help children report their diets more accurately, applying a cognitive-processing approach, is emerging (Baranowski and Domel, 1994).

Examples of the most commonly reported retrieval responses indicating how children remember items they have eaten are shown in Table 5.2. In this study, children appeared to recall most readily foods they liked the most. Whether the retrieval responses for children differ with age, the various components of a meal, number of foods consumed, ethnicity, sex, and time period between the actual intake and recall have not been extensively investigated (Domel, 1997).

Category and item remembered	Responses indicating how student remembered item
Visual imagery	
Corn	"It was yellow."
Green salad	"The cucumber was round and has seeds in it ...the carrots [were] all shredded up like [they] came from a salad shooter or something ...then the lettuce was just a little leaf ...tomatoes were sliced up in big cubes ...onions were curved."
Usual practice	
Milk	"We have milk every day"
Green salad	"Every time we have pizza, they serve salad."
Behavior chaining	
Mashed potatoes	"I put a little bit of some ...potatoes on my tray, so I put them on my nuggets and tried that with the honey dip."
Cornbread	" ...was the second thing I ate."
Preference	
Low-fat milk	"It was good."
Jello	"It wasn't good ...I didn't like it."

Table 5.2: Examples of the most commonly reported retrieval response categories. From Domel, American Journal of Clinical Nutrition 65: 1148S–1152S, 1997 © Am J Clin Nutr. American Society for Clinical Nutrition.

Warren et al. (2003) concluded that children aged 5–7 y were unable to provide an accurate dietary recall of their school lunch, especially when they consumed a dinner provided by the school rather than eating their own packed lunch, as shown in Figure 5.2. Nevertheless, prompts and cues enhanced recall by all children in this study. Main dishes were remembered best by the children; leftovers were not readily reported. A series of recommendations and suggestions for future studies on children have been compiled by these investigators and are shown in Box 5.2 (Warren et al., 2003). There is no doubt that more work is needed on methods to determine more accurately what children aged less than 8 y are eating.

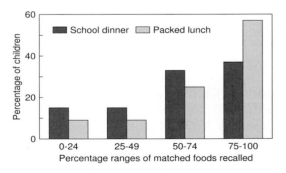

Figure 5.2: Distribution of percentage of correct recall in children eating packed lunch and school dinner. Data from Warren et al., Public Health Nutrition 6: 41–47, 2003, with permission of the authors.

A **free uninterrupted recall** of foods eaten should be allowed when interviewing children aged 5–7 y. Prompts should be employed at the end of the recall.

The main dish and their familiarity with and preference for the foods recalled should be the focus of the child's recall. Prompts should not overburden the child.

Side dishes, fruit, vegetables, and sweets may need specific inquiry.

Leftover food should be inquired about afterwards in a nondirective manner.

The time lag between the meal and the recall, and environmental factors, may both impact on the accuracy of recall and their effects need to be established.

Portion size estimation, using aids appropriate to the cognitive development of the child, should be carefully assessed.

Box 5.2. Recommendations and suggestions to aid the recall of food eaten by children. From Warren et al., Public Health Nutrition 6: 41–47, 2003, with permission of the authors.

5.2.5 Incorrect estimation of portion size consumed

The errors associated with quantifying the portion of food consumed are probably the largest measurement error in most dietary assessment methods. They can arise from respondents failing to quantify accurately the amount of food consumed, or from misconceptions of an "average" portion size. Unfortunately, very few studies have attempted to quantify these sources of error.

Respondents differ in their ability to accurately estimate portion sizes visually. In general, such discrepancies appear to be independent of age, body weight, social status, and gender of the respondent, but they do vary with the type and size of food (Young and Nestle, 1995). Large errors may occur, for example, for estimates of foods high in volume but low in weight (Gittelsohn et al., 1994) and for intact cuts of meat of irregular shape (Godwin et al., 2001). Furthermore, respondents appear to have greater difficulty estimating the size of large portions than they do small portions, irrespective of their body weight (Young and Nestle, 1995).

Guthrie (1984) assessed the accuracy with which young adults could describe portion sizes of foods consumed, in terms of common household measures or weights. No food models were used in this study. The ability of the respondents to describe the amounts of food consumed was poor. For 13 food items, from 6% to 75% of respondents estimated portion sizes that varied by more than 50% of their actual weight. Of the respondents, 26% consistently over- or underestimated all food items in the meal. Reported intakes of orange juice and milk were closer to actual intakes than reported amounts of foods such as breakfast cereals and butter.

5.2.6 Measurement aids to quantify portion sizes

Several types of portion-size measurement aids have been developed for use in dietary studies, in an effort to enhance the accuracy of portion size estimates when weighing methods cannot be used. They have been classified into two- and three-dimensional memory aids as listed in Box 5.3.

The measurement aids most commonly used are household measures, drawings and photographs, and food models employing abstract shapes and geometrical models. In low-income countries, salted replicas of actual staple foods may be useful (Gibson and Ferguson, 1999). In all cases, measurement aids

Two-dimensional memory aids

- Drawings of real foods, abstract shapes, household measures
- Food photographs
- Computer graphics
- Food package labels

Three-dimensional memory aids

- Household measures
- Real food samples
- Food replicas (models of real foods)
- Food models (abstract models)

Box 5.3. A classification of memory aids into two- and three-dimensional types. From Cypel et al., Validity of portion-size measurement aids: a review. Journal of the American Dietetic Association 97: 289–292, 1997 © with permission from Elsevier.

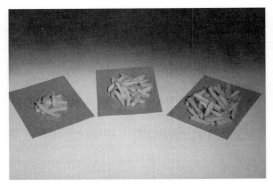

Chipped fried potatoes

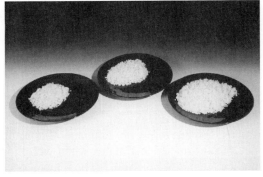

Boiled rice

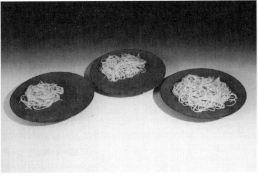

Noodles

Figure 5.3: Photographs of three different foodstuffs with small, medium and large portion sizes.

that depict a range of portion sizes should be used to avoid the tendency to "direct" responses; details are given in Section 3.2.3.

The effects of portion-size measurement aids on the accuracy of the quantity estimates are sometimes difficult to interpret. Some studies have not provided clear descriptions of the portion-size measurement aids

(Kirkcaldy-Hargreaves et al., 1980; Posner et al., 1992; Kuehneman et al., 1994). Others have not examined the errors specifically associated with the portion-size measurement aids, but instead have assessed errors associated with the combination of procedures used in the dietary methods (Pietinen et al., 1988).

Photographs are being increasingly used to assist respondents in estimating portion sizes (Nelson et al., 1994); several approaches have been used, and are discussed in Section 3.2.2. Photographs that depict a range of portion sizes (Figure 5.3) are often used to aid in the estimation of portion size in 24-h recalls and food frequency questionnaires (Bohlscheid-Thomas et al., 1997; Slimani et al., 2000).

Photographs for quantifying portion sizes should be standardized with respect to several factors; these are discussed in Section 3.2.1. They should also portray the range of portion sizes consumed by the subjects of the study (Lucas et al., 1995). In the multi-country EPIC study, for example, the choice of the smallest and largest portions of each series of photographs for each food was based on data collected during the EPIC pilot study phase (van Kappel et al., 1994). When used in this way, photographs appear to be associated with relatively small errors in portion size estimation compared to the use of a single photograph (Nelson et al., 1994). Nevertheless, potentially important confounders such as age, sex, and body mass index (BMI) should be investigated when estimating food intakes using photographs (Nelson et al., 1996).

Graduated food models and household measures have been used in several national food consumption surveys (Section 3.2.3). Cleveland and Ingwersen (2001) compared the portion-size reporting accuracy of two-dimensional (2-D) food models and a range of 3-D measurement aids now used as a tool in the dietary component of NHANES. The 2-D food models are 32 life-size drawings of household vessels (glasses, mugs, bowls), abstract shapes (mounds and spreads), and geometric models (circles, a grid, wedges, and thickness bars). The 3-D measurement aids are actual measuring cups, spoons, and a ruler. Overall, both the 2-D and the 3-D guides helped generate relatively good estimates of food amounts, although in this study, more accurate estimates were obtained on average with the 2-D than the 3-D guides, especially for mounded foods. Other investigators have reported that 2-D pictures are just as effective as 3-D models (Pietinen et al., 1988; Posner et al., 1992).

Portion-size estimates for meat are especially difficult because of the irregular shape of intact cuts of meat. Indeed, in a study by Weber et al. (1997), errors in the estimation of meat (steak) portions of up to 80% were found. Godwin et al. (2001) have investigated the use of various portion-size estimation aids for meat (e.g., bean bag, peg board, ruler, sausage diagram, and size grid). The greatest source of error was noted for estimates of thickness rather than length or width, attributed to perceptual factors. Large portion-size estimation errors (30% – 73.2%) were reported for portion-size estimates of intact meat with more than one irregular dimension (e.g., ribs), irrespective of the measurement aids used to estimate portion sizes. Because of these inaccuracies, the researchers recommended the use of predetermined standardized weights based on portion-size categories (i.e., small, medium, and large) for estimating intact irregular cuts of meat such as ribs. For intact, more regular, meat portions, a ruler should be used to estimate length and width, together with food-specific, standardized measures for thickness. For link-type sausages, use of a sausage diagram instead of a ruler, is recommended (Godwin et al., 2001).

More research comparing the accuracy of portion-size measurement aids in controlled testing environments is urgently required. Nelson and Haraldsdóttir (1998a,b) provide details on the design of such studies, with particular reference to the use of photographs for quantifying portion sizes. Use of such studies will assist in identifying both foods that cannot be measured reliably, and population subgroups for whom the use of 2-D drawings or photographs is inappropriate.

In addition to training interviewers (Section 5.2.3), some studies have investigated whether it is helpful to train respondents to use portion-size measurement aids such as graduated food models or household measures. In general, the use of short group training sessions for respondents using food models or household measures should be encouraged. Training sessions enhance the ability of both children and adults to estimate food portion sizes accurately, although for children, more than one training session is probably necessary (Bolland et al., 1990; Weber et al., 1999). Training using a combination of food models and life-sized food photographs may be best (Howat et al., 1994).

Quantifying standard reference portion sizes

Semiquantitative food frequency questionnaires, used to rank individuals according to food or nutrient intake, often specify a standard reference portion size for each specific food. Typically this is intended to represent the median amount consumed during a single meal. The values may be generated from country-specific national nutrition surveys (e.g., Block et al., 1986) or other large surveys (e.g., Willett et al., 1985), as shown in Table 5.3. Respondents appear to have difficulty relating what they consumed to such predefined standard reference portion sizes, (Friedenreich et al., 1992), and inconsistent results and large errors have been reported (Willett, 1994).

Many factors affect actual food portion sizes, including age, gender, activity level, the appetite of the individual, household utensils used, and where and when the food is obtained and eaten. Table 5.4 compares the actual weights of portion sizes of certain foods (e.g., slice of bread, butter, cheese) and the volume of various household utensils (e.g., teacup and drinking glass) used in 30 households with standard reference portion sizes used in the Netherlands at that

	Standard reference serving		Standard reference portion size	
	USDA (1992) Pyramid	FDA (1993) Food label	Food frequency questionnaires Willett et al. (1985)	Block et al. (1986)
Grains and cereals				
Bread	1 slice	1–3 slices	Slice	2 slices
Crackers	3–4 small	5–18	1	3
Rice, cooked	$^1/_2$ cup	1 cup	1 cup	$^3/_4$ cup
Cereal, ready-to-eat	1 oz	$^1/_2 - 1^1/_4$ cup	1 cup	1 medium bowl
Cereal, cooked	$^1/_2$ cup	1 cup	1 cup	1 medium bowl
Fruit				
Whole fruit	1 medium	—	1	1 medium
Juice	$^3/_4$ cup	8 oz	Small glass	6-oz glass
Fresh, frozen, or canned	$^1/_2$ cup	$^1/_2$ cup	$^1/_2$ cup	$^1/_2$ cup
Vegetables				
Raw leafy	1 cup	—	Serving	1 medium bowl
Carrots, raw	$^1/_2$ cup	—	$^1/_2$ cup or 2–4 sticks	$^1/_2$ cup
Potato	$^1/_2$ cup	—	1 or 1 cup	1 or $^1/_2$ cup
French fries	10	3 oz	4 oz	$^3/_4$ cup
Tomato juice	$^3/_4$ cup	8 oz	Small glass	6 oz
Meat				
Beef	2–3 oz	—	4–6 oz	4 oz
Hamburger	3 oz	—	1 patty	1 medium
Poultry	2–3 oz	—	4–6 oz	2 small or 1 large piece

Table 5.3: Examples of standard reference serving sizes and standard reference portion sizes. Note that in some cases, FDA food label standard serving sizes vary by weight or size of items. From Young and Nestle (1995) Nutrition Reviews 53, 149–158, ILSI Press.

time (van Staveren and Hulsof, 1980). Results emphasize the large between-subject variation in portion sizes for these Dutch households. Even in institutional settings such as a school canteen, the actual weights of food served can vary by as much as 18% (Comstock and Symington, 1982).

Guthrie (1984) compared the amount of food selected as a usual portion size by young adults, in relation to the U.S. standard ref-

	n	Mean	Med.	Range	Std.
Slice of bread (g)	30	30	30	25–38	30
Butter/margarine (g)	60	4	4	2–12	5
Gouda cheese (g)	34	21	20	9–42	20
Teaspoon sugar (g)	43	5	4	2–13	3
Teacup (mL)	30	136	128	110–175	125
Drinking glass (mL)	19	184	173	85–300	150

Table 5.4: The mean, median (Med.), range, and standard size (Std.) of portions of bread, butter, cheese, and sugar and two household measures. From van Staveren and Burema, Näringsforskning 29: 38–42, 1985.

erence portion sizes at that time. The latter were based on median portions derived from USDA Nationwide Food Consumption Survey data (Pao et al., 1982). Items such as butter on toast, sugar on cereal, milk as a beverage, and tossed salad corresponded closely with standards, whereas others such as dry cereals, orange juice, and fruit salad did not. Men tended to select larger portions than women.

In view of these findings, the use of standard reference portion sizes in food frequency questionnaires is still hotly debated. Some investigators have argued that because variations in food intake are mainly determined by frequency of consumption, obtaining information on portion sizes in semiquantitative food frequency questionnaires is not always justified (Samet et al., 1984; Noethlings et al., 2003). Others recommend the use of small, medium, and large portions, based on age- and gender-specific median portion sizes as standards (Cummings et al., 1987). Japanese

Food	FGP serving sizes	20–29 years		40–49 years		60+ years	
		Men	Women	Men	Women	Men	Women
		Number of FGP servings					
Apples, raw	1 medium	1.0	1.0	1.0	1.0	0.9	0.9
Orange juice	$^3/_4$ cup	1.3	1.3	1.3	1.1	1.1	1.0
String beans, cooked	$^1/_2$ cup	1.5	1.0	1.0	1.0	1.4	1.0
Broccoli, cooked	$^1/_2$ cup	1.3	1.0	1.6	1.3	0.8	1.1
Fluid milk	1 cup	1.0	0.9	1.0	0.7	0.8	0.7
Cheese	1 $^1/_2$ oz	0.7	0.6	0.7	0.7	0.7	0.7
White bread	1 slice	2.0	1.6	1.9	1.7	1.8	1.5
Rice, cooked	$^1/_2$ cup	1.7	1.5	1.6	1.3	1.4	1.2
RTE cereals	1 oz	2.1	1.5	1.8	1.3	1.7	1.2
Pasta, cooked	$^1/_2$ cup	2.2	1.5	2.0	1.5	1.7	1.5
Muffins	1 oz (approx.)	2.3	1.9	2.1	1.8	2.0	2.0
		Number of 1-ounce meat equivalents					
Beef steak, cooked	1 oz	5.7	4.9	5.3	4.3	4.9	3.8
Ham, cured cooked	1 oz	1.9	1.5	2.0	1.6	2.0	1.9
Eggs, fried	1 large	1.8	1.4	1.8	1.0	1.6	0.9
Dry beans, cooked	$^1/_2$ cup	1.9	1.0	1.5	1.0	1.3	1.0

Table 5.5: Comparison of the median number of food guide pyramid (FGP) servings consumed by men and women in the three age groups in the U.S. Continuing Survey of Food Intakes by Individuals. From Hogbin et al., Nutrition Insights No. 11, 1999, USDA.

investigators have cautioned that the relative contributions of within- and between-subject variations in portion size vary among food items, so that whether separate questions on portion size should be included will depend on the food groups relevant to the diet–disease association being studied (Tsubono et al., 1997).

There is some confusion in the literature between the use of standard reference portion sizes and standard reference serving sizes. Two examples of standard reference serving sizes established for use in the Food Guide Pyramid (FGP) by USDA (USDA, 1992), and for food labels by the U.S. Food and Drug Administration (FDA, 1993), are shown in Table 5.3, and compared with standard reference portion sizes generated by Willett et al. (1985) and Block et al. (1986). Inconsistencies occur between the standard reference serving sizes and standard reference portion sizes.

Table 5.5 depicts the typical amounts of selected foods, expressed in the number of food guide pyramid servings (FGPS), consumed by three age groups of adult men and women in the USDA Continuing Survey of Food Intakes by Individuals (CSFII). For men, the number of FGPS consumed at each eating occasion is greater on average than those for women, consistent with their larger energy needs. In general, the number of FGPS consumed decreases with age, especially for meats and grain products. These findings highlight the need to compile different standard portion sizes for each specific food, based on age and sex.

5.2.7 Omission of information on nutrient supplement usage

The correct recording of dietary supplement use in any nutrition survey conducted in industrialized countries is now critically important. In the United States, for example, approximately 40% of the population sampled during NHANES III between 1988 and 1994 used a dietary supplement during the month prior to the interview (Ervin et al., 1999). In New Zealand, 51% of the population surveyed reportedly consumed a vitamin or mineral supplement at some time during the year 1996 to 1997 (Russell et al., 1999).

Table 5.6 shows the mean daily iron intakes by females from diet alone and from diet plus supplements in NHANES III (Heimbach, 2001). These results emphasize that failure to collect accurate data on supplement use may result in a systematic underestimate of intakes of certain nutrients, and thus an overestimate of the prevalence of nutrient inadequacy.

Discrepancies exist in the terminology and the methods used to measure dietary supplements and the criteria used to define dietary supplement users, thus limiting comparisons across studies (Brownie and Myers, 2004). In addition, the optimal time period over which dietary supplement usage should be recorded has not yet been established. In NHANES III, detailed information on the frequency and amount of seven categories of vitamin and mineral supplements used over the past month were collected (Balluz et al., 2000; Briefel et al., 2000), whereas in the New Zealand national survey, data on the level and type of vitamin and mineral supplements used only during the preceding 24 h are available (MOH, 1997; Russell et al., 1999).

The U.K. National Diet and Nutrition Sur-

Population	Mean daily iron intake from diet alone	Mean daily iron intake from diet plus supplements
Age 9–13 y	13.7	15.0
Age 14–18 y	12.1	13.6
Age 19–30 y	12.8	18.2
Age 31–50 y	12.8	18.9
Age 51–70 y	12.8	18.1
Age 71 +	12.8	17.8
Pregnant /Lactating	16.3	48.2

Table 5.6: NHANES III data for mean daily iron intakes (mg) by females from diet alone and from diet plus supplements. From Heimbach, Journal of Nutrition 131: 1335S–1338S, 2001, with permission of the American Society for Nutritional Sciences.

vey of people aged 65 y or over obtained information on supplement usage from responses on a health and lifestyle questionnaire and a 7-d weighed diet record. A comparison of the total nutrient intakes and the corresponding blood biochemical indices suggested that the 7-d record was not long enough to record customary dietary supplement use. Instead, a structured questionnaire probing for supplement use over a longer time period was recommended. This included close-ended questions about the specific brand taken, the amount per pill, the frequency of use, and the duration of use (Bates et al., 1998; Bates, 2000). A similar conclusion was reached by Patterson et al. (1998b). These investigators also emphasized that measurement errors associated with long-term supplemental vitamin and mineral intake may be responsible for the lack of any observed association between vitamin supplements and the risk of cancer.

Accurate information on brand names is critical for dietary supplements because interbrand variability is large. Indeed, failure to correctly quantify the dose of a supplement can have a greater impact on the estimation of nutrient intakes than from any source of food intake underreporting. Additionally, the chemical form of the dietary supplements can affect their bioavailability, so it is preferable to record the chemical characteristics of the dietary supplements, whenever possible (Heimbach, 2001). This can be achieved by asking participants to have the dietary supplements that they take available. In this way, the interviewer can ensure the type and amounts recorded are correct (Patterson et al., 1998a).

In Australia, a detailed database on the composition of various dietary supplements sold has been compiled. The database can be queried by the Australian Register of Therapeutic Goods (ARTG) identification number, brand, product title, or a variety of other fields (Ashton et al., 1997). In the United States, the database on the composition of branded dietary supplements was expanded in 2001 for use within the NHANES/CSFII. This survey now places more emphasis on consumer use of dietary supplements than in the past. Adoption of the dietary supplement definition of the Dietary Supplement Health and Education Act (DSHEA) of 1994 would also avoid some of the difficulties that have arisen in the past in the interpretation of data on supplement use (Brownie and Myers, 2004).

5.2.8 Coding errors

Establishing a standardized coding system is especially critical for nutritional surveillance, and for cross-cultural studies involving international comparisons (Arab, 1985). In such cases, discrepancies in coding, either over time or among countries, can confound potential changes or between-country differences in dietary intakes (Buzzard and Sievert, 1994; Slimani et al., 2000). In the original SENECA study, for example, some difficulties were encountered in comparing the food intake data across the European sites, attributed to problems in classifying the foods by the Eurocode system (Kohlmeier, 1992; Schroll et al., 1997). The latter has since been revised, and the new system is now more satisfactory.

To overcome problems with coding systems used during between-country comparisons, INFOODS has developed rules and guidelines for the identification of foods, the definition of food components, and the description of food component data (See Section 4.5 and the publication by Klensin et al. (1989) for further details). Also INFOODS maintains a database of software related to food composition and nutrition. Information can be obtained on their Web site.

http://www.fao.org/infoods/

In the past, duplicate coding of recalls or records by independent coders has been used as a quality control for coding. Beaton et al. (1979) reported that coding errors arising exclusively from inadequate descriptions of foods rather than weight errors resulted in coefficients of variation ranging from 3% for protein and 8% for total fat to 17% for the ratio of polyunsaturated : saturated fatty acids. Gross errors in coding can be reduced if "coding rules" are established to deal with incomplete or ambiguous descriptors of the foods (Anderson, 1986), and large databases are used, with a comprehensive range of food items (Dwyer and Suitor, 1984). The latter enable the coder to select the appropriate food item more readily.

Food code errors have been greatly reduced by automating and integrating the data collection and coding processes (as described in Section 3.2.5) and by allowing food codes to be generated automatically by the coder selecting the food item from a computer-based pull-down menu. Both of these strategies were used for identifying and describing foods in the EPIC-SOFT program used for the EPIC study, in an effort to minimize subjective interpretations and coding errors. First, a predefined country-specific list of foods and mixed dishes was compiled, classified by common foods and food subgroups. These lists also included "non-specified" generic foods which were used when respondents were not able to describe the foods adequately. Use of these generic foods minimized arbitrary decisions by the interviewers. Second, the level of detail for describing each of the foods and mixed dishes was standardized across countries. Details are given in Slimani et al. (2000). The USDA also uses an automated food coding system for their nutrition surveys called SURVEY NET (Tippett and Cypel, 1997). As an example, a standardized approach used to describe a food such as salmon is shown in Figure 5.4.

When the dietary assessment is carried out in the home, bar-code scanners can be used to reduce errors in coding product name information for branded items. Such scanners also decrease the time spent on data entry. They were used in both the New Zealand 1997 National Nutrition Survey (MOH, 1997) and the Children's Nutrition Survey (Parnell et al., 2003). A bar-code reader has also been incorporated into a nutrient analysis system developed by U.K. researchers. Comparison with the conventional manual system revealed that data entry for nutrient analysis was faster with the bar-code system (29 versus 47 min per 7-d record), but differences between the two methods for mean intakes for macro- and micronutrients were small (Anderson et al., 1999). These findings suggest that the main advantage of bar-code scanners may be in reducing the time spent on data entry.

Meal code errors can be avoided by standardizing the codes prior to the study, and by adhering to their assignment. Frank et al. (1984) noted that the use of quantity of food consumed as a basis for defining meal codes, rather than time of consumption, led to some discrepancies in meal code assignment by different interviewers. In the EPIC-SOFT program developed for the European EPIC study, the 24-h recall period was divided into 11 common food consumption occasions during the day from "breakfast" to "after dinner" and during the night. A checklist was also devised and was adapted to the local dietary habits of each participating country, so that the interviewer could ensure that no major component of the food consumption occasion was forgotten (Slimani et al., 2000).

Weight code errors may also be made during the coding of food items. Their detection can be facilitated by including a routine in the

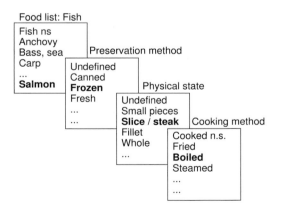

Figure 5.4: Food description in EPIC-SOFT using the facet/descriptor approach. Boiled steak of frozen salmon is used as an example. From Slimani et al., *European Journal of Clinical Nutrition* 54: 900–917, 2000 © with permission of Nature Publishing Group.

computer program that flags the subjects with the 10 highest and 10 lowest daily intakes of energy and selected nutrients, such as protein, calcium, and iron. Checks can then be made for weight errors in the coded data for these selected subjects (Sabry et al., 1984).

The EPIC-SOFT system was also designed to check for outliers arising from weight errors, as well as for missing information, while the subject was still present. This was achieved by calculating the energy and macronutrient intakes from the 24-h recall immediately after the interview. Calculated values were then checked against standard requirements based on the subject's age, sex, weight, and height. Such a strategy limits a posteriori arbitrary decisions on outlier values or unlikely food data (Slimani et al., 2000).

5.2.9 Errors in the handling of mixed dishes

There are two major sources of error during the handling of mixed dishes. First, errors may occur during the breakdown of mixed dishes into raw ingredients and their subsequent conversion to an "as consumed" form. The conversion usually involves applying adjustment factors for both changes in weight due to cooking and for nutrient retention. These adjustment factors are generally derived from the literature, and are discussed in Section 4.1.5. Sources for yield and retention factors include Matthews and Garrison (1975), Paul and Southgate (1978), Bergström (1994), and USDA (2003). After applying the appropriate adjustments, the "as consumed" form is used, along with the estimate of the quantity of the mixed dish consumed by the subject. An example of this calculation is given in Table 5.7.

The second major source of error may arise during the assignment of the mixed dish to an appropriate food group. Conventionally, this has been based on the primary ingredient in each mixed dish. Such an approach, however, often yields incorrect estimates for the contribution of major food groups to energy and nutrient intakes. For example, the fat and oil group may more than double its energy contribution from 5% to 12% when mixed dishes are incorrectly assigned in this way (Krebs-Smith et al., 1990). To avoid this source of error, all mixed dishes should be broken down into simple ingredients (i.e., single foods), as described earlier, which can then classified into their appropriate food groups. Nonetheless, when this approach is used, it is still necessary to define systematically which items need to be classified as prepared foods per se (i.e., bread, biscuits, soup, drinks) and thus not broken down into ingredients, a procedure followed during the EPIC study (Slimani et al., 2000).

5.3 Implications of measurement errors in dietary assessment

The existence of both random and systematic measurement errors is a major challenge to the design of all types of nutritional assessment systems. The existence of such errors in dietary assessment can have serious consequences when interpreting dietary data:

- Underreporting of energy intake will result in serious overestimates of nutrient inadequacies and hence the prevalence of

Egg custard ingredient	Wt (g)	Amounts contributed		
		Protein (g)	Fat (g)	Carb. (g)
Milk	500	16.5	19.0	23.5
Egg	100	12.3	10.9	Tr.
Sugar	30	0	0	31.5
Vanilla essence	Tr.	Ignored for calculation		
Total	630	28.8	29.9	55.0
Cooked weight	500			
per 100 g	100	5.8	6.0	11.0

Table 5.7: An example of the calculation of the nutrient composition of a mixed dish. The loss in weight during cooking is the result of water loss. The calculation of the composition per 100 g uses the cooked weight. Losses (destruction) of these particular nutrients during cooking is assumed to be zero. Thus, for protein, $(28.8 / 500) \times 100 = 5.8$. Carb., Carbohydrate; Tr., Trace. From Cameron and van Staveren (1988) with permission of Oxford University Press.

inadequate nutrient intakes in a population (Smith et al., 1994).

- Selective underreporting of certain foods will hamper the usefulness of dietary data for developing food-based dietary guidelines (Section 8.4) (Becker and Welten, 2001).

- The existence of dietary measurement error attenuates correlations between nutrient intake and the outcome parameters (e.g., biomarkers), so that important associations between diet and disease may be obscured. This phenomenon is termed "attenuation bias."

Efforts to overcome the problem of energy underreporting have led some investigators to exclude underreporters from the data set (Shortt et al., 1997). However, such an approach introduces a source of unknown bias into the data set and is not recommended. Others advocate the inclusion of all the respondents, but the use of statistical methods that control for energy intake. Several methods for energy adjustment exist, and their choice (Kipnis et al., 1993, 1997; Mackerras, 1996; Hu et al., 1999), as well as the justification for their use, is hotly debated (Kohlmeier and Bellach, 1995). Most corrections for energy intake are appropriate only if the underreporting is occurring at the whole-diet level. They are not sufficient to eliminate the biases arising from selective underreporting of certain food types (e.g., foods of low social desirability). Clearly, the selection of an appropriate model for energy adjustment depends on the particular research question of interest; readers are advised to consult a statistician on this issue.

More research is needed to understand when energy adjustment methods are appropriate and the choice of appropriate models for different study questions. Complex comprehensive statistical models are also being developed to overcome other sources of bias in dietary intake data, but more research is needed before they can be used (Kipnis et al., 2002). Indeed, several investigators suggest that the results of nutrition–disease relationships should be interpreted cautiously until

Sources of error	24-h recall	Dietary history	Estimated record	Weighed record
Omitting foods	●	●	⊙	⊙
Adding foods	●	●	○	○
Estimating food weights	●	●	●	○
Estimating frequency of food consumption	○	●	○	○
Day-to-day variation	●	○	●	●
Changes in diet	○	○	⊙	●
Coding errors	●	●	●	●

Table 5.8: Sources of error in techniques estimating food consumption. ● error is likely; ⊙ error is possible; ○ error is unlikely. From van Staveren WA and Burema J, Näringsforskning 29: 38–42, 1985.

the structure of dietary measurement error is better understood (Samaras et al., 1999; Kipnis et al., 2002).

5.4 Summary

This chapter outlines the systematic and random errors that may occur during all stages of the collection and recording of food consumption data; the more important sources of error are summarized in Table 5.8.

Quality-control procedures that minimize possible sources of measurement error include training the interviewing and coding staff and developing standard interviewing techniques and questionnaires during the pilot survey. Increasingly, sources of error arising from both respondent and interviewer biases and respondent memory lapses can be reduced by computerizing probing questions, standardized prompts, and built-in cues during automated dietary interviews. Nevertheless, underreporting of energy and selective underreporting of certain food types remain important sources of respondent biases.

A variety of portion-size measurement aids are now available for use when weighing methods are not possible. These include the use of 2-D graduated food models or photographs and 3-D measurement guides (e.g., household measures) to quantify portions of foods consumed. Training respondents to use these measurement guides to estimate food portion sizes will also improve

accuracy. Collection of accurate data on consumer use of dietary supplements is now essential; information on brand, dosage, chemical form, and time period over which use of the dietary supplement has been recorded is required. Adoption of a standard definition of a dietary supplement is urgently needed.

Establishing a computerized standard coding system for both foods and meals to avoid coding errors is critical, especially for surveillance and cross-country comparisons. This is now facilitated by the use of INFOODS tag names for foods and, in some studies, use of bar-code scanners for branded items. Systematic detection of wrongly coded weights of foods is more difficult, although computer-calculation of energy and macronutrient intakes from 24-h recall interviews, while the subject is still present, allows the correction of any gross errors. Finally, care must be taken to avoid errors during the handling of data for mixed dishes, by using software that breaks down the recipes into simple ingredients. These are then converted from the raw form to an "as consumed" form.

Despite all efforts to minimize sources of random and systematic errors that may occur during the measurement of food and nutrient intakes, some errors remain difficult to predict and to prevent and, as a result, may introduce a differential bias in reported food intakes. Further studies are needed to investigate the specific type and nature of measurement errors, especially those related to underreporting, so that these can be minimized or corrected statistically. In this way, the analysis and interpretation of dietary data can be improved. The existence of dietary measurement error attenuates the estimates of disease relative risk, and thus has major implications in epidemiological studies of dietary risk factors and disease.

References

Anderson AS, Maher L, Ha TK, Cooney J, Eley S, Martin M, Vespasiani G, Bruni M, Lean ME. (1999). Evaluation of a bar-code system for nutrient analysis in dietary surveys. Public Health Nutrition 2: 579–586.

Anderson AS (ed.). (1986). Guidelines for Use of Dietary Intake Data. Life Sciences Research Office, Federation of American Societies for Experimental Biology, Bethesda, MD.

Arab L. (1985). Summary of survey of food composition tables and nutrient data banks in Europe. Annals of Nutrition and Metabolism 29(suppl. 1): 39–45.

Ashton BA, Ambrosini GL, Marks GC, Harvey PW, Bain C. (1997). Development of a dietary supplement database. Australian and New Zealand Journal of Public Health 21: 699–702.

Ballard-Barbash R, Graubard I, Krebs-Smith SM, Schatzkin A, Thompson FE. (1996). Contribution of dieting to the inverse association between energy intake and body mass index. European Journal of Clinical Nutrition 50: 98–106.

Balluz LS, Kieszak SM, Philen RM, Mulinare J. (2000). Vitamin and mineral supplement use in the United States: results from the third National Health and Nutrition Examination Survey. Archives of Family Medicine 9: 258–262.

Baranowski T, Domel SB. (1994). A cognitive model of children's reporting of food intake. American Journal of Clinical Nutrition 59: 212S–217S.

Bates CJ. (2000). Dietary supplement use at the population level: recent experience from the 1994–5 British National Diet and Nutrition Survey: people aged 65 years and over. Journal of Nutrition, Health and Aging 4: 51–53.

Bates CJ, Prentice A, van der Pols JC, Walmsley C, Pentieva KD, Finch S, Smithers G, Clarke PC. (1998). Estimation of the use of dietary supplements in the National Diet and Nutrition Survey: people aged 65 years and over: an observed paradox and a recommendation. European Journal of Clinical Nutrition 52: 917–923.

Bathalon GP, Tucker KL, Hays NP, Vinken AG, Greenberg AS, McCrory MA, Roberts SB. (2000). Psychological measures of eating behavior and the accuracy of three common dietary assessment methods in healthy postmenopausal women. American Journal of Clinical Nutrition 71: 739–745.

Beaton GH, Milner J, Corey P, McGuire V, Cousins M, Stewart E, de Ramos M, Hewitt D, Grambsch PV, Kassim N, Little JA. (1979). Sources of variance in 24-hour dietary recall data: implications for nutrition study design and interpretation. American Journal of Clinical Nutrition 32: 2546–2559.

Beaton GH, Burema J, Ritenbaugh C. (1997). Errors in the interpretation of dietary assessments. American Journal of Clinical Nutrition 65: 1100S–1107S.

Becker W, Welten D. (2001). Under-reporting in dietary surveys: implications for development of food-based dietary guidelines. Public Health Nutrition 4: 683–687.

Bergström L. (1994). Nutrient Losses and Gains in Preparation of Foods. Rapport 32/1994. Livsmedelsverket (National Food Administration), Uppsala, Sweden.

Bingham SA, Cassidy A, Cole TJ, Welch A, Runswick SA, Black AE, Thurnham D, Bates C, Khaw K, Key TJA, Day NE. (1995). Validation of weighed records and other methods of dietary assessment using the 24-h urine nitrogen technique and other biological markers. British Journal of Nutrition 73: 531–550.

Block G, Hartman AM, Dresser CM, Carroll MD, Gannon J, Gardner L. (1986). A data-based approach to diet questionnaire design and testing. American Journal of Epidemiology 124: 453–469.

Bohlscheid-Thomas S, Hoting I, Boeing H, Wahrendorf J. (1997). Reproducibility and relative validity of a food group intake in a food frequency questionnaire developed for the German part of the EPIC project. International Journal of Epidemiology 26: S59–S70.

Bolland JE, Ward JY, Bolland TW. (1990). Improved accuracy of estimating food quantities up to 4 weeks after training. Journal of the American Dietetic Association 90: 1402–1404.

Braam LA, Ocké MC, Bueno-de-Mesquita HB, Seidell JC. (1998). Determinants of obesity-related underreporting of energy intake. American Journal of Epidemiology 147: 1081–1086.

Briefel RR, Sempos CT, McDowell MA, Chien S, Alaimo K. (1997). Dietary method research in the third National Health and Nutrition Examination Survey: underreporting of energy intake. American Journal of Clinical Nutrition 65: 1203S–1209S.

Briefel RR, Bialostosky K, Kennedy-Stepehnson J, McDowell MA, Ervin RB, Wright JD. (2000). Zinc intake of the U.S. population: findings from the Third National Health and Nutrition Examination Survey, 1988–94. Journal of Nutrition 130: 1367S–1373S.

Brown JE, Tharp TM, Dahlberg-Luby EM, Snowdon DA, Ostwald SK, Buzzard IM, Rysavy SM, Wieser SM. (1990). Videotape dietary assessment: validity, reliability, and comparison of results with 24-hour dietary recalls from elderly women in a retirement home. Journal of the American Dietetic Association 90: 1675–1679.

Brownie S, Myers S. (2004). Wading through the

quagmire: making sense of dietary supplement utilization. Nutrition Reviews 62: 276–282.

Buzzard IM, Sievert YA. (1994). Research priorities and recommendations for dietary assessment
methodology. American Journal of Clinical Nutrition 59: 275S–280S.

Cameron ME, van Staveren WA. (1988). Manual on
Methodology for Food Consumption Studies. Oxford University Press, New York.

Campbell VA, Dodds ML. (1967). Collecting dietary
information from groups of older people. Journal of
the American Dietetic Association 51: 29–33.

Cleveland LE, Ingwersen LA. (2001). Was it a slab, a
slice, or a sliver? High-tech innovations take food
survey to new levels. Agricultural Research, March
2001: 4–7.

Comstock EM, Symington LE. (1982). Distributions
of serving sizes and plate waste in school lunches.
Implications for measurement. Journal of the American Dietetic Association 81: 413–422.

Cummings SR, Block G, McHenry K, Baron RB.
(1987). Evaluation of two food frequency methods of measuring dietary calcium intake. American
Journal of Epidemiology 126: 796–802.

Cypel YS, Guenther PM, Petot GJ. (1997). Validity of
portion-size measurement aids: a review. Journal of
the American Dietetic Association 97: 289–292.

de Vries JHM, Zock PL, Mensink RP, Katan MB.
(1994). Underestimation of energy intake by 3-d
records compared with energy intake to maintain
body weight in 269 nonobese adults. American
Journal of Clinical Nutrition 60: 855–860.

Domel SB. (1997). Self-reports of diet: how children
remember what they have eaten. American Journal
of Clinical Nutrition 65: 1148S–1152S.

Dwyer J, Suitor CW. (1984). Caveat emptor: assessing
needs, evaluating computer options. Journal of the
American Dietetic Association 84: 302–312.

Ervin RB, Wright JD, Kennedy-Stephenson J. (1999).
Use of dietary supplements in the United States,
1988–94. Vital Health Statistics 11(244): 1–14.

FDA (Food and Drug Administration). (1993). Food
labeling: serving sizes. Federal Register 58: 2229–
2291.

Fowler FJ, Mangione TW. (1990). Standardized Survey Interviewing: Minimizing Interviewer-Related
Error. Sage Publications, Thousand Oaks, CA.

Frank GC, Berenson GS, Schilling PE, Moore MC.
(1977). Adapting the 24-hr recall for epidemiologic
studies of school children. Journal of the American
Dietetic Association 71: 26–31.

Frank GC, Hollatz AT, Webber LS, Berenson GS.
(1984). Effect of interviewer recording practices on
nutrient intake: Bogalusa Heart Study. Journal of
the American Dietetic Association 84: 1432–1439.

Friedenreich CM, Slimani N, Riboli E. (1992). Measurement of past diet: review of previous and proposed methods. Epidemiological Review 14: 177–
196.

Gibson RS. Ferguson EL. (1999). An Interactive 24-
hour Recall for Assessing the Adequacy of Iron and
Zinc Intakes in Developing Countries. International
Life Sciences Institute Press, Washington, DC.

Gittelsohn J, Shankar AV, Pokhrel RP, West KP Jr.
(1994). Accuracy of estimating food intake by
observation. Journal of the American Dietetic Association 94: 1273–1277.

Godwin S, McGuire B, Chambers E, McDowell M,
Cleveland L, Edwards-Perry E, Ingwersen L. (2001).
Evaluation of portion size estimation aids used for
meat in dietary surveys. Nutrition Research 221:
1217–1233.

Goldberg GR, Black AE, Jebb SA, Cole TJ, Murga-
troyd PR, Coward WA, Prentice AM. (1991). Critical evaluation of energy intake data using fundamental principles of energy physiology. 1: Derivation of
cut-off limits to identify under-recording. European
Journal of Clinical Nutrition 45: 569–581.

Goris AHC, Westerterp KR. (1999). Underreporting of
habitual food intake is explained by undereating in
highly motivated lean women. Journal of Nutrition
129: 878–882.

Goris AHC, Westerterp-Plantenga MS, Westerterp KR.
(2000). Undereating and underreporting of habitual
food intake in obese men: selective underreporting
of fat intake. American Journal of Clinical Nutrition
71: 130–134.

Gregory J, Foster K, Tyler H, Wiseman M. (1990). The
Dietary and Nutritional Survey of British Adults.
The Stationery Office, London.

Guthrie HA. (1984). Selection and quantification of
typical food portions by young adults. Journal of
the American Dietetic Association 84: 1440–1444.

Habicht J-P, Mason JB, Tabatabai H. (1984). Basic
concepts in the design of evaluation during programme implementation. In: Sahn DE, Lockwood
R, Scrimshaw NS (eds.). Methods for the Evaluation
of the Impact of Food and Nutrition Programmes.
United Nations University, Tokyo, Japan, pp.1–24.

Hankin JH, Wilkens LR. (1994). Development and validation of dietary assessment methods for culturally
diverse populations. American Journal of Clinical
Nutrition 59: 198S–200S.

Hebert JR, Clemow L, Pbert L, Ockene IS, Ockene JK.
(1995). Social desirability bias in dietary self-report
may compromise the validity of dietary intake measures. International Journal of Epidemiology 24:
389–398.

Hebert JR, Ma Y, Clemow L, Ockene IS, Saperia G,
Stanek EJ 3rd, Merriam PA, Ockene JK. (1997).
Gender differences in social desirability and social
approval bias in dietary self-report. American Journal of Epidemiology 146: 1046–1055.

Heerstrass DW, Ocké MC, Bueno-de-Mesquita HB,
Peeters PH, Seidell JC. (1998). Underreporting of
energy, protein and potassium intake in relation to
body mass index. International Journal of Epidemiology 27: 186–193.

Heimbach JT. (2001). Using the national nutrition
monitoring system to profile dietary supplement use.
Journal of Nutrition 131: 1335S–1338S.

Heitmann BL. (1993). The influence of fatness, weight

change, slimming history and other lifestyle variables on diet reporting in Danish men and women aged 35–65 years. International Journal of Obesity and Related Metabolic Disorders 17: 329–336.

Heitmann BL, Lissner L. (1995). Dietary underreporting by obese individuals: is it specific or non-specific? British Medical Journal 311: 986–989.

Hogbin M, Shaw A, Anand RS. (1999). Food Portions and Servings: How do They Differ. Nutrition Insights No. 11, Center for Nutrition Policy and Promotion, Washington, DC. <www.usda.gov/cnpp>

Howat PM, Mohan R, Champagne C, Monlezun C, Worniak P, Bray GA. (1994). Validity and reliability of reported dietary intake data. Journal of the American Dietetic Association 94: 169–173.

Hu FB, Stampfer MJ, Rimm E, Ascherio A, Rosner BA, Spiegelman D, Willett WC. (1999). Dietary fat and coronary heart disease: a comparison of approaches for adjusting for total energy intake and modeling repeated dietary measurements. American Journal of Epidemiology 149: 531–540.

Hughes BA. (1986). Nutrition interviewing and counseling in public health: the North Carolina experience. Topics in Clinical Nutrition 1: 43–50.

Johansson G, Wikman A, Ahren AM, Hallmans G, Johansson I. (2001). Underreporting of energy intake in repeated 24-hour recalls related to gender, age, weight status, day of interview, educational level, reported food intake, smoking habits and area of living. Public Health Nutrition 4: 919–927.

Johansson L, Solvoll K, Bjørneboe GE, Drevon CA. (1998). Under- and overreporting of energy intake related to weight status and lifestyle in a nationwide sample. American Journal of Clinical Nutrition 68: 266–274.

Johnson RK, Goran MI, Poehlman ET. (1994). Correlates of over- and underreporting of energy intake in healthy older men and women. American Journal of Clinical Nutrition 59: 1286–1290.

Karvetti RL, Knuts LR. (1985). Validity of the 24-hour dietary recall. Journal of the American Dietetic Association 85: 1437–1442.

Kipnis V, Freedman LS, Brown CC, Hartman AM, Schatzkin A, Wacholder S. (1993). Interpretation of energy-adjustment models for nutritional epidemiology. American Journal of Epidemiology 137: 1376–1380.

Kipnis V, Freedman LS, Brown CC, Hartman AM, Schatzkin A, Wacholder S. (1997). Effect of measurement error on energy-adjustment models in nutritional epidemiology. American Journal of Epidemiology 146: 842–855.

Kipnis V, Midthune D, Freedman L, Bingham S, Day N, Riboli E, Ferrari P, Carroll RJ. (2002). Bias in dietary-report instruments and its implications for nutritional epidemiology. Public Health Nutrition 5: 915–923.

Kirkcaldy-Hargreaves M, Lynch GW, Santor C. (1980). Assessment of the use of four food models. Journal of the Canadian Dietetic Association 41: 102–110.

Klensin JC, Feskanich D, Lin V, Truswell AS, Southgate DAT. (1989). Identification of Food Components for INFOODS Data Interchange. United Nations University, Tokyo, Japan.

Klesges RC, Eck LH, Ray JW. (1995). Who underreports dietary intake in a dietary recall? Evidence from the second National Health and Nutrition Examination Survey. Journal of Consulting and Clinical Psychology 63: 438–444.

Kohlmeier L. (1992). The Eurocode 2 food coding system. European Journal of Clinical Nutrition 46: S9–S24.

Kohlmeier L, Bellach B. (1995). Exposure assessment error and its handling in nutritional epidemiology. Annual Review of Public Health 16: 43–59.

Krall EA, Dwyer JT, Coleman KA. (1988). Factors influencing accuracy of dietary recall. Nutrition Research 8: 929–941.

Krantzler NJ, Mullen BJ, Schutz HG, Grivetti LE, Holden CA, Meiselman HL. (1982). Validity of telephoned diet recalls and records for assessment of individual food intake. American Journal of Clinical Nutrition 36: 1234–1242.

Krebs-Smith SM, Cronin FJ, Haytowitz DB, Cook DA. (1990). Contributions of food groups to intakes of energy, nutrients, cholesterol, and fiber in women's diet: effect of method of classifying food mixtures. Journal of the American Dietetic Association 90: 1541–1546.

Krebs-Smith SM, Graubard BI, Kahle LI, Subar AF, Cleveland LE, Ballard-Barbash R. (2000). Low energy reporters vs others: a comparison of reported food intakes. European Journal of Clinical Nutrition 54: 281–287.

Kretsch MJ, Fong AKH, Green MW. (1999). Behavioral and body size correlates of energy intake underreporting by obese and normal-weight women. Journal of the American Dietetic Association 99: 300–306.

Kuehneman T, Stanek K, Eskridge K, Angle C. (1994). Comparability of four methods for estimating portion sizes during a food frequency interview with caregivers of young children. Journal of the American Dietetic Association 94: 548–551.

Lafay L, Basdevant A, Charles M-A, Vray M, Balkau B, Borys JM, Eschwège E, Romon M. (1997). Determinants and nature of dietary underreporting in a free-living population: the Fleurbaix Laventie Ville Santé (FLVS) Study. International Journal of Obesity and Related Metabolic Disorders 21: 567–573.

Livingstone MBE, Black AE. (2003). Markers of the validity of reported energy intake. Journal of Nutrition 133: 895S–920S.

Livingstone MBE, Prentice AM, Strain JJ, Coward WA, Black AE, Barker ME, Mckenna PG, Whitehead RG. (1990). Accuracy of weighed dietary records in studies of diet and health. British Medical Journal 300: 708–712.

Lucas F, Niravong M, Villeminot S, Kaaks R, Clavel-Chapelon F. (1995). Estimation of food portion size using photographs: validity, strengths, weaknesses and recommendations. Journal of Human Nutrition and Dietetics 8: 65–74.

Macdiarmid JI, Blundell JI. (1997). Dietary under-reporting: what people say about recording their food intake. European Journal of Clinical Nutrition 51: 199–200.

Mackerras D. (1996). Energy adjustment: the concepts underlying the debate. Journal of Clinical Epidemiology 49: 957–962.

Matthews RH, Garrison YJ. (1975). Food Yields Summarized by Different Stages of Preparation. Agriculture Handbook No. 102. U.S. Department of Agriculture, Washington, DC.
http://www.nal.usda.gov/fnic/foodcomp/

McCrory MA, Hajduk CL, Roberts SB. (2002). Procedures for screening out inaccurate reports of dietary energy intake. Public Health Nutrition 5: 873–882.

Mela DJ, Aaron JI. (1997). Honest but invalid: what subjects say about recording their food intake. Journal of the American Dietetic Association 97: 791–793.

MOH (Ministry of Health). (1997). Food Comes First: Methodologies for the National Nutrition Survey of New Zealand. Public Health Report No. 2. Public Health Group, Ministry of Health, Wellington, New Zealand.

NCHS (National Center for Health Statistics). (1994). Plan and Operation of the Third National Health and Nutrition Examination Survey, 1988–94. Vital and Health Statistics 1(32).

Nelson M, Haraldsdóttir J. (1998a). Food photographs — practical guidelines. I: Design and analysis of studies to validate portion size estimates. Public Health Nutrition 1: 219–230.

Nelson M, Haraldsdóttir J. (1998b). Food photographs — practical guidelines. II: Development and use of photographic atlases for assessing food portion size. Public Health Nutrition 1: 231–237.

Nelson M, Atkinson M, Darbyshire S. (1994). Food photography. I: The perception of food portion size from photographs. British Journal of Nutrition 72: 649–663.

Nelson M, Atkinson M, Darbyshire S. (1996). Food photography. II: Use of food photographs for estimating portion size and the nutrient content of meals. British Journal of Nutrition 76: 31–49.

Noethlings U, Hoffmann K, Bergmann MM, Boeing H. (2003). Portion size adds limited information on variance in food intake of participants in the EPIC-Potsdam study. Journal of Nutrition 133: 510–515.

Pao EM, Fleming KH, Guenther PM, Mickle SJ. (1982). Foods Commonly Eaten by Individuals: Amount per Day and per Eating Occasion. Home Economics Research Report No. 44. U.S. Department of Agriculture, Hyattsville, MD.

Parnell W, Scragg R, Wison N, Schaaf D, Fitzgerald E. (2003). NZ Food and NZ Children: Key Results of the 2002 National Children's Nutrition Survey. Ministry of Health, Wellington, New Zealand.

Patterson RE, Kristal A, Levy L, McLerran D, White E. (1998a). Validity of methods used to assess vitamin

and mineral supplement use. American Journal of Epidemiology 148: 643–649.

Patterson RE, Neuhouser ML, White E, Kristal AR, Potter JD. (1998b). Measurement error from assessing use of vitamin supplements at one point in time. Epidemiology 9: 567–569.

Paul AA, Southgate DAT. (1978). McCance and Widdowson's "The Composition of Foods". 4th edition. Her Majesty's Stationery Office, London.

Pietinen P, Hartman AM, Haapa E, Rasanen L, Haapakoski J, Palmgren J, Albanes D, Virtamo J, Huttunen JK. (1988). Reproducibility and validity of dietary assessment instruments. I: A self-administered food use questionnaire with a portion size picture booklet. American Journal of Epidemiology 128: 655–666.

Poppitt SD, Swann D, Black AE, Prentice AM. (1998). Assessment of selective under-reporting of food intake by both obese and nonobese women in a metabolic facility. International Journal of Obesity and Related Metabolic Disorders 22: 303–311.

Posner BM, Smigelski C, Duggal A, Morgan J, Cobb J, Cupples LA. (1992). Validation of two-dimensional models for estimation of portion size in nutrition research. Journal of the American Dietetic Association 92: 738–741.

Price GM, Paul AA, Cole TJ, Wadsworth MEJ. (1997). Characteristics of the low-energy reporters in a longitudinal national dietary survey. British Journal of Nutrition 77: 833–851.

Pryer JA, Vrijheid M, Nichols R, Kiggins M, Elliott P. (1997). Who are the "low energy reporters" in the dietary and nutritional survey of British adults? International Journal of Epidemiology 26: 146–154.

Roth DL, Snyder CR, Pace LM. (1986). Dimensions of favourable self- presentation. Journal of Personality and Social Psychology 51: 867–874.

Rowland ML, Forthofer RN. (1993). Adjusting for nonresponse bias in a health examination survey. Public Health Reports 108: 380–386.

Russell D, Parnell W, Wilson N, Faed J, Ferguson E, Herbison P, Horwath C, Nye T, Walker R, Wilson B. (1999). New Zealand Food, New Zealand People: Key Results of the 1997 National Nutrition Survey. Ministry of Health, Wellington, New Zealand.

Rutishauser IHE, Wheeler CE, Conn JA, O'Dea K. (1994). Food and nutrient intake in a randomly selected sample of adults: demographic and temporal influences on energy and nutrient intake. Australian Journal of Nutrition and Dietetics 51: 157–166.

Sabry JH, Gibson RS, Pen C. (1984). Nutrient Intake System: User's Guide for the Program. Department of Family Studies, University of Guelph, Guelph, ON, Canada.

Samaras K, Kelly PJ, Campbell LV. (1999). Dietary underreporting is prevalent in middle-aged British women and is not related to adiposity (percentage body fat). International Journal of Obesity and Related Metabolic Disorders 23: 881–888.

Samet JM, Humble CG, Skipper BE. (1984). Alternatives in the collection and analysis of food frequency interview data. American Journal of Epidemiology 120: 572–581.

Schoeller DA. (1990). How accurate is self-reported dietary energy intake? Nutrition Reviews 48: 373–379.

Schroll K, Moreiras-Varela O, Schlettwein-Gsell D, Decarli B, de Groet L, van Staveren W. (1997). Cross cultural variations and changes in food group intake among elderly women in Europe: results from the Survey in Europe on Nutrition and the Elderly — Concerted Action (SENECA). American Journal of Clinical Nutrition 65: 1282S–1289S.

Shortt CT, Duthie GG, Robertson JD, Morrice PC, Nicol F, Arthur JR. (1997). Selenium status of a group of Scottish adults. European Journal of Clinical Nutrition 51: 400–404.

Sichert-Hellert W, Kersting M, Schoch G. (1998). Underreporting of energy intake in 1- to 18-year-old German children and adolescents. Zeitschrift für Ernährungswissenschaft 37: 242–251.

Slimani N, Deharveng G, Charrondière RU, van Kappel AL, Ocké MC, Welch A, Lagiou A, van Liere M, Agudo A, Pala V, Brandstetter B, Andrén C, Stripp C, van Staveren WA, Riboli E. (1999). Structure of the standardized computerized 24-hour diet recall interview used as reference method in the 22 centres participating in the EPIC project. Computer Methods and Programs in Biomedicine 53: 251–266.

Slimani N, Ferrari P, Ocké M, Welch A, Boeing H, van Liere M, Pala V, Amiano P, Lagiou A, Mattisson I, Stripp C, Engeset D, Charrondiere R, Buzzard M, van Staveren W, Riboli E. (2000). Standardization of the 24-hour diet recall calibration method used in the European prospective investigation into cancer and nutrition (EPIC): general concepts and preliminary results. European Journal of Clinical Nutrition 54: 900–917.

Smith AF, Jobe JB, Mingay DJ. (1991). Retrieval from memory of dietary information. Applied Cognitive Psychology 5: 269–296.

Smith WT, Webb KL, Heywood PF. (1994). The implications of underreporting in dietary studies. Australian Journal of Public Health 18: 311–314.

Stunkard AJ, Messick S. (1985). The three-factor eating questionnaire to measure dietary restraint, disinhibition and hunger. Journal of Psychosomatic Research 29: 71–83.

Taren DL, Tobar M, Hill A, Howell W, Shissiak C, Bell I, Ritenbaugh C. (1999). The association of energy intake bias with psychological scores of women. European Journal of Clinical Nutrition 53: 570–578.

Tippett KS, Cypel YS (eds.). (1997). Design and Operation: The Continuing Survey of Food Intakes by Individuals and the Diet and Health Knowledge Survey, 1994–96. Nationwide Food Surveys Report No. 96-1. U.S. Department of Agriculture and Agricultural Research Service, Hyattsville, MD.

Tomoyasu NJ, Toth MJ, Poehlman ET. (2000). Misreporting of total energy intake in older African Americans. International Journal of Obesity Related Metabolic Disorders 24: 20–26.

Tonstad S, Gorbitz C, Sivertsen M, Ose L. (1999). Under-reporting of dietary intake by smoking and non-smoking subjects counselled for hypercholesterolaemia. Journal of Internal Medicine 245: 337–344.

Tsubono Y, Kobayashi M, Takahashi T, Iwase Y, Ilitoi Y, Akabane M, Tsugane S. (1997). Within- and between-person variations in portion sizes of foods consumed by the Japanese population. Nutrition and Cancer 29: 140–145.

USDA (U.S. Department of Agriculture). (1992). The Food Guide Pyramid. Home and Garden Bulletin No. 252. U.S. Department of Agriculture, Washington, DC.

USDA (U.S. Department of Agriculture). (2003). Table of Nutrient Retention Factors. Release 5. U.S. Department of Agriculture, Washington DC.

van Staveren WA, Burema J. (1985). Food consumption surveys: frustrations and expectations. Näringsforskning 29: 38–42.

van Staveren WA, Hulshof KFAM. (1980). De voedingsanamnese in het voedingsonderzoek, mogelijkheden en beperkingen. Voeding 41: 228–233.

van Staveren WA, de Groot LC, Blauw YH, van der Wielen RPJ. (1994). Assessing diets of elderly people: problems and approaches. American Journal of Clinical Nutrition 59: S128–S136.

van Strien T, Frijters JER, Bergers GPA, Defares PB. (1986). The Dutch Eating Behaviour Questionnaire (DEBQ) for assessment of restrained, emotional, and external eating behavior. International Journal of Eating Disorders 5: 295–315.

van't Hof MA, Hautvast JGAJ, Schroll M, Vlachonikolis IG. (1991). Design, methods and participation: Euronut SENECA investigators. European Journal of Clinical Nutrition 45: 5–22.

Voss S, Kroke A, Lipstein-Grosbusch K, Boeing H. (1998). Is macronutrient composition of dietary intake data affected by underreporting? Results from the EPIC-Potsdam study. European Journal of Clinical Nutrition 52: 119–126.

Wakefield LM. (1966). The interview technique in research: source of bias. Journal of Home Economics 58: 640–642.

Warren JM, Henry CJK, Livingstone MBE, Lightowler HJ, Bradshaw SM, Perwaiz S. (2003). How well do children aged 5–7 years recall food eaten at school lunch? Public Health Nutrition 6: 41–47.

Weber JL, Tinsley AM, Houtkooper LB, Lohman TG. (1997). Multi-method training increased portion-size estimation accuracy. Journal of the American Dietetic Association 97: 176–179.

Weber JL, Cunningham-Sabo L, Skipper B, Lytle L, Stevens J, Gittelsohn J, Anliker J, Heller K, Pablo JL. (1999). Portion-size estimation training in second- and third-grade American Indian children. American Journal of Clinical Nutrition 69: 782S–787S.

Willett WC, Sampson L, Stampfer MJ, Rosner B,

Bain C, Witschi J, Hennekens CH, Speizer FE. (1985). Reproducibility and validity of a semiquantitative food frequency questionnaire. American Journal of Epidemiology 122: 51–65.

Worsley A, Baghurst KI, Leitch DR. (1984). Social desirability response bias and dietary inventory responses. Human Nutrition: Applied Nutrition 38: 29–35.

Wynder EL. (1994). Investigator bias and interviewer bias: the problem of reporting systematic error in epidemiology. Journal of Clinical Epidemiology 47: 825–827.

Young LR, Nestle M. (1995). Portion sizes in dietary assessment: issues and policy implications. Nutrition Reviews 53: 149–158.

Zhang J, Temme EH, Sasaki S, Kesteloot H. (2000). Under- and overreporting of energy intake using urinary cations as biomarkers: relation to body mass index. American Journal of Epidemiology 152: 453–462.

6

Reproducibility in dietary assessment

A dietary assessment method is considered reproducible if it gives very similar results when used repeatedly in the same situation. The reproducibility of any dietary method is a function of the measurement errors (discussed in Chapter 5), uncertainty resulting from true variation in daily nutrient intakes (Section 3.3.2), and variability introduced by a variety of other confounding factors (e.g., age and sex, season, chronic illness or dieting). Even if the measurement errors and confounding factors are minimized, uncertainty in the estimation of usual nutrient intakes remains. Consequently, although the dietary survey results from two separate occasions may disagree, the method may not have poor reproducibility; the food intakes of the individuals may indeed have changed. Therefore, only an estimate of reproducibility can be made. True reproducibility cannot be determined because replicate observations in dietary assessment are impossible.

For a group of individuals, true variability arises because dietary intakes differ among individuals (between- or intersubject variation) and within one individual over time (within- or intrasubject variation). Unlike measurement errors, no attempt should be made to try to minimize between- and within-subject variation because they characterize the true usual intake of a group of individuals. Instead, the dietary assessment protocol should allow these two sources of variability to be separated and estimated statistically using analysis of variance. In this way, the magnitude of the effect of within-subject ver-

sus between-subject variation can be taken into account during the interpretation of the dietary data. This is important because one of the effects of this variation is to attenuate correlations and the other measures of association, thus obscuring diet–disease relationships (Section 5.3). An additional effect of within-subject variation that is less well recognized is on the prevalence of "inadequate" or "excess" intakes in a population (Section 3.3.2).

This chapter describes the assessment of reproducibility in the most commonly used dietary assessment methods. Some notes on the statistical techniques used to assess reproducibility are also included.

6.1 Assessment of reproducibility in dietary methods

Conventionally, reproducibility has been determined using a "test–retest" design, in which the same dietary method is repeated on the same subjects over the same time period, after a preselected time interval. The selection of the time interval depends on the time frame of the dietary method used. More research is needed to establish the optimal time interval between the two administrations of the dietary method: Block and Hartman (1989) recommend a time interval of 4–8 wk. Care must be taken to avoid the second measurement being influenced by the earlier one, through recollection of the first interview. The effects of season or changes in food habits over time must also be avoided. In low-income countries, the effects of season on food availability, and thus nutrient intakes, may be marked.

Assessment of reproducibility using a test–retest design has other limitations. Reproducibility is a function of both the uncertainty resulting from true variation in daily nutrient intakes within individuals and random errors in measurement. Normally, these sources of uncertainty cannot be distinguished. However, random measurement errors can be reduced by incorporating various quality control procedures into the dietary assessment method (Section 5.2): increasing the number of observations decreases the effect of random measurement error on the mean.

There will always be a tendency for some dietary assessment methods to have higher reproducibility than others because some designs limit the recording of variability in food and, hence, nutrient intakes. An example is a food frequency questionnaire in which estimates of portion size are based on a single set of "standard reference" portions (Hankin et al., 1978). Moreover, because a food frequency questionnaire (and a dietary history) is designed to assess the usual food intake of an individual over a relatively long time period, they are not sensitive to day-to-day variations in intake (Burema et al., 1988).

Reproducibility may also be high, even if some subjects consistently under- or overestimate the portion sizes consumed. Thus, even if the dietary assessment method appears to have high reproducibility using a test–retest design, it does not necessarily produce the correct answers. Conversely, a lack of agreement between two sets of nutrient intake results may not reflect poor reproducibility in the method: the nutrient intake may have changed in the interval between the two measurements as a result of usual daily variation in food intake. Perfect reproducibility at the individual level is unlikely.

In general, the reproducibility of a dietary assessment method depends on the time frame of the method, the population group under study, the nutrient of interest, the technique used to measure the foods and quanti-

	Mean		%
	Summer	Winter	Diff.
Energy (kcal)	2221	2256	−2
Protein (g)	71	72	1
Fat (g)	103	103	0
Carbohydrate (g)	267	272	−2
Calcium (mg)	1095	1080	1
Iron (mg)	11.2	13.0	−14
Vitamin A (RE µg)	1004	1431	−30
Thiamin (mg)	1.3	1.4	−7
Riboflavin (mg)	2.4	2.6	−8
Niacin (mg)	11.7	12.0	−2
Ascorbic acid (mg)	81	104	−22

Table 6.1: Comparison of mean daily intakes of energy and nutrients in two 24-h recalls ($n = 158$). Differences are expressed as percentages of the values obtained in the winter. Significant differences were observed for vitamin A ($0.01 < p < 0.05$), iron, and ascorbic acid ($0.001 < p < 0.01$), based on the results of the paired t-test. From Räsänen, American Journal of Clinical Nutrition 32: 2560–2567, 1979 © Am J Clin Nutr. American Society for Clinical Nutrition.

ties consumed, and the between- and within-subject variances, as noted above.

6.1.1 Twenty-four-hour recalls

Many researchers have examined the reproducibility of the 24-h recall when used to estimate the mean nutrient intake of a group. In general, results based on paired t-tests (Table 6.1) have suggested that this method can provide a relatively reproducible estimate of the mean usual intakes of a group, provided days in all parts of the week are represented in the final sample and many subjects are interviewed (Räsänen, 1979). When repeated 24-h recalls are used, nonconsecutive days are preferred, because eating behaviors on consecutive days are correlated (Hartman et al., 1990).

The exact number of subjects required to estimate the average usual intake of a group with a specified degree of precision can be calculated, provided that the between-subject variation is known; an example is given in Section 3.3.1. Basiotis et al. (1987) calculated that only four 1-d records were required to estimate the average protein intake over 1 y within ± 10% of true usual intake 95%

of the time for a group of 16 adult women, compared to 44 1-d records for the average intake of vitamin A for the group over 1 y for the same degree of precision.

Single 24-h recalls have sometimes been used to assess usual intakes of individuals, presumably on the assumption that the intake over one 24-h period adequately represents the habitual intake. This assumption is not correct. Any estimate of an individual's usual intake, based on a single 24-h recall, has low reproducibility because of relatively large within-subject variation in food intake. Nevertheless, single 24-h recalls can be used to assess actual intakes of food and nutrients, sometimes required for metabolic studies, or for counseling purposes.

The reproducibility of the measurement of the usual intake of an individual can be improved by obtaining several 24-h recalls or records for the same individual, preferably on nonconsecutive days.

Several authors have developed equations for calculating the number of replicate days required to characterize the average intake of an individual with a desired level of precision (Liu et al., 1978; Beaton et al., 1979; Black et al., 1983; Marr and Heady, 1986; Basiotis et al., 1987; Nelson et al., 1989), as noted in Section 3.3.4. Obtaining an estimate within ± 10% of the true usual intake requires more days of intake data per individual than when an estimate within ± 20% is required. For example, using dietary data from the Food Habits of Canadians Survey, Palaniappan et al. (2003) calculated that 30 × 24-h recalls per person were required to obtain an estimate of the energy intake of an individual within ± 10% of the true usual intake 95% of the time, compared to 8 × and 3 × 24-h recalls per person when estimates within ± 20% and ± 30% respectively are required.

The number of days required also depends on the variability of the nutrient, the study group, and the dietary methodology used (Beaton et al., 1979; Basiotis et al., 1987; Nelson et al., 1989; IOM, 2000). Among pregnant women in Indonesia, for example, only 6 × 24-h recalls were needed to esti-

mate the intake of energy, carbohydrate, vitamin A, iron, and vitamin C for an individual within ± 20% of the true usual intake, whereas for calcium 24 replicates would be required (Persson et al., 2001). In both the study of Palaniappan et al. (2003) and Persson et al. (2001), the equation developed by Beaton et al. (1979) (Section 3.3.4) was used. In the Indonesian study, the between-subject variation for energy and nutrients was greater relative to the within-subject variation, perhaps because of the limited number of foods consumed. In more affluent countries, the within-subject variation for nutrients is generally greater than the between-subject variation (Palaniappan et al., 2003). As a result, more observational days are needed to characterize the average intake of an individual with a desired level of precision.

Only a few studies using repeated 24-h recalls have reported the within-subject variation in nutrient intakes, despite its importance in calculating the number of days needed to characterize the average usual intake at the individual level with a specified level of precision.

6.1.2 Food records

To minimize errors resulting from memory lapses and inadequate estimation of portion size, a weighed food record is sometimes used. A 7-d weighed record has often been considered appropriate for estimating the average usual nutrient intakes of individuals. Indeed, this was the method selected for all the U.K National Diet and Nutrition Surveys (Gregory et al., 1990; Finch et al., 1998; Henderson et al., 2002). However, the respondent burden is high, and problems with compliance may arise. Consequently, shorter periods, ranging from 2 to 5 d, are often used. Sometimes, 1-d weighed food records are collected to assess actual food intakes of individuals participating in laboratory studies or for counseling purposes.

In general, studies of the reproducibility of a 7-d weighed record have found good agreement between group mean values obtained for energy and most nutrients on two sep-

Principles of Nutritional Assessment

arate occasions, except when subjects have been on special diets. For example, Adelson (1960) found no significant differences between group mean weekly intakes derived from weighed records of 39 professional men collected for each of two consecutive weeks. Average intakes for individuals, compared by paired difference tests, were also similar in this study, with the exception of vitamin C.

In a later study of nurses living in the United States (Table 6.2), Pearson's and intraclass correlation coefficients were used at the individual level to assess the reproducibility of two 7-d weighed records (Section 6.3.5). As shown in Table 6.2, intraclass correlation coefficients ranged from 0.41 to 0.79, the lowest being for total vitamin A without supplements ($r_i = 0.41$) and polyunsaturated fat ($r_i = 0.45$) (Willett et al., 1985). These studies suggest that, in some circumstances, the 7-d record can provide a relatively reproducible estimate of the usual intake of an individual, but only for certain nutrients.

| | Correlation Coefficients Record 1 vs. 4 | |
	Pearson r	Intraclass r_i
Protein	0.56	0.56
Total fat	0.57	0.54
Saturated fat	0.57	0.56
Polyunsaturated fat	0.44	0.45
Cholesterol	0.54	0.53
Total carbohydrate	0.74	0.72
Sucrose	0.60	0.66
Crude fiber	0.65	0.65
Total vitamin A	0.47	0.56
Without suppl.	0.34	0.41
Vitamin B_6	0.68	0.79
Without suppl.	0.60	0.60
Vitamin C	0.67	0.70
Without suppl.	0.63	0.68
Total calories	0.67	0.63

Table 6.2: Reproducibility of 7-d weighed food records. The data were obtained on two occasions 1 y apart from 173 female registered nurses, aged 34 to 59, residing in the Boston area, 1980–1981. Correlation coefficients were calculated on log-transformed data to improve normality. From Willett et al., American Journal of Epidemiology 122: 51–65, 1985, with permission of the Society for Epidemiologic Research.

Sempos et al. (1985) were among the first investigators to use analysis of variance estimates of the within- and between-subject variation to assess the reproducibility of food records at the individual level. In this study, 2-d food records were collected on two randomly selected days per sampling month over a 2-y period. The subjects were 151 middle-aged women. Estimates of the ratios of within- to between-subject variance were calculated for 15 nutrients from the diet. For all 15 nutrients examined, within-subject variation in the dietary intake was greater than between-subject variation.

Even in some low-income countries where diets are often less varied, high within- to between-subject variance ratios have sometimes (Nyambose et al., 2002), but not always (Persson et al., 2001), been reported. For example, in a study of energy and nutrient intakes of pregnant women in rural Malawi, weighed intakes were collected on average for six consecutive days per women. Variance ratios (i.e., ratios of within- to between-subject variances) (Section 6.2.3) were then calculated; they ranged from 1.1 for fat to 10 for vitamin B_{12}, for women during the second trimester of pregnancy. Indeed, in this study, only individual intakes of energy, protein, carbohydrate, and fiber could be determined within ± 30% of their true usual intakes, with 10 replicate days of weighed intake (Nyambose et al., 2002). To obtain estimates within 20% of the true usual intakes of energy, protein, carbohydrates, and fiber, from 8 to 23 record days were needed. For the micronutrients, from 95 to 213 record days were required. This shows how difficult it may be to obtain precise estimates of an individual's usual intake of micronutrients.

6.1.3 Dietary histories

The reproducibility of a dietary history when used to assess usual mean intakes at the group level depends on the time frame used, its method of administration (e.g., face-to-face or telephone interviews), the time lag of the method, the technique of measuring amounts of foods consumed, and the population group.

	1st interview (mean)	2nd interview (mean)	SD of differences	Intraclass correlation r_I
Energy (kcal)	2352	2327	434	0.86
Protein (g)	82	79	14	0.80
Fat (g)	101	103	26	0.81
Saturated fat (g)	45	46	9	0.89
Linoleic acid (g)	12	14	7	0.67
Carbohydrate (g)	256	248	46	0.87
Dietary fiber (g)	24	23	6	0.75
Alcohol (g)	12	12	8	0.91

Table 6.3: Reproducibility of a dietary history based on interviews with 47 Dutch adults. Data were collected 1 mo apart. From van Staveren et al., American Journal of Clinical Nutrition 42: 554–559, 1985 © Am J Clin Nutr. American Society for Clinical Nutrition.

Normally, the dietary history yields good reproducibility when used to obtain group mean intake information, especially over a relatively short time frame. For example, van Staveren et al. (1985) concluded that their dietary history method, covering 1 mo, provided reproducible estimates of the mean energy and nutrient intakes for an average weekday (Table 6.3). On an individual level, high intraclass correlations also suggested good overall agreement between the two dietary histories. For weekend days, reproducibility was poorer, especially for saturated fat, carbohydrate, and linoleic acid, because of greater dietary variability on weekends.

In a case-control study on breast cancer in a group of Caucasian and Japanese-Hawaiian women, a dietary history questionnaire covering a typical week was repeated after 3 mo (Hankin et al., 1983). The amounts of food consumed were estimated using photographs of three serving sizes (small, medium, and large) of each food. Mean intakes of total fat, saturated fat, cholesterol, and animal protein for all subjects on the two occasions were not significantly different, as tested by the paired *t*-test. Furthermore, the extent of the variability in the nutrient intake, as measured by the standard deviation, was also similar in both interviews. Hence, the questionnaire yielded a reproducible estimate of the usual mean intake of total and saturated fat, cholesterol, and animal protein for the entire group. Nevertheless, when the mean intakes for the two interviews were examined by ethnicity, significant differences for the healthy Caucasian controls were found. These investigators suggested that a longer period was required to estimate the usual food intake of Caucasians because of greater variability in their usual diets compared with Japanese-Hawaiian women.

Note that the use of only three possible portion sizes in the dietary history questionnaire of Hankin et al. (1983) may have contributed in part to the lower variability, and thus higher reproducibility (Block and Hartman, 1989). Certainly, intraclass correlation coefficients obtained after repeated administrations ($n = 3$) of a dietary history questionnaire based on variable portion sizes compared to one without variable portion sizes, on the same study group, were lower (Pietinen et al., 1988a, 1988b).

Dutch investigators evaluated the reproducibility of a cross-check dietary history method covering one year, by repeating the survey four times over a 4-y period (van Beresteyn et al., 1987). They noted that mean daily intakes of energy and most nutrients (total protein, vegetable and animal protein, total fat, saturated fat, mono- and polyunsaturated fat, carbohydrate, dietary fiber, calcium, phosphorus, cholesterol, iron, and sodium) for the group of 246 women were very similar over each of the 4 y, with correlation coefficients ranging from 0.70 to 0.84. Vitamin A and vitamin C were exceptions, with lower correlation coefficients (0.63 and 0.67, respectively), attributed to variation in intakes of foods containing relatively high concentrations of these vitamins.

Question no.	no. of possible answers	Percentage of no. of pairs of answers				Total no. of pairs of answers
		Identical	Within one grade of one another	Separated by more than one grade	Incomplete or not applicable	
2	5	39.6	46.0	14.2	0.0	63
3	5	58.2	30.7	9.3	1.8	3087
4	5	60.1	30.2	5.8	4.0	504
7	4	65.0	31.7	3.2	0.0	63
8	5	45.2	30.2	4.0	20.6	126

Table 6.4: Reproducibility of the answers to questions in a food frequency questionnaire administered twice, with a 3-mo time lag. Subjects were 10 cancer patients and 53 controls from the United Kingdom, all under the age of 75 y. From Acheson and Doll, Gut 5: 126–131, 1964, with permission of the BMJ Publishing Group.

Slightly lower correlation coefficients (0.54 to 0.75 depending on the nutrient) were reported by a French group using a self-administered dietary history questionnaire with 238 food items structured according to the French meal pattern (van Liere et al., 1997). This dietary history was administered twice to 110 subjects, with an interval of approximately 1 y.

6.1.4 Food frequency questionnaires

Several studies have investigated the reproducibility of food frequency questionnaires. One of the first was conducted by Acheson and Doll in 1964. These investigators repeated a food frequency questionnaire after 3 mo had elapsed. Respondents were asked to identify the frequency with which they consumed 48 foods and 8 types of drinks, using a five-point scale. After 3 mo, 90% of the responses differed by less than one point from the original measurement, suggesting that the reproducibility of this food frequency questionnaire for classifying the frequency of food use was good (Table 6.4). However, the limited number of both food items (i.e., 48) and response categories (i.e., 5) may have led to an overstatement of the reproducibility for this instrument (Block and Hartman, 1989).

Willett et al. (1985) evaluated the reproducibility of a self-administered, semiquantitative food frequency questionnaire on 173 female registered nurses, after a time lapse of 1 y. Portion sizes of 99 foods were specified using household measures (e.g., one slice of bread, 8-ounce glass of milk), where possible. Mean daily nutrient intakes were similar. Intraclass correlation coefficients for nutrient intake scores, adjusted for total energy intake, ranged from 0.49 for total vitamin A (without supplements) to 0.71 for sucrose (Table 6.5).

Several investigators have examined the reproducibility of food frequency question-

	Correlation coefficients questionnaire 1 vs. 2	
	Pearson r	Intraclass r_I
Protein	0.54	0.52
Total fat	0.57	0.57
Saturated fat	0.55	0.55
Polyunsaturated fat	0.64	0.64
Cholesterol	0.64	0.63
Total carbohydrate	0.70	0.70
Sucrose	0.71	0.71
Crude fiber	0.67	0.64
Total vitamin A	0.57	0.58
Without suppl.	0.52	0.49
Vitamin B_6	0.60	0.60
Without suppl.	0.57	0.52
Vitamin C	0.59	0.58
Without suppl.	0.62	0.59
Total calories	0.63	0.63

Table 6.5: Reproducibility of a semiquantitative food frequency questionnaire. Data obtained on two occasions 1 y apart from 173 female registered nurses, aged 34 to 59, residing in the Boston area, 1980–1981. Correlation coefficients were calculated on log-transformed data to improve normality. From Willett et al., American Journal of Epidemiology 122: 51–65, 1985, with permission of the Society for Epidemiologic Research.

naires developed for the EPIC study. In the Dutch (Ocké et al., 1997a) and U.K. (Bingham et al., 2001) cohorts, self-administered food frequency questionnaires with questions on the habitual consumption frequency of 178 and 130 food items, respectively, were tested. Frequency of consumption categories were number of times per day, per week, per month, or per year. For most of the food items in the Dutch food frequency questionnaire, questions on portion size were specified in the questionnaire, although for 28 items, color photographs depicted a range of portion sizes (Ocké et al., 1997b). The U.K. food frequency questionnaire did not include specific questions on portion sizes. Instead, medium servings were defined by natural (e.g., apple, slice of bread) or household units, with no distinction according to age or sex (McKeown et al., 2001).

To assess the reproducibility, the Dutch food frequency questionnaire was administered three times — at baseline and 6 and 12 mo later — to 121 subjects, whereas the U.K. EPIC food frequency questionnaire was administered twice to 146 subjects over 9 mo. In both studies, Pearson's correlation coefficients on log-transformed data were used to test the reproducibility of the nutrient intakes calculated from the food frequency questionnaires. Reproducibility was moderate to high, with correlation ranging from 0.59 to 0.94 in the Dutch study, and from 0.50 to 0.80 in the U.K. study, depending on the nutrient. In these studies, energy adjustment (Sections 5.3 and 7.4.2) did not consistently increase the correlation coefficients on the test–retest results. In contrast, Baumgartner et al. (1998) noted higher reproducibility correlation coefficients after an energy adjustment with an interviewer-administered, semiquantitative food frequency questionnaire used with Hispanic and non-Hispanic women aged 35–74 y.

In general, the correlations noted in the literature between repeat administrations of food frequency questionnaires in adults range from $r = 0.5$–0.8, depending on the study group and its size, the nutrient of interest, and certain design features and instructions associated with the instrument. A food frequency questionnaire may limit responses about consumption frequency and portion size, as noted earlier for dietary histories. If less variability is permitted in these two response categories, correlations between repeat administrations of the food frequency questionnaire will be higher.

The quality of the food frequency questionnaire design, and the adequacy of the instructions to the respondent, can also have a significant influence on reproducibility. Optical scanning can reduce coding errors and thus improve the apparent reproducibility of a food frequency questionnaire (Block and Hartman, 1989).

Several food frequency questionnaires have been developed and tested for use with children (Hammond et al., 1993) and adolescents (Rockett et al., 1997). Reproducibility of food frequency questionnaires administered to children may be poor because the children may have difficulty conceptualizing the time frame used and averaging out consumption frequencies and portion sizes over time (Frank, 1994). Field et al. (1999) in a 1-y food frequency questionnaire reproducibility study, noted that U.S. children in the fourth and fifth grades experienced more difficulty completing a food frequency questionnaire than students in the sixth and seventh grades. Female subsistence farmers in rural Malawi had similar difficulties conceptualizing the time frame and averaging consumption frequencies (Ferguson et al., 1995).

Studies examining the reproducibility of food frequency questionnaires assessing the frequency of consumption of specific food items, rather than nutrient intakes, may generate more variable correlation coefficients (Hartman et al., 1990). This arises because there is often a large number of days when a given food or food group is not consumed at all. Converting the data to nutrients tends to smooth out this variation. For example, in rural areas of Malawi, animal source foods are consumed only very occasionally, and then irregularly (Nyambose et al., 2002). Therefore, in such settings the within-subject

	Mean	Total	Between-subject CV	Within-subject CV	Ratio
Energy (kcal/day)	2639	35.8	24.9	25.7	1.0
Protein (g/day)	98.2	46.1	29.1	35.7	1.2
Carbohydrate (g/day)	264.6	37.7	23.4	29.5	1.3
Fat (g/day)	113.9	41.7	28.1	30.8	1.1
Cholesterol (mg/day)	521.1	59.4	28.2	52.3	1.9
Calcium (mg/1000 kcal)	356.1	49.7	26.4	42.1	1.6
Iron (mg/1000 kcal)	5.99	27.6	12.7	24.5	1.9
Thiamin (mg/1000 kcal)	0.674	39.9	16.9	36.2	2.1
Riboflavin (mg/1000 kcal)	0.929	48.5	18.7	44.8	2.4
Vitamin C (mg/1000 kcal)	42.4	71.5	31.7	64.1	2.0
Crude fiber (g/1000 kcal)	1.43	50.5	23.6	44.7	1.9

Table 6.6: Estimated coefficients of variation for total, between-subject, and within-subject variability, and the ratio of within- to between-subject coefficients of variation. Within-subject variability is taken as the residual in the analysis of variance and includes both within-subject variation and variability of the methodology. Data from a study of 30 Toronto male subjects using a 24-h dietary recall, repeated for six days. From Beaton et al., American Journal of Clinical Nutrition 32: 2546–2559, 1979; Beaton et al., American Journal of Clinical Nutrition 37: 986–995, 1983 © Am J Clin Nutr. American Society for Clinical Nutrition.

to between-subject variance (i.e., variance ratios) for foods and food groups may often be greater than for nutrients.

6.2 Sources of true variability in nutrient intakes

If measurement errors are minimized using the strategies described in Chapter 5, the reproducibility of any method for assessing the nutrient intake at the group or individual level is a function of the overall true variability in intake. This is determined by the between- and within-subject variation. In any dietary assessment procedure, replicate observations are not possible; hence, as noted previously, within-subject variation cannot be separated statistically from the measurement errors described in Chapter 5. Nevertheless, if the quality-control procedures outlined in Section 5.2 are used, the confounding effects of measurement error on within-subject variability will be small. Both within- and between-subject variability can be estimated statistically using analysis of variance, as long as two or more days of intake are available on at least a subsample of the population. Hence, within- and between-subject variability cannot be calculated when a food

frequency questionnaire or a dietary history is used.

Other sources of variance, discussed below, can also be estimated using analysis of variance techniques, provided that the initial design of the dietary assessment protocol allowed for their occurrence. Selecting the correct initial study design is thus of great importance.

6.2.1 Between-subject variation

Subjects differ from each other in their usual daily food intake. The between-subject variation is a measure of these differences, which, in turn, depend on the nutrient and the characteristics of the study group. If between-subject variation is large relative to within-subject variation, subjects can be readily distinguished so that the usual nutrient intakes of individuals can be characterized.

Unfortunately, for most nutrients, there is more variability in nutrient intakes within subjects than between them (Beaton et al., 1979, 1997) (Table 6.6). Hence, the within- to between-subject variance ratio is greater than 1.0. This partly explains why the mean intake of a group can usually be assessed more readily than the usual mean intake of an individual. To allow for the effect of between-

	Group size, assuming one observation per individual					
	5	15	25	50	100	200
Energy (kcal/d)	± 32%	± 18%	± 14%	± 10%	± 7.2%	± 5.1%
Cholesterol (mg/d)	± 53%	± 31%	± 24%	± 17%	± 12%	± 8.4%

Table 6.7: Theoretical 95% confidence ranges for the percentage deviation of the group sample mean from the group usual intake, for groups of similar composition but different size. Data derived from a study of 30 Toronto male subjects using a 24-h dietary recall. From Beaton et al., American Journal of Clinical Nutrition 32: 2546–2559, 1979 © Am J Clin Nutr. American Society for Clinical Nutrition.

subject variation on group mean nutrient intakes, the sample size should be as large as possible, and representative of the group to be studied. For example, Table 6.7 shows that for any male study group with between- and within-subject variance comparable to the Toronto subjects, it would be necessary to include 50 or more subjects to be 95% certain that the observed group mean energy intake was within 10% of the true group mean.

6.2.2 Age and sex effects

Variation in nutrient intakes resulting from age and sex differences of the subjects contributes to between-subject variation. Maisey et al. (1995), for example, demonstrated significant differences in the intakes of some nutrients between elderly men and women subjects (Table 6.8). As a result, energy and nutrient intakes should always be presented separately by sex. If the variation in age is very large, the results will also need to be broken down into a number of separate age groups.

Sex differences appear to be largely associated with differences in the amounts of food consumed, rather than the pattern of food consumption (Beaton et al., 1979). If the nutrient intakes are expressed in terms of nutrient densities, differences between males and females tend to disappear, and between-subject variation is often reduced (see example in Table 6.11 and Beaton et al., 1979). This approach does not reduce the within-subject variation, however, or the ratio of within- to between-subject variation (variance ratio) (Section 6.3.1).

6.2.3 Within-subject variation

The within-subject variance is a measure of the true day-to-day variation in the dietary intake of a subject. When estimated by analysis of variance, it represents the sum of true variation in the day-to-day intake of a person, plus all remaining random variation, including measurement error, that remain in the data set. The within-subject variance (s_w^2) may be expressed as a standard deviation (s_w) or as a coefficient of variation (CV_w), where

$$CV_w = s_w / (\text{mean level of intake})$$

The only way to reduce the effect of the

Nutrient	Men ($n = 340$)	Women ($n = 492$)	p
Retinol (µg)	408 (386–457)	355 (333–384)	< 0.001
Carotene (µg)	851 (741–977)	838 (747–939)	0.870
Retinol equ. (µg)	645 (588–706)	567 (518–594)	0.001
Thiamin (mg)	1.10 (1.05–1.16)	1.10 (1.06–1.15)	0.923
Pantothenate (mg)	3.74 (3.59–3.89)	3.18 (3.08–3.30)	< 0.001

Table 6.8: Intakes of selected vitamins by sex for elderly subjects. 95% confidence intervals are shown in parentheses, along with the significance of the differences, p. Geometric means are shown for carotene, thiamin, and pantothenate and are from a general linear model applied to log-transformed data. The Kruskal-Wallis test was applied to the data for retinol and retinol equivalent and the values shown are medians. Data from Maisey et al., British Journal of Nutrition 73: 359–373, 1995, with permission of the Nutrition Society.

	Replicate measures per individual			
	1	2	5	Infinite
Energy	± 55%	± 39%	± 25%	± 10%
Protein	± 64%	± 45%	± 29%	± 12%

Table 6.9: The theoretical 95% confidence ranges for the percentage deviation of the observed mean intake of an individual from the true usual mean intake of the individual, for different numbers of replicate observations. Data calculated from 15-d weighed food intakes of 18 healthy, male California subjects, recorded on tape. From Todd et al., American Journal of Clinical Nutrition 37: 139–146, 1983 © Am J Clin Nutr. American Society for Clinical Nutrition.

within-subject variance on the mean daily intake is to increase the number of measurement days on each individual. The number of measurement days required depends on the desired precision of the estimate. Table 6.9 shows that for male subjects comparable to those from the study in California, it would be necessary to make weighed observations on at least 5 d to be 95% certain that the observed mean energy intake of an individual was within ± 25% of their true usual energy intake.

Measurement days should represent the population of days to be studied. For example, the days can be closely spaced to eliminate bias from seasonal changes, and the days should be selected such that weekend days as well as weekdays are proportionately included (Sempos et al., 1985). Most researchers suggest that nonadjacent days should be chosen to avoid the effects of autocorrelation of consecutive daily intakes (NRC, 1986; Hartman et al., 1990; IOM, 2000).

Minimizing within-subject variation by increasing the number of measurement days does not affect the between-subject variation; it simply enables the usual intake of individuals to be characterized more precisely.

The extent of within-subject variation recorded during dietary assessment depends, in part, on the variety versus monotony in the food choices of an individual (Baisotis et al., 1987; Tarasuk and Beaton, 1991,1992). For example, in Indonesia where a more limited number of foods is consumed, and where the consumption is more closely linked with income than with food availability, within-subject variation is less than between-subject variation (Persson et al., 2001). In contrast, in Malawian female subsistence farmers, higher within- than between-subject variance ratios were reported, and these higher ratios were attributed to the occasional and irregular use of animal foodstuffs (Nyambose et al., 2002). Physiological factors may also influence the within-subject variation. Studies have shown that energy intakes in women vary across the menstrual cycle (Tarasuk and Beaton, 1991; Barr et al., 1995).

Within-subject (and between-subject) variation is a function of the nutrient of interest. Generally, for nutrients found in high concentrations in a few foods that are consumed only occasionally, such as vitamin A, vitamin D, sodium, cholesterol, and linoleic acid, within-subject variation is high, making it more difficult to obtain precise estimates of the usual intakes of these nutrients for individuals; conversely, within-subject variation is lower for nutrients found in many foods, such as carbohydrate and protein (Gibson et al., 1985) (Table 6.6).

Consideration of within-subject variation is particularly important for assessing the prevalence of inadequate intakes in a population group (level two studies, Section 3.3.2), for ranking individuals within a group (level three studies, Section 3.3.3), or when data on usual intakes of individuals are required for correlation or regression analysis with biochemical or clinical parameters at the individual level (level four studies, Section 3.3.4) (Carriquiry, 1999).

Prevalence estimates of inadequate intakes for a specific nutrient are influenced by within-person variation, particularly when the observed distribution of nutrient intakes is based on a single measurement for each subject (e.g., one 24-h recall). In such cases, the mean or median intake for the group may be adequately estimated, but the within-subject variability distorts estimates of the percentiles above and below the mean by increasing the total variance of the distribution. As

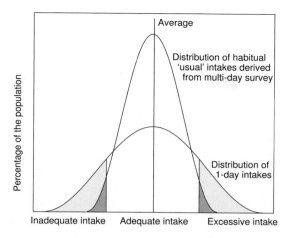

Figure 6.1: Prevalence estimates of excessive and inadequate intakes in both 1-d and multiday surveys of the same population. The prevalence estimated from multiday surveys (dark-shaded areas) is much less than the prevalence estimated from the 1-day survey.

a result, the distribution of observed intakes is wider and flatter.

Figure 6.1 shows the effect of using a single day's intake versus multiple days to characterize usual intakes of individuals. In this example, estimates based on a single day's intake will exaggerate the prevalence of both "inadequate" and "excess" intakes in the population (Beaton, 1982). The extent of the bias in the prevalence estimates depends on the within-subject variation in intake; it cannot be diminished by increasing the sample size.

Disease-diet relationships tend to be obscured and appear less significant if within-subject variation in nutrient intake is ignored. Correlations at the individual level between diet and disease are lowered by within-subject variation. The theoretical reduction in the absolute value of the correlation coefficient can be calculated from the ratio of the within-subject to between-subject variance and the number of replicate observations, provided that the sample size is large (i.e., >100). For example, if the observed variance ratio is 2.0, as determined from three separate dietary intake measurements (such as three 24-h recalls), the correlation coefficient (r) between the estimated intake and some biochemical

parameter is 77% of the true correlation. This figure represents the theoretical attenuation factor from Table 6.10. Hence, the calculated correlation coefficient can be corrected by dividing by 0.77 before testing the significance of the r value. However, with small sample sizes (i.e., < 100), this correction is not advised because the sampling error associated with the correlation coefficient may be too large.

Attenuation may also reduce the significance of regression. Attenuation factors corresponding to different ratios of within- to between-subject variance and different numbers of measurements are also available for simple linear regression. As an example, if the variance ratio equals 2.0 and three measurements of dietary intake (e.g., three 24-h recalls) are used, the regression coefficient of a biological variable on the estimated value of the dietary factor is 60% of the true coefficient. Such a correction must be made with caution, as noted for correlation coefficients. The complete data tables for the attenuation factors for simple correlation and linear regression coefficients are given in Appendices 6.1 and 6.2.

| Variance | No. of replicates per individual | | | | | |
ratio	1	3	5	7	10	14
0.0	1.00	1.00	1.00	1.00	1.00	1.00
0.5	0.82	0.93	0.95	0.97	0.98	0.98
1.0	0.71	0.87	0.91	0.94	0.95	0.97
1.5	0.63	0.82	0.88	0.91	0.93	0.95
2.0	0.58	0.77	0.85	0.88	0.91	0.94
2.5	0.53	0.74	0.82	0.86	0.89	0.92
3.0	0.50	0.71	0.79	0.84	0.88	0.91
3.5	0.47	0.68	0.77	0.82	0.86	0.89
4.0	0.45	0.65	0.75	0.80	0.85	0.88
4.5	0.43	0.63	0.73	0.78	0.83	0.87
5.0	0.41	0.61	0.71	0.76	0.82	0.86

Table 6.10: Attenuation factors for simple correlation coefficients, as determined by the number of replicate observations per individual and the variance ratio (the ratio of the within- to between-subject variances). Abstracted from a more complete data table given in Anderson SA (1986), Guidelines for Use of Dietary Data (Life Sciences Research Office, Federation of American Societies for Experimental Biology).

Finally, within-subject variation and the use of only a limited number of record or recall days, will result in errors when the individuals are classified into terciles, quartiles, or quintiles, based on their nutrient intakes (Anderson, 1986). This classificatory approach is frequently used to examine associations of dietary intake and chronic disease (Section 3.3.3). For example, in cross-sectional studies, relative risks can be computed for each of the four lower quintiles by treating the uppermost quintile of intake as the reference quintile (Table 3.4) (Holick et al., 2002). However, as a result of misclassification, the relative risks are attenuated, and it becomes more difficult to detect the strength of association between diet and disease. Only when the classification is based on sound estimates of the usual daily intake of the nutrient, will the relative risks be more meaningful.

6.2.4 Day-of-the-week effects

Group mean nutrient intakes per day and individual usual intakes per day may both vary with the day of the week. Beaton et al. (1979) demonstrated that women, not men, ate more food on Sundays than weekdays. However, such sex differences have not always been observed subsequently. For example, van Staveren et al. (1982) demonstrated that both sexes had lower intakes of dietary fiber on weekends (Table 6.11).

Not all nutrients exhibit a weekend effect: for those where there are large within- and between-subject fluctuations in daily intakes (e.g., cholesterol, vitamin A, and sodium), a weekend effect may not always be evident (Gibson et al., 1985). Maisey et al. (1995), however, reported increased intakes on Sundays of vegetable-derived micronutrients in their elderly population, especially for the intakes of carotene, retinol equivalents, folate, vitamin C, pantothenate, and zinc.

The weekend effect on nutrient intakes sometimes disappears when nutrients are expressed in terms of nutrient densities (Beaton et al., 1979; Gibson et al., 1985). This finding suggests that the food consumption patterns

are comparable for weekdays and weekend days, but that the total energy intakes differ. Again, this is not always the case. In the study of Maisey et al. (1995), the increased intake of vegetable-derived micronutrients on Sundays was still observed when these nutrients were expressed in terms of the nutrient density.

Any day-of-the-week effect on usual intakes of an individual or group can be accounted for by representing all days of the week in the study design (Beaton et al., 1979; Sempos et al., 1985). It is probably not sufficient to just proportionally include weekend days and weekdays, especially for studies among the elderly whose intakes for some nutrients may vary over the course of the week (Maisey et al., 1995). In such cases, it is preferable to include each day of the week equally in the final study design.

6.2.5 Seasonal and other effects

The effects of the different seasons of the year on food or nutrient intake depend on the population group, its socioeconomic status, and the country. In general, seasonal effects tend to be greater for food items than for

	Fiber intake (mean $\pm$ SD)	
	g/day	g/1000 kcal
	Men ($n=44$)	
Weekdays	28.7 ± 8.5	10.7 ± 2.8
Weekends	24.5 ± 10.2	8.8 ± 3.7
Sig. of differences	$p < 0.01$	$p < 0.01$
	Women ($n=56$)	
Weekdays	21.9 ± 5.0	11.4 ± 2.7
Weekends	19.7 ± 6.7	9.6 ± 3.5
Sig. of differences	$p < 0.05$	$p < 0.01$

Table 6.11: Comparison of the mean daily dietary fiber intakes of male and female subjects on weekdays (Monday to Friday) with weekends (Saturday and Sunday). Data from the intakes of 150 Dutch adults, calculated from 7-d estimated food records. From van Staveren WA et al., Dietary fiber consumption in an adult Dutch population: a methodological study using a seven-day record. Journal of the American Dietetic Association 80: 324–330, 1982 © with permission from the American Dietetic Association.

energy or nutrient intakes (Hartman et al., 1990; Joachim, 1997).

Small seasonal effects have been demonstrated for energy intakes in studies in industrialized countries (Kim et al., 1984; Sempos et al., 1984; van Staveren et al., 1986; Hartman et al., 1990; Palaniappan et al., 2003), whereas marked effects have been noted in less industrialized countries (Ross et al.,1986; Kigutha, 1997). Intakes of certain nutrients — such as vitamin A, vitamin C, iron, and in some cases fat — appear to show seasonal variation in both low-income and industrialized countries (van Staveren et al., 1986; Hartman et al., 1990; Kigutha, 1997).

A seasonal effect can be taken into account by administering the survey over a long interval of time (e.g., 1 y) and including randomly selected days representative of all seasons of the year (Hartman et al., 1990; Ocké et al., 1997b). If this is not done, investigators should be wary of applying the results obtained at one particular season to the rest of the year.

The existence of chronic illness or dieting in certain subgroups of the population may adversely affect dietary intakes. This may lead to a bias in the prevalence of inadequate intakes in a population presumed to be normal and healthy (van Staveren et al., 1994).

6.2.6 Sequence effect

Subjects may react to repeated interviews, showing a sequence or training effect that may result in changing reported nutrient intakes over time (Frank et al., 1984). This effect may be severe if subjects complete the recall or records on consecutive days (Sharma et al., 1998). The presence or absence of a sequence effect on group mean or individual intakes can be assessed by completing the interviews or records on randomly selected days of the week and recording their order. Beaton et al. (1979) did not observe a sequence effect in their study involving highly trained, standardized interviewers. Other investigators have also found no evidence of a sequence effect (Gibson et al., 1985; Maisey et al., 1995).

6.3 Statistical assessment of reproducibility

The following sections provide only a brief account of the statistical methods for assessing reproducibility. Readers are advised to consult a standard statistics text for further information (e.g., Altman, 1991).

Reproducibility is affected by between- and within-subject variation, as noted earlier, and hence investigators should always try to design the dietary assessment protocol in such a way that these two sources of variability can be separated and estimated statistically. Normally this is achieved by using analysis of variance techniques (see below).

Many of the earlier reproducibility studies of dietary assessment methods did not include any consideration of between- and within-subject variability, and they did not use analysis of variance. Instead, as noted earlier, reproducibility was assessed using a test–retest design, in which the same dietary method was repeated on the same individuals after a preselected time interval. Other statistical procedures, some of which are described below, were then used to examine the extent of agreement at the group and individual level.

6.3.1 Analysis of variance

The preferred statistical approach to estimate reproducibility of any dietary method involves analysis of variance (ANOVA). This procedure assesses the differences, if any, in the group mean intake of each nutrient between the replicates, and it can be used to identify and estimate between- and within-subject variability. The variance ratio (the ratio of within-subject (s_w^2) to the between-subject (s_b^2) variation) can then be calculated. Variance ratios depend critically on the nutrient, sample size, number of measurement days per subject, dietary methodology, and probably the age, sex, and sociocultural group (NRC, 1986; Hartman et al., 1990). Hence, when comparing variance ratios from different studies, these factors should be taken into consideration.

The NRC (1986) Report on Nutrient Adequacy presents a summary table of reported variance ratios for dietary studies of adults, compiled from the literature (Table 6.12). A ratio of 1.0 indicates that the within-subject and between-subject variances are equal. As stated previously, the within-subject variation is usually larger than between-subject variation. Nutrients such as cholesterol, polyunsaturated fatty acids, and, in most cases, vitamin A, have larger variance ratios than other dietary components. In general, energy intake tends to have the smallest variance ratio (approximately 1.0), with those for protein, carbohydrate, total fat, and saturated fats ranging approximately from 1.0 to 2.0.

Once estimates of the between- and within-subject variability have been calculated using analysis of variance, they can be used in the following equations to calculate, based on the standard error of the mean: (*a*) the reproducibility of the dietary method to estimate the usual intake of a group and (*b*) the reproducibility of the dietary method to estimate the usual intake of an individual (Cole and Black, 1984):

(a) standard error of the group mean intake

$$= \sqrt{\frac{s_b^2}{n} + \frac{s_w^2}{mn}}$$

(b) standard error of the individual's mean intake

$$= \sqrt{\frac{s_w^2}{m}}$$

where n = sample size, m = number of days measured, s_b^2 = between-subject variance, and s_w^2 = within-subject variance.

6.3.2 Paired tests on the mean or median intake

Paired t-tests or the nonparametric Wilcoxon matched-pairs signed-rank test for nonnormally distributed data are commonly used to assess agreement between nutrient intakes on a group basis. No significant difference between the group mean or median intakes for the two sets of data is taken to indicate satisfactory agreement, and hence reproducibility (Table 6.1). In the example given in Table 6.13, there were no significant differences between the median intake of any of the dietary components listed, assessed by the two administrations of the food frequency questionnaire, with the single exception of vitamin C.

The confounding effect of within-subject variation on usual nutrient intakes is not taken into account when a paired t-test or the Wilcoxon's signed-rank test is used. When the within-subject variation is large relative to the between-subject variation, the power of the t-test will be reduced. As a result, nonsignificant differences in group mean intakes may not necessarily indicate good reproducibility but the confounding effect of large within-subject variation, apparent in a large coefficient of variation (NRC, 1986).

6.3.3 Degree of misclassification

Assessment of the degree of misclassification is the simplest method of quantifying the extent of agreement on an individual basis. This approach is often used for qualitative food frequency questionnaires in which the data have been classified according to frequency of food use. The percentage of pairs with exact agreement or within a selected number of units is calculated. An example is shown in Table 6.4.

Alternatively, if a semiquantitative food frequency questionnaire has been used, permitting nutrient intakes to be calculated, they can be classified into quartiles, for example, to assess the ability of a food frequency questionnaire to assign individuals to the same quartile of intake on both occasions. Next the following percentages may be calculated: percentage correctly classified into the same quartile, percentage correctly classified into the extreme quartiles, percentage correctly classified within one quartile, and the percentage grossly misclassified (i.e., classified into opposite quartiles). This approach, however, ignores the fact that a certain amount of

Nutrient	24-hour recall by young adults [a]	3-day record by older adults [b]	1-day recall by women [c] Year 1	1-day recall by women [c] Year 2	7-day record by men [d]	24-hour recall by pregnant women [e]
Males:						
Energy	1.1	1.0			0.8	
Protein	1.5	1.2			1.4	
Carbohydrate	1.6	2.1			0.6	
Fat	1.2	1.2			1.3	
SFA [f]	1.1	2.2			1.4	
PUFA [g]	2.8	3.5			1.9	
Cholesterol	3.4	5.6			1.9	
Vitamin A	[h]	1.6				
Vitamin C	3.5	2.3				
Thiamin	2.5	0.9				
Riboflavin	2.4	0.9				
Niacin equivalent	1.6	2.2				
Calcium	2.2	1.1				
Iron	1.7	1.8				
Females:						
Energy	1.4	0.8	1.6	1.6		1.1
Protein	1.5	1.3	2.1	2.1		1.4
Carbohydrate	1.4	1.2	NR [i]	NR		1.2
Fat	1.6	0.9	NR	NR		1.2
SFA [f]	1.4	1.7	NR	NR		NR
PUFA [g]	4.0	2.2	NR	NR		NR
Cholesterol	4.3	4.2	NR	NR		NR
Vitamin A	24.3	2.5	7.7	10.9		NR
Vitamin C	2.0	2.8	2.3	2.5		NR
Thiamin	4.4	1.6	3.3	3.9		NR
Riboflavin	2.2	1.8	3.0	3.3		NR
Niacin equivalent	4.0	2.5	NR	NR		NR
Calcium	0.9	1.7	1.1	1.2		1.0
Iron	2.5	1.5	2.7	2.5		NR

Table 6.12: Observed ratios of within-subject to between-subject variances. A ratio of 1.0 indicates that the within-subject and between-subject variances are equal. A ratio greater than 1.0 indicates that within-subject variance is greater than between-subject variance. The original papers contain additional data. Only those nutrient variables examined in two or more papers are included here. [a] From Beaton et al. (1979, 1983). [b] From Hunt et al. (1983). [c] From Sempos et al. (1985). [d] From McGee et al. (1982). [e] From Rush and Kristal (1982). [f] Saturated fatty acids. [g] Polyunsaturated fatty acids. [h] None of the variance could be assigned to subjects. [i] NR, not reported. Reproduced from NRC (1986) Nutrient Adequacy: Assessment Using Food Consumption Surveys, with permission of the National Academy Press, Washington, DC.

agreement invariably occurs by chance alone. This limitation can be overcome by using Cohen's weighted kappa statistic (Cohen, 1968).

6.3.4 Mean and standard deviation of the difference

Bland and Altman (1986) have recommended the use of the mean and standard deviation of the differences between the two replicates for comparing nutrient intakes at an individual level. They also suggested calculating the 95% confidence limits (i.e., mean difference $\pm 2\,\mathrm{SDs}$) for the difference between the two replicates. They refer to these as the "limits of agreement" (LOA). A judgment can then be made as to whether the agreement reached between the two replicates is acceptable.

	First FFQ	Second FFQ	Mean difference (LOA)	Correlation
Iron (mg)	9.0 (7.9, 12)	9.2 (8.4, 12)	−0.4 (−4.8, 4.0)	0.65
Nonheme iron (mg)	8.0 (6.8, 10)	8.5 (7.8, 10)	−0.4 (−4.2, 3.4)	0.67
Heme iron (mg)	1.0 (0.4, 1.3)	0.8 (0.5, 1.3)	0.1 (−0.9, 1.1)	0.71
Meat iron (mg)	2.5 (1.0, 3.3)	1.9 (1.2, 3.3)	0.2 (−2.0, 2.4)	0.71
Vitamin C (mg)	82 (69, 120)	99 (70, 149)*	−22 (−116, 72)	0.61
Phytate (mg)	1031 (636, 1429)	963 (720, 1368)	75 (−781, 931)	0.86
Calcium (mg)	672(476, 924)	641 (527, 841)	4.1 (−326, 334)	0.90
Meat/fish/poultry (g)	126 (55,159)	114 (54,141)	14 (−68, 96)	0.71
Tea (g)	0.0 (0.0, 168)	22 (0.0 276)	−32 (−202, 138)	0.89
Coffee (g)	134 (0.0, 365)	74 (0.0, 562)	−65 (−417, 287)	0.84

Table 6.13: Comparison of intakes of iron, iron enhancers, and iron inhibitors from two administrations of an iron food frequency questionnaire; $n = 22$, mean (25th and 75th percentiles). Also shown are the mean differences and the associated 95% CI, and the correlation coefficients. *Significant differences between first and second administration of the food frequency questionnaire (Wilcoxon: $p \leq 0.05$). From Heath et al., European Journal of Clinical Nutrition 54: 592–599, 2000 © with permission of the Nature Publishing Group.

Table 6.13 illustrates the use of the Bland and Altman (1986) approach for comparing the intakes of iron and selected iron absorption modifiers, obtained from repeat administrations of a computer-administered food frequency questionnaire (Heath et al., 2000). Here the mean difference between the iron intakes reported in the two administrations of the iron food frequency questionnaire was −0.4 mg (LOA −4.8, 4.0). As the 95% LOA include 0.0 (no difference), the results suggest that the listed nutrients and food qualities estimated from the food frequency administered on the two occasions are in agreement and that the method is reproducible.

Calculating the mean difference provides information immediately about the direction of bias. A plot of the individual differences against the mean level of intake can indicate if the bias is constant across levels of intake. Calculating the LOA provides a way of assessing the differences between the measurements.

Ambrisoni et al. (2001) also followed this approach when examining differences between β-carotene and retinol intakes obtained from a brief food frequency questionnaire administered twice, 1 y apart, to former workers and residents (n = 83) of an asbestos mining and milling town in Western Australia. The differences between the two measures were plotted against the average of the two. Any

dependency was then formally tested by fitting the regression line of differences (H_0 : $\beta = 0, \alpha = 0.05$).

However, the appropriateness of this approach is disputed. Willett (1998) argues that the mean and standard deviation of the difference between two methods tends to be a cumbersome way of evaluating intakes of many nutrients, and they are difficult to interpret because the between-subject variability varies from nutrient to nutrient. Burema et al. (1988) also discourage the use of this approach as an indication of reproducibility at the group level.

6.3.5 Correlation analysis

Either Pearson's product moment correlation coefficients for normally distributed data or Spearman's nonparametric rank correlation coefficients and/or intraclass correlation coefficients are often calculated to assess agreement on an individual (within-pair) basis. Intraclass correlation coefficients (r_i) correct for the number of chance expected agreements (Tables 6.2, 6.3, and 6.5). High correlation coefficients relating nutrient intakes measured on the two separate occasions are taken as indicative of good overall agreement between the two sets of nutrient data (Ocké et al., 1997b).

In fact, both parametric and nonparametric

correlation coefficients quantify the extent of the linear trend relating the two sets of results, and not agreement. Additionally, sources of bias in one of the replicates may not be revealed by correlation analysis. For example, assume that results for the second replicate were exactly 10% higher than those obtained on the first occasion. Analysis will indicate perfect correlation ($r = 1.0$) between the two replicates, but there is far from perfect agreement. Altman et al. (1983) also stressed that the correlation coefficients cannot be judged on a null hypothesis basis of no correlation because there is an a priori reason to believe that the results correlate. People tend to eat similar foods from day to day; some agreement is to be expected.

Notwithstanding the frequent use of correlation analysis, caution is needed when it is applied to evaluate the extent of the agreement in a test–retest design for measuring reproducibility. If the line of equality is drawn, the plot of the test against the retest results can be useful in indicating bias and the presence of outliers. However, the numerical value of r should be interpreted with caution and other statistical measures used to assess reproducibility (see analogous discussion in relation to validity in Section 7.4.2).

6.4 Summary

Reproducibility of dietary surveys refers to the extent to which a specific dietary method used repeatedly in the same situation gives similar results. In general, reproducibility of a dietary assessment method depends on the time frame of the method, the population group under study, the nutrient of interest, the technique used to measure the foods and quantities consumed, and the between- and within-subject variances. True reproducibility cannot be measured in dietary assessment because nutrient intakes vary daily. Instead, it is conventionally estimated using a test–retest design, followed by an assessment of the extent of the agreement between the nutrient intakes obtained on the two separate occasions, by the same method.

Reproducibility studies suggest that the 24-h recall and dietary histories over a short time frame can provide a relatively reproducible estimate of the average usual intake for most nutrients for a large group, but not for individuals. For the latter, weighed dietary records, especially those completed for 7 d, yield nutrient intakes that are more reproducible, with the notable exception of vitamins A and C, and polyunsaturated fat. The reproducibility of qualitative food frequency questionnaires for classifying individuals according to the frequency of use of certain foods or food groups depends on the frequency with which the foods are consumed. For foods consumed less frequently, reproducibility tends to be less than for those eaten frequently. The reproducibility of semi-quantitative food frequency questionnaires depends on their design, the study group, and the nutrients under study. For some food frequency questionnaires, reproducibility may be high because their design limits the recording of variability in food and, hence, nutrient intakes.

The preferred method of estimating reproducibility in dietary assessment is to calculate the within- and between-subject variance, using analysis of variance. Such an approach can only be used for recalls or records. The variance ratios (the ratios of within- to between-subject variance) cannot be compared among different studies because they depend critically on the nutrient, sample size, number of measurement days per subject, dietary methodology, age, sex, and sociocultural group.

Statistical methods for assessing reproducibility on a group average (aggregate) basis using a test–retest design include paired tests on the mean (paired t-tests), or the median (Wilcoxon matched-pairs signed-rank test) intakes.

At the individual level, the simplest method for testing agreement is to calculate the percentage of misclassification, by comparing the number of pairs, with exact agreement or within a selected numbers of units. For foods, this may be based on frequency of use or amount (in grams), whereas for nutrients, scores (intakes per 1000 kcal) may be used. Cohen's weighted kappa statistic should then be calculated.

Additional methods for testing agreement between the results at the individual level include the mean and standard deviation of the differences between the two replicates, referred to as the limits of agreement (LOA) by Bland and Altman. They also suggest calculating the 95% confidence interval. Alternatively, for individual agreement, correlation analysis can be performed, although it must be used with caution. The use of intraclass correlation coefficients (r_i) are preferred because they correct for the amount of chance-expected agreements.

References

Acheson ED, Doll R. (1964). Dietary factors in carcinoma of the stomach: a study of 100 cases and 200 controls. Gut 5: 126–131.

Adelson SF. (1960). Some problems in collecting dietary data from individuals. Journal of the American Dietetic Association 36: 453–461.

Altman DG. (1991). Practical Statistics for Medical Research. Chapman & Hall, London.

Altman DG, Gore SM, Gardner MJ, Pocock SJ. (1983). Statistical guidelines for contributors to medical journals. British Medical Journal 286: 1489–1495.

Ambrisoni GI, de Klerk NH, Musk AW, Mackerras D. (2001). Agreement between a brief food frequency questionnaire and diet records using two statistical methods. Public Health Nutrition 4: 255–264.

Anderson SA (ed.). (1986). Guidelines for Use of Dietary Data. Life Sciences Research Office, Federation of American Societies for Experimental Biology, Bethesda, MD.

Barr SI, Janelle KC, Prior JC. (1995). Energy intakes are higher during the luteal phase of ovulatory menstrual cycles. American Journal of Clinical Nutrition 61: 39–43.

Basiotis PP, Welsh SO, Cronin FJ, Kelsay JL, Mertz W. (1987). Number of days of food intake records required to estimate individual and group nutrient intakes with defined confidence. Journal of Nutrition 117: 1638–1641.

Baumgartner KB, Gilliland F, Nicholson CS, McPherson RS, Hunt WC, Pathak DR, Samet JM. (1998). Validity and reproducibility of a food frequency questionnaire among Hispanic and non-Hispanic white women in New Mexico. Ethnicity and Disease 8: 81–92.

Beaton GH. (1982). What do we think we are estimating. In: Beal VA, Laus MJ (eds.) Proceedings of the Symposium on Dietary Data Collection, Anal-

ysis and Significance. Research Bulletin No. 675. Massachusetts Agricultural Research Station, University of Massachusetts, Amherst, pp. 36–48.

Beaton GH, Milner J, Corey P, McGuire V, Cousins M, Stewart E, de Ramos M, Hewitt D, Grambsch PV, Kassim N, Little JA. (1979). Sources of variance in 24-hour dietary recall data: implications for nutrition study, design and interpretation. American Journal of Clinical Nutrition 32: 2546–2559.

Beaton GH, Milner J, McGuire V, Feather TE, Little JA. (1983). Sources of variance in 24-hour dietary recall data; implications for nutrition study design and interpretation: carbohydrate sources, vitamins, and minerals. American Journal of Clinical Nutrition 37: 986–995.

Beaton GH, Burema J, Ritenbaugh C. (1997). Errors in the interpretation of dietary assessments. American Journal of Clinical Nutrition 65: 1100S–1107S.

Bingham SA, Welch AA, McTaggart A, Mulligan AA, Runswick SA, Luben R, Oakes S, Khaw KT, Wareham N, Day NE. (2001). Nutritional methods in the European Prospective Investigation of Cancer in Norfolk. Public Health Nutrition 4: 847–858.

Black AE, Cole TJ, Wiles SJ, White F. (1983). Daily variation in food intake of infants from 2 to 18 months. Human Nutrition: Applied Nutrition 37: 448–458.

Bland JM, Altman DG. (1986). Statistical methods for assessing agreement between two methods of clinical measurement. Lancet 1(8476): 307–310.

Block G, Hartman AM. (1989). Issues in reproducibility and validity of dietary studies. American Journal of Clinical Nutrition 50: 1133–1138.

Burema J, van Staveren WA, van den Brandt PA (1988). Validity and reproducibility. In: Cameron ME, van Staveren WA (eds.). Manual on Methodology for Food Consumption Studies. Oxford University Press, Oxford. pp. 171–181.

Carriquiry AL. (1999). Assessing the prevalence of nutrient inadequacy. Public Health Nutrition 2: 23–33.

Cohen J. (1968). Weighted kappa, nominal scale agreement with provision for scaled disagreement or partial credit. Psychological Bulletin 70: 213–220.

Cole T, Black A. (1984). Statistical aspects in the design of dietary surveys. In: The Dietary Assessment of Populations. Medical Research Council Scientific Report No. 4. Southampton General Hospital, Medical Research Council, pp. 5–8.

Ferguson EL, Gadowsky SL, Huddle J-M, Cullinan TR, Lehrfeld J, Gibson RS. (1995). An interactive 24-h recall technique for assessing the adequacy of trace mineral intakes of rural Malawian women: its advantages and limitations. European Journal of Clinical Nutrition 49: 565–578.

Field AE, Peterson KE, Gortmaker SL, Cheung L, Rockett H, Fox MK, Colditz GA. (1999). Reproducibility and validity of a food frequency questionnaire among fourth to seventh grade inner-city school children: implications of age and day-to-day variation in dietary intake. Public Health Nutrition 2: 293–300.

Finch S, Doyle W, Lowe C, Bates CJ, Prentice A, Smithers G, Clarke PC. (1998). National Diet and Nutrition Survey: People Aged 65 Years and Over. Volume 1: Report of the Diet and Nutrition Survey. The Stationery Office, London.

Frank GC. (1994). Environmental influences on methods used to collect dietary data from children. American Journal of Clinical Nutrition 59: 207S–211S.

Frank GC, Farris RP, Berenson GS. (1984). Comparison of dietary intake by two computerized analysis systems. Journal of the American Dietetic Association 84: 818–820.

Gibson RS, Gibson IL, Kitching J. (1985). A study of inter- and intra-subject variability in seven-day weighed dietary intakes with particular emphasis on trace elements. Biological Trace Element Research 8: 79–91.

Gregory J, Foster K, Tyler H, Wiseman M. (1990). The Dietary and Nutritional Survey of British Adults. The Stationery Office, London.

Hammond J, Nelson M, Chinn S, Rona RJ. (1993). Validation of a food frequency questionnaire for assessing dietary intake in a study of coronary heart disease risk factors in children. European Journal of Clinical Nutrition 47: 242–250.

Hankin JH, Rawlings V, Nomura A. (1978). Assessment of a short dietary method for a prospective study on cancer. American Journal of Clinical Nutrition 31: 355–359.

Hankin JH, Nomura AMY, Lee J, Hirohata T, Kolonel LN. (1983). Reproducibility of a diet history questionnaire in a case-control study of breast cancer. American Journal of Clinical Nutrition 37: 981–985.

Hartman AM, Brown CC, Palmgren J, Pietinen P, Verkasalo M, Myer D, Virtamo J. (1990). Variability in nutrient and food intakes among older middle-aged men: implications for design of epidemiology and validation studies using food recording. American Journal of Epidemiology 132: 999–1012.

Heath A-LM, Skeaff CM, Gibson RS. (2000). The relative validity of a computerized food frequency questionnaire for estimating intake of dietary iron and its absorption modifiers. European Journal of Clinical Nutrition 54: 592–599.

Henderson L, Gregory J, Swan G. (2002). National Diet and Nutrition Survey: Adults aged 19 to 64. Volume 1: Types and Quantities of Foods Consumed. The Stationery Office, London.

Holick CN, Michaud DS, Stolzenberg-Solomon R, Mayne ST, Pietinen P, Taylor PR, Virtamo J, Albanes D. (2002). Dietary carotenoids, serum β-carotene, and retinol and risk of lung cancer in the α-tocopherol, β-carotene cohort study. American Journal of Epidemiology 156: 536–547.

Hunt WC, Leonard AG, Garry PJ, Goodwin JS. (1983). Components of variance in dietary data for an elderly population. Nutrition Research 3: 433–444.

IOM (Institute of Medicine). (2000). Dietary Reference Intakes: Applications in Dietary Assessment. Institute of Medicine, National Academy Press, Washington, DC.

Joachim G. (1997). The influence of time on dietary data: differences in reported summer and winter food consumption. Nutrition and Health 12: 33–43.

Kigutha HN. (1997). Assessment of dietary intake in rural communities in Africa: experiences in Kenya. American Journal of Clinical Nutrition 65: 1168S–1172S.

Kim WW, Kelsay JL, Judd JT, Marshall MW, Mertz W, Prather ES. (1984). Evaluation of long-term dietary intakes of adults consuming self-selected diets. American Journal of Clinical Nutrition 40: 1327–1332.

Liu K, Stamler J, Dyer A, McKeever J, McKeever P. (1978). Statistical methods to assess and minimize the role of intra-individual variability in obscuring relationships between dietary lipids and serum cholesterol. Journal of Chronic Diseases 31: 399–418.

Maisey S, Loughridge J, Southon S, Fulcher R. (1995). Variation in food group and nutrient intake with day of the week in an elderly population. British Journal of Nutrition 73: 359–373.

Marr JW, Heady JA. (1986). Within- and between-person variability in dietary surveys: number of days needed to classify individuals. Human Nutrition: Applied Nutrition 40A: 347–364.

McGee D, Rhoads G, Hankin J, Yano K, Tillotson J. (1982). Within-person variability of nutrient intake in a group of Hawaiian men of Japanese ancestry. American Journal of Clinical Nutrition 36: 657–663.

McKeown NM, Day NE, Welch AA, Runswick SA, Luben RN, Mulligan AA, McTaggart A, Bingham SA. (2001). Use of biological markers to validate self-reported dietary intake in a random sample of the European Prospective Investigation into Cancer United Kingdom Norfolk cohort. American Journal of Clinical Nutrition 74: 188–196.

Nelson M, Black AE, Morris JA, Cole TJ. (1989). Between- and within-subject variation in nutrient intake from infancy to old age: estimating the number of days required to rank dietary intakes with desired precision. American Journal of Clinical Nutrition 50: 155–167.

NRC (National Research Council). (1986). Nutrient Adequacy: Assessment using Food Consumption Surveys. National Academy Press, Washington, DC.

Nyambose J, Koski KG, Tucker KL. (2002). High intra/interindividual variance ratios for energy and nutrient intakes of pregnant women in rural Malawi show that many days are required to estimate usual intake. Journal of Nutrition 132: 1313–1318.

Ocké MC, Bueno-de-Mesquita H, Goddijn HE, Jansen A, Pols MA, van Staveren WA, Kromhout D. (1997a). The Dutch EPIC food frequency questionnaire. I: Description of the questionnaire and relative validity and reproducibility for food groups. International Journal of Epidemiology 26: S37–S48.

Ocké MC, Bueno-de-Mesquita H, Pols MA, Smit HA, van Staveren WA, Kromhout D. (1997b). The Dutch EPIC food frequency questionnaire. II: Relative validity and reproducibility for nutrients. International Journal of Epidemiology 26: S49–S58.

Palaniappan U, Cue RI, Payette H, Gray-Donald K. (2003). Implications of day-to-day variability on measurements of usual food and nutrient intakes. Journal of Nutrition 133: 232–235.

Persson V, Winkvist A, Ninuk T, Hartini S, Greiner T, Hakimi M, Stenlund H. (2001). Variability in nutrient intakes among pregnant women in Indonesia: implications for the design of epidemiological studies using the 24-h recall method. Journal of Nutrition 131: 325–330.

Pietinen P, Hartman AM, Haapa E, Rasanen L, Haapakoski J, Palmgren J, Albanes D, Virtamo J, Huttenen JK. (1988a). Reproducibility and validity of dietary assessment instruments. I: A self-administered food use questionnaire with a portion size picture booklet. American Journal of Epidemiology 128: 655–666.

Pietinen P, Hartman AM, Haapa E, Rasanen L, Haapakoski J, Palmgren J, Albanes D, Virtamo J, Huttenen JK. (1988b). Reproducibility and validity of dietary assessment instruments. II: A qualitative food frequency questionnaire. American Journal of Epidemiology 128: 667–676.

Räsänen L. (1979). Nutrition survey of Finnish rural children. VI: Methodological study comparing the 24-hour recall and the dietary history interview. American Journal of Clinical Nutrition 32: 2560–2567.

Rockett HR, Breitenbach M, Frazier Al, Witschi J, Wolf AM, Field AE, Colditz GA. (1997). Validation of a youth/adolescent food frequency questionnaire. Preventive Medicine 26: 808–816.

Ross J, Gibson RS, Sabry JH. (1986). A study of seasonal trace element intakes and hair trace element concentrations in selected households from the Wosera, Papua New Guinea. Tropical and Geographical Medicine 38: 246–254.

Rush D, Kristal AR. (1982). Methodologic studies during pregnancy: the reliability of the 24-hour dietary recall. American Journal of Clinical Nutrition 35: 1259–1268.

Sempos CT, Johnson NE, Smith EL, Gilligan C. (1984). A two-year dietary survey of middle-aged women: repeated dietary records as a measure of usual intake. Journal of the American Dietetic Association 84: 1008–1013.

Sempos CT, Johnson NE, Smith EL, Gilligan C. (1985). Effects of intraindividual and interindividual vari-

ation in repeated dietary records. American Journal of Epidemiology 121: 120–130.

Sharma M, Rao M, Jacob S, Jacob CK. (1998). Validation of a 24-hour dietary recall: a study on hemodialysis patients. Journal of Renal Nutrition 8: 199–202.

Tarasuk V, Beaton GH. (1991). The nature and individuality of within-subject variation in energy intake. American Journal of Clinical Nutrition 54: 464–470.

Tarasuk V, Beaton GH. (1992). Statistical estimation of dietary parameters: implications of patterns in within-subject variation — a case study of sampling strategies. American Journal of Clinical Nutrition 55: 22–27.

Todd KS, Hudes M, Calloway DH. (1983). Food intake measurement: problems and approaches. American Journal of Clinical Nutrition 37: 139–146.

van Beresteyn ECH, van't Hof MA, van der Heiden-Winkel-dermaat HJ, ten Have-Witjes A, Neeter R. (1987). Evaluation of the usefulness of the cross-check dietary history method in longitudinal studies. Journal of Chronic Diseases 40: 1051–1058.

van Liere M, Lucas F, Clavel F, Slimani N, Villeminot S. (1997). Relative validity and reproducibility of a French dietary history questionnaire. International Journal of Epidemiology 26: S128–S136.

van Staveren WA, Hautvast JGAJ, Katan MB, van Montfort MAJ, van Oosten-Van Der Goes HGC. (1982). Dietary fiber consumption in an adult Dutch population: a methodological study using a seven-day record. Journal of the American Dietetic Association 80: 324–330.

van Staveren WA, de Boer JO, Burema J. (1985). Validity and reproducibility of a dietary history method estimating the usual food intake during one month. American Journal of Clinical Nutrition 42: 554–559.

van Staveren WA, Deurenberg P, Burema J, de Groot LCPGM, Hauvast JGAJ. (1986). Seasonal variation in food intake, pattern of physical activity and change in body weight in a group of young adult Dutch women consuming self-selected diets. International Journal of Obesity 10: 133–145.

van Staveren WA, De Groot LC, Blauw YH, van der Wielen RP. (1994). Assessing diets of elderly people: problems and approaches. American Journal of Clinical Nutrition 59: 221S–223S.

Willett W. (1998). Nature of variation in diet. In: Willett W (ed.) Nutrition Epidemiology. Oxford University Press, New York, pp.33–49, 1998.

Willett W, Sampson L, Stampfer M, Rosner B, Bain C, Witschi J, Hennekens CH, Speizer FE. (1985). Reproducibility and validity of a semiquantitative food frequency questionnaire. American Journal of Epidemiology 122: 51–65.

7

Validity in dietary assessment methods

Validity describes the degree to which a dietary method measures what it is intended to measure (Block and Hartman, 1989). Dietary methods designed to characterize usual intakes of individuals are the most difficult to validate because the "truth" is never known with absolute certainty. Even if the actual food intake, monitored from the results of unobtrusive weighed observations, compares favorably with results obtained from food records maintained by the subjects during the same period, there is no guarantee that the records represent the subjects' true usual food intake (Block, 1982). To detect any changes in usual intake during the study, observations of actual food intake during, and either before or after the study period should be compared. Such a procedure attempts to measure absolute validity, but it is very time consuming and presents overwhelming practical difficulties. Consequently, absolute validity is generally determined in dietary studies that involve a limited number of subjects or only cover a relatively short time frame.

Relative validity, however, can be assessed on dietary methods covering both short- and long-term time frames. Relative validity can be defined as the comparison of the "test" method with another method, termed the "reference" method, which has a greater degree of demonstrated validity (Bailey, 1978). Ideally, the reference is generally a dietary method, chosen in such a way that errors in the two dietary methods are independent. In practice, however, reference dietary methods seldom meet this criterion.

An alternative approach involving external independent markers of intake, termed "biomarkers," is being increasingly used to overcome the limitations of "reference" dietary methods. To be a valid measure of relative validity, biomarkers must provide an independent assessment of the intake of the nutrient and respond to the intake of the nutrient, preferably in a dose-dependent manner. As a result, biomarkers are only available for a limited number of nutrients. Most biomarkers are measured in body fluids or tissues; their use in dietary assessment has highlighted important sources of bias in all dietary methods.

In general, the errors that affect the validity of a dietary method are systematic; those associated with reproducibility are random. Systematic errors are much more difficult to control than the sources of random measurement errors discussed in Chapter 5. Subjects may eat atypically during a dietary period, or systematically misreport certain foods, even though every effort is made to discourage this.

This chapter discusses the measurement of relative validity of dietary methods using a second dietary method as the reference, as well as the newer methods that employ biomarkers.

7.1 Design of relative validity studies

Because of the difficulties in measuring the absolute validity of dietary intake data, researchers have adopted an approach that measures relative validity. In this approach, the "test" dietary method is evaluated against another "reference" dietary method performed on the same subjects. Several factors must be taken into account in the design of such a validation study; these factors are outlined below. For a more detailed discussion of these factors, see Block and Hartman (1989) and Nelson (1997).

7.1.1 Selection of subjects for a validation study

The test dietary method should be validated on subjects who are representative of the population under study. This is particularly important in multicenter trials, when cultural or language differences may influence the way in which subjects respond to a dietary assessment method. All too often, the volunteers who participate in validation studies are self-selected; they may provide more accurate responses and have different dietary habits than the study population (Riboli et al., 1997). Other characteristics of subjects that may influence subject selection include overweight (Braam et al., 1998), history of dieting or restrained eating (Lafay et al., 1997), depression (Kretsch et al., 1999), body image (Taren et al., 1999), and social desirability (Hebert et al., 1995; Taren et al., 1999).

7.1.2 Study objective and time frame

The reference dietary method chosen must have the same objective and must measure similar parameters over the same time frame (i.e., the current, past, or usual intake), as the test method. Four possible levels of objectives for dietary assessment protocols have been defined, and these are discussed in detail in Section 3.3. For example, if a single 24-h recall has been chosen to achieve a level one objective (i.e., mean intake of a group), then a 1-d weighed food record is the reference method of choice, because it is designed to assess intakes over the same time frame as the 24-h recall. The equations needed for calculating the number of recalls or records required to achieve each

of the four possible levels of objectives are also given in Section 3.3.

Assessment of the relative validity of a method designed to determine usual food or nutrient intakes of individuals over the distant past is especially difficult. Indeed, it may not be possible to validate a test method designed to look at the past diet. As an alternative, validation studies of the current diet have sometimes been conducted as a proxy for past diet, on the assumption that it is related to the past diet. However, this may not be the case. Several studies have reported a tendency for the recall of past diet to be affected by recent consumption, termed a "recency" effect (Byers et al., 1983; Rohan and Potter, 1984). This effect may be especially important for seriously ill patients: retrospective reports of diets obtained from such subjects may be biased by recent dietary changes (Friedenreich et al., 1992).

7.1.3 Sequence and spacing of test and reference methods

In general, the test method should be administered prior to the reference method in a validation study, so as to mimic the situation that will actually take place in the proposed study. Furthermore, the test and reference methods must be carefully spaced so that completion of the test method does not influence the responses to the reference method (Table 7.1). Too long a time interval between the test and reference methods, however, may introduce seasonal effects on food intake. Such an effect may be especially evident for dietary studies in low-income countries.

Willett et al. (1985) showed that food frequency questionnaire results correlated better with those from a reference method based on four 1-wk weighed records completed over the course of a year, if the food frequency questionnaire was administered after, rather than before, the reference method (Table 7.1). Similar findings were observed in a Finnish validation study which used six 3-d weighed records as the reference method (Elmståhl et al., 1996). Perhaps the process of weighing and recording the food intakes over four

	Before food record r	After food record r
Protein	0.18	0.33
Total fat	0.27	0.39
Saturated fat	0.31	0.44
Polyunsaturated fat	0.31	0.40
Cholesterol	0.46	0.52
Total carbohydrate	0.48	0.53
Vitamin A	0.37	0.41
Vitamin B_6	0.44	0.54
Vitamin C	0.53	0.73

Table 7.1: Pearson correlation coefficients for the comparison of a food frequency questionnaire with the mean of four 1-wk diet records. Data from Willett WC, et al., American Journal of Epidemiology 122: 51–65, 1985, with permission of the Society for Epidemiologic Research.

1-wk periods sensitized participants with respect to food consumption, so that they were able to complete the food frequency questionnaire more accurately on the second occasion.

7.1.4 Independent errors

Errors in the reference dietary method should be independent of those in the test method and also of the true intake (Nelson, 1997; Kipnis et al., 2001, 2002). As a result, the selected reference dietary method must be different from the test method. For example, both methods should not rely on memory or use the same method for estimating portion sizes. Some examples of ways to reduce measurement errors in dietary assessment are given in Chapter 5.

Recent studies have emphasized that even when precautions are taken, the reference dietary method is rarely free from all sources of error (Kaaks and Riboli, 1997; Kaaks et al., 1997; Kipnis et al., 2001; 2002). Systematic error made up of both intake-related and person-specific biases may exist. An intake-related bias usually reveals itself in a "flattened" slope of the regression of reported intake on the true intake. As an example of an intake-related bias, persons with a low consumption of supposedly "good" foods may be tempted to overreport their true intake.

In contrast, those with a high intake of supposedly "bad" foods may tend to underreport (Section 5.2).

Person-specific bias may be caused by certain personality characteristics. Indeed, it is possible that some subjects may under- or overreport in both dietary methods, leading to artificially high correlation coefficients between the two different methods.

New statistical models can now be used which measure and take into account any systematic errors in the test method, as long as the validation study includes a biochemical marker as an additional reference measure (Ocké and Kaaks, 1997; Kipnis et al., 2001). Further details of the use of biochemical markers to validate dietary intakes are given in Section 7.3.

7.1.5 Sex and age

The relative validity of a dietary method should be tested separately on both men and women. Studies have shown that the response of women to dietary assessment differs from that of men (Johnson et al., 1994). In contrast, age does not appear to influence the validity of a dietary method for adults ranging in age from 18 to 64 y. However, not surprisingly, memory and conceptualization skills affect the response of both younger (i.e., < 18 y) (Domel 1997; Field et al., 1999) and older individuals (Brown et al., 1990; Nelson et al., 1994). For example, elderly persons tend to overestimate portion sizes when photographs are used (Nelson et al., 1994). Therefore, the validation design should take these factors into account.

7.1.6 Socioeconomic status, ethnicity, and health status

Socioeconomic status and ethnicity may affect the outcome of a relative validity study, through a link with dietary diversity (Kristal et al., 1997; Stallone et al., 1997). Certainly, in a study of Mexican-Americans, the high correlation reported for estimates of energy, fat, and cholesterol derived from a food frequency questionnaire and food records was linked to low dietary diversity (McPherson et al., 1995).

The health status of the subjects is also important, especially in case-control studies. Here, attempts should be made to validate the dietary method with representatives of both the cases and the healthy controls.

7.1.7 Other factors

A variety of external factors, including those of day of the week, season, training, and the use of vitamin and mineral supplements, should also be taken into account, when appropriate, in the design of a relative validity study. These sources of variance are discussed in Section 6.2.

The examples discussed above emphasize the importance of taking all these factors into account in the design of any dietary validation study. In particular, the importance of selecting a target population for the validation that is similar to that of the study population cannot be overemphasized.

7.2 Relative validity in dietary studies

No reference method provides a true measure of the dietary intake. Instead, the extent of the agreement between the test and reference method is used to indicate the relative validity of the test method, as well as the extent to which the reference method is believed to yield the truth.

Statistically, the extent of the agreement can be expressed as a comparison of the group means (or medians), differences between measurements within individuals, rankings, correlation or regression analysis, and use of Bland-Altman analysis (Nelson, 1997). Further details of these statistical methods are given in Section 7.4; examples are given in the discussions below.

Table 7.2 provides the recommended combinations of the test and reference dietary methods to use in relative validity studies, taking into account the various factors outlined in Section 7.1. The number of 1-d

Test method	Reference method
Single 24-h recall	Single 1-d weighed record
Multiple 24-h recalls	Multiple 1-d weighed records
Food frequency question-naire over 1 y	Four 7-d weighed records at 3-mo intervals over 1 y and spaced to account for seasonal variation
Dietary history over 1 mo	Single 1-d weighed records spaced evenly over 1 mo, the number depending on the nutrient

Table 7.2: Appropriate combinations of test and reference dietary methods for use in validation studies.

weighed records used to validate a dietary history will depend on the nutrient of interest and the study group. For any of these combinations, good agreement does not necessarily indicate validity: agreement may merely reflect similar errors in both methods. Indeed, recent research has highlighted widespread underreporting of energy intakes, using a variety of dietary assessment methods (Sawaya et al., 1996). Alternatively, poor agreement between the two methods does not necessarily indicate that the test dietary method has failed to assess the intake correctly. Such uncertainties emphasize the importance of careful interpretation of the dietary data from relative validity studies.

Numerous studies of the relative validity of dietary assessment methods are reported in the literature; examples for each of the major dietary assessment methods follow. Examples of the use of biomarkers to validate dietary assessment methods are given in Section 7.3.

7.2.1 Relative validity of 24-h recalls

Unlike the other dietary assessment methods, it is possible in some settings to determine the absolute validity of a 24-h recall.

Methods used include surreptitious observation or weighing of duplicate portions of the actual intake of foods recalled by the same subjects, over the same 24-h period or for one meal. This procedure has been employed in institutional settings such as congregate meal

	Mean observed	Mean recalled	Mean ± SE difference	*t*-value	*p*
Energy (kcal)	2348	1896	452 ± 144	3.13	≤ 0.002
Protein (g)	82	66	16 ± 5.8	2.83	≤ 0.004

Table 7.3: Comparison of average observed and recalled energy and protein intakes of twenty-eight 10- to 12-year-old children attending a summer camp. From Carter, et al., Journal of the American Dietetic Association 79: 542–547, 1981 © with permission of the American Dietetic Association.

sites (Madden et al., 1976; Gersovitz et al., 1978), school lunch programs (Emmons and Hayes, 1973; Warren et al., 2003), college cafeterias (Krantzler et al., 1982), a metabolic unit (Greger and Etnyre, 1978; Poppitt et al., 1998), hospitals (Linusson et al., 1974), and summer camps (Carter et al., 1981).

In general, for the studies that have compared recalled with the observed intake, the agreement for mean intakes of energy has been acceptable (Gersovitz et al., 1978; Greger and Etnyre, 1978; Basch et al., 1990; Baranowski et al., 1991). Exceptions noted have included studies on the elderly (Madden et al., 1976), U.K. women (Poppitt et al., 1998), and sometimes children (Table 7.3) (Carter et al., 1981). In the U.K. metabolic study, it was the total energy from snack foods, rather than the meals, that was consistently and significantly underestimated during the 24-h recall by both nonobese and obese women (Figure 7.1) (Poppitt et al., 1998).

Agreement for intakes of nutrients among these studies has been less consistent. For example, Greger and Etnyre (1978) observed no significant differences between actual intakes and the mean recalled intakes of protein, calcium, and zinc for adolescent girls. In contrast, average recalls of vitamin A, thiamin, riboflavin, niacin, vitamin C, and iron were significantly less than actual intakes (Table 7.4). In the U.K. metabolic study of both obese and nonobese women, reported daily intakes of total carbohydrate and added sugar were significantly lower than the measured intakes, suggesting a bias in underreporting of high carbohydrate foods (Poppitt et al., 1998). There was no evidence of bias in reporting of high-fat or protein foods (Table 7.5).

More recently, the results of a videotape

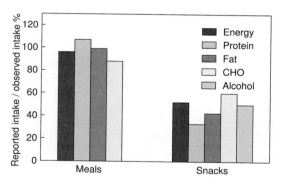

Figure 7.1: The mean proportion of energy and macronutrients reported or observed in meal foods and snack foods in a group of 33 women. CHO, carbohydrate; standard error of the mean values were < 10%. Data from Poppitt et al., International Journal of Obesity and Related Metabolic Disorders 22: 303–311, 1998 © with permission of the Nature Publishing Group.

	Mean daily intake Actual	Recall (± SD)	*p*
Energy (kcal)	2172	2000 ± 408	ns
Protein (g)	44	51 ± 13	ns
Vitamin A (IU)	7663	3377 ± 2278	< 0.001
Thiamin (mg)	2.3	1.4 ± 0.7	< 0.001
Riboflavin (mg)	2.7	1.6 ± 0.8	< 0.001
Niacin (mg)	29	16 ± 9	< 0.001
Vitamin C (mg)	116	78 ± 31	< 0.001
Calcium (mg)	391	418 ± 118	ns
Iron (mg)	25.5	14 ± 8	< 0.001
Zinc (mg)	6.7	8 ± 2	ns

Table 7.4: Comparison of actual observed intakes with recalled intakes. Data from 17 female subjects, aged 12.5 to 14.5 y. Statistical significance of the mean differences were assessed using the paired *t*-test; ns, significant. From Greger and Etnyre, American Journal of Public Health 68: 70–72, 1978, with permission of the American Public Health Association.

Nutrient	Observed	Reported	p
Energy (MJ)	15.4 ± 4.8	13.3 ± 4.6	< 0.01
Carbohydrate (g)	425 ± 131	333 ± 121	< 0.01
Fat (g)	163 ± 61	147 ± 67	ns
Protein (g)	122 ± 37	121 ± 44	ns
Alcohol (g)	14 ± 19	9 ± 12	ns
Added sugar (g)	131 ± 103	95 ± 80	< 0.05
Meals (MJ)	11.7 ± 3.5	11.2 ± 4.2	ns
Snacks (MJ)	3.8 ± 2.6	2.1 ± 1.2	< 0.001

Table 7.5: Underestimation of energy and macronutrient intake in a group of 33 women during 24 h in a metabolic facility. Significance of differences (p) tested using a paired t-test. Data from Poppitt et al., International Journal of Obesity and Related Metabolic Disorders 22: 303–311, 1998 © by permission of the Nature Publishing Group.

method used to assess the validity of 24-h recalls have again highlighted that 24-h recalls may be an inappropriate method for the elderly. Brown et al. (1990) used this method to assess nutrient intakes of 37 retired elderly nuns (76–91 years of age), with intact mental functioning. Results are shown in Table 7.6. The mean differences between the two methods were $\geq 10\%$ for energy and 6 of the 14 nutrients, with differences being significant for energy, protein, fat, cholesterol, and iron. Errors in both the types and amounts of food recalled occurred. The recall errors arose from both the omission of foods and erroneously recalling foods that were not consumed, although the former errors were more common.

Novotny et al. (2001) used an alternative approach to assess the accuracy of descriptions of reported food items in 24-h recall interviews. In this study, they compared qualitative descriptions of the same food items by subjects who normally consumed at least two meals together (11 pairs), using a 24-h recall interview conducted twice. The potential error in energy intakes produced by the mistakes in reporting the food items was also determined. They noted both frequent omissions of food items (mainly snacks or side dishes), especially in the male subjects, and discrepancies in food descriptions, both of which decreased from recall 1 to recall 2.

The discrepancies in the descriptions resulted in marked differences in the energy density of the food described. Because of the design of this study, the test and reference methods were not independent, limiting its usefulness.

Several other researchers have assessed the relative validity of the 24-h recall method by comparing recalled intakes with those derived from a reference dietary method. In some cases, a dietary history (Räsänen, 1979) or a 7-d weighed record (Young et al., 1952) has been used to assess the relative validity of recalled intakes, based on single 24-h recalls. These two methods of validation are not appropriate because the test and reference methods do not measure intakes over the same time frame. Instead, the most appropriate choice for the reference method is a single weighed record (Table 7.2), sometimes (Ferguson et al., 1994), but not always (Iannotti et al., 1994), carried out on the same day as the recall. The latter procedure assumes that, at the group level, individual differences between the intakes on the two days will not be significant.

Nutrient	Videotape	24-h recall	Sig.
Energy (kcal)	1138 ± 251	1013 ± 334	x
Protein (g)	41 ± 13	36 ± 15	x
Fat (g)	48 ± 15	41 ± 17	x
Cholesterol (mg)	325 ± 137	186 ± 125	x
Carbohydrate (g)	140 ± 30	130 ± 46	
Fiber (g)	11 ± 5.4	9.6 ± 4.1	
Calcium (mg)	530 ± 291	520 ± 382	
Sodium (mg)	1931 ± 505	1829 ± 686	
Zinc (mg)	4.9 ± 1.5	4.5 ± 1.9	
Iron (mg)	8.2 ± 3.6	6.6 ± 2.2	x
Vitamin A (IU)	4279 ± 3927	3804 ± 3735	
Thiamin (mg)	0.7 ± 0.3	0.7 ± 0.4	
Riboflavin (mg)	1.0 ± 0.4	1.0 ± 0.6	
Niacin (mg)	8.0 ± 3.4	8.0 ± 3.6	
Vitamin C (mg)	53 ± 32	58 ± 34	

Table 7.6: Comparison of the mean ($\pm$ SD) nutrient values of three meals among 37 subjects determined by videotape and by 24-h dietary recall. Differences are significant for energy and the indicated nutrients (paired t-test; $p < 0.05$). From Brown et al., Journal of the American Dietetic Association 90: 1675–1679, 1990 © with permission of the American Dietetic Association.

7.2.2 Relative validity of food records

A few studies have attempted to determine the absolute validity of weighed or estimated food records. Gersovitz et al. (1978) compared the noon meals recorded in 7-d weighed food records with actual intakes, weighed surreptitiously during lunch at a congregate meal site for the elderly. Although the record tended to underestimate the actual mean intakes, differences were only significant for energy and thiamin. Regression analysis showed that, because of a deterioration in the accuracy of recording, records from the first 2 d of record keeping were more valid for assessing group comparisons than those from the last 3 d. Usable records during days 5 to 7 were from the more highly educated respondents, resulting in a sample bias. These results question the apparent validity of the 7-d record to assess usual intakes of the elderly, because of the high respondent burden.

A similar approach was used by Crawford et al. (1994) to investigate the validity of a 3-d estimated food record completed by 20 nine- and ten-year-old U.S. school-girls. In this study, unobtrusive observers recorded the types and amounts of foods eaten for school lunch during the 3-d period, and these amounts were compared with the foods reported for the school lunch by the girls in a 3-d estimated food record. A comparison of actual observed intakes for lunch was also made with recalled intakes from a 24-h recall (Table 7.7), and those made with a 5-d food frequency questionnaire for the lunchtime portion of the day in the following week. Not surprisingly, agreement between observed and reported intakes was best for the 3-d record in this study, based on least significant differences (LSD) (Table 7.7). The latter represent the smallest difference that would be statistically significant with a paired t-test at the 5% level.

Intermittent duplicate diet collections have also been used to validate weighed and estimated food records (Gibson and Scythes, 1982; Holbrook et al., 1984; Kim et al., 1984). For example, in a U.S. study, 29 subjects consuming self-selected diets kept detailed

| | 24 h recall, $n = 18$ | | |
	Observed	Recall	LSD
Energy (kcal)	564 ± 209	610 ± 274	120
Carbohydrate (g)	68 ± 30	75 ± 31	16
Protein (g)	22 ± 8	21 ± 8	4
Fat (g)	24 ± 11	26 ± 17	8
Saturated fat (g)	10 ± 5	11 ± 6	2
Cholesterol (mg)	67 ± 34	60 ± 36	15

| | Mean of 3 days, $n = 20$ | | |
	Observed	Record	LSD
Energy (kcal)	489 ± 200	490 ± 232	55
Carbohydrate (g)	66 ± 26	67 ± 29	8
Protein (g)	16 ± 9	16 ± 10	2
Fat (g)	19 ± 9	19 ± 10	3
Saturated fat (g)	8 ± 5	7 ± 4	1
Cholesterol (mg)	47 ± 34	49 ± 41	8

Table 7.7: Means ± standard deviations and least significant differences (LSD) between observed and reported energy and nutrient intakes from lunch using a 24-h recall and a 3-d record. Data from Crawford et al., Journal of the American Dietetic Association 94: 626–630, 1994 © with permission of the American Dietetic Association.

weighed food records for 1 y and periodically made duplicate diet collections (Kim et al., 1984). The daily energy and nutrient intakes calculated from the 1-y food records were significantly higher than those calculated from the records made during collection of the duplicate diets.

Gibson and Scythes (1982) also demonstrated a decrease in energy intake associated with the collection of duplicate diets for analysis. Unfortunately, it is not possible from these studies to establish whether this bias arises from overestimation of food intake during recording or from an underestimation during collection of the duplicate diets. Hence, duplicate diets are not an ideal method for validating food record methods (Stockley, 1985).

Weighed food records are often regarded as the "gold" standard against which other dietary assessment methods are compared. Hence, the relative validity of weighed food records cannot be determined in the normal way; potential reference dietary methods are *less* accurate and their use inappropriate. As an alternative, the doubly labeled water method has been used in several studies to validate mean energy intakes based on weighed food records; details are given in Section 7.3.1. Again, results in selected small samples of adults have highlighted a systematic bias toward underestimation of energy intake, when these reported mean energy intakes are compared with energy expenditure (Livingstone and Black, 2003). There is also some evidence that even when weighed food records have been used, low-energy reporters have lower intakes of most nutrients as well (Pryer et al., 1997). Moreover, weighed food records have not consistently provided more accurate average estimates of energy intake when compared with doubly labeled water measurements of total energy expenditure, than multiple 24-h recalls, dietary histories (Section 7.2.3), or food frequency questionnaires (Section 7.2.4) (Livingstone et al., 1992; Sawaya et al., 1996; Bathalon et al., 2000).

Clearly, the use of weighed records as the gold standard method for dietary assessment has been challenged. Underreporting does occur and probably results from the combined effects of incomplete recording and undereating arising from the impact of the recording process on food choices (Bathalon et al., 2000).

7.2.3 Relative validity of dietary histories

One of the major advantages of the dietary history method is its ability to assess meal patterns and specific details about the preparation and consumption of food over an extended period of time. However, some respondents find the task of reporting their usual food intake and the amounts eaten difficult. Further, for certain sub-populations or age groups (e.g., adolescents), who may lack set meal patterns, such a meal-based approach is not useful.

Very few studies have measured the absolute validity of the dietary history method by comparison with actual food intake. This is not surprising, in view of the difficulties of monitoring an individual's usual long-term intake. Bray et al. (1978), in a study of 15 obese patients hospitalized in a metabolic unit, compared the actual food intake for 1 wk with the results of three retrospective dietary histories, conducted subsequently at monthly intervals. Energy intakes were underestimated in the first dietary history, but by the third history, the correlation between actual and reported energy intakes had increased. The improvement was attributed to more accurate reporting of alcohol intake.

Weighed or estimated food records have been most frequently used as the reference dietary method in studies of the relative validity of dietary histories. Early studies used 7-d food records (Young et al., 1952; Jain et al., 1980). In general, the dietary history produces *higher* estimates of group mean intakes than the food record (Nes et al., 1991; Jain et al., 1996; van Liere et al., 1997), especially if the time frame for the dietary history is long (6 mo to 1 y) (Young et al., 1952; Jain et al., 1980). In cases where a shorter time frame for the dietary history has been used, smaller differences in mean intakes have been reported (Livingstone et al., 1992). Unfortunately, in most of these early studies it is not possible to establish whether this bias arises from underestimation of food intake by recording or from overestimation by the diet history.

A few studies have also tested the agreement between dietary histories and weighed records by ranking subjects using correlation coefficients (Mahalko et al., 1985). It appears that for those nutrients for which day-to-day variation in individual diets is usually high, notably vitamin A, cholesterol, and linoleic acid, agreement by ranking is poor, regardless of the time frame of the dietary history used (Table 7.8) (Mahalko et al., 1985; Liu et al., 1994).

Finnish investigators have examined the relative validity of a modified diet history for measuring food rather than nutrient intakes. Six 3-d weighed records were used as the reference method evenly distributed over 1 y (Elmståhl et al., 1996). The diet history method combined a 2-wk food record measuring lunch and dinner meals with a

	Dietary history	Food record	% diff.	Pearson's *r*	Intraclass *r_I*	% with diff. < 20%	% in same tertile	% in opposite tertile
Energy (kcal)	1634	1745	−6	0.59	0.58	67	54	15
Carbohydrate (g)	194	200	−3	0.25	0.25	44	43	15
Protein (g)	72	73	−1	0.56	0.56	56	46	17
Fat (g)	65	74	−12*	0.74	0.70	46	59	11
Vitamin A (IU)	6147	6908	−11	0.22	0.21	30	41	19
Ascorbic acid (mg)	106	90	+18*	0.45	0.39	37	59	7
Niacin eq. (mg)	31	31	0	0.56	0.57	63	52	9
Riboflavin (mg)	1.6	1.7	−6	0.45	0.45	43	54	11
Thiamin (mg)	1.3	1.2	+8	0.47	0.46	48	52	11
Calcium (mg)	754	725	+4	0.69	0.69	48	50	7
Phosphorus (mg)	1221	1206	+1	0.68	0.68	57	56	4
Iron (mg)	13.8	13.7	+1	0.43	0.44	50	50	9
Zinc (mg)	10.5	10.2	+3	0.59	0.59	43	48	11
Potassium (g)	2.8	2.6	+8**	0.51	0.49	46	43	11
Sat. fatty acids (g)	25	27	−7*	0.75	0.73	48	59	7
Oleate (g)	23	27	−15*	0.76	0.71	43	56	6
Linoleate (g)	10	11	−9**	0.57	0.54	37	46	9
Cholesterol (mg)	260	315	−17*	0.42	0.34	17	35	20

Table 7.8: Comparison of the dietary history and 7-d food record results from 54 older U.S. adults aged 55 to 95 years. % difference = (dietary history − food record) ÷ dietary history × 100%. *paired *t*-test indicates that differences are significant at $p < 0.05$; **$p < 0.01$. From Mahalko et al., American Journal of Clinical Nutrition 42: 542–553, 1985 © Am J Clin Nutr. American Society for Clinical Nutrition.

130-item food frequency questionnaire for average consumption of foods, snacks, and beverages during the past year. Portion sizes in the diet history were estimated using a booklet with 120 photographs. Indeed, the modified diet history method overestimated the intake of most food groups compared with the weighed record reference method. Pearson correlation coefficients for 14 major food groups ranged from 0.32 for fish to 0.88 for meat. Classification of food intake into quartiles revealed that, on average, for all food groups, 55% of the subjects in the lowest quartile and 57%–59% of those in the highest quartile were correctly classified; gross misclassification was small for most food groups.

Relative validity of dietary histories has also been assessed by comparing the respondent's results with those collected from another person, such as a spouse or parent (Kolonel at al., 1977; Jain et al., 1980; Marshall et al., 1980). Good agreement between spouses has been found. In general, however, the results of the spouse cannot be assumed to be any more accurate than those of the original respondent. Furthermore, because the same method has been used for both the respondent and the spouse, the spouse's recall is not an appropriate reference method.

Interest in diet in relation to disease has prompted several studies of the validity of dietary history methods to determine dietary intakes over a long time span. In such methods, as noted earlier, there is a danger that long-term information may be distorted by the current intake — termed a "recency" effect — so that validity is reduced (Dwyer and Coleman, 1997). For instance, Jain et al. (1980), in a prospective study of diet and cancer, showed that newly diagnosed cancer patients who were asked to recall their food intake 6 mo ago underestimated the earlier intakes that had also been recorded 6 mo previously. Among the controls, however, there was little difference between reported and recalled intakes. The authors concluded that the recalled intakes of the cancer patients in this study were influenced by the current intakes, distorting the recall.

In their study of contemporaneous and retrospective estimates of food intake using a dietary history, Van Staveren et al. (1986b) also concluded that current food intake affected the reporting of past food intake. These studies emphasize the difficulties of obtaining unbiased estimates of retrospective food intakes, and such difficulties must be taken into account when interpreting the results of studies of diet and cancer (Hebert and Miller, 1988).

7.2.4 Relative validity of food frequency questionnaires

Numerous food frequency questionnaires exist for use among different populations and for a variety of purposes. Studies of the absolute validity of food frequency methods are limited, despite their frequent use in epidemiological studies. Mullen et al. (1984) tested the absolute validity of a food frequency questionnaire by comparison with actual food consumption surreptitiously observed at each meal for 28 consecutive days. Respondents recorded food items and number of servings selected on a form designed to measure food preferences. Forms were later checked for accuracy against returned trays by staff. The focus on the food preferences served to lessen the emphasis on food selection in an effort to prevent changes in usual food intake. Correlation analysis indicated that a large proportion of individuals could accurately estimate their own food intake using the food frequency questionnaire.

Decker et al. (1986) also observed actual food intake directly at a potluck lunch, by recording intakes using a video recorder and camera. The recorded intakes were then used to assess the validity of responses from a questionnaire that was administered 2–3 d later to assess intakes of specific foods. Associations between actual recorded and reported intakes were high, although only 10 out of the 32 respondents made no mistakes.

In a study of the carefully monitored food intake of hospital patients (Krall and Dwyer, 1987), intakes of energy, macronutrients, and vitamins A and C were underreported, based on a food frequency questionnaire covering

1 wk. In a more recent trial, subjects completed a food frequency questionnaire when consuming high- or low-fat diets of known composition. When the food frequency questionnaire was used, the intake of fat was underestimated on the high-fat diet but overestimated on the low-fat diet (Schaefer et al., 2000).

The relative validity of food frequency questionnaires has been evaluated using a variety of dietary assessment methods chosen, in most cases, to provide an independent assessment of nutrient intake. The approach used by several investigators is to use multiple food records, preferably weighed, over a designated time period, as the reference method (Russell-Briefel et al., 1985; Willett et al., 1985; Elmståhl et al., 1996) (Table 7.2). Sometimes, multiple 24-h recalls have been used as the reference dietary method (Ocké et al., 1997; Field et al., 1999). Use of the latter combination will, however, yield portion size recall errors. Further, care must be taken to ensure that the measurement days selected cover the same time frame as the food frequency questionnaire.

In a study by Willett et al. (1985), the relative validity of a semiquantitative food frequency questionnaire designed to estimate food intake during a 1-y period was assessed. The study compared the average nutrient intakes derived from the food frequency questionnaire with those estimated from four 1-wk weighed records. The degree to which subjects were classified into the same lowest or highest quintiles by the two dietary methods was also examined. The weighed food records were collected at 3-mo intervals and spaced to account for seasonal and short-term variability. Hence the two methods were independent and assessed food and nutrient intake over the same time frame. Nutrient intake results assessed by the two methods, with the exception of vitamin A and polyunsaturated fat, correlated strongly, especially when expressed as nutrient densities. Overall agreement for the two dietary methods, for subjects within the lowest and highest quintiles for all the nutrients examined, was 48% and 49%, respectively. On average,

	Lowest quintile on food record			Highest quintile on food record		
	Quintile of questionnaire			Quintile of questionnaire		
	Lowest (%)	Lowest 2 (%)	Highest (%)	Highest (%)	Highest 2 (%)	Lowest (%)
Protein	44	68	0	47	71	9
Total fat	53	71	3	33	70	3
Saturated fat	47	88	3	47	82	0
Polyunsaturated fat	47	71	9	41	79	3
Cholesterol	53	76	6	50	68	6
Total carbohydrate	47	71	9	46	71	0
Sucrose	38	62	9	50	82	0
Crude fiber	41	69	3	41	79	3
Vitamin A	44	68	3	44	79	3
Vitamin B_6	47	88	0	74	88	3
Vitamin C	68	85	0	62	79	0
Mean	48	74	4	49	77	3

Table 7.9: Comparison of semiquantitative food frequency questionnaire scores with mean daily intakes derived from four 1-wk food records, based on joint classification by quintiles. Both intake scores adjusted for total energy intake. Data from 173 Boston-area registered nurses aged 34 to 59 y. From Willett et al., American Journal of Epidemiology 122: 51–65, 1985, with permission of the Society for Epidemiologic Research.

only 3% of subjects were misclassified into extreme quintiles (Table 7.9). For the intermediate (second and fourth quintiles), and the center quintile, however, agreement was significantly lower.

A comparable approach was used to validate the food frequency questionnaire in the Dutch component of the EPIC study, although 12 monthly standardized 24-h recalls were used in this study instead of weighed records (Ocké et al., 1997). Crude correlation coefficients between nutrient intakes assessed by the questionnaire and 24-h recalls varied widely, ranging from 0.25 to 0.83 for men and from 0.35 to 0.90 for women, emphasizing the difficulties of designing a food frequency questionnaire that performs equally well for all nutrients.

In this Dutch study, the correlation coefficients were deattenuated to remove the effects of the within-subject variance in nutrient intakes, as discussed in Section 6.2.3. Table 7.10 compares the deattenuated coefficients with the crude nonadjusted correlation coefficients. The adjustment increased the median correlation coefficients from 0.59 to 0.66 for men and from 0.58 to 0.63 for

women. Biomarkers were also used in this study (Section 7.3).

Mayer-Davis et al. (1999) selected a series of 24-h dietary recalls collected over 1 y as the reference method for assessing the relative validity of a food frequency question-

Nutrient	Males ($n = 63$)	
	Crude	Deattenuated
Energy	0.71	0.77
Protein	0.61	0.68
Fat	0.69	0.74
Carbohydrate	0.72	0.75
Alcohol	0.83	0.87
Dietary fiber	0.51	0.56
Retinol	0.57	0.61
β-carotene	0.26	0.34
Vitamin C	0.39	0.45
Vitamin E	0.57	0.63

Table 7.10: Pearson correlation coefficients between daily intake of nutrients assessed by the Dutch EPIC food frequency questionnaire and by twelve 24-h dietary recalls. All variables were $\log_e$-transformed before analysis. The deattenuated coefficients are corrected for within-subject variation in the 24-h dietary recalls. From Ocké et al., International Journal of Epidemiology 26: S49–S58, 1997, by permission of the International Epidemiological Association.

naire for a multicultural insulin resistance atherosclerosis study. However, in this validation, the eight recalls were administered by telephone.

It is now recognized that when carrying out relative validity studies of food frequency questionnaires among adults, it is advisable to ask respondents to complete them twice, both before and after the reference method. In this way, a conservative estimate (provided by the first questionnaire) and an optimistic estimate (provided by the second questionnaire) of the true correlation between the food frequency questionnaires and the reference method will be provided (Willett, 1998). Certainly in a Finnish validation study, higher correlation coefficients were obtained when a food frequency questionnaire was completed after the reference method (six 3-d weighed records) than at the beginning of the study, as noted earlier (Elmståhl et al., 1996).

Several studies have used a dietary history as the reference method for testing the relative validity of a food frequency questionnaire (Table 7.11), assuming it also estimates food intake over a longer time period (Jain et al., 1982; Feunekes et al., 1993). However, because the two methods rely on the memories of the respondents and on their ability to estimate amounts, the correlations obtained may be inflated (Block and Hartman, 1989). Therefore, a dietary history is best not used as the reference method for assessing the validity of a food frequency questionnaire.

Increasingly, computer-administered food frequency questionnaires are being used to standardize the interviews, reduce respondent burden, and facilitate data analyses. Heath et al. (2000) assessed the relative validity of a computerized food frequency questionnaire in comparison with weighed records collected on 11 specific days over 1 mo. The recording days were divided into blocks of no more than 3 consecutive days to minimize recording fatigue. The food frequency questionnaire had a meal-based format designed to estimate usual intakes of dietary iron and its absorption modifiers over the previous month. Results indicated that the food frequency questionnaire was appropriate for assessing group

intakes for total, nonheme, and heme iron; calcium; vitamin C; and phytate and for ranking individuals according to these specific nutrients.

Sometimes investigators have used weighed diet records to select the key foods and the corresponding average portion size for a food frequency questionnaire (Hankin et al., 1970). In such cases, if the food frequency questionnaire is administered to the same group of subjects who completed the diet records, then the relative validity based on correlation coefficients is likely to be overestimated.

Haile et al. (1986) used a different approach, involving regression analysis. They showed that each of three lists of a limited number of carefully selected foods had a strong ability to predict total intakes of fat, dietary fiber, and vitamins A, C, and E calculated from an original extensive dietary questionnaire. Whether the same limited lists of foods predict subsequent intakes of these nutrients in another group comparable to that of the target population under study

	Same category	Same or adjacent category	Grossly misclass-ified[a]
Energy (kJ)	38.2	81.7	0.5
Total fat			
(g)	37.7	68.6	1.6
(% of energy)	37.7	58.6	2.1
Saturated			
Fatty acids (g)	44.5	80.6	0.5
(% of energy)	34.0	71.7	0.0
Monounsaturated			
Fatty acids (g)	46.1	84.3	0.5
(% of energy)	38.7	72.3	1.0
Polyunsaturated			
fatty acids (g)	41.4	62.8	2.6
(% of energy)	32.5	62.8	2.6
Cholesterol			
(mg)	35.1	77.5	0

Table 7.11: Percentage of 191 subjects classified into five categories using a food frequency questionnaire compared with the results obtained from a dietary history. [a]Classified from one extreme category to the other extreme category. From Feunekes et al., American Journal of Clinical Nutrition 58: 489–496, 1993 © Am J Clin Nutr. American Society for Clinical Nutrition.

with equal confidence was not tested. This is unfortunate, because the assessment of relative validity should always be performed on a sample population independent of that used to develop the questionnaire (Nelson, 1997). Indeed, only a few investigators have had success with methods based on prediction equations, in terms of their generalizability to other population groups (Wakai et al., 1999).

More recently, studies of the validity of all the dietary assessment methods discussed in Section 7.1 have incorporated biomarkers — such as doubly labeled water for energy expenditure and urinary nitrogen for protein intake — in addition to a reference dietary method; details are given in Sections 7.3.1 and 7.3.4. Results of these biomarker studies have emphasized that energy underreporting occurs in all dietary assessment methods. Further, the performance of any dietary assessment method is markedly influenced by the motivation and compliance of the respondents. At present, no firm conclusions about the comparative validity of these different dietary methods on different population groups can be made. Interested readers are referred to the U.S. National Cancer Institute register of dietary assessment validation studies and publications (Thompson et al., 1997). This information can be accessed at

http://www-dacv.ims.nci.nih.gov/

7.3 Use of biomarkers to validate dietary intakes

As stated earlier, good agreement between the dietary intake results of the test and reference methods does not necessarily indicate validity. It may merely indicate similar errors in both methods. Recognition of this problem has prompted the development of objective and accurate procedures, independent of the measurement of food intake, to validate dietary assessment methods. The approach uses external variables, termed "biomarkers," to measure the relative validity of the dietary

assessment methods prior to their use in a research study. Alternatively, biomarkers can be used to calibrate dietary data collected in prospective multicenter cohort studies so that adjustments for possible sources of bias can be made (Section 7.3.5). The use of biomarkers as a surrogate for actual dietary intake in epidemiological studies of chronic disease is discussed elsewhere (Toniolo et al., 1997).

Most biomarkers are components of body fluids or tissues that have a strong direct relationship with dietary intakes of one or more dietary components. Nevertheless, their sensitivity to intake is generally low, so many biomarkers only have the capacity to discriminate between the extremes of the intake ranges (i.e., very low or very high intakes). Examples of exceptions that reflect intakes over the entire range are urinary nitrogen, sodium, and potassium. Bates et al. (1997) provide a summary of the range of intakes over which biomarkers of micronutrients are likely to predict intakes. Several criteria must be considered before adopting a biomarker for use in dietary validation and calibration studies. A brief account of these considerations follows below.

Temporal relations with the dietary intake must be considered, when selecting a suitable biomarker. The latter must reflect the intake of the dietary constituent of interest over the same time period as the dietary method. Nutrient levels in serum or plasma and urine, for example, tend to reflect recent dietary intake, and thus they are only appropriate biomarkers for validating dietary methods that are designed to cover short time periods, such as recalls or records. Nutrients in serum or plasma that can be used in this way include vitamin B_6, vitamin C, and the fat-soluble vitamins. Twenty-four-hour urine samples can be used for vitamin C, the B vitamins (except folate and B_{12}), nitrogen, and certain inorganic ions (e.g., Na^+ and K^+), provided kidney function is normal. For some nutrients (e.g., vitamin A and iodine), breast milk samples can be used as biomarkers of recent intake, provided an appropriate sampling protocol is used. In some cases, the

Disease	Nutrient indices that may be altered (usually lowered)
Pernicious anemia	Vitamin B_{12} (secondary effect on folate)
Vitamin-responsive metabolic errors	Usually B-vitamins (e.g., vitamins B_{12}, vitamin B_6, riboflavin, biotin, folate)
Tropical sprue	Vitamin B_{12} and folate (local deficiencies), protein
Steatorrhea	Fat-soluble vitamins, lipid levels, energy
Diabetes	Possibly vitamin C, zinc, and several other nutrients, lipid levels
Infections, inflammation, acute phase reaction	Vitamin C, vitamin A, and several other nutrients, lipids, protein, energy
Measles, upper respiratory tract infections, diarrheal disease	Especially vitamin A, lipid levels, protein
Renal disease	Increased retention or increased loss of many circulating nutrients, lipid levels, protein
Cystic fibrosis	Especially vitamin A, lipid levels, protein
Various cancers	Lowering of vitamin indices
Acute myocardial infarction	Lipid levels affected for about 3 mo
Huntingdon's chorea	Energy
Acrodermatitis enteropathica; various bowel, pancreatic, or liver diseases	Zinc, lipid levels, protein.
Hormone imbalances	Minerals, parathyroid hormone, thyrocalcitonin (effects on alkali metals and calcium), lipid levels affected by oral contraception and estrogen therapy

Table 7.12: Some disease states that may affect nutrient status indices independently of intake. From Bates et al. (1997). Biochemical markers of nutrient intake. In: Margetts BM, Nelson M (eds.) Design Concepts in Nutritional Epidemiology. 2nd ed. By permission of Oxford University Press.

stage of lactation can be a complicating factor, as discussed for breast milk retinol levels (Section 18.1.5).

Medium-term biomarkers include levels of certain nutrients (e.g., fatty acids; folate; selenium; and vitamins B_1, B_2, and B_6) in erythrocytes, whereas examples of long-term biomarkers are nutrient levels in hair, fingernails, and toenails (e.g., selenium), and adipose tissue (e.g., fatty acids).

Biomarkers that respond over months or years (e.g., hair, toenails, adipose tissue) are especially useful for validating retrospective dietary intakes over an extended time period (e.g., food frequency questionnaires or dietary histories) and are often used in epidemiological studies. In some circumstances, the time integration of exposure of the biomarker can be enhanced by obtaining samples

(e.g., plasma) at several points in time. For more specific details, see Bates et al. (1997).

Within-subject variation of a biomarker, if large in relation to between-subject variation, may obscure relationships with the usual nutrient intakes of an individual. In such cases, replicate samples of the biomarker should be obtained, where possible, so that misclassification can be minimized. Correlation and regression coefficients can then be adjusted for within-subject variation (i.e., deattenuated), as described for 24-h recalls (Table 7.10) (Section 6.2.3). Such short-term fluctuations are more likely to occur for nutrient concentrations in plasma than in erythrocytes or adipose tissue, and may be exacerbated by time of day, exercise, medication, and other factors; details are given in the specific chapters dealing with the vitamins and minerals.

Biological confounders may cause considerable variation in biomarker levels unrelated to the dietary component of interest. Confounders attenuate the association between the biomarker and true dietary intake levels; they have been reviewed in detail by Bates et al. (1997). Confounding factors may include the genetic background of the individual, the nutritional status of the subject, the presence of other environmental constituents (e.g., cigarette smoke), marked homeostatic regulation of biomarker levels (e.g., plasma retinol levels), metabolism and excretion of the biomarker, interactions of the biomarker in the gut or during absorption and metabolism, and medication use of the subject. Details of the effects of some of these confounders on biomarkers of nutrient status are given in Chapters 16–26.

Disease states may also affect biomarker levels independent of intake: these have also been summarized by Bates et al. (1997) and examples are shown in Table 7.12. In some cases, measures of disease status or infection should be measured concurrently with the biomarkers of interest. More specific details of the effect of disease processes on biomarkers of nutrient status are also given in the nutrient-specific chapters.

Sample collection, transport, and storage of biological fluids and tissues for analyses of biomarkers must be carried out using trained staff and standardized protocols and conditions appropriate for the chosen biomarker. Examples of details that must be considered include the correct choice of anticoagulant, preservative, specimen vials, and clotting time; a more extensive list is given in Box 7.1. Attention to such details will minimize variations related to both sampling, and deterioration of sample quality. This is especially critical for certain nutrients (e.g., vitamin C, folate, zinc, homocysteine) in serum or specific cell types and for all biomarkers used in multicenter trials. Careful storage and use of aliquots of a pooled sample are es-

---

The correct specimen type (e.g., plasma, serum, urine, blood spots) must be collected.

The collection method (e.g., capillary sample, venipuncture, midstream urine) must be appropriate.

Instructions to the subjects may be required (e.g., to request fasting).

Vials used must hold appropriate volumes, be stable when frozen, and not leak.

Labels and markings must have long-term adhesion and stability over a wide temperature range.

Anticoagulants or preservatives may need to be added to the sample.

Sample volume/size must be appropriate.

Dilution, aliquoting, or hemolysate preparation may be necessary prior to sample storage.

Sample aliquots should be of a size to efficiently use the sample and meet the requirements of the laboratory assay.

Light-, oxygen-, and temperature-sensitive samples may require special handling, vials, or storage.

A local laboratory may provide facilities for biomarker collection. Alternatively, resources including, where appropriate, a centrifuge, refrigerator, freezer, wet or dry ice, gloves, alcohol, gauze, bandages, vacutainers and needles, sample tubes, and biohazard disposal containers must be transported to the field.

Sufficient supplies to allow the preparation of duplicate samples must be provided.

Sample stability under field conditions must be considered. Shipping of refrigerated or frozen samples with wet or dry ice within 24 h may be required.

Sample storage should be at a temperature to minimize sample loss.

Box 7.1: Considerations in biomarker specimen collection and processing. From Blanck et al., Journal of Nutrition 133: 888S–894S, 2003, with permission of the American Society for Nutritional Sciences.

---

sential for all multicenter trials to monitor the sampling, subsequent storage, and handling of the samples.

Analytical measurement error may result from failure to comply with the appropriate protocols. Guidelines for the internal quality control of analytical results are available in Petersen et al. (1996). The analytical accuracy and precision must be closely monitored. This should involve the routine analysis of suitable certified reference materials, determination of recoveries, use of internal standards, comparison with analyses by a second laboratory or another previously validated method, as well as some statistical quality-control procedures (e.g., calculation and consideration of CVs). More details are given in Sections 15.4.1 and 15.4.2. Care must be taken to ensure that the assay methodology is precise and accurate over the range expected for the study population.

Biomarkers can be used to assess the validity of energy intake, a surrogate measure of the total amount of food consumed, as well as several other dietary constituents; some specific examples are discussed below. Poor agreement between the biomarker and the dietary intake of the nutrient of interest does not necessarily indicate that the dietary method has failed to assess the intake correctly. Lack of agreement may also occur because of biological confounders and laboratory measurement errors associated with the biomarker, as noted above (Blanck et al., 2003).

7.3.1 Use of doubly labeled water to validate reported energy intake

The underreporting of total energy intake in community-based studies has gained increasing recognition with the development of the doubly labeled water method for the measurement of energy expenditure in humans (Black et al., 1993). When the total energy intake is underestimated, then it is likely that the intakes of all the nutrients correlated with the energy intake (e.g., macronutrients, most minerals, B vitamins) are also underestimated. Hence, by evaluating the validity of reported energy intakes, the general quality of the dietary intake data collected can assessed (Livingstone and Black, 2003).

Figure 7.2 summarizes the frequency distribution of the ratio of energy intake : energy expenditure derived from 43 studies of adults

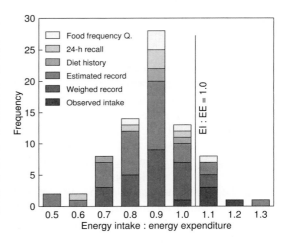

Figure 7.2: Frequency distribution of energy intake : energy expenditure (EI:EE) according to dietary assessment method in 43 studies of adults, comprising 77 subgroups (men and women separately). From Livingstone and Black, Journal of Nutrition 133: 895S–920S, 2003, with permission of the American Society for Nutritional Sciences.

using five dietary assessment methods. Note how the distribution is not centered about the line of EI:EE = 1.0, almost certainly indicating significant underreporting of intakes. Table 7.13 provides a more detailed comparison of the results of several studies in which doubly labeled water has been used to validate self-reported energy intake in adults, obtained using a variety of dietary assessment methods (Hill and Davies, 2001). Both Figure 7.2 and Table 7.13 emphasize the widespread nature of energy underreporting in dietary assessment methods.

Measuring energy expenditure

The doubly labeled water method is based on the simple principal of energy balance: energy expenditure and metabolizable energy intake are equal under conditions of stable body weight and composition. The method can be used to measure total energy expenditure over about 2 wk.

The method involves the administration, after a fast of at least 6 h, of an oral loading dose of water labeled with both deuterium, a stable isotope of hydrogen, and the stable oxygen isotope ^{18}O. These tracers quickly

Author	Subjects	EI method	EI (MJ/day)	EE (MJ/day)	% Difference
Bathalon et al. (2000)	60 F classified as RE (mean age 60 y; $n=26$) and URE (mean age 59 y; $n=34$)	FFQ, three 24-h recalls and 7-d weighed record	URE 8.30 (WR) 7.60 (24 h) 7.40 (FFQ) RE 7.10 (WR) 6.60 (24 h) 6.50 (FFQ)	URE 8.52 (WR) 8.44 (24 h) 8.64 (FFQ) RE 8.12 (WR) 8.11 (24 h) 8.23 (FFQ)	URE +7% (WR) −2% (24 h) −8% (FFQ) RE −6% (WR) −13% (24 h) −14% (FFQ)
Black et al. (1997)	18 F aged 50–65 y; 27 M aged 55–87 y	4-d weighed record in each of four seasons	8.30 F 10.06 M	9.50 F 11.67 M	−11% F −12% M
Johnson et al. (1996)	35 low-income F aged 19–46 y	Four multiple-pass recalls	9.19	11.23	−17%
Jones et al. (1997)	29 F aged 49 y	7-d weighed record	7.08	9.56	−26%
Kroke et al. (1999)	28 M + F aged 35–67 y	3 × 24-h recalls/season (total 12); self-administered FFQ	9.05 (FFQ)	11.23 (FFQ)	−22% (FFQ)
Martin et al. (1996)	29 F aged 49 y	7-d weighed record	6.98	9.00	−20%
Rothenberg et al. (1998)	9 F and 3M mean age 73 y	Diet history	8.62	9.90	−12%
Sawaya et al. (1996)	10 F aged 25 y (Y) and 10 F aged 74 years (O)	7-d weighed record; two 24-h recalls; and two FFQ (Willett, F1; Fred Hutchinson Cancer Research Centre, F2)	7.96 (Y,WR) 5.85 (O,WR) 8.51 (Y,24 h) 5.66 (O,24 h) 7.89 (Y,F1) 7.41 (O,F1) 6.78 (Y,F2) 5.66 (O,F2)	9.82 (Y) 7.52 (O)	−19% (Y,WR) −22% (O,WR) −13% (Y,24 h) −16% (O,24 h) −16% (Y,F1 +7% (O,F1) −29% (Y,F2) −16% (O,F2)
Seale and Rumpler (1997)	11 F aged 52 y, 8 M aged 50 y	7-d weighed record	7.88 (F) 8.96 (M)	9.57 (F) 12.91 (M)	−18% (F) −30% (M)
Taren et al. (1999)	37 F aged 44 y	3-d weighed records used with models	6.86 (F) 8.73 (M)	8.35 (F) 11.30 (M)	−18% (F) −23% (M)
Tomoyasu et al. (1999)	39 M aged 70 y 43 F aged 68 y	3-d weighed records	6.86 (F) 8.73 (M)	8.35 (F) 11.30 (M)	−18% (F) −23%
Velthuis-te Wierik et al. (1995)	8 M aged 35–50 y (mean 43 y)	7-d food record	11.80	14.3	−17%

Table 7.13: Summary of some studies where self-reported energy intakes of adults are compared with energy expenditure measured using doubly labeled water. EI, energy intake; EE, energy expenditure; FFQ, food frequency questionnaire; RE, restrained eaters; URE, unrestrained eaters; WR, weighed record; M, males; F, females; Y, young; O, old. From Hill and Davies, British Journal of Nutrition 85: 415–430, 2001, with permission of the authors.

equilibrate with the body water. The deuterium is eliminated from the body in the urine, and the ^{18}O is eliminated both in the urine and as carbon dioxide. The elimination of deuterium provides a measure of water turnover; the elimination of ^{18}O provides a measure of the sum of water turnover and carbon dioxide production. The difference between these two elimination rates is therefore proportional to carbon dioxide production over the measurement period (usually 10–14 d). The total energy expenditure by the subject can be calculated from the carbon dioxide production by using standard equations for indirect calorimetry (de V Weir, 1949). An error in the assumed macronutrient composition of the diet can introduce a bias in the results at this step. Detailed guidelines for this method are given by Prentice (1990).

The doubly labeled water technique is safe and noninvasive. The subjects are required to drink a dose of isotope-labeled water and collect a single casual urine sample on that day and again at the end of the 10–14-d measurement period. Hence, there is little disruption to the daily activities of the subjects. In some protocols, additional urine samples are collected at 2, 3, and 4 h post-dose, and two casual urine samples after 14 d, at the same time of day as the post-dose specimen. In tropical regions, an interval of 7 d instead of 14 d should be used because high water turnover can result in excessive tracer elimination.

Individuals who have traveled a significant distance away from the study site during the 2 wks prior to administration of the dose should not participate because of possible regional variation in the ^2H and ^{18}O background abundances (Horvitz and Schoeller, 2001). Subjects with malabsorption must also be excluded because such conditions might reduce the metabolizable energy value of foods.

Urine specimens must be at least 25 mL, capped after collection, and an aliquot (4 mL) transferred to an O-ring-sealed plastic tube and preferably frozen at −10°C. Specimens can be shipped without freezing if they are cooled with sealed frozen gel coolants. Isotopic analysis must be performed by isotope ratio mass spectrometry. Calculation methods are given in Schoeller (2002).

The laboratory reproducibility (CV, 5%) and accuracy (1%) of the doubly labeled water method can be high, although they often vary markedly among analytical centers. The method is based on some assumptions, including the constancy of the water pool throughout the measurement period, the rate of H_2O and CO_2 fluxes, isotopic fractionation, and no label re-entering the body; details are available in Prentice (1990). The method is expensive.

Comparing measured energy expenditure and reported energy intake

Increasingly, doubly labeled water has been used to assess the validity of reported energy intakes from a variety of dietary assessment methods, as noted earlier. Studies using this marker have highlighted a systematic bias toward underestimation of energy intake that may occur in all dietary assessment methods (Figure 7.2) and among males and females (Figure 5.1) (Table 7.13) of all age groups (Livingstone and Black, 2003). For example, underreporting of energy often occurs in 24-h recalls (Sawaya et al., 1996; Bathalon et al., 2000), although among younger children, this finding is less consistent (Livingstone et al., 1992; Johnson et al., 1996). Livingstone and Black (2003) provide a summary of the validation studies using 24-h recalls in children and adolescents aged 1–18 y.

Similarly, energy intakes based on diet histories can be underreported. In studies of adults, mean energy intakes assessed by diet histories have been underreported compared to energy expenditure measured using doubly labeled water (Livingstone et al., 1992; Rothenberg et al., 1998), although in some cases the differences have been small. Indeed, Livingstone et al. (1992) concluded that energy intakes assessed by a dietary history method provided a better estimate of habitual intake than self-reported weighed records, especially among adolescents.

The performance of several food frequency

questionnaires has also been compared using doubly labeled water studies. The food frequency questionnaire developed by Willett et al. (1985) (Table 7.9) has been reported to perform better (Sawaya et al., 1996) than that of either the Block et al. (1990) or Kristal et al. (1990) food frequency questionnaires, when mean energy intakes have been compared with energy expenditure.

Even when weighed food records are used, underreporting may still occur among some age groups (Livingstone and Black, 2003). Indeed, weighed food records have not consistently provided more accurate average estimates of energy intake than multiple 24-h recalls, dietary histories, or food frequency questionnaires (Livingstone et al., 1992; Sawaya et al., 1996; Bathalon et al., 2000; Black et al., 2000). Moreover, there is also some evidence that when weighed food records are used, low-energy reporters have lower intakes of most nutrients as well (Pryer et al., 1997). These findings are important because weighed food records are often regarded as the gold standard against which other dietary assessment methods are compared in studies of relative validity.

In most of the doubly labeled water studies, the validity of the mean energy intake and not the ability of the dietary assessment method to rank individuals has been measured. Black (2000), however, has investigated the correlation between energy intake (EI) and energy expenditure (EE) in 429 individuals who participated in 22 studies. Energy intakes were calculated mainly from 7-d weighed records (15 studies). Although the reported correlation for all individuals in these studies was low ($r = 0.425$), if misreporters were excluded (based on the ratio of EI:EE < 0.76 and > 1.24), the correlation improved ($r = 0.83$).

Several factors have been associated with underreporters: weight status, age and sex, health-related activities, and certain behavioral and psychological effects. These characteristics of energy-intake underreporters in dietary assessment methods have been discussed in detail in Section 5.2.2. At present, very few studies have characterized overreporters of energy intake.

7.3.2 Basal metabolic rate as a biomarker for energy intakes

Goldberg et al. (1991) proposed an alternative approach to identifying underreporting in community-based studies — the Goldberg cutoff method. It can be used at both the individual and group levels. The method is simple, less expensive, and more practical than using doubly labeled water but it excludes only the most biased records. It is based on the principle that an individual of a given sex, age, and body weight needs a minimum energy intake. Intakes below this level are considered to be an unacceptable representation of the habitual intake and incompatible with long-term survival.

Use of Goldberg cutoff method

The Goldberg cutoff method compares the daily mean reported energy intake (EI_{rep}) with FAO/WHO/UNU (1985) recommended energy intakes for a sedentary lifestyle of

Age (y)	Basal metabolic rate (kJ) (kcal$_{th}$ in parentheses)	r	Residual SD
Men			
10–18	69.4W + 322.2H + 2392 (16W + 77H + 572)	0.89	418 (100)
18–30	64.4W − 113.0H + 3000 (15.4W − 27H + 717)	0.65	632 (151)
30–60	47.2W + 66.9H + 3769 (11.3W + 16H + 901)	0.60	686 (164)
> 60	36.8W + 4719.5H − 4481 (8.8W + 1128H − 1071)	0.84	552 (132)
Women			
10–18	30.9W + 2016.6H + 907 (7.4W + 482H + 217)	0.77	473 (113)
18–30	55.6W + 1397.4H + 146 (13.3W + 334H + 35)	0.73	502 (120)
30–60	36.4W − 104.6H + 3619 (8.7W − 25H + 865)	0.70	452 (108)
> 60	38.5W + 2665.2H − 1264 (9.2W + 637H − 302)	0.82	393 (94)

Table 7.14: Equations for the prediction of basal metabolic rate from weight (W) in kg and height (H) in m. From FAO/WHO/UNU (1985) with permission.

1.55 × basal metabolic rate (BMR). The BMR is the energy expenditure of an individual, lying at rest, in a thermoneutral environment and fasted state; it is expressed in MJ/d. Whole-body calorimetry can be used to measure the BMR directly. Alternatively, BMR can be predicted from standard age- and sex-specific equations derived by Schofield (1985) and given in FAO/WHO/ UNU (1985) (Table 7.14), using either body weight plus height or body weight alone.

At the individual level, underreporters can be identified by calculating for each individual the ratio $EI_{rep} : BMR_{est}$. These ratios are then compared with the cutoffs given in Table 7.15 for $n = 1$, and the appropriate number of days of dietary assessment used to calculate the EI_{rep}.

The cutoffs depicted in Table 7.15 represent the value below which it is statistically unlikely that the reported ratio $EI_{rep} : BMR_{est}$ reflects "habitual" long-term intake. The cutoffs shown, set at the 95% confidence limit, are based on an energy requirement of 1.55 × BMR for a person with a sedentary lifestyle, adjusted for the number of days of the survey. The cutoffs rise with increases in the number of dietary assessment days.

The Goldberg cutoff method can also be used to identify whether underreporting exists at the group level. First, the average BMR for the group is calculated from the BMR_{est} for each individual, using the data in Table 7.14. Then the overall mean energy intake is divided by the average BMR for the group. Finally, this ratio is compared with the appropriate cutoff for the study group, based on the number of subjects and number of dietary assessment days used in the study. Use of this approach at the group level can identify the existence of an overall underreporting bias and indicate whether it is mild or severe (Ferrari et al., 2002).

Several limitations are associated with the Goldberg cutoff method. These include:

- Use of 1.55 × BMR assumes a sedentary lifestyle for all individuals, which may not be appropriate for those with a high energy expenditure. However, use of this universal

	No. of days				
n	1	4	7	14	28
1	0.90	1.06	1.10	1.12	1.14
2	1.05	1.19	1.21	1.23	1.24
3	1.13	1.25	1.27	1.29	1.30
4	1.18	1.28	1.30	1.32	1.33
5	1.21	1.31	1.33	1.34	1.35
10	1.30	1.38	1.39	1.40	1.40
15	1.34	1.41	1.42	1.43	1.43
20	1.37	1.42	1.43	1.44	1.45
25	1.39	1.44	1.45	1.45	1.46
30	1.40	1.45	1.46	1.46	1.46
40	1.42	1.46	1.47	1.47	1.48
50	1.43	1.47	1.48	1.48	1.48
100	1.47	1.49	1.50	1.50	1.50
200	1.49	1.51	1.51	1.51	1.52
300	1.50	1.52	1.52	1.52	1.52
500	1.51	1.52	1.53	1.53	1.53
750	1.52	1.53	1.53	1.53	1.53
1000	1.52	1.53	1.53	1.53	1.53
1500	1.53	1.53	1.54	1.54	1.54
2000	1.53	1.54	1.54	1.54	1.54

Table 7.15: Predicted cutoffs for assessing reported energy intakes. Values in the table are for y, where reported energy intake of less than (y × Basal Metabolic Rate) are not plausible, at the 95% confidence limit, according to the number of subjects (*n*) in the sample and the number of days for which the intake was estimated. Data from Goldberg et al. European Journal of Clinical Nutrition 45: 569–581, 1991 © with permission of the Nature Publishing Group.

cutoff (i.e., 1.55 × BMR) will not overestimate the extent of underreporting.

- Subjects with a high energy expenditure and a relatively high intake may report intakes that are too low, yet their EI_{rep}: BMR_{est} are not below the cutoff of 1.55 × BMR. Because of this problem, all subjects with reported intakes below the cutoff are sometimes termed "low energy reporters" rather than "underreporters."

- If a large proportion of the population has a body weight > 84 kg, the equations for estimating basal metabolic rate cannot be safely applied at the individual level.

- The cutoffs are only appropriate for individuals who are in energy balance. Hence, they are not useful for growing children, or for adults who are dieting to lose weight. Inevitably, in any large-scale survey of adults, there are always subjects claiming

to be trying to lose weight. To identify weight-conscious persons, a questionnaire on restrained eating might also be
included in the survey (Stunkard and Messick, 1985).

- Some invalid data at the upper end of the
distribution (i.e., overreporters) may also
exist, but they are not identified.

Application of Goldberg cutoff method

Several investigators have used this approach
to identify and, in some cases, characterize underreporters at the individual level in
both national dietary surveys (Briefel et al.,
1997; Price et al., 1997) and some smaller
studies (Haraldsdóttir and Sandström, 1994;
Rutishauser et al., 1994). In all these studies, the cutoff for a sample size of $n = 1$ has
been used, but the actual cutoff has varied
depending on the number of days of dietary
assessment and whether the data for the 95%
(Table 7.15) or 99% confidence limits (data
not shown) were chosen.

The sensitivity and specificity of the Goldberg cutoff for identifying diets of poor validity has been assessed by Black (2000). Data
for 429 subjects from 22 studies in which
reported energy intake and energy expenditure determined by doubly labeled water were
measured simultaneously, were used for this
analysis. Results indicated that when the cutoff factor for physical activity of 1.55 was
used for men and women, the sensitivity was
0.50 and 0.52 and the specificity was 1.00 and
0.95, respectively. Use of a higher physical
activity factor cutoff of 1.95 in both men and
women increased the sensitivity (0.76 and
0.85, respectively), but resulted in decreased
specificity (0.87 and 0.78, respectively).

Subjects can also be classified into low,
medium, and high activity levels, based on
their individual EE:BMR ratio. Different
cutoffs can then be applied for each activity level. When this approach was used,
the sensitivity was 0.74 and 0.67 and the
specificity was 0.97 and 0.98, respectively, in
men and women. As a result, this approach
was recommended by Black (2000) as a reasonable compromise between sensitivity and
specificity. The approach, however, does necessitate that the investigator chooses suitable
physical activity factor values for each activity level.

Black (2000) has also emphasized that applying the Goldberg cutoff method to identify
"Low Energy Reporters" does not exclude
biased underreporting at the upper end of the
distribution of energy intake and expenditure.
The approach, however, is useful to identify the existence and magnitude of underreporting at a group level. At the individual
level, the method can also provide valuable
information on the characteristics of underreporters (Macdiarmid and Blundell, 1997).

7.3.3 Cutoffs based on predicted total energy expenditure

Recognition of the limitations of the Goldberg cutoff approach has prompted McCrory
et al. (2002) to develop a new method for
identifying inaccurate reports of dietary energy intake. This new method examines the
difference between predicted total energy expenditure (pTEE) from published equations
and EI_{rep}. It also takes into account the
within-subject errors in the methods used to
quantify pTEE and EI_{rep}. The pTEE is calculated from the age, weight, height, and sex of
the subjects; the activity levels are not taken
into account. The equation used by McCrory
et al. (2002) to calculate pTEE is

$$pTEE = 7.377 - (0.073 \times age) + (0.0806 \times weight) \\ + (0.0135 \times height) - (1.363 \times sex)$$

where age is in years, weight is in kg, height
is standing height in cm, and sex is 0 for men
and 1 for women. The equation, derived from
a study of 93 subjects ranging in age from
18 to 81 y, has an r^2 of 0.64. This approach
was applied to data from the U.S. Continuing Survey of Food Intakes by Individuals,
1994–1996 for men and non-pregnant, nonlactating women aged 21–45 y ($n = 3755$).
Cutoffs for excluding EI_{rep} at both ± 1 SD
and ± 2 SD for the agreement between EI_{rep}
and pTEE were computed, although those
based on ± 1 SD are preferred; details are
given in McCrory et al. (2002).

	Total group (n = 44)	Men (n = 22)	Women (n = 22)
Nitrogen intake from dietary history (N_I)	13.3 ± 0.51	14.6 ± 0.77	11.9 ± 0.55
Nitrogen intake from nitrogen excretion in the urine (including 2 g allowance for extra-renal losses (N_E)	13.3 ± 0.46	14.4 ± 0.60	12.1 ± 0.63
(N_I) − (N_E)	0.0 ± 0.50	0.2 ± 0.94	-0.2 ± 0.57
95% confidence limits (N_I) − (N_E)	−1.1 and 1.1	−1.6 and 2.0	−1.5 and 1.1

Table 7.16: Comparison of nitrogen intake (g/day; mean ± SE) as assessed by a dietary history and daily urinary nitrogen excretion in young adults. From van Staveren et al., American Journal of Clinical Nutrition 42: 554–559, 1985 © Am J Clin Nutr. American Society for Clinical Nutrition.

7.3.4 Twenty-four-hour urinary nitrogen excretion to validate protein intake

Isaksson (1980) was one of the first investigators to use nitrogen excretion levels in 24-h urine samples to validate 24-h protein intake estimated by record or recall. This procedure was adopted because of the positive correlation observed between daily nitrogen intake and daily nitrogen excretion when the dietary intake is kept constant in metabolic studies of adults with stable body weights.

The early studies used urinary nitrogen based on only one or two 24-h urine samples per individual to validate the mean protein intake of a group (Isaksson, 1980). For example, in a study by van Staveren et al. (1985), 24-h urine samples were collected by each subject, on a preselected day, so that for the group as a whole, urine collections for all days of the week were evenly represented. The mean urine nitrogen excretion of an average weekday was calculated, with the addition of a correction factor of 2 g for extrarenal nitrogen losses. The results suggested that there was no difference between mean excretion and mean intake of nitrogen for the group, as shown in Table 7.16. Hence in this study the dietary history method had made a valid assessment of the group mean intake of foods containing protein.

Later studies have used 24-h urine nitrogen to validate estimates of protein intake on an individual basis. In such cases, repeat collections of consecutive 24-h urine samples are necessary. Indeed, in a 28-d metabolic study of Bingham and Cummings (1985), eight 24-h urine collections, verified for completeness, were necessary to estimate dietary nitrogen intakes of individuals to within 5% (Table 7.17). In general, correlations between 24-h urine nitrogen based on repeat 24-h urine collections, and estimates of protein intake have been higher for weighed or estimated records than for food frequency questionnaires (Bingham et al., 1995; Porrini et al., 1995; McKeown et al., 2001). There are several limitations to the use of urinary nitrogen as a biomarker of dietary protein intake:

Stable nitrogen balance is assumed, with subjects retaining no nitrogen for growth or the repair of lost muscle tissue. No allowances are made for losses as a result of starvation, dieting, or injury.

Extra-renal losses of nitrogen via the skin and feces are not measured directly, and thus 24-h urinary nitrogen underestimates nitrogen output. To account for these extra-renal losses, 2 g of nitrogen are added to each 24-h nitrogen excretion in the urine. Hence if the 24-h protein intake is 24Prot and the subject is in nitrogen balance, the following relationship is said to apply:

24Prot (g)/6.25 = N excretion in 24 hours (g) + 2 (g)

The use of a universal correction of 2 g is probably not appropriate because of a large

Subject	1	2	3	4	5	6	7	8	Mean
Dietary N (g)	13.2	21.7	21.2	15.8	15.7	11.7	12.7	14.0	—
Urinary N (g)	12.1	15.6	16.6	13.8	13.2	9.6	10.2	10.8	—
% Urine N / diet N	88	72	78	87	84	82	80	77	81 ± 5

Table 7.17: Comparison of nitrogen intake as assessed by 18 days of observation and urinary nitrogen output after 8 days of complete 24-h collections. From Bingham and Cummings, American Journal of Clinical Nutrition 42: 1276–1289, 1985 © Am J Clin Nutr. American Society for Clinical Nutrition.

variation in fecal nitrogen excretion among individuals. Further, dermal losses, when measured directly, appear to range from 100 to 500 mg rather than the 1 g assumed (Calloway et al., 1971). Moreover, intakes of dietary fiber, as well as exercise, all affect the level of the external losses of nitrogen (Cummings et al., 1981). Hence, an alternative approach that assumes the extra-renal losses account for a fixed proportion (i.e., 80%) of total nitrogen excretion, is often used (Bingham, 2003), although this might not apply to all subjects.

Complete 24-h urine collections are required. Note that the use of repeat overnight urine collections cannot replace the necessity for 24-h urine collections. In the past, creatinine excretion in the 24-h urine samples was often used to measure the completeness of urine collections, based on the assumption that creatinine excretion is constant from day to day in an individual. Creatinine excretion, however, depends on creatinine intake (primarily from meat in the diet) and creatinine production. The latter is proportional to the fat-free mass. Within subjects, the coefficient of variation (CV) in the 24-h output of creatinine may be 10%, but between subjects, it may be as large as 23%, even when urine collections are known to be complete (Bingham, 2003).

British investigators have confirmed that 4-aminobenzoic acid (PABA) is a safe, reliable, exogenous marker that can be used to validate the completeness of urine collections (Bingham and Cummings, 1983). PABA can be easily administered in capsules (3×80 mg tablets) and analyzed with a maximum intersubject variation in excretion of only 15%.

Urine collections containing $< 85\%$ of the PABA marker are probably incomplete (Figure 15.2). Overcollection of urine cannot be detected using PABA. Further details on the use of PABA are given in Section 15.2. Use of lithium to assess the completeness of 24-h urine collections is discussed in Section 7.3.6.

Concentrations of PABA in urine were used to verify the completeness of 24-h urine samples in studies designed to evaluate the validity (and reproducibility) of the dietary assessment methods for the U.K., Dutch, and German EPIC studies (Bingham et al., 1997; Ocké et al., 1997; Kroke et al., 1999; McKeown et al., 2001).

Within-subject variation in daily nitrogen excretion of individuals may be large, and repeat collections of consecutive 24-h urine samples are necessary if the method is to be used to validate the protein intakes of individuals, as noted earlier. For example, when data based on a single day are used, the expected correlation between nitrogen intake and 24-h urine nitrogen is approximately 0.5 with a CV of 24%, whereas when eight 24-h urine collections, validated for completeness, and 18 d of dietary intake data are available as shown in Table 7.17, the correlation increases to 0.95, and the CV declines to 5% (Bingham, 2003). The exact number of days needed to validate protein intakes of individuals varies according to the degree of precision required.

7.3.5 Other uses of 24-h urine nitrogen in validation studies

As the collection of 24-h urine samples is a relatively noninvasive procedure, urinary nitrogen has been used in a variety of other ways to validate dietary assessments.

Changes in usual dietary intakes may occur during relatively long-term dietary studies designed to assess the usual intakes of individuals. Such changes may influence validity. Twenty-four-hour urinary nitrogen excretion has been used to detect such changes in usual dietary intake, by comparing the nitrogen excretion in 24-h urine samples collected both during the dietary assessment period and at a time either before or after the assessment is completed (Bingham et al., 1982; McKeown et al., 2001).

McKeown et al. (2001) correlated nitrogen intakes from two 7-d food records with corresponding urinary nitrogen excretion results, based on at least two 24-h urine collections per subject (verified for completeness). However, in this study, the 24-h urine samples were not collected during the two 7-d food record periods, so that any errors between the dietary assessment method and the biomarkers were completely independent. Nitrogen intakes from the first 7-d diet record correlated strongly with urinary nitrogen excretion ($r = 0.67$). However, correlation for the second set of intakes was weaker ($r = 0.57$), suggesting that the recording of intake had indeed changed during the validation study.

Assessment of measurement error is critical in studies of diet and disease. The error assessment can be achieved by using a reference method with errors that are both independent of true intake and any error component in the "test" dietary method. Urinary nitrogen excretion satisfies both these criteria as a reference biomarker of protein intake, and was used in the EPIC study to identify the most valid dietary method (Ocké et al., 1997; Kroke et al., 1999; McKeown et al., 2001).

McKeown et al. (2001) described a study in which 134 subjects who participated in the EPIC U.K. Norfolk cohort, collected up to six complete 24-h urine collections over a 9-mo period, during which they also completed two food frequency questionnaires and two 7-d estimated food records. The dietary

assessment methods were completed at random times and not in concordance with the collection of the 24-h urines as noted earlier, in an effort to ensure that errors between the dietary method and biomarker were independent. Higher correlations were observed between the estimates of nitrogen intake based on the 24-h urine nitrogen excretion and the two 7-d food records (i.e., 0.57 and 0.67), compared to the two food frequency questionnaires (i.e., 0.21 and 0.29).

Use of the repeated 24-h urine collections and repeated dietary intake data also permitted calculation of within-subject error variance for each of the dietary methods used in the U.K. EPIC study. Not surprisingly, the estimated food records were associated with a smaller variance ratio so that correction factors for correlation and regression were markedly less than those for the other dietary methods (Section 6.2.3) (Day et al., 2001). Further details of the statistical models that can be used to calculate the sources of error variance are given in Kipnis et al. (2001).

It is noteworthy that individuals judged as underreporters by the 24-h urine nitrogen method also tend to be classified as underreporters by the doubly labeled water method (Bingham, 2003). This characteristic highlights that repeat dietary intake measurements do not necessarily provide valid measures of individual intake. Indeed, extreme intakes may reflect under- and overreporting rather than true low or high intakes. Further, individuals who are most prone to reporting bias may be repeatedly misclassified in quantiles of the distribution (Black and Cole, 2001).

Calibration of dietary data is becoming increasingly important in multisite cohort studies to adjust for any between-center biases in the test dietary method. Twenty-four-hour urine nitrogen can be used to calibrate the dietary data collected in these multisite studies. It serves as a standardized reference measurement to correct for any systematic errors in the collection of the dietary intakes (Kaaks and Riboli, 1997).

EPICSOFT, a computerized 24-h recall

method (Section 5.2.4) was developed and used to assess dietary intakes in a representative subsample within each EPIC cohort (Slimani et al., 2000, 2003). Some respondents in each cohort (100–350) also collected a single 24-h urine sample verified for completeness using PABA. A high correlation between the mean intake and excretion of nitrogen was observed across the populations studied, confirming the validity of the 24-h recall calibration method across all countries.

7.3.6 Excretion of nutrients in urine

The urinary excretion of certain other nutrients for which the urine is the major excretory route has also been used as a biomarker of dietary intake and is discussed below.

Sodium excretion in urine is often used as a measure of dietary sodium intake instead of calculating sodium intake from food intake and food composition data. Losses of sodium via the feces and sweat are probably minimal in temperate climates, although they may be increased by vigorous physical activity or diarrhea. Diurnal and day-to-day fluctuations in sodium excretion are larger than those for nitrogen. Hence, even more collections are required to correctly characterize sodium excretion in an individual than for nitrogen (McKeown et al., 2001).

Simpson et al. (1983) estimated that fifteen 24-h urine collections are required to characterize an individual's sodium output with 95% accuracy. Hence, it is not surprising that only a weak association between sodium intake (assessed via two 7-d estimated food records) and excretion was reported in the EPIC study ($r = 0.48$), when some of the subjects only provided two or three complete 24-h urine samples (McKeown et al., 2001). Even when the mean of six urine collections and 16-d weighed records are used to estimate sodium intake, the relationship between the two measures may still be only moderate (Bingham et al., 1995).

Correlations between sodium intake and excretion can be strengthened if the within-subject variability in urinary sodium excre-

tion is estimated from replicate 24-h urine samples collected from the entire study population, or from a random subsample only (e.g., 8% of the subjects) (see Section 6.2.3). The latter approach was used in the INTER-SALT study, a large international collaborative investigation of the relation between blood pressure and dietary intake. This study measured several urinary biomarkers of dietary intake, including urinary sodium, potassium, and nitrogen (Dyer et al., 1997). It appears, however, that the use of urinary sodium to validate self-reported dietary intakes is limited.

Potassium excretion in urine can also be used as a biomarker of potassium intake; approximately 77% of dietary potassium is reportedly excreted in the urine (Holbrook et al., 1984; Caggiula et al., 1985). Like urinary sodium, there is considerable within-subject variation in urinary potassium excretion (Dyer et al., 1997). Hence, again in the U.K. EPIC cohort, only a weak correlation ($r = 0.58$) between potassium intake (based on two 7-d estimated food records) and urinary potassium excretion (based on two to six 24-h urine collections) was noted (McKeown et al., 2001). This was in contrast to the earlier validation studies in which subjects provided eight 24-h urine samples per subject, when not surprisingly, higher correlations were observed ($r = 0.74–0.82$) (Bingham and Day, 1997).

Belgium investigators used ratios of dietary intake to urinary excretion of potassium as a measure of the prevalence of under- and overreporting of potassium intake in a large survey of nutrition and health (Zhang et al., 2000). The ratio, based on the assumption that 77% of dietary potassium is excreted in the urine, was calculated as:

$$(\text{dietary potassium} \times 0.77) / \text{urinary potassium}$$

The subjects with ratios < 1 were defined as underreporters and those with ratios > 1 were defined as overreporters.

Lithium excretion in urine is used to monitor dietary sources of lithium-tagged foodstuffs such as table salt (Sanchez-Castillo et al., 1987). Lithium is almost completely excreted in urine so that excretion of this element in a 24-h urine sample reflects the daily dose. Lithium can also be used to determine the completeness of 24-h urine collections. When used for this purpose, the lithium-tagged food must be given daily to subjects some days before the intended urine collection to achieve equilibrium (Bingham, 2003).

Serum lithium concentrations can be used to distinguish between intake and no intake of lithium-tagged foods or supplements (de Roos et al., 2001).

Selenium, chromium, and iodine all have urine as their main excretory route. Research on the use of 24-h urinary excretion of selenium and chromium as biomarkers of dietary intake is limited. In contrast, urinary iodine has been extensively studied as a biomarker of dietary iodine intake (Wild et al., 2001). Approximately 90% of dietary iodine is excreted in the urine. Hence

$$I_{intake} = (\text{24-h urinary iodide}) / 0.90$$

Alternatively, assuming a median 24-h urine volume of about 0.0009 L/h/kg and an average bioavailability of iodine in the diet of 92%, then daily iodine intake (in μg) can be calculated from urinary iodine based on casual urine samples as follows:

$$I_{intake} = (0.0009 \times 24 / 0.92) \times Wt \times Ui$$
$$= 0.0235 \times Wt \times Ui$$

where Wt is the body weight (kg) and Ui is the urinary iodine (μg/L) (IOM, 2001).

More than one 24-h urine sample per subject should be collected, where possible, to assess the iodine status of individuals. Thomson et al. (2001) used two 24-h urine samples to assess the iodine status of New Zealand adults. When information at the group level is required, single void fasting urine specimens can be used (Section 25.1.3.)

7.3.7 Fatty acids in adipose tissue

Currently there is no suitable biomarker for quantifying the usual dietary intake of total fat, although serum apolipoprotein A-IV concentrations may be useful to monitor short term changes (days or weeks) in total fat intake (Weinburg et al., 1990). The lack of a biomarker is unfortunate because the intake of total fat is difficult to quantify using conventional methods of dietary assessment (Chapter 3). In addition, reported total fat intakes are especially prone to bias; individuals tend to underreport fat intake because of its social undesirability.

In contrast, levels of certain fatty acids can be used as biomarkers and related to dietary intakes. Fatty acids form the basic structural components of triglycerides and are also found in phospholipids and cholesterol esters. They rarely exist as free fatty acids in vivo. The structure of fatty acids is simple: they consist of an even-numbered chain of carbon atoms, with a carboxyl group at one end and a methyl group at the other.

Fatty acid biomarkers in adipose tissue measure long-term dietary intakes, generally reflecting fatty acid intake over the preceding 1–2 y. When selecting fatty acids for use as biomarkers, consideration must be given to how ingested fatty acids are handled by the body. In general, only those fatty acids that are absorbed and stored in adipose tissue without modification, and that are not synthesized endogenously, are used. Several other factors that influence the measurement of fatty acid profiles in adipose tissue must also be taken into account, and are summarized in Box 7.2.

Three classes of fatty acids have been studied in relation to dietary intakes: some specific n-3 and n-6 polyunsaturated fatty acids, *trans* unsaturated fatty acids, and some odd-numbered and branched-chain saturated fatty acids which are found in dairy products (e.g., pentadecanoic acid and heptadecanoic acid). None of these fatty acids are produced endogenously, so they all possess the necessary characteristics for a biomarker.

Table 7.18 provides examples of the correlation coefficients linking concentrations of fatty acids determined from dietary assessment and those in adipose tissue samples. Not surprisingly, the reported correlations vary

Reference	Dietary method	PUFA	LA	EPA	DHA	TUFA
Godley et al. (1996)	FFQ	–	–	0.41	0.43	–
van Staveren et al. (1986a)	19 × 24-h recall	0.68	0.70	–	–	–
Hunter et al. (1992)	FFQ	0.50	0.48	0.47	–	0.29
Hunter et al. (1992)	2 × 7-d record	0.49	–	–	–	–
London et al. (1991)	19 × 24-h recall	0.37	0.35	0.48*	–	0.51
Feunekes et al. (1993)	FFQ	0.24	0.28	–	–	–
Garland et al. (1998)	2 × FFQ	0.40	0.37	–	–	0.40
Garland et al. (1998)	1 week diet record	0.37	–	–	–	–
Marckmann et al. (1995)	3 × 7-d record	0.38	–	0.40	0.66	–
Tjønneland et al. (1993)	2 × 7-d record	0.57	0.51	0.44	0.55	–
Tjønneland et al. (1993)	FFQ	0.44	0.44	0.47	0.41	–
Lemaitre et al. (1998)	FFQ	–	–	–	–	0.55–0.67

Table 7.18: Correlation coefficients of dietary estimates of fatty acid intake (g/100 g fatty acids) versus adipose-tissue-biopsy concentrations (g/100 g fatty acids). PUFA, polyunsaturated fatty acids; LA, linoleic acid; EPA, eicosapentaenoic acid; DHA, docosahexaenoic acid; TUFA, *trans* unsaturated fatty acids; FFQ, food frequency questionnaire; *average of EPA and DHA. From Cantwell, Proceedings of the Nutrition Society 59: 187–191, 2000, with permission of the Nutrition Society.

markedly across studies. The extent of the correlation depends on numerous factors, including the biomarker itself and the factors itemized in Box 7.2, and discussed in detail by Arab (2003). The between-subject varia-

tion in dietary intake, the dietary assessment method used, the quality of the food composition database, the population group under study, and the statistical treatment of the data are all additional sources of variance. Only in some studies have adjustments been made for attenuation due to within-subject variance in the adipose tissue biomarker and dietary intakes (Section 6.2.3). Examples of the three classes of fatty acids used as biomarkers are discussed below.

Dietary intake of the respondent

Relative amounts of other fatty acids in the adipose tissue samples

Supplement use (such as fish-oil capsules) by the respondent

Genetic polymorphisms of elongase and desaturase enzymes

Tissue-sampling site

Tissue sampling procedures and subsequent sample handling and storage

Amount sampled in relation to the analytical method and detection limit

Lipolysis or the breakdown of fat stored in fat cells

Nutritional status (Fe, Zn, Cu, and Mg sufficiency)

Lipogenesis or the production of fat from the metabolism of protein and carbohydrate

Diseases: cystic fibrosis, malabsorption, liver cirrhosis, diabetes, Zellweger syndrome

Fat oxidation abnormalities

Box 7.2: Factors influencing measured fatty acid biomarker levels in adipose tissue. From Arab, Journal of Nutrition 133: 925S–932S, 2003, with permission of the American Society for Nutritional Sciences.

n-3 polyunsaturated fatty acids

Polyunsaturated fatty acids (PUFAs) contain more than two double bonds and are generally liquid at room temperature. They can be subdivided into three families based on the position of their first double bond: n-3, n-6, and n-9 fatty acids. In the n-3 fatty acids, the first double bond is three carbon atoms from the methyl end of the carbon chain. The n-3 family cannot be synthesized de novo in the human body, or interconverted in humans, because of the lack of an appropriate enzyme. Therefore, in humans, the diet is the only source of body stores of the n-3 family of PUFAs.

Two common examples of very long chain n-3 PUFAs, typically found in marine oils, are described below. Both eicosapentaenoic

Fatty acid	Spearman	Pearson	Corrected
	Food frequency questionnaire		
20:5n-3 (EPA)	0.55	0.47	
22:6n-3 (DHA)	0.42	0.41	
	two 7-d diet records		
20:5n-3 (EPA)	0.57	0.44	0.63
22:6n-3 (DHA)	0.56	0.55	0.80

Table 7.19: Correlations between fatty acid composition of adipose tissue from 86 subjects (both sexes) and fatty acid dietary intake, expressed as percentage of total fat intake, using a food frequency questionnaire and 7-d record dietary methodologies. The corrected correlations were calculated on the basis of the within- to between-person variance ratio. This correction is not possible with the food frequency questionnaire. Data from Tjønneland et al., American Journal of Clinical Nutrition 57: 629–633, 1993 © Am J Clin Nutr. American Society for Clinical Nutrition.

acid (EPA) and docosahexaenoic acid (DHA) have a direct impact on eicosanoid production. Eicosanoids are high-potency, fast-acting hormones that are produced from free fatty acids locally and serve as second messengers. Examples of eicosanoids are prostacyclin, an inhibitor of platelet aggregation, and thromboxane A2, a stimulator of platelet aggregation. Interest in the use of biomarkers for intakes of these two n-3 PUFAs has stemmed from their preventive role in cardiovascular disease and cancer.

Eicosapentaenoic acid (EPA) has been studied by several investigators. In a U.S. study by Hunter et al. (1992), EPA concentrations in subcutaneous fat aspirates from the lateral buttock were measured in 115 men aged 40–75 y, and dietary intakes were determined from a food frequency questionnaire, administered twice. These investigators also calculated the within- to between-person variance for the EPA measures in the fat biopsy samples collected on two occasions from 17 of the subjects. This permitted the calculation of the theoretical reduction in the absolute value of the correlation coefficient (Section 6.2.3). After deattenuation, the Spearman correlation coefficients between the estimates of EPA intake, when expressed as percentage of total

fat intake, and concentrations in fat aspirates were $r = 0.47$ and $r = 0.49$ for the food frequency questionnaires I and II, respectively. Correlations ranging from 0.41 to 0.47 have also been reported by other investigators (Tjønneland et al., 1993; Godley et al., 1996) based on estimates of EPA intake (g/100 g fatty acids) from food frequency questionnaires versus adipose tissue biopsy concentrations, as shown in Table 7.18 and Table 7.19.

Even higher Spearman correlations were noted when EPA intakes were measured by two 7-d diet records in a study of Danish men and women ($r = 0.57$), after deattenuation and correction for the variance (Table 7.19). The results emphasize the large daily variation in the intake of this n-3 polyunsaturated fatty acid (Tjønneland et al., 1993).

Docosahexaenoic acid (DHA) content of adipose tissue and diets has also been studied. In general, stronger correlations have been reported between dietary intakes and adipose tissue concentrations for DHA compared with that for EPA (Table 7.18), especially after deattenuation and correction for the variance (Table 7.19) (Tjønneland et al., 1993; Marckmann et al., 1995). Indeed, adipose tissue DHA content appears to be the biomarker of choice in epidemiological studies for the assessment of the long-term habitual dietary intakes of n-3 PUFAs derived from coldwater and marine fish (Markmann et al., 1995; Baylin et al., 2002).

n-6 polyunsaturated fatty acids

The first double bond in the n-6 fatty acids is next to the sixth carbon atom from the methyl end of the carbon chain. The n-6 fatty acid family, like the n-3 family, cannot be synthesized de novo in the human body, or interconverted in humans, because of the lack of the appropriate enzymes. Therefore, the diet is the only source of body stores of the n-6 PUFAs in humans.

Linoleic acid is an essential n-6 PUFA, required for the structural integrity of all cell membranes. Numerous studies have confirmed that the composition of linoleic acid in adipose tissue is a good biomarker for linoleic acid intake. For example, long-term dietary intervention studies (i.e., 5 y) with diets high in linoleic acid have led to increases in the linoleic acid content of adipose tissue ranging from 11% to 32% (Dayton et al., 1966).

Reported correlations between the linoleic acid composition of adipose tissue and the diet, however, have varied, ranging from 0.28 to 0.70, depending on the study group, gender, and dietary method used (Table 7.18). In a Danish study, for example, the correlation for men ($r = 0.76$) was higher than that for women ($r = 0.36$), when two 7-d weighed records were used to assess intakes (Tjønneland et al., 1993).

Table 7.20 presents data from a study conducted on 59 young adult Dutch women (van Staveren et al., 1986a). A highly significant correlation between the linoleic acid composition of adipose tissue and the diet ($r = 0.77$) was reported. Dietary intakes in this study were calculated from the mean of 19 repeat 24-h recalls administered over a period of 30 mo. Moreover, when only a single 24-h recall was used to assess the dietary intake in this Dutch study, the correlation for linoleic acid fell to 0.28, emphasizing the importance of obtaining dietary information

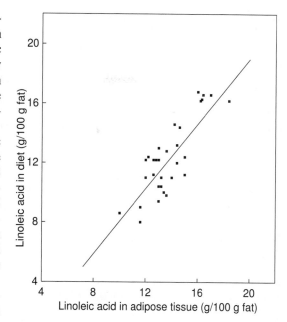

Figure 7.3: Linear regression ($y = 1.10x - 3.12$) of linoleic acid (g/100 g fat) in the diet of 32 Dutch female subjects, assessed with a 24-h recall repeated nineteen times over 30 mo, on the corresponding value in adipose tissue. From van Staveren et al., American Journal of Epidemiology 123: 455–463, 1986, by permission of the Society for Epidemiologic Research.

on the long-term habitual intake (Katan et al., 1991). The same group of Dutch investigators also confirmed, using linear regression analysis, that the linoleic acid composition of the diet could be predicted from the linoleic acid composition of the adipose tissue, as shown in Figure 7.3.

In this Dutch study, when women whose weight changed by 3 kg or more were excluded, the correlation coefficient for linoleic acid rose from $r = 0.77$ to $r = 0.82$. Stronger correlations have also been reported by others for subjects with stable weight (London et al., 1991). These findings emphasize the large effect of fluctuations in body weight on the relationship between the fatty acid profile of adipose tissue and the average fatty acid composition of the diet. This effect may be due to the more accurate reporting of usual diet by persons with a stable body weight. Alternatively, weight fluctuations may alter the fatty acid content of adipose tissue.

Fatty acid or ratio of fatty acids	Correlation coefficient observed	Correlation coefficient unattenuated
P/S	0.57	0.63
M/P	0.63	0.69
P	0.68	0.75
L/S	0.62	0.68
M/L	0.63	0.69
L	0.70	0.77

Table 7.20: Observed and unattenuated correlation coefficients between the fatty acid composition of the diet and of the adipose tissue. Subjects were 59 adult Dutch women. P, polyunsaturated fatty acids; L, linoleic acid; M, mono-unsaturated fatty acids; S, saturated fatty acids. All correlation coefficients quoted are significant ($p < 0.05$). From van Staveren et al., American Journal of Epidemiology 123: 455–463, 1986, with permission of the Society for Epidemiologic Research.

Trans unsaturated fatty acids

In most unsaturated fatty acids in the diet, the two hydrogen atoms (attached to the double-bond carbon atoms) are in the *cis* configuration — on the same side of the molecule. In *trans* fatty acids, the two hydrogen atoms, are on opposite sides of the molecule. Most *trans* fatty acids in the diet occur through industrial hydrogenation of PUFAs to enhance their stability and prevent their oxidation. This practice has increased, so the dietary intake of *trans* unsaturated fatty acids has risen dramatically in recent years. In the United States, for example, many margarines now contain as much as 15% to 25% of their fat as *trans* fatty acids. Hydrogenated vegetable oils are also a major source of *trans* fatty acids in the United Kingdom and in many other European countries.

Results of studies that have examined the relationships between *trans* fatty acid levels in the diet and adipose tissue concentrations have been mixed. Both the total *trans* fatty acid content and the concentrations of only elaidic acid, the most common *trans* fatty acid, have been investigated. In general, correlations have ranged from 0.5 to 0.67 for total *trans* fatty acids (Table 7.18) (London et al., 1991; Garland et al., 1998; Lemaitre et al., 1998; van de Vijver et al., 2000), although sometimes they have been much lower (Hunter et al., 1992; Cantwell, 2000; Pedersen et al., 2000).

There are several possible reasons for the marked variation in the strength of the correlations observed. They may be related in part to inaccuracies in food composition values for *trans* unsaturated fatty acids. Alternatively, there may be difficulties with the analysis of certain *trans* fatty acids in adipose tissue, so results may be unreliable, especially for the longer-chain *trans* fatty acids from marine oils. In addition, absorption of *trans* fatty acids appears to decrease with increasing chain length (Peters et al., 1991). As a result, the long-chain *trans* fatty acids may be taken up into tissues in disproportionately low amounts compared to their level in dietary fat (Webb et al., 1991).

Odd-numbered and branched-chain saturated fatty acids

The saturated fatty acids have carbon–carbon bonds that are fully saturated with hydrogen atoms: there are no double bonds. Pentadecanoic acid (15:0) and heptadecanoic acid (17:0) are two saturated fatty acids with an odd number of carbon atoms that cannot be synthesized in the human body: they are produced by bacterial flora in the rumen of ruminants (Wu and Palmquist, 1991). Therefore, their content in adipose tissue can be used as a biomarker of dairy fat intake. Use of a biomarker of dairy fat intake is important; dairy fat has atherogenic and thrombogenic properties, which have been linked to the development of artery disease.

Pentadecanoic acid (PDA) content of adipose tissue correlates with intakes of PDA and total dairy fat, the strength of the association again varying with the dietary method used. For example, in a study of Swedish women, the correlation with total dairy fat intake calculated using food records completed over the previous 4 wks was $r = 0.63$, but only $r = 0.40$ when a food frequency questionnaire was used (Wolk et al., 1998). However, in a study of Swedish men using two 1-wk

| Adipose tissue fatty acid | 2 × 1-wk dietary record | | |
	Total dairy fat	Fatty acid 15:0	Fatty acid 17:0
PDA 15:0	0.71	0.58	0.51
HDA 17:0	0.16	0.22	0.24

| Adipose tissue fatty acid | 14 × 24-h diet recall | | |
	Total dairy fat	Fatty acid 15:0	Fatty acid 17:0
PDA 15:0	0.74	0.67	0.60
HDA 17:0	0.23	0.22	0.20

Table 7.21: Pearson correlation coefficients of relative total dairy fat and pentadecanoic acid (PDA) and heptadecanoic acid (HDA) intakes with the corresponding fatty acid content of adipose tissue among 114 men. Data abstracted from a more comprehensive table of results in Wolk et al., Journal of Nutrition 131: 828–833, 2001, with permission of the American Society for Nutritional Sciences.

food records, 6 months apart, and 14 telephone-administered 24-h recalls distributed
evenly throughout the year, correlations between the PDA content of adipose tissue and
total dairy-fat intake for both dietary methods were comparable and relatively high,
as shown in Table 7.21 (Wolk et al., 2001).
These findings for PDA are consistent with
those noted for other high dairy-fat consuming populations (e.g., the Netherlands and
Denmark) (van Staveren et al., 1986a; Tjønneland et al., 1993). Note, however, that
lower correlations might be observed for population groups with a high intake of ruminant
fat (beef and lamb) and a low intake of milk
fat because PDA is also present in the fat from
ruminants, as noted earlier.

Lower correlations ($r = 0.31$) of dairy product intake, assessed by a food frequency
questionnaire, and adipose PDA levels were
noted in Costa Rican men and women (Baylin
et al., 2002). Figure 7.4 shows the correlation between mean content of PDA in adipose
tissue (as percentage of total fatty acids) plotted against daily intake of dairy products by
decile, assessed by a food frequency questionnaire in this study. Age, sex, body mass
index, and smoking status were taken into
account in this analysis. The lower correlations observed probably reflect a much lower

intake of dairy products in Costa Rica than in
Sweden, Denmark, and the Netherlands.

Heptadecanoic acid (HDA) content of adipose tissue has also been investigated as a
biomarker of intake of HDA and total dairy
fat. In general, low correlations have been
reported, irrespective of the dietary method
used, as shown for the study of Swedish men
presented in Table 7.21 (Wolk et al., 2001). In
the Costa Rican study, for example, no correlation between HDA in adipose tissue (as
percentage of total fatty acids) and the corresponding dietary fatty acid was noted, most
likely partly due to the paucity of food composition data for this fatty acid (Baylin et al.,
2002).

Sampling, analysis, and interpretation of fatty acids in adipose tissue

Samples of adipose tissue (5–10 mg) can be
collected by aspiration with a 15-gauge needle, with or without local anesthesia. The
safety of this procedure is similar to that of
phlebotomy. Several sites can be used, although throughout an investigation, the same
site should be sampled: within an individual, fatty acid profiles may vary across
sites (Table 7.22). In general, exogenously
produced PUFA profiles tend to be less site-
specific than the profiles for the endogenous
saturated fatty acids. Subcutaneous fat samples from the outer upper arm are often used
because of ease of access (Smith et al., 1985),

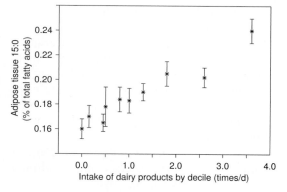

Figure 7.4: Mean (SEM) adipose tissue pentadecanoic
acid (PDA) levels plotted against median daily intake
of dairy products by decile after adjustment for age,
sex, body mass index, and smoking status: $r = 0.31$,
$p < 0.01$; $n = 503$. From Baylin et al., American Journal
of Clinical Nutrition 76: 750–757, 2002 © Am J Clin
Nutr. American Society for Clinical Nutrition.

Fatty acid	Perirenal	Abdomen	Buttock
C14:0	2.58 ± 0.82	2.43 ± 0.75	2.16 ± 0.73
C16:0	23.76 ± 2.40	23.13 ± 2.11	21.79 ± 2.51
C16:1	4.90 ± 2.05	5.61 ± 2.16	7.22 ± 2.68
C18:0	6.54 ± 1.54	5.28 ± 1.73	4.00 ± 1.60
C18:1	45.59 ± 2.92	46.97 ± 2.75	48.26 ± 2.83
C18:2	15.36 ± 2.93	15.32 ± 2.85	15.37 ± 2.82
C18:3	0.62 ± 0.20	0.61 ± 0.19	0.61 ± 0.20

Table 7.22: Mean ($\pm$ SD) concentrations of fatty acids
(% of total fatty acids) in adipose tissue samples from
the perirenal region, abdomen, and buttock of adults
($n = 143$). Data from Arab and Akbar, Public Health
Nutrition 5: 865–871, 2002, by permission of the
authors.

although abdominal or gluteal fat is also frequently sampled.

The standardization of the sampling techniques, and the correct handling and storage of the sample is critical (Beynen and Katan, 1985). However, adipose tissue samples can be stored for long periods without major changes to the fatty acid composition, even at temperatures of −20°C. Where possible, multiple adipose tissue samples and multiple measures of the dietary intake should be collected from at least a subsample of subjects. This will allow the effects of within-subject variance to be reduced, or at least taken into account. The deattenuation of the correlation coefficients can be very significant and lead to more meaningful results (Table 7.19).

Analysis of fatty acids is complex and usually involves separation, identification, and quantification (Nightingale et al., 1999). Hydrolyis of fatty acids to unesterified forms is often required. First the lipid fractions are separated by thin layer chromatography or silica cartridges. Then, the individual fatty acids are separated and measured by high-performance liquid chromatography, gas-liquid chromatography, or gas chromatography–mass spectrometry (Kohlmeier and Kohlmeier, 1995). Of these techniques, gas-liquid chromatography is the most popular (Arab and Akbar, 2002).

Measurement errors for the analysis of fatty acids can be large; coefficients of variation may exceed 25% for the analysis of minor fatty acids by gas chromatography. Several factors have a role in this variation, including the sampling techniques and the handling and storage of the sample. The more important factors are itemized in Box 7.2. Note that the concentrations of individual fatty acids in biomarkers are conventionally expressed as a proportion of the total fatty acid profile and not as an absolute amount. This means that an increased intake of one specific fatty acid can decrease the relative percentage of other fatty acids, without any change in the general intake. For this reason, quantifiable standards of defined amounts of specific fatty acids must be included during analysis.

7.3.8 Fatty acids in blood fractions

Use of plasma/serum or cellular components of blood as biomarkers of fatty acid intake has been extensively studied because blood samples are often more readily available than adipose tissue in epidemiological studies. Fatty acids can be measured as free fatty acids in serum, plasma, or the cellular components of blood (e.g., erythrocytes, erythrocyte membranes, or platelets). Individual fatty acids can also be measured in several lipid subfractions found in plasma. These include the cholesteryl ester and the phospholipid or triglyceride fractions of plasma. Measurement of free fatty acids is the least time consuming method.

The concentrations of the different fatty acids in the various plasma lipid fractions and the cellular components of the blood varies markedly. For example, in the cholesteryl fraction of plasma, the concentration of linoleic acid is typically about two to three times higher than that of oleic acid, whereas in triglycerides, oleic acid predominates. Arachidonic acid tends to be particularly variable, but strongly controlled, across tissues; it can represent only 2.3% of total fatty acids in plasma triglycerides, 11.5% in plasma phospholipids, and 27% in platelet phospholipids (Arab, 2003). Such differences are attributed to the specific physiological functions of fat in the different cell constituents.

The turnover of the different cells from which the fatty acids are extracted control the timing of the relationship to the dietary intake: concentrations in platelets or red cell membranes may reflect the intake over the last few days, whereas erythrocyte concentrations reflect intake over recent months (Arab, 2003).

Plasma levels of the fatty acid composition of cholesteryl esters : phospholipids also tend to reflect intake over the past few days, whereas plasma triglycerides reflect the intake of the past few hours to days. Some exchange takes place, however, between membranes and plasma lipids and lipoproteins throughout the life cycle of the cell. Clearly, the choice of biomarker will depend on the time frame of interest: the dietary methodology must be appropriately matched to that time frame.

Experimental trials and epidemiological studies have confirmed associations between the fatty acid composition of plasma, plasma phospholipids, or the cellular components of blood such as erythrocytes, erythrocyte membranes, and platelets and the dietary intake of fatty acids. Of the fatty acids, linoleic acid, and n-3 PUFAs (i.e., EPA and DHA) have been studied most frequently (Dyerberg et al., 1975; Andersen et al., 1996; Kobayashi et al., 2001), although some saturated fatty acids (e.g., serum PDA levels) have also been studied (Wolk et al., 2001). The strength of the associations have varied, as described for adipose tissue. Many factors influence the level of fatty acids in blood fractions, even when dietary intakes are unaltered. These may include smoking, exercise, stress, pregnancy, oral contraceptives and estrogen therapy, obesity, alcohol intake, and certain disease states (see Table 7.12). The effects of de novo synthesis should also be considered when assessing the relationship between intake and fatty acid levels in blood fractions. Again, sampling, handling, storage, and analysis of the blood fraction samples must be rigorously standardized and controlled.

In some cases, fatty acid levels in plasma and components of blood have been used as indirect biomarkers of the consumption of certain foods or food groups, as described earlier. Examples include the levels of EPA or DHA in plasma phospholipids (Andersen et al., 1996; Hjartaker et al., 1997) and erythrocyte membranes (Godley et al., 1996) as biomarkers of cold-water fish intake, and levels of PDA in serum, cholesterol esters, or phospholipids as a marker for the intake of dairy fat (Smedman et al., 1999; Wolk et al., 2001).

Connor (1996) recommends that when dealing with fatty acids, data for both the biomarkers and intakes should be expressed in comparable units. In a study by Andersen et al. (1996), the correlation between dietary and plasma phospholipid linoleic acid in-creased significantly when both plasma phospholipids and dietary fatty acids were expressed as a percentage of total fatty acids ($r = 0.33$, $p < 0.001$) but not when dietary data were expressed as g/d and when plasma phospholipid concentrations were expressed as μmol/L ($r = 0.01$, ns). This approach may be especially important when combining dietary data for men and women because their energy needs are so different. In the study by Andersen et al. (1996), the ratio of linoleic acid intake was 1.10 between men and women when expressed as g/d, but 0.94 when expressed as a percentage of fat intake.

Plasma carotenoid concentrations

Evidence for a protective effect of carotenoid-rich foods against cancer has prompted work on the use of plasma carotenoid levels as biomarkers of carotenoid intake (Holick et al., 2002). Plasma carotenoid concentrations are not closely regulated by homeostatic mechanisms and thus are said to be sensitive to dietary intake. The magnitude of the correlations between diet and plasma carotenoids varies with the specific carotenoid, the population group studied, the dietary assessment tool used, the quality of the carotenoid food composition database, and the presence or absence of potential confounders.

Intakes of total energy and alcohol, plasma lipid concentrations, and body mass index have all been identified as potential confounders of the diet–plasma carotenoid relationship and, hence, should always be taken into account. Factors related to the absorption and post-absorption metabolism of carotenoids may also play a part.

Likewise, smoking is known to have a significant effect on carotenoid concentrations in plasma, as well as other tissues (e.g., buccal mucosa cells and skin). Those carotenoid concentrations most affected appear to be β-carotene, *cis*-β-carotene and α-carotene, as shown in Table 7.23 (Peng et al., 1995).

Studies have reported correlations between specific dietary and plasma carotenoids ranging from 0.09 to 0.31 for lutein, 0.10 to 0.51 for β-carotene, and 0.58 to 0.62 for α-carotene, again the strength of the relationships depending on the dietary assessment tool (Yong et al., 1994; Bingham et al., 1997).

Plasma carotenoids have also been used as biomarkers of the dietary intake of fruit and vegetables. Research by van Kappel et al. (2001) on women from New York suggests that a single measurement of α-carotene, β-carotene, and lutein in serum could accurately rank subjects according to their usual serum level, in accordance with the findings of Scott et al. (1996). Nevertheless, correlations of these serum levels with estimated intake of fruits and vegetables derived from a dietary history questionnaire were low. More work is required to identify factors associated with the low correlations observed, before serum carotenoids can be considered a valid biomarker of fruit and vegetable consumption.

7.4 Statistical assessment of validity

There is a lack of consensus on the most appropriate statistical methods for assessing the relative validity of dietary assessment method (Burema et al., 1995; Margetts and Thompson 1995). Readers are therefore advised to seek statistical advice before undertaking this task.

The statistical methods used will depend on the objectives of the study (Section 3.3). For the level one objective, only the extent of the agreement on a group basis is of concern, whereas for higher level two to four objec-

	Smokers	Nonsmokers
Lutein	89 ± 36	106 ± 53
Zeaxanthin	19 ± 10	23 ± 13
Cryptoxanthin	84 ± 74	110 ± 68
Lycopene	325 ± 167	325 ± 138
α-carotene	38 ± 21	73 ± 64
β-carotene	116 ± 62	266 ± 259
cis-β-carotene	9 ± 4	19 ± 18

Table 7.23: Mean ($\pm$ SD) plasma carotenoid concentrations (ng/mL) in smokers and nonsmokers. Data from Peng et al., Nutrition and Cancer 23: 233–246, 1995.

tives, an assessment of the validity of the dietary intake data at the individual level is required. There are several methods that can be used to accomplish this task. They have been summarized by Nelson (1997) and are discussed only briefly in this section. Care must be taken when conducting validation studies to ensure that they are conducted on a representative subgroup drawn from the population in which the methods are to be used.

Any assessment of relative validity should consider each of the nutrients of interest separately. Particular attention should be given to those present in high concentrations in relatively few foods (e.g., vitamin A). As well, the effect of potential confounders such as gender, age, weight loss, or certain lifestyle factors (e.g., vegetarian diet, smoking) on the interpretation of the results must also be considered.

The statistical methods most frequently used to assess relative validity are itemized in turn below. In general, several different statistical methods should be used; the results should be compared and then interpreted with caution.

7.4.1 Tests on the means or medians

To assess relative validity at the group level (i.e., level one), a paired *t*-test should be used to examine if the two means are statistically different at some predetermined probability level, provided that the data are "normally" distributed (Tables 7.4, 7.5). If, however, the distribution of nutrient intakes is skewed, attempts should be made to normalize the data before testing the means.

If the intake data are not amenable to log-transformation, the median (50th percentile) and selected percentiles (e.g., 25th and 75th percentiles) should be used to describe the intakes and their variability. The Wilcoxon's signed rank test for paired data can then be used to test the comparability of the medians and, hence, the relative validity of the test method. This procedure is more appropriate than the paired *t*-test for testing for statistical differences for nonnormally distributed data (Snedecor and Cochran, 1989).

If differences between the means for the test and reference methods are significant for multiple nutrients and if the differences are all in the same direction, bias in the test method may be indicated. Alternatively, the means for the test and reference methods may be similar — not significantly different — even when the relative validity at the level of the individual (for example, as measured by correlation) is poor; plots of the test versus reference results for each nutrient or food group of interest should always be drawn to highlight these relationships.

7.4.2 Pearson correlation coefficients

Correlation analysis is the most commonly used method to measure the strength of the relationship at the individual level, between the intakes from the test and the reference dietary method. Usually Pearson correlation coefficients are calculated, although other measures of correlation can also be used (see Section 7.4.3). The data should be transformed, if it is nonnormally distributed, to increase normality before the correlation coefficients are computed.

As noted in Section 6.2.3, intakes of food and nutrients differ within one individual over time: that is, within-subject variation is usually significant. The effect of large within-subject variation in nutrient intakes is to lower and make less significant correlations between the test and a reference method. Such an effect can be taken into account by deattenuating the correlation coefficients using the ratio of within- to between-subject variation (the variance ratio), calculated from the replicate observations in the reference dietary method (Table 7.24). This can be achieved by dividing the correlation coefficients by the appropriate attenuation factors given in Table 6.10, as described in Section 6.2. Rosner and Willet (1988) also recommend calculating the 95% confidence intervals for the deattenuated correlation coefficients.

Within-subject variation also exists for biomarkers of dietary intake. Its effect can also be "removed" from the correlation co-

	Pearson r	Deattenuated r
Energy	0.71	0.77
Protein	0.61	0.68
Fat	0.69	0.74
Carbohydrates	0.72	0.75
Alcohol	0.83	0.87
Dietary fiber	0.51	0.56
Retinol	0.57	0.61
β-carotene	0.26	0.34
Vitamin C	0.39	0.45
Vitamin E	0.57	0.63

Table 7.24: Pearson correlation coefficients between daily intake of nutrients assessed by the Dutch EPIC food frequency questionnaire and by twelve 24-h dietary recalls. Data for males ($n = 63$). All variables were $\log_e$-transformed before analysis. Deattenuated correlation coefficients were based on a correction for within-subject variation in 24-h dietary recalls. Data from Ocké et al., American Journal of Epidemiology 26: S49–S58, 1997, with permission of the Society for Epidemiologic Research.

efficients by deattenuation, as described for the study of EPA levels in adipose tissue by Hunter et al. (1992). In general, however, deattenuation in relation to biomarker levels is seldom performed.

Several investigators have recommended energy-adjusting the nutrient intakes prior to correlation analysis (Bingham et al., 1997; McKeown et al., 2001). Such an approach may allow for the underreporting of intakes. Sometimes (Bingham and Day, 1997; McKeown et al. 2001), but not always (Bohlscheid-Thomas et al., 1997), depending on the dietary method, higher correlation coefficients result from applying an energy adjustment. Beaton et al. (1997) caution that where differential biases in the reporting of intakes of certain macronutrients exist, such as food sources of fat, energy-adjustment procedures will not alleviate the problem.

In its simplest form, the energy adjustment involves calculating the nutrient densities by dividing nutrient values for each subject by the energy content of the diet for that subject. These nutrient densities are then used instead of the original nutrient intake values. Data for both the test and reference methods may be transformed in this way before examining correlations.

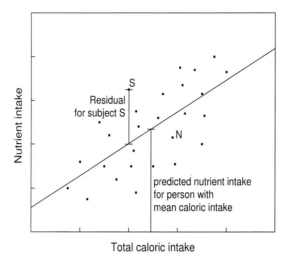

Figure 7.5: The calculation of the energy-adjusted intake using the regression line with the nutrient of interest as the dependent variable. The residual for each subject is added to the predicted nutrient intake for a subject with an energy intake equal to the mean for the group. Note that subjects such as "N" have negative residuals. After Willett (1998).

An alternative and sometimes preferable procedure is to use linear regression with total energy intake as the independent variable (x) and intake of the nutrient of interest as the dependent variable (y) (Willett, 1998). In cases where the nutrient variables are skewed, they should be transformed to improve normality prior to their use in the regression. The energy-adjusted nutrient intake of each subject is determined by adding the residual — that is, the difference between the observed nutrient values for each subject and the values predicted from the regression equation — to the nutrient intake corresponding to mean energy intake of the study population (Figure 7.5). Again, data for both the test and reference methods may be recalculated in this way. Bingham and Day (1997) used this approach to energy-adjust intakes of nitrogen derived from a food frequency questionnaire, and weighed and estimated records. Only the correlations between 24-h urine nitrogen and nitrogen intakes from the food frequency questionnaire improved after the energy adjustment from $r = 0.24$ to $r = 0.48$.

Limitations of Pearson *r* in validity

Bland and Altman (1986) have noted several limitations associated with using Pearson correlation coefficients as a measure of agreement in dietary validation studies. These limitations are summarized in below.

An over-optimistic or inflated measure of agreement between the test and reference method may be given by the Pearson (or Spearman) correlation coefficient. This is because a positive correlation is to be expected when two methods are used to measure the same variable, whereas the conventional basis (null hypothesis) for the test is that there is no such expected correlation. As a result, the conventional significance values often calculated along with the Pearson correlation coefficients are best ignored in the context of the assessment of relative validity.

The strength of the relationship between the test and reference method is indicated by the Pearson correlation coefficient; it does not measure the extent of the agreement. Indeed, poor agreement can exist between a test and reference method even when correlation coefficients are very high. Perfect agreement will only occur if the two methods yield identical results. There is also perfect correlation under these circumstances. However, perfect correlation will also occur if the test method generates results which are exactly a fixed proportion greater or less than the reference method. For example, if the test results are exactly 24% higher than the reference method, the correlation will be perfect and highly significant, yet the agreement is unsatisfactory — the test method is biased, generating spuriously high results. Such a bias will not be evident using correlation analysis.

Characteristics of the study population, as well as the quality of the dietary methods, affects the degree of correlation, and the calculated r. For example, when the between-subject variation in the measured nutrient intakes is large, then the correlation generated

Nutrient	Pearson r	Pearson (95% CI)	r_s	Spearman (95% CI)	% in tertiles: Same	% in tertiles: Opposite	κ_w
Energy	0.40	(0.11, 0.63)	0.39	(0.09, 0.62)	58	13	0.37
Fat	0.83	(0.70, 0.91)	0.64	(0.41, 0.79)	53	8	0.37
Cholesterol	0.51	(0.23, 0.71)	0.39	(0.09, 0.62)	35	15	0.09
Alcohol	0.70	(0.50, 0.83)	0.79	(0.63, 0.88)	60	0	0.54
Vitamin D	0.39	(0.09, 0.62)	0.37	(0.06, 0.61)	48	13	0.26
Riboflavin	0.82	(0.68, 0.90)	0.69	(0.48, 0.82)	65	5	0.54
Iron	0.64	(0.41, 0.79)	0.54	(0.27, 0.73)	58	8	0.43
Calcium	0.78	(0.63, 0.88)	0.75	(0.57, 0.86)	70	5	0.60
Zinc	0.61	(0.37, 0.77)	0.57	(0.31, 0.75)	55	5	0.43

Table 7.25: Pearson r and Spearman r_s correlation coefficients, percentages of subjects classified into the same and opposite thirds of intake, and weighted kappa (κ_w). Results assess the validity of a food frequency questionnaire relative to a 4-d weighed record completed by 40 women. Pearson coefficients were calculated on $\log_e$-transformed, energy-adjusted nutrient intakes. Spearman coefficients were calculated on energy-adjusted nutrient intakes. Data abstracted from a larger table of nutrients in Masson et al., Public Health Nutrition 6: 313–321, 2003, with permission of the authors.

will be higher than that for a group with a more limited range of intakes and thus give a lower between-subject variation. Such an effect may be apparent when comparing the strength of correlations between the test and reference method for males versus females. Because males tend to eat more than females, their nutrient intakes tend to have a wider range than females, resulting in an apparently higher correlation between intakes for the test and reference methods. However, the higher correlation is spurious and provides no indication as to whether agreement between the test and reference method is better for the males or females.

In view of these limitations, relative validity of a dietary assessment method should not be described using Pearson correlation coefficients alone. Other measures of agreement between the test and reference methods must also be used. Table 7.25 compares three statistical methods for assessing the level of agreement of energy-adjusted nutrient intakes derived from a semiquantitative food frequency questionnaire (test method) and a 4-d weighed diet record (reference method) (Masson et al., 2003).

7.4.3 Other measures of correlation

Spearman rank correlation coefficients can be calculated for nonnormally distributed data,

although the same limitations apply as those itemized for the Pearson correlation coefficients. They can also be used when the primary objective of the validation study is to investigate how well the test method ranks the subjects, rather than to assess the level of agreement between the test and reference methods.

The intraclass correlation (r_I) can also be used and is a better measure of association for interval measurements than the Pearson coefficient r (Lee, 1980). The intraclass correlation takes into account the extent of the disagreement within pairs and the degree of correlation:

$$r_I = \frac{s_b^2 - s_w^2}{s_b^2 + s_w^2}$$

where s_b^2 is the variance of the sum of the pairs of observations, and s_w^2 is the variance of the differences between pairs. Values for r_I are normally less that those for r: values above 0.4 indicate good agreement (Nelson, 1997).

7.4.4 Regression analysis

Regression analysis can be viewed as an extension of correlation and is especially appropriate when validity is being assessed using biomarkers. In the simplest case, the aim of regression analysis is to find the best mathematical model for predicting the dependent variable (y) from the independent variable (x). In Figure 7.3 the linoleic acid content of the diet is treated mathematically as the dependent variable, on the basis that one is trying to predict, or validate, the reported dietary intake from the biochemical marker. Linear regression is the most common form of regression used, in which the mathematical model is a straight line, described as:

$$y = a + mx$$

where y is the dependent variable, x the independent variable, a the intercept value of y for $x = 0$, and m the slope of regression line. A t-test can be used to assess whether the slope of the regression line is statistically significantly different from zero and, hence, that the biomarker has some validity. An indication of how well the data fit the regression line can be obtained by calculating r^2, which varies between 0 and 1. The value of r^2, expressed as a percentage, gives the proportion of the variance in y, which is explained by the regression line. More complex multiple regression models can also be applied which take into consideration the effects of confounders (smoking, body mass index, total energy intake, etc).

7.4.5 Cross-classification

Often subjects are classified into categories, usually thirds (tertiles), fourths (quartiles), or fifths (quintiles), of intake by the test and reference method. The percentage of subjects correctly classified into the same category and grossly misclassified into the opposite category is calculated. This provides an indication of how well the dietary method, such as a food frequency questionnaire, separates the subjects into classes of intake and thus provides an estimate of the relative validity of the test method.

Cross-classification, however, has limitations. In particular, the percentage agreement will include agreement that occurs by chance. This limitation is best circumvented by using Cohen's weighted kappa statistic (κ_w) (Co-

hen, 1968). However, the magnitude of κ_w depends on the number of categories used and what weightings are applied, as well as the relative validity (or reproducibility); its use has been questioned by both Maclure and Willet (1987) and Bellach (1993). Finally, values for κ_w, like the correlation coefficient, also depend on the characteristics of the study population.

Table 7.25 compares the use of Pearson r and Spearman r_s correlation coefficients, percentages of subjects classified into the same and opposite thirds of intake, and weighted kappa (κ_w). These data emphasize how different measures of agreement do not necessarily yield the same relative result.

7.4.6 Mean and standard deviation of the difference

Bland and Altman (1986) discourage the use of correlation coefficients for comparing two measures, for the reasons outlined in Section 7.4.2. Instead, they advocate using the mean and standard deviation of the difference between the test and reference method for each nutrient. This approach does not make any assumption about whether the test or reference method is better.

To apply the Bland and Altman approach, first the results of the test method for the nutrient of interest should be plotted against those of the reference method, and the line of equality (but not a regression line) drawn. The plot will highlight any outliers in the data and indicate any bias in the test method. Bias will be apparent if the data for the nutrient of interest in the test method falls preferentially either above or below the line of equality, rather than being scattered along the line.

Next, a second plot should be drawn for each nutrient, depicting the mean of the test and reference intake for each subject plotted against the difference between each pair of observations. If there is no bias in the test method, the differences will cluster along the horizontal line, $y = 0$, and the mean difference should be close to zero. This second plot will also reveal whether the differences between the two methods become progressively larger

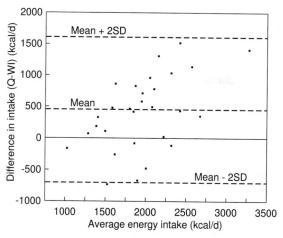

Figure 7.6: Bland and Altman plot of energy intake showing differences against mean of energy intake estimated by questionnaire and 7-d weighed inventory in 14 men and 15 women aged 50–70 y. Data from Nelson (1997).

or smaller with increasing intake. Bland and Altman (1986) recommend calculating the 95% confidence limits for the difference between the two methods. A judgment can then be made as to whether the agreement between the test and reference methods is acceptable.

An example of a Bland and Altman plot of energy intake is shown in Figure 7.6. This example shows a large variation in energy intake about the mean, indicating that in this case the food frequency questionnaire is likely to have generated large errors and should not be used to assess an individual's energy intake. In addition, there is a trend whereby increases in energy intake are associated with increasing differences between the measurements. These results emphasize that the two methods are not interchangeable in relation to assessing the energy intake of an individual.

7.4.7 Analysis of surrogate categories

To use analysis of surrogate categories, the individuals are assigned to a category (e.g., a quintile or quartile), according to the intake of a specific nutrient as estimated by the test method. Next, the mean intake in each quintile is calculated, using the nutrient intake for each subject as determined by the refer-

ence method. This gives an indication of the "true," or reference method nutrient intakes that are equivalent to the test method quintiles. One-way analysis of variance followed by Tukey's test can then be used to determine whether the mean intakes of the quintiles are statistically significantly different. If the test method is valid, the differences should be significantly different, and the means should change regularly from the top to the bottom category.

Because this method involves calculating the mean intakes for a group — each quintile or quartile — it does not require multiple replicate days of intake per individual to represent the "truth." Even a single day of intake will provide unbiased estimates of the actual values for these categories (Willett, 1998).

7.4.8 New approaches

New models have been developed to estimate the level of agreement between a test method and the truth. These include the method of triads (Ocké and Kaaks, 1997) and multivariate regression models. Readers are advised to consult a statistician before using these approaches.

7.5 Summary

Validity describes the degree to which a dietary method measures what it is intended to measure. Absolute validity is usually assessed in institutional settings by surreptitiously weighing or observing food items subsequently recalled by the subjects over the same time period. In general, the 24-h dietary recall tends to underestimate mean dietary intakes in the elderly, and in children when they are the respondents, but it may produce valid mean intakes for other population groups. For most other dietary methods, relative, rather than absolute, validity is assessed by evaluating the "test" dietary method against another reference dietary method, chosen for its accuracy, reproducibility, and ability to measure similar parameters over the same time frame. Furthermore, errors in the reference dietary method should be independent of both the true intake and any errors present in the test method.

The appropriate reference dietary method for validating a dietary history is the use of 1-d weighed food records, spaced evenly over the same time frame as the dietary history, the number of weighed record days depending on the nutrient of interest. Food records themselves have been validated, with limited success, by collecting intermittent duplicate diets. For food frequency questionnaires or repeated 24-h recalls, weighed food records should be used, their number and spacing depending on the nutrient of interest and the time frame involved. Prediction equations, based on 7-d weighed records, have been developed to validate food frequency questionnaires but have often not been successful.

The relative validity of dietary intake data can also assessed by using biomarkers, chosen because of their strong direct relationship with dietary intakes and their ability to provide an independent assessment of the dietary intake of the nutrient of interest. Examples of important biomarkers include the use of doubly labeled water as a marker of dietary energy intake, and the use of urinary nitrogen as a marker of dietary protein. Biomarkers for other dietary components include the measurement of sodium and potassium in 24-h urine samples to reflect intakes of sodium and potassium, respectively, and fatty acids in adipose tissue and various blood fractions. In general, only fatty acids that are absorbed and stored in adipose tissue without modification, and that are not synthesized endogenously are used. Examples include some specific n-3 and n-6 polyunsaturated fatty acids, *trans* unsaturated fatty acids, and pentadecanoic and heptadecanoic acid found in dairy products. Fatty acid levels in adipose tissue measure long-term fatty acid intakes whereas those in blood fractions reflect intakes that range over the past few days (e.g., plasma or platelets) to recent months (erythrocytes). In some cases, levels reflect intakes of certain foods (e.g., cold-water and marine fish, dairy fat). Use of biomarkers has highlighted the problem of underreporting that occurs with all

dietary assessment methods and among various population groups.

Statistical methods used to measure validity include paired *t*-tests and Wilcoxon's signed rank test for testing aggregate agreement. For quantifying agreement at the individual level, correlation and regression analysis and analysis of surrogate categories can be used. Bland and Altman advocate using the mean and standard deviation of the difference between the test and reference method for each nutrient instead of using correlation coefficients. Increasingly, energy-adjusted nutrient intakes are calculated prior to carrying out correlation analysis in validity studies in an attempt to adjust for underreporting.

References

Andersen LF, Solvoll K, Drevon CA. (1996). Very-long-chain n-3 fatty acids as biomarkers for intake of fish and n-3 fatty acids concentrates. American Journal of Clinical Nutrition 64: 305–311.

Arab L. (2003). Biomarkers of fat and fatty acid intake. Journal of Nutrition 133: 925S–932S.

Arab L, Akbar J. (2002). Biomarkers and the measurement of fatty acids. Public Health Nutrition 5: 865–871.

Bailey KD. (1978). Methods of Social Research. The Free Press, Collier Macmillan Publishers, London.

Baranowski T, Sprague D, Baranowski JH, Harrison JA. (1991). Accuracy of maternal dietary recall for preschool children. Journal of the American Dietetic Association 91: 669–674.

Basch CE, Shea S, Arliss R, Contento IR, Rips J, Gutin B, Irigoyen M, Zybert P. (1990). Validation of mothers' reports of dietary intake by four to seven year-old children. American Journal of Public Health 80: 1314–1317.

Bates CJ, Thurnham DI, Bingham SA, Margetts BM, Nelson M. (1997). Biochemical markers of nutrient intake. In: Margetts BM, Nelson M (eds.) Design Concepts in Nutritional Epidemiology. 2nd ed. Oxford University Press, New York, pp 170–240.

Bathalon GP, Tucker KL, Hays NP, Vinken AG, Greenberg AS, McCrory MA, Roberts SB. (2000). Psychological measures of eating behavior and the accuracy of three common dietary assessment methods in healthy postmenopausal women. American Journal of Clinical Nutrition 71: 739–745.

Baylin A, Kabagambe EK, Siles X, Campos H. (2002). Adipose tissue biomarkers of fatty acid intake. American Journal of Clinical Nutrition 76: 750–757.

Beaton GH, Burema J, Ritenbaugh C. (1997). Errors in the interpretation of dietary assessments. American Journal of Clinical Nutrition 65: 1100S–1107S.

Bellach B. (1993). Remarks on the use of Pearson's correlation coefficient and other association measures in assessing validity and reliability of dietary assessment methods. European Journal of Clinical Nutrition 47: S42–S45.

Beynen AC, Katan MB. (1985). Rapid sampling and long-term storage of subcutaneous adipose-tissue biopsies for determination of fatty acid composition. American Journal of Clinical Nutrition 42: 317–322.

Bingham SA. (2003). Urine nitrogen as a biomaker for the validation of dietary protein intake. Journal of Nutrition 133: 921S–924S.

Bingham S, Cummings JH. (1983). The use of 4-amino-benzoic acid as a marker to validate the completeness of 24-h urine collections in man. Clinical Science 64: 629–635.

Bingham SA, Cummings JH. (1985). Urine nitrogen as an independent validatory measure of dietary intake: a study of nitrogen balance in individuals consuming their normal diet. American Journal of Clinical Nutrition 42: 1276–1289.

Bingham SA, Day NE. (1997). Using biochemical markers to assess the validity of prospective dietary assessment methods and the effect of energy adjustment. American Journal of Clinical Nutrition 65: 1130S–1137S.

Bingham S, Wiggins HW, Englyst H, Seppanen R, Helms P, Strand R, Burton R, Jorgensen IM, Poulsen L, Paerrgaard A, Bjerrum L, James WPT. (1982). Methods and validity of the dietary assessments in four Scandinavian populations. Nutrition and Cancer 4: 23–33.

Bingham SA, Cassidy A, Cole TJ, Welch A, Runswick SA, Black AE, Thurnham D, Bates C, Khaw K, Key TJ, Day NE. (1995). Validation of weighed records and other methods of dietary assessment using the 24 h urine nitrogen technique and other biological markers. British Journal of Nutrition 73: 531–550.

Bingham SA, Gill C, Welch A, Cassidy A, Runswick SA, Oakes S, Lubin R, Thurnham DI, Key TJ, Roe L, Khaw KT, Day NE. (1997). Validation of dietary assessment methods in the UK arm of EPIC using weighed records, and 24-hour urinary nitrogen and potassium and serum vitamin C and carotenoids as biomarkers. International Journal of Epidemiology 26: S137–S151.

Black AE. (2000). The sensitivity and specificity of the Goldberg cut-off for EI:BMR for identifying diet reports of poor validity. European Journal of Clinical Nutrition 54: 395–404.

Black AE, Cole TJ. (2001). Biased over- or under-reporting is characteristic of individuals whether over time or by different assessment methods. Journal of the American Dietetic Association 101: 70–80.

Black AE, Prentice AM, Goldberg GR, Jebb SA, Bingham SA, Livingstone MBE, Coward WA. (1993). Measurements of total energy expenditure provide insights into the validity of dietary measurements of energy intake. Journal of the American Dietetic Association 93: 572–579.

Black AE, Bingham SA, Johansson G, Coward WA. (1997). Validation of dietary intakes of protein and energy against 24 hour urinary N and DLW energy expenditure in middle-aged women, retired men and post-obese subjects: comparisons with validation against presumed energy requirements. European Journal of Clinical Nutrition 51: 405–413.

Black AE, Welch AA, Bingham SA. (2000). Validation of dietary intakes measured by diet history against 24 h urinary nitrogen excretion and energy expenditure measured by the doubly-labeled water method in middle-aged women. British Journal of Nutrition 83: 341–354.

Blanck HM, Bowman BA, Cooper GR, Myers GL, Miller DT. (2003). Laboratory issues: uses of nutritional biomarkers. Journal of Nutrition 133: 888S–894S.

Bland JM, Altman DJ. (1986). Statistical methods for assessing agreement between two methods of clinical measurement. Lancet 1(8476): 307–310.

Block G. (1982). A review of validations of dietary assessment methods. American Journal of Epidemiology 115: 492–505.

Block G, Hartman AM. (1989). Issues in reproducibility and validity of dietary studies. American Journal of Clinical Nutrition 50: 1133–1138.

Block G, Woods M, Potosky A, Clifford C. (1990). Validation of a self-administered diet history questionnaire using multiple diet records. Journal of Clinical Epidemiology 43: 1327–1335.

Bohlscheid-Thomas S, Hoting I, Boeing H, Wahrendorf J. (1997). Reproducibility and relative validity of energy and macronutrient intake of a food frequency questionnaire developed for the German part of the EPIC project. International Journal of Epidemiology 26: S71–S81.

Braam LA, Ocké MC, Bueno-de-Mesquita HB, Seidell JC. (1998). Determinants of obesity-related underreporting of energy intake. American Journal of Epidemiology 147: 1081–1086.

Bray GA, Zachary B, Dahms WT, Atkinson RL, Oddie TH. (1978). Eating patterns of massively obese individuals. Journal of the American Dietetic Association 72: 24–27.

Briefel RR, Sempos CT, McDowell MA, Chien S, Alaimo K. (1997). Dietary methods research in the third National Health and Nutrition Examination Survey: underreporting of energy intake. American Journal of Clinical Nutrition 65S: 1203S–1209S.

Brown JE, Tharp TM, Dahlberg-Luby EM, Snowdon DA, Ostwald SK, Buzzard IM, Rysavy SM, Wieser SM. (1990). Videotape dietary assessment: validity, reliability, and comparison of results with 24-hour dietary recalls from elderly women in a retirement home. Journal of the American Dietetic Association 90: 1675–1679.

Burema J, van Staveren WA, Feunekes GIJ. (1995). Guidelines for reports on validation studies. European Journal of Clinical Nutrition 49: 932–933.

Byers TE, Rosenthal RI, Marshall JR, Rzepka TF, Cummings KM, Graham S. (1983). Dietary history from the distant past: a methodological study. Nutrition and Cancer 5: 69–77.

Caggiula AW, Wing RR, Nowalk MP, Milas NC, Lee S, Langford H. (1985). The measurement of sodium and potassium intake. American Journal of Clinical Nutrition 42: 391–398.

Calloway DH, Odell ACF, Margen S. (1971). Sweat and miscellaneous nitrogen losses in human balance studies. Journal of Nutrition 101: 775–786.

Cantwell MM. (2000). Assessment of individual fatty acid intake. Proceedings of the Nutrition Society 59: 187–191.

Carter RL, Sharbaugh CO, Stapell CA. (1981). Reliability and validity of the 24-hour recall. Journal of the American Dietetic Association 79: 542–547.

Cohen J. (1968). Weighted kappa, nominal scale agreement with provision for scaled disagreement or partial credit. Psychological Bulletin 70: 213–220.

Connor SL. (1996). Biomarkers and dietary intake data are mutually beneficial. American Journal of Clinical Nutrition 64: 379–380.

Crawford PB, Obarzanek E, Morrison J, Sabry ZI. (1994). Comparative advantage of 3-day food records over 24-hour recall and 5-day food frequency validated by observation of 9- and 10-year-old girls. Journal of the American Dietetic Association 94: 626–630.

Cummings JH, Stephen AM, Branch WJ. (1981). Implications of dietary fiber breakdown in the human colon. In: Bruce RW, Correa P, Lipkin P, Tannenbaum SR, Wilkins TC. (eds.) Gastrointestinal Cancer: Endogenous Factors. Banbury Report 7. Cold Spring Harbor Laboratory, Cold Spring Harbor, NY, pp. 71–81.

Day NE, McKeown N, Wong MY, Welch A, Bingham S. (2001). Epidemiological assessment of diet: a comparison of a 7-day diary with a food frequency questionnaire. International Journal of Epidemiology 30: 309–317.

Dayton S, Hashimoto S, Dixon W, Pearce ML. (1966). Composition of lipids in human serum and adipose tissue during prolonged feeding of a diet high in saturated fat. Journal of Lipid Research 7: 103–111.

Decker MD, Booth AL, Dewey MJ, Fricker RS, Hutcheson RH Jr, Schaffner W. (1986). Validity of food consumption histories in a foodborne outbreak investigation. American Journal of Epidemiology 124: 859–863.

de Roos NM, de Vries JHM, Katan MB. (2001). Serum lithium as a compliance marker for food and supplement intake. American Journal of Clinical Nutrition 73: 75–79.

de V Weir JB. (1949). New methods for calculating metabolic rate with special reference to protein metabolism. Journal of Physiology 109: 1–9.

Domel SB. (1997). Self-reports of diet: how children remember what they have eaten. American Journal of Clinical Nutrition 65: 1148S–1152S.

Dwyer JT, Coleman KA. (1997). Insights into dietary recall from a longitudinal study: accuracy over four decades. American Journal of Clinical Nutrition 65S: 1153S–1158S.

Dyer A, Elliott P, Chee D, Stamler J. (1997). Urinary biochemical markers of dietary intake in the INTERSALT Study. American Journal of Clinical Nutrition 65: 1246S–1253S.

Dyerberg J, Bang HO, Hjørne N. (1975). Fatty acid composition of the plasma lipids in Greenland Eskimos. American Journal of Clinical Nutrition 28: 958–966.

Elmståhl S, Riboli E, Lindgärde F, Gullberg B, Saracci R. (1996). The Malmö Food Study: the relative validity of a modified diet history method and an extensive food frequency questionnaire for measuring food intake. European Journal of Clinical Nutrition 50: 143–151.

Emmons L, Hayes M. (1973). Accuracy of 24-h recalls of young children. Journal of the American Dietetic Association 62: 409–415.

EPIC Group of Spain. (1997). Relative validity and reproducibility of a diet history questionnaire in Spain. III: Biochemical markers. International Journal of Epidemiology 26(Suppl.1): S110–S117.

FAO/WHO/UNU (Food and Agricultural Organization / World Health Organization / United Nations University). (1985). Energy and Protein Requirements. WHO Technical Report Series No. 724. World Health Organization, Geneva.

Ferguson EL, Gibson RS, Opare-Obisaw C. (1994). The relative validity of the repeated 24-h recall for estimating energy and selected nutrient intakes of rural Ghanian children. European Journal of Clinical Nutrition 48: 241–252.

Ferrari P, Slimani N, Ciampi A, Trichopoulou A, Naska A, Lauria C, Veglia F, Bueno-de-Mesquita HB, Ocké MC, Brustad M, Braaten T, Jose Tormo M, Amiano P, Mattisson I, Johansson G, Welch A, Davey G, Overvad K, Tjonneland A, Clavel-Chapelon F, Thiebaut A, Linseisen J, Boeing H, Hemon B, Riboli E. (2002). Evaluation of under- and overreporting of energy intake in the 24-hour diet recalls in the European Prospective Investigation into Cancer and Nutrition (EPIC). Public Health Nutrition 5: 1329–1345.

Feunekes GIJ, van Staveren WA, De Vries JHM, Burema J, Hautvast JGAJ. (1993). Relative and biomarker-based validity of a food-frequency questionnaire estimating intake of fats and cholesterol. American Journal of Clinical Nutrition 58: 489–496.

Field AE, Peterson KE, Gortmaker SL, Cheung L, Rockett H, Fox MK, Colditz GA. (1999). Reproducibility and validity of a food frequency questionnaire among fourth to seventh grade inner-city school children: implications of age and day-to-day variation in dietary intake. Public Health Nutrition 2: 293–300.

Friedenreich CM, Slimani N, Riboli E. (1992). Measurement of past diet: a review of previous and proposed methods. Epidemiological Review 14: 177–196.

Garland M, Sacks FM, Colditz GA, Rimm EB, Sampson LA, Willett WC, Hunter DJ. (1998). The relation between dietary intake and adipose tissue composition of selected fatty acids in US women. American Journal of Clinical Nutrition 67: 25–30.

Gersovitz M, Madden JP, Smiciklas-Wright H. (1978). Validity of the 24-h dietary recall and seven-day record for group comparisons. Journal of the American Dietetic Association 73: 48–55.

Gibson RS, Scythes CA. (1982). Trace element intakes of women. British Journal of Nutrition 48: 241–248.

Godley PA, Campbell MK, Miller C, Gallagher P, Martinson FE, Moher JL, Sandler RS. (1996). Correlation between biomarkers of omega-3 fatty acid consumption and questionnaire data in African American and Caucasian United States males with and without prostatic carcinoma. Cancer Epidemiology, Biomarkers & Prevention 5: 115–119.

Goldberg GR, Black AE, Jebb SA, Cole TJ, Murgatoroyd PR, Coward WA, Prentice AM. (1991). Critical evaluation of energy intake data using fundamental principles of energy physiology. 1: Derivation of cut-off limits to identify under-recording. European Journal of Clinical Nutrition 45: 569–581.

Greger JL, Etnyre GM. (1978). Validity of 24-hour dietary recalls by adolescent females. American Journal of Public Health 68: 70–72.

Haile RW, Hunt IF, Buckley J, Browdy BL, Murphy NJ, Alpers D. (1986). Identifying a limited number of foods important in supplying selected dietary nutrients. Journal of the American Dietetic Association 86: 611–616.

Hankin JH, Messinger HB, Stallones RA. (1970). A short dietary method for epidemiological studies. IV: Evaluation of questionnaire. American Journal of Epidemiology 91: 562–567.

Haraldsdóttir J, Sandström B. (1994). Detection of underestimated energy intake in young adults. International Journal of Epidemiology 23: 577–582.

Hartman AM, Brown CC, Palmgren J, Pietinen P, Verkasalo M, Myer D, Virtamo J. (1990). Variability in nutrient and food intakes among older middle-aged men. Implications for design of epidemiologic and validation studies using food recording. American Journal of Epidemiology 132: 999–1012.

Heath A-LM, Skeaff CM, Gibson RS. (2000). The relative validity of a computerized food frequency questionnaire for estimating intake of dietary iron and its absorption modifiers. European Journal of Clinical Nutrition 54: 592–599.

Hebert JR, Miller DR. (1988). Methodologic considerations for investigating the diet–cancer link. American Journal of Clinical Nutrition 47: 1068–1077.

Hebert JR, Clemow L, Pbert L, Ockene IS, Ockene JK. (1995). Social desirability bias in dietary self-report may compromise the validity of dietary intake measures. International Journal of Epidemiology 24: 389–398.

Hill RJ, Davies PSW. (2001). The validity of self-reported energy intake as determined using the doubly labelled water technique. British Journal of Nutrition 85: 415–430.

Hjartaker J, Lund E, Bjerve KS. (1997). Serum phospholipid fatty acid composition and habitual intake of marine foods registered by a semi-quantitative food frequency questionnaire. European Journal of Clinical Nutrition 51: 736–742.

Holbrook JT, Patterson KY, Bodner JE, Douglas LW, Veillon C, Kelsay JL, Mertz W, Smith JC. (1984). Sodium and potassium intake and balance in adults consuming self-selected diets. American Journal of Clinical Nutrition 40: 786–793.

Holick CN, Michaud DS, Stolzenberg-Solomon R, Mayne ST, Pietinen P, Taylor PR, Virtamo J, Albanes D. (2002). Dietary carotenoids, serum β-carotene, and retinol and risk of lung cancer in the α-tocopherol, β-carotene cohort study. American Journal of Epidemiology 156: 536–547.

Horvitz MA, Schoeller DA. (2001). Natural abundance deuterium and 18-oxygen effects on the precision of the doubly labeled water method. American Journal of Physiology, Endocrinology and Metabolism 280: E965–E972.

Hunter DJ, Rimm EB, Sacks FM, Stampfer MJ, Colditz GA, Litin LB, Willett WC. (1992). Comparison of measures of fatty acid intake by subcutaneous fat aspirate, food frequency questionnaire, and diet records in a free-living population of US men. American Journal of Epidemiology 135: 418–427.

Iannotti RJ, Zuckerman AE, Blyer EM, O'Brien RW, Finn J, Spillman DM. (1994). Comparison of dietary intake methods with young children. Psychology Reports 74: 883–889.

IOM (Institute of Medicine). (2001). Dietary Reference Intakes for Vitamin A, Vitamin K, Arsenic, Boron, Chromium, Copper, Iodine, Iron, Manganese, Molybdenum, Nickel, Silicon, Vanadium, and Zinc. National Academy Press, Washington, DC.

Isaksson B. (1980). Urinary nitrogen output as a validity test in dietary surveys. American Journal of Clinical Nutrition 33: 4–5.

Jain MG, Howe GR, Johnson KC, Miller AB. (1980). Evaluation of a diet history questionnaire for epidemiologic studies. American Journal of Epidemiology 111: 212–219.

Jain MG, Harrison L, Howe GR, Miller AB. (1982). Evaluation of a self-administered dietary questionnaire for use in a cohort study. American Journal of Clinical Nutrition 36: 931–935.

Jain MG, Howe GR, Rohan T. (1996). Dietary assessment in epidemiology: comparison of a food frequency and a diet history questionnaire with a 7-day food record. American Journal of Epidemiology 143: 953–960.

Johnson RK, Goran MI, Poehlman ET. (1994). Correlates of over- and underreporting of energy intake in healthy older men and women. American Journal of Clinical Nutrition 59: 1286–1290.

Johnson RK, Driscoll P, Goran MI. (1996). Comparison of multiple-pass 24-h recall estimates of energy intake with total energy expenditure determined by the doubly labeled water method in young children. Journal of the American Dietetic Association 96: 1140–1144.

Jones PJ. Martin LJ, Su W, Boyd NF. (1997). Canadian recommended nutrient intakes underestimate true energy requirements in middle-aged women. Canadian Journal of Public Health 88: 314–319.

Kaaks R, Riboli E. (1997). Validation and calibration of dietary intake measurements in the EPIC project: methodological considerations. International Journal of Epidemiology 26: S15–S25.

Kaaks R, Riboli E, Sinha R (1997). Biochemical Markers of Dietary Intake. In: Toniolo P, Bofetta P, Shuker D, Rothman N, Bulka B, Pearce N (eds.) Application of Biomarkers in Cancer Epidemiology. Scientific Publication No. 142, International Association for Research on Cancer, Lyon, pp. 103–126.

Kark JD, Kaufmann NA, Binka F, Goldberger N, Berry EM. (2003). Adipose tissue n-6 fatty acids and acute myocardial infarction in a population consuming a diet high in polyunsaturated fatty acids. American Journal of Clinical Nutrition 77: 796–802.

Katan MB, van Birgelen A, Deslypere JP, Penders M, van Staveren WA. (1991). Biological markers of dietary intake, with emphasis on fatty acids. Annals of Nutrition and Metabolism 35: 249–252.

Kim WW, Mertz W, Judd JT, Marshall MW, Kelsay JL, Prather ES. (1984). Effect of making duplicate food collections on nutrient intakes calculated from diet records. American Journal of Clinical Nutrition 40: 1333–1337.

Kipnis V, Midthune D, Freedman LS, Bingham S, Schatzkin A, Subar A, Carroll RJ. (2001). Empirical evidence of correlated biases in dietary assessment instruments and its implications. American Journal of Epidemiology 153: 394–403.

Kipnis V, Midthune D, Freedman L, Bingham S, Day NE, Riboli E, Ferrari P, Carroll RJ. (2002). Part E: new statistical approaches to dealing with bias associated with dietary data. Bias in dietary-report instruments and its implications for nutritional epidemiology. Public Health Nutrition 5: 915–923.

Kobayashi M, Sasaki S, Kawabata T, Hasegawa K, Akabane M, Tsugane S. (2001). Single measurement of serum phospholipid fatty acid as a biomarker of specific fatty acid intake in middle-aged Japanese men. European Journal of Clinical Nutrition 55: 643–650.

Kohlmeier L, Kohlmeier M. (1995). Adipose tissue as a medium for epidemiologic exposure assessment. Environmental Health Perspectives 103(Suppl 3): 99–106.

Kolonel LN, Hirohata T, Nomura AMY. (1977). Adequacy of survey data collected from substitute respondents. American Journal of Epidemiology 106: 476–484.

Krall EA, Dwyer JT. (1987). Validity of a food frequency questionnaire and a food diary in a short-term recall situation. Journal of the American Dietetic Association 87: 1374–1377.

Krantzler NJ, Mullen BJ, Schutz HG, Grivetti LE, Holden CA, Meiselman HL. (1982). Validity of

telephoned diet recalls and records for assessment of individual food intake. American Journal of Clinical Nutrition 36: 1234–1242.

Kretsch MJ, Fong AKH, Green MW. (1999). Behavioral and body size correlates of energy intake underreporting by obese and normal-weight women. Journal of the American Dietetic Association 99: 300–306.

Kristal AR, Shattuck AL, Henry HJ, Fowley AS.(1990). Rapid assessment of dietary intake of fat, fiber and saturated fat: validity of an instrument suitable for community intervention research and nutritional surveillance. American Journal of Health Promotion 4: 288–295.

Kristal AR, Feng Z, Coates RJ, Oberman A, George V. (1997). Associations of race/ethnicity, education, and dietary intervention with the validity and reliability of a food frequency questionnaire: the Women's Health Trial Feasibility Study in minority populations. American Journal of Epidemiology 146: 856–869. Erratum in American Journal of Epidemiology 148: 820.

Kroke A, Klipstein-Grobusch K, Voss S, Möseneder J, Thielecke F, Noack R, Boeing H. (1999). Validation of a self-administered food-frequency questionnaire administered in the European prospective Investigation into Cancer and Nutrition (EPIC) Study: comparison of energy, protein, and macronutrient intakes estimated with the doubly labeled water, urinary nitrogen, and repeated 24-h dietary recall methods. American Journal of Clinical Nutrition 70: 439–447

Lafay L, Basdevant A, Charles MA, Vray M, Balkau B, Borys JM, Eschwege E, Romon M. (1997). Determinants and nature of dietary underreporting in a free-living population: the Fleurbaix Laventie Ville Sante (FLVS) Study. International Journal of Obesity and Related Metabolic Disorders 21: 567–573.

Lee J. (1980). Alternate approaches for quantifying aggregate and individual agreements between two methods for assessing dietary intakes. American Journal of Clinical Nutrition 33: 956–964.

Lemaitre RN, King IB, Patterson RE, Psaty BM, Kestin M, Heckbert SR. (1998). Assessment of *trans*-fatty acid intake with a food frequency questionnaire and validation with adipose tissue levels of *trans*-fatty acids. American Journal of Epidemiology 148: 1085–1093.

Linusson EEI, Sanjur D, Erickson EC. (1974). Validating the 24-hour recall as a dietary survey test. Archivos Latinoamericanos de Nutrición 24: 277–294.

Liu K, Slattery M, Jacobs DJ, Cutter G, McDonald A, Van Horn L, Hilner JE, Caan B, Bragg C, Dyer A. (1994). A study of the reliability and comparative validity of the Cardia Dietary History. Ethnicity and Disease 4: 15–27.

Livingstone MBE, Black AE. (2003). Markers of the validity of reported energy intake. Journal of Nutrition 133: 895S–920S.

Livingstone MBE, Prentice AM, Coward WA, Strain JJ,

Black AE, Davies PSW, Stewart CM, McKenna PG, Whitehead RG. (1992). Validation of estimates of energy intake by weighed dietary record and diet history in children and adolescents. American Journal of Clinical Nutrition 56: 29–35.

London SJ, Sacks FM, Caesar J, Stampfer MJ, Siguel E, Willett WC. (1991). Fatty acid composition of subcutaneous adipose tissue and diet in postmenopausal US women. American Journal of Clinical Nutrition 54: 340–345.

Macdiarmid JI, Blundell JE. (1997). Dietary under-reporting: what people say about recording their food intake. (1997). European Journal of Clinical Nutrition 51:199–200.

Maclure M, Willett WC. (1987). Misinterpretation and misuse of the kappa statistic. American Journal of Epidemiology 126: 161–169.

Madden JP, Goodman SJ, Guthrie HA. (1976). Validity of the 24-h recall: analysis of data obtained from elderly subjects. Journal of the American Dietetic Association 68: 143–147.

Mahalko JR, Johnson LK, Gallagher SK, Milne DB. (1985). Comparison of dietary histories and seven-day food records in a nutritional assessment of older adults. American Journal of Clinical Nutrition 42: 542–553.

Marckmann P, Lassen A, Haraldsdóttir J, Sandström B. (1995). Biomarkers of habitual fish intake in adipose issue. American Journal of Clinical Nutrition 62: 956–959.

Margetts BM, Thompson RL. (1995). Validation of dietary intake estimation. European Journal of Clinical Nutrition 49: 934.

Marshall J, Priore R, Haughey B, Rzepka T, Graham S. (1980). Spouse-subject interviews and the reliability of diet studies. American Journal of Epidemiology 112: 675–683.

Martin LJ, Su W, Jones PJ, Lockwood GA, Tritchler D, Boyd NF. (1996). Comparison of energy intakes determined by food records and doubly labeled water in women participating in a dietary-intervention trial. American Journal of Clinical Nutrition 63: 483–490.

Masson LF, McNeill G. Tomany JO, Simpson JA, Peace HS, Wei L, Grubb DA, Bolton-Smith C. (2003). Statistical approaches for assessing the relative validity of a food-frequency questionnaire: use of correlation coefficients and the kappa statistic. Public Health Nutrition 6: 313–321.

Mayer-Davis EJ, Vitolins MZ, Carmichael SL, Hemphill S, Tsaroucha G, Rushing J, Levin S. (1999). Validity and reproducibility of a food frequency interview in a Multi-Cultural Epidemiology Study. Annals of Epidemiology 9: 314–324.

McCrory MA, Hajduk CL, Roberts SB. (2002). Procedures for screening out inaccurate reports of dietary energy intake. Public Health Nutrition 5: 873–882.

McKeown NM, Day NE, Welch AA, Runswick SA, Luben RN, Mulligan AA, McTaggart A, Bingham SA. (2001). Use of biological markers to validate self-reported dietary intake in a random sample of the European Prospective Investigation into Cancer United Kingdom Norfolk cohort. American Journal of Clinical Nutrition 74: 188–196.

McPherson RS, Kohl HW 3rd, Garcia G, Nichaman MZ, Hanis CL. (1995). Food-frequency questionnaire validation among Mexican-Americans: Starr County, Texas. Annals of Epidemiology 5: 378–385.

Mullen BJ, Krantzler NJ, Grivetti LE, Schutz HG, Meiselman HL. (1984). Validity of a food frequency questionnaire for the determination of individual food intake. American Journal of Clinical Nutrition 39: 136–143.

Nelson M. (1997). The validation of dietary assessment. In: Margetts BM, Nelson M (eds.) Design Concepts in Nutritional Epidemiology, 2nd ed. Oxford University Press, New York, pp. 241–272.

Nelson M, Atkinson M, Daryshire S. (1994). Food photography. I: The perception of portion size from photographs. British Journal of Nutrition 72: 649–663.

Nes M, van Staveren WA, Zajkas G, Inelmen EM, Moreiras-Varela O. (1991). Validity of the dietary history method in elderly subjects. European Journal of Clinical Nutrition 45(Supp. 3): 97–104.

Nightingale ZD, Blumberg JB, Handelman GJ. (1999). Purification of fatty acid methyl esters by high-performance liquid chromatography. Journal of Chromatography B: Biomedical Sciences and Applications. 732: 495–500.

Novotny JA, Rumpler WV, Judd JT, Riddick PH, Rhodes D, McDowell M, Briefel R. (2001). Diet interviews of subject pairs: how different persons recall eating the same foods. Journal of the American Dietetic Association 101: 1189–1193.

Ocké MC, Kaaks RJ. (1997). Biomarkers as additional measurements in dietary validity studies: application of the method of triads with examples from the European Prospective investigation into cancer and nutrition. American Journal of Clinical Nutrition 65S: 1240S–1245S.

Ocké MC, Bueno-de-Mesquita HB, Pols MA, Smit HA, van Staveren WA, Kromhout D. (1997). The Dutch EPIC food frequency questionnaire. II: Relative validity and reproducibility for nutrients. International Journal of Epidemiology 26: S49–S58.

Pedersen JI, Ringstad J, Almendingen K, Haugen TS, Stensvold I, Thelle DS. (2000). Adipose tissue fatty acids and risk of myocardial infarction: a case-control study. European Journal of Clinical Nutrition 54: 618–625.

Peng YM, Peng YS, Lin Y, Moon T, Roe DJ, Ritenbaugh C. (1995). Concentrations and plasma-tissue-diet relationships of carotenoids, retinoids, and tocopherols in humans. Nutrition and Cancer 23: 233–246.

Peters JC, Holcombe BN, Hiller LK, Webb DR. (1991). Caprenin 3: absorption and caloric value in adult humans. Journal of the American College of Toxicology 10: 357–367.

Petersen PH, Ricos C, Stockl D, Libeer JC, Baadenhuijsen H, Fraser C, Thienpont L. (1996). Proposed guidelines for the internal quality control of analytical results in the medical laboratory. European Journal of Clinical Chemistry and Clinical Biochemistry 34: 983–999.

Poppitt SD, Swann D, Black AE, Prentice AM. (1998). Assessment of selective under-reporting of food intake by both obese and nonobese women in a metabolic facility. International Journal of Obesity and Related Metabolic Disorders 22: 303–311.

Porrini M, Gentile MG, Fidanza F. (1995). Biochemical validation of a self administered FFQ. British Journal of Nutrition 74: 323–333.

Prentice AM (ed.). (1990). The Doubly-Labelled Water Method for Measuring Energy Expenditure: A Consensus Report by the IDECG Working Group, NAHRES-4. International Atomic Energy Agency, Vienna, Austria.

Price GM, Paul AA, Cole TJ, Wadsworth MEJ. (1997). Characteristics of the low-energy reporters in a longitudinal national dietary survey. British Journal of Nutrition 77: 833–851.

Pryer JA, Vrijheid M, Nichols R, Kiggins M, Elliot P. (1997). Who are the "low energy reporters" in the dietary and nutritional survey of British adults? International Journal of Epidemiology 26: 146–154.

Räsänen L. (1979). Nutrition survey of Finnish rural children. VI: Methodological study comparing the 24-hour recall and the dietary history interview. American Journal of Clinical Nutrition 32: 2560–2567.

Riboli E, Toniolo P, Kaaks R, Shore RE, Casagrande C, Pasternack BS. (1997). Reproducibility of a food frequency questionnaire used in the New York University Women's Health Study: effect of self-selection by study subjects. European Journal of Clinical Nutrition 51: 437–442.

Rohan TE, Potter JD. (1984). Retrospective assessment of dietary intake. American Journal of Epidemiology 107: 876–887.

Rosner B, Willett WC. (1988). Interval estimates for correlation coefficients corrected for within-person variation. Implications for study design and hypothesis testing. American Journal of Epidemiology 127: 377–386.

Rothenberg E, Bosaeus I, Lernfelt B, Landahl S, Steen B. (1998). Energy intake and expenditure: validation of a diet history by heart rate monitoring, activity diary and doubly labeled water. European Journal of Clinical Nutrition 52: 832–838.

Russell-Briefel R, Caggiula AW, Kuller LH. (1985). A comparison of three dietary methods for estimating vitamin A intake. American Journal of Epidemiology 122: 628–636.

Rutishauser IHE, Wheeler CE, Conn JA, O'Dea K. (1994). Food and nutrient intake in a randomly selected sample of adults: demographic and temporal influences on energy and nutrient intake. Australian Journal of Nutrition and Dietetics 51: 157–166.

Sanchez-Castillo CP, Branch WJ, James WP. (1987). A test of the validity of the lithium-marker technique for monitoring dietary sources of salt in man. Clinical Science 72: 87–94.

Sawaya AL, Tucker K, Tsay R, Willett W, Saltzman E, Dallal GE, Roberts SB. (1996). Evaluation of four methods for determining energy intake in young and older women: comparison with doubly labeled water measurements of total energy expenditure. American Journal of Clinical Nutrition 63: 491–499.

Schaefer EJ, Augustin JL, Schaefer MM, Rasmussen H, Ordovas JM, Dallal GE, Dwyer JT. (2000). Lack of efficacy of a food-frequency questionnaire in assessing dietary micronutient intakes in subjects consuming diets of known composition. American Journal of Clinical Nutrition 71: 746–751.

Schoeller DA. (2002). Validation of habitual energy intake. Public Health Nutrition 5: 883–888.

Schofield WN. (1985). Predicting basal metabolic rate: new standards and review of previous work. Human Nutrition Clinical Nutrition 39C(Suppl. 1): 5–41.

Scott KJ, Thurnham DI, Hart DJ, Bingham SA, Day K. (1996). The correlation between the intake of lutein, lycopene and beta-carotene from vegetables and fruits and blood plasma concentrations in a group of women aged 50–65 years in the UK. British Journal of Nutrition 75: 409–418.

Seale JL, Rumpler WV. (1997). Comparison of energy expenditure measurements by diet records, energy intake balance, doubly labeled water and room calorimetry. European Journal of Clinical Nutrition 51: 856–863.

Simpson FO, Paulin JM, Phelan EL. (1983). Repeated 24-hour urinary electrolyte estimations in the community. New Zealand Medical Journal 96: 910–911.

Slimani N, Ferrari P, Ocké M, Welch A, Boeing H, van Liere M, Pala V, Amiano P, Lagiou A, Mattisson I, Stripp C, Engeset D, Charrondière R, Buzzard M, van Staveren W, Riboli E. (2000). Standardization of the 24-hour diet recall calibration method used in the European prospective investigation into Cancer and Nutrition (EPIC): general concepts and preliminary results. European Journal of Clinical Nutrition 54: 900–917.

Slimani N, Bingham S, Runswick S, Ferrari P, Day NE, Welch AA, Key TJ, Miller AB, Boeing H, Sieri S, Veglia F, Palli D, Panico S, Tumino R, Bueno-De-Mesquita B, Ocké MC, Clavel-Chapelon F, Trichopoulou A, van Staveren WA, Riboli E. (2003). Group level validation of protein intakes estimated by 24-hour diet recall and dietary questionnaires against 24-hour urinary nitrogen in the European Prospective Investigation into Cancer and Nutrition (EPIC) calibration study. Cancer Epidemiology Biomarkers & Prevention. 12: 784–795.

Smedman AEM, Gustafsson IB, Berglund LGTM, Vessby BOH. (1999). Pentadecanoic acid in serum as a marker for intake of milk fat: relations between intake of milk fat and metabolic risk factors. American Journal of Clinical Nutrition 69: 22–29.

Smith WCS, Crombie IK, Irving JM, Kenicer MB,

Tunstall-Pedoe H, Tavendale R. (1985). The Scottish Heart Health Study. European Heart Journal 6(Suppl.1): 105.

Snedecor GW, Cochran WG. (1989). Statistical Methods. 8th ed. Iowa State University Press, Ames.

Stallone DD, Brunner EJ, Bingham SA, Marmot MG. (1997). Dietary assessment in Whitehall II: the influence of reporting bias on apparent socioeconomic variation in nutrient intakes. European Journal of Clinical Nutrition 51: 815–825.

Stockley L. (1985). Changes in habitual food intake during weighed inventory surveys and duplicate diet collections: a short review. Ecology of Food and Nutrition 17: 263–269.

Stunkard AJ, Messick S. (1985). The three-factor eating questionnaire to measure dietary restraint, disinhibition and hunger. Journal of Psychosomatic Research: 29: 71–83.

Taren DL, Tobar M, Hill A, Howell W, Shisslak C, Bell I, Ritenbaugh C. (1999). The association of energy intake bias with psychological scores of women. European Journal of Clinical Nutrition 53: 570–578.

Thomson CD, Woodruffe S, Colls A, Joseph J, Doyle T. (2001). Urinary iodine and thyroid status of New Zealand residents. European Journal of Clinical Nutrition 55: 387–392.

Thompson FE, Moler JE, Freedman LS, Clifford CK, Stables GJ, Willett WC. (1997). Register of dietary assessment calibration-validation studies: a status report. American Journal of Clinical Nutrition 65: 1142S–1147S.

Tjønneland A, Overvad K, Thorling E, Ewertz M. (1993). Adipose tissue fatty acids as biomarkers of dietary exposure in Danish men and women. American Journal of Clinical Nutrition 57: 629–633.

Tomoyasu NJ, Toth MJ, Poehlman ET. (1999). Misreporting of total energy intake in older men and women. Journal of the American Geriatrics Society 47: 710–715.

Toniolo P, Boffetta P, Shuker DEG, Rothman N, Hulka B, Pearce N (eds.) (1997). Application of Biomarkers in Cancer Epidemiology. IARC Scientific Publications No. 142. International Agency for Research on Cancer, Lyon.

van de Vijver LP, Kardinaal AF, Couet C, Aro A, Kafatos A, Steingrimsdottir L, Amorim Cruz JA, Moreiras O, Becker W, van Amelsvoort JM, Vidal-Jessel S, Salmanin I, Moschandreas J, Sigfusson N, Martins I, Carbajal A, Ytterfors A, Poppel G. (2000) Association between *trans* fatty acid intake and cardiovascular risk factors in Europe: the TRANSFAIR study. European Journal of Clinical Nutrition 54: 126–135.

van Kappel AL, Steghens J-P, Zeleniuch-Jacquotte A, Chajès V, Toniolo P, Riboli E. (2001). Serum carotenoids as biomarkers of fruit and vegetable consumption in the New York Women's Health Study. Public Health Nutrition 4: 829–835.

van Liere M, Lucas F, Clavel F, Slimani N, Villeminot S. (1997). Relative validity and reproducibility of a French dietary history questionnaire. International Journal of Epidemiology 26(Suppl. 1): S128–S136.

van Staveren WA, de Boer JO, Burema J. (1985). Validity and reproducibility of a dietary history method estimating the usual food intake during one month. American Journal of Clinical Nutrition 42: 554–559.

van Staveren WA, Deurenberg P, Katan MB, Burema J, de Groot LCPGM, Hoffmans MDAF. (1986a). Validity of the fatty acid composition of subcutaneous fat tissue microbiopsies as an estimate of the long-term average fatty acid composition of the diet of separate individuals. American Journal of Epidemiology 123: 455–463.

van Staveren WA, West CE, Hoffmans MDAF, Bos P, Kardinaal AFM, van Poppel GAFC, Schipper HJ-A, Hautvast JGAJ, Hayes RB. (1986b). Comparison of contemporaneous and retrospective estimates of food consumption made by a dietary history method. American Journal of Epidemiology 123: 884–893.

Velthuis-te Wierik EJ, Westerterp KR, van den Berg H. (1995). Impact of a moderately energy-restricted diet on energy metabolism and body composition in nonobese men. International Journal of Obesity and Related Metabolic Disorders 19: 318–324.

Wakai E, Egami I, Kato K, Lin Y, Kawamura T, Tamakoshi A, Aoki R, Kojima M, Nakayama T, Wada M, Ohno Y. (1999). A simple food frequency questionnaire for Japanese diet. Part I: Development of the questionnaire, and reproducibility and validity for food groups. Journal of Epidemiology 9: 216–226.

Warren JM, Henry CJ, Livingstone MBE, Lightowler HL, Bradshaw SM, Perwaiz S. (2003). How well do children aged 5–7 years recall food eaten at school lunch? Public Health Nutrition 6: 41–47.

Webb DR, Peters JC, Jandacek RJ, Fortier NE. (1991). Caprenin 2: short-term safety and metabolism in rats and hamsters. Journal of the American College of Toxicology 10: 341–356.

Weinburg RB, Dantzker C, Patton CS. (1990). Sensitivity of serum apolipoprotein A-IV levels to change in dietary fat content. Gastroenterology 98: 17–24.

Wild CP, Andersson C, O'Brien N, Wilson L, Woods J. (2001). A critical evaluation of the application of biomarkers in epidemiological studies on diet and health. British Journal of Nutrition 86: S37–S53.

Willett WC. (1998). Nutritional Epidemiology. 2nd ed. Oxford University Press, New York.

Willett WC, Sampson L, Stampfer MJ, Rosner B, Bain C, Witschi J, Hennekens CH, Speizer FE. (1985). Reproducibility and validity of a semiquantitative food frequency questionnaire. American Journal of Epidemiology 122: 51–65.

Wolk A, Vessby B, Ljung H, Barrefors P. (1998). Evaluation of a biological marker of daily fat intake. American Journal of Clinical Nutrition 68: 291–295.

Wolk A, Furuheim M, Vessby B. (2001). Fatty acid composition of adipose tissue and serum lipids are valid biological markers of dairy fat intake in men. Journal of Nutrition 131: 828–833.

Wu Z, Palmquist L. (1991). Synthesis and biohydrogenation of fatty acids by ruminal microorganisms in vitro. Journal of Dairy Science 74: 3035–3046.

Yong L-C, Forman MR, Beecher GR, Graubard BI, Campbell WS, Reichman ME, Taylor PR, Lanza E, Holden JM, Judd JT. (1994). Relationship between dietary intake and plasma concentrations of carotenoids in premenopausal women: application of the USDA-NCI carotenoid food-composition data-base.

American Journal of Clinical Nutrition 60: 223–230.

Young CM, Hagan GC, Tucker RE, Foster WD. (1952). A comparison of dietary study methods. II: Dietary history vs. seven-day records vs. 24-hour recall. Journal of the American Dietetic Association 28: 218–221.

Zhang J, Temme EHM, Sasaki S, Kesteloot H. (2000). Under- and overreporting of energy intake using urinary cations as biomarkers: relation to body mass index. American Journal of Epidemiology 152: 453–462.

8

Evaluation of nutrient intakes and diets

Dietary intake data resulting from nutritional assessment systems have been severely criticized in the past because both random and systematic errors occur in measuring intakes of food and calculating their nutrient content. The data are also frequently misinterpreted. This is particularly unfortunate because the careful evaluation of food- and nutrient-intake data has important applications, provided that the limitations of the methods are clearly understood.

This chapter describes two ways for evaluating the adequacy of diets — quantitative and qualitative — that can be used at both the individual and the population levels. The target audience for the quantitative method is the nutrition professional. In the quantitative approach, nutrient adequacy is based on comparison of nutrient intakes per day with tables of nutrient reference levels. In some countries, tables of nutrient reference levels have been expanded to include "non-nutritive" components such as dietary fiber, carotenoids, and lycopene, and not just essential nutrients. In addition, the revised tables often focus on optimizing health and reducing the risk of chronic disease, and not only on the prevention of nutritional deficiencies. In some cases, tolerable upper-intake levels have been defined to help people avoid harm from ingesting too much of a nutrient.

More reliable methods have also been developed to assess the risk of inadequate or excessive intakes of nutrients for individuals and population groups. As a result, the more vulnerable individuals and subgroups

in the population can now be more accurately identified and targeted during intervention programs.

In contrast, the qualitative approach is based on foods rather than nutrients and provides guidelines for healthy food choices. These food-based dietary guidelines focus on diet-related public health issues specific to a country and address the consumer, either directly or indirectly, through educators, health professionals, and policy-makers. Food-based guidelines are being used increasingly in both developed and low-income countries.

None of the evaluation methods described in this chapter provides information on the nutritional status of individuals or population groups. Such information can only be obtained when dietary intake data are combined with biochemical, anthropometric, and clinical indices.

8.1 Nutrient reference levels

The first set of nutrient reference levels was produced by the Technical Commission on Nutrition (League of Nations, 1938). These reference levels formed the basis for the first Canadian Dietary Standard compiled by the Canadian Council on Nutrition (1940). The U.S. Food and Nutrition Board prepared the first U.S. Recommended Dietary Allowances (RDAs) in 1941 (Food and Nutrition Board, 1943). Later, tables of nutrient reference levels were developed by WHO/FAO and a number of individual countries.

8.1.1 Underlying principles

Many of the underlying principles used by the expert committees developing nutrient reference levels are similar. These are that reference levels

- Are always set for a particular group of individuals with specified characteristics, consuming a specified diet
- Refer to the average daily need over a reasonable period of time, although the latter has seldom been defined; hence, the suggested amounts do not have to be consumed every day, but omissions or short-falls must be balanced by increased intake on other occasions
- Refer to levels of intake needed to maintain health in already healthy individuals; they do not allow for illnesses or stresses in life
- Are based on the typical dietary pattern of the country and may not be appropriate for persons following atypical diets
- Generally ignore possible interactions that involve nutrients and other dietary components because, at present, these interactions and their effect on requirements cannot be adequately quantified
- Assume that requirements for energy and all the other nutrients are met.

Some countries have expanded their tables of nutrient reference levels to include additional "non-nutritive" components that are not conventionally considered to be essential nutrients but which may have a possible benefit to health. Examples include dietary fiber, choline, carotenoids, and lycopenes. In addition, expert groups are now defining multiple nutrient-based levels for different purposes, each associated with a defined level of nutrient adequacy. These levels no longer focus solely on the nutrient requirements to correct or prevent a clinical deficiency: requirement levels necessary to optimize health and prevent chronic disease are also considered. In some cases (e.g., the United States and Canada), the revised tables also include tolerable upper intake levels to help people avoid harm from taking too much of a nutrient. In other countries (e.g., the United Kingdom), a lower reference level has been defined, below which habitual intakes are almost certainly inadequate for most individuals.

Establishing the EAR

At present, the nutrient reference levels are based on measurements of the nutrient requirements of individuals from a specific sex and life-stage group. For certain groups (e.g., the elderly), the requirements may be extrapolated from measurements made on young adults. In the future, additional factors, other than sex and life stage, may be taken into account when compiling nutrient requirements; these include race and ethnicity, activity level, environment and lifestyle, family history, and genetic predisposition to disease (Hoolihan, 2003).

A nutrient requirement has been defined by Yates (1998) as

> the lowest continuing intake level of a nutrient that will maintain a defined level of nutriture in an individual.

The requirements for a specific nutrient vary from individual to individual and thus form a distribution of requirements valid for a defined level of nutrient adequacy and a specific sex and life-stage group. For most nutrients, the requirements are generally considered to follow a normal symmetrical distribution, except for iron requirements which are said to be positively skewed for some age/sex groups. The median of this requirement distribution represents the Estimated Average Requirement (EAR) for that particular group of individuals (Figure 8.1). Therefore, the EAR is:

> the amount of nutrient that is estimated to meet the nutrient requirement of half the healthy individuals in a life-stage and sex group.

Strenuous efforts are now made to establish the EAR for each nutrient because it is the basis for the multiple nutrient-based reference levels in use in several countries.

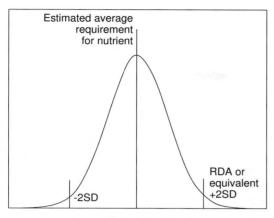

Figure 8.1: Estimated average requirement (EAR) for a nutrient. The nutrient requirements are defined in relation to a frequency distribution of individual requirements. The Recommended Dietary Allowance (RDA) or equivalent is defined as two standard deviations above the EAR.

The intake of a nutrient:

- Which induces marginally low or deficient levels of a nutrient, followed by correction of the deficit with measured amounts of that nutrient (i.e., depletion/repletion studies)

- Needed to maintain balance, taking into account that the period over which the balance needs to be measured varies, depending on the nutrient and individual

- Needed to maintain a given circulating concentration or degree of enzyme saturation, tissue saturation, or adequacy of molecular function

- Needed to cure clinical signs of deficiency

- Associated with optimal physiological, psychological, or immune function, and performance

The nutrient intakes of fully breastfed infants

The observed nutrient intakes in healthy populations

The intakes associated with chronic diseases based on epidemiological studies

Extrapolation of data from animal studies

Box 8.1: Examples of data used by expert committees to derive nutrient requirement estimates.

However, there is still no agreement by expert groups on the criteria used to define the requirements for each nutrient. Indeed, a range of criteria, selected on the basis of a careful review of the literature, are often used and the strengths and weaknesses of each of the sources of data are considered. Examples of the data used by expert committees to derive the nutrient requirements are shown in Box 8.1

There is increasing emphasis on the selection of physiological functional criteria for defining nutrient requirements. Functional endpoints are especially needed to establish an intake that reduces the risk of chronic disease. Unfortunately, at present, there is no consensus on the choice of a physiological functional criterion for each nutrient or on the appropriate indices or markers of this function. Functional indices are discussed in detail in Section 15.3. They include, for example, the activity of an enzyme dependent on a specific nutrient, or they may be less specific and measure more general functions that are directly related to disease mechanisms or ill health. Some examples include indices of immune function, antioxidant status, muscle strength, glucose metabolism, nerve function, and work capacity (Lukaski and Penland, 1996).

Once the criteria for defining the requirement of a nutrient have been selected, then appropriate cutoffs must be chosen that differentiate between adequate and inadequate levels of nutritional status for a specific nutrient. In some cases, more than one cutoff point for the same criterion may be chosen, or the criterion for a specific nutrient may differ for different life-stage groups (e.g., adolescents or the elderly). The reliability of the data used to select the criterion (or criteria) to define the requirements varies with the nutrient.

Establishing requirements for energy

The requirements for energy differ from those for the nutrients because they are set at a level to meet the average requirement for energy for a group of comparable individuals, as shown in Figure 8.2. This means that approximately 50% of a specific sex and life-stage group will have requirements above, and 50%

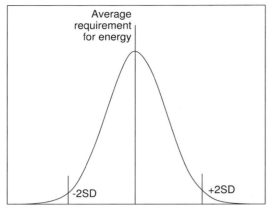

Figure 8.2: Estimated Average Requirement (EAR) for energy. The requirement for energy is defined in relation to a frequency distribution of individual requirements. Only the EAR is defined.

requirements below the EAR for energy. This approach has been adopted for energy by all the expert groups because of the potential adverse consequences to an individual from intakes that fall below their requirement (weight loss) or that exceed their requirement (weight gain). Furthermore, the body's regulatory mechanisms maintain energy intakes near requirements over long periods.

Energy needs are determined by energy expenditure so that theoretically measurements of energy expenditure should be used to estimate energy requirements. In the past, for some life-stage groups, such estimates were based on measurements of habitual energy intake. This approach assumes that in healthy persons with appropriate body composition and levels of physical activity, measurements of mean habitual energy intake will yield an estimate of their mean energy expenditure. This procedure was used by FAO/WHO/UNU (1985), and the United Kingdom (COMA, 1990) to set the energy requirement for young children.

For older children and adults, FAO/WHO/ UNU (1985) used an alternative approach to calculate energy requirement. This involved estimating energy expenditure as multiples of the basal metabolic rate (BMR) predicted from regression equations based on age, sex, and weight, or weight and height. An example of these equations derived by Schofield (1985) is given in Table 7.14. Data on the energy costs of various physical and discretionary activities are also available in FAO/WHO/UNU (1985) together with examples on how to calculate the energy requirements for adults engaged in light, moderate, and heavy activity work. Separate examples are also given for children that take into account the additional energy requirements for growth. Estimates for energy requirements that include an estimate of the variance of energy requirements have also been developed by the FAO/WHO/UNU (1985).

Increasingly, in many countries (e.g., the United Kingdom, France, Germany, Austria, Switzerland, the Netherlands, Canada, and the United States), the estimates of energy requirements are based on energy expenditure measured with doubly labeled water (Section 7.3.1) in an effort to improve the accuracy of the estimates (Prentice, 1988; COMA, 1991; Butte, 1996; Butte et al., 2000; IOM, 2002; Prentice et al., 2004; Spaaij and Pijls, 2004). The doubly labeled water method measures all components of energy expenditure, including basal metabolism, thermogenesis, physical activity, and the energy cost of synthesizing new tissue (Prentice et al., 1988). Details of the doubly labeled water method are given in Section 7.3.1.

The reference level at EAR+2SD

Once the EAR and associated standard deviation have been set, most expert groups then define a reference level at two standard deviations (2 SDs) above the EAR. This means that this higher level is sufficient to meet the daily requirements of that nutrient for almost all (about 97%) of the healthy individuals in that particular life-stage and sex group (Figure 8.1). When the standard deviation is unknown, a coefficient of variation (CV) of 10% or 15% of the EAR is often assumed (IOM, 2000c), and the standard deviation is calculated from the EAR and assumed CV.

Unfortunately, there is a lack of consensus among countries on the terminology used

	Protein (g)	Vit. A RE (μg)	Vit. C (mg)	Thiamin (mg)	Vit. B$_6$ (mg)	Folate (μg)	Calcium (mg)	Iron (mg)
Indonesia								
Male	55	400	60	1.2		190	500	10
Female	42	500	60	1.0		160	500	24
Malaysia								
Male	45	750	30	1.0		200	450	9
Female	37	750	30	0.8		200	450	28
Philippines								
Male	60	525	75	1.3		170	500	12
Female	52	450	70	1.0		150	500	26
Singapore								
Male		750	30	1.0	2.0		500	10
Female		750	30	1.0	2.0		500	10
Thailand								
Male	50	800	60	1.5	2.0	200	800	15
Female	50	800	60	1.5	2.0	200	800	15

Table 8.1: Representative reference levels in 1998 set at two standard deviations above the Estimated Average Requirement (EAR) for men and women 19–59 years of age in Indonesia, Malaysia, the Philippines, Singapore, and Thailand. Data from Lachance, Nutrition Reviews 56: S34–S39, 1998, with permission of the International Life Sciences Institute.

for the reference nutrient intake level set at 2 SDs above the EAR. The United Kingdom has adopted the term "Reference Nutrient Intake" (RNI) (COMA, 1991), the United States uses the term "Recommended Dietary Allowances" (RDA) (Anonymous, 1997a), and Australia and New Zealand currently employ the term "Recommended Dietary Intake" (RDI) (Truswell et al., 1990).

The reference level at 2 SDs above the EAR should not be used as a cutoff value for assessing the prevalence of inadequate intakes in a group. As the RDA, or its equivalent, is set at an intake level that exceeds the requirements of 97%–98% of all individuals, such an approach will always result in a gross overestimate of the proportion of the group at risk of inadequate intakes. However, one can conclude that an individual with a usual intake at or above the RDA has a low risk of inadequacy (i.e., 2–3%).

Sources of discrepancies in nutrient requirement estimates

In light of the preceding discussion, it is not surprising that the nutrient requirement esti-mates and the derived reference levels vary among countries. Table 8.1 compares nutrient reference levels for selected nutrients set at 2 SDs above the EAR in six countries in 1998. Sources of some of the discrepancies noted in Table 8.1 are summarized in Box 8.2.

Some discrepancies arise because of differences in judgment by the expert groups

---

Interpretation of data on which EAR's are based

Selection of physiological criteria used to define nutrient adequacy

Limited data on requirements for certain nutrients and life-stage groups

Unknown factors influencing nutrient requirements

Uncertain extent of metabolic adaptation during pregnancy and lactation due to limited data

Varying bioavailability factors, depending on the composition of habitual national diet

Number of life-stage groupings differing among countries

Uncertain SD of the requirement estimates

Box 8.2: Sources of discrepancies in the EAR and thus reference level set at EAR + 2SD.

setting the requirement estimates, especially in relation to the selection of the criteria used to define nutrient adequacy, the measures or markers of the physiological function selected, and the interpretation of the data. Such discrepancies may be especially large for those nutrients and specific age groups for which the available data on requirements are very limited (e.g., children, adolescents, and the elderly). In such cases, requirements are often extrapolated from data for other age groups, or they are not compiled at all. In addition, during pregnancy and lactation, maternal metabolic adaptation for certain nutrients may occur, but because the adaptation has not been firmly characterized, the additional nutrient needs are still equivocal.

A further source of discrepancy in the reference levels among countries and expert groups arises from the adjustments made to the physiological requirement estimates of certain nutrients to yield a dietary requirement estimate. The latter takes into account the bioavailability of nutrients such as iron and zinc in the habitual national diet. Such adjustments depend on the nature of the diet ingested, the chemical form of the nutrient in the diet, and a variety of systemic factors known to affect the absorption and utilization of the nutrient.

For many nutrients, factors affecting their bioavailability have yet to be established, so appropriate adjustments to yield dietary requirement estimates cannot be made. For others, fixed bioavailability factors are applied, even though the efficiency of absorption may vary with the dietary level of the nutrient or the life-stage group (Turnland, 1994). For example, in U.K. diets, iron is assumed to have a fixed bioavailability of 15%, irrespective of the age and life-stage group (COMA, 1991), whereas in the United States a factor of 18% is used for the bioavailability of iron for the mixed diets of both children and non-pregnant adults, but 25% for women in the second and third trimester of pregnancy (IOM, 2001). Similarly, the United Kingdom uses a fixed bioavailability factor of 30% for zinc, irrespective of the age and

life-stage group, but the United States applies a factor of 40% for the bioavailability of zinc from adult diets ($\geqslant 19$ y) and 30% for preadolescent children (IOM, 2001). Other expert groups such as FAO/WHO (2002) employ several factors to adjust for bioavailability, depending on the composition of the diet, as discussed in Section 8.1.5.

Several other factors besides sex and life-stage group are known to influence the requirements for many nutrients. Examples include body size, lean body mass, and activity level. For this reason, the requirement estimates are often set using a standard height and weight, and/or energy intake for a particular age and life-stage group. The values for standard height, weight, and energy intake vary across countries. Therefore, those nutrients with requirements expressed per kg body weight or per MJ, may also differ. In the future, factors such as race or ethnicity, lifestyle (e.g., smokers, vegetarians, oral contraceptive users), the existence of chronic disease (e.g., asthma, diabetes), environment, family history, and genetic predisposition to disease may also be taken into account when setting requirement estimates (Hoolihan, 2003). Indeed, in the United States and Canada, vegetarianism and some other lifestyle factors are already considered. For example, the EAR for iron for vegetarians is higher than that for persons consuming a mixed Western diet to take into account the lower bioavailability of iron from a vegetarian diet (i.e., 10% vs 18%) (IOM, 2001), whereas the EAR for vitamin C for smokers is higher than for nonsmokers (IOM, 2000a).

The life-stage groupings are not defined in the same way among countries. North America has 22 such groups. Fewer groupings are defined in Europe: the United Kingdom, Germany, and the Netherlands have 14 each, but the number is presently not standardized, even within the EEC (Trichopoulou and Vassilakou, 1990).

Finally, knowledge of the SD associated with the EAR is required to set the reference level at two SDs above the EAR. In many cases, however, the SD is calculated from the EAR and an assumed CV, because the

SD is unknown. Although a CV of 10% or 15% is often assumed, this is not always the case. FAO/WHO (2002), for example, has assumed a CV of 25% for the dietary zinc requirement estimate, resulting in a further source of discrepancy for the reference levels for zinc set at EAR + 2SD.

Setting a reference level for nutrients with a limited scientific basis

For certain nutrients, there is still not enough information to establish an EAR. In such cases, the nutrient reference levels are often based on observed intakes for the nutrient, and these levels are judged to be adequate for the specific life-stage group but not so large as to cause undesirable effects. This is an approach often adopted for infants < 6 mo, when the reference levels are usually based on the varying content of the nutrient in breast milk and the average amount of breast milk consumed.

Again, the terminology used for reference levels set in this way varies. The United Kingdom has adopted the term "Safe Intake" (SI) for seven nutrients defined in this way, whereas the U.S. Food and Nutrition Board use the term "Adequate Intake" (AI). FAO/WHO (2002) have adopted the term "Acceptable Intake" for nutrients (e.g., vitamin E) for which data were considered insufficient to set an EAR.

Clearly, there is an urgent need to harmonize the nutrient requirement estimates among countries, and the nomenclature used. This requires agreement on the physiological criteria of "adequacy" for each nutrient, as well as data on the physiological, behavioral, and environmental factors (e.g., ultraviolet light, altitude, extremes in ambient temperature, and genetic variance) that may influence nutrient requirements so that they can be adjusted to local situations, where necessary (King, 1998). More precise information on local dietary factors that influence the absorption and utilization of certain nutrients must also be obtained so that their effects on dietary requirements can be taken into account. Finally, consensus must be reached

on how the different nutrient-based reference levels should be used (Beaton, 1998). Details of their correct use with individuals and populations groups are given in Sections 8.2 and 8.3, respectively.

8.1.2 U.K. Dietary Reference Values

The United Kingdom was the first country to adopt a framework for developing the Dietary Reference Values (COMA, 1991); the framework is depicted in Figure 8.3.

The generic term "Dietary Reference Values" (DRVs) was used to embrace three reference levels: the Lower Reference Nutrient Intake (LRNI), the Estimated Average Requirement (EAR), and the Reference Nutrient Intake (RNI). The term "reference values" was adopted by the U.K. panel in an effort to prevent users interpreting the figures as recommended or desirable intakes. Instead, the expert panel hoped that users would select the figure most appropriate for its intended use (Beaton, 1998).

Lower Reference Nutrient Intakes are set at two standard deviations below the EAR

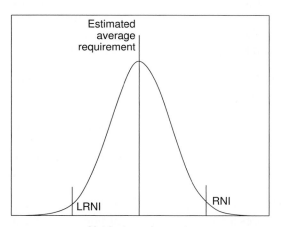

Figure 8.3: Dietary reference values for the United Kingdom. The nutrient requirements are defined in relation to a frequency distribution of individual requirements. The Lower Reference Nutrient Intake (LRNI) is defined as two standard deviations below the Estimated Average Requirement (EAR). The Reference Nutrient Intake (RNI) is defined as two standard deviations above the EAR (COMA, 1991).

for each nutrient and represent the lowest intakes that will meet the needs of some individuals in the group. Habitual intakes below this level are almost certainly inadequate for most individuals. For confirmation, however, biological parameters should be measured, especially when the nutrient intake of the individual lies between the LRNI and the EAR (COMA, 1991).

Estimated Average Requirements represent the level of the nutrients that are estimated to meet the nutrient requirement of 50% of the healthy individuals in a particular sex and life-stage group.

Reference Nutrient Intakes are defined as 2 SDs above the EAR for each nutrient (Appendix A8.1, A8.2). When data about variability in requirements are insufficient to calculate a SD, a coefficient of variation for the EAR of 10% is ordinarily assumed. Habitual intakes above the RNI will almost certainly be adequate for all but 2% to 3% of individuals in a specific sex and life-stage group.

For some nutrients with important functions in humans, but for which the expert committee considered there were insufficient data to set DRVs (e.g., biotin, pantothenic acid, vitamin E, vitamin K, manganese, molybdenum, and chromium), the United Kingdom set a Safe Intake (SI) value. This SI was judged to be a level or range of intake at which there is no risk of deficiency and below a level where there is a risk of undesirable effects (COMA, 1991).

The United Kingdom also proposed DRVs for starches, sugars, fats, and fatty acids. This group of DRVs are not defined in the same way as those for the other nutrients. They represent average intakes for populations and not for individuals, which are consistent with good health, and are expressed as a percentage of daily total energy intake and as a percentage of food energy (i.e., excluding the contribution from alcohol). Table 8.2 summarizes the current U.K. recommendations for the macronutrients (COMA, 1991, 1994) and compares them with the WHO

(2003) population nutrient intake goals for the prevention of diet-related chronic diseases (Section 8.1.7). The U.S. and Canadian Acceptable Macronutrient Distribution Ranges (AMDRs) for adults (IOM, 2002) are also given for comparison. Note that these U.S. and Canadian recommendations, unlike those set by WHO and the United Kingdom, are intended for use by individuals.

The Expert Group on Vitamins and Minerals (EVM) in the United Kingdom has recently set new recommendations for Safe Upper Levels for certain nutrients (EVM, 2003). The Safe Upper Level represents an intake that can be consumed daily over a lifetime without significant risk to health. Intakes from all sources were taken into account. Safe Upper Levels for vitamin B_6, β-carotene, vitamin E, boron, copper, nickel, selenium, zinc, and silicon were set.

The EVM group also provided guidance for those nutrients for which the database was inadequate to establish a Safe Upper Level. Nutrients in this category included biotin, folic acid, vitamin B_{12}, niacin, pantothenic acid, riboflavin, thiamin, vitamin C, vitamin A, vitamin D, vitamin K, chromium, cobalt, iodine, manganese, molybdenum, tin, calcium, iron, magnesium, and potassium. Suggested levels for these nutrients would not be expected to be associated with any adverse effects. Nevertheless, the EVM acknowledged that the suggested levels may not be applicable to all life stages or for lifelong intake, and should not be used as Safe Upper Levels. The EVM group could not provide Safe Upper Levels or guidance for germanium, vanadium, and sodium chloride, and two minerals were not considered at all: sulfur and fluoride.

8.1.3 U.S. and Canadian Dietary Reference Intakes

The United States and Canada have also adopted a paradigm for nutrient reference levels that incorporates data to optimize health, prevent risk of chronic disease and avoid deficiency. Their approach also provides multiple reference levels for each nutrient to meet the

	UK DRVs for total energy and food energy (COMA, 1991, 1994, 1998)[a]	WHO (2003)[b]	U.S./Canadian AMDRs for adults (IOM, 2002)
Total fat	33% or 35% of FE	15%–30%	20%–35%
Saturated fatty acids	10% or 11% of FE	< 10%	UL not set
PUFAs	6% or 6.5% of FE	6%–10%	
n-6 PUFAs		5%–8%	5%–10%
n-3 PUFAs		1%–2%	
α-linolenic acid			0.6%–1.2%
Trans fatty acids	2% or 2% of FE	< 1%	UL not set
MUFAs	2% or 2% of FE	By difference[c]	UL not set
Total carbohydrate	47% or 50% of FE	55%–75%	45%–65%
Sugars	10% or 11% of FE[d]	< 10%[e]	Maximal intake of 25% energy or less from added sugars
Protein	15%	10%–15%	10%–35%
Cholesterol		< 300 mg/d	UL not set

Table 8.2: U.K. dietary reference values (DRVs) and the WHO population nutrient intake goals for the energy-supplying macronutrients for the prevention of diet-related chronic diseases. Figures are for percentage of total energy, unless otherwise stated. The U.S. and Canadian Acceptable Macronutrient Distribution Ranges (AMDRs) intended for individual adults are shown for comparison. [a]Recommendations apply to adults and children over 5 y of age; [b]Represent the population average intake that is judged to be consistent with the maintenance of health in a population; [c]This is calculated as total fat – (saturated fatty acids + unsaturated fatty acids + *trans* fatty acids); [d]Refers to non-milk extrinsic sugars; PUFAs, Polyunsaturated fatty acids; MUFAs, Monounsaturated fatty acids; [e]Refers to "free sugars," a term that includes all monosaccharides and disaccharides added to foods by the manufacturer, cook, or consumer, plus sugars naturally present in honey, syrups, and fruit juices; FE, Food Energy (excludes contribution from alcohol); UL, Upper Limit.

expanding list of uses. Specifically, the U.S. Food and Nutrition Board has expanded their definition of requirements to:

- Consider reduction in the risk of chronic degenerative disease, where possible
- Establish an upper level of intake designed to avoid risk of adverse health effects, where data exist
- Include components of food not conventionally considered to be essential nutrients (e.g., choline, carotenoids, lycopenes, boron, vanadium) but which may have a possible benefit to health

These new nutrient reference levels were established by a joint committee of both Canadian and U.S. scientists set up by the U.S. Food and Nutrition Board with the aim of harmonizing the U.S. Recommended Dietary Allowances (RDAs) and the Canadian Recommended Nutrient Intakes (RNIs).

The committee adopted the generic term "Dietary Reference Intakes" for a set of reference values for each life-stage and sex group. The U.S. Dietary Reference Intakes (DRIs), unlike the U.K. DRVs, encompass Tolerable Upper Intake Levels (ULs), which are designed to avoid adverse health effects from consuming excessive amounts of a nutrient. Figure 8.4 shows the relationship of the observed level of intake to the risk of inadequacy and toxicity for each of the U.S. and Canadian reference values.

The criterion chosen by the U.S. Food and Nutrition Board to define nutrient adequacy differs for each nutrient and, sometimes, within the life-stage groups for the

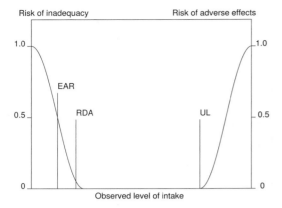

Figure 8.4: United States and Canadian dietary reference intakes — definitions showing the relationship of the observed level of intake to the risk of inadequacy/toxicity. The Estimated Average Requirement (EAR) is the intake at which the risk of inadequacy is 0.5 (50%) to an individual. The Recommended Dietary Allowance (RDA) is the intake at which the risk of inadequacy is very small — only 0.02 to 0.03 (2% to 3%). At intakes above the Tolerable Upper Intake Level (UL), the risk of adverse effects increases. From Health and Welfare, Canada. (1983).

same nutrient, as noted in Section 8.1.1; details are given in the separate reports published by the Food and Nutrition Board (IOM, 1997, 2000a, 2000b, 2001, 2002). Further, each nutrient-based reference intake refers to the average daily nutrient intake of apparently healthy persons over time, and does not have to be consumed every day. The set of reference values defined by the Food and Nutrition Board are as follows.

Estimated Average Requirement (EAR) or the median requirement for a specified criterion of adequacy for individuals of a certain life-stage and sex group. When the mean usual intake of the group is equal to the EAR, 50% of the healthy individuals in that particular life-stage and sex group, meet their requirement and the other half of the group do not. Hence, the EAR is *not* used as an intake goal for individuals: usual intake at this level is associated with a 50% risk of inadequacy (Barr et al., 2003).

The EAR is based on a specific criterion of adequacy, defined by a specific function or biochemical measurement, which varies

with the nutrient. It is especially useful for evaluating the possible adequacy of nutrient intakes of population groups (Table 8.8).

Recommended Dietary Allowance (RDA) refers to the intake level that meets the daily nutrient requirements of almost all (97 to 98%) of the individuals in a specific life-stage and sex group (Appendix A8.3, A8.4). If the variation in requirement is well defined and symmetrically distributed, then the RDA is set at two standard deviations above the EAR:

$$RDA = EAR + (2\ SD)$$

If a coefficient of variation (CV) for the EAR of 10% is assumed (the CV is equal to the SD / EAR), then:

$$RDA = 1.2 \times EAR$$

Alternatively, if the CV is 15%, then:

$$RDA = 1.3 \times EAR$$

No RDA is proposed if there is not enough data to establish an EAR for that nutrient. Because the usual intake at the level of the RDA is, by definition, associated with a very low (2%–3%) risk of inadequacy to an individual, the RDA is used as a recommended intake when planning diets for individuals (Barr et al., 2003). For example, the appropriate target for phosphorus intake for a woman aged 31–50 y is the RDA of 700 mg. The RDA should not be used to assess the intakes of groups.

Adequate Intake (AI) refers to a recommended average daily nutrient intake level based on observed or experimentally derived approximations or estimates of the nutrient intake by a group (or groups) of apparently healthy people. The observed or derived intakes are assumed to be adequate. The AI is used when there are not enough scientific data to establish an EAR, and is used as an intake goal for individuals (Table 8.8). For example, the appropriate target for calcium intake for a woman age 31–50 y is the AI of 1000 mg/d.

Tolerable Upper Intake Level (UL) is the highest usual daily nutrient intake level likely

Physical activity category	PAL (multiples of basal energy expenditure)	Description	Physical Activity Coefficient (PA)	
			Men $\geqslant 19$ y	Women $\geqslant 19$ y
Sedentary	1.0 to < 1.4	Activities of daily living (ADL) only	1.00	1.00
Low active	$\geqslant 1.4$ to < 1.6	ADL plus walking about 2 miles/d (1.5/2.9)* or equivalent	1.11	1.12
Active	$\geqslant 1.6$ to < 1.9	ADL plus walking about 7 miles/d (5.3/9.9)* or equivalent	1.25	1.27
Very active	$\geqslant 1.9$ to < 2.5	ADL plus walking about 17 miles/d (12.3/22.5)* or equivalent	1.48	1.45

Table 8.3: Description of physical activity level (PAL) categories. *Walking distance is estimated for the midpoint of the range (i.e., PAL = 1.5 for low active, 1.75 for active, and 2.2 for very active) and for midweight individuals weighing 70 kg. Values in parentheses reflect walking distances at the same PAL for relatively heavy weight (120 kg) and relatively light weight (44 kg) individuals, respectively. From Barr et al., Nutrition Reviews 61: 352–360, 2003, with permission of the International Life Sciences Institute.

to pose no risk of adverse health effects for almost all individuals in a life-stage and sex group. ULs were not set for some nutrients with limited scientific data. Details of the adverse health effects used to set the ULs are given in the U.S. Institute of Medicine (IOM) reports. For some nutrients such as calcium, phosphorus, copper, zinc, selenium, and iodine, the UL refers to the total intake from all sources, including food, fortified food, water, supplements, and medications, where relevant. For others such as niacin, vitamin B_6, folate, and magnesium, the UL applies only to intake from supplements, fortificants, and medications. In some cases, the form of the nutrient for the UL differs from that used for the RDA; examples include vitamin E, niacin, and folate.

The UL should be used by health professionals to ensure that nutrient intakes are not too high. As intake increases above the UL, the risk of adverse health effects increases. The UL is based on risk-assessment methodologies similar to those used in toxicological studies (Anonymous, 1997b; IOM, 1998).

Estimated Energy Requirement (EER) is defined as the average energy intake required to maintain current body weight and activity level (and to allow for growth or milk pro-

duction, where relevant) in healthy, normal-weight individuals of a specified age, sex, height, weight, and physical activity level.

The estimated energy requirements (EER) compiled by the IOM (2002) were based on doubly labeled water measurements of energy expenditure, and where relevant, energy deposition from protein and fat accretion in growing infants and children. Several regression equations have been developed for estimating the energy requirements of different life-stage and sex groups, with separate equations for individuals with a normal body weight (i.e., BMI 18.5–24.9 kg/m^2) and those overweight or obese (BMI $\geqslant 25$). An example of the regression equation for men aged $\geqslant 19$ y of normal weight is given below:

EER (kcal) = 661.8 − [9.53 × Age (y)] +
PA × {[15.91 × Weight (kg)] + [539.6 × Height (m)]}

where PA = physical activity coefficient corresponding to a given physical activity level (PAL). Details of the different physical activity level categories are given in Table 8.3.

For individuals with a BMI $\geqslant 25$, the estimated energy intake required to maintain current weight and activity level is termed the Total Energy Expenditure (TEE) and not the EER. This practice has been adopted because overweight is not consistent with long-term good health (Barr et al., 2003).

Acceptable Macronutrient Distribution Range (AMDR) is defined as a range of intakes for a particular energy source associated with reduced risk of chronic disease, while providing adequate levels of essential nutrients (IOM, 2002). They are intended for use by individuals, and have been established for carbohydrate, protein, total fat, *n*-6 polyunsaturated fats, and α-linolenic acid, as shown in Table 8.4. Individuals should have intakes that fall within the limits of the AMDRs. If the usual intake of an individual is below or above the AMDR, there is a potential for increased risk of both inadequate intakes of essential nutrients and chronic diseases (IOM, 2002).

8.1.4 European reference values

The Scientific Committee for Food of the European Community (CEC, 1993) has proposed three reference values for each nutrient:

- Lowest Threshold Intake
- Average Requirement
- Population Reference Intake

The nutrient requirements of individuals are again assumed to have a normal or symmetrical distribution, with the exception of the iron needs of menstruating women.

Lowest Threshold Intake (LTI) is defined as the intake below which almost all individuals

Macronutrient	AMDR (as % of energy)
Carbohydrate	45–65
Protein	10–35[a]
Fat	20–35[b]
n-6 polyunsaturated fatty acids	5–10[c]
α-linolenic acid	0.6–1.2[c]

Table 8.4: Acceptable Macronutrient Distribution Ranges (AMDRs) for adults. [a]For children 1–3 y and 4–18 y, the AMDR for protein is 5%–20% and 10%–30% respectively. [b]For children 1–3 y and 4–18 y, the AMDR for fat is 30%–40% and 25%–35%, respectively. [c]Included within the AMDR for total fat. From Barr et al., Nutrition Reviews 61: 352–360, 2003, with permission of the International Life Sciences Institute.

in the population will be unable to maintain metabolic integrity according to the criterion of adequacy chosen. The LTI represents the mean −2SD.

Average Requirement (AR) for a specific sex and life-stage group is defined in the conventional way.

Population Reference Intake (PRI) is defined as the intake that will meet the needs of almost all healthy people in the population or group. It corresponds conceptually with the RNI or equivalent, and hence represents the mean + 2 SD.

These reference values for adults are shown in Table 8.5; the CEC (1993) report also presents comprehensive values for infants (6–11 mo), children and adolescents 1–17 y, and pregnant and lactating women (Appendix A8.5, A8.6). Only values for protein and energy are given for infants < 6 mo. For those nutrients for which the data are deemed inadequate to set an AR (i.e., pantothenic acid, biotin, vitamin D, sodium, magnesium, manganese), an acceptable range of intakes is given. No reference values are given for vitamin K, molybdenum, chromium, and fluoride, or for infants < 6 mo. A detailed discussion of these reference values is given in several publications (Anonymous, 1993; CEC, 1993; Aggett et al., 1997).

More recently, the Scientific Committee on Food for the European Commission have also defined an Upper Level of Intake (ULI) for certain vitamins and minerals. Details are available at:

http://www.europa.eu.int/comm/food/index_en.html

A comparison of the various methodological approaches and nutrient recommendations for children aged 2–18 y in 29 countries in Europe is available (Prentice et al., 2004).

8.1.5 FAO/WHO nutrient requirements

When vitamin and mineral requirements for a specific country are not available, the FAO/

Nutrient	Average Requirement (AR)	Population Reference Intake (PRI)	Lowest Threshold Intake (LTI)
Protein (g)	0.6/kg body weight	0.75/kg body weight	0.45/kg body weight
Vitamins			
Vitamin A (μg)	500 (400)	700 (600)	300 (250)
Thiamin (μg)	72/MJ	100/MJ	50/MJ
Riboflavin (mg)	1.3 (1.1)	1.6 (1.3)	0.6
Niacin (mg niacin equivalents)	1.3/MJ	1.6/MJ	1.0/MJ
Vitamin B_6 (μg)	13/g protein	15/g protein	
Folate (μg)	140	200	85
Vitamin B_{12} (μg)	1.0	1.4	0.6
Vitamin C (mg)	30	45	12
Vitamin E (mg α-tocopherol equivalents)		0.4/g PUFA	4 (3)/d regardless of PUFA intakes
Fatty acids			
n-6 PUFA (as % energy)	1	2	0.5
n-3 PUFA (as % energy)	0.2	0.5	0.1
Minerals			
Calcium (mg)	550	700	400
Phosphorus (mg)	400	550	300
Potassium (mg)		3100	1600
Trace elements			
Iron (mg)	7 (10, 6^a)	9 (16^b, 8^a)	5 (7, 4^a)
Zinc (mg)	7.5 (5.5)	9.5 (7)	5.5 (4)
Copper (mg)	0.8	1.1	0.6
Selenium (μg)	40	55	20
Iodine (μg)	100	13	70

Table 8.5: European Community Reference Values for adults. Amounts are per day unless given in other terms. Data for women, where different from that for men, are given in parentheses. [a]Postmenopausal women, [b]PRI to cover 90% of women, PUFA, polyunsaturated fatty acids. In addition, for the following, acceptable ranges of intake are: pantothenic acid, 3–12 mg; biotin, 15–100 μg; vitamin D, 0–10 μg; sodium, 0.575–3.5 g; magnesium, 150–500 mg; manganese, 1–10 mg. From Anonymous, Nutrition Reviews 51: 209–212, 1993, with permission of the International Life Sciences Institute.

WHO (2002) report can be used. FAO/WHO (2002) have defined four levels:

- Requirement
- Recommended Nutrient Intake
- Tolerable Upper Nutrient Intake Level
- Protective Nutrient Intake

Requirement is defined as an intake level, which will meet specified criteria of adequacy, preventing risk of deficit or excess. Where necessary, an allowance for variations in nutrient bioavailability has been included (FAO/WHO, 2002).

Recommended Nutrient Intake (RNI) is defined as the daily nutrient intake which meets the nutrient requirements of almost all (97.5%) apparently healthy individuals in an age and sex-specific population group. Thus it is based on 2 SDs above the nutrient requirement and is equivalent to, and derived in the same way as both the U.K. RNI (COMA, 1991) and the RDA of the IOM (2001). When the standard deviation for the nutrient requirement is unknown, FAO/WHO (2002) has generally assumed a CV of 10%–12.5%, although there are exceptions for some nutrients (e.g., zinc), when a CV of 25% is assumed. Appendix A8.7 and A8.8 summarize the FAO/WHO (2002) Recommended Nutrient Intakes for minerals and vitamins.

Tolerable Upper Nutrient Intake Levels have only been defined for some nutrients as the maximum intake from food of that nutrient that is unlikely to pose risk of adverse health effects from excess in almost all (97.5%) apparently healthy individuals in an age and sex-specific population group. Exposure from both food and fortified food products were considered. The ULs were developed using the model outlined in Anonymous (1997b).

Protective Nutrient Intake is a concept introduced by FAO/WHO (2002) for certain circumstances. It is used when an amount of a nutrient greater than the RNI may be protective against a specified health or nutritional risk of public health relevance. Examples include the consumption of vitamin C with a meal to enhance nonheme iron absorption, and the intake of folic acid necessary to lower the risk of neural tube defects.

FAO/WHO (2002) adopted alternative terms for certain nutrients (e.g., vitamin A and vitamin E). For vitamin A, for example, they adopted the term "Recommended Safe Intake," as used in their earlier report (FAO/WHO, 1988) because of the lack of data for deriving a mean requirement for any group. The Recommended Safe Intake level is set to prevent clinical signs of deficiency and allow normal growth, but it does not allow for prolonged periods of infection or other stresses. As such, it represents the normative storage requirement plus 2 SDs. For vitamin E, "Acceptable Intakes" are listed because there was not enough data to formulate RNIs for this vitamin.

The FAO/WHO (2002) RNIs for dietary iron and zinc are also based on estimates that meet the normative storage requirements, and are adapted from earlier reports (FAO/WHO, 1988; WHO, 1996a). In these reports the normative requirement was defined as "the amount needed to generate reserve capacity." Table 8.6 provides an example of the average individual normative requirements for zinc expressed in terms of µg/kg of body weight per day from diets of three levels of zinc bioavailability: high (i.e., 50%), moderate (i.e., 30%), and low (i.e., 15%).

In Table 8.7, the Recommended Nutrient Intakes for dietary zinc (mg/d) are presented from diets with three levels of zinc bioavailability. For these derivations, a CV for the dietary zinc requirement of 25% is assumed.

8.1.6 WHO Safe Range of Population Intakes for Trace Elements

In 1996, the WHO expert group on trace elements (WHO, 1996a) incorporated a new concept to derive estimates of the necessary group mean intakes that would be associated with low risk of inadequacy in the population as a whole. Such estimates are very different from those used for individuals. They are derived from epidemiological data and represent estimates of the safe range of population mean intakes.

The lower limit of the safe range of the population mean intakes (Figure 8.5) represents the lowest population mean intake

Age range (y)	Sex	Bioavailability		
		High	Mod.	Low
0.5–1	M and F	186	311	621
1–3	M and F	138	230	459
3–6	M and F	114	190	380
6–10	M and F	90	149	299
10–12	F	68	113	227
12–15	F	64	107	215
15–18	F	56	93	187
18–60+	F	36	59	119
10–12	M	80	133	267
12–15	M	76	126	253
15–18	M	61	102	205
18–60+	M	43	72	144

Table 8.6: Average individual normative dietary requirements for zinc (µg/kg of body weight per day) from diets of differing zinc bioavailability. High bioavailability = 50%, moderate bioavailability = 30%, low bioavailability = 15%. From FAO/WHO (2002) with permission.

Age group	Assumed weight (kg)	Bioavailability		
		High	Mod.	Low
Infants and children				
0–6 mo	6	1.1[a]	2.8[b]	6.6[c]
7–12 mo	9	0.8[a]	—	—
7–12 mo	9	2.5[d]	4.1	8.4
1–3 y	12	2.4	4.1	8.3
4–6 y	17	2.9	4.8	9.6
7–9 y	25	3.3	5.6	11.2
Adolescents				
F. 10–18 y	47	4.3	7.2	14.4
M. 10–18 y	49	5.1	8.6	17.1
Adults				
F. 19–65 y	55	3.0	4.9	9.8
M. 19–65 y	65	4.2	7.0	14.0
F. 65+ y	55	3.0	4.9	9.8
M. 65+ y	65	4.2	7.0	14.0
Pregnant women				
1st trimester	—	3.4	5.5	11.0
2nd trimester	—	4.2	7.0	14.0
3rd trimester	—	6.0	10.0	20.0
Lactating women				
0–3 mo	—	5.8	9.5	19.0
3–6 mo	—	5.3	8.8	17.5
6–12 mo	—	4.3	7.2	14.4

Table 8.7: Recommended nutrient intakes for dietary zinc (mg/d) to meet the normative storage requirements from diets differing in zinc bioavailability. Unless otherwise specified, the within-subject variation of zinc requirements is assumed to be 25%. [a]For infants receiving maternal milk only, assumed CV = 12.5%. [b]Formula-fed infants; moderate bioavailability for whey-adjusted milk formula and for partly breastfed infants or given low-phytate feeds supplemented with other milks; assumed CV = 12.5%. [c]Formula-fed infants; low bioavailability applicable to phytate-rich vegetable-protein based formula with or without whole-grain cereal; assumed CV = 12.5%. [d]Not applicable to infants consuming human milk only. From FAO/WHO (2002) with permission.

that is accompanied by the acceptable risk of functional impairment, arising from a deficiency in the diet of a specific trace element. WHO (1996a) set this lower limit of the safe range of the population mean intake at 2 SD of intake above the average requirement for an individual in the same specific age and sex group. They assumed that the typical intake distribution for any nutrient would be approximately Gaussian. Applying the lower limit as a cutoff, the expected prevalence of individuals with inadequate intakes in a group with

a mean intake at the cutoff would be about 2%–3%, as shown in Figure 8.5.

Theoretically, the upper limit of the population mean intake could also be derived in a similar way such that only 2%–3% of individuals within the population subgroup would have intakes above the average threshold for toxicity. Further details of this approach can be found in WHO (1996a). It is not clear whether these estimates for the population mean intakes are applicable to all populations; it may be preferable to derive population-specific estimates in the future (Beaton, 1998).

8.1.7 WHO Recommendations for prevention of diet-related chronic diseases

The WHO (2003) population dietary recommendations for total carbohydrate, protein and fat, n-3 and n-6 polyunsaturated fatty acids, α-linoleic acid, *trans* fatty acids, and free sugars are included in Table 8.2. These WHO recommendations are termed population nutrient intake goals and are expressed as a proportion of the daily total energy in-

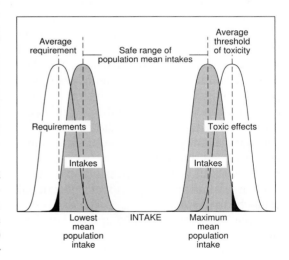

Figure 8.5: Safe range of population mean intakes: definitions. For diagrammatic purposes, the distribution of intakes (light shading) is assumed to have the same variance as the distribution of requirements; in general this is almost certainly not the case. Again, in the absence of specific information, the threshold of toxicity is assumed to be similarly distributed.

take rather than the absolute amount, except for cholesterol which is given in mg/d. The range of intakes given are said to be consistent with the maintenance of health and the prevention of diet-related chronic diseases. In general, most of the ranges set are comparable to those of the United Kingdom and the United States and Canada, but the meaning and application of the ranges differ. The WHO (2003) recommendations, like those of the United Kingdom, are intended as population average intakes, as noted earlier (Section 8.1.2), whereas those of the United States and Canada are intended for use by individuals. For further details see WHO (2003).

8.2 Evaluating the nutrient intakes of individuals

None of the methods of evaluating nutrient-intake data described below identify actual individuals in the population who have a specific nutrient inadequacy. This uncertainty arises because the actual nutrient requirement of an individual is not known. In addition, the nutrient-intake data recorded only approximate the individual's *usual* nutrient intake, because of normal day-to-day variation in the diet (Sections 6.2.1 and 6.2.3) combined with measurement errors (Chapter 5). For these reasons, dietary data alone can only provide an estimate of the *risk* of a nutrient inadequacy. The reliability of this risk estimate depends on the method used for its calculation. Only when biochemical, anthropometric, and clinical assessments are combined with the dietary investigation can a valid assessment of an individual's nutritional status be made.

Table 8.8 summarizes the appropriate nutrient-based reference levels for evaluating nutrient intakes of individuals and groups, using the U.S. Food and Nutrition Board Dietary Reference Intakes as an example. More specific details of these applications are given in Sections 8.2.1 and 8.3. In the past, nutrient-based reference levels have not always been applied correctly and the outline

Application to individuals
EAR: use to examine the probability that the usual intake of an individual is inadequate
RDA: a usual intake by an individual at or above the RDA has a low probability of inadequacy
AI: usual intake by an individual $\geqslant$ this level has a low probability of inadequacy (used when there is not enough evidence to set an RDA)
UL: usual intakes above this level may place an individual at risk of adverse effects from excessive nutrient intake

Applications with groups
EAR: use to estimate the prevalence of inadequate intakes within a group
RDA: do not use to assess the intakes of groups
AI: group mean usual intakes $\geqslant$ this level suggest a low prevalence of inadequate intakes[a]
UL: use to estimate the percentage of the group at potential risk of adverse effects from excessive nutrient intake

Table 8.8: Uses of Dietary Reference Intakes (DRIs) for assessing intakes of individuals and groups. [a]When the Adequate Intake (AI) for a nutrient is not based on mean intakes of healthy populations, this assessment is made with less confidence. From IOM (2000c).

in this table should be followed when interpreting nutrient intakes.

8.2.1 Using the EAR

It is not possible to compare the intake of an individual with his or her own requirement, because the actual requirement for any given individual is rarely known. Moreover, the reported nutrient intake of an individual is unlikely to represent their usual intake because of within-subject variation in nutrient intakes, as discussed in Section 6.2.3. In view of these limitations, the IOM (2000c) has developed a statistical approach to provide an estimate of the level of confidence that the usual intake of an individual meets their requirement. In this approach, both the variability of the requirement and the day-to-day variability of nutrient intake within an individual (i.e., within-subject variability) are taken into account.

The new statistical approach is based on the following assumptions:

- The EAR is the best estimate of an individual's requirement.
- There is person-to-person variation in the requirements (i.e., between-subject variation), which can be described by the SD of the requirement estimate. Hence, the latter indicates how much the individual's requirement for a nutrient can deviate from the median requirement in the population. In the absence of data for the SD of the requirement estimate, IOM (2000c) has assumed a CV of 10% for most nutrients, with the exception of niacin, when a CV of 15% has been estimated. The SD is then calculated from the EAR and assumed CV, as noted earlier (Section 8.1.1).
- Mean reported intake of an individual is the best estimate of the usual intake of an individual.
- Day-to-day variation in intake for an individual exists and can be estimated by the within-subject standard deviation of intakes. Hence, the latter indicates how much the reported intake might deviate from usual intake.

Inferences about the adequacy of the nutrient intake of an individual can be made by examining the difference between the individual's reported intake (the best estimate of their usual intake) and the median requirement (i.e., the EAR or the best estimate of their requirement). The difference is then standardized by dividing by its standard deviation, which reflects uncertainty in both the estimated usual intake and the estimated requirement.

The result of this comparison is a Z-score, from which a probability value (p) reflecting the degree of confidence that the individual's usual intake meets their requirement can be determined. For example, when $Z = 0.50$, $p = 70\%$; when $Z = 1.0$, then $p = 85\%$, and when $Z = 2.0$, then $p = 98\%$ (Barr et al., 2002). To evaluate nutrient intakes for individuals in this way, consult IOM (2000c) for details of the equations and worked examples using

the EARs. A detailed review is also available in Barr et al. (2002) and Murphy and Poos (2002).

8.2.2 Using the AI

By definition, the AI is used for those nutrients for which there is insufficient available information to set an EAR and thus an RDA. Therefore, the approach described above cannot be used for nutrients with an AI. Instead, a statistically based hypothesis testing procedure can be used to compare an individual's intake to the AI. Details are given in IOM (2000c). Again, the procedure consists of a simple Z-test based on the within-subject standard deviation of daily intake of the nutrient of interest (Barr et al., 2002).

If the usual nutrient intake of an individual equals or exceeds the AI, the diet is almost certainly adequate in a given nutrient. In contrast, no evaluation can be made of the probability of an inadequate nutrient intake when the intake of the nutrient falls below the AI because the requirement is unknown. In such cases, the interpretation must rely solely on the judgment of nutrition professionals. In general, to eliminate the possibility of nutrient inadequacy, individuals should be encouraged to increase their nutrient intakes to meet the AIs (Barr et al., 2002; Murphy and Poos, 2002).

8.2.3 Using the UL

The UL can be used to determine whether the usual intake of an individual is so high that it poses a risk of adverse health effects. Another statistical test can be used to determine the level of confidence that the usual intake of an individual is below the UL; details of this test are also given in IOM (2000c). Whether the UL applies to the intake from supplements, fortificants, or medications or to the total intake from all sources depends on the nutrient (Barr et al., 2002; Murphy and Poos, 2002).

The statistical approaches outlined above cannot be used when the distribution of daily nutrient intakes for an individual is not nor-

---

Recommended Dietary Allowance (RDA)

If the intake ⩾**RDA** there is a high level of confidence that intake is adequate if observed over a large number of days

If the intake is between the **Estimated average requirement (EAR)** and the **RDA**, the intake probably needs to be improved because the probability of adequacy is less than 97.5%

If the intake ⩽**EAR**, then the intake very likely needs to be improved because the probability of adequacy is less than 50%

Adequate Intake (AI)

If the intake ⩾**AI**, then the mean intake is likely adequate if observed over a large number of days

If the intake < **AI**, then the adequacy of intake cannot be determined

Tolerable Upper Intake Level (UL)

If the intake ⩾**UL**, there is a potential risk of adverse effects if observed over a large number of days

If the intake < **UL**, the intake is likely safe if observed over a large number of days

---

Table 8.9: Guidelines for the qualitative interpretation of individual intakes. Compiled from IOM (2000c).

mal. Examples include those nutrients for which the within-subject CV of the intake is above 60%–70% (e.g., often folate, and vitamins A, B_{12}, C, and E, and possibly others). Likewise, the methods cannot be used when the distribution of requirements for a nutrient is skewed (e.g., iron requirements).

It is anticipated that, in the future, computer programs will be developed to perform the calculations described above. In the interim, a qualitative interpretation of individual intakes in relation to the EAR, RDA, AI, and UL can be made, using the guidelines given in Table 8.9. Hypothetical examples are given in Barr et al. (2002) and Murphy and Poos (2002).

8.3 Evaluating the nutrient intakes of population groups

Information is often required on the proportion of a group with usual intake of a nutrient below their own requirement. An estimate of the proportion of the group with an excessive usual nutrient intake is also important, as it exposes that portion of the group to the risk of adverse effects.

In the past, to assess the adequacy of nutrient intakes for groups, the intakes of members of the group have been compared directly with the RDA or equivalent. This approach is not appropriate and should not be used. By definition, the RDA or equivalent is set at an intake level that exceeds the requirements of 97%–98% of all individuals, as noted in Section 8.1.1. Hence, use of the RDA as a cutoff, to calculate the proportion of individuals in the group with inadequate intakes, results in a serious overestimate of the proportion at risk (Murphy and Poos, 2002).

Another approach used in the past to evaluate intakes of groups, has been to compare the mean nutrient intake of the group with the corresponding RDA (or equivalent) for that nutrient. When the mean nutrient intake was ⩾RDA, the diets of the group were considered adequate. Again, this approach should not be used because it is misleading. Even when the mean nutrient intake of a group equals the RDA, a proportion of persons in the group will still have usual intakes below the EAR because of the wide variation in nutrient intakes. Indeed, to ensure a low prevalence of intakes below the EAR, the mean nutrient intake of a group should exceed the RDA, often by a considerable amount. Moreover, to compare the adequacy of nutrient intakes of two groups, the prevalence of inadequate intakes should be determined, and not the mean intakes. The latter can be the same, despite different proportions with inadequate intakes in the two groups (Figure 8.6). This occurs when the intakes in one group are much more variable than in the other group (Murphy and Poos, 2002).

The recommended approach for evaluating the adequacy of nutrient intakes of population groups is to use the estimated average requirement (EAR). Two methods based on the EAR have been developed: the probability approach and the EAR cutpoint method; they are described below.

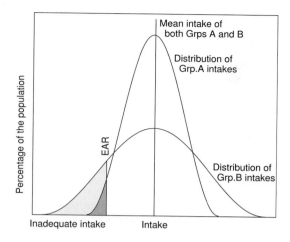

Figure 8.6: Groups A and B have the same mean intake, but the intakes of Group A are less varied. As a result many fewer subjects in Group A have intakes below the EAR (dark shaded area), relative to Group B (total shaded area on low-side of EAR).

8.3.1 Probability approach

The probability approach was first described by Beaton (1972); it combines the distributions of requirements and individual usual nutrient intakes for the group to estimate the proportion of individuals at risk for inadequate intakes. Normally, there is no information about the actual requirements of each individual and, as a result, the procedure does not identify with certainty which individuals are "at risk."

To adopt the probability approach for evaluating nutrient intakes, the following information is required:

- The EAR for each nutrient for the particular sex and life-stage group of individuals
- The distribution of requirements for each nutrient among similar individuals: for most nutrients, this is not precisely known; in the absence of such information, the distribution of requirements for most nutrients is assumed to be symmetrical (not necessarily normal) with a coefficient of variation of 10% (or 15% for niacin) about the EAR — a notable exception is the iron requirement distribution for menstruating women, which is positively skewed
- Reliable data on the distribution of *usual*

nutrient intakes for the group being assessed
- Knowledge of the expected correlation between intakes and requirements among individuals: for all nutrients (except energy), this is assumed to be very low.

Reliable information on the distribution of usual intakes of the nutrient in the group can be obtained by adjusting the distribution of observed intakes statistically in an attempt to partially remove the effects of day-to-day variability in intakes (i.e., within-subject variation) (Section 6.2.3). This yields an adjusted intake distribution, as discussed in detail in Section 3.3.2. Such an adjustment can be applied, provided at least two independent days or three consecutive days of dietary intake data for a representative subsample of individuals in the group, have been collected.

Figure 8.7 shows an example of observed (unadjusted) and adjusted zinc intakes for a group of Malawian women. The intakes were obtained from two independent 24-h recalls from each woman and adjusted to remove the effects of day-to-day (within-subject) variability in intake following the procedure outlined in Section 6.2.3. Note that the adjustment process has yielded a distribution with the same mean (6.6 mg/d) but reduced variability. Further, in this example, the number of women with adjusted intakes below the as-

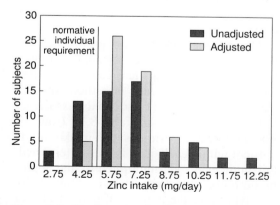

Figure 8.7: Unadjusted and adjusted zinc intakes of some rural Malawian women. From Gibson and Ferguson, American Journal of Clinical Nutrition 68: 430S–434S, 1998 © Am J Clin Nutr. American Society for Clinical Nutrition.

	Class 1	Class 2	Class 3	Class 4	Class 5	Class 6
A. Individual's intake in terms of the distribution of requirements	< −2 SD	−2 SD to −1 SD	−1 SD to mean	mean to +1 SD	+1 SD to +2 SD	> +2 SD
B. Probability that individual intake doesn't meet requirement	1.0	0.93	0.69	0.31	0.07	0.0

Table 8.10: Assignment of 'risk' or probability statements to six classes of observed intakes expressed as proportions of the Estimated Average Requirement. An assumption in this model is that the distribution of requirements for most nutrients is symmetrical with the coefficient of variation at 10% or 15%. Compiled from Beaton, American Journal of Clinical Nutrition 41: 155–164, 1985 © Am J Clin Nutr. American Society for Clinical Nutrition.

sumed normative EAR for zinc is markedly reduced, emphasizing that without the adjustment, the estimate obtained for the prevalence of inadequate zinc intakes would have been incorrect. This effect is also highlighted in Figures 3.3 and 6.1. Any bias arising from under- or overreporting of food intakes is not removed by this adjustment process.

In this statistical approach, a probability of inadequacy can be calculated for any level of usual intake because information on the distribution of requirements for the group is known. The risk of inadequate intakes associated with the usual intake of each individual in the group is determined first, followed by the average risk for the group as a whole. The latter is estimated as the weighted average of the risks to each individual, as outlined below (Barr et al., 2002).

The calculations for the probability approach can be performed manually or by a computer. For the manual calculation, first the nutrient intakes are classified into six classes defined by the EAR and the associated SD limits as shown in Table 8.10 (row A). The number of individuals with intakes of the nutrient within each class is then determined; this number is then multiplied by the appropriate probability for each class (Table 8.10, row B) to give the number of individuals per class who were likely to have intakes below their own requirements. The numerical probabilities are derived from the area beneath the "normal" curve between the stated SD lim-

its. The sum of these numbers gives the total number of individuals in the population group who are at risk of inadequate intakes for the nutrient. This sum can be expressed as a percentage of the total population group to give a probability estimate for the population group as a whole. For example, assume that in a population group of $n = 4600$, the numbers of individuals with usual intakes of vitamin C within classes one to six, respectively, are 300, 500, 800, 900, 1400, and 700. When multiplied by the appropriate probabilities for each class (Table 8.10, row B), the number of individuals per class likely to have vitamin C intakes below their own requirements becomes 300, 465, 552, 279, 98, and 0. The sum of these numbers equals 1694, and this represents the total number of individuals who are at risk of inadequate intakes for vitamin C. When expressed as a percentage, 37% of the total population are predicted to have intakes of vitamin C below their own requirements.

Alternatively, these calculations can be carried out using a function like PROBNORM in the statistical package SAS. The relevant equation to calculate the individual probability of inadequacy is:

$$1 - \mathrm{PROBNORM}((O_\mathrm{I} - \mathrm{EAR})/\mathrm{SD_R})$$

where O_I = observed intake of the individual, EAR = estimated average requirement of the group, and $\mathrm{SD_R}$ = standard deviation of the requirement.

The iron requirement curve for menstruating women is highly skewed because some women have high menstrual iron losses. As a result, the EAR and data on usual iron intakes for this group must be normalized before the probability approach is applied. Further details are given in Gibson and Ferguson (1999).

At present, the absence of reliable estimates of the EARs for all nutrients limits the general applicability of the probability approach to estimate the prevalence of inadequacy for every nutrient. Table 8.11 summarizes the nutrients for which an EAR and CV% of the requirement have been set by the U.S. Food and Nutrition Board (IOM, 2000c). In the United Kingdom, EARs have been documented for iron, calcium, zinc, vitamin C, vitamin B_{12}, folate, riboflavin, and vitamin A

Nutrient	EAR	RDA	AI	UL
Copper	✓	✓		✓
Iodine	✓	✓		✓
Magnesium	✓	✓		✓
Molybdenum	✓	✓		✓
Phosphorus	✓	✓		✓
Selenium	✓	✓		✓
Thiamin	✓	✓		
Riboflavin	✓	✓		
Niacin	✓	✓		✓
Vitamin B_6	✓	✓		✓
Folate	✓	✓		✓
Vitamin B_{12}	✓	✓		
Vitamin C	✓	✓		✓
Vitamin A	✓	✓		✓
Vitamin E	✓	✓		✓
Calcium			✓	✓
Fluoride			✓	✓
Sodium			✓	✓
Potassium			✓	
Biotin			✓	
Choline			✓	✓
Vitamin D			✓	✓
Pantothenic Acid			✓	

Table 8.11: List of nutrients with dietary reference intakes (DRIs) for the United States and Canada. The ✓ indicates that the specific DRI has been defined for that nutrient. EAR, Estimated Average Requirement; RDA, Recommended Dietary Allowance; AI, Adequate Intake; UL, Tolerable Upper Intake Level. Note that only the nutrients for which the RDA is defined meet the assumptions of the cutpoint method. From IOM (2000a; 2000b; 2001).

(COMA, 1991). The FAO/WHO (2002) report also provides EARs for selected nutrients.

In theory, the probability approach also could be applied to assess the proportion of the population potentially at risk of adverse health effects from excessive nutrient intakes, defined by the IOM (2000c) as exceeding the Tolerable Upper Intake level (UL) (Section 8.1.3). In practice, only some nutrients have a defined UL, as shown in Table 8.11. Uncertainty factors were used in the derivation of these ULs in an effort to reflect inaccuracies in the data on nutrient intakes and other sources of uncertainty. Examples of the latter include the dose–response data on adverse health effects and the severity of the adverse effects, extrapolation of data based on animal studies, and variation in individual susceptibility (Murphy et al., 2002). Details are given in IOM (1998).

8.3.2 EAR cutpoint method

A shortcut to the probability approach has been developed by Beaton (1994) for assessing the proportion of inadequate intakes in a group. This simpler version is termed the EAR cutpoint method and does not require information on the exact requirement distribution. The EAR cutpoint method can be used providing the following conditions are met:

- Intakes and requirements of the nutrient are independent (assumed to be true for all nutrients, but is not true for energy).
- The variance of the distribution of intakes in the population group is larger than the variance of their requirements (generally the case in free-living populations).
- The distribution of requirements in the group is symmetrical about the EAR (but this is not the case for the iron requirements of premenopausal women).

Again, data on the usual nutrient intakes are required, and these are best obtained by statistically adjusting the observed intakes for day-to-day variation (i.e., within-subject variation), as discussed in Section 3.3.2. In this simplified version, instead of estimating the risk of inadequacy for the intake level of each individual separately, the prevalence of inadequate intakes within the group is simply estimated by counting the number of individuals in the group with usual intakes below the EAR. This prevalence is represented by the shaded area to the left of the EAR under the curve showing the distribution of usual intakes, as shown in Figure 8.8. The larger area to the right of the EAR represents the majority with usual intakes above the EAR. Further theoretical justification for this approach can be found in Carriquiry (1999) and IOM (2000c).

This EAR cutpoint method is especially useful when the actual prevalence of inadequate intakes in the group is close to 50%. As the true prevalence approaches zero, or 100%, the performance of this method declines, even if the conditions listed above are met. Some examples of simulations used to assess the performance of the EAR cutpoint method in different situations are given in IOM (2000c).

Currently, the EAR cutpoint method based on the U.S Food and Nutrition Board DRIs can be applied to assess the prevalence of inadequate intakes among population subgroups for the following nutrients: copper, iodine, magnesium, molybdenum, phosphorus, selenium, zinc, thiamin, riboflavin, niacin, vitamin B_6, folate, vitamin B_{12}, vitamin C, vitamin A, and vitamin E (Table 8.11). As noted earlier the EAR cutpoint method cannot be used for assessing iron intakes for menstruating women because their distribution of iron requirements is skewed, although it can be used with this group for the other nutrients listed above. Moreover, in the model used by the U.S. Food and Nutrition Board, the iron requirements for all the life-stage and sex groups are skewed, so the probability approach is recommended for assessing iron intakes of all the groups (IOM, 2001).

8.3.3 Using 77% percent of the RDA as a cutoff value

In some tables of nutrient reference levels, estimated average requirements (i.e., EARs) for nutrients are not specified. In such cases, approximations for the estimated average requirements can be calculated, provided the RDAs or equivalent for each nutrient approximate the mean requirement estimate plus two standard deviations, with a specified coefficient of variation (NRC, 1986). The proportion of the population with *usual* intakes below the derived EAR is then calculated, as described in Section 8.3.2.

Use of 77% of the RDA as a cutoff value assumes a CV for the nutrient of 15% about the EAR. Such an assumption will yield a conservative estimate of nutrient inadequacy compared to that based on a CV for the nutrient of 10% about the EAR. Use of the latter CV corresponds to a cutoff of approximately 83% of the RDA instead of 77%, and hence will yield a larger percentage of the group likely to have inadequate intakes. Briefel et al. (2000) used 77% of the 1989 U.S. RDA values for zinc as a cutoff to evaluate the zinc intakes of the U.S. population in the National Health and Nutrition Examination Survey (NHANES) III, 1988–1994, prior to the release of the EAR for Zinc by the IOM (2001).

8.3.4 Use of AI for groups

Use of the AI for assessing the nutrient adequacy of groups is limited. It can only be

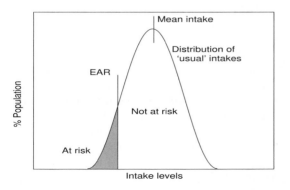

Figure 8.8: The estimated average requirement cutpoint method for estimating the proportion of individuals with intakes below the EAR.

Nutrient (mg)	Mean intake	Requirement	Inadequacy (%)	UL	Excessive intakes (%)
Thiamin	1.44	0.5 (EAR)	< 1	None set	Unknown
Magnesium	212	110 (EAR)	5	110	Unknown (supps. only)
Calcium	838	800 (AI)	Low	2500	< 1
Vitamin C	96	22 (EAR)	< 1%	650	< 1
Iron	14	10 (1989 RDA)	? No DRIs yet	? no DRIs yet	Unknown

Table 8.12: Evaluation of a hypothetical group's diet. Data for children 4–8 y, from 1994–1996 Continuing Survey of Food Intakes by Individuals. UL, Tolerable Upper Intake Level; EAR, Estimated Average Requirement; AI, Adequate Intake; RDA, Recommended Dietary Allowance; Inadequacy, percentage of intakes below the EAR; Excessive intakes, percentage of intakes above the UL. The intakes were adjusted to remove the effects of day-to-day variation before these assessments were made. From Murphy and Poos, Public Health Nutrition 5: 843–849, 2002, with permission of the authors.

used with confidence when the AI represents the mean or median intake of a group similar to that being evaluated. In such cases, mean intakes at or above the AI can be assumed to have a low prevalence of inadequate intakes (Table 8.8). It cannot be used in this way when other criteria have been used to set the AI. No assumptions can be made about the prevalence of inadequate intakes when the mean intake of a group falls below the AI (Barr et al., 2002; Murphy and Poos, 2002).

8.3.5 Use of UL for groups

When any comparison is made with the UL, it is important to note if the UL assessment for the nutrient of interest is based on information on usual daily intakes from all sources or only from supplements, fortificants, and medications. At present, because uncertainty factors have been used to set the ULs in an effort to take into account inaccuracies in all the sources of data used, the UL should be used only as a cutoff. In such cases, a low proportion of a group with intakes above the Ul is an appropriate goal (Barr et al., 2002; Murphy and Poos, 2002).

Table 8.12 provides an example of the use of all the approaches described above for assessing nutrient intakes of a group derived from a national nutrition survey. Further details are given in Murphy and Poos (2002).

8.3.6 WHO lower limits of safe ranges of population mean intakes

As discussed in Section 8.1.5, WHO (1996a) has established a safe range of population mean intakes for copper, zinc, and selenium. The lower limits are defined as the lowest population mean intake at which the population's risks of depletion remain acceptable when judged by normative criteria. The upper limits of the safe range of population mean intakes are defined by the maximum population group mean intake at which risks of toxicity remain tolerable.

WHO (1996a) set the lower limits at two standard deviations of intake above the corresponding average for the normative requirement estimates for individuals, as shown in Figure 8.5. Applying the lower limit as a cutoff, the expected prevalence of individuals with inadequate intakes in a group with a mean intake at the cutoff would be about 2%–3%, as shown in Figure 8.5. Table 8.13 provides an example of the lower limits of the safe ranges of population group mean intakes for copper and selenium based on the normative requirement estimates; those for zinc are given in WHO (1996a).

Theoretically, the upper limit of the safe range of the population mean intakes could be derived in a similar way such that only 2%–3% of individuals within the population

Age (y)	Sex	Wt (kg)	Copper (mg/d)	Selenium (μg/d)
0–0.25	M + F	5	0.33–0.55[a]	6
0.25–0.5	M + F	7	0.37–0.62[a]	9
0.5–1	M + F	9	0.60	12
1–3	M + F	12	0.56	20
3–6	M + F	17	0.57	24
6–10	M + F	25	0.75	25
10–12	F	37	0.77	30
12–15	F	48	1.00	30
15–18	F	55	1.15	30
18–60+	F	55	1.15	30
10–12	M	35	0.73	30
12–15	M	48	1.00	36
15–18	M	64	1.33	40
18–60+	M	65	1.35	40
Pregnancy			1.15[b]	39
Lactation			1.25	42–52[c]

Table 8.13: Lower limits of the safe ranges of population mean intakes of dietary copper and selenium, based on the normative requirement estimates. Unless otherwise specified, the CV of the usual dietary copper intakes is assumed to be 20%. It is assumed that 80% of dietary selenium is available and that the CV of the usual dietary intake of selenium is 16%. [a]For formula-fed infants only; CV of intake is assumed to be 12.5%. The bioavailability of copper is in the range 30%–50%. [b]From evidence of other species, it is assumed that the small increase in demand during pregnancy is met by an increased efficiency of copper absorption. [c]To meet requirements of milk-fed infants on the assumption that 80% of milk selenium is bioavailable and that the CV of milk selenium intake is 12.5%. From WHO (1996a) with permission.

subgroup would have intakes above the average threshold for toxicity.

8.4 Food-based dietary guidelines

Food-based dietary guidelines provide the consumer with a general description of a healthy dietary pattern. The guidelines give advice on the consumption of types of foods or food components for which there are diet-related public health issues specific to a country. The guidelines usually relate to the total diet. They are expressed in qualitative terms and are less technical and more easily understood than the nutrient recommendations discussed in Section 8.1. However, food-based dietary guidelines lack precision because recommendations such as "eat less of . . ." and "increase consumption of . . ." are interpreted differently by different individuals.

The first set of food-based dietary guidelines, termed "dietary goals" at that time, were developed in 1968 for the Nordic countries. They focused on replacing sources of "empty calories" with a variety of nutritious foods to enhance the nutrient density of Scandinavian diets. In the early 1970s, these were followed by dietary goals prepared by several other countries, including Australia, New Zealand, the Netherlands, the United Kingdom, West Germany, Canada, and the United States. These food-based dietary guidelines emphasized dietary modification to reduce the risk of coronary heart disease by decreasing the intake of total fat, restricting dietary cholesterol, and increasing the proportion of polyunsaturated fats (Truswell, 1989). Unfortunately, within some countries, multiple guidelines have since been published by different expert groups, some with conflicting advice, causing confusion among the public.

The aim of food-based dietary guidelines is to promote overall health, control specific nutritional diseases (whether they are induced by deficiency or excess), and reduce the risk of multifactorial diet-related diseases. Food-based dietary guidelines should be specific for a given ecological setting and appropriate in terms of the sociodemographic profile of the target groups, and they should take into account the customary dietary patterns within a country. Different guidelines within the same country may be required, depending on the target group. New Zealand, for example, has separate dietary guidelines for infants, children, and adolescents, whereas Australia has a report for children of all ages and another for persons over 65 y of age. India has two sets of dietary guidelines, one for the "relatively poor" majority and a second for affluent Indians. A detailed description of the food-based dietary guidelines for the

European Union member states is given in Williams et al. (1999).

8.4.1 Characteristics of food-based dietary guidelines

Food-based dietary guidelines should provide a framework for a healthy diet based on current nutrition research and dietary recommendations. Thus the guidance system needs a set a range of goals and objectives that are clearly defined. Food-based dietary guidelines should:

- Embrace the total diet, including all foods in daily meals and snacks
- Be based on foods commonly eaten by the population, and all types of foods should be accommodated
- List foods classified by food groups recognizable by consumers
- Describe food servings in terms of common household measures
- Permit the maximum flexibility in food choices to accommodate the many different eating styles within a country
- Be designed to accommodate most healthy persons > 2 y; as an alternative, separate guidelines for specific age and sex segments of the target population may be compiled
- Be evaluated to confirm that they meet the dietary recommendations for the country; use of current food consumption patterns and food composition data for the evaluation is essential
- Evolve to reflect new research and recommendations.

WHO (1996b) has developed a document on the preparation and use of food-based dietary guidelines in collaboration with FAO. The report focuses on the scientific basis for food-based dietary guidelines, along with their development, implementation, and evaluation. It also emphasizes that relationships between diet and disease of particular relevance to the country should determine the direction and relevance of food-based dietary guidelines. In a review of the dietary guidelines available in 1998, Truswell (1998) noted there was almost complete agreement on six recommendations:

- Eat a nutritionally adequate diet composed of a variety of foods.
- Eat less fat, particularly saturated fat.
- Adjust energy balance for body weight control — reduce energy intake, exercise more.
- Eat more whole grain cereals, vegetables, and fruits.
- Reduce salt intake.
- If you drink alcohol, do so in moderation.

A few food-based dietary guidelines specify the presence or absence of certain food-processing characteristics (e.g., whole grain, smoked, full cream, salt-cured, fresh) and sometimes eating behaviors (e.g., eat happily for a happy family life). Care must be taken to ensure that the food-based dietary guidelines are tested appropriately with the general public by using focus groups to determine the appropriateness and cultural acceptability of their content and visual presentation, followed by an in-depth evaluation of the consumer's understanding of the guidelines. Finally, the validity of the content should be carefully checked.

Several countries have produced graphic representations of their food-based dietary guidelines that aim to integrate essential food groups and dietary guidelines. Generally, the area (or volume) in these graphic representations represents the amount that should be consumed. Supplemental information on serving sizes, subgroups within food groups, and information about sources of fat and sugars in foods is often provided.

In some countries, food circles have been used with a varying number of sectors representing the food groups, sometimes each with a different area. These often range from the smallest for fats to the largest for the cereals and the vegetable and fruit groups. Other countries have used a pyramid that shows different groups on one face only (e.g., USDA's Food Guide Pyramid) or two faces (e.g., New Zealand Heart Foundation). Alternatively, a

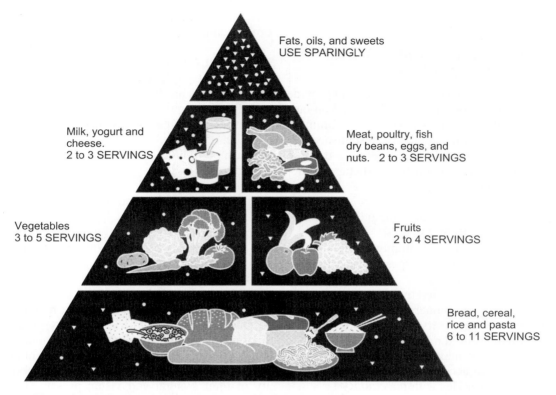

Figure 8.9: U.S. Food Guide Pyramid, a guide to daily food choices. From U.S. Department of Agriculture / U.S. Department of Health and Human Services (2000).

triangle (Sweden), a quarter rainbow (Canada's Food Guide), or a health food plate (U.K. Food Guide) have been used. An example of this type of graphic representation currently used by the USDA is shown in Figure 8.9. The figure depicts the U.S. Food Guide Pyramid (USDA, 1992), developed to assist the U.S. public to make healthy food choices.

These tools and strategies must be continuously revised as the science base evolves, lifestyles change, and to some extent, as the food supply changes. They must also be continuously evaluated to enhance understanding of how to communicate the messages more effectively to diverse audiences (Hogbin et al., 2002). The United States, for example, revised their dietary guidelines in 2000 (Table 8.14) and again in January, 2005. The new guidelines can be obtained from:

http:/www.healthierus.gov/dietaryguidelines/

8.4.2 Evaluating intakes using food-based dietary guidelines

Several indices based on food-based dietary guidelines have been developed to evaluate the overall quality of the diet. They generally combine food groups and nutrients, sometimes focusing only on certain components such as total fat or total saturated fat, cholesterol, and sodium; some examples are given below.

The Healthy Eating Index

The Healthy Eating Index (HEI) was developed from food-based dietary guidelines and data from the USDA 1989–1990 Continuing

Aim for fitness	Aim for a healthy weight. Be physically active each day.
Build a healthy base	Let the Pyramid guide your food choices. Choose a variety of grains daily, especially whole grains. Choose a variety of fruits and vegetables daily. Keep food safe to eat.
Choose sensibly	Choose a diet low in saturated fat and cholesterol and moderate in total fat. Choose beverages and foods to moderate your intake of sugars. Choose and prepare foods with less salt. If you drink alcoholic beverages, do so in moderation.

Table 8.14: ABC Dietary guidelines for Americans. From Home and Garden Bulletin No. 232, 2000, U.S. Government Printing Office, Washington, DC.

Survey of Food Intake by Individuals. This survey involved a 2-d food record and a 24-h dietary recall from 7500 individuals $\geqslant 2$ y. The HEI provides an overall picture of the type and quantity of foods consumed by an individual and their compliance with the dietary guidelines, by combining information on certain nutrients and food groups.

The index consists of 10 components, as shown in Table 8.15, each representing different aspects of a healthy diet. In components 1 to 5, scores are assigned for consumption of the suggested number of servings of each of the five food groups recommended in the USDA's Food Guide Pyramid: grains (bread, cereal, rice, and pasta), vegetables, fruits, milk (milk, yogurt, and cheese), and meat (meat, poultry, fish, dry beans, eggs, and nuts). Components 6 and 7 measure consumption of total fat and saturated fat respectively, as a percentage of total food energy intake, and components 8 and 9 measure intakes of total cholesterol and total sodium, respectively. Component 10 measures dietary variety. Each component of the HEI has a maximum score of 10 and a minimum score of zero, yielding a maximum of

100 for the combined scores of all components. Intermediate scores are computed proportionately and expressed as percentages. The HEI is thus computed as a continuous variable, facilitating statistical analysis. High component scores indicate intakes close to recommended ranges or amounts, whereas low component scores indicate less compliance with recommended ranges or amounts. USDA has assigned the following descriptors to HEI scores:

> Above 80: good diet
> 51–80: diet needs improvement
> Below 51: poor diet

Further details on computing the HEI scores are available in Kennedy et al. (1995) and Bowman et al. (1998).

The HEI tool has been used to evaluate the quality of the diets of U.S. children 2–9 y in 1989 and 1998, based on data from USDA's Continuing Survey of Food Intakes by Individuals. The overall HEI score for the diets of the children in both 1989 and 1998, was approximately 70, indicating that the diets "need improvement." As well, there were no differences in the scores for the individual components of the HEI scores for children's diets in 1989 and 1998. In 1998, however, the HEI scores varied with age: they were highest (74.4) for children aged 2 to 3 years and significantly lower (68.0) for children aged 7 to 9 years (Carlson et al., 2001).

The HEI has also been used to evaluate the quality of diets in NHANES III, using data from the 1999–2001 survey. Only 10% of the U.S. population had a good diet, 16% had a poor diet, and the remainder had a diet that needs improvement, based on the HEI. Several subgroups of the population were particularly at risk for lower quality diets. These were males aged 15–18 y, low-income groups, non-Hispanic Americans of African descent, and persons with less education (Basiotis et al., 2002).

Dubois et al. (2000) also used the HEI to evaluate the quality of the diets from the 1990 Canadian Quebec Nutrition Survey. In this study, the HEI was adjusted to the 1990

Component	Criteria for score of 10	Criteria for score of 0
Food group		
1. Grains	6–11 servings	0 servings
2. Vegetables	3–5 servings	0 servings
3. Fruits	2–4 servings	0 servings
4. Milk	2–3 servings	0 servings
5. Meat	2–3 servings	0 servings
Dietary guidelines		
6. Total fat	30% or less energy from fat	40% or greater energy from fat
7. Saturated fat	Less than 10% energy from saturated fat	15% or greater energy from saturated fat
8. Cholesterol	Less than 300 mg	Greater than or equal to 450 mg
9. Sodium	Less than 2400 mg	Greater than or equal to 4800 mg
10. Variety over 3-d period	16 different food items	6 or fewer different food items

Table 8.15: Components of the Healthy Eating Index. Persons with component scores between the maximum and minimum cutoff points are assigned scores proportionately. The optimal number of servings in the food group components depends on the recommended energy intakes. Three milk servings are required for pregnant and breast-feeding women and for teenagers and young adults up to age 24 years. Adapted from Kennedy et al., Journal of the American Dietetic Association 95: 1103–1108, 1995 © with permission of the American Dietetic Association.

Canadian nutrition recommendations (Health Canada, 1990).

Most recently, the HEI has been validated by using plasma biomarkers (Section 7.3). In a study by Hann et al. (2001), diets with a high HEI score correlated positively with plasma concentrations of several carotenoids and vitamin C, indicating that food choices based on the Food Guide Pyramid lead to a healthier diet. Nevertheless, elevated concentrations of these biomarkers do not necessarily indicate a reduced risk of disease. Confirmation is still required for the existence of a positive relationship between food intakes, plasma biomarkers, and disease outcomes. Up to now, only weak correlations between HEI scores and chronic disease risk (cardiovascular disease and cancer) have been reported (McCullough et al., 2000a, 2000b).

Healthy Diet Indicator

The Healthy Diet Indicator (HDI) is based on the dietary guidelines for the prevention of chronic diseases as defined by WHO (1996b). It consists of nine components depicted in Table 8.16 (Huijbregts et al., 1997). Total fat and total carbohydrate are not included in Table 8.16. Further modifications are the exclusion of salt because of the limitations of accurately determining salt intake from food consumption data, and the replacement of the free sugars component by mono- and disaccharides. The latter modification was recognized to lead to an overestimate of free sugars in countries where the intake of milk products and thus lactose is high (e.g., Finland).

When using the HDI, a dichotomous variable is generated for each food group or nutrient included in the nine WHO guidelines: individuals score one point if their diet meets the recommended criteria for each component and zero if it does not. The final score is based on the sum of all the scores for each of the nine components. Hence, using this model, a total of nine points indicates an excellent score.

Huijbregts et al. (1997) used this HDI to evaluate the relationship between dietary patterns and mortality in elderly men (50–70 y) in Finland, Italy, and the Netherlands, using dietary data based on dietary histories from

Nutrient or food group	Score	Criteria
1. Saturated fatty acids (% of energy intake)	0 1	> 10% 0%–10%
2. Polyunsaturated fatty acids (% of energy intake)	0 1	< 3% or > 7% 3%–7%
3. Protein (% of energy intake)	0 1	< 10% or > 15% 10%–15%
4. Complex carbohydrates (% of energy intake)	0 1	< 50% or > 70% 50%–70%
5. Dietary fiber (g)	0 1	< 27 or > 40 27–40
6. Fruit and vegetables (g)	0 1	< 400 ⩾ 400
7. Pulses, nuts & seeds (g)	0 1	< 30 ⩾ 30
8. Mono- and disaccharides (% of energy intake)	0 1	> 10% 0%–10%
9. Cholesterol (mg)	0 1	> 300 0–300

Table 8.16: The calculation of the Healthy Diet Indicator (HDI). Scores (0,1) are summed across the nine criteria. From Huijbregts et al., British Medical Journal 315: 13–17, 1997, with permission of the BMJ Publishing Group.

the 1969–1970 Seven Countries Study. They showed a significant inverse association of the HDI with all-cause mortality after a 20-y follow-up in all three countries. This relationship was even stronger when mortality from cardiovascular diseases alone was examined.

The HDI was also used by Dubois et al. (2000) to examine the quality of the diets in the Canadian 1990 Quebec Nutrition Survey. In this survey, 24-h recalls were conducted on a representative sample of males and females (n = 2103) 18–74 y in the province of Quebec. The HDI was adjusted in this study to the 1990 Canadian nutrition recommendations and then modified by replacing complex carbohydrates with total carbohydrates and omitting mono- and disaccharides. As a result, in this Canadian modification of the HDI, an excellent diet is represented by a total score of eight instead of nine points.

Diet Quality Index

The Diet Quality Index (DQI) is based on eight of the U.S. diet and health recommendations and is shown in Table 8.17. It incorporates an ad hoc weighting scheme in which the first and most important diet and health recommendation on dietary lipids is based on measures of three components (total fat, saturated fat, and dietary cholesterol), resulting in a weight of three. The carbohydrate recommendation is represented by two index

Recommendation	Score	Intake
1. Reduce total fat intake to 30% or less of energy	0 1 2	⩽ 30% 30%–40% > 40%
2. Reduce saturated fatty acid intake to less than 10% of energy	0 1 2	⩽ 10% 10%–13% > 13%
3. Reduce cholesterol intake to less than 300 mg daily	0 1 2	⩽ 300 mg 300–400 mg > 400 mg
4. Eat five or more servings daily of a combination of vegetables and fruits	0 1 2	5+ servings 3–4 servings 0–2 servings
5. Increase intake of starches and other complex carbohydrates by eating six or more servings daily of breads, cereals, and legumes	0 1 2	6+ servings 4–5 servings 0–3 servings
6. Maintain protein intake at moderate levels (i.e., less than twice the RDA)	0 1 2	⩽ 100% RDA 100%–150% RDA > 150% RDA
7. Limit total daily intake of sodium to 2400 mg or less	0 1 2	⩽ 2400 mg 2400–3400 mg > 3400 mg
8. Maintain adequate calcium intake (approximately RDA levels)	0 1 2	⩾ RDA 66%–100% RDA ⩽ 66% RDA

Table 8.17: Calculation of the Diet Quality Index (DQI). Scores (0, 1 or 2) are summed across the eight recommendations to develop a score for an individual. RDA, Recommended Dietary Allowance. From Patterson et al., Journal of the American Dietetic Association 94: 57–64, 1994 © with permission of the American Dietetic Association.

Index	Author(s)	Year	Validation
Nutrient-based indices examined for relation to nutrient intake			
Diet quality score	Hulshof et al.	1992	Dietary fat
Diet quality	Murphy et al.	1992	Nutrient adequacy, fat intake
Nutrient-based indices examined for relation to health outcome			
Nutrient adequacy ratio	Philipps and Johnson	1977	Pregnancy outcome
Diet clusters	Farchi et al.	1989	All-cause & cause-specific mortality
Food- and food-group-based indices examined for relation to nutrient intake and nutritional status			
Dietary score	Krebs-Smith and Clark	1989	Nutrient adequacy
Food group pattern score	Wolfe and Campbell	1993	Sociodemographic
Food- and food-group-based indices examined for relation to risk reduction and health outcome			
Dietary patterns	Randall et al.	1991	Health behaviours
Total diet diversity	Fernandez et al.	1996	Colorectal cancer
Nutrient and food- and food-group-based indices combined examined for relation to nutrient intake			
Diet quality index	Patterson et al.	1994	Nutrient adequacy, fat intake
Healthy eating index	Kennedy et al.	1995	Nutrient adequacy
Nutrient and food- and food-group-based indices combined examined for relation to health outcome			
Risk Score	Kune et al.	1987	Colorectal cancer

Table 8.18: Selected Indices of diet Quality. From Kant, Journal of the American Dietetic Association 96: 785–791, 1996 © with permission of the American Dietetic Association.

measures — numbers 4 and 5 — the fourth related to servings of fruits and vegetables and the fifth to servings of grains and legumes. For each of the diet and health recommendations related to protein, calcium, and sodium, only one index measure is used. The recommendations for use of supplements, alcohol usage, and fluoride intake, and those balancing food intake with physical activity to maintain an appropriate body weight, were excluded in the DQI (Patterson et al., 1994).

For each of these eight components, the cutoffs selected for the scaling correspond to the goals for the dietary intake recommended by the U.S. Committee on Diet and Health, plus an additional cutoff separating "poor" from "fair" diets, with the exception of the recommendation for dietary protein. For the latter, the RDA for protein was selected as the cutoff point, because the Diet and Health Committee recommendation emphasizes that protein intakes should be maintained at less than twice the RDA for protein or 1.6 g/kg body weight. Individuals who meet this goal are assigned a score of zero; those who do not meet the goal but have a fair diet are given one point; and those who have a poor diet are given two points. These points are then summed across the eight diet variables, resulting in an index score from zero (excellent diet) to 16 (poor diet).

Other indices of dietary quality

Other indices have also been used that are not based exclusively on the food-based dietary guidelines. In such cases, the definition of dietary quality varies, depending on the attributes selected by the investigator. These attributes can be classified into three main groups: those based on foods or food groups, those derived from nutrients only, and those based on a combination of nutrients and foods (Kant, 1996); some examples are shown in Table 8.18.

The choice of the most appropriate dietary quality index depends on the dietary assessment method, the needs of the population to be assessed, and the resources available for the data analysis. With increasing emphasis on reducing the risk of chronic diseases, indices of dietary quality are now being defined according to attributes of the diet associated with risk reduction. Examples include the following:

- A low-fat diet with high fruit, vegetable, and grain intake (Davenport et al., 1995)
- A low intake of energy-dense, nutrient-poor foods such as visible fats, nutritive sweeteners, sweetened beverages, desserts, and snacks (Kant, 2000)
- A relatively low-fat diet that meets energy and selected nutrient needs (Dixon et al., (2000)

Studies to validate dietary quality indices against biochemical, anthropometric, or clinical indices of nutritional status are limited (Kant, 2000). Some dietary quality indices have been examined in relation to health outcomes such as risk of all-cause mortality (Kant et al., 1993), heart disease (Miller et al., 1992), and cancer (McCann et al., 1994). In general, those indices of dietary quality based on a combination of food groups and selected nutrients have been related more strongly to disease risk than those based on individual nutrients or foods. More work is urgently required to validate indices of overall dietary quality against a variety of indices of nutritional status, as well as with health outcomes. A comprehensive review of indices that have been used to examine overall dietary quality in earlier studies is available in Kant (1996).

8.5 Summary

Both quantitative and qualitative methods are available for defining and evaluating the adequacy of a diet. In the quantitative approach, the diet is expressed in terms of nutrients per day and the nutrient adequacy evaluated by comparison with tables of nutrient reference levels. The latter are based on measurements of nutrient requirements of individuals from a specific sex and life-stage group. A nutrient requirement is defined as the lowest continuing intake level of a nutrient that will maintain a defined level of nutrient adequacy in an individual. The measurements of nutrient requirements generate a distribution of requirements that are valid for a specific sex and life-stage group. No single criterion exists to define the requirement estimates for all nutrients. In several countries (e.g., the United Kingdom and the United States), the criterion used is no longer based on its ability to correct or avoid a nutrient deficiency but on its ability to define optimal health and reduce risk of chronic disease. Hence, a range of criteria for each nutrient or life-stage group (or both) are often used to define nutrient requirements. Discrepancies exist among expert groups in different countries over the choice of these criteria.

Expert groups now define multiple levels of nutrient adequacy for different purposes, each associated with a defined level of nutrient adequacy. The multiple reference levels in the United Kingdom and the United States are collectively termed Dietary Reference Values (DRVs) and Dietary Reference Intakes (DRIs), respectively. They both define an Estimated Average Requirement (EAR) and a reference level set at two standard deviations (2 SDs) above the EAR, termed the Reference Nutrient Intake (RNI) in the United Kingdom and the Recommended Dietary Allowance (RDA) in the United States. In addition, the United Kingdom has defined a reference value at 2 SDs below the EAR, termed the Lower Reference Nutrient Intake (LRNI), whereas the United States has defined a Tolerable Upper Intake Level (UL). For nutrients for which an EAR cannot be defined, the United Kingdom has set a Safe Intake (SI) and the United States an Adequate Intake (AI). The Scientific Committee for Food of the European Community has also adopted three reference values for selected nutrients: the Average Requirement, the Population Reference Intake, and the Lowest Threshold Intake Level. For some nutrients, only an acceptable range of intakes is given. In the most recent FAO/WHO vitamin and mineral requirement estimates, four levels were defined: Requirement, Recommended Nutrient Intake, Upper Tolerable Nutrient Intake Level, and Protective Nutrient Intake. Again, for certain nutrients, only Acceptable Intakes are listed. All these reference levels are always set for a particular group of healthy individuals with specified characteristics, consuming a typical dietary pattern of the country over a reasonable period of time. They generally do not take into account possible interactions involving nutrients and other dietary components.

The requirements of energy are always defined as the energy intake estimated to meet the average requirement for a group of comparable individuals. Increasingly, estimated energy requirements are based on doubly labeled water measurements of energy expenditure. Expert groups in the United Kingdom, the United States, and FAO/WHO have also compiled dietary recommendations for total carbohydrate, protein, total fat, free sugars, saturated fatty acids, PUFAs, α-linoleic acid, α *trans* fatty acids, *n*-3 and *n*-6 PUFAs, and cholesterol, consistent with good health and for the prevention of diet-related chronic diseases. These macronutrient recommendations set by the United Kingdom and WHO apply to populations, but those set by the IOM for the United States and Canada apply to individuals.

Discrepancies among countries in the reference levels arise because of differences in the sources and interpretation of the nutrient requirement data, incomplete or nonexistent data for some nutrients and specific age groups, different life-stage groups, different criteria used to define the levels of nutrient adequacy, differences in judgment by the committees, and differences in the characteristics of the diets and, hence, bioavailability factors for certain nutrients among countries.

New methods have been developed by the U.S. Food and Nutrition Board to evaluate nutrient intakes of individuals, based on comparison of individual intakes with the EAR, AIs, and ULs. For population groups, probability analysis and the EAR cutpoint method can be used for selected nutrients, provided certain assumptions are met. Both methods assess more reliably the prevalence of inadequate intakes within a group. In cases

where the level of the EAR is not specified, but an RDA or equivalent is provided, then the mean nutrient requirement estimate can be calculated as 77% of the RDA or equivalent and the EAR cutpoint method applied, where appropriate. When using the WHO requirements for populations, the lower limit of the population mean estimates for normative requirement estimates for copper, selenium, and zinc can be applied.

The qualitative approach to evaluating the adequacy of a healthy diet is food-based, with guidelines that provide advice on the optimal mixture of locally available foods or food components for which there are diet-related public health issues specific to a country. In some countries, several sets of food-based dietary guidelines may exist, depending on the target group. WHO has developed guidelines on the preparation and use of food-based dietary guidelines. They must be tested appropriately, first with the general public to determine their appropriateness and cultural acceptability, then by an in-depth evaluation of their understanding by consumers. Finally, the validity of the content must be checked.

Several indices based on food-based dietary guidelines have been developed to evaluate the overall quality of the diet. These include the Healthy Eating Index (HEI) developed by USDA. This combines information on certain nutrients and food groups to provide an overall picture of the type and quantity of foods consumed by an individual and compliance with the dietary guidelines. The HEI has been validated by using plasma biomarkers. WHO has developed a Healthy Diet Indicator (HDI) based on the dietary guidelines for the prevention of chronic diseases. Relationships between scores for the HDI and mortality from all causes and from cardiovascular diseases alone have been reported. Finally, a Diet Quality Index (DQI) has been developed based on the U.S. Diet and Health Recommendations. Several other indices of diet quality are available, which vary according to the attributes under investigation. Some are based on foods or food groups, some are based on nutrients only, and some are based on a combination of nutrients and foods. Indices of the latter type are related most strongly to disease risk. More work is required to validate the indices of overall dietary quality.

References

Aggett PJ, Bresson J, Haschke F, Hernell O, Koletzko B, Lafeber HN, Michaelsen KF, Micheli J, Ormisson A, Rey J, Salazar de Sousa J, Weaver L. (1997). Recommended Dietary Allowances (RDAs), Recommended Dietary Intakes (RDIs), Recommended Nutrient Intakes (RNIs), and Population Reference Intakes (PRIs) are not "Recommended Intakes." Journal of Pediatric Gastroenterology and Nutrition 25: 236–241.

Anonymous. (1993). Proposed nutrient and energy intakes for the European Community: a report of the scientific committee for food of the European Community. Nutrition Reviews 51: 209–212.

Anonymous. (1997a). Origin and framework of the development of Dietary Reference Intakes. Nutrition Reviews 55: 332–334.

Anonymous. (1997b) A model for the development of tolerable upper intake levels. Nutrition Reviews 55: 342–351.

Barr SI, Murphy SP, Poos MI. (2002). Interpreting and using the Dietary Reference Intakes in dietary assessment of individuals and groups. Journal of the American Dietetic Association 102: 780–788.

Barr SI, Murphy SP, Agurs-Collins TD, Poos MI. (2003). Planning diets for individuals using the dietary reference intakes. Nutrition Reviews 61: 352–360.

Basiotis PP, Carlson A, Gerriror SA, Juan WY, Lino M. (2002). The Healthy Eating Index: 1999–2000. CNPP-12. U.S. Department of Agriculture, Center for Nutrition and Promotion, Washington, DC. www.cnpp.usda.gov.

Beaton GH. (1972). The use of nutritional requirements and allowances. In: Proceedings of Western Hemisphere Nutrition Congress II. Futura Publishing Co., Mt. Kisco, NY, pp. 356–363.

Beaton GH. (1985). Uses and limits of the use of the Recommended Dietary Allowances for evaluating dietary intake data. American Journal of Clinical Nutrition 41: 155–164.

Beaton GH. (1994). Criteria of an adequate diet. In: Shils ME, Olson JA, Shike M (eds.) Modern Nutrition in Health and Disease, 8th ed. Lea & Febiger, Philadelphia. pp. 1491–1505.

Beaton GH. (1998). What nutrient values should be estimated and why. In: Fitzpatrick DW, Anderson JE, L'Abbé ML (eds.) Proceedings of the 16th International Congress of Nutrition. Canadian Federation of Biological Societies, Ottawa, pp. 164–167.

Bowman SA, Lino M, Gerrior SA, Basiotis PP. (1998). The Healthy Eating Index: 1994–96. CNPP-5, U.S. Department of Agriculture, Center for Nutrition Policy and Promotion, Washington, DC.

Briefel RR, Bialostosky K, Kennedy-Stephenson J, McDowell MA, Ervin RB, Wright JD. (2000). Zinc intake of the U.S. population: findings from the third National Health and Nutrition Examination Survey, 1988–1994. Journal of Nutrition 130: 1367S–1373S.

Butte NF. (1996). Energy requirements of infants. European Journal of Clinical Nutrition 50(Suppl.1): S24–S36.

Butte NF, Wong WW, Hopkinson JM, Heinz CJ, Mehta NR, Smith EO. (2000). Energy requirements derived from total energy expenditure and energy deposition during the first 2 y of life. American Journal of Clinical Nutrition 72: 1558–1569.

Canadian Council on Nutrition. (1940). The Canadian Dietary Standard. National Health Review 8: 1–9.

Carlson A, Lino M, Gerrior S, Basiotis PP. (2001). Report card on the diet quality of children ages 2 to 9. Nutrition Insight 25. Center for Nutrition Policy and Promotion, USDA, Washington, DC. www.cnpp.usda.gov.

Carriquiry AL. (1999). Assessing the prevalence of nutrient inadequacy. Public Health Nutrition 2: 23–33.

CEC (Commission of the European Communities) (1993). Nutrient and Energy Intakes for the European Community. Reports of the Scientific Committee for Food, Thirty-first series. Office for Official Publications of the European Communities, Luxembourg.

COMA (Committee on Medical Aspects of Food Policy). (1991). Dietary reference values for food energy and nutrients for the United Kingdom. Report of the panel on Dietary Reference Values. Report on Health and Social Subjects No. 41. Her Majesty's Stationery Office, London.

COMA (Committee on Medical Aspects of Food Policy). (1994). Nutritional Aspects of Cardiovascular Disease. Report on Health and Social Subjects No. 46. Her Majesty's Stationery Office, London.

COMA (Committee on Medical Aspects of Food Policy). (1998). Nutritional Aspects of the Development of Cancer. Report on Health and Social Subjects No. 48. The Stationery Office, London.

Davenport M, Roderick P, Elliott L, Victor C, Geissler C. (1995). Monitoring dietary change in populations and the need for specific food targets: lessons from the North West Thames Regional Health Survey. Journal of Human Nutrition and Dietetics 8: 119–128.

Dixon LB, Sundquist J, Winkleby M. (2000). Differences in energy, nutrient, and food intakes in a U.S. sample of Mexican-American women and men: findings from the Third National Health and Nutrition Examination Survey, 1988–1994. American Journal of Epidemiology 152: 548–557.

Dubois L, Girard M, Bergeron N. (2000). The choice of a diet quality indicator to evaluate the nutritional health of populations. Public Health Nutrition 3: 357–365.

EVM (Expert Group on Vitamins and Minerals).(2003). Safe Upper Levels for Vitamins and Minerals. Food Standards Agency, The Stationery Office, London.

FAO/WHO (Food and Agriculture Organization / World Health Organization). (1988). Requirements of Vitamin A, Iron, Folate and Vitamin B_{12}. FAO Food and Nutrition Series No. 23. FAO, Rome.

FAO/WHO (Food and Agriculture Organization / World Health Organization). (2002). Human Vitamin and Mineral Requirements. Food and Nutrition Division, FAO, Rome.

FAO/WHO/UNU (Food and Agriculture Organization / World Health Organization / United Nations University). (1985). Energy and Protein Requirements. WHO Technical Report Series No. 274. WHO, Geneva.

Farchi G, Mariotti S, Menotti A, Seccareccia F, Torsello S, Fidanza F. (1989). Diet and 20-y mortality in two rural population groups of middle-aged men in Italy. American Journal of Clinical Nutrition 50: 1095–1103.

Fernandez E, D'Avanzo B, Negri E, Franceschi S, La Vecchia C. (1996). Diet diversity and the risk of colorectal cancer in northern Italy. Cancer Epidemiology Biomarkers and Prevention 5: 433–436.

Food and Nutrition Board. (1943). Recommended Dietary Allowances. Reprint and Circular Series No. 115, National Academy of Sciences, National Research Council, Washington, DC.

Gibson RS, Ferguson EL. (1998). Assessment of dietary zinc in a population. American Journal of Clinical Nutrition (Suppl)68: 430S–434S.

Gibson RS, Ferguson EL. (1999). An interactive 24-hour recall for assessing the adequacy of iron and zinc intakes in developing countries. International Life Sciences Institute Press, Washington, DC.

Hann CS, Rock CL, King I, Drewnowski A. (2001). Validation of the Healthy Eating Index with use of plasma biomarkers in a clinical sample of women. American Journal of Clinical Nutrition 74: 479–486.

Health and Welfare, Canada. (1983). Recommended Nutrient Intakes for Canadians. Compiled by the Committee for the Revision of the Dietary Standard for Canada. Bureau of Nutritional Sciences, Food Directorate, Health Protection Branch, Department of National Health and Welfare. Canadian Government Publishing Centre, Ottawa.

Health Canada. (1990). Nutrition Recommendations: Report of the Scientific Review Committee. Minister of Supplies and Services Canada, Ottawa.

Hogbin M, Lyon J, Davis C. (2002). Comparison of dietary recommendations using the Dietary Guidelines for Americans as a framework. Nutrition Today 38: 204–217.

Hoolihan LE. (2003). Individualization of nutrition recommendations and food choices. Nutrition Today 38: 225–231.

Huijbregts P, Feskens E, Rasanen L, Fidanza F, Nissinen A, Menotti A, Kromhout D. (1997). Dietary pattern and 20 year mortality in elderly men in Finland, Italy, and the Netherlands: longitudinal cohort study. British Medical Journal 315: 13–17.

Hulshof KF, Wedel M, Lowik MR, Kok FJ, Kistemaker C, Hermus RJ, ten Hoor F, Ockhuizen T. (1992). Clustering of dietary variables and other lifestyle factors (Dutch Nutritional Surveillance System). Journal of Epidemiology and Community Health 46: 417–424.

IOM (Institute of Medicine). (1997). Dietary Reference Intakes for Calcium, Phosphorus, Magnesium, Vitamin D, and Fluoride. National Academy Press, Washington, DC.

IOM (Institute of Medicine). (1998). Dietary Reference Intakes: A Risk Assessment Model for Establishing Upper Intake Levels for Nutrients. National Academy Press, Washington, DC.

IOM (Institute of Medicine). (2000a). Dietary Reference Intakes for Vitamin C, Vitamin E, Selenium and Carotenoids. National Academy Press, Washington, DC.

IOM (Institute of Medicine). (2000b). Dietary Reference Intakes for Thiamin, Riboflavin, Niacin, Vitamin B_6, Folate, Vitamin B_{12}, Pantothenic Acid, Biotin, and Choline. National Academy Press, Washington, DC.

IOM (Institute of Medicine). (2000c). Dietary Reference Intakes: Applications in Dietary Assessment. National Academy Press, Washington, DC.

IOM (Institute of Medicine). (2001). Dietary Reference Intakes for Vitamin A, Vitamin K, Arsenic, Boron, Chromium, Copper, Iodine, Iron, Manganese, Molybdenum, Nickel, Silicon, Vanadium, and Zinc. National Academy Press, Washington, DC.

IOM (Institute of Medicine). (2002). Dietary Reference Intakes for Energy, Carbohydrate, Fiber, Fat, Fatty Acids, Cholesterol, Protein, and Amino Acids (Macronutrients). National Academy Press, Washington, DC.

Kant AK. (1996). Indexes of overall diet quality: a review. Journal of the American Dietetic Association 96: 785–791.

Kant AK. (2000). Consumption of energy-dense, nutrient-poor foods by adult Americans: nutritional and health implications. The third National Health and Nutrition Examination Survey, 1988–1994. American Journal of Clinical Nutrition 72: 929–936.

Kant AK, Schatzkin A, Harris TB, Ziegler RG, Block G. (1993). Dietary diversity and subsequent mortality in the First National Health and Nutrition Examination Survey Epidemiologic Follow-up Study. American Journal of Clinical Nutrition 57: 434–440.

Kennedy ET, Ohls J, Carlson S, Fleming K. (1995). The Healthy Eating Index: design and applications. Journal of the American Dietetic Association 95: 1103–1108.

King J. (1998). From experiment to reality: accounting for body size, dietary patterns, and environmental factors. In: Fitzpatrick DW, Anderson JE, L'Abbé ML (eds.) Proceedings of the 16th International

Congress of Nutrition. Canadian Federation of Biological Societies, Ottawa, pp. 161–163.

Krebs-Smith SM, Clark LD. (1989). Validation of a nutrient adequacy score for use with women and children. Journal of the American Dietetic Association 89: 775–783.

Kune S, Kune GA, Watson LF. (1987). Case-control study of dietary etiological factors: the Melbourne Colorectal Cancer Study. Nutrition and Cancer 9: 21–42.

Lachance PA. (1998). Overview of key nutrients: micronutrient aspects. Nutrition Reviews 56: S34–S39.

League of Nations. (1938). Report by the Technical Commission on Nutrition as the work of its third session. Bulletin of the League of Nations Health Organization 7: 461–492.

Lukaski HC, Penland JG. (1996). Functional changes appropriate for determining mineral element requirements. Journal of Nutrition 126: 2354S–2364S.

McCann SE, Randall E, Marshall JR, Graham S, Zielezny M, Freudenheim JL. (1994). Diet diversity and the risk of colon cancer in western New York. Nutrition and Cancer 21: 133–141.

McCullough ML, Feskanich D, Stampfer MJ, Rosner BA, Hu FB, Hunter DJ, Variyam JN, Colditz GA, Willet WC. (2000a). Adherence to the Dietary Guidelines for Americans and risk of major chronic disease in women. American Journal of Clinical Nutrition 72: 1214–1222.

McCullough ML, Feskanich D, Rimm EB, Giovannucci EL, Ascherio A, Variyam JN, Spiegelman D, Stampfer MJ, Willet WC. (2000b). Adherence to the Dietary Guidelines for Americans and risk of major chronic disease in men. American Journal of Clinical Nutrition 72: 1223–1231.

Miller WL, Crabtree BF, Evans DK. (1992). Exploratory study of the relationship between hypertension and diet diversity among Saba Islanders. Public Health Reports 107: 426–432.

Murphy SP, Poos MI. (2002). Dietary reference intakes: summary of applications in dietary assessment. Public Health Nutrition 5: 843–849.

Murphy SP, Rose D, Hudes M, Viteri FE. (1992). Demographic and economic factors associated with dietary quality for adults in the 1987–88 Nationwide Food Consumption Survey. Journal of the American Dietetic Association 92: 1352–1357.

NRC (National Research Council). (1986). Nutrient Adequacy: Assessment using Food Consumption Surveys. National Academy Press, Washington, DC.

Patterson RE, Haines PS, Popkin BM. (1994). Diet quality index: capturing a multidimensional behavior. Journal of the American Dietetic Association 94: 57–64.

Philipps C, Johnson NE. (1977). The impact of quality of diet and other factors on birth weight of infants. American Journal of Clinical Nutrition 30: 215–225.

Prentice AM, Lucas A, Vasquez-Velasquez L, Davies PS, Whitehead RG. (1988). Are current dietary guidelines for young children a prescritpion for overfeeding? Lancet

Prentice A, Branca F, Decsi T, Michaelson KF, Fletcher RJ, Guesry P, Manz F, Vidailhet M, Pannemans D, Samartin S. (2004). Energy and nutrient dietary reference values for children in Europe: methological approaches and current nutritional recommendations. British Journal of Nutrition 92: S83–S146.

Randall E, Marshall JR, Graham S, Brasure J. (1991). High-risk health behaviors associated with various dietary patterns. Nutrition and Cancer 16: 135–151.

Raper NR, Rosenthal JC, Woteki CE. (1984). Estimates of available iron in diets of individuals 1 year old and older in the Nationwide Food Consumption Survey. Journal of the American Dietetic Association 84: 783–787.

Schofield WN. (1985). Predicting basal metabolic rate: new standards and review of previous work. Human Nutrition Clinical Nutrition 39C(Suppl. 1): 5–41.

Spaaij CJK, Pijls LTJ. (2004). New dietary reference intakes in the Netherlands for energy, proteins, fats and digestible carbohydrates. European Journal of Clinical Nutrition 58: 191–194.

Trichopoulou A, Vassilakou T. (1990). Recommended dietary intakes in the European community member states: an overview. European Journal of Clinical Nutrition 44(Suppl. 2): 51–125.

Truswell AS. (1989). Dietary goals and guidelines in affluent countries. In: Latham MC, van Veen MS (eds.) Proceedings of an International Conference on Dietary Guidelines. International Nutrition Monograph Series No. 21. Cornell University, Ithaca, NY, pp. 9–27.

Truswell AS. (1998). Nutrition recommendations for the general population. In: Mann J, Truswell AS (eds.) Essentials of Human Nutrition. Oxford University Press, Oxford, pp. 523–537.

Truswell AS, Dreosti IE, English RM, Rutishauser IHE, Palmer N. (1990). Recommended Nutrient Intakes. Australian Papers. Australian Professional Publications, Sydney.

Turnland JR. (1994). Future directions for establishing mineral/trace element requirements. Journal of Nutrition 124: 1765S–1770S.

USDA (U.S. Department of Agriculture). (1992). The Food Guide Pyramid. Home and Garden Bulletin No. 252. U.S. Government Printing Office, Washington, DC.

USDA (U.S. Department of Agriculture) and U.S. Department of Health and Human Services. (2000). Dietary Guidelines for Americans. 5th ed. Home and Garden Bulletin No. 232. U.S. Government Printing Office, Washington, DC.

WHO (World Health Organization). (1996a). Trace Elements in Human Nutrition and Health. World Health Organization, Geneva.

WHO (World Health Organization). (1996b). Preparation and Use of Food-based Dietary Guidelines: Report of a Joint FAO/WHO Consultation, Nicosia,

Cyprus. Technical Report Series No. 880. World Health Organization, Geneva.

WHO (World Health Organization). (2003). Nutrition and the Prevention of Chronic Diseases. Report of a Joint WHO/FAO Expert Consultation. Technical Report Series No. 916. World Health Organization, Geneva.

Williams C, Wiseman M, Buttris J. (1999). Food-based dietary guidelines: a staged approach. British Jour-

nal of Nutrition 81(Suppl. 2): S31–S153.

Wolfe WS, Campbell CC. (1993). Food pattern, diet quality, and related characteristics of school children in New York State. Journal of the American Dietetic Association 93: 1280–1284.

Yates AA. (1998). Process and development of dietary reference intakes: basis, need, and application of recommended dietary allowances. Nutrition Reviews 56: S5–S9.

9

Anthropometric assessment

The term "nutritional anthropometry" first appeared in "Body Measurements and Human Nutrition" (Brožek, 1956) and was later defined by Jelliffe (1966) as

> measurements of the variations of the physical dimensions and the gross composition of the human body at different age levels and degrees of nutrition.

Subsequently, a number of publications made recommendations on specific body measurements for characterizing nutritional status, standardized measurement techniques, and suitable reference data (Jelliffe, 1966; WHO, 1968; Weiner and Lourie, 1969). Today, anthropometric measurements are widely used in the assessment of nutritional status, at both the individual and population levels. One of their main advantages is that anthropometric measurements may be related to past exposures, to present processes, or to future events (WHO, 1995).

For individuals in low-income countries, anthropometry is particularly useful when there is a chronic imbalance between intakes of protein and energy. Such disturbances modify the patterns of physical growth and the relative proportions of body tissues such as fat, muscle, and total body water. Anthropometry is also used in clinical settings in developed countries to diagnose both failure to thrive and overweight in children. At the population level, anthropometry has an important role in targeting interventions through screening, in assessing the response to interventions, in identifying the determinants and

consequences of malnutrition, and in conducting nutritional surveillance.

Anthropometric measurements are of two types. One group of measurements assesses body size (Section 10.1), the other group determines body composition. Measurements in the latter group can be further subdivided into measurements of body fat (Section 11.1) and the fat-free mass (Section 11.2), the two major components of body mass.

Anthropometric indices are derived from combinations of raw measurements. Examples include weight-for-age, sum of triceps and subscapular skinfolds, and waist–hip circumference ratio. Indices are essential for the interpretation of measurements. The combination of triceps skinfold and mid-upper-arm circumference can be used to estimate the mid-upper-arm muscle area and mid-upper-arm fat area, surrogates for the muscle mass and total body fat content of the body, respectively. Other combinations, such as the body mass index (wt/ht^2) and the waist–hip circumference ratio, are used in population studies as indicators of obesity and intra-abdominal fat mass, respectively.

An alternative approach involves using anthropometric measurements or indices in regression equations to predict body density and to calculate body fat and the fat-free mass (Section 11.1.5). However, most of these prediction equations were developed on young, healthy, lean Caucasian population groups and, hence, are less appropriate for malnourished, obese, or elderly subjects or for other ethnic and racial groups.

The selection of anthropometric indices for nutritional assessment systems depends on the factors discussed in detail in Section 1.4. Consideration of the sensitivity, specificity, and predictive value of anthropometric indices is especially critical. Sensitive indices exhibit large changes during nutritional deprivation and after a nutritional intervention and correctly identify those individuals who are truly malnourished. Consequently, anthropometric indices with high sensitivity should be selected for nutritional assessment systems involving screening, surveillance, or an intervention (Ruel et al., 1995). Anthropometric indices with high specificity are desirable to identify healthy persons correctly and thereby avoid unnecessary nutritional intervention. Both the sensitivity and specificity of an anthropometric index will vary according to the age of the subjects, the cutoff point used, and the severity and prevalence of the nutritional problem in the population, as discussed in Section 1.5. All these factors must be considered when selecting an anthropometric index.

9.1 Advantages and limitations of anthropometric assessment

Anthropometric measurements are of increasing importance in nutritional assessment as they have many advantages (Box 9.1). However, anthropometric measures are relatively insensitive and cannot detect disturbances in nutritional status over short periods of time. Furthermore, nutritional anthropometry cannot identify any specific nutrient deficiency and, therefore, is unable to distinguish disturbances in growth and body composition induced by nutrient deficiencies (e.g., zinc) from those caused by imbalances in protein and energy intake. Nevertheless, nutritional anthropometry can be used to monitor changes in both growth and body composition in individuals (e.g., hospital patients) and in population groups, provided sources of measurement error and the effects of confounding factors are minimized (Ulijaszek and Kerr, 1999).

Certain non-nutritional factors (such as disease, genetic influences, diurnal variation, and reduced energy expenditure) can lower the specificity and sensitivity of anthropometric measurements (Section 1.4), although such effects generally can be excluded or taken into account by appropriate sampling and experimental design.

9.2 Errors in anthropometry

Errors can occur in nutritional anthropometry which may affect the precision, accuracy, and validity of the measurements and indicators. Three major sources of error are significant: measurement errors, alterations in the composition and physical properties of certain tissues, and the use of invalid assumptions in the derivation of body composition from anthropometric measurements (Heymsfield and Casper, 1987).

Both random and systematic measurement errors may occur in nutritional anthropometry, and they have been extensively reviewed by Ulijaszek and Kerr (1999). Random errors limit precision or the extent to which repeated

---

Simple, safe, noninvasive techniques are involved, which can be used at the bedside of a single patient, but are also applicable to large sample sizes.

Inexpensive equipment is required. It is portable, and durable and can be made or purchased locally.

Relatively unskilled personnel can perform the measurement procedures.

Methods can be precise and accurate, if standardized techniques and trained personnel are used.

Retrospective information is generated on past long-term nutritional history, which cannot be obtained with equal confidence using other techniques.

Mild to moderate undernutrition, as well as severe states of under- or overnutrition, can be identified.

Changes in nutritional status over time and from one generation to the next, a phenomenon known as the secular trend, can be evaluated.

Screening tests that identify individuals at high risk to under- or overnutrition can be devised.

Box 9.1: The advantages of anthropometric measurements in nutritional assessment.

Measurements and common error	Proposed solution
All measurements	
Inadequate instrument	Select method appropriate to resources
Restless child	Postpone measurement or involve parent in procedure or use culturally appropriate procedures
Reading	Training and refresher exercises stressing accuracy and intermittent revision by supervisor
Recording	Record results immediately after measurement and have results checked by second person
Length	
Incorrect method for age	Use only when subject is $< 2\,y$
Footwear/headwear not removed	Remove as local culture permits (or make allowances)
Head not in correct plane	Correct position of child before measuring
Child not straight along board and/or feet not parallel with movable board	Have assistant and child's parent present; don't take the measurement while the child is struggling; settle child
Board not firmly against heels	Correct pressure should be practiced
Height	
Incorrect method for age	Use only when subject is $\geq 2\,y$
Footwear/headware not removed	Remove as local culture permits (or make allowances)
Head not in correct plane, subject not straight, knees bent, or feet not flat on floor	Correct technique with practice and retraining; provide adequate assistance; calm noncooperative children
Board not firmly against head	Move head board to compress hair
Weight	
Room cold, no privacy	Use appropriate clinic facilities
Scale not calibrated to zero	Re-calibrate after every subject
Subject wearing heavy clothing	Remove or make allowances for clothing
Subject moving or anxious as a result of prior incident	Wait until subject is calm or remove the cause of anxiety (e.g., scale too high)

Table 9.1: Common errors and possible solutions when measuring length, height, and weight. From Zerfas AJ (1979) In Jelliffe DB, Jelliffe EFP (eds.), Human Nutrition: A Comprehensive Treatise. Volume 2: Nutrition and Growth. Plenum Press, New York.

measurements give the same value. Systematic measurement errors affect accuracy or the degree to which the measurements depart from "true" values (Section 1.4.8). Measurement errors arise from examiner error resulting from inadequate training, instrument error, and difficulties in making the measurement (e.g., skinfold thicknesses). The major sources of measurement error in anthropometry are shown in Tables 9.1 and 9.2.

9.2.1 Random measurement errors and precision

Random measurement errors can be minimized by training personnel to use standardized techniques and precise, correctly calibrated instruments (Lohman et al., 1988). Furthermore, the precision (and accuracy)

of each measurement technique should be firmly established prior to use. To improve precision, multiple measurements on each individual should be completed.

Poor precision often reflects within-examiner error, but between-examiner error may be significant in surveys with multiple examiners. The precision of a measurement technique can be assessed by calculating

- Technical error of the measurement (TEM)
- Percentage technical error (%TEM)
- Coefficient of reliability (R)

These parameters can be calculated for each anthropometric measurement technique from repeated measurements on each subject made within a few minutes to avoid physiological fluctuations. A minimum of 10 subjects is recommended.

Measurements and common error	Proposed solution
Arm circumference	
Subject not standing in correct position	Position subject correctly
Tape too thick, stretched, or creased	Use correct instrument
Wrong arm	Use left arm
Mid-arm point incorrectly marked	Measure midpoint carefully
Arm not hanging loosely by side during measurement, examiner not comfortable or level with subject, tape around arm not at midpoint: too tight (causing skin contour indentation), too loose	Correct techniques with training, supervision, and regular refresher courses; take into account any cultural problems, such as wearing of arm band
Head circumference	
Occipital protuberance / supraorbital landmarks poorly defined	Position tape correctly
Hair crushed inadequately, ears under tape, or tension position poorly maintained at time of reading	Correct technique with training, supervision, and regular refresher courses
Headwear not removed	Remove as local culture permits
Triceps fatfold	
Wrong arm	Use left arm
Mid-arm point or posterior plane incorrectly measured or marked	Measure midpoint carefully
Arm not loose by side during measurement	
Finger-thumb pinch or caliper placement too deep (muscle) or too superficial (skin)	Correct technique with training, supervision, and regular refresher courses and workshops
Caliper jaws not at marked site; reading done too early, pinch not maintained, caliper handle not released	
Examiner not comfortable or level with subject	Ensure examiner is correctly positioned

Table 9.2: Common errors and possible solutions when measuring mid-upper-arm circumference, head circumference, and triceps skinfold. From Zerfas AJ (1979) In Jelliffe DB, Jelliffe EFP (eds.), Human Nutrition: A Comprehensive Treatise. Volume 2: Nutrition and Growth. Plenum Press, New York.

Technical error of the measurement

The square root of the measurement error variance is known as the technical error of the measurement (TEM). It is expressed in the same units as that of the anthropometric measurement under study. Technical error of the measurement is age dependent, and the value is also related to the anthropometric characteristics of the study group. The calculation varies according to the number of replicate measurements made. For one examiner making two measurements,

$$\text{TEM} = \sqrt{(\Sigma D^2)/2N}$$

where D = the difference between two measurements and N = number of subjects. For more than two measurements, the equation is more complex, and TEM =

$$\sqrt{\Sigma_1^N [(\Sigma_1^K M^2) - ((\Sigma_1^K M)^2/K)] / [N(K-1)]}$$

where N = number of subjects, K is the number of determinations of the variable taken on each subject, and M_n is the nth replicate of the measurement, where n varies from 1 to K. Table 9.3 shows the calculation of TEM from measurements of stature performed four times on 10 subjects by a single anthropometrist.

Note that the size of the measurement also influences the size of the associated TEM, so that comparisons of precision of different anthropometric measures using TEM cannot be made easily.

Percentage TEM

The use of percentage TEM has been recommended (Norton and Olds, 1996) to overcome the difficulty of the TEM being dependent on the size of the original measurement. The percentage technical error of the measurement is

Subject no.	Stature (m) as determined on repeat				(1) ΣM^2	(2) $(\Sigma M)^2/K$	Diff. (1) − (2)
	1	2	3	4			
1	0.865	0.863	0.863	0.864	2.984259	2.984256	0.000003
2	1.023	1.023	1.027	1.025	4.198412	4.198401	0.000011
3	0.982	0.980	0.989	0.985	3.873070	3.873024	0.000046
4	0.817	0.816	0.812	0.817	2.660178	2.660161	0.000017
5	0.901	0.894	0.900	0.903	3.236446	3.236401	0.000045
6	0.880	0.876	0.881	0.881	3.094098	3.094081	0.000017
7	0.948	0.947	0.947	0.946	3.587238	3.587236	0.000002
8	0.906	0.905	0.907	0.908	3.286974	3.286969	0.000005
9	0.924	0.924	0.926	0.924	3.418804	3.418801	0.000003
10	0.969	0.987	1.002	0.993	3.942343	3.942210	0.000133
							$\Sigma = 0.000282$

$$\text{TEM} = \sqrt{0.000282/[N(K-1)]} = \sqrt{0.000282/[10(4-1)]} = 0.00307$$

Table 9.3: Sample calculation of technical error of measurement (TEM) from repeat measurements of stature (m) carried out by one anthropometrist on 10 subjects. M = measurement, K = number of replicates, N = number of subjects.

analogous to the coefficient of variation and is calculated as

$$\%\text{TEM} = (\text{TEM/mean}) \times 100\%$$

Note that %TEM has no units and can be used to make direct comparisons of all types of anthropometric measurements. It cannot be used, however, when more than one examiner is involved, as then both within- and between-examiner errors are involved. Uljaszek and Kerr (1999) describe ways to deal with this more complex case.

Coefficient of reliability

An alternative approach that is widely used for comparing measurement errors among anthropometric measurements is to calculate the coefficient of reliability (R), which ranges from 0 to 1. This coefficient can be calculated using the following equation:

$$R = 1 - ((\text{TEM})^2/s^2)$$

where s^2 is the between-subject variance. The coefficient indicates the proportion of between-subject variance in a measured population which is free from measurement error. Hence, a measurement with $R = 0.95$ indicates that 95% of the variance is due to factors other than measurement error.

Whenever possible, a coefficient of reliability > 0.95 should be sought. Coefficients of reliability can be used to compare the relative reliability of different anthropometric measurements, and the same measurements in different age groups, as well as for calculating sample sizes in anthropometric surveys. More details of standardization procedures and calculation of precision using TEM, percentage TEM, and coefficient of reliability are given in Lohman et al. (1988).

In general, the precision of weight and height measurements is high. However, for waist and hip circumferences, between-examiner error tends to be large and it is preferable for only one examiner to take these measurements. Because skinfolds are notoriously imprecise, both within- and between-examiner errors can be large. Therefore, rigorous training using standardized techniques and calibrated equipment are critical when skinfold measurements are taken.

9.2.2 Systematic measurement errors and accuracy

Systematic measurement errors affect the accuracy of anthropometric measurements or how close the measurements are to the true value. The most common form of systematic error in anthropometry results from equipment bias. For example, apparent discrepancies in skinfold measurements performed on the same person but with different calipers may be due to compression differences arising from variations in spring pressure and surface area of the calipers (Schmidt and Carter, 1990); Harpenden and Holtain skinfold calipers consistently yield smaller values than Lange calipers (Gruber et al., 1990).

The timing of some anthropometric measurements of body size and composition is also known to be critical, particularly for short-term growth studies: progressive decreases in the height of an individual during the day as a consequence of compression of the spinal column, for example, may seriously compromise the accuracy of height velocity measurements.

The determination of accuracy in anthropometry is difficult because the correct value of any anthropometric measurement is never known with absolute certainty. In the absence of absolute reference standards, the accuracy of anthropometric measurements is estimated by comparing them with those made by a criterion anthropometrist (Ulijaszek and Kerr, 1999), a person who has been highly trained in the standardized measurement techniques and whose measurements compare well to those from another criterion anthropometrist.

Zerfas (1985) gives targets for anthropometric assessment using a repeat-measures protocol that can be used for training anthropometrists for length, height, weight, arm circumference, and skinfolds (Table 11.3). In this way, both measurement differences between trainee and criterion anthropometrist and systematic biases in measurement are reduced. Targets for sports anthropometrists are also available (Gore et al., 1996).

Attempts should always be made to minimize measurement errors. In longitudinal studies involving sequential anthropometric measurements on the same group of individuals (e.g., surveillance), it is preferable, whenever possible, to have one person carrying out the same measurements throughout the study to eliminate between-examiner errors. This is particularly critical when increments in growth and body composition are calculated; such increments are generally small and are associated with two error terms, one on each measurement occasion. Recommen-

dations for the minimum intervals necessary to provide reliable data on growth increments during infancy and early childhood (Guo et al., 1991) and adolescence (WHO, 1995) are available.

In large regional surveillance studies, it is often necessary to use several well-trained anthropometrists. In such circumstances, the between-examiner differences among anthropometrists must be monitored throughout the study to maintain the quality of the measurements and thereby to identify and correct systematic errors in the measurements.

In studies involving two longitudinal measurements, the TEM can be calculated to estimate the proportion of the difference that can be attributed to measurement error. For example, with a TEM of 0.3 for a given anthropometric measurement, the TEM for the difference between two measurements is

$$\sqrt{(0.3)^2 + (0.3)^2} = 0.42$$

because both TEM values contribute to the variance in the difference. Only if the difference exceeds $2 \times 0.42 = 0.84$ is there a 95% probability that the difference exceeds the measurement error alone.

Once assured that such differences are not a function of measurement error, then any changes in growth and body composition can be correlated with factors such as age, the onset of disease, response to nutrition intervention therapy, and so on.

The collection of longitudinal anthropometric data is more time consuming, expensive, and laborious than are cross-sectional surveys, and, as a result, the sample size is generally smaller. Hence, the probability of systematic sampling bias (Section 1.4.2) is generally greater than in more extensive cross-sectional surveys.

For cross-sectional studies, the examiners should be rotated among the subjects to reduce the effect of measurement bias of the individual examiners. Statistical methods exist for removing anthropometric measurement error from cross-sectional anthropometric data; details are given in Ulijaszek and Lourie (1994).

Cross-sectional surveys are useful for comparing population groups, provided that probability sampling techniques have been used to ensure that the samples are representative of the populations from which they are drawn (Section 1.4.2).

9.2.3 Errors from changes in tissue composition and properties

Variation in the composition and physical properties of certain tissues may occur in both healthy and diseased subjects, resulting in inaccuracies in certain anthropometric measurements. Even among healthy individuals, body weight may be affected by variations in tissue hydration with the menstrual cycle (Heymsfield and Casper, 1987).

Skinfold thickness measurements may be influenced by variations in compressibility and skin thickness with age, gender, and the level of tissue hydration (Martin et al., 1992; Ward and Anderson, 1993). For example, repeated measurements of skinfolds, over a short period (i.e., 5 min), may actually decrease accuracy of skinfolds because later measurements are more compressed due to the expulsion of water from the adipose tissue at the site of the earlier measurement (Ulijaszek and Kerr, 1999). In addition, during aging, demineralization of the bone and changes in body water may result in a decrease in the density of the fat-free mass (Visser et al., 1994). Generally, anthropometric measurements are not corrected to account for these effects.

9.2.4 Invalid models and errors in body composition

Invalid assumptions may lead to erroneous estimates of body composition when these are derived from anthropometric measurements, especially in obese or elderly patients and those with protein-energy malnutrition or certain disease states. For instance, use of skinfold thickness measurements to estimate total body fat assumes that (*a*) the thickness of the subcutaneous adipose tissue reflects a constant proportion of the total body fat and (*b*) the sites selected represent the average thickness of the subcutaneous adipose tissue. In fact, the relationship between subcutaneous and internal fat is nonlinear and varies with body weight, age, and disease state. Very lean subjects have a smaller proportion of body fat deposited subcutaneously than do obese subjects, and in malnourished persons there is probably a shift of fat storage from subcutaneous to deep visceral sites. Variations in the distribution of subcutaneous fat also occur with age, sex, and ethnicity or race (Wagner and Heyward, 2000; He et al., 2002).

Estimates of mid-upper-arm muscle area are used as an index of total body muscle and the fat-free mass (Section 11.2.3), regardless of age and health status of the subjects. Such estimates are made, despite the known changes in the relationship between arm muscle and fat-free mass with age and certain disease states (Heymsfield and McManus, 1985), and the questionable accuracy of the algorithms used (Martine et al., 1997). Moreover, even the corrected algorithms developed for adults overestimate arm muscle area in obese persons when compared with the determination by computerized tomography (Forbes et al., 1988).

Increasingly, body composition is assessed by laboratory methods; these are described in Chapter 14. Even laboratory methods are based on certain assumptions that have been challenged in recent years. For example, until recently, densitometry, frequently using underwater weighing, has been the gold standard reference method for the determination of the percentage of body fat. The assumptions used in densitometry are that the densities of the fat mass and fat-free mass are constant at 0.90 and 1.10 kg/L, respectively (Section 11.1.5). Several researchers have questioned the validity of using a constant density of the fat-free mass for groups who vary in age, gender, levels of body fatness, and race or ethnicity (Visser et al., 1997). During aging, the density of the fat-free mass may decrease due to demineralization of the bone and changes in body water, leading to a 1%–2% overestimate of the body fat content in such subjects (Deurenberg et al., 1989).

In contrast, persons of African descent have a larger fat-free mass because they have a greater bone mineral density and body protein content compared to Caucasians (Wagner and Heyward, 2000). This results in an underestimate of body fat, when generalized equations developed for Caucasians are used.

Percentage of body fat can also be determined using an isotope dilution technique (Section 14.3) and dual-energy X-ray absorptiometry (DXA) (Section 14.11). Both of these methods assume a constant hydration of the fat-free mass, despite knowledge that it varies with age (Wang et al., 1999). When the actual hydration of fat-free mass is higher than the assumed value, then the percentage of body fat is underestimated by isotope-dilution techniques (Section 14.3) (Deurenberg-Yap et al., 2001). In contrast, hydration effects on estimates of fat by DXA are not significant (Pietrobelli et al., 1998). Fortunately, the advent of multiple-compartment models for assessing body composition circumvent the use of older methods, which use assumptions that may not be valid for certain ethnic groups or the elderly. Nevertheless, use of multicompartmental models is expensive, requiring more time and facilities.

9.3 Interpretation and evaluation of anthropometric data

Anthropometric indices are derived from two or more raw measurements, as noted earlier. Normally, it is these indices that are interpreted and evaluated — not the raw measurements. For children, weight-for-height and height-for-age are the preferred anthropometric indices of body size. In combination, they can be used as indicators to identify wasting, that arises from gaining insufficient weight relative to height (i.e., low weight-for-height), and stunting (i.e., gaining insufficient height relative to age) (WHO, 1995); they are discussed in detail in Sections 10.2.3 and 10.2.4.

Anthropometric indices can be used at both the individual and the population levels to assess nutritional status and to screen and assess a response during interventions. In addition, in populations, anthropometry can be used to identify the determinants and consequences of malnutrition and for nutritional surveillance. To achieve these objectives, knowledge of factors that may modify or "condition" the interpretation of abnormal anthropometric indices is generally required. These conditioning factors are briefly discussed below, together with reference data and associated methodologies and classification systems that identify individuals as "at risk" for malnutrition.

9.3.1 Conditioning factors

A variety of factors are known to modify or condition the interpretation of anthropometric data and must be taken into account. Some important examples include age, birthweight, birth length, gestational age, sex, parental stature, and feeding mode during infancy. Maturation during adolescence, prepregnancy weight, maternal height, parity, and pregnancy are major conditioning factors for adults (WHO, 1995).

Information on some of these conditioning factors can be obtained by physical examinations, questionnaires, or self-reports. An accurate assessment of age is especially critical for the derivation of many anthropometric indices used to identify abnormal anthropometry, notably height-for-age and weight-for-age. Age is also important for categorizing the data into the age groups recommended by WHO for analysis and interpretation. In more affluent countries, the assessment of age using birth certificates is generally easy, but in some low-income countries, local calendars of special events are often constructed to assist in identifying the birth date of a child.

Alternatively, for young children, age is sometimes assessed by counting deciduous teeth. This method is most appropriate at the population level because of the wide variation among individuals in the timing of deciduous eruption (Delgado et al., 1975). For individuals, bone age can be estimated from the left-hand-wrist radiograph using the Tanner

Whitehouse II method (Tanner et al., 1983). Gorstein (1989) has highlighted the marked discrepancies that may occur in the prevalence estimates of undernutrition during infancy when different methods are used to determine age.

With infants, an accurate assessment of birth weight, and, if possible, birth length and gestational age, is also important (Hediger et al., 1999). Assessment of gestational age is especially important for the interpretation of both size-for-age measurements during infancy and the neurodevelopmental progress of preterm infants. It is also essential for the management of pregnancy and the treatment of newborn infants. Several strategies are available for estimating gestational age. Prenatal measures of gestational age include calculating the number of completed weeks since the beginning of the last menstrual period, prenatal ultrasonography, and clinical methods; they are all described in Section 10.1.2.

For studies of the adolescent age group, defined by WHO (1995) as 10–19 y, information on maturation should also be collected. There is marked variation in the timing of the maturational changes during adolescence. The best measure of maturity is bone age — often termed skeletal maturation — because it can be obtained for both sexes over a wide age range. However, special equipment and expertise are required for the assessment of bone age. Hence, instead, surrogate measures of somatic maturation are generally used in nutrition surveys. WHO (1995) recommends the use of two maturational events for each sex to assist in interpreting anthropometric data during adolescence: one marker signaling the beginning of the adolescent growth spurt in each sex, and one indicating that the peak velocity for height and associated changes have passed (Figure 12.16).

When an assessment of somatic maturation cannot be obtained by physical examination, then a self-administered questionnaire containing drawings illustrating Tanner's stages of development of breasts and pubic hair for females, or pubic hair and male genitalia, may be used. Adolescents are requested to select the drawing closest to their stage of development, as described in Morris and Udry (1980).

9.3.2 Appropriate reference data

There is lack of agreement regarding the use of local versus international reference data. Some investigators advocate the use of local growth reference data derived from ethnically similar but privileged groups living in the same country, to minimize genetic influences; others suggest that the advantages of one universal reference drawn from a well-defined and accurately sampled population outweigh the problems of genetic influence (WHO, 1995; Ulijaszek, 2001). At present, the World Health Organization (WHO, 1995) recommends the use of the National Center of Health Statistics (NCHS)/WHO reference growth data (WHO, 1983) as an international growth reference for comparisons of health and nutritional status of children among countries. These growth data were selected because they meet the criteria suggested by the International Union of Nutritional Sciences (IUNS, 1972), described in Chapter 12.

Revised childhood growth charts have been prepared for U.S. children (Kuczmarski et al., 2000). They are designed to replace the widely used 1977 NCHS growth percentiles but have not been recommended for use by WHO. Instead, WHO is compiling a new international growth reference for young children which will represent the best standard possible of optimal growth for all children < 5 y (Garza and de Onis, 1999); details are given in Section 12.4.2. WHO anticipates that this new growth reference will be available in 2005. In the interim, growth curves based on the WHO (1994) pooled analyses should be used in research settings to assess the growth of infants (WHO, 1995).

Use of international reference data for the indices of body composition is not considered appropriate. These indices are more influenced by ethnic and genetic differences than those for growth (Wagner and Heyward, 2000; He et al., 2002) (Section 12.6), but only a few countries have local body composition reference data. In the absence of such local data, WHO (1995) provisionally recommends the use during childhood of the NCHS reference data based on National Health and Nutrition Examination Surveys (NHANES I and NHANES II) for subscapular and triceps skinfold thicknesses, and mid-upper arm circumference (MUAC) (de Onis et al., 1997) (Section 12.13). Body composition measurements derived from the new international WHO growth reference study should become available in 2005.

In population studies, anthropometric indices can be evaluated by comparison with the distribution of the reference data using standard deviation scores (Z-scores) or percentiles. The percentiles are not appropriate for use in low-income countries where many children may fall below the lowest percentile, making it difficult to quantify the degree of risk (WHO, 1995). Instead, Z-scores should be used because they can be calculated accurately beyond the limits of the original reference data. Z-scores can be readily calculated using user-friendly microcomputer software (Sullivan et al., 1990).

For some growth indices, the percentage of the reference median can be used to categorize children. This method is especially useful when the distribution of the reference data has not been normalized, such as the earlier Harvard reference growth data (Gorstein et al., 1994). However, calculation of the percentage of the median does not take into account either the distribution of the data within the reference set or the variability in the relative width of the distributions of the different growth indices (Dibley et al., 1987).

9.3.3 Classification systems

Several systems are available for classifying individuals as "at risk" to malnutrition based on anthropometric information. All use at least one anthropometric index and one or more reference limits derived from appropriate reference data. Alternatively, cutoff points are used.

In developing countries, anthropometric

reference limits based on standard deviation scores (Z-scores) are preferred. Often anthropometric values more than 2 SDs below or above the reference data mean are used to designate individuals with either unusually low or unusually high anthropometric indices (WHO, 1995). Selection of −2 SD scores as a reference limit means that the proportion of children below −2 SD in the reference population will be 2.3%. This percentage can be compared with the prevalence of low scores in the study population. In industrialized countries, the 3rd or 5th and 95th or 97th percentiles are often used as reference limits (Sections 13.1 and 13.2.2).

Cutoff points, unlike reference limits, are established by a review of the anthropometric characteristics of individuals with either clinically moderate or severe malnutrition or who subsequently die. Several investigators have examined relationships between low growth indices and morbidity and mortality in children (Vella et al., 1992; Schroeder and Brown, 1994). In practice, defining such cutoffs is difficult because the relationship between the indices and the biological factors cannot be generalized from one region to another.

The use of universal cutoff points for anthropometric indices of body composition is also limited. Relationships between indices of body composition and health risks are more likely to vary with age, gender, race, and environmental hazards than those for growth. For example, in Pakistan as a whole, the cutoff for low body mass index associated with higher morbidity was < 18.5, whereas in Calcutta it was < 16.0 (Campbell and Ulijaszek, 1994; Kennedy and Garcia, 1994).

In population studies, cutoff points may be combined with "trigger levels" to define criteria for an intervention. WHO has proposed epidemiological criteria for assessing and comparing the severity of undernutrition in children < 60 mo across populations, based on the prevalence of underweight, stunting, and wasting (Gorstein et al., 1994). For example, an intervention may only be initiated if at least 10% of the population have a specific anthropometric index (e.g., weight-for-age) below the established cutoff point (WHO, 1976). In this case, 10% is the trigger level for that specific anthropometric index and cutoff.

Details of the techniques used to measure body size and body composition, together with the indices derived from these measurements, are discussed in Chapters 10 and 11. Sources of reference data available for comparison of both body size and body composition indices are presented in Chapter 12, whereas Chapter 13 includes a discussion of methods used for evaluation of anthropometric indices and their application in studies of individuals and populations. Laboratory techniques used to measure body composition are discussed in Chapter 14.

References

Brožek JF. (ed.). (1956). Body Measurements and Human Nutrition. Wayne State University Press, Detroit.

Campbell P, Ulijaszek SJ. (1994). Relationships between anthropometry and retrospective morbidity in poor men in Calcutta, India. European Journal of Clinical Nutrition 48: 507–512.

Delgado H, Habicht JP, Yarbrough C, Lechtig A, Martorell R, Malina RM, Klein RE. (1975). Nutritional status and the timing of deciduous tooth eruption. American Journal of Clinical Nutrition 28: 216–224.

de Onis M, Yip R, Mei Z. (1997). The development of MUAC-for-age reference data recommended by a WHO Expert Committee. Bulletin of the World Health Organization 75: 11–18.

Deurenberg P, Weststrate JA, van der Kooy K. (1989). Is an adaptation of Siri's formula for the calculation of body fat percentage from body density in the elderly necessary? European Journal of Clinical Nutrition 43: 559–567.

Deurenberg-Yap M, Schmidt G, van Staveren WA, Hautvast JG, Deurenberg P. (2001). Body fat measurement among Singaporean Chinese, Malays and Indians: a comparative study using a four-compartment model and different two-compartment models. British Journal of Nutrition 85: 491–498.

Dibley MJ, Goldsby JB, Staehling NW, Trowbridge FL. (1987). Development of normalized curves for the international growth reference: historical and technical considerations. American Journal of Clinical Nutrition 46: 736–748.

Forbes GB, Brown MR, Griffiths HJ. (1988). Arm muscle plus bone area: anthropometry and CAT scan compared. American Journal of Clinical Nutrition 47: 929–931.

Garza C, de Onis M. (1999). A new international growth reference for young children. American Journal of Clinical Nutrition 70: 169S–172S.

Gore C, Norton K, Olds T, Whittingham N, Birchall K, Clough M, Dickerson B, Downie L. (1996). Accreditation in anthropometry: an Australian model. In: Norton K, Olds T (eds.) Anthropometrica: A Textbook of Body Measurement for Sports and Health. University of New South Wales Press, Sydney, pp. 395–411.

Gorstein J. (1989). Assessment of nutritional status: effects of different methods to determine age on classification of undernutrition. Bulletin of the World Health Organization 67: 143–150.

Gorstein J, Sullivan K, Yip R, de Onis M, Trowbridge F, Fajans P, Clugston G. (1994). Issues in the assessment of nutritional status using anthropometry. Bulletin of the World Health Association 72: 273–283.

Gruber JJ, Pollock ML, Graves JE, Colvin A, Braith R. (1990). Comparison of Harpenden and Lange calipers in predicting body composition. Research Quarterly for Exercise and Sport 61: 184–190.

Guo SM, Roche AF, Fomon SJ, Nelson SE, Chumlea WC, Rogers RR, Baumgartner RN, Ziegler EE, Siervogel RM. (1991). Reference data on gains in weight and length during the first two years of life. Journal of Pediatrics 119: 355–362.

He Q, Horlick M, Thornton J, Wang J, Pierson RN Jr, Heshka S, Gallagher D. (2002). Sex and race differences in fat distribution among Asian, African-American and Caucasian prepubertal children. Journal of Clinical Endocrinology and Metabolism 87: 2164–2170.

Hediger ML, Overpeck M, McGlynn A, Kuczmarski R, Maurer KR, Davis WW. (1999). Growth and fatness at three to six years of age of children born small- or large-for-gestational age. Pediatrics 104: e33.

Heymsfield SB, Casper K. (1987). Anthropometric assessment of the adult hospitalized patient. Journal of Parenteral and Enteral Nutrition 11: 36S–41S.

Heymsfield SB, McManus CB. (1985). Tissue components of weight loss in cancer patients: a new method of study and preliminary observations. Cancer 55: 238–249.

IUNS (International Union of Nutritional Sciences). (1972). The creation of growth standards: a committee report. American Journal of Clinical Nutrition 25: 218–220.

Jelliffe DB. (1966). The Assessment of the Nutritional Status of the Community. WHO Monograph No. 53. World Health Organization, Geneva.

Kennedy E, Garcia M. (1994). Body mass index and economic productivity. European Journal of Clinical Nutrition 48(Suppl. 3): S45–S53.

Kuczmarski RJ, Ogden CL, Grummer-Strawn LM, Flegal KM, Guo SS, Wei R, Mei Z, Curtin LR, Roche AF, Johnson CL. (2000a). CDC Growth Charts: United States. Advance Data 314: 1–27.

Lohman TG, Roche AF, Martorell R (eds.). (1988).

Anthropometric Standardization Reference Manual. Human Kinetics Books, Champaign, IL.

Martin AD, Drinkwater DT, Clarys JP, Daniel M, Ross WD. (1992). Effects of skin thickness and skinfold compressibility on skinfold thickness measurements. American Journal of Human Biology 4: 453–460.

Martine T, Claessens AL, Vlietinck R, Marchal G, Beunen G (1997). Accuracy of anthropometric estimation of muscle cross-sectional area of the arm in males. American Journal of Human Biology 9: 73–86.

Morris NM, Udry JR. (1980). Validation of a self-administered instrument to assess stage of pubertal development. Journal of Youth and Adolescence. 9: 271–280.

Norton K, Olds T (eds.). (1996). Anthropometrica: A Textbook of Body Measurement for Sports and Health. University of New South Wales Press, Sydney.

Pietrobelli A, Wang Z, Formica C, Heymsfield SB. (1998). Dual-energy X-ray absorptiometry: fat estimation errors due to variation in soft tissue hydration. American Journal of Physiology, Endocrinology and Metabolism 274: E808–E816.

Ruel MT, Rivera J, Habicht JP. (1995). Length screens better than weight in stunted populations. Journal of Nutrition 125: 1222–1228.

Schmidt PK, Carter JE. (1990). Static and dynamic differences among five types of skinfold calipers. Human Biology 62: 369–388.

Schroeder DG, Brown KH. (1994). Nutritional status as a predictor of child survival: summarizing the association and quantifying the impact. Bulletin of the World Health Organization 72: 569–579.

Sullivan KM, Gorstein J, Dean AG, Fichtner R. (1990). Use and availability of anthropometry software. Food and Nutrition Bulletin 12: 116–119.

Tanner JM, Whitehouse RH, Cameron N, Marshall W, Healy MJR, Goldstein H. (1983). The assessment of skeletal maturity and the prediction of adult height (TW2 method). 2nd ed. Academic Press, London.

Ulijaszek SJ. (2001). Ethnic differences in patterns of human growth in stature. In: Martorell R, Haschke F (eds.) Nutrition and Growth. Lippincott-Williams & Wilkins, Philadelphia, pp. 1–20.

Ulijaszek SJ, Kerr DA. (1999). Anthropometric measurement error and the assessment of nutritional status. British Journal of Nutrition 82: 165–177.

Ulijaszek SJ, Lourie JA. (1994). Intra- and inter-observer error in anthropometric measurements. In: Ulijaszek SJ, Mascie-Taylor CGN (eds.) Anthropometry: The Individual and the Population. Cambridge University Press, Cambridge, pp. 30–55.

Vella V, Tomkins A, Borghesi A, Migliori G, Adriko B, Crevatin E. (1992). Determinants of child nutrition and mortality in north-west Uganda. Bulletin of the World Health Organization 70: 637–643.

Visser M, van den Heuvel E, Deurenberg P. (1994). Prediction equations for the estimation of body composition in the elderly using anthropometric data. British Journal of Nutrition 71: 823–833.

Visser M, Gallagher D, Deurenberg P, Wang J, Pierson RN Jr, Heymsfield SB. (1997). Density of fat-free body mass: relationship with race, age, and level of body fatness. American Journal of Physiology 272: E781–E787.

Wagner DR, Heyward VH. (2000). Measures of body composition in blacks and whites: a comparative review. American Journal of Clinical Nutrition 71: 1392–1402.

Wang Z, Deurenberg P, Wang W, Pietrobelli A, Baumgartner RN, Heymsfield SB. (1999). Hydration of fat-free body mass: review and critique of a classic body-composition constant. American Journal of Clinical Nutrition 69: 833–841.

Ward R, Anderson G. (1993). Examination of the skinfold compressibility and skinfold thickness relationship. American Journal of Human Biology 5: 541–548.

Weiner JS, Lourie JA. (1969). Human Biology: A Guide to Field Methods. International Biological Programme IBP Handbook No. 9. Blackwell Scientific, Oxford.

WHO (World Health Organization). (1968). Nutritional Status of Populations: A Manual on Anthropometric Appraisal of Trends. WHO/Nutr/70.129. World Health Organization, Geneva.

WHO (World Health Organization). (1976). Report on Methodology of Nutritional Surveillance. FAO/ UNICEF/WHO Expert Committee. WHO Technical Report Series No. 593. World Health Organization, Geneva.

WHO (World Health Organization). (1983). Measuring Change in Nutritional Status: Guidelines for Assessing the Nutritional Impact of Supplementary Feeding Programmes for Vulnerable Groups. World Health Organization, Geneva.

WHO (World Health Organization). (1994). An Evaluation of Infant Growth. WHO/NUT/94.8. World Health Organization, Geneva.

WHO (World Health Organization). (1995). Physical Status: The Use and Interpretation of Anthropometry. Report of a WHO Expert Committee. WHO Technical Report Series No. 854. World Health Organization, Geneva.

Zerfas AJ. (1979). Anthropometric field methods: general. In: Jelliffe DB, Jelliffe EFP (eds.) Human Nutrition: A Comprehensive Treatise. Volume 2: Nutrition and Growth. Plenum Press, New York, pp. 339–364.

Zerfas AJ. (1985). Checking Continuous Measures: Manual for Anthropometry. Division of Epidemiology, School of Public Health, University of California, Los Angeles.

10

Anthropometric assessment of body size

The most widely used anthropometric measurements of body size are those of stature (height or length) and body weight. These measurements can be made quickly and easily and, with care and training, accurately. Head circumference measurements are often taken in association with stature. Details of standardized procedures for these measurements of body size are summarized below and are given in detail in Lohman et al. (1988).

Indices such as head-circumference-for-age, weight-for-age, weight-for-stature, and stature-for-age and the ratio of weight:stature are derived from these measurements. Of these, stature-for-age and weight-for-stature have been recommended by the World Health Organization (WHO, 1995a) for use in low-income countries. In combination, they can distinguish between stunting and wasting. Increasingly, body mass index (BMI) (wt/ht^2, usually kg/m^2) is used in epidemiological studies as the recommended indicator for defining overweight and obesity in adults, children, and adolescents. In hospital, anthropometric indices of body size are used primarily to identify under- or overnutrition and obesity, and to monitor changes after a nutrition intervention.

10.1 Measurements of body size

Of the various measurements of body size, head circumference is important because it is closely related to brain size. It is often used with other measurements to detect the pathological conditions associated with either an unusually large (macrocephalic) or small (microcephalic) head.

Recumbent length is measured in infants and children < 2 y. Height is measured in older children and adults. Interpretation of weight and length at birth and during later infancy requires a valid and precise measure of gestational age: making such an estimate is often difficult in many low-income countries. Measurement of lower-leg length in infants and children can be used to assess growth over short time periods. In adults, knee-height measurements are used to estimate height in those persons with severe spinal curvature and in those who are unable to stand. Alternatively, arm span can be measured when actual height cannot be used.

Weight in infants and young children can be measured using a suspended scale and a weighing sling, or a pediatric scale. For older children and adults, a beam balance with nondetachable weights is recommended. Elbow breadth is used as a measure of frame size, which is relatively independent of adiposity and age (Frisancho, 1990); it should be measured with flat-bladed sliding calipers.

10.1.1 Head circumference

For the measurement of head circumference, a narrow, flexible, nonstretch tape made of fiberglass or steel about 0.6 cm wide should be used. The subject stands with the left side facing the measurer, with arms relaxed and legs apart. The subject must look straight

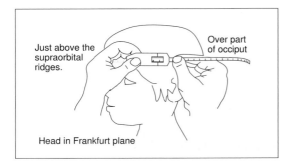

Figure 10.1: Measurement of head circumference.

ahead so the line of vision is perpendicular to the body and the Frankfurt plane — that is, an imaginary plane which passes through the external auditory meatus (the small flap of skin on the forward edge of the ear) and over the top of the lower bone of the eye socket immediately under the eye — is horizontal. The tape is placed just above the supraorbital ridges covering the most prominent part of the frontal bulge and over the part of the occiput that gives the maximum circumference (Figure 10.1). Care must be taken to ensure that the tape is at the same level on each side of the head and pulled tightly to compress the hair. Measurements are made to the nearest millimeter.

10.1.2 Gestational age

The assessment of gestational age is necessary for the interpretation of any size-for-age measurement of infants and for following the neurodevelopmental progress of preterm infants. It is also essential for the management of pregnancy and treatment of the newborn.

Several strategies are available for estimating gestational age. Prenatal measures of gestational age include calculating the number of completed weeks since the beginning of the last menstrual period, prenatal ultrasonography, and clinical methods. Of these, the definition of gestational age on the basis of the last menstrual period is most frequently used, but it is associated with several problems: errors may occur because of irregular menses, bleeding early in pregnancy, and incorrect recall by mothers.

Prenatal ultrasonography during the first or second trimester is considered by many to be the gold standard for assessment of gestational age. Estimates are based on different ultrasonic measures of fetal size, such as the biparietal diameter, crown-rump length, femoral length, and abdominal circumference (Reece et al., 1989). Measurements are most accurate when made early in gestation. Unfortunately, ultrasonography is not universally available, especially in low-income countries, and the quality of both the equipment used and the technical training varies.

Clinical methods of prenatal assessment involve measurement of fundal height, the auscultation of fetal heart tones, and recording of fetal movements (Belizan et al., 1978; Alexander and Allen, 1996).

Several scoring systems, based on external and neurological criteria, have been developed to estimate maturity — and thus gestational age — postnatally. The scoring systems initially devised by Dubowitz et al. (1970) and later modified by Ballard et al. (1979) have been widely adopted. Both methods appear to have limited accuracy at the extremes of gestation, and the measurement of gestational age postnatally at the individual and population levels continues to be problematic (Alexander and Allen, 1996).

10.1.3 Recumbent length

For infants and children ≤ 85 cm, recumbent length is measured (WHO, 1995a), generally with a wooden or Perspex measuring board (Figure 10.2). Two examiners are required to correctly position the subject and ensure accurate and reliable measurements of length. The subject is placed face upward, with the head toward the fixed end of the board and the body parallel to the board's axis (Figure 10.3). The shoulders should rest against the surface of the board. One examiner applies gentle traction to bring the crown of the child's head into contact with the fixed headboard and positions the head so that the Frankfurt plane is vertical. The second examiner holds the subject's feet, without shoes, toes pointing directly upward, and keeping

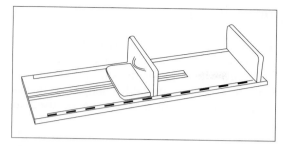

Figure 10.2: Device for the measurement of recumbent length.

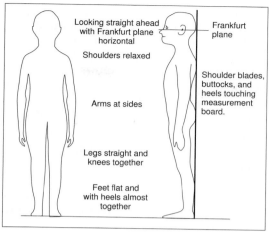

Figure 10.4: Positioning of subject for height measurement. Horizontal line is the Frankfurt plane, which should be in a horizontal position when height is measured. Reproduced from Robbins GE, Trowbridge FL, in: Nutrition Assessment: A Comprehensive Guide for Planning Intervention by M.D. Simko, C. Cowell, and J.A. Gilbride (eds.), p.77, with permission of Aspen Publishers, Inc., © 1984.

the subject's knees straight, brings the movable footboard to rest firmly against the heels. The reading is taken to the nearest millimeter. If the subject is restless, only the left leg should be positioned for the measurement.

For field use, a portable infant length measuring scale can be used. This device is assembled from four separate plastic sections that lock together to form head and foot plates, with a strong, 2-m metal tape insert. Suppliers of measuring devices and scales are listed in Appendix A10.1.

10.1.4 Height

Children > 85 cm and adults should be measured in the standing position, if possible (WHO, 1995a), using a free-standing stadiometer, sometimes termed an "anthropometer". Alternatively, a right-angle headboard

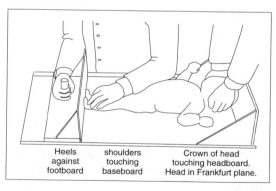

| Heels against footboard | shoulders touching baseboard | Crown of head touching headboard. Head in Frankfurt plane. |

Figure 10.3: Measurement of recumbent length. Reproduced from Robbins GE, Trowbridge FL, in: Nutrition Assessment: A Comprehensive Guide for Planning Intervention by M.D. Simko, C. Cowell, and J.A. Gilbride (eds.), p.75, with permission of Aspen Publishers, Inc., © 1984.

and a measuring rod or nonstretchable tape fixed to a vertical surface can be used. In the field, vertical surfaces are not always available. In such circumstances, modified tape measures such as the Microtoise, which measure up to 2 m, can be used. Platform scales with movable measuring rods are not suitable for research measurements because they can be inaccurate. Clothing should be minimal when measuring height so that posture can be clearly seen. Shoes and socks should not be worn.

Modern digital devices can measure stature to 0.1 mm. To take full advantage of this precision, the equipment must be calibrated and used carefully. The subject is asked to stand straight with the head in the Frankfurt plane (Figure 10.4), feet together, knees straight, and heels, buttocks, and shoulder blades in contact with the vertical surface of the stadiometer, anthropometer, or wall. Arms should be hanging loosely at the sides with palms facing the thighs; the head is not necessarily in contact with the vertical surface. For younger subjects, it may be necessary to hold the heels to ensure they do not leave the ground.

Some investigators recommend applying gentle upward pressure to the mastoid processes to stretch the spine and minimize effects produced by diurnal variation (Tanner et al., 1966). Subjects are asked to take a deep breath and stand tall to aid the straightening of the spine. Shoulders should be relaxed. The movable headboard is then gently lowered until it touches the crown of the head. The height measurement is taken at maximum inspiration, with the examiner's eyes level with the headboard to avoid parallax errors. Height is recorded to the nearest millimeter, or even more precisely with more modern digital equipment.

The time at which the measurement is made should be recorded; diurnal variations in height occur due to compression of the spine as the day progresses. Consequently, for cross-sectional and longitudinal studies, heights should be measured at the same time of day, preferably in the afternoon. In cases where large amounts of adipose tissue prevent the heels, buttocks, and shoulders from simultaneously touching the wall, subjects should simply be asked to stand erect.

When the Microtoise tape is used, it is first placed on the floor. The tape is then pulled out to its fullest extent and released, and the end is fixed with a nail to a door or doorway. The subject is then instructed to stand erect directly below the point of attachment. An anthropometrist should position the subject's head correctly in the Frankfurt plane, as described in Section 10.1.1, before the tape is lowered by a second person until the head-bar touches the crown of the head and compresses the hair. A direct reading of height to the nearest millimeter may then be obtained.

Recumbent length for a child of about 2 y is approximately 5 mm greater on average than standing height for the same child (Haschke and van't Hof, 2000). Hence, if standing height rather than recumbent length is measured, 5 mm must be added to the standing height value when recumbent length reference data are used. Self-reported heights tend to produce slightly higher estimates of height and should be avoided (Millar, 1986).

10.1.5 Knee height in children

The measurement of knee height in children is termed "knemometry." Two similar devices are available for the measurement — a knemometer and a portable knee height measuring device. Both models can be used to measure knee height in children > 3 y who are able to sit quietly and cooperate. For children $\leqslant 3$ y, a mini-knemometer can be used to measure lower leg length (Section 10.1.6).

Knemometer

The knemometer was first developed in 1971 by Valk, and modified in 1983 to improve its accuracy. The instrument enables the distance between the heel and knee of the right leg — termed the lower leg length — of a sitting child to be estimated with a technical error of the measurement (TEM) of 0.09–0.16 mm (Hermanussen, 1988). Figure 10.5 depicts the technique of lower leg length measurement using this newer device.

To take the measurement, the child is asked to sit on the chair. The sitting height (A) and the chair back (B) and chair position can be adjusted. The foot of the child is placed on the foot rest (C) and the angle and the length of the foot are recorded. The sitting position of the child is standardized by recording the following:

- sitting height of the child
- distance between the chair and the measuring board
- individual sitting position of the child (i.e., distance between the lateral condyle [X] and the back of the chair [B]).

Next, the measuring board (D) is lowered onto the child's knee, and then the chair on which the child is sitting is gently moved forward and backward. The knee is moved passively under the measuring board (D) and the foot plate (C), while the length is displayed continuously on an electronic display. A counterweight (E) ensures a constant pressure of the measuring board of about 200 g.

The actual lower leg length is defined as

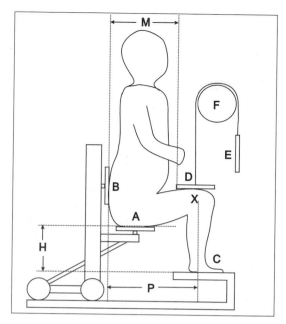

Figure 10.5: Diagram of the knemometer. Movable chair with adjustable height (A) and back (B); foot plate (C); Measuring board (D); Counterweight (E); Visual electronic display (F). The coordinates of the child's sitting position are defined by: the sitting height (H); the distance between the chair and the measuring board (M); and the distance between the lateral condyle (marked "X") and the back of the chair (P). From Hermanussen et al., Annals of Human Biology 15: 1–16, 1988.

the maximum distance that can be reached during the movements of the child's knee. The minimum distance that can be discriminated by this instrument is 0.1 mm. Six knemometric measurements are preferred for an accurate determination of the lower leg length in a child, although three have been used (Hermanussen et al., 1988). Children should be lightly dressed when these measurements are taken.

Knee height measurement device

The portable instrument — the knee height measurement device (KHMD) — is also designed to measure short-term growth of the lower leg. This device is less costly and easier to use than the knemometer. Again, the measurements are taken while the child is sitting. The chair used with this device should

have a seat height of 33 cm and a seat length of 26 cm.

The KHMD consists of a standard industrial electronic height gauge (precision of 0.01 mm) to measure the distance between the knee and foot plate. A Plexiglas knee plate is mounted on the height gauge. A dial indicator is attached to the height gauge, so accurate and repeatable force can be applied to the knee during each measurement. The reading on the dial indicator corresponds to the torque flexion of the knee plate during the measurement.

The height gauge with the knee plate attached is mounted on a base comprised of a foot plate, wheels, and a handgrip to move the device. Both heel and toe plates are mounted on the foot plate to ensure that the position of the foot is reproducible for each measurement. The knee is also fixed in position during the measurement by an adjustable knee brace. The knee brace position is recorded by the operator from a numerical scale attached to the upright support. This allows the operator to position the subject reproducibly at each measurement session.

The position of the chair relative to the KHMD must also be fixed for each subject at each measurement session. This is achieved by placing the chair on a Plexiglas grid with numbered and lettered squares. This marked grid, together with the braces for the knee, foot, and toe, ensure that the position of the subject at each measurement session can be replicated (Cronk et al., 1989).

For the measurement, subjects should sit with buttocks and the small of the back firmly in contact with the chair back, with the foot on the foot plate flush with the heel brace. The top of the knee brace is then adjusted until it has contact with the nonboney space between the patella and the tibial tuberosity. The chair is then pushed forward so that the knee is in full contact with the knee brace, with the leg centered in relation to the knee plate. The opposite foot is positioned so it is flush with the instrument and parallel with the foot plate. Next, the knee plate is lowered onto the top of the knee until it is deflected 0.03 mm (equivalent to about 2 kg of pressure on the knee which yields the smallest degree of error without causing discomfort). The knee height measurement is electronically recorded. Subjects should remain seated between measurements but remove their foot from the foot plate and then return it again. The position of the child in the chair and the foot on the foot plate should be readjusted, and three additional independent measurements should be taken.

The performance of the KHMD has been compared with that of the Valk knemometer on 103 children 6–10 y. Growth was measured at 28-d intervals with both devices. The within-observer error for the measurements was 0.295 mm for the KHMD and 0.206 mm for the knemometer. The correlation between devices for measurements of growth rate on each child was 0.73 ($p < 0.002$) (Cronk et al., 1989).

Several factors other than growth influence the measurement of lower leg length, and, hence, must be controlled. For example, as diurnal variation influences the measurement, it is preferable for all measurements to be performed during the afternoon, and by one trained observer. Before the measurement, children should avoid vigorous physical activity for at least 2-h, and, instead, stand or walk slowly for 5–10 min.

Knee height appears to be a valid index of linear growth in well-nourished children (Wales and Milner, 1987), although its use in children recovering from severe malnutrition is uncertain (Doherty et al., 2001). Knee height is of increasing importance as it appears to be possible to detect growth increments in children — more readily and over a shorter time frame — by measuring knee height than by conventional height measurements. Moreover, knee height measurements can be made with greater precision.

10.1.6 Lower leg length in infants

The lower leg length of infants can be measured using mini-knemometry. Earlier studies used a handheld knemometer to measure short term changes in lower leg length in infants. The TEM using this device, how-

ever, was moderately high, ranging from 0.82 down to 0.31 mm (Michaelsen et al., 1991; Gibson et al., 1993).

A new measuring device has been developed for accurate measurements of the lower leg length in prematures, newborns, and infants, with a TEM of 0.144 mm (Hermanussen and Seele, 1997). The device contains a commercially available electronic slide that discriminates intervals of 10 μm. The slide is connected to two measuring arms (A, B) with metallic holders, as shown in Figure 10.6. The infant's knee and heel are placed between the holders. Knee and heel holders of different sizes can be fitted, depending on the age of the infant.

When serial measurements are being taken, care must be observed to ensure that the infant is always measured in the same position. A spring mounted within the instrument between the arms ensures a constant soft-tissue pressure between 2.0 and 3.0 N. The measurement is painless for the infant and is best made during breast-feeding. Four independent measurements of leg length should be taken on each child within 1–3 min. Lower leg growth appears to be nonlinear, with periods of slow and then accelerated growth (Hermanussen and Seele, 1997).

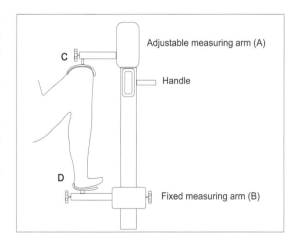

Figure 10.6: Diagram of a mini-knemometer: measuring arms (A and B); metallic holders for knee and heel (C and D). The arms are spring-loaded so that a constant pressure is applied during measurement. From Hermanussen and Seele, Annals of Human Biology 24: 307–313, 1997.

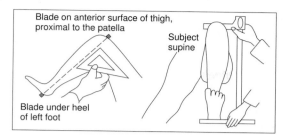

Figure 10.7: Measurement of knee height in adults.

10.1.7 Knee height in adults

Knee height is highly correlated with stature and may be used to estimate height in persons with severe spinal curvature or who are unable to stand. Knee height is measured with a caliper consisting of an adjustable measuring stick with a blade attached to each end at a 90° angle. Suppliers of knee height calipers are listed in Appendix A10.2.

Recumbent knee height is measured on the left leg, which is bent at the knee at a 90° angle, while the subject is in a supine position (Figure 10.7). One of the blades is positioned under the heel of the left foot and the other is placed over the anterior surface of the left thigh above the condyles of the femur and just proximal to the patella. The shaft of the caliper is held parallel to the shaft of the tibia, and gentle pressure is applied to the blades of the caliper. Some of the knee-height calipers are equipped with a locking mechanism to retain the measurement after removing the caliper from the leg. At least two successive measurements should be made, and they should agree within 5 mm; the mean is then calculated. Details for measuring knee height in elderly persons seated in wheel chairs are given in WHO (1995a).

Formulae are used to estimate stature from knee height. Separate equations are available for Caucasian and African American elderly persons 60–80 y (Chumlea and Guo, 1992). The equations shown here were generated using a selected population living in the United States: their appropriateness for estimating stature among other ethnic groups has been questioned. Population-specific equations may be necessary (Prothro and Rosen-

bloom, 1993; Zhang et al., 1998).

Height (Caucasian men, cm) =
$$(2.08 \times \text{knee height}) + 59.01$$
Height (Caucasian women, cm) =
$$1.91 \times \text{knee height} - (0.17 \times \text{age}) + 75.00$$
Height (African-American men, cm) =
$$1.37 \times \text{knee height} + 95.79$$
Height (African-American women, cm) =
$$1.96 \times \text{knee height} + 58.72$$

Cockram and Baumgartner (1990) evaluated the accuracy and reliability of three models of knee-height calipers for measuring recumbent knee height in the elderly. They reported that the equations based on knee height given above predicted subject's stature to ± 2.3 cm. Nonetheless, these investigators emphasize that an assessment of stature based on knee height should be used only for individuals for whom a direct measurement of stature is not possible, or is likely to be inaccurate, because of vertebral flexions or other skeletal deformities.

10.1.8 Arm span

Arm span, like knee height, is also highly correlated with stature and, hence, can be used as an alternative measurement when actual height cannot be used (Jarzem and Gledhill, 1993). It is especially useful for assessing retrospective stature at young adulthood — that is stature prior to any age-associated loss in the elderly — rather than the current (reduced) height.

The measurement of arm span is easier if carried out against a flat wall (Figure 10.8), to which is attached a fixed marker board at the zero end of a horizontal scale. Sliding

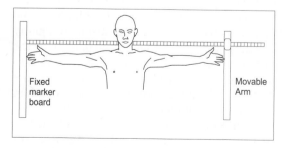

Figure 10.8: Measurement of arm span.

on the scale is a vertical movable arm. The horizontal scale should be positioned so that it is just above the shoulders of the subject. Two examiners are needed to measure arm span: one is at the fixed end of the scale; the other positions the movable arm and takes the readings. For the measurement, the individual should stand with feet together, back against the wall, with the arms extended laterally in contact with the wall, and with the palms facing forward. The arms should be kept at shoulder height and outstretched maximally. The measurement is taken when the tip of the middle finger (excluding the fingernail) of the right hand is kept in contact with the fixed marker board, while the movable arm is set at the tip of the middle finger (excluding the fingernail) of the left hand. Two readings are taken for each measurement, which is recorded to the nearest 0.1 cm (Lohman et al., 1988).

Arm span is difficult to measure in non-ambulatory elderly persons and in individuals with significant chest and spinal deformities. Zhang et al. (1998) concluded that in a group of elderly Chinese, for example, knee height provided a more valid estimate of maximum stature during early adulthood than arm span.

10.1.9 Weight in infants and children

In field surveys, a suspended scale and a weighing sling may be used for weighing infants and children < 2 y (Figure 10.9). They should be weighed naked or with the minimum of clothing. After slipping the subject into the sling, the weight is recorded as soon as the indicator on the scale has stabilized.

Alternatively, a pediatric scale with a pan may be used (Figure 10.10a). Care must be taken to ensure that the infant is placed on the pan scale so the weight is distributed equally on each side of the center of the pan. Once the infant is lying quietly, weight is recorded to the nearest 10 g. If there is no alternative, the mother and subject can be weighed together, and then the mother alone, using a beam balance or battery-operated precision electronic scales. The subject's weight can then be calculated by subtraction.

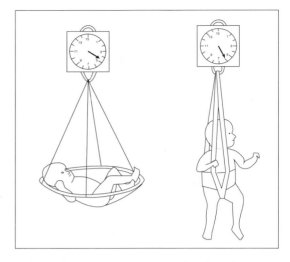

Figure 10.9: Measurement of weight in infants and children using a spring balance. The bowl for the baby is made from a metal or bamboo ring and netting.

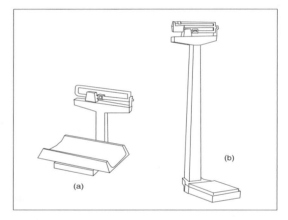

Figure 10.10: Measurement of weight: (a) pediatric scale for infants, (b) beam balance for a child or adult.

10.1.10 Weight in older children and adults

The measurement of weight in older children and adults should be done preferably after the bladder has been emptied and before a meal. A beam balance (Figure 10.10b) with nondetachable weights should be used, where possible. Unfortunately, beam balances tend to be heavy and bulky and therefore unsuitable for field use. In such cases, a spring balance or, preferably, electronic scales can be used.

The balance should be placed on a hard, flat surface (not carpet) and checked and adjusted for zero-balance before each measurement. The subject should stand in the center of the platform and look straight ahead, standing unassisted, relaxed but still, and preferably nude. If nudity is not possible, the subject can wear light underclothing or a paper examination gown, and the weight of these garments should be recorded for later subtraction; standard corrections for clothing should not be used. The presence of visible edema should also be recorded. Body weight should be recorded to the nearest 0.1 kg. Again, the time at which the measurement is made should be recorded because diurnal variations in weight occur.

The balance should be calibrated with a set of weights, both regularly throughout the year and whenever it is moved to another location. Special equipment, such as a movable wheelchair balance beam scale or bed scales, is needed for weighing nonambulatory persons (Chumlea et al., 1984).

Estimates of weight for the U.S. elderly population can be derived from calf circumference (calf circ), knee height (knee ht), mid-upper-arm circumference (MUAC), and subscapular skinfold (subscap), using equations developed by Chumlea et al. (1989); examples are given below:

Weight (M) = $(0.98 \times \text{calf circ}) + (1.16 \times \text{knee ht})$
$\quad + (1.73 \times \text{MUAC}) + (0.37 \times \text{subscap}) - 81.69$
Weight (F) = $(1.27 \times \text{calf circ}) + (0.87 \times \text{knee ht})$
$\quad + (0.98 \times \text{MUAC}) + (0.40 \times \text{subscap}) - 62.35$

As the above equations were developed from a selected population living in the United States, these formulae may be inappropriate for estimating weights of other populations. Instead, population-specific equations may be required. Use of self-reported weights in adults leads to bias and should be avoided (Millar, 1986).

10.1.11 Elbow breadth

Elbow breadth is a good measure of skeletal dimensions and, hence, frame size. The measure is less affected by adiposity than

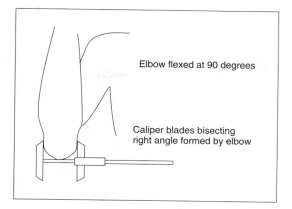

Elbow flexed at 90 degrees

Caliper blades bisecting right angle formed by elbow

Figure 10.11: Measurement of elbow breadth.

many other anthropometric dimensions and is highly associated with lean body mass and muscle size (Frisancho, 1990).

Elbow breadth is measured as the distance between the epicondyles of the humerus. For the measurement, the right arm is raised to the horizontal and the elbow is flexed to 90°, with the back of the hand facing the measurer (Figure 10.11). The measurer then stands in front of the subject and locates the lateral and medial epicondyles of the humerus. The two blades of a flat-bladed sliding caliper are applied to the epicondyles, with the blades pointing upward to bisect the right angle formed at the elbow. Care must be taken to ensure that the caliper is held at a slight angle to the epicondyles and that firm pressure is exerted to minimize the influence of soft tissue on the measurement. The latter is taken to the nearest millimeter (Lohman et al., 1988).

10.2 Growth indices

The correct interpretation of anthropometric measurements requires the use of anthropometric indices (WHO, 1995a). They are usually calculated from two or more raw anthropometric measurements. In the simplest case the indices are numerical ratios such as weight/(height)^2 (kg/m^2). Combinations such as weight-for-age, height-for-age, and weight-for-height are more complex (Section 1.5). These latter indices are not ratios and, to avoid confusion with numerical ratios, should *not* be written as "wt/age," "ht/age," and "wt/height." Combinations such as weight-for-age are expressed, instead, as *Z*-scores, percentiles, or percentage of the median (Section 13.1), relative to appropriate reference data. They can then be used to compare an individual or a group with a reference population. Deficits in one or more anthropometric indices of body size are frequently regarded as evidence of malnutrition. The influence of nutrition and health on indices of body size depends on the index and the circumstances, and thus it may vary across or within populations.

10.2.1 Head circumference-for-age

Head circumference-for-age can be used as an index of chronic protein-energy deficiency for children < 2 y. Chronic malnutrition during the first few months of life, or intrauterine growth retardation, may hinder brain development and result in an abnormally low head circumference. Beyond 2 y, growth in head circumference is slow and its measurement is no longer useful (Table 10.1) (Nellhaus, 1968). Head circumference-for-age is not sensitive to less extreme malnutrition (Yarbrough et al., 1974).

Certain non-nutritional factors, including some diseases and pathological conditions, genetic variation, and cultural practices such as binding of the head during infancy, as well as a difficult or forceps-assisted delivery at birth, may also influence head circumference.

10.2.2 Weight-for-age

Weight-for-age reflects body mass relative to chronological age. Low weight-for-age is described as "lightness" and reflects a pathological process referred to as "underweight," arising from gaining insufficient weight relative to age, or losing weight (WHO, 1995a). Because of its simplicity and the availability of scales in most health centers in low-income countries, weight-for-age is widely used in children from 6 mo to 7 y to assess under- and overnutrition.

A major limitation of weight-for-age is that

Age	Boys (cm)	Girls (cm)
Birth – 3 mo	5.9	5.7
3 – 6 mo	3.2	3.0
6 mo – 1 y	3.2	3.1
1 – 2 y	2.2	2.2
2 – 4 y	1.7	2.1
4 – 6 y	0.5	0.5
6 – 8 y	1.0	1.1
8 – 10 y	0.7	0.5
10 – 12 y	0.6	0.9
12 – 14 y	0.9	1.0
14 – 16 y	0.8	0.6
16 – 18 y	0.5	0.3

Table 10.1: Mean increment in head circumference. From Nellhaus, Pediatrics 211: 106–114, 1968 © with permission of Pediatrics.

it reflects both weight-for-height and height-for-age. It fails to distinguish tall, thin children from those who are short with adequate weight. Thus, children with a low weight-for-age may be genetically short, or their low weight-for-age may result from "stunting" or nutritional growth failure. This condition is characterized by low height-for-age but a weight appropriate to their short stature. Consequently, the prevalence of undernutrition in small children may be overestimated if only weight-for-age is used. Conversely, in populations where the prevalence of stunting is high but wasting is very low (e.g., Sub-Saharan Africa and Latin America), the use of weight-for-age to estimate the prevalence of undernutrition leads to a gross underestimate of the problem (WHO, 1995a).

To interpret any single measurement of either weight or height in relation to the reference data, the exact age of the child at the date of the measurement must be calculated from the date of birth. Software, such as Epi-Info 2004, can calculate exact ages in decimal fractions of a year, from birth and visit dates. EpiInfo 2004 is available from

http://www.cdc.gov/epiinfo/

Even when information on the date of birth is available, ages are sometimes calculated by rounding off to the most recently attained whole month. This practice should not be followed, because it results in systematic errors

(Gorstein, 1989). Details of alternative methods that can be used to assess the age of children in low-income countries where birth certificates are often not available are given in Section 9.3.1.

10.2.3 Weight-for-height

Weight-for-height measures body weight relative to height. Low weight-for-height in children is described as "thinness" and reflects a pathological process referred to as "wasting." It arises from a failure to gain sufficient weight relative to height or from losing weight. High weight-for-height in children is termed "overweight" and arises from gaining excess weight relative to height or from gaining insufficient height relative to weight (WHO, 1995a).

In stunted children, weight may be appropriate for length or height (i.e., stature), whereas in wasting, weight is very low for stature as a result of marked deficits in both tissue and fat mass. Children with poor linear growth should not be classified as "normal," based on weight-for-stature alone. In a study in Guatemala, for example, only a small percentage of children were identified as malnourished on the basis of low weight-for-length alone. As a result, policy-makers concluded that food aid was not necessary, despite Guatemala having the highest rates of stunting in all of Latin America (Ruel et al., 1995). A combination of weight-for-stature and height-for-age (Section 10.2.4) should always be used for children in those low-income countries where the prevalence of stunting is generally much higher than that of wasting.

Population studies of infants have shown that older infants at a given length tend to be heavier. Hence, during the first year, weight-for-length should be classified into narrow age groupings. Between 1 and approximately 10 y, however, weight-for-stature is relatively independent of age, enhancing its usefulness in areas where the ages of the children are uncertain. Weight-for-stature may also be independent of ethnic group, particularly for children 1–5 y (Waterlow et al., 1977).

During adolescence, the weight-for-height relationship changes dramatically with age and also with maturational status. For this reason the National Center for Health Statistics/WHO (NCHS/WHO) weight-for-height reference data extend only to 145 cm for boys and 137 cm for girls (Section 12.4.1). The new U.S. CDC 2000 growth charts provide weight-for-height reference data that range from 77 to 121 cm for both boys and girls (Kuczmarski et al., 2000) (Section 12.4). In most industrialized countries, these weight-for-height reference data can only be used for younger, preadolescent children.

Wasting often develops very rapidly but can be reversed quickly with an appropriate intervention. As a result, weight-for-stature is the preferred index for identifying young children who are most likely to benefit from a feeding program or for evaluating the benefits of intervention programs. It is more sensitive to changes in nutritional status than height-for-age. Weight-for-height is also frequently used in the nutritional assessment of hospital patients to identify wasting.

Seasonal, geographical, and age differences in the prevalence of wasting occur and are usually associated with both variations in food supply and the prevalence of infectious diseases. Nevertheless, in most low-income countries, with the notable exception of the Indian subcontinent, the prevalence of low weight-for-stature for children 0.5–5 y is said to be less than 5%, despite a high prevalence of stunting. The highest prevalence of low weight-for-stature often occurs during the postweaning period (12–23 mo) (WHO, 1986).

It is unclear why there is a low prevalence of weight-for-stature deficits in some regions with a high prevalence of stunting. Post and Victoria (2001) have argued that, in Brazilian children, the difference in body proportions — specifically the high circumference measurements of head, chest, and particularly abdomen — may account for their apparently adequate weight-for-stature. More detailed studies of body composition in stunted children in developing countries are needed to clarify the reasons for these apparent discrepancies. More appropriate anthropometric indices of thinness and overweight in stunted children are required.

In many of the industrialized countries, overweight in young children, defined by weight-for-height > 2 Z-scores, is becoming increasingly common. Overweight is also a problem among children in some emerging countries of Latin America and Asia and is discussed in more detail in Section 10.2.6.

10.2.4 Height-for-age

Height-for-age is a measure of achieved linear growth that can be used as an index of past nutritional or health status. Low height-for-age is defined as "shortness" and reflects either a normal variation or a pathological process involving failure to reach linear growth potential. The outcome of the latter process is termed "stunting," or the gaining of insufficient height relative to age (WHO 1995a).

Stunting results from extended periods of inadequate food intake, poor dietary quality, increased morbidity, or a combination of these factors. It is generally found in countries where economic conditions are poor. In some low-income countries, the prevalence of low height-for-age in children can be very high, ranging from 18% in South America to 60% in Southern Asia (de Onis et al., 1993). In such circumstances, most short children can be assumed to be stunted. However, when the prevalence is much lower and approximates the expected level, then those with low height-for-age are likely to be genetically short.

The prevalence of low stature-for-age, unlike wasting, is generally highest during the second or third year of life (WHO, 1986), although, in some settings, low length-for-age may occur as early as the first 3–6 mo. In these circumstances, low length-for-age is said to reflect a continuous process of "failing to grow" or "stunting," whereas in older children, it reflects "having failed to grow" or "being stunted" (WHO, 1995a).

In populations with a high prevalence of stunting but not wasting (e.g., Guatemala)

(Ruel et al., 1995), length-for-age at 3 mo can be used to screen for children at risk for stunting by 3 y. Identification of such children is important because stunting during childhood results in a reduction in adult size, which, in turn, has been associated with reduced work capacity and, in women, adverse reproductive outcomes.

The distribution of height measurements at a given age within most populations is often narrow, so that accurate measuring techniques are essential. During infancy, length can be assessed at 1-mo intervals for the first 6 mo, and at 2-mo intervals from 6 to 12 mo (Guo et al., 1991). A deficit in length takes some time to develop, so assessment of nutritional status based on length-for-age alone may underestimate malnutrition in infants in some settings. The influence of any possible genetic and ethnic differences must also be considered when evaluating stature-for-age.

10.2.5 Selecting the appropriate growth indices

Table 10.2 summarizes the information that can be obtained from each of the three growth indices discussed above. The choice of index depends on whether the information is required for diagnosing malnutrition at the individual or the population level, as well as

	Wt.-for-Ht.	Ht.-for-age	Wt.-for-age
Usefulness in populations where age is unknown or uncertain	1	4	4
Usefulness in identifying wasted children[a]	1	4	3
Sensitivity to weight change over a short period of time	1	4	2
Usefulness in identifying stunted children	4	1	2

Table 10.2: The relative usefulness of different anthropometric indices on a scale from 1 (excellent) to 4 (poor). [a]Depends to some extent on the prevalence of stunting and wasting in the population. From Gorstein et al., Bulletin of the World Health Organization 72: 273–283, 1994, with permission.

the study objectives. At the individual level, weight-for-height is the index of choice when the main objective is to identify and treat wasted children, whereas for stunted children stature-for-age is more appropriate.

At the population level, a combination of weight-for-stature and stature-for-age is preferred for identifying subgroups with a high prevalence of wasting (low weight-for-stature) and stunting (low stature-for-age), enabling necessary resources to be targeted to combat the problem.

Additional factors that must be considered when selecting an index or combination of indices, include the availability of accurate measuring equipment, the training of examiners to collect accurate information and to interpret the results correctly, and the time required to take the measurements. Finally, often overlooked are the costs of not identifying undernourished children or incorrectly identifying adequately nourished children as undernourished (Gorstein et al., 1994).

10.2.6 Weight changes

Body weight is the sum of the protein, fat, water, and bone mass in the body. Changes in body weight do not provide any information on the relative changes among these components. In normal adults, there is a tendency to increased fat deposition with age, concomitant with a reduction in muscle protein. Such changes are not evident in body weight measurements but can be seen by determining either body fat or the fat-free mass. In healthy persons, the daily variations in body weight are generally small (i.e., less than $\pm 0.5\,\mathrm{kg}$). In conditions of acute or chronic illness, however, negative energy-nitrogen balance may occur as the body can use endogenous sources of energy (including protein) as fuel for metabolic reactions. Consequently, body weight declines. In conditions of total starvation, the maximal weight loss is approximately 30% of initial body weight, at which point death occurs. In chronic semistarvation, body weight may decrease to approximately 50%–60% of ideal weight. In contrast, when persistent positive

energy balance occurs, there is an accumulation of adipose tissue, and body weight increases.

Body weight can only be used to assess the severity of undernutrition in subjects with relatively uncomplicated, nonedematous forms of semistarvation (Heymsfield et al., 1984). In disease conditions in which edema, ascites (fluid in the abdominal cavity), dehydration, diuresis, massive tumor growth, and organomegaly occur, or in obese patients undergoing rapid weight loss, body weight is a poor measure of body energy-nitrogen reserves. In such conditions, a relative increase in total body water, for example, may mask actual weight loss that results from losses of fat or skeletal muscle. Massive tumor growth may also mask losses of fat and muscle tissue, which may occur during severe undernutrition. Hence, additional anthropometric measurements (e.g., mid-upper-arm circumference and triceps skinfold thickness) should be taken to obtain more information on the origin of any change in body weight (Heymsfield et al., 1984).

To assess weight changes, the actual and usual weight of a subject must be known. From these two measurements, the percentage of usual weight, percentage of weight loss, and rate of change can be calculated (Table 10.3). The patient's actual weight can also be compared with appropriate age- and sex-specific reference data (Section 12.8).

Weight change indicator	Calculation method
% usual wt.	$\dfrac{\text{actual wt.}}{\text{usual wt.}} \times 100\%$
% wt. loss	$\dfrac{\text{usual wt.} - \text{actual wt.}}{\text{usual wt.}} \times 100\%$
Rate of change	$\dfrac{BW_p - BW_i}{Day_p - Day_i}\ (\text{kg/d})$

Table 10.3: Calculation of weight change indicators. BW_p and BW_i indicate present and initial body weights on the respective days.

Duration	Significant weight loss (%)	Severe weight loss (%)
1 wk	1–2	> 2
1 mo	5	> 5
3 mo	7.5	> 7.5
6 mo	10	> 10

Table 10.4: Evaluation of percentage of weight changes. From Blackburn et al., Journal of Parenteral and Enteral Nutrition 1: 11–22, 1977 © American Society for Parenteral and Enteral Nutrition.

Percentage of weight change can be evaluated in hospitalized patients using the guidelines of Blackburn et al. (1977) (Table 10.4). A weight loss of more than 10% of initial weight in 6 mo, or more than 5% in the 1 mo before admission to the hospital, is often clinically significant. Physiological impairment (e.g., reduced respiratory function) invariably accompanies a weight loss of more than 20% body weight (Hill, 1992). Such weight losses reflect an energy deficit that may arise from a combination of factors, including the clinical disease state, depression, loss of appetite, pain, and possibly swallowing difficulties (Corish and Kennedy, 2000).

The clinical outcome may be significantly affected in patients with a weight loss of between 10% and 20%. Indeed, the rate and timing of weight loss, rather than the underlying diagnosis, may be a more important predictive factor for the development of postoperative complications (Detsky et al., 1987). Moreover, preadmission weight loss of 10% may be a better indicator of prognostic performance in any preoperative nutritional assessment than multiple biochemical indices (e.g., total lymphocyte count, serum albumin, iron-binding capacity, and serum cholinesterase activity) (Gianotti et al., 1995). Weight loss in the preceding year was found to correlate significantly with the need for in-patient treatment in those patients with chronic obstructive airways disease (Braun et al., 1984), whereas in patients with chronic heart failure, wasting was an independent risk factor for mortality (Anker et al., 1997).

Marton et al. (1981) evaluated 91 patients with involuntary weight loss (> 5% of their

usual body weight during the previous 6 mo) in a prospective study. They estimated the prognosis of patients with weight loss: 25% of their patients had died, and another 15% had deteriorated clinically 1 y after the initial visit. They also developed a diagnostic strategy for weight loss to distinguish patients with a physical cause of weight loss from patients with no physical cause of weight loss. Six attributes were identified as significant independent diagnostic predictors of weight loss, all of which were based on medical history and physical examination. In population studies, however, it is not possible to define universal cutoff points for weight changes (either loss or gain) to identify high risk population groups (WHO, 1995a).

In low-income countries where there is a high prevalence of malnutrition, weekly weight gain is often used to monitor the short-term response to a feeding program. Maternal weight gain is also monitored routinely in pregnancy, in part because of the strong associations observed between pregnancy weight gain and infant size (Abrams et al., 2000). The U.S. Food and Nutrition Board (IOM, 1990) have compiled guidelines for recommended total weight gain ranges for U.S. women, according to prepregnancy body mass index (BMI in kg/m^2). These are given in Table 10.5.

In the United States, a weight gain of 0.4 kg/wk during both the second and third trimesters is recommended for women with a normal prepregnant BMI, 0.5 kg for those who are underweight, and 0.3 kg for overweight women (IOM, 1990). These recom-

BMI category (kg/m^2)	IOM (1990) recommended total gain (kg)[a]
Low (BMI < 19.8)	12.5–18
Normal (BMI 19.8–26.0)	11.5–16
High (BMI 26.0–29.0)[b]	7–11.5

Table 10.5: Recommended total weight gain in pregnant women by prepregnancy BMI. [a]Adolescents and African-American women should strive for gains at the lower end of the range. [b]The recommended target weight gain for obese women (BMI > 29.0) is ⩾ 6.0.

mendations are consistent with the findings of the WHO Collaborative Study; therefore, at present, WHO (1995b) recommends using the U.S. IOM (1990) guidelines for both total weight gain and weekly weight gain for low-income populations, until specific country cutoff values are available.

Marked changes in body weight with age have been documented in healthy adults in several recent national surveys conducted in industrialized countries (e.g., NHANES III). Weight tends to increase through early adulthood and then decreases with advancing age in the elderly.

10.3 Body mass index in adults

Weight to height ratios indicate body weight in relation to height and are particularly useful for providing a measure of overweight and obesity in adult populations. Hence these ratios are sometimes referred to as obesity indices.

At the present time, the ratio most commonly used in this way is the body mass index (BMI) (also termed Quetelet's index), calculated as weight (kg) / height (m)^2. Body mass index is used in preference to other weight/height indices, including the weight/height ratio, the Ponderal index, and Benn's index (Table 10.6). It is now used extensively internationally to classify overweight and obesity in adults.

Body mass index is relatively unbiased by height and appears to correlate reasonably well with laboratory-based measures of adiposity in most younger and older adults, as shown in Table 10.7 and Figure 10.12. Body

Age (y) and (n)	Partial corr. (r) of BMI with:		
	Fat mass	Lean mass	Total mass
Females			
16–49 (119)	0.81	0.44	0.81
50–84 (34)	0.93	0.43	0.85
All (153)	0.85	0.47	0.81
Males			
15–49 (48)	0.76	0.63	0.78
50–86 (25)	0.83	0.75	0.90
All (73)	0.77	0.63	0.84

Table 10.7: Partial correlations (r) of BMI with fat, lean, and total masses determined by dual-energy X-ray absorptiometry in male and female subjects of different ages. Correlations with fat mass hold lean mass, bone mass, and age constant. Correlations with lean mass hold fat mass, bone mass, and age constant. Correlations with total mass hold age constant. Data from Morabia et al., British Journal of Nutrition 82: 49–55, 1999, with permission of the Nutrition Society.

mass index is employed in large-scale nutrition surveys and epidemiological studies as a measure of overweight and obesity; measurements of weight and height are easy, quick, relatively noninvasive, and more precise than skinfold thickness measurements.

Nevertheless, BMI does not distinguish

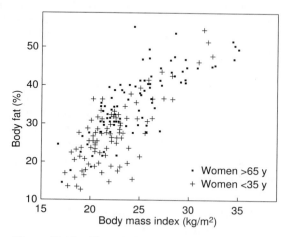

Figure 10.12: The relationship between body mass index and percentage of body fat in both younger and older women from New York City. Body fat determinations based on a four-compartment body-composition model. Data from Gallagher et al., American Journal of Epidemiology 143: 228–239, 1996, with permission of the Society for Epidemiologic Research.

Index	Formula
Weight/height ratio	wt/ht
Body Mass Index	wt/(ht)^2
Ponderal index	ht/$\sqrt[3]{\text{wt}}$
Benn's index	wt/(ht)^p

Table 10.6: Indices for weight relative to height. The power p in Benn's index is calculated to minimize the direct relationship with height (Benn, 1971).

between weight associated with muscle and weight associated with body fat. Hence, in some circumstances, an elevated BMI may result from excessive adiposity, muscularity, or edema. Further, BMI gives no indication about the distribution of body fat. Anomalies in the distribution of abdominal fat are now recognized to be as great a risk factor for disease as is excess body fat per se. Hence, when practical, it is often better to include a more direct measure of obesity, such as skinfold thickness measurements, with the BMI (WHO, 1995a). Waist circumference can also be used as a surrogate estimate of abdominal fat (Section 11.1.3), and is used to predict risk of cardiovascular disease. A high skinfold thickness or waist circumference would suggest that an elevated BMI is indeed from excessive adiposity.

Differences in body proportions and in the relationship between BMI and body fat content may result in certain population groups being misclassified as overweight or obese, based on BMI. Polynesians, for example, tend to be leaner with a lower percentage of body fat than are Caucasians at any given body size (Swinburn et al., 1996, 1999), but in some Asian populations, the reverse is true (Section 10.3.1) (Deurenberg et al., 1998; WHO Expert Consultation 2004). Other examples include athletic populations and individuals who are very short (<150 cm) or very muscular. Abnormal relationships between leg and trunk length can also lead to some misclassification, although BMI can now be corrected to take into account unusual leg length based on the ratio of sitting height to standing height (Norgan and Jones, 1995). Such adjustments are necessary for example, among Australian Aboriginals.

10.3.1 BMI and measures of body fat and disease risk

The validity of BMI as an index of the percentage body fat in adults has been assessed by correlating BMI with body fatness derived from the application of the best criterion models (Chapter 14). Examples of the latter include the four-compartment body-

composition model, based on densitometry, total body water via isotope dilution (Figure 10.12), and dual-energy X-ray absorptiometry (DXA) (Table 10.7). Use of such a multicomponent body-composition model reduces any bias introduced by the assumptions of the individual methods (Wells et al., 1999).

A major assumption of BMI is that it is an independent index of body fat. This means that after adjusting for body weight-for-stature, all subjects with the same BMI have the same relative fatness, irrespective of their age, sex, or ethnicity. Results of numerous recent studies have challenged the validity of this assumption. Several factors confound the relationship between BMI and body fat, all of which have implications for the use of BMI as an index of body fatness.

First, it is recognized that the relationship between BMI and body fat is both age- and sex-dependent (Deurenberg et al., 1991; Gallagher et al., 1996). For example, in the study shown in Figure 10.12, older women tend to have a relatively greater percentage of body fat than younger women of comparable BMI. A similar age-related trend was noted for men in this study (Gallagher et al., 1996); these trends persist up to 60–65 y of age in both sexes. Further, women have significantly greater amounts of total body fat than do men for an equivalent BMI. These sex differences are substantial and are maintained throughout the entire adult lifespan (Gallagher et al., 1996) and can be seen in children as young as 3–8 y (Taylor et al., 1997).

Second, the relationship between BMI and the percentage of body fat appears to differ among certain ethnic groups, as noted earlier. Figure 10.13 shows results of a meta-analysis among different ethnic groups conducted by Deurenberg et al. (1998). Of the 15 studies included in the meta-analyses, 11 used a "reference criterion method" for the measurement of body fat. The methods included DXA, densitometry, deuterium oxide dilution, and three or four multi-compartment models. Results of the meta-analysis indicate that in some populations (e.g., some Chinese, urban Thais, Indonesians), levels of obesity in terms of percentage of body fat will be greater at the $30 \, \text{kg/m}^2$ obesity cutoff suggested by WHO (2000) than for Europeans. The existence of such ethnic-related differences has been confirmed by several other investigators (Gurrici et al., 1999; Dudeja et al., 2001). For example, Asian Indians are also reported to have more body fat than Europeans at any given BMI (Wang et al. 1994; Dudeja et al., 2001), whereas for Chinese from Beijing and rural Thais, values are similar to those of Europeans (WHO Expert Consultation, 2004). In contrast, in some Pacific populations, the percentage of body fat at a given BMI is lower (Figure 10.13) (Swinburn et al., 1999). These ethnic-related discrepancies may be linked to differences in energy intake, dietary patterns, and amount of physical activity, as well as body build (e.g., leg length) or frame size (Norgan, 1994; Gurrici et al., 1999; Deurenberg-Yap et al., 2000).

Body mass index has been used in several international population studies to assess disease risk among adults. Increasing BMI is clearly associated with a higher risk of high blood pressure, type 2 diabetes mellitus, other cardiovascular disease risk factors, and increased mortality (Figure 10.14) (Manson et

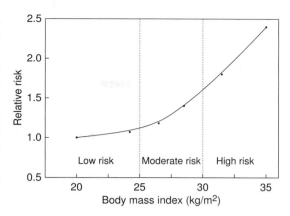

Figure 10.14: Relationship between BMI and the relative risk of mortality. Data from WHO (2000), with permission.

al., 1995; WHO 2000; Song and Sung, 2001; WHO Expert Consultation, 2004). Indeed, the relative risk for cardiovascular disease risk factors and cardiovascular disease incidence increases in a graded fashion with increasing BMI in all population groups. In addition, associations between musculoskeletal disorders, impairments in respiratory and physical functioning, and quality of life have been reported (Seidall et al., 2001). As a result, in epidemiological studies, BMI is the preferred index to classify overweight and obesity in adults and to estimate relative risk of disease (NHLBI, 1998).

10.3.2 WHO classification of overweight and obesity in adults

The WHO International Obesity Task Force has defined obesity as a condition in which excess body fat adversely affects health and well-being (WHO, 2000). They have recommended the use of a graded classification of overweight and obesity to:

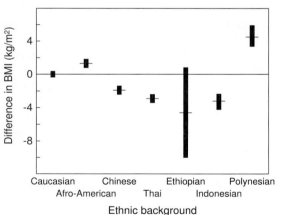

Figure 10.13: Ethnic differences in calculated values for body mass index (BMI) (mean and 95% confidence interval) which reflect equal levels of body fat, adjusted for age and sex. The means are relative to the results for Caucasians (set to 0.0). Data from Deurenberg et al., International Journal of Obesity and Related Metabolic Disorders 22: 1164–1171, 1998 © with permission of the Nature Publishing Group.

- Compare weight status within and between populations
- Identify individuals and groups who are at increased risk of morbidity and mortality
- Identify priorities for intervention at both the individual and community levels
- Allow interventions to be evaluated appropriately

Table 10.8 shows the classification of adults according to BMI recommended for international use by WHO (2000). It is based primarily on the association between BMI and mortality. The general term "overweight" is used by WHO (2000) to describe all subjects with BMI ≥ 25 kg/m^2. Subjects with BMI from 25.0 to 29.9 are further termed "pre-obese." Three classes of obesity are defined based on BMI cutoffs of 30, 35, and 40 kg/m^2. This classification system is not intended for use with pregnant and lactating women, or persons < 18 y.

WHO (1995a) suggested that a universal cutoff point of BMI ≥ 30 could be used to estimate and compare the prevalence of obesity within and between populations. The results shown in Table 10.9 emphasize the wide variation in the prevalence across countries. Similar differences among populations exist when the BMI cutoffs for defining overweight (i.e., ≥ 25 and < 30) are used.

WHO (2000, 2004) recognizes that these BMI cutoff points for overweight and obesity may not correspond to the same degree of fatness and health risks across different populations, as noted earlier. In particular, in their 2004 report, WHO emphasizes the mounting evidence that Asian populations have a particularly high risk of type 2 diabetes, cardiovascular disease, and mortality from other causes at relatively low BMIs. Nevertheless, more prospective studies are needed in Asian countries to clarify these

Country and date	Age (y)	Prevalence (%) Men	Women
Australia 1989	25–64	11.5	13.2
Brazil 1989	25–64	6	13
Canada 1986–1990	18–74	15.0	13.0
China 1992	20–45	1.20	1.60
Cyprus 1989–1990	35–64	19	24
England 1995	16–64	15	16.5
Finland 1991–1993	20–75	14	11
Japan 1993	20+	1.7	2.7
Kuwait 1994	18+	32	41
Netherlands 1995	20–59	8	8
New Zealand 1989	18–64	10	13
Saudi Arabia 1990-1993	15+	16	24
USA 1988–1994	20–74	19.9	24.9

Table 10.9: Obesity prevalence (BMI ≥ 30) in selected countries. Data from WHO (2000), with permission.

issues. A recent evaluation of the effect of BMI on mortality among several Asian cohorts, for example, provided no evidence for a need for lower cutoff points for Asians (Stevens and Nowicki, 2003).

In light of the ethnic differences discussed above, WHO (2004) has now proposed the use of four new intermediate public health action points at BMI values of 23.0, 27.5, 32.5, and 37.5 kg/m^2. These values are for use by Asian populations, in whom the existing WHO BMI cutoff points shown in Table 10.8 for risks related to overweight and obesity may not apply. Justification for these new action points is given in WHO (2004). In the future, waist circumference (Section 11.1.3) may be a useful measurement to refine these new WHO action levels based on BMI in populations with a predisposition to central obesity and the related increased risk of developing metabolic disturbances.

10.3.3 Canadian classification of overweight and obesity in adults

The BMI classification system for adults used by Health Canada (Table 10.10) has been adapted from that of WHO (2000). Health Canada (2003) cautions that the classification system may misclassify certain population groups such as adults with a very lean body build or who are highly muscular, young

Classification	BMI (kg/m^2)	Risk of comorbidities
Underweight	< 18.50	Low (but risk of other clinical problems is increased)
Normal range	18.50–24.99	Average
Overweight	≥ 25.00	
Preobese	25.00–29.99	Increased
Obese class I	30.00–34.99	Moderate
Obese class II	35.00–39.99	Severe
Obese class III	≥ 40.00	Very severe

Table 10.8: WHO classification of overweight in adults according to body mass index (BMI). From WHO (2000), with permission.

Health Canada Classification	BMI	Risk of developing health problems
Underweight	< 18.50	Increased
Normal weight	18.50–24.99	Least
Overweight	25.00–29.99	Increased
Obese		
Class I	30.00–34.99	High
Class II	35.00–39.99	Very high
Class III	≥ 40.00	Extremely high

Table 10.10: Health Canada (2003) classification of adults according to BMI. For persons ≥ 65 y, the "normal" range may begin slightly above BMI 18.5 and extend into the "overweight" range.

adults who have not reached full growth, those over 65 years of age, and certain ethnic and racial groups. Several health problems associated with overweight and obesity are also specified. They include coronary heart disease, type 2 diabetes, hypertension, dyslipidemia, gallbladder disease, obstructive sleep apnea, and certain cancers.

10.3.4 U.S. classification of overweight and obesity in adults

The cutoff points that define normal weight, overweight, and the various levels of obesity in the United States are the same as those used by WHO (2000). Differences exist in the terms used to describe overweight and the levels of obesity in the United States, as shown in Table 10.11. Individuals with BMIs ranging from 25.0 to 29.9 are desig-

Classification	BMI	Disease risk
Underweight	< 18.50	—
Normal weight	18.50–24.99	—
Overweight	25.00–29.99	Increased
Obese		
Class I	30.00–34.99	High
Class II	35.00–39.99	Very high
Class III (Extreme obesity)	≥ 40.00	Extremely high

Table 10.11: U.S. classification of overweight and obesity by BMI. From NHLBI, Obesity Research 6: 51S–209S, 1998.

nated as "overweight" instead of "preobese," and class III (i.e., BMI ≥ 40) is termed "extreme obesity" rather than "very severe obesity" (Table 10.8) (NHLBI, 1998). Such differences are potentially confusing.

10.3.5 BMI and chronic energy deficiency in adults

In low-income countries, low values for BMI in adults have been consistently associated with a decline in work output, productivity, and income-generating ability, as well as a compromised ability to respond to stressful conditions (Ferro-Luzzi et al., 1992). In some more affluent countries, underweight has been associated with osteoporosis, infertility, and impaired immunocompetence (Health Canada, 2003). A cutoff point of < 18.5 kg/m^2 is used to define low BMI values, indicative of underweight in both men and women in both low-income and more affluent countries (James et al., 1988; Ferro-Luzzi et al., 1992; Health Canada, 2003).

In 1994, FAO adopted the term "chronic energy deficiency" for underweight (Shetty and James, 1994). They categorized three degrees of underweight on the basis of BMI; the cutoffs used are shown in Table 10.12. WHO (1995a, 2004) has adopted these same cutoffs to define three grades of low BMI, referred to as "thinness" in WHO (1995a) and as "underweight" in WHO (2004), rather than "chronic energy deficiency." In WHO (2004), Grade I (17.0–18.4) is termed "mild underweight," Grade II (16.0–16.9) "moderate underweight," and Grade III (< 16 kg/m^2) "severe underweight."

Chronic energy deficiency grade	BMI (kg/m^2)
Normal	> 18.5
Grade I	17.0–18.4
Grade II	16.0–16.9
Grade III	< 16.0

Table 10.12: Simple classification of adult chronic energy deficiency using BMI (kg/m^2). From Shetty and James, FAO (1994), with permission.

WHO (1995a) has also devised a classification system to identify populations with a public health problem on the basis of low BMI; details are shown in Table 10.13. In any healthy adult population, 3%–5% can be expected to have a BMI $< 18.5\,\mathrm{kg/m^2}$. However, in countries with food insecurity, an excessive proportion of the population may have BMIs < 18.5, with very few obese subjects. In contrast, as the proportion of thin individuals decreases, the proportion with BMI $\geqslant 25$ increases. Indeed, generally, as socio-economic conditions improve, there is a tendency for a population to shift from thinness to overweight (de Onis and Habicht, 1996). This relationship can be seen in the probability density functions drawn in Figure 10.15, generalized from 52 surveys in 32 countries and in Figure 10.16.

Although somewhat arbitrary, the low BMI classification system shown in Table 10.13 reflects the situation in the adult population of several developing countries. In Singapore, however, in the National Health Survey (Ministry of Health, 1999), 11% of females and 7% of males had a BMI < 18.5. As it is unlikely that undernutrition is a significant problem in Singapore, this finding suggests that the cutoff point for underweight, like overweight, noted earlier (Section 10.3.3), might also differ with ethnicity and environment, as well as age, sex, and duration of undernutrition. Indeed, in a study of African

women, Gartner et al. (2001) proposed a new category of "normal but vulnerable" women based on a BMI of between 17.0 and 18.5 and MUAC $\geqslant 23.0\,\mathrm{cm}$. Clearly, challenges still exist in relation to the use of low BMI cutoffs for defining thinness or chronic energy deficiency in adult populations, and more research is required.

10.4 BMI in children and adolescents

Body mass index is now also the internationally recommended indicator of overweight and obesity in both children and adolescents (WHO, 1995a). The recommendation arises from the following observations:

- Strong positive correlations between BMI and body fatness (measured in children by densitometry, magnetic resonance imaging, or DXA) (Figure 10.17) (Deurenberg et al., 1991; Goran et al., 1996; Goulding et al., 1996; Daniels et al., 1997; Pietrobelli et al., 1998; Ellis et al., 1999)
- Associations between BMI or changes in BMI in children and several major risk factors for subsequent heart disease and other chronic diseases; risk factors include increased blood pressure, adverse lipoprotein

Situation	% of population with BMI <18.5
Low prevalence (warning sign, monitoring required)	5–9
Medium prevalence (poor situation)	10–19
High prevalence (critical situation)	20–39
Very high prevalence (critical situation)	$\geqslant 40$

Table 10.13: WHO classification of populations on the basis of low BMI. Compiled from WHO (1995), with permission.

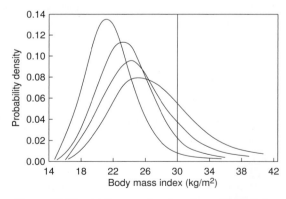

Figure 10.15: A diagram showing the pattern of the shifting distribution of BMI in adult populations. As the mean population BMI increases, the level of obesity (BMI $\geqslant 30$) increases at an even faster rate because of the skewing of the distribution to higher BMIs. From WHO (2000).

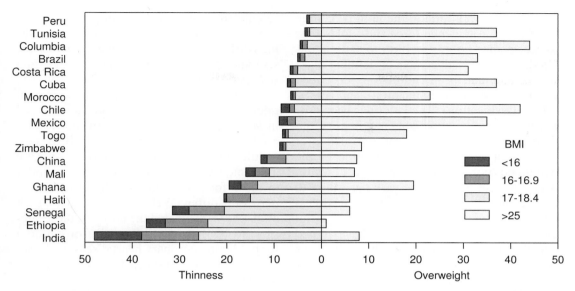

Figure 10.16: BMI distribution of various adult populations worldwide (both sexes). For each country, the percentage of the population who are overweight and thin is shown: normal subjects (BMI from 18.5 to 25) are not shown. From WHO (1995), with permission.

profiles, late-onset diabetes and early atherosclerotic lesions (Zwiauer et al., 1990; McGill et al., 1995; Dwyer and Blizzard, 1996)

- BMI in childhood correlating more significantly with BMI in young adulthood (i.e., tracks more closely) than the corresponding skinfold measures (Clarke and Lauer, 1993; Guo et al., 1994)
- Boys with BMI > 75th percentile having increased risk of mortality from all causes, coronary heart disease, atherosclerosis, and cerebrovascular diseases (Ellis, 2001)

Notwithstanding the correlation in some children of BMI and body fatness measured by DXA, BMI is not a perfect indicator of body fatness. Dietz and Bellizzi (1999) have cautioned that BMI will falsely classify some children of normal fatness as overweight and some overweight children as not overweight. Although errors in the measurement of percentage of body fat may account for some of the variability in the relationship between BMI and body fatness in children, several other factors may be implicated. These include enhanced muscular development, large

head size, and a high torso-to-leg ratio. All these factors may falsely elevate BMI into an overweight range in some "nonoverweight" children (Roberts and Dallal, 2001).

Defining overweight and obesity in children is more difficult than in adults, and the age-independent adult BMI classifica-

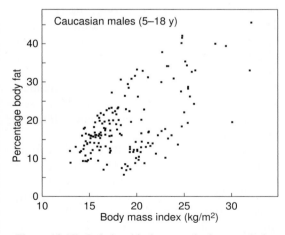

Figure 10.17: Relationship between body mass index (BMI) and percentage body fat (via DXA) for boys ages 5–18 y. Data from Ellis, Journal of Nutrition 131: 1589S–1595S, 2001, with permission of the American Society for Nutritional Sciences.

tions are not appropriate: the 50th percentile for BMI for younger children and adolescents increases markedly from birth to early adulthood. Two alternative ways of defining overweight and obesity in children are described in 10.4.1 (WHO classification) and 10.4.2 (U.S. classification). The latter has been criticized because overweight and obesity are defined statistically, with the prevalence of overweight set at a fixed proportion of the childhood population at any age. Moreover, because BMI values vary according to degree of sexual maturity, even in adolescents of the same chronological age (Bini et al., 2000), some investigators have argued that the stage of sexual maturity, as well as age, should be taken into account when assessing overweight in adolescents. Taylor et al. (2003) concluded, however, that the additional burden of securing information on pubertal status, did not justify the use of age- and sexual maturity-specific cutoffs.

10.4.1 WHO classification of overweight and obesity in children

In 1998, WHO convened an International Task Force on Obesity to define overweight and obesity in children and adolescents. This expert group agreed to recommend the adoption of an earlier approach developed by the European Childhood Obesity group (Poskitt, 1995). The approach links the adult BMI definitions of both overweight (BMI $\geqslant 25$) and obesity (BMI $\geqslant 30$) to BMI percentiles for children to provide child cutoff points. The WHO (2000) Task Force also recommended that the BMI percentiles for children used should be based on an international reference population.

In response to this WHO (2000) recommendation, Cole et al. (2000) compiled data for BMI from six large nationally representative cross-sectional growth studies (Brazil, Great Britain, Hong Kong, the Netherlands, Singapore, and the United States). For each country, the two percentile values equivalent to a BMI of 25 and 30 kg/m^2 at 18 y were determined for each sex. The BMI values at different childhood ages were then

calculated for the same pair of percentiles for each of the six national data sets. The resulting BMI values were then averaged across the six data sets to provide international age- and sex-specific cutoff points from 2 to 18 y.

The adoption of this approach has several important advantages, which are summarized in Box 10.1. However, it is still not clearly established if these age-specific BMI percentile cutoffs in childhood (Table 10.14) are associated with health risks that are similar to those for adults: the health consequences may well differ (WHO, 2000). Katzmarzyk et al. (2003) evaluated the utility of these age-specific BMI percentile cutoffs for children for predicting coronary heart disease risk factors. Overweight French Canadian children had between 1.6 and 9.1 times the risk of elevated risk factors compared to their normal-weight counterparts. Hence, these results support the adoption of these age-dependent international cutoffs among youth. Nevertheless, more research is required on the validity of these new cutoff points, especially among Hispanic and Asian populations and those with a high prevalence of stunting: factors other than increased body fat may be responsible for increased weight-for-height in such populations, as noted in Section 10.2.3.

10.4.2 U.S. classification of overweight and obesity in children

The approach of Cole et al. (2000) has not been widely adopted in the United States. Instead, an earlier U.S. Expert Committee (Himes and Dietz, 1994) recommended that the 85th percentile of BMI-for-age be used to

---

International comparisons of the prevalence of overweight and obesity in children and adolescents can be made.

Weight-for-stature charts, which cover only a restricted age range, and may omit adolescence entirely, are eliminated.

Obesity assessment in adults is integrated with that for children and adolescents.

Box 10.1: Advantages of the age-dependent international cutoffs for BMI for children for overweight and obesity.

Age (y)	BMI = 25 kg/m²		BMI = 30 kg/m²	
	Males	Females	Males	Females
2.0	18.41	18.02	20.09	19.81
2.5	18.13	17.76	19.80	19.55
3.0	17.89	17.56	19.57	19.36
3.5	17.69	17.40	19.39	19.23
4.0	17.55	17.28	19.29	19.15
4.5	17.47	17.19	19.26	19.12
5.0	17.42	17.15	19.30	19.17
5.5	17.45	17.20	19.47	19.34
6.0	17.55	17.34	19.78	19.65
6.5	17.71	17.53	20.23	20.08
7.0	17.92	17.75	20.63	20.51
7.5	18.18	18.03	21.09	21.01
8.0	18.44	18.35	21.60	21.57
8.5	18.76	18.69	22.17	22.18
9.0	19.10	19.07	22.77	22.81
9.5	19.46	19.45	23.39	23.46
10.0	19.84	19.86	24.00	24.11
10.5	20.20	20.29	24.57	24.77
11.0	20.55	20.74	25.10	25.42
11.5	20.89	21.20	25.58	26.05
12.0	21.22	21.68	26.02	26.67
12.5	21.56	22.14	26.43	27.24
13.0	21.91	22.58	26.84	27.76
13.5	22.27	22.98	27.25	28.20
14.0	22.62	23.34	27.63	28.57
14.5	22.96	23.66	27.98	28.87
15.0	23.29	23.94	28.30	29.11
15.5	23.60	24.17	28.60	29.29
16.0	23.90	24.37	28.88	29.43
16.5	24.19	24.54	28.14	29.56
17.0	24.46	24.70	29.41	29.69
17.5	24.73	24.85	29.70	29.84
18.0	25.00	25.00	30.00	30.00

Table 10.14: International cutoff points for BMI for children for overweight and obesity by sex from 2 to 18 y, defined to pass through BMI = 25 kg/m² and BMI = 30 kg/m² at 18 y obtained by averaging data from Brazil, Great Britain, Hong Kong, the Netherlands, Singapore, and the United States. Data from Cole et al., British Medical Journal 320: 1240–1243, 2000, with permission of the BMJ Publishing Group.

diagnose "at risk of overweight" and the 95th percentile of BMI-for-age to identify "overweight," as shown in Table 10.15. Originally, the 85th and 95th percentiles for BMI-for-age were developed by Must et al. (1991), based on the NHANES I data for children 6–19 y. Today, use of the 85th and 95th percentiles for BMI-for-age, from the Centers for Disease Control and Prevention (CDC) 2000 growth charts, is preferred (Kuczmarski et al., 2000).

Overweight category	Percentile limits
Normal	< 85th percentile
At risk of overweight	≥ 85th and < 95th percentile
Overweight	≥ 95th percentile

Table 10.15: BMI cutoffs for overweight in children and adolescents for use in the United States. Data from Himes and Dietz, American Journal of Clinical Nutrition 59: 307–316, 1994 © Am J Clin Nutr. American Society for Clinical Nutrition.

The NHANES III data for children ≥ 6 y were not included in the data set used to calculate the updated CDC 2000 BMI percentiles because of the marked increases in weight of children ≥ 6 y in NHANES III compared with earlier U.S surveys (Section 12.4.4). Without this exclusion, overweight would be underdiagnosed in U.S. children and adolescents.

As BMI changes with age, the definition of overweight (i.e., 95th percentile values) based on the CDC 2000 growth charts varies from a low of 17.5 and 18.5 (in boys and girls at 4.25 y and 4 y, respectively) to 30.5 and 31.7 (in boys and girls at 20 y).

10.4.3 Comparisons of overweight and obesity among countries

At present, countries vary in the choice of the indicator, the reference data, the cutoff points, and the nomenclature used to define overweight and obesity in children (Guillaume, 1999). The United Kingdom, the United States, and most countries in Europe now use the 85th and 95th percentiles to define overweight, but retain their own BMI reference data. In Latin America and Asia, however, weight-for-height is still more frequently used. Hence, caution must be used when examining the prevalence of overweight and obesity across countries. For example, Table 10.16 compares the prevalence (as percent) of overweight in U.S. children in NHANES III, when the CDC 2000 definition of overweight (95th percentile) is used, with the corresponding prevalence calculated using the sex- and age-specific cutoff points of Cole et al. (2000) equivalent to an adult BMI of 30 kg/m². Relative to the CDC 2000

Age group reference values	NHANES III Boys	Girls
2–5 y		
CDC 2000	6.2	8.2
Cole et al., 2000	2.5	4.2
6–8 y		
CDC 2000	10.8	11.0
Cole et al., 2000	7.7	7.8
9–11 y		
CDC 2000	12.8	11.0
Cole et al., 2000	6.5	8.8
12–14 y		
CDC 2000	11.9	11.7
Cole et al., 2000	6.9	10.1
15–17 y		
CDC 2000	12.0	8.7
Cole et al., 2000	8.9	6.6
18–19 y		
CDC 2000	9.2	8.1
Cole et al., 2000	9.3	11.7

Table 10.16: Prevalence of BMIs $\geqslant$ 95th percentile in children in NHANES based on two different reference data sets. From Flegal et al., American Journal of Clinical Nutrition 73: 1086–1093, 2001 © Am J Clin Nutr. American Society for Clinical Nutrition.

growth charts, use of the method of Cole et al. (2000) results in lower prevalence estimates for overweight for young children but higher estimates for older children (i.e., aged 18–19 y).

Clearly, an international consensus must be reached before meaningful comparisons can be made. Hopefully, if further research demonstrates that the BMI cutoffs derived by Cole et al. (2000) can predict morbidity and mortality across countries, they will become accepted for international use.

10.5 Summary

Standardized methods for measuring stature (height or length), knee height, head circumference, body weight, and elbow breadth in infants, children, and adults are available and should always be used to ensure accurate and precise measurements. Indices can then be constructed from these raw measurements. Such indices include either simple numerical ratios (e.g., weight/height^2) (BMI), or combinations such as weight-for-age, height-for-

age, weight-for-height, and head circumference-for-age. The latter is closely related to brain size and is used as an index of chronic protein-energy deficiency during the first 2 y of life, provided non-nutritional effects have been excluded.

Low weight-for-age is described as "lightness" and reflects "underweight." It tends to overestimate undernutrition in children who are either genetically short, or "stunted," as it does not take into account height differences. Low weight-for-height is described as "thinness" and reflects "wasting." High weight-for-height is usually termed "overweight." Weight-for-height is relatively independent of age in children 1–10 y. The presence of edema, obesity, or poor linear growth may complicate the interpretation of this index, and, as a result, a combination of weight-for-height and height-for-age is often recommended at the population level.

Height-for-age reflects the achieved linear growth and is used as an index of past nutritional or health status in both children and adults, although genetic and ethnic influences must be taken into account. Low height-for-age is defined as "shortness" and reflects a failure to reach linear growth potential, the outcome of which is termed "stunting."

Weight/height ratios measure body weight corrected for height, but cannot distinguish between excessive weight produced by adiposity, muscularity, or edema. The BMI (wt/ht^2) is the indicator of choice for defining overweight and obesity in epidemiological studies among adults, as well as children and adolescents. It correlates strongly in both adults and children with body fatness as measured by reference criterion methods (e.g., densitometry and DXA) and also with many health-related indices including cardiovascular disease risk factors such as high blood pressure, type 2 diabetes mellitus, as well as the risk of mortality.

WHO has defined obesity as a condition in which excess body fat adversely affects health and well-being. In adults, WHO has recommended the use of universal BMI cutoff points for overweight (BMI $\geqslant$ 25) and obesity (BMI $\geqslant$ 30); three levels of obesity are defined. This classification has been adopted by several countries. In the U.S. and Canadian classifications, the same cutoff points for overweight and three levels of obesity are used, although some of the terms used to describe the levels of overweight and obesity differ from those used by WHO. In the WHO, U.S. and Canadian classifications, the highest grade is represented by BMI ≥ 40.

FAO and WHO have also recommended cutoffs to define three grades of low BMI values, indicative of underweight in adults. This is termed "chronic energy deficiency" by FAO and "thinness" by WHO. WHO has also developed a classification to identify populations with a public health problem on the basis of low BMI.

At present, no consensus exists among countries about the indicator, reference data, cutoff points, or nomenclature used to define overweight and obesity in children. In children and adolescents, universal cutoffs for overweight and obesity cannot be applied because BMI increases with age. Instead, WHO recommends the use of internationally derived, age-specific BMI values for children that are equivalent to the adult BMI definitions of overweight (BMI ≥ 25) and obesity (BMI ≥ 30). Currently, in the United States, the diagnosis of overweight is based on $\geq$ 95th percentile, and the risk of overweight on $\geq$ 85th and $\leq$ 95th percentiles of the CDC 2000 BMI reference data. Countries in Europe and the United Kingdom use these same percentile cutoffs but their own BMI reference data. In the future, it is hoped that the international BMI cutoffs for overweight and obesity derived by Cole et al. (2000) will become accepted for international use for children and adolescents.

References

Abrams B, Altman SL, Pickett KE. (2000). Pregnancy weight gain: still controversial. American Journal of Clinical Nutrition 71: 1233S–1241S.

Alexander GR, Allen MC. (1996). Conceptualization, measurement, and use of gestational age. I. Clinical and public health practice. Journal of Perinatology 16: 53–59.

Anker SD, Ponikowski P, Varney S, Chua TP, Clark AL, Webb-Peploe KM, Harrington D, Kox WJ, Poole-Wilson PA, Coats AJS. (1997). Wasting as independent risk factor for mortality in chronic heart failure. Lancet 349: 1050–1053.

Ballard JL, Novak KK, Driver M. (1979). A simplified score for assessment of fetal maturation of newly born infants. Journal of Pediatrics 95: 769–774.

Belizan JM, Villar J, Nardin JC, Malamud J, De Vicuna LS. (1978). Diagnosis of intrauterine growth retardation by a simple clinical method: measurement of uterine height. American Journal of Obstetrics and Gynecology 131: 643–646.

Benn RT. (1971). Some mathematical properties of weight-for-height indices used as measures of adiposity. British Journal of Preventive and Social Medicine 25: 42–50.

Bini V, Celi F, Berioli MG, Bacosi ML, Stella P, Giglio P, Tosti L, Falorni A. (2000). Body mass index of children and adolescents according to age and pubertal stage. European Journal of Clinical Nutrition 54: 214–218.

Blackburn GL, Bistrain BR, Maini BS, Schlamm HT, Smith MF. (1977). Nutritional and metabolic assessment of the hospitalized patient. Journal of Parenteral and Enteral Nutrition 1: 11–22.

Braun SR, Dixon RM, Keim NL, Luby M, Anderegg A, Shrago ES. (1984). Predictive clinical value of nutritional assessment factors in COPD. Chest 85: 353–357.

Chumlea WC, Guo S. (1992). Equations for predicting stature in white and black elderly individuals. Journal of Gerontology 47: M197–M203.

Chumlea WC, Roche AF, Mukherjee D. (1984). Nutritional Assessment of the Elderly through Anthropometry. Ross Laboratories, Columbus, Ohio.

Chumlea WC, Roche AF, Steinbaugh ML. (1989). Anthropometric approaches to the nutritional assessment of the elderly. In: Munro HN (ed.) Human Nutrition and Aging, Plenum Publishing, New York, pp. 335–361.

Clarke WR, Lauer RM. (1993). Does childhood obesity track into adulthood? Critical Review of Food Science and Nutrition 33: 423–430.

Cockram DB, Baumgartner RN. (1990). Evaluation of accuracy and reliability of calipers for measuring recumbent knee height in elderly people. American Journal of Clinical Nutrition 52: 397–400.

Cole TJ, Bellizzi MC, Flegal KM, Dietz WH. (2000). Establishing a standard definition for child overweight and obesity worldwide: international study. British Medical Journal 320: 1240–1243.

Corish CA, Kennedy NP. (2000). Protein-energy undernutrition in hospital in-patients. British Journal of Nutrition 83: 575–591.

Cronk CE, Stallings VA, Spender QW, Ross JL, Widdoes H. (1989). Measurement of short-term growth with a new knee height measuring device. American Journal of Human Biology 1: 421–428.

Daniels SR, Khoury PR, Morrison JA. (1997). The utility of body mass index as a measure of body fatness in children and adolescents: differences by race and gender. Pediatrics 99: 804–807.

de Onis M, Habicht J-P. (1996). Anthropometric reference data for international use: recommendations from a World Health Organization Expert Committee. American Journal of Clinical Nutrition 64: 650–658.

de Onis M, Monteiro C, Akré J, Clugston G. (1993). The worldwide magnitude of protein-energy malnutrition: an overview from the WHO Global Database on Child Growth. Bulletin of the World Health Organization 71: 703–712.

Detsky AS, McLaughlin JR, Baker JP, Johnson N, Whittaker S, Mendelson RA, Jeejeebhoy K. (1987). What is subjective global assessment of nutritional status? Journal of Parenteral and Enteral Nutrition 11: 8–13.

Deurenberg P, Westrate JA, Seidell JC. (1991). Body mass index as a measure of body fatness: age- and sex-specific prediction formulas. British Journal of Nutrition 65: 105–114.

Deurenberg P, Yap M, van Staveren WA. (1998). Body mass index and percent body fat: a meta analysis among different ethnic groups. International Journal of Obesity and Related Metabolic Disorders 22: 1164–1171.

Deurenberg-Yap M, Schmidt G, van Staveren WA, Deurenberg P. (2000). The paradox of low body mass index and high body fat percentage among Chinese, Malays and Indians in Singapore. International Journal of Obesity and Related Metabolic Disorders 24: 1011–1017.

Dietz WH, Bellizzi MC. (1999). Introduction: the use of body mass index to assess obesity in children. American Journal of Clinical Nutrition 70: 123S–125S.

Doherty CP, Sarkar MA, Shakur MS, Ling SC, Elton RA, Cutting WA. (2001). Linear and knemometric growth in the early phase of rehabilitation from severe malnutrition. British Journal of Nutrition 85: 755–759.

Dubowitz LM, Dubowitz V, Goldberg C. (1970). Clinical assessment of gestational age in the newborn infant. Journal of Pediatrics 77: 1–10.

Dudeja V, Misra A, Pandey RM, Devina G, Kumar G, Vikram NK. (2001). BMI does not accurately predict overweight in Asian Indians in northern India. British Journal of Nutrition 86: 105–112.

Dwyer T, Blizzard CL. (1996). Defining obesity in children by biological endpoint rather than population distribution. International Journal of Obesity and Related Metabolic Disorders 20: 472–480.

Ellis KJ. (2001). Selected body composition methods can be used in field studies. Journal of Nutrition 131: 1589S–1595S.

Ellis KJ, Abrams SA, Wong WW. (1999). Monitoring childhood obesity: assessment of the weight/height^2 index. American Journal of Epidemiology 150: 939–946.

Ferro-Luzzi A, Sette S, Franklin M, James WP. (1992). A simplified approach to assessing adult chronic energy deficiency. European Journal of Clinical Nutrition 46: 173–186.

Flegal KM, Ogden CL, Wei R, Kuczmarski RL, Johnson CL. (2001). Prevalence of overweight in U.S. children: comparison of U.S. growth charts from the Centers for Disease Control and Prevention with other reference values for body mass index. American Journal of Clinical Nutrition 73: 1086–1093.

Frisancho AR. (1990). Anthropometric Standards for the Assessment of Growth and Nutritional Status. University of Michigan Press, Ann Arbor.

Gallagher D, Visser M, Sepulveda D, Pierson RN, Harris T, Heymsfield SB. (1996). How useful is body mass index for comparison of body fatness across age, sex, and ethnic groups? American Journal of Epidemiology 143: 228–239.

Gartner A, Maire B, Kameli Y, Traissac P, Delpeuch F. (2001). Body composition unaltered for African women classified as "normal but vulnerable" by body mass index and mid-upper-arm-circumference criteria. European Journal of Clinical Nutrition 55: 393–399.

Gianotti L, Braga M, Radaelli G, Mariani L, Vignali A, Di Carlo V. (1995). Lack of improvement in prognostic performance of weight loss when combined with other parameters. Nutrition 11: 12–16.

Gibson AT, Pearse RG, Wales JK. (1993). Knemometry and the assessment of growth in premature babies. Archives of Disease in Childhood 69: 498–504.

Goran MI, Driscoll P, Johnson R, Nagy TR, Hunter G. (1996). Cross-calibration of body-composition techniques against dual-energy X-ray absorptiometry in young children. American Journal of Clinical Nutrition 63: 299–305.

Gorstein J. (1989). Assessment of nutritional status: effects of different methods to determine age on the classification of undernutrition. Bulletin of the World Health Organization 67: 143–150.

Gorstein J, Sullivan K, Yip R, de Onis M, Trowbridge F, Fajans P, Clugston G. (1994). Issues in the assessment of nutritional status using anthropometry. Bulletin of the World Health Organization 72: 273–283.

Guillaume M. (1999). Defining obesity in childhood: current practice. American Journal of Clinical Nutrition 70: 126S–130S.

Guo SM, Roche AF, Fomon SJ, Nelson SE, Chumlea WC, Rogers RR, Baumgartner RN, Ziegler EE, Siervogel RM. (1991). Reference data on gains in weight and length during the first two years of life. Journal of Pediatrics 119: 355–362.

Guo SS, Roche AF, Chumlea WC, Gardner JD, Siervogel RM. (1994). The predictive value of childhood body mass index values for overweight at age 35 y. American Journal of Clinical Nutrition 59: 810–819.

Gurrici S, Hartriyanti Y, Hautvast JG, Deurenberg P. (1999). Differences in the relationship between body fat and body mass index between two different Indonesian ethnic groups: the effect of body build. European Journal of Clinical Nutrition 53: 468–472.

Haschke F, van't Hof MA. (2000). Euro-Growth references for length, weight, and body circumferences. Euro-Growth Study Group. Journal of Pediatric Gastroenterology and Nutrition 31: S14–S38.

Health Canada. (2003). Canadian Guidelines For Body Weight Classification in Adults. Health Canada, Ottawa.

Hermanussen M. (1988). Knemometry, a new tool for the investigation of growth. European Journal of Pediatrics 147: 350–355.

Hermanussen M, Seele K. (1997). Mini-knemometry: an accurate technique for lower leg length measurements in early childhood. Annals of Human Biology 24: 307–313.

Hermanussen M, Geiger-Benoit K, Burmeister J, Sippell WG. (1988). Knemometry in childhood: accuracy and standardization of a new technique of lower leg length measurement. Annals of Human Biology 15: 1–16.

Heymsfield SB, McManus CB, Seitz SB, Nixon DW, Smith J. (1984). Anthropometric assessment of adult protein-energy malnutrition. In: Wright RA, Heymsfield S (eds.) Nutritional Assessment of the Hospitalized Patient. Blackwell Scientific Boston, pp. 27–82.

Hill GL. (1992). Body composition research: implications for the practice of clinical nutrition. Journal of Parenteral and Enteral Nutrition 16: 197–218.

Himes JH, Dietz WH. (1994). Guidelines for overweight in adolescent preventive services: recommendations from an expert committee: the Expert Committee on Clinical Guidelines for Overweight in Adolescent Preventive Services. American Journal of Clinical Nutrition 59: 307–316.

IOM (Institute of Medicine). (1990). Nutrition during Pregnancy: Report of the Subcommittee on Nutritional Status and Weight Gain during Pregnancy. National Academy Press, Washington, DC.

James WPT, Ferro-Luzzi A, Waterlow JC. (1988). Definition of chronic energy deficiency in adults: report of a working party of the International Dietary Energy Consultative Group. European Journal of Clinical Nutrition 42: 969–981.

Jarzem PF, Gledhill RB. (1993). Predicting height from arm measurements. Journal of Pediatric Orthopaedics 13: 761–765.

Katzmarzyk PT, Tremblay A, Pérusse L, Despreés J-P, Bouchard C. (2003). The utility of the international child and adolescent overweight guidelines for predicting coronary heart disease risk factors. Journal of Clinical Epidemiology 56: 456–462.

Kuczmarski RJ, Ogden CL, Grummer-Strawn LM, Flegal KM, Guo SS, Wei R, Mei Z, Curtin LR, Roche AF, Johnson CL. (2000a). CDC Growth Charts: United States. Advance Data 314: 1–27.

Lohman TG, Roche AF, Martorell R (eds.). (1988). Anthropometric Standardization Reference Manual. Human Kinetics Books, Champaign, IL.

Manson JE, Willett WC, Stampfer MJ, Colditz GA, Hunter DJ, Hankinson SE, Hennekens CH, Speizer FE. (1995). Body weight and mortality among women. New England Journal of Medicine 333: 677–685.

Marton KI, Sox HC Jr, Krupp JR. (1981). Involuntary weight loss: diagnostic and prognostic significance. Annals of Internal Medicine 95: 568–574.

McGill HC Jr, McMahan CA, Malcom GT, Oalmann MC, Strong JP. (1995). Relation of glycohemoglobibin and adiposity to atherosclerosis in youth. Arteriosclerosis, Thrombosis, and Vascular Biology 15: 431–440.

Michaelson KF, Skov L, Badsberg JH, Jorgensen M. (1991). Short-term measurement of linear growth in preterm infants: validation of a hand-held knemometer. Pediatric Research 30: 464–468.

Millar WJ. (1986). Distribution of body weight and height: comparison of estimates based on self-reported and observed measures. Journal of Epidemiology and Community Health 40: 319–323.

Ministry of Health. (1999). National Health Survey 1998. Epidemiology and Disease Control Department, Ministry of Health, Singapore.

Morabia A, Ross A, Curtin F, Pichard C, Slosman DO. (1999). Relation of BMI to a dual-energy X-ray absorptiometry measure of fatness. British Journal of Nutrition 82: 49–55.

Must A, Dallal GE, Dietz WH. (1991). Reference data for obesity: 85th and 95th percentiles of body mass index (wt/ht^2) and triceps skinfold thickness. American Journal of Clinical Nutrition 53: 839–846. Correction in: 54: 773.

Nellhaus G. (1968). Head circumference from birth to eighteen years: practical composite international and interracial graphs. Pediatrics 41: 106–114.

NHLBI (National Heart, Lung, and Blood Institute) (1998). Obesity Education Initiative Expert Panel on the Identification, Evaluation, and Treatment of Overweight and Obesity in Adults. Clinical guidelines on the identification, evaluation, and treatment of overweight and obesity in adults: the evidence report. Obesity Research 6: 51S–209S.

Norgan NG. (1994). Population differences in body composition in relation to body mass index. European Journal of Clinical Nutrition 48(suppl. 3): S10–S27.

Norgan NG, Jones PR. (1995). The effect of standardising the body mass index for relative sitting height. International Journal of Obesity and Related Metabolic Disorders 19: 206–208.

Pietrobelli A, Faith MS, Allison DB, Gallagher D, Chiumello G, Heymsfield SB. (1998). Body mass index as a measure of adiposity among children and adolescents: a validation study. Journal of Pediatrics 132: 204–210.

Poskitt EM. (1995). Defining childhood obesity: the relative body mass index (BMI). European Childhood Obesity Group. Acta Paediatrica 84: 961–963.

Post CL, Victora CG. (2001). The low prevalence of weight-for-height deficits in Brazilian children is related to body proportions. Journal of Nutrition 131: 1290–1296.

Prothro JW, Rosenbloom CA. (1993). Physical measurements in an elderly black population: knee height as the dominant indicator of stature. Journal of Gerontology 48: M15–M18.

Reece EA, Gabrielli S, Degennaro N, Hobbins JC. (1989). Dating through pregnancy: a measure of growing up. Obstetrical and Gyneocological Survey 44: 544–555.

Robbins GE, Trowbridge FL. (1984). Anthropometric techniques and their application. In: Simko MD, Cowell C, Gilbride JA (eds.) Nutrition Assessment: A Comprehensive Guide for Planning Intervention. Aspen Corporation, Rockville, MD, pp. 69–92.

Roberts SB, Dallal GE. (2001). The new childhood growth charts. Nutrition Reviews 59: 31–36.

Ruel MT, Rivera J, Habicht JP. (1995). Length screens better than weight in stunted populations. Journal of Nutrition 125: 1222–1228.

Seidall JC, Kahn HS, Williamson DF, Lissner L, Valdez R. (2001). Report from a Centers for Disease Control and Prevention workshop on use of adult anthropometry for public health and primary health care. American Journal of Clinical Nutrition 73: 123–126.

Shetty PS, James WPT. (1994). Body Mass Index. A Measure of Chronic Energy Deficiency in Adults. FAO Food and Nutrition Paper No. 56. Food and Agriculture Organization, Rome.

Song Y-M, Sung J. (2001). Body mass index and mortality: a twelve-year prospective study in Korea. Epidemiology 12: 173–179.

Stevens J, Nowicki EM. (2003). Body mass index and mortality in Asian populations: implications for obesity cut-off points. Nutrition Reviews 61: 104–107.

Swinburn BA, Craig PL, Daniel R, Dent DP, Strauss BJ. (1996). Body composition differences between Polynesians and Caucasians assessed by bioelectrical impedance. International Journal of Obesity and Related Metabolic Disorders 20: 889–894.

Swinburn BA, Ley SJ, Carmichael HE, Plank LD. (1999). Size and composition in Polynesians. International Journal of Obesity 23: 1178–1183.

Tanner JM, Whitehouse RH, Takaishi M. (1966). Standards from birth to maturity for height, weight, height velocity, and weight velocity: British children, 1965 II. Archives of Disease in Childhood 41: 613–625.

Taylor RW, Gold E, Manning P, Goulding A. (1997). Gender differences in body fat content are present well before puberty. International Journal of Obesity and Related Metabolic Disorders 21: 1082–1084.

Taylor RW, Falomi A, Jones IE, Goulding A. (2003). Identifying adolescents with high percentage body fat: a comparison of BMI cutoffs using age and stage puberty development compared BMI cutoffs using age alone. European Journal of Clinical Nutrition 57: 764–769.

Wales JK, Milner RD. (1987). Knemometry in assessment of linear growth. Archives of Disease in Childhood 62: 166–171.

Wang J, Thornton JC, Russell M, Burastero S, Heymsfield S, Pierson RN Jr. (1994). Asians have lower body mass index (BMI) but higher percent body fat than do whites: comparisons of anthropometric measurements. American Journal of Clinical Nutrition 60: 23–28.

Waterlow JC, Buzina R, Keller W, Lane JM, Nichaman MZ, Tanner JM. (1977). The presentation and use of height and weight data for comparing the nutritional status of groups of children under the age of 10 years. Bulletin of the World Health Organization 55: 489–498.

Wells JCK, Fuller NJ, Dewit O, Fewtrell MS, Elia M, Cole TJ. (1999). Four-component model of body composition in children: density and hydration of fat-free mass and comparison with simpler models. American Journal of Clinical Nutrition 69: 904–912.

WHO (World Health Organization Working Group). (1986). Use and interpretation of anthropometric indicators of nutritional status. Bulletin of the World Health Organization 64: 929–941.

WHO (World Health Organization). (1995a). Physical Status: The Use and Interpretation of Anthropometry: Report of a WHO Expert Committee. Technical Report Series No. 854. World Health Organization, Geneva.

WHO (World Health Organization). (1995b). Maternal anthropometry and pregnancy outcomes: a WHO collaborative project. Bulletin of the World Health Organization 73(Suppl.): 1–98.

WHO (World Health Organization). (2000). Obesity: Preventing and Managing the Global Epidemic: Report on a WHO Consultation. Technical Report Series No. 894. World Health Organization, Geneva.

WHO (World Health Organization) Expert Consultation. (2004). Appropriate body-mass index for Asian populations and its implications for policy and intervention strategies. Lancet 363: 157–163.

Yarbrough C, Habicht J-P, Martorell R, Klein RE. (1974). Anthropometry as an index of nutritional status. In: Roche AF, Falkner R (eds.) Nutrition and Malnutrition: Identification and Measurement. Plenum Press, New York, pp. 15–26.

Zhang H, Hsu-Hage BH, Wahlqvist ML. (1998). The use of knee height to estimate maximum stature in elderly Chinese. Journal of Nutrition, Health and Aging 2: 84–87.

Zwiauer K, Widhalm K, Kerbl B. (1990). Relationship between body fat distribution and blood lipids in obese adolescents. International Journal of Obesity and Related Metabolic Disorders 14: 271–277.

11

Anthropometric assessment of body composition

Most anthropometric methods used to assess body composition are based on a model in which the body consists of two chemically distinct compartments: fat and fat-free mass. The latter — also referred to as the body cell mass — consists of the skeletal muscle, non-skeletal muscle, soft lean tissues, and the skeleton. Anthropometric techniques can indirectly assess fat and the fat-free mass, and variations in their amount and proportion can be used as indices of nutritional status. For example, fat is the main storage form of energy in the body and is sensitive to acute malnutrition. Thus, alterations in body fat content provide indirect estimates of changes in energy balance. Body muscle, composed largely of protein, is a major component of the fat-free mass and serves as an index of the protein reserves of the body; these reserves become depleted during chronic undernutrition, resulting in muscle wasting.

The anthropometric measurement of body composition is both fast and noninvasive, and it requires the minimum of equipment compared to laboratory techniques. Details of the standardized procedures used for anthropometric measurements of body composition, and the derivation of the more important indices, are summarized in this chapter and are given in Lohman et al. (1988).

Indices of body composition are used in clinical settings to identify hospital patients with chronic under- or overnutrition and to monitor long-term changes in body composition during nutritional support. In public health they can identify individuals who are vulnerable to under- or overnutrition and help evaluate the effectiveness of nutrition intervention programs.

11.1 Assessment of body fat

The body fat content is the most variable component of the body, differing among individuals of the same sex, height, and weight. On average, the fat content of women is higher than that of men, representing 26.9% of their total body weight compared with 14.7% for men. Table 11.1 presents data for the distribution of body fat in reference man and woman.

Body fat is deposited in two major types

Fat location	man	woman
Essential fat (lipids of the bone marrow, central nervous systems, mammary glands and other organs)	2.1	4.9
Storage fat (depot)	8.2	10.4
Subcutaneous	3.1	5.1
Intermuscular	3.3	3.5
Intramuscular	0.8	0.6
Fat of thoracic and abdominal cavity	1.0	1.2
Total fat	10.5	15.3
Body weight	70.0	56.8
Percentage fat	14.7	26.9

Table 11.1: Distribution of body fat in reference man and women. Data in kilograms. Weights for total fat and body weight in reference man and woman from Behnke (1969). Other weights from Allen et al. (1956), Alexander (1964), and Wilmore and Brown (1974).

273

of sites: one for essential lipids, and the other for storage of fat. Essential lipids are found in the bone marrow, central nervous system, mammary glands, and other organs and are required for normal physiological functioning; fat from these sites makes up about 9% (4.9 kg) of body weight in reference woman and 3% (2.1 kg) in reference man. Storage fat consists of inter- and intramuscular fat, fat surrounding the organs and gastrointestinal tract, and subcutaneous fat (Lohman, 1981). The proportion of storage fat in males and females is relatively constant, averaging 12% of total body weight in males and 15% in females.

Of the total body fat, over one-third in reference man and woman is estimated to be subcutaneous fat. Body fat can be expressed either in absolute terms (the weight of total body fat in kilograms) or as a percentage of the total body weight. It is highly correlated with many health-related indices such as risk of mortality or morbidity, specifically coronary heart disease, high blood pressure, and type 2 diabetes (Kissebah et al., 1989).

In population studies, body fat is often assessed by anthropometry. Skinfold thickness determinations, either alone or in association with limb circumference measurements, are frequently used to estimate the percentage body fat. More recently, this percentage is estimated from the body mass index (BMI).

Estimates of body fat, together with the rate of change in the body fat content, are recommended to assess the presence and severity of undernutrition. A large and rapid loss of body fat is indicative of severe negative energy balance. Small changes in body fat (i.e., < 0.5 kg) cannot be measured accurately using anthropometry.

At the present time, there is increasing emphasis on the assessment of both the amount of body fat and its distribution: the amount of intra-abdominal visceral fat often correlates significantly with metabolic disturbances that can be linked to the risk of cardiovascular disease. Waist-hip circumference ratio and the waist circumference alone are used as anthropometric surrogates for intra-abdominal visceral fat (Sections 11.1.2 and 11.1.3).

11.1.1 Skinfold thickness measurements

Skinfold thickness measurements provide an estimate of the size of the subcutaneous fat depot, which, in turn, provides an estimate of total body fat. Such estimates are based on two assumptions: (*a*) the thickness of the subcutaneous adipose tissue reflects a constant proportion of the total body fat, and (*b*) the skinfold sites selected for measurement, either singly or in combination, represent the average thickness of the entire subcutaneous adipose tissue. Neither of these assumptions is true. In fact, the relationship between subcutaneous and internal fat is nonlinear and varies with body weight and age: very lean subjects have a smaller proportion of body fat deposited subcutaneously than obese subjects have. Moreover, variations in the distribution of subcutaneous fat occur with sex, race or ethnicity, and age (Wagner and Heyward, 2000). The following sites, described in detail in Lohman et al. (1988), are commonly used:

- Triceps skinfold is measured at the midpoint of the back of the upper arm (Figure 11.1).

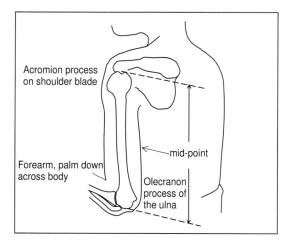

Figure 11.1: Location of the midpoint of the upper arm. Reproduced from Robbins GE, Trowbridge FL, in: Nutrition Assessment: A Comprehensive Guide for Planning Intervention by M.D. Simko, C. Cowell, and J.A. Gilbride (eds.), p. 87, with permission of Aspen Publishers, Inc., © 1984.

- Biceps skinfold is measured as the thickness of a vertical fold on the front of the upper arm, directly above the center of the cubital fossa, at the same level as the triceps skinfold.
- Subscapular skinfold is measured below and laterally to the angle of the shoulder blade, with the shoulder and arm relaxed. Placing the subject's arm behind the back may assist in identification of the site. The skinfold should angle 45° from horizontal, in the same direction as the inner border of the scapula (i.e., medially upward and laterally downward) (Figure 11.2A).
- Suprailiac skinfold is measured in the midaxillary line immediately superior to the iliac crest. The skinfold is picked up obliquely just posterior to the midaxillary line and parallel to the cleavage lines of the skin (Figure 11.2B).
- Midaxillary skinfold is picked up horizontally on the midaxillary line, at the level of the xiphoid process.

Skinfold thickness measurements are best made using precision thickness calipers; they measure the compressed double fold of fat plus skin. As a result of the compression, they always underestimate actual subcutaneous fat thickness. The skinfold is always grasped at the marked site with the fingers on top, thumb below, and forefinger on the marked site. Three types of precision calipers can be used: Harpenden, Lange, and Holtain (Figure 11.3). Some suppliers of these calipers

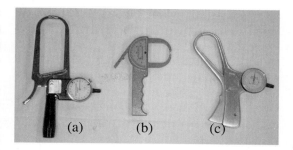

Figure 11.3: Harpenden (a), Lange (b), and Holtain (c) precision skinfold thickness calipers.

are listed in Appendix A10.2. Low-cost plastic calipers are also available, but will have a reduced precision and accuracy.

Precision calipers are designed to exert a defined and constant pressure throughout the range of measured skinfolds and to have a standard contact surface area or "pinch" area of 20–40 mm^2. The skinfold calipers must be recalibrated at regular intervals using a calibration block. Both the Harpenden and Holtain skinfold calipers, which have a standard jaw pressure of 10 g/mm^2, give smaller skinfold values than Lange calipers, which are fitted with a lighter spring (Gruber et al., 1990).

For all the skinfold measurements, the subject should stand erect with the weight evenly distributed and feet together, shoulders relaxed, and arms hanging freely at the sides. The measurement technique is described in detail for the triceps skinfold, as the latter is the site most frequently used to obtain a single indirect measure of body fat; the technique used for the other skinfold sites is similar. There is no consensus as to whether the left or right side of the body should be used. The current practice of the National Health and Nutrition Examination Survey (NHANES) is that skinfold sites are measured on the right side of the body.

Measurement of triceps skinfold

The measurement of the triceps skinfold is performed at the midpoint of the upper right arm, between the acromion process and the tip of the olecranon, with the arm hanging relaxed. To mark the midpoint, the right

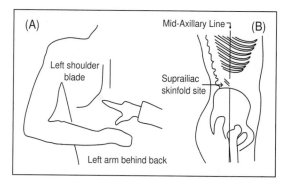

Figure 11.2: Location of the subscapular (A) and suprailiac (B) skinfold sites.

arm is bent 90° at the elbow, and the fore-arm is placed palm down across the body. Then the tip of the acromion process of the shoulder blade at the outermost edge of the shoulder and the tip of the olecranon process of the ulna are located and marked. The distance between these two points is measured using a nonstretchable tape, and the midpoint is marked with a soft pen or indelible pencil, directly in line with the point of the elbow and acromion process. The right arm is then extended so that it is hanging loosely by the side. The examiner grasps a vertical fold of skin plus the underlying fat, 2 cm above the marked midpoint, in line with the tip of the olecranon process (Figure 11.1), using both the thumb and forefinger. The skinfold is gently pulled away from the underlying muscle tissue, and then the caliper jaws are applied at right angles, exactly at the marked midpoint (Figure 11.4). The skinfold remains held between the fingers while the measurement is taken.

When using the Lange, Harpenden, or Holtain calipers, pressure must be applied to open the jaws before the instrument is placed on the skinfold; the jaws will then close under spring pressure. As the jaws compress the tissue, the caliper reading generally diminishes for 2–3 s, and then the measurements are taken. Skinfolds should be recorded to

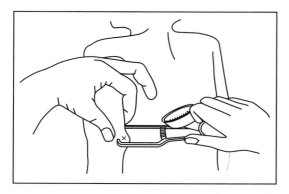

Figure 11.4: Measurement of the triceps skinfold in the upright position using the Harpenden caliper. From Robbins GE, Trowbridge FL, in: Nutrition Assessment: A Comprehensive Guide for Planning Intervention by M.D. Simko, C. Cowell, and J.A. Gilbride (eds.) p. 90, with permission of Aspen Publishers, Inc., © 1984.

0.1 mm on the Harpenden and Holtain skinfold calipers and to 0.5 mm on the Lange. Duplicate skinfold measurements made with precision calipers should normally agree to within 1 mm.

Triceps skinfold measurements can also be made with the subject lying down. The subject lies on the left side with legs bent, the head supported by a pillow, and the left hand tucked under the pillow. The right arm rests along the trunk, with the palm down. The measurement is taken at the marked midpoint of the back of the upper right arm, as described above. The examiner should be careful to avoid parallax errors by bending down to read the calipers while taking the measurements (Chumlea et al., 1984).

Precision of skinfold measurements

Both within-examiner and between-examiner measurement errors can occur when measuring skinfolds, particularly for subjects with flabby, easily compressible tissue or with very firm tissue that is not easily deformed (Lukaski, 1987).

Within-examiner errors can occur when an examiner fails to obtain identical results on repeated skinfolds on the same subject; such errors are a function of the skinfold site, the experience of the examiner, and the fatness of the subject. Within-examiner measurement errors can be small when measuring triceps skinfolds, provided that training in standardized procedures is given; the errors in these circumstances typically range from 0.70 to 0.95 mm.

Between-examiner errors arise when two or more examiners measure the same subject and site; such errors are usually larger than within-examiner errors, but they can be reduced to not more than 2 mm with training and care (Burkinshaw et al., 1973). Within- and between-examiner measurement errors tend to be greater if very large (>15 mm) or small (< 5 mm) skinfolds are measured (Edwards et al., 1955). Table 11.2 lists some reported values for both within- and between-examiner technical error of the measurement (TEM) (Section 9.2.1) for biceps, triceps,

Skinfold measurement	No. of studies	Mean (mm)	Range (mm)
Within-observer TEM			
Biceps	3	0.17	0.1–0.2
Triceps	21	0.84	0.1–3.7
Subscapular	19	1.26	0.1–7.4
Suprailiac	10	1.16	0.1–3.2
Between-observer TEM			
Biceps	8	0.84	0.2–2.1
Triceps	28	1.06	0.2–4.7
Subscapular	28	1.21	0.1–3.3
Suprailiac	11	2.28	0.3–6.4

Table 11.2: Reported values for within-observer and between-observer technical error of the measurement (TEM) for skinfold measurements. From Ulijaszek and Kerr, British Journal of Nutrition 82: 165–177, 1999, with permission of the Nutrition Society.

subscapular, and suprailiac skinfold measurements, compiled by Ulijaszek and Kerr (1999).

Zerfas (1985) has evaluated the measurement error for skinfolds from any site using a repeat-measures protocol and recommended target values for the differences between the trainee and a criterion anthropometrist; the target training values are shown in Table 11.3. A difference of more than 5 mm between the measurements of the criterion anthropometrist and the trainee indicates a gross error related to the reading or recording; a difference between the measurement of the criterion anthropometrist and the trainee of 0.0–0.9 mm indicates that the trainee has reached an acceptable level of proficiency in the measurement technique. Sports anthro-

Measurement	Trainee-trainer difference		
	Good	Fair	Poor
Height or length (mm)	0–5	6–9	10–19
Weight (kg)	0–0.1	0.2	0.3–0.4
Arm circ. (mm)	0–5	6–9	10–19
Skinfolds (any) (mm)	0–0.9	1.0–1.9	2.0–4.9

Table 11.3: Evaluation of measurement error in anthropometric measurements. After Zerfas (1985). Differences greater than those noted under "Poor" are taken to indicate a gross error. From Ulijaszek and Kerr, British Journal of Nutrition 82: 165–177, 1999, with permission of the Nutrition Society.

pometrists have set target values for training which also include skinfolds and arm circumference measurements (Gore et al., 1996); these could be adopted by nutritionists. Suggested target values are expressed as TEM (as a percentage), and for skinfolds are 7.5 (level 1) and 5.0 (levels 2 and 3). Criterion anthropometrists should be expected to achieve a %TEM of 5.0 for skinfolds.

Assessing body fat with single skinfolds

Skinfold measurements at a single site are sometimes used to estimate total body fat or the percentage of body fat. If this single measurement approach is used, it is critical to select the skinfold site that is most representative of the whole subcutaneous fat layer, because subcutaneous fat is not uniformly distributed about the body. Unfortunately, the most representative site is not the same for both sexes, nor is it the same for all age and ethnic groups. For example, Siervogel et al. (1982) concluded that the triceps skinfold was most representative of the total subcutaneous layer for boys < 16 y, whereas for adult males both subscapular and midaxillary sites were equally representative. Hence, it is not surprising that there is no general agreement as to the best single skinfold site as an index of total body fat.

The assessment of total body fat from a single skinfold is particularly difficult in adult females, for whom the distribution of subcutaneous fat is more variable than in males. Sloan et al. (1962) reported that the suprailiac skinfold was the best single index of total skinfold thickness for young women, whereas Siervogel et al. (1982) recommended the triceps skinfold.

Roche et al. (1981) emphasized that the most appropriate skinfold site also depends on whether total body fat or percentage body fat is the parameter of interest. They found that the triceps skinfold provided the best estimate of percentage body fat, in children and adult women (Table 11.4), but not in adult men. In contrast, the subscapular skinfold was recommended if total body fat in boys was to be estimated. For assessment of total

| | Correlation Coefficients | | | |
| | % Body fat | | Total body fat | |
	Men	Women	Men	Women
Weight	0.67	0.70	0.82	0.91
Relative weight	0.64	0.69	0.78	0.89
Weight/(height)^2	0.77	0.76	0.87	0.92
Weight/(height)^3	0.75	0.75	0.83	0.88
Triceps skinfold	0.70	0.77	0.73	0.80
Subscap. skinfold	0.75	0.71	0.79	0.80
Suprailiac skinfold	0.69	0.59	0.73	0.69

Table 11.4: Correlations between selected anthropometric variables and percentage of body fat or total body fat in 276 adults 18–49 y. All correlations are significant ($p < 0.01$). From Roche et al., American Journal of Clinical Nutrition 34: 2831–2838, 1981 © Am J Clin Nutr. American Society for Clinical Nutrition.

body fat in girls and adults, no single skinfold measurement was regarded as adequate; instead, body mass index was preferred (Section 10.2.7).

The discussion above emphasizes the problems of using single skinfolds to assess total body fat or percentage of body fat. In general, the triceps skinfold thickness has been the site most frequently selected by nutritionists for a single, indirect estimate of body fat. This site, however, appears to be suitable for the assessment of percentage of body fat in women and children only.

Assessing body fat with multiple skinfolds

The optimum combination of skinfold measurement sites for assessing subcutaneous fat and, by inference, total body fat has not been extensively investigated. No single region of the body (for example, upper or lower trunk or limbs) appears to have sites that are consistently representative of the whole subcutaneous fat layer (Siervogel et al., 1982). Moreover, the proportion of total body fat that is distributed subcutaneously in adults varies with age, sex, degree of adiposity, and race or ethnicity (Malina, 1996). Similar relationships probably exist among children, although research on this age group is limited.

In general, when studying both children and adults, investigators recommend taking

one limb skinfold (right triceps) and one body skinfold measurement (right subscapular) to account for the differing distribution of subcutaneous fat. Persons of African descent tend to have less subcutaneous fat in the extremities than in the trunk relative to Caucasians, irrespective of age and athletic status (Wagner and Heyward, 2000). As a result, Frisancho (1990) compiled separate percentile curves by race or ethnicity and by age and sex for the sum of triceps and subscapular for U.S. persons 1–74.9 y, drawn from the NHANES I and NHANES II data.

When estimating body fat, multiple skinfolds, not just a single skinfold measurement, are particularly advisable when individuals are undergoing rapid and pronounced weight gain. Changes in the energy balance are known to alter the rate of fat accumulation differently among skinfold sites (Heymsfield et al., 1984).

Assessing the distribution of body fat using multiple skinfolds

Variations in the distribution of body fat are known to be associated with genetic differences among individuals. Ethnicity, age, sex, and certain disease states may also be important factors in fat distribution. The location of adipose tissue on the body is probably a more important predictor of any metabolic alterations than total adiposity per se, and, in turn can indicate the risk of developing certain obesity-related illnesses (Kissebah et al., 1989; Després et al., 1990).

Of the body adipose tissue, it is the deposition of excess fat in the abdomen as a proportion of total body fat that is strongly associated with metabolic and cardiovascular disease risk and a variety of chronic diseases (Després et al., 1990; Björntorp, 1993).

Attempts to measure the intra-abdominal depots of fat led to the development of trunk (T) to extremity (E) skinfold thickness ratios. The ratios typically involve measurements of the subscapular skinfold (i.e., trunk) and the triceps skinfold (i.e., extremity). Such ratios classify individuals according to whether they have more subcutaneous fat deposited on the

Age (y)	Mexican			Caucasian		
	n	$\overline{x}$	SD	n	$\overline{x}$	SD
Men						
25–34	236	1.75	0.52	90	1.52	0.58
35–44	208	1.96	0.68	115	1.63	0.52
45–54	144	1.85	0.54	88	1.77	0.68
55–69	123	1.83	0.60	79	1.74	0.58
Women						
25–34	288	1.18	0.30	115	0.96	0.31
35–44	292	1.18	0.31	158	0.94	0.30
45–54	215	1.15	0.27	89	0.95	0.27
55–69	157	1.13	0.33	86	0.96	0.31

Table 11.5: Ratios of subscapular to triceps skinfolds (mm/mm) in Mexican and Caucasian Americans from San Antonio, Texas. From Malina RM (1996). Regional Body Composition: Age, Sex, and Ethnic Variation. In: Human Body Composition. Adapted with permission from Human Kinetics (Champaign, IL).

trunk than on the limbs (i.e., a centripetal fat pattern with a high T/E ratio), or vice versa (more peripheral fat with a low T/E ratio).

Table 11.5 compares a T/E ratio (subscapular/triceps) of some Mexican and Caucasian Americans, 25–69 y, from Texas, using data from NHANES II and the Hispanic Health and Nutrition Survey. This ratio is consistently higher in Mexican Americans, and indicates a more central distribution of subcutaneous adipose tissue. The difference is especially marked in females (Malina, 1996). A more central distribution of subcutaneous adipose tissue (as indicated by T/E ratios) has also been reported in both children and youth of African, Mexican, and Japanese ancestry compared to Caucasian American children. The latter have a more peripheral pattern (Najjar and Rowland, 1987; Najjar and Kuczmarski, 1989; Ryan et al., 1990).

More recently, the waist-hip circumference ratio and waist-circumference have been used as anthropometric surrogates of intra-abdominal fat; they are discussed below.

11.1.2 Waist-hip circumference ratio

The waist-hip circumference ratio (waist circumference divided by hip circumference) (WHR) is a simple method for distinguishing between fatness in the lower trunk (hip

and buttocks) and fatness in the upper trunk (waist and abdomen areas). Lower trunk fatness (i.e., lower waist to hip ratio) is often referred to as "gynoid obesity" because it is more typical of females. Upper trunk or central fatness (higher waist to hip ratio) is called "android obesity" and is more characteristic of males. Nevertheless, obese men and women can be, and often are, classified into either group.

The fat depots assessed by the WHR are mainly subcutaneous (external or outer) and visceral (internal or deep). The subcutaneous adipose tissue is found largely in the lower trunk. The WHR correlates strongly with total body fat mass (Figure 11.5).

Use of the WHR has risen dramatically with the recognition that central obesity is a critical risk factor in the development of certain diseases, independent of overall obesity. Several prospective cohort studies have confirmed that in both men and women an elevated WHR is strongly associated with an increased risk of developing coronary heart disease, stroke, and type 2 diabetes mellitus (Larsson et al., 1984; Lapidus et al., 1984).

With the application of new laboratory methods including computerized tomography and magnetic resonance imaging, semiquantitative estimates of the total fat stored within the abdomen have been obtained (Ashwell et al., 1985; Heymsfield et al., 1998).

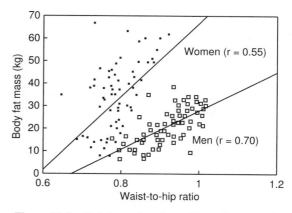

Figure 11.5: Relation of waist-to-hip ratio to total body fat mass determined by densitometry in men and women. Data from Pouliot et al., American Journal of Cardiology 73: 460–468, 1994 © with permission from Excerpta Medica Inc.

These results have indicated that the intra-abdominal (visceral) fat content may be the key variable that explains the correlation of an elevated WHR with the increased risk of developing certain obesity-related illnesses and metabolic disorders. Indeed, some metabolic consequences of obesity such as disturbances in lipoprotein metabolism and plasma insulin-glucose homeostasis are much more likely to be associated with an android distribution of adipose tissue (upper trunk fatness) than a gynoid distribution of adipose tissue (lower trunk fatness) (Kalkhoff et al., 1983; Krotkiewski et al. 1983; Després et al., 1990; Björntorp, 1993).

Several studies in adults have shown that the WHR varies with race or ethnicity, age, sex, geographic region, and the degree of overweight. Jones et al. (1986) measured the waist-hip ratio of a semi-random, age-stratified sample of 4349 British Caucasian men 20–64 y. They noted that the ratio increased with both age (curvilinearly) and excessive weight.

In the WHO Multinational MONItoring of trends and determinants of CArdiovascular disease (MONICA) project, the WHR was

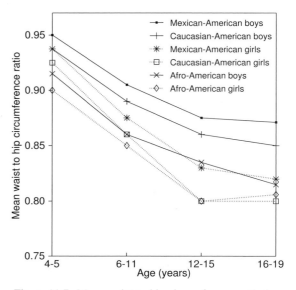

Figure 11.7: Mean waist-to-hip circumference ratio in male and female children and young adults of three racial groups. NHANES III data (1988-1994) from Gillum, International Journal of Obesity and Related Metabolic Disorders 23: 556–563, 1999 © with permission of the Nature Publishing Group.

also reported to increase with age, the increase being more pronounced in women, as shown in Figure 11.6. This study used a standard protocol to measure waist and hip circumferences in men and women 25–64 y in 19 countries (Molarius et al., 1999). Mean waist-hip ratio in the 19 countries varied considerably among the study populations, ranging from 0.87 to 0.99 for men and from 0.76 to 0.84 for women.

Relationships between the WHR and age, sex, and race or ethnicity have also been investigated in children. In the NHANES III, mean WHR varied consistently with age, sex, and ethnic group in children and adolescents aged 4–19 y, as shown in Figure 11.7. Ratios were highest in Mexican American boys (Gillum, 1999).

The relationship between the WHR and plasma high-density lipoprotein (HDL)-cholesterol concentrations, one risk factor for cardiovascular morbidity, was also investigated in these U.S. children. Gillum (1999) recorded consistent negative associations of HDL-cholesterol levels and WHR across age, sex, and ethnic subgroups in the sample,

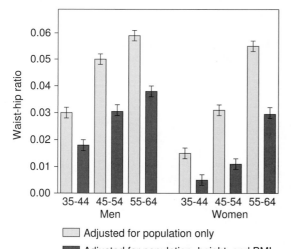

Figure 11.6: Effect of age on the waist-hip ratio in a pooled dataset of 19 male and 18 female populations from the second MONICA survey. Data from Molarius et al., International Journal of Obesity and Related Metabolic Disorders 23: 116–125, 1999 © with permission of the Nature Publishing Group.

including an association of WHR with HDL-cholesterol in prepubertal girls. These findings are important because earlier studies had suggested that the distribution of body fat was only an important correlate of blood lipids in children after sexual maturity. In younger children, overall obesity was thought to be more important (Sangi and Mueller, 1991). The NHANES III results of Gillum (1999) suggest that both body fat distribution and HDL-cholesterol concentrations should be assessed as a risk factor for atherosclerosis in childhood and adolescence.

Measurement of waist-hip ratio

Currently, no universally accepted procedure exists for defining the site for the measurement of waist circumference. Two sites are frequently used: (*a*) at the natural waist, i.e., mid-way between the tenth rib (the lowest rib margin) and the iliac crest, as recommended by WHO (2000) and Lohman et al. (1988), and (*b*) at the umbilicus level (van der Kooy and Seidell, 1993). The latter site is preferred for obese subjects because it is sometimes difficult to identify a waist narrowing. Hip circumference is measured at the widest point over the buttocks (Lohman et al., 1988).

Subjects should be asked to fast overnight prior to measurement and wear little clothing to allow the tape to be correctly positioned. Subjects should stand erect with the abdomen relaxed, arms at the sides, feet together, and their weight equally divided over both legs.

To perform the measurement at the natural waist, the lowest rib margin is first located and marked with a felt tip pen. The iliac crest is then palpated in the midaxillary line and also marked. An elastic tape is then applied horizontally midway between the lowest rib margin and the lateral iliac crest: it is tied firmly so that it stays in position around the abdomen about the level of the umbilicus. The elastic tape thus defines the level of the waist circumference, which can then be measured by positioning a flexible nonstretch fiberglass tape over the elastic tape (Jones et al., 1986). Subjects are asked to breathe normally and to breathe out gently at the time of the measurement to prevent them from contracting their muscles or from holding their breath. The measurement is taken without the tape compressing the skin. The reading is taken to the nearest millimeter.

For the hip circumference measurement, the subject should stand erect with arms at the side and feet together. The measurement should be taken at the point yielding the maximum circumference over the buttocks (Jones et al., 1986), with the tape held in a horizontal plane, touching the skin but not indenting the soft tissue (Lohman et al., 1988). The measurement is taken to the nearest millimeter. The degree to which factors such as postprandial status, standing position, and depth of inspiration contribute to error in the measurement of waist-hip circumference ratio is uncertain.

In some epidemiological studies, respondents have measured their own body circumferences and then mailed their responses back to the investigators. In general, the reproducibility and validity of such self-assessed circumference measurements, based on correlations for repeated self-measurements, as well as those between self measurements and trained anthropometrists, have been high (Rimm et al., 1990; Roberts et al., 1997).

Interpretive criteria

Björntorp (1987) was the first to suggest that waist-hip ratios > 1.0 for men and > 0.85 for women indicated abdominal fat accumulation and an increased risk of cardiovascular complications and related deaths. These cutoffs have now been widely accepted for international use (Han et al., 1997a; WHO, 2000).

Nevertheless, the appropriateness of using universal cutoffs to assess health risk across ethnic groups has been questioned, in view of the known ethnic variations in body fat distribution (Wagner and Heyward, 2000). Further, different contributions of muscle mass and bone structure, as well as stature and abdominal muscle tone, may all lead to different associations between WHR and visceral fat accumulation. More research is needed to establish whether ethnic-specific cutoffs for WHR are required.

In addition, the validity of serial measurements of WHR to measure changes in intra-abdominal visceral fat over time is uncertain and requires more investigation. Any beneficial reductions in abdominal fat will not be evident as a decrease in the waist-hip ratio if fat is also lost from the hips. In such cases, waist circumference alone is the preferred index for monitoring fat loss. This is discussed briefly below.

11.1.3 Waist circumference

Several studies have shown that waist circumference alone is a better correlate of abdominal fat content, measured by computer tomography or by dual X-ray absorptiometry (DXA), than waist-hip ratio (Després et al., 1989; Pouliot et al., 1994; Daniels et al., 2000). In a Canadian study of 151 adults, Pouliot et al. (1994) reported higher correlations between abdominal visceral fat area and waist circumference compared to correlations with WHR (Table 11.6). Waist circumference was also more strongly associated with total body fat, measured by densitometry, than was WHR (Figures 11.5 and 11.8). Further, because the WHR is a ratio, it suffers from problems in relation to its use in statistical analyses and its interpretation (Allison et al., 1995).

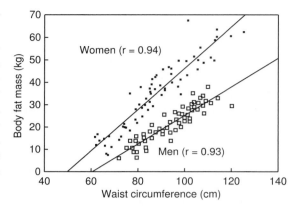

Figure 11.8: Relation of waist circumference to total body fat mass obtained by densitometry in men and women. Data from Pouliot et al., American Journal of Cardiology 73: 460–468, 1994 © with permission from Excerpta Medica Inc.

Waist circumference is also more closely related to potentially atherogenic metabolic disturbances associated with abdominal obesity than is the waist-to-hip ratio. For example, when the Canadian subjects of Pouliot et al. (1994) were divided into quintiles of waist circumference or WHR (Figure 11.9), an increasing waist circumference was more consistently associated with increases in fasting plasma insulin levels than increasing val-

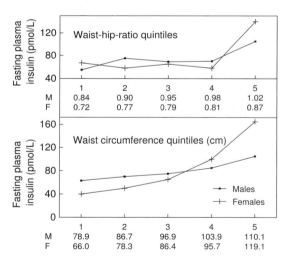

Figure 11.9: Relation of waist-to-hip ratio quintiles and waist circumference quintiles to fasting plasma insulin concentrations in males and females. Data from Pouliot et al., American Journal of Cardiology 73: 460–468, 1994 © with permission from Excerpta Medica Inc.

	Men (n = 70)		Women (n = 81)	
	Waist	WHR	Waist	WHR
Body mass index	0.92	0.78	0.94	0.58
Body fat mass	0.93	0.70	0.94	0.55
Total abdominal TA	0.94	0.76	0.94	0.53
Abdominal visc. TA	0.77	0.71	0.87	0.67
Abdominal subcut. TA	0.90	0.68	0.91	0.47

Table 11.6: Correlation coefficients relating waist circumference and waist-hip ratio (WHR) to various measures of body fat in men and women. TA, tissue area from computer tomography; visc., visceral; subcut., subcutaneous. Body fat mass determined by hydrostatic weighing. Data from Pouliot et al., American Journal of Cardiology 73: 460–468, 1994 © with permission from Excerpta Medica Inc.

ues of WHR, especially in the women of this study. A similar trend was also noted for plasma triglyceride and HDL-cholesterol levels, and in postglucose insulin levels (data not shown).

Hence, waist circumference is now the preferred anthropometric measurement for the assessment of abdominal fat (WHO, 2000). It is a simple and cheap method of assessment, and it is unrelated to height (Han et al., 1997b). It is also considered to be the most practical anthropometric measurement for assessing the abdominal fat content of a patient before and during weight loss treatment.

There is considerable variation in waist circumference among populations. In the WHO MONICA project involving 19 countries, the difference between the populations with the highest and lowest age standardized mean value for waist circumference was 13–15 cm. Increases with age were reported in both men and women among all the 19 populations, with about one-half of the increase in waist circumference in men and as much as three-quarters in women being explained by an increasing degree of overweight. In all countries, men had higher values of waist circumference than women in all age groups. Physical stature, as indicated by height, contributed very little to the variance in waist circumference. Not surprisingly, however, BMI was a major contributor, as shown in Figure 11.10 (Molarius et al., 1999).

These findings indicate that use of universally applicable cutoff values for waist circumference to delineate health risk among adults is probably not appropriate. The level of risk associated with a particular waist circumference appears to vary by sex and across populations. Women, for example, have a greater relative risk of cardiovascular disease at lower waist circumference values than do men (WHO, 2000). The health risk appears to be less for women of African descent, however, than for Caucasian women (Dowling and Pi-Sunyer, 1993). Therefore, the development of sex- and ethnic-specific cutoffs may be warranted.

Only a few studies have examined the use

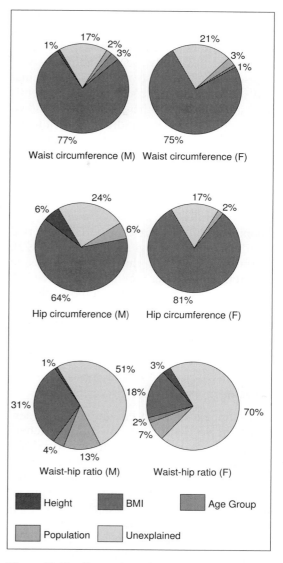

Figure 11.10: Proportion of variance in waist circumference, hip circumference, and waist-hip ratio, explained by height, BMI, age group, and population. Pooled data set of 19 male and 18 female populations from the second MONICA survey. Data from Molarius et al., International Journal of Obesity and Related Metabolic Disorders 23: 116–125, 1999 © with permission of the Nature Publishing Group.

of waist circumference as a screening tool for assessing abdominal fat distribution in children (Flodmark et al., 1994; Goran et al., 1998; Freedman et al., 1999; Taylor et al., 2000). Results of a study of 580 New Zealand children aged 3–19 y suggest that waist circumference performs well as an index of central adiposity in both children and adolescents and, indeed, better than WHR (Taylor et al., 2000). In this study, central adiposity was measured by DXA, so that intra-abdominal and subcutaneous fat could not be differentiated. Nevertheless, other studies have shown strong correlations in children between intra-abdominal fat (measured with computerized tomography) and trunk fat mass or central adiposity (measured by DXA) (Goran and Gower, 1999). Moreover, relationships in children between abdominal fat indicated by waist circumference and adverse atherogenic lipoprotein profiles have also been reported (Flodmark et al., 1994; Freedman et al.,1999).

Further studies of these relationships in children from other countries are needed, preferably using computer tomography or magnetic resonance imaging, so that abdominal adipose tissue located intra-abdominally can be distinguished between that located subcutaneously.

Measurement of waist circumference

Measurement of waist circumference is described in Section 11.1.2. A "waist-watcher" tape measure has also been developed for self-measurement, marked in both centimeters and inches. Step by step photographic instructions based on the WHO (1995) guidelines are supplied with the tape measure; details are given in Han and Lean (1998).

To use the waist-watcher tape, it is first made into a complete loop and fitted firmly around the waist by a spring mechanism, which is controlled by a pushbutton. This enables the subjects to have both hands free for adjusting the position of the tape. The tape is then read, either while in place or after removal from the waist. Removal is particularly helpful to overweight subjects who may find it hard to read the tape while it is in position.

The waist-watcher tape measure is also color coded with three color bands — green, amber, and red — each corresponding to an action level. The green band shows the waist circumference for normal subjects who are below level 1 (<94 cm in men; <80 cm in women); the amber band is for action level 1 (94–102 cm in men; 80–88 cm in women); and the red band for action level 2 (>102 cm in men; >88 cm in women). The cutoffs used to delineate the three action levels correspond to the WHO cutoffs.

Han and Lean (1998) evaluated the accuracy of self-reported home-assessed and self-measured waist circumference using the waist-watcher tape measure in subjects aged 28–76 y ($n = 194$). They noted that, although both men and women tend to underreport their waist circumference, use of the waist-watcher tape measure and photographic instructions enabled most subjects to identify themselves correctly in different categories of waist circumference according to the action levels.

Interpretive criteria

Waist circumference cutoffs have been developed to identify the increased risk associated with excess abdominal fat in adults. These cutoffs are $\geqslant 102$ cm for men and $\geqslant 88$ cm for women (NIH, 1998; WHO, 2000; Health Canada, 2003). The cutoffs are based on studies of Caucasian populations. WHO (2000) recognizes that additional population-specific cutoffs are also warranted because populations differ in the level of risk associated with a particular cutoff, depending on levels of obesity and other risk factors for cardiovascular disease and type 2 diabetes.

The World Health Organization, the International Association for the Study of Obesity, and the International Obesity Task Force (2000) jointly recommend the use of lower cutoffs for urban Asians (i.e., >80 cm for women and >90 cm for men), because they have high rates of obesity-related disorders and are more prone to central adiposity than other ethnic groups (McKeigue, 1996; Ramachandran et al., 1997). Certainly, McNeely et al. (2001) showed that the U.S. cutoffs were insensitive predictors of diabetes in a study of 466 nondiabetic Japanese American adults.

None of these cutoffs for waist circumference were chosen on the basis of their empirical relation to risk factors; they were derived by identifying waist circumference values corresponding to BMI cutoffs for overweight (BMI = 25) or obesity (BMI = 30). In an effort to overcome this limitation, Zhu et al. (2002) determined the waist circumference thresholds with degrees of cardiovascular disease risk equivalent to those of the conventional BMI cutoffs of 25 and 30. In this study, the obesity-associated risk factors were based on high LDL cholesterol, low HDL cholesterol, high blood pressure, and high plasma glucose determined in Caucasians in NHANES III. Waist circumferences of 90 cm for men and 83 cm for women were reported to be equivalent in risk to a BMI of 25, whereas waist circumferences of 100 cm for men and 93 cm for women were equivalent in risk to a BMI of 30. Note that cross-sectional, not longitudinal, data were used to compute these waist circumference threshold levels. As the waist circumference cutoffs were developed from studies on Caucasian subjects, there are limitations to applying them to assess health risks of individuals in diverse populations, as discussed earlier for waist-hip ratios.

Limited data are available to define cutoffs for waist circumference for children. It appears that ethnic differences in intra-abdominal fat mass also exist for children. African American children, like their adult counterparts, have lower mean values for the intra-abdominal fat mass (based on computerized tomography) than Caucasians have (Goran et al., 1997). In the interim, the 85th and 95th waist circumference percentiles derived from population-specific data have been used to classify overweight and obesity in children (McCarthy et al., 2001).

More research is needed to establish race- and ethnic-specific cutoffs for waist circumference for both adults and children. If it is confirmed that waist circumference is a better predictor of obesity-related diseases than either BMI or WHR, then its use as a simple and effective clinical and public health tool could dramatically increase, especially if ongoing U.S. longitudinal studies show that low intra-abdominal fat in childhood tracks with a reduced risk in adulthood.

11.1.4 Limb fat area

The calculated cross-sectional area of limb fat, derived from skinfold thickness and limb circumference measurements, may be used as an anthropometric index. It correlates more significantly with total body fat (i.e., fat weight) than does a single skinfold thickness at the same site. In contrast, the estimation of *percentage* of body fat from limb fat area is no better than the corresponding estimation from the skinfold measurement, particularly in males (Himes et al., 1980).

The advantage of using limb fat area to estimate body fat is expected; more fat is needed to cover a large limb with a given thickness of subcutaneous fat than to cover a smaller limb with the same thickness of fat. Subcutaneous fat, however, is not evenly distributed around the limbs or trunk. For example, triceps skinfolds are consistently larger than the corresponding biceps skinfold, and, as a result, either the sum or the average of these should theoretically be used for the calculation of mid-upper-arm fat area (Himes et al., 1980). In practice, current reference data are based only on triceps skinfold and mid-upper-arm circumference (MUAC) measurements.

Reference data for mid-upper-arm fat area show little variation between 1–7 y, so that mid-upper-arm fat area in adequately nourished children provides an age-independent assessment of total body fat for this age range (Gurney and Jelliffe, 1973).

The determination of mid-upper-arm fat area as a measure of total body fat should not be attempted in patients with edema or ascites (fluid in the abdominal cavity), and the appropriateness of this technique for severely undernourished hospital patients has not been adequately evaluated.

The sites commonly selected for the calculation of limb fat area are the mid-upper arm, mid-thigh, and mid-calf. Both skinfold thickness and the corresponding limb circumference should be measured by trained examiners using standard techniques. The calf and thigh skinfolds are taken on the lateral aspects of the right calf and thigh, at the point of their largest circumference. Measurements of circumferences for the calf, thigh, and arm are taken at the same level as the skinfolds, using the technique described for MUAC (Section 11.2.1). The equation for calculating mid-upper-arm fat area is:

$$A = (\text{SKF} \times \text{MUAC}/2) - (\pi \times (\text{SKF})^2/4)$$

where A = mid-upper-arm fat area (mm^2), MUAC = mid-upper-arm circumference (mm), and SKF = triceps skinfold thickness (mm). Arm fat area calculated from this equation was reported to agree within 10% to values measured by computerized axial tomography in adults (Heymsfield et al., 1982).

The equation used for the calculation of mid-upper-arm fat area is based on several assumptions, each of which may result in inaccuracies, leading to an underestimate of the degree of adiposity (Rolland-Cachera et al., 1997). The equation assumes that the limb is cylindrical, with fat evenly distributed about its circumference, and also makes no allowance for variable skinfold compressibility. This compressibility probably varies with age, sex, and site of the measurement, as well as among individuals, and is a source of error in population studies when equal compressibility of skinfolds is assumed. A correction for skinfold compressibility may be advisable in future studies. Reference data compiled from NHANES I and II are available for mid-upper-arm fat area (Section 12.9) (Frisancho, 1990).

A simplified index has also been proposed, the upper arm fat estimate (UFE in cm^2). This is also based on MUAC (in cm) and triceps skinfold thickness (TSF in cm)

$$\text{UFE} = \text{MUAC} \times \text{TSF}/2$$

This equation was validated by comparing arm fat areas assessed by magnetic resonance imaging (MRI) and anthropometry in 11 obese and 17 control children. Both the traditional upper arm fat area and the upper arm fat estimate were calculated. Results indicated that the UFE measurements were close to the MRI estimates (Rolland-Cachera et al., 1997). This index should be validated in studies involving larger numbers of both ap-

parently healthy and undernourished children before it is used.

11.1.5 Calculation of body fat from skinfolds via body density

Skinfold thickness measurements from multiple anatomical sites are also used to estimate body density, the percentage of body fat, and total body fat. The method involves:

1. Determination of appropriate skinfolds and other anthropometric measurements for the prediction of body density; the selection of the sites depends on the age, sex, race, and population group under investigation
2. Calculation of body density, using an appropriate regression equation
3. Calculation of the percentage of body fat from body density, using population-specific or generalized regression equations
4. Calculation of total body fat and/or the fat-free mass:

$$\text{Total body fat (kg)} = \frac{\text{body wt. (kg)} \times \% \text{ body fat}}{100}$$

$$\text{Fat-free mass (kg)} = \text{body wt. (kg)} - \text{body fat (kg)}$$

Choice of appropriate skinfold sites

Numerous studies have investigated the best combination of skinfolds and other anthropometric measurements from which to derive a regression equation for the estimation of body density. Population groups ranging from sedentary to athletic and from children to the elderly have been studied. Rarely have the studies recommended the same combination, particularly for young men. In general, a combination of skinfolds (such as triceps, subscapular, suprailiac, thigh or abdomen) are used for young adult men and women. For the elderly, the biceps, triceps, suprailiac, and subscapular skinfolds are preferred as these sites are closely associated with body density (Lohman, 1981; Visser et al., 1994).

Calculation of body density using population-specific regression equations

Population-specific prediction equations have been published for college students, soldiers, male and female athletes (e.g., high school long-distance runners or wrestlers), different ethnic groups, and ballet dancers. Some equations are also available for children (Slaughter et al., 1988), although the sources of biological variability in children are not clearly defined (Lohman, 1992).

Caution is needed when selecting one of these regression equations. Many have been derived from small samples, homogeneous in terms of age, sex, and body fatness. Hence, they should not be applied to other age groups and populations (Sinning, 1978). For example, the regression equation developed by Sloan (1967) was based on 50 college men and is only applicable to studies of young men and male adolescents. The equation is not valid for young women and middle-aged men.

In general, population-specific regression equations tend to overestimate body fat for leaner groups but underestimate body fat in fatter groups (Sinning, 1978), although the errors may be largely a statistical artifact of the regression procedure.

A detailed discussion of the merits of different population-specific regression equations can be found in Brodie (1988). In addition, guidelines on how to select regression equations for specific population groups are given in Heyward and Stolarczyk (1996). Clearly, no matter which equation is selected, it should have been cross-validated on other samples from the same population (internal validity) and from other populations (external validity). Moreover, a criterion (or reference) method for determining body density, such as underwater weighing, should also be used. Alternatively, the criterion value for percentage fat mass can be calculated using a four-compartment model, on the basis of measurements of body density, body water, and bone mineral content (Wong et al., 2000).

Other selection factors that must also be considered include the experience of the an-thropometrist, the type of skinfold caliper used, and the hydration status of the subjects under study. In the future, with the advent of more accurate and less invasive criterion methods for assessing body density, better population-specific regression equations will be developed for use on children, the elderly, and populations who are acutely or chronically ill.

Calculation of body density using generalized regression equations

Generalized regression equations have been developed based on large heterogeneous samples, varying in age and degree of body fatness (Durnin and Womersley, 1974; Jackson and Pollock, 1978; Jackson et al., 1980). These more complex equations allow the calculation of body density for the specified age and sex groups from selected skinfold thickness measurements and, sometimes, waist and forearm circumference measurements. In some of these equations, age is included as an independent variable. Either logarithmic (or quadratic) transformations or curvilinear equations (or both) are used, because the relationship between skinfold fat and body density is curvilinear over a wide range of densities. For example, in more obese subjects, relatively large increments in skinfold thickness are associated with only small changes in body density. If more complex generalized regression equations are used, their applicability to other specific population groups should first be established by cross-validation analysis.

The failure of a single simple equation to relate skinfold measurements to body density for subjects of a wide age range is not surprising: the ratio of internal fat to subcutaneous fat, fat patterning, and bone density changes with age. The direction of these changes is controversial, however. Differences in skinfold compressibility may be partly responsible for the necessity for different equations for the sexes.

Two examples of these generalized regression equations for the calculation of body density are given below. They are both based on the two-compartment model, assume constant density of the fat-free mass with age, and have been validated for use in adult Caucasian populations (Lohman, 1981). The first equation, from Durnin and Womersley (1974), is valid for male subjects 20–29 y and calculates the body density (D):

$$D \text{ (kg/m}^3) = 1.1631 - (0.0632 \times \log_{10}(\text{SK4 [mm]}))$$

SK4 represents the sum (in mm) of the skinfold measurements for the biceps, triceps, subscapular, and suprailiac skinfolds. The second equation is valid for adult male subjects 18–61 y of varying fatness and is taken from Jackson and Pollock (1978):

$$D = 1.10938 - (8.267 \times 10^{-4} \times \text{SK3}) + (1.6 \times 10^{-6} \times (\text{SK3})^2) - (2.574 \times 10^{-4} \times \text{AGE})$$

This second equation uses SK3, the sum (mm) of the chest, abdomen, and thigh skinfolds, and the age in years to calculate the body density (D) (kg/m^3). A similar equation was also developed for women (Jackson et al., 1980). The two equations take into account changes with age in bone density and in the ratio of internal to external fat. A nonlinear relationship linking skinfold thickness and body density is also considered. The equation of Jackson et al. (1980) appears to provide valid estimates of body density and the percentage of body fat, even in some formerly obese adults (Scherf et al., 1986), but not in adolescent girls (Wong et al., 2000).

The degree to which these equations are generalizable to other ethnic groups is equivocal. Zillikens and Conway (1990) concluded that the Durnin and Womersley equation successfully predicted percentage of body fat (estimated by total body water using isotope dilution [Section 14.3]) in persons of African descent, provided the Holtain caliper is used. A similar conclusion was reached for healthy Chinese adults (Yao et al., 2002). Immink et al. (1992), however, reported that in rural adults from Guatemala with chronic energy deficiency, the Durnin and Womersley equation could not be used to predict percentage of body fat as determined by densitometry.

Calculation of percentage body fat

In most cases, the final stage in the calculation of the percentage of body fat (F) from multiple skinfold measurements is the selection of an empirical equation relating fat content to body density (D). Several equations have been derived based on the classic two-compartment model for body composition. In this model the body is divided into two compartments — fat and fat-free mass. All the equations assume: (*a*) the density of the fat-free mass is relatively constant; (*b*) the density of fat for normal persons does not vary among individuals; (*c*) the water content of the fat-free mass is constant; and (*d*) the proportion of bone mineral (i.e., skeleton) to muscle in the fat-free body is constant. Different authors use different values for the density of fat and the fat-free mass:

$$\%F = ((4.950/D) - 4.500) \times 100\% \qquad \text{(Eq. A)}$$
$$\%F = ((4.570/D) - 4.142) \times 100\% \qquad \text{(Eq. B)}$$
$$\%F = ((5.548/D) - 5.044) \times 100\% \qquad \text{(Eq. C)}$$

The Siri (1961) equation (Eq. A) assumes that the densities of fat and the fat-free mass are 0.90 and 1.10 kg/L respectively. Brožek et al. (1963) (Eq. B) and Rathburn and Pace (1945) (Eq. C) used the concept of a reference man of a specified density and composition; these equations avoid the requirement of estimating the density of fat-free mass. They were developed from the chemical analysis of cadavers.

The equation of Brožek et al. (1963), originally developed for use in nonathletic young adult males, has subsequently been applied to various other populations, including the elderly, women, children, athletes, and various racial groups. The equations of Siri (1961) and Brožek et al. (1963) yield similar values for percentage of body fat for normal subjects with $<30\%$ body fat (Lohman, 1981), but, as body fatness increases, the equation of Siri yields increasingly higher estimates of percentage of body fat than does that of Brôzek et al. (1963). Hence, with the increasing prevalence of overweight and obesity in the more affluent countries, use of the equation by Brožek et al. (1963) may now be preferable (Yao et al., 2002).

These empirical equations should not be used for undernourished individuals, as there is a decreasing correlation between skinfold thickness and total body fat content with increasing severity of undernutrition. This change in correlation may arise from a shift of fat storage from the regions represented by the subscapular and triceps skinfolds to other subcutaneous sites. Alternatively, a shift from subcutaneous to deep visceral sites may occur (Spurr et al., 1981).

The empirical equations are also unsuitable for use with patients undergoing hyperalimentation with high-sodium fluids, or with congestive heart failure or liver disease, as total body water content as a fraction of fat-free mass may be markedly higher in these patients. Large errors then arise when the body fat content is calculated indirectly from skinfold measurements, via body density (Heymsfield and Casper, 1987). Nevertheless, the method is sufficiently reliable to allow study of changes in the body fat content of an individual.

Not surprisingly, for patients with known abnormalities in mineral mass, variations in the density of the fat-free mass can be extreme (Werdein and Kyle, 1960). Even for healthy individuals, errors in body density ranging from 0.003 to 0.005 kg/L result from variations in bone density (Siri, 1956; Bakker and Struikenkamp, 1977). When these classical empirical equations are used, these errors may result in a variation in percentage of body fat of approximately 2% (Werdein and Kyle, 1960).

Increasingly, researchers are trying modifications of these empirical equations with specific population groups. For example, Lohman (1989) has proposed an adjustment to the Siri equation for calculating percentage of body fat in children, based on age- and sex-specific values for the density of the fat-free mass. The specific equations for each age and sex group are shown in Table 11.7. Such adjustments are needed because of the known changes in body water and bone mineral content in growing children. When applying this modification in populations where delays in maturation are significant, skeletal age

Age (y)	DFFM	k_1	k_2
Females			
7–9	1.079	5.451	5.052
9–11	1.082	5.376	4.968
11–13	1.086	5.279	4.861
13–15	1.092	5.141	4.708
15–17	1.094	5.098	4.660
17–20	1.095	5.076	4.636
20–25	1.096	5.055	4.612
Males			
7–9	1.081	5.400	4.996
9–11	1.084	5.327	4.914
11–13	1.087	5.255	4.835
13–15	1.094	5.098	4.660
15–17	1.096	5.055	4.612
17–20	1.098	5.002	4.554
20–25	1.100	4.971	4.519

Table 11.7: Calculation for children of percentage of fat from body density (BD) using age- and sex-specific values for the density of the fat-free mass (DFFM). Percent fat = $((k_1/\text{BD}) - k_2) \times 100\%$. Data from Conlisk et al., American Journal of Clinical Nutrition 55: 1051–1060, 1992 © Am J Clin Nutr. American Society for Clinical Nutrition.

should be used to select the appropriate age-specific values. Skeletal age can be estimated from the left-hand-wrist radiograph using the Tanner Whitehouse II method (Tanner et al., 1983) (Section 9.3.1).

Similar concerns have been raised over the use of Siri's formula to calculate body fat content in the elderly. With increasing age, the density of the fat-free mass is not constant but may decrease due to demineralization of the bone and changes in body water. Hence, the assumption that the density of the fat-free mass is 1.100 kg/L could result in a systematic overestimation of the body fat content of elderly subjects by 1%–2% (Deurenberg et al., 1989a). Moreover, with increasing fatness, the relative amounts of minerals and protein in the fat-free mass may decrease (Deurenberg et al., 1989b). Even after an adjustment to Siri's formula, individual values should be interpreted cautiously (Visser et al., 1994). Some of this uncertainty may be resolved in the future by using a four-compartment model (fat, protein, water, minerals) (Chapter 14) to establish reference data for body composition in the elderly.

11.2 Assessment of the fat-free mass

The fat-free mass is a mixture of water, minerals, and protein, with most of the protein being stored in the muscle. Assessment of muscle mass can therefore provide an index of the protein reserves of the body. Both the mid-upper-arm muscle circumference and the mid-upper-arm muscle area correlate with measures of total muscle mass and are therefore used to predict changes in the protein nutritional status. Unfortunately, the ratios of mid-upper-arm muscle circumference or area to total skeletal muscle mass, and of mid-upper-arm muscle circumference or area to the fat-free mass, are not constant but change with age and certain disease states (Heymsfield and McManus, 1985). As a result, these anthropometric indices do not provide a simple, direct measure of body protein and cannot be used to detect small changes. Arm muscle circumference and arm muscle area are both derived from the mid-upper-arm circumference (MUAC) and triceps skinfold measurements.

11.2.1 Mid-upper-arm circumference

The arm contains both subcutaneous fat and muscle; a decrease in MUAC may therefore reflect a reduction in either muscle mass or subcutaneous tissue (or both). In some less industrialized countries, where the amount of subcutaneous fat is often small, changes in MUAC tend to parallel changes in muscle mass and, hence, are particularly useful in the diagnosis of protein-energy malnutrition or starvation. The changes in the MUAC measurements can also be used to monitor progress during nutritional therapy.

Arm circumference changes are easy to detect and require a minimal amount of time and equipment. Some investigators claim that MUAC-for-age can differentiate normal children from those with protein-energy malnutrition as reliably as weight-for-age (Shakir and Morley, 1974). As a result, MUAC has been used for screening for protein-energy malnutrition in emergencies such as famines and refugee crises. In such situations, the

measurement of weight or height may not be feasible, and ages of the children are often uncertain (de Onis et al., 1997). Consequently, a single MUAC cutoff of 12.5 cm has sometimes been used in the past for children < 5 y as a proxy for low weight-for-height (i.e., wasting), on the assumption that MUAC measurements are relatively independent of age and sex from 1 to 4 y (Shakir and Morley, 1974).

More recently, the age- and sex-independence of MUAC has been questioned (Hall et al., 1993; Bern and Nathanail, 1995). Data from both affluent and low-income countries indicate that MUAC is age-dependent, so that when a fixed cutoff point is used, wasting is overestimated among younger children and underestimated among older ones (de Onis et al., 1997). Instead, the use of MUAC Z-scores, which adjust for age and sex differences, has been advocated, whenever possible, for nutritional surveillance (Hall et al., 1993) (Section 13.3.1).

Measurement of MUAC

Measurements of MUAC should be made using a flexible, nonstretch tape made of fiberglass or steel; alternatively, a fiberglass insertion tape can be used. The subject should stand erect and sideways to the measurer, with the head in the Frankfurt plane, arms relaxed, and legs apart. If the subject is wearing a sleeved garment, it should be removed or the sleeves should be rolled up. The measurement is taken at the midpoint of the upper arm, between the acromion process and the tip of the olecranon (Figure 11.1). After locating the midpoint, the arm is extended so that it is hanging loosely by the side, with the palm facing inward. The tape is then wrapped gently but firmly around the arm at the midpoint (Figure 11.11), care being taken to ensure that the arm is not squeezed. MUAC is often measured at the same time as triceps skinfold.

If necessary, MUAC can be measured with subjects in the recumbent position. In this case, a sandbag is placed under the elbow to raise the arm slightly off the surface of the

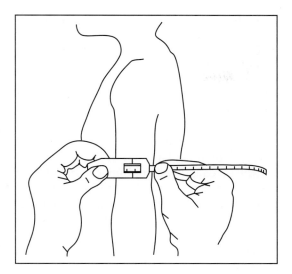

Figure 11.11: Use of insertion tape to measure mid-upper-arm circumference. From Robbins GE, Trowbridge Fl, in: Nutrition Assessment: A Comprehensive Guide for Planning Intervention by M.D. Simko, C. Cowell, and J.A. Gilbride (eds.), p. 88, with permission of Aspen Publishers, Inc., © 1984.

bed (Chumlea et al., 1984). Measurements are taken to the nearest mm.

Precision of MUAC measurements, both within and between examiners, can be high, even if the subjects are obese, provided that trained examiners and standardized methods are used. High precision is critical as MUAC varies little at any given age, with measurements tending to form a narrow symmetrical distribution, so that even small errors are significant.

11.2.2 Mid-upper-arm muscle circumference

The muscle circumference of the mid-upper arm is derived from measurements of both the MUAC and triceps skinfold thickness, and is the calculated circumference of the inner circle of muscle surrounding a small central core of bone (Gurney and Jelliffe, 1973). Mid-upper-arm muscle circumference can be used to assess total body muscle mass, and is frequently used for this purpose in field surveys. It is also used in hospitals to assess protein-energy malnutrition, as the size of the muscle mass is an index of protein reserves.

Nevertheless, it is important to realize that the mid-upper-arm muscle circumference is a one-dimensional measurement, whereas mid-upper-arm muscle area is two-dimensional, and mid-upper-arm muscle volume is three-dimensional. Consequently, if the volume of the mid-upper-arm muscle declines during protein-energy malnutrition or enlarges following a program of nutritional support, the mid-upper-arm muscle circumference change will be proportionally smaller than the change in the mid-upper-arm muscle area (Heymsfield et al., 1982). Hence, arm muscle circumference is insensitive to small changes of muscle mass that might occur, for example, during a brief illness.

Calculation of mid-upper-arm muscle circumference

Mid-upper-arm muscle circumference is calculated using the following equation:

$$\text{MUAMC} = \text{MUAC} - (\pi \times \text{TSK})$$

where MUAMC = mid-upper-arm muscle circumference, MUAC = mid-upper-arm circumference, and TSK = triceps skinfold thickness (Figure 11.12). Note that this equation is only valid when all measurements are in the same units (preferably mm).

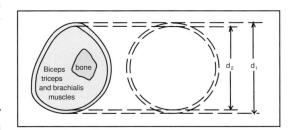

Figure 11.12: Calculation of mid-upper-arm muscle circumference. Let MUAC = mid-upper-arm circumference, TSK = triceps skinfold, d_1 = arm diameter, and d_2 = muscle diameter. Then TSK = $2 \times$ subcutaneous fat = $d_1 - d_2$ and MUAC = πd_1. But mid-upper-arm muscle circumference (MUAMC) = $\pi d_2 = \pi[d_1 - (d_1 - d_2)] = \pi d_1 - \pi(d_1 - d_2)$. Hence MUAMC = MUAC $- \pi \times$ TSK. From Jelliffe DB, The Assessment of the Nutritional Status of the Community. Geneva, World Health Organization (1966). WHO Monograph Series, No. 53, page 77, Figure 44, with permission.

The equation for the calculation of mid-upper-arm muscle circumference is based on the same assumptions as those described for mid-upper-arm fat area (Section 11.1.4). As variations in skinfold compressibility are ignored, and as the triceps skinfold of females is generally more compressible than that of males, female mid-upper-arm muscle circumferences may be underestimated (Clegg and Kent, 1967). As a further complication, the mid-upper-arm muscle circumference equation does not take into account between-subject variation in the diameter of the humerus relative to MUAC (Frisancho, 1981).

11.2.3 Mid-upper-arm muscle area

Mid-upper-arm muscle area is preferable to mid-upper-arm muscle circumference as an index of total body muscle mass because it more adequately reflects the true magnitude of muscle tissue changes (Frisancho, 1981). Studies of adults and children have consistently demonstrated higher correlations of mid-upper-arm muscle area and the creatinine/height ratio (an index of body mass), compared to mid-upper-arm muscle circumference (Trowbridge et al., 1982).

Calculation of mid-upper-arm muscle area

The following equation may be used to estimate mid-upper-arm muscle area:

Arm muscle area $= ((MUAC - (\pi \times TSK))^2)/4\pi$

where MUAC = mid-upper-arm circumference and TSK = triceps skinfold thickness (Frisancho, 1981). Consistent units, preferably mm, should be used throughout. The index is based on the following assumptions:

- The mid-upper-arm cross-section is circular.
- The triceps skinfold is twice the average adipose tissue rim diameter at the middle of the upper arm.
- The mid-upper-arm muscle compartment is circular in cross-section.
- Bone atrophies in proportion to muscle

wastage during protein-energy malnutrition.
- The cross-sectional areas of neurovascular tissue and the humerus are relatively small and ignored.

The first three assumptions are those used in the calculations of mid-upper-arm fat area and muscle circumference.

Heymsfield et al. (1982) examined the accuracy of calculated mid-upper-arm muscle area values by comparing them with computed axial tomography measurements (Section 14.9). They showed that the equation overestimated the mid-upper-arm muscle area by between 20% and 25% in adults and, as a result, may underestimate the severity of muscle atrophy. As an alternative, they suggested a revised equation, which calculates absolute bone-free arm muscle area (Heymsfield et al., 1982).

$$cAMA = \frac{(MUAC - (\pi \times TSK))^2}{4\pi} - 6.5 \quad (women)$$

$$cAMA = \frac{(MUAC - (\pi \times TSK))^2}{4\pi} - 10.0 \quad (men)$$

where cAMA = corrected mid-upper-arm muscle area, MUAC = mid-upper-arm circumference, and TSK = triceps skinfold thickness. This equation assumes that the measurements have been made in cm, and not mm, for conformity with the original reference.

This revised equation takes into account errors resulting from the noncircular nature of the muscle compartment and the inclusion of nonskeletal muscle tissue (e.g., the neurovascular tissue and bone). It reduces the average intraindividual error for a given subject to 7% to 8% for the calculated mid-upper-arm muscle area. Nevertheless, the authors caution that even the corrected mid-upper-arm muscle area equation is only an approximation (e.g., ±8%) of the actual mid-upper-arm muscle area.

These revised equations have not been validated for use with elderly persons and are not appropriate for obese patients because they overestimate arm muscle area when compared with the determination by computerized tomography scan (Forbes et al., 1988).

The estimated coefficient of variation for measurements of mid-upper-arm muscle area made by trained examiners is 7% (Heymsfield et al., 1982). Therefore, this index is not appropriate for detecting small changes in mid-upper-arm muscle area such as those which may follow short-term nutritional support or deprivation.

Heymsfield et al. (1982) also developed an equation to predict total body muscle mass from corrected mid-upper-arm muscle area (cAMA), using estimates of muscle mass derived from urinary creatinine excretion (Section 16.1.1) (Forbes and Bruining, 1976). The total body muscle mass (kg) =

$$\text{height (cm)} \times (0.0264 + [0.029 \times \text{cAMA}])$$

The error of this prediction ranges from 5% to 9%.

To avoid overestimating arm muscle area in obese persons, use of a new index — upper arm muscle area estimate — (UME) may be useful

$$\text{UME} = (\text{MUAC}^2/4\pi) - \text{UFE}$$

where MUAC is the mid-upper-arm circumference and UFE is upper arm fat area estimate (Section 11.1.4). The percentage of fat in the upper arm can be obtained from (UFE/TUA) × 100%. This equation for UME was validated on a small group of obese and control French children, as described for UFE. Results indicate that use of the conventional AFA equation overestimates the arm muscle area, as noted earlier (Heymsfield et al., 1982; Forbes et al., 1988). Application of this new index for undernourished children requires validation, however (Rolland-Cachera et al., 1997).

11.3 Summary

An indirect assessment of both body fat and the fat-free mass can be made from selected skinfold thickness and circumference measurements, taken by standardized techniques. Skinfold thickness measurements at one or more sites (e.g., triceps, biceps, subscapular, suprailiac, and midaxillary skinfold thickness) provide estimates of the subcutaneous fat depot, and hence total body fat. No consensus exists on the best single, or combination of, skinfold site(s) to assess body fat. The most appropriate site(s) depend(s) on the age, sex, and race or ethnicity of the subject, and on whether an estimate of total body fat or percentage of body fat is required. In general, a combination of skinfolds provides a more valid assessment of body fat content and can indicate the distribution of subcutaneous fat.

Recognition that the regional distribution of body fat, specifically the abdominal fat mass, is a critical factor for obesity-related illnesses, independent of overall obesity, has led to the search for anthropometric surrogates of abdominal fat mass. Ratios of trunk (T) to extremity (E) skinfold thicknesses based on the subscapular and triceps have been used, as well as the waist-hip ratio (WHR), and more recently waist circumference. Of these, a high WHR (WHR > 1.0 in men and > 0.85 in women) indicates abdominal fat accumulation and is associated with increased risk of cardiovascular morbidity and mortality. Nevertheless, more research is needed to set ethnic-specific cutoffs for WHR because abdominal fatness may imply different health risks for different racial groups. Currently, no universally standardized procedure exists to measure the WHR.

The measurement of waist circumference alone is now said to provide the best simple and practical indicator of the intra-abdominal fat mass. It correlates closely with BMI and WHR, is unrelated to height, and is also more closely related to potentially atherogenic metabolic disturbances than WHR. A color-coded "waist-watcher" tape measure can be used for self-measurement with three action levels. Tentative sex-specific waist circumference cutoffs are available for adult Caucasians to assess the risk of metabolic consequences associated with obesity (i.e., ≥ 88 cm for women and ≥ 102 cm for men). They are not appropriate for persons with a BMI > 35 or other ethnic groups;

lower cutoffs have been proposed for Asians (> 80 cm for Asian women and > 90 cm for Asian men).

Mid-upper-arm fat area, derived from triceps skinfold thickness and mid-upper-arm circumference measurements, also provides a better estimate of total body fat than a single skinfold at the same site. The mid-upper-arm fat area equation assumes that the limb is cylindrical, with fat evenly distributed about its circumference; no allowance is made for differences in skinfold compressibility. Such assumptions limit the accuracy of body fat estimates from mid-upper-arm fat areas.

A combination of skinfold measurements and either population-specific or generalized regression equations can be used to estimate body density and, in turn, the percentage of body fat using one of three empirical equations. Increasingly, these original empirical equations are being adjusted for use with specific population groups (e.g., children, elderly). Once the percentage of body fat is calculated, total body fat content and the fat-free mass can be derived.

Measurements of mid-upper-arm circumference, either alone or combined with triceps skinfold thickness to calculate mid-upper-arm muscle circumference or muscle area, provides estimates of varying accuracy of the protein reserves of the body and, hence, protein nutritional status. Mid-upper-arm muscle area is preferable to circumference because it more adequately reflects the true magnitude of tissue changes. Nevertheless, the equation overestimates mid-upper-arm muscle area by 20% to 25%. Revised equations have not been validated for use with the elderly and are inappropriate for the obese. None of the anthropometric indices are sensitive enough to monitor small changes in body fat or fat-free mass that may arise after short-term nutritional support or deprivation.

References

Alexander ML. (1964). The postmortem estimation of total body fat, muscle and bone. Clinical Science 26: 193–202.

Allen TH, Peng MT, Owen KP, Huang TF, Chang C, Fung HS. (1956). Prediction of total adiposity from skinfolds and the curvilinear relationship between external and internal adiposity. Metabolism 5: 346–352.

Allison DB, Paultre F, Goran MI, Poehlman ET, Heymsfield SB. (1995). Statistical considerations regarding the use of ratios to adjust data. International Journal of Obesity and Related Metabolic Disorders 19: 644–652.

Ashwell M, Cole TJ, Dixon AK. (1985). Obesity: new insight into the anthropometric classification of fat distribution shown by computer tomography. British Medical Journal 290: 1692–1694.

Bakker HK, Struikenkamp RS. (1977). Biological variability and lean body mass estimates. Human Biology 49: 187–202.

Behnke AR. (1969). New concepts of height-weight relationships. In: Wilson NL (ed.) Obesity. FA Davis, Philadelphia, pp. 25–53.

Bern C, Nathanail L. (1995). Is mid-upper-arm circumference a useful tool for screening in emergency settings? Lancet 345(8950): 631–633.

Björntorp P. (1987). Classification of obese patients and complications related to the distribution of surplus fat. American Journal of Clinical Nutrition 45: 1120–1125.

Björntorp P. (1993). Visceral obesity: a "civilization syndrome." Obesity Research 1: 206–222.

Brodie DA. (1988). Techniques of measurement of body composition, part I. Sports Medicine 5: 11–40.

Brožek J, Grande F, Anderson JT, Keys A. (1963). Densitometric analysis of body composition: revision of some quantitative assumptions. Annals of the New York Academy of Sciences 110: 113–140.

Burkinshaw L, Jones PRM, Krupowicz DW. (1973). Observer error in skinfold thickness measurements. Human Biology 45: 273–279.

Chumlea WC, Roche AF, Mukherjee D. (1984). Nutritional Assessment of the Elderly through Anthropometry. Ross Laboratories, Columbus, Ohio.

Clegg EJ, Kent C. (1967). Skinfold compressibility in young adults. Human Biology 39: 418–429.

Conlisk EA, Haas JD, Martinez EJ, Flores R, Rivera JD, Martorell R. (1992). Predicting body composition from anthropometry and bioimpedance in marginally undernourished adolescents and young adults. American Journal of Clinical Nutrition 55: 1051–1060.

Daniels SR, Khoury PR, Morrison JA. (2000). Utility of different measures of body fat distribution in children and adolescents. American Journal of Epidemiology 152: 1179–1184.

de Onis M, Yip R, Mei Z. (1997). The development of MUAC-for-age reference data recommended by a WHO Expert Committee. Bulletin of the World Health Organization 75: 11–18.

Després JP, Nadeau A, Tremblay A, Ferland M, Moorjani S, Lupien PJ, Théiault G, Pinault S, Bouchard C. (1989). Role of deep abdominal fat in the association between regional adipose tissue distribution and glucose tolerance in obese women. Diabetes 38: 304–309.

Després JP, Moorjani S, Lupien PJ, Tremblay A, Nadeau A, Bouchard C. (1990). Regional distribution of body fat, plasma lipoproteins, and cardiovascular disease. Arteriosclerosis 10: 497–511.

Deurenberg P, Weststrate JA, van der Kooy K. (1989a). Is an adaptation of Siri's formula for the calculation of body fat percentage from body density in the elderly necessary? European Journal of Clinical Nutrition 43: 559–567.

Deurenberg P, Leenen R, van der Kooy K, Hautvast JGAJ. (1989b). In obese subjects the body fat percentage calculated with Siri's formula is an overestimation. European Journal of Clinical Nutrition 43: 569–575.

Dowling HJ, Pi-Sunyer FX. (1993). Race-dependent health risks of upper body obesity. Diabetes 42: 537–543.

Durnin JVGA, Womersley J. (1974). Body fat assessed from total body density and its estimation from skinfold thickness: measurements on 481 men and women aged from 16 to 72 years. British Journal of Nutrition 32: 77–97.

Edwards DA, Hammond WH, Healy MJ, Tanner JM, Whitehouse RH. (1955). Design and accuracy of calipers for measuring subcutaneous tissue thickness. British Journal of Nutrition 9: 133–143.

Flodmark CE, Sveger T, Nilsson-Ehle P. (1994). Waist measurement correlates to a potentially atherogenic lipoprotein profile in obese 12–14 year-old children. Acta Paediatrica 83: 941–945.

Forbes GB, Bruining GJ. (1976). Urinary creatinine excretion and lean body mass. American Journal of Clinical Nutrition 29: 1359–1366.

Forbes GB, Brown MR, Griffiths HJL. (1988). Arm muscle plus bone area: anthropometry and CAT scan compared. American Journal of Clinical Nutrition 47: 929–931.

Freedman DS, Serdula MK, Srinivasan SR, Berenson GS. (1999). Relation of circumferences and skinfold thicknesses to lipid and insulin concentrations in children and adolescents: the Bogalusa Heart Study. American Journal of Clinical Nutrition 69: 308–317.

Frisancho AR. (1981). New norms of upper limb fat and muscle areas for assessment of nutritional status. American Journal of Clinical Nutrition 34: 2540–2545.

Frisancho AR. (1990). Anthropometric standards for the assessment of growth and nutritional status. University of Michigan Press, Ann Arbor.

Gillum RF. (1999). Distribution of waist-to-hip ratio, other indices of body fat distribution and obesity and associations with HDL cholesterol in children and young adults aged 4–19 years: the Third National Health and Nutrition Examination Survey. International Journal of Obesity and Related Metabolic Disorders 23: 556–563.

Goran MI, Gower BA. (1999). Relation between visceral fat and disease risk in children and adoles-

cents. American Journal of Clinical Nutrition 70: 149S–156S.

Goran MI, Nagy TR, Treuth MS, Trowbridge C, Dezenberg C, McGloin A, Gower BA. (1997). Visceral fat in white and African American prepubertal children. American Journal of Clinical Nutrition 65: 1703–1708.

Goran MI, Gower BA, Treuth M, Nagy TR. (1998). Prediction of intra-abdominal and subcutaneous abdominal adipose tissue in healthy prepubertal children. International Journal of Obesity and Related Metabolic Disorders 22: 549–558.

Gore C, Norton K, Olds T, Whittingham N, Birchall K, Clough M, Dickerson B, Downie L. (1996). Accreditation in anthropometry: an Australian model. In: Anthropmetrica. Norton K, Olds T (eds.) University of New South Wales Press, Sydney.

Gruber J, Pollock M, Graves J, Colvin A, Braith R. (1990). Comparison of Harpenden and Lange calipers in predicting body composition. Research Quarterly for Exercise and Sport 61: 184–190.

Gurney JM, Jelliffe DB. (1973). Arm anthropometry in nutritional assessment: nomogram for rapid calculation of muscle circumference and cross-sectional muscle and fat areas. American Journal of Clinical Nutrition 26: 912–915.

Hall G, Chowdhury S, Bloem M. (1993). Use of mid-upper-arm circumference Z-scores in nutritional assessment. Lancet 341(8858): 1481.

Han TS, Lean MEJ. (1998). Self-reported waist circumference compared with the "Waist Watcher" tape measure to identify individuals at increased health risk through intra-abdominal fat accumulation. British Journal of Nutrition 80: 81–88.

Han TS, McNeill G, Seidell JC, Lean MEJ. (1997a). Predicting intra-abdominal fatness from anthropometric measures: the influence of stature. International Journal of Obesity and Related Metabolic Disorders 21: 587–593.

Han TS, Seidell JC, Currall JEP, Morrison CE, Deurenberg P, Lean MEJ. (1997b). The influence of height and age on waist circumference as an index of adiposity in adults. International Journal of Obesity and Related Metabolic Disorders 21: 83–89.

Health Canada. (2003). Canadian guidelines for body weight classification in adults. Health Canada, Ottawa.

Heymsfield SB, Casper K. (1987). Anthropometric assessment of the adult hospitalized patient. Journal of Parenteral and Enteral Nutrition 11: 36S–41S.

Heymsfield SB, McManus CB. (1985). Tissue components of weight loss in cancer patients: a new method of study and preliminary observations. Cancer 55: 238–249.

Heymsfield SB, McManus CB, Smith J, Stevens V, Nixon DW. (1982). Anthropometric measurement of muscle mass: revised equations for calculating bone-free arm muscle area. American Journal of Clinical Nutrition 36: 680–690.

Heymsfield SB, McManus CB, Seitz SB, Nixon DW, Smith J. (1984). Anthropometric assessment of adult protein-energy malnutrition. In: Wright RA, Heymsfield SB (eds.) Nutritional Assessment of the Adult Hospitalized Patient. Blackwell Scientific, Boston, pp. 27–82.

Heymsfield SB, Allison DB, Wang ZM, Baumgartner RM, Ross R. (1998). Evaluation of total and regional body composition. In: Bray GA, Bouchard C, James WPT (eds.) Handbook of Obesity. Marcel Dekker, New York, pp. 41–77.

Heyward VH, Stolarczyk LM. (1996). Applied Body Composition Assessment. Human Kinetics, Champaign, IL.

Himes JH, Roche AF, Webb P. (1980). Fat areas as estimates of total body fat. American Journal of Clinical Nutrition 33: 2093–2100.

Immink MD, Flores R, Diaz EO. (1992). Body mass index, body composition and the chronic energy deficiency classification of rural adult populations in Guatemala. European Journal of Clinical Nutrition 46: 419–427.

Jackson AS, Pollock ML. (1978). Generalized equations for predicting body density of men. British Journal of Nutrition 40: 497–504.

Jackson AS, Pollock ML, Ward A. (1980). Generalized equations for predicting body density of women. Medicine and Science in Sports and Exercise 12: 175–181.

Jelliffe DB. (1966). The Assessment of the Nutritional Status of the Community. WHO Monograph Series No. 53. World Health Organization, Geneva.

Jones PRM, Hunt MJ, Brown TP, Norgan NG. (1986). Waist-hip circumference ratio and its relation to age and overweight in British men. Human Nutrition: Clinical Nutrition 40: 239–247.

Kalkhoff RK, Hartz AH, Rupley D, Kissebah AH, Kelber S. (1983). Relationship of body fat distribution to blood pressure, carbohydrate tolerance, and plasma lipids in healthy obese women. Journal of Laboratory and Clinical Medicine 102: 621–627.

Kissebah AH, Freedman DS, Peiris AN. (1989). Health risks of obesity. Medical Clinics of North America 73: 111–138.

Krotkiewski M, Björntorp P, Sjöström L, Smith U. (1983). Impact of obesity on metabolism in men and women: importance of regional adipose tissue distribution. Journal of Clinical Investigation 72: 1150–1162.

Lapidus L, Bengtsson C, Larsson B, Pennert K, Rybo E, Sjostrom L. (1984). Distribution of adipose tissue and risk of cardiovascular disease and death: a 12-year follow-up of participants in the population study of women in Gothenburg, Sweden. British Medical Journal 289: 1257–1261.

Larsson B, Svardsudd B, Welin L, Wilhelmsen L, Björntorp P, Tibblin G. (1984). Abdominal adipose tissue distribution, obesity and risk of cardiovascular disease and death: 13-year follow-up of participants in the study of men born in 1913. British Medical Journal 288: 1401–1404.

Lohman TG. (1981). Skinfolds and body density and their relation to body fatness: a review. Human Biology 53: 181–225.

Lohman TG. (1989). Assessment of body composition in children. Pediatric Exercise Science 1: 19–30.

Lohman TG. (1992). Advances in Body Composition Assessment. Current Issues in Exercise Science Series Monograph No. 3. Human Kinetics, Champaign, IL.

Lohman TG, Roche AF, Martorell R (eds.). (1988). Anthropometric Standardization Reference Manual. Human Kinetics, Champaign, IL.

Lukaski HC. (1987). Methods for the assessment of human body composition: traditional and new. American Journal of Clinical Nutrition 46: 537–556.

Malina RM. (1996). Regional body composition: age, sex, and ethnic variation. In: Roche AF, Heymsfield SB, Lohman TG (eds.) Human Body Composition. Human Kinetics, Champaign, IL, pp. 205–216.

McCarthy HD, Jarrett KV, Crawley HF. (2001). The development of waist percentiles in British children aged 5.0–16.9 y. European Journal of Clinical Nutrition 55: 902–907.

McKeigue PM. (1996). Metabolic consequences of obesity and body fat pattern: lessons from migrant studies. In: Chadwick DJ, Cardew GC (eds.) The Origins and Consequences of Obesity: Ciba Foundation Symposium 201. Wiley, Chichester, pp. 54–67.

McNeely MJ, Boyko EJ, Shofer JB, Newell-Morris L, Leonetti DL, Fujimoto WY. (2001). Standard definitions of overweight and central adiposity for determining diabetes risk in Japanese Americans. American Journal of Clinical Nutrition 74: 101–107.

Molarius A, Seidell JC, Sans S, Tuomilehto J, Kuulasmaa K. (1999). Waist and hip circumferences, and waist-hip ratio in 19 populations of the WHO MONICA Project. International Journal of Obesity and Related Metabolic Disorders 23: 116–125.

Najjar MF, Kuczmarski RJ. (1989). Anthropometric Data and Prevalence of Overweight for Hispanics, 1982–1984. Vital and Health Statistics 11(239): 1–106.

Najjar MF, Rowland M. (1987). Anthropometric data and prevalence of overweight, United States, 1976–1980. Vital and Health Statistics 11(238): 1–73.

NIH (National Institutes of Health). (1998). Clinical guidelines on the identification, evaluation and treatment of overweight and obesity in adults: the evidence report. Obesity Research 6: 51S–209S.

Pouliot M-C, Després J-P, Lemieux S, Moorjani S, Bouchard C, Tremblay A, Nadeau A, Lupien PJ. (1994). Waist circumference and abdominal sagittal diameter: best simple anthropometric indexes of abdominal visceral adipose tissue accumulation and related cardiovascular risk in men and women. American Journal of Cardiology 73: 460–468.

Ramachandran A, Snehalatha C, Viswanathan V, Viswanathan M, Haffner SM. (1997). Risk of noninsulin dependent diabetes mellitus conferred by obesity and central adiposity in different ethnic groups: a comparative analysis between Asian Indians, Mexican Americans and Whites. Diabetes Research and Clinical Practice 36: 121–125.

Rathburn EN, Pace N. (1945). Studies on body composition I: The determination of total body fat by means of the body specific gravity. Journal of Biological Chemistry 158: 667–676.

Rimm EB, Stampfer MJ, Colditz GA, Chute CG, Litin LB, Willett WC. (1990). Validity of self-reported waist and hip circumferences in men and women. Epidemiology 1: 466–473.

Robbins GE, Trowbridge FL. (1984). Anthropometric techniques and their application. In: Simko MD, Cowell C, Gilbride JA (eds.) Nutrition Assessment. Aspen Systems, Rockville, MD, pp. 69–92.

Roberts CA, Wilder LB, Jackson RT, Moy TF, Becker DM. (1997). Accuracy of self-measurement of waist and hip circumference in men and women. Journal of the American Dietetic Association 97: 534–536.

Roche AF, Siervogel RM, Chumlea WC, Webb P. (1981). Grading body fatness from limited anthropometric data. American Journal of Clinical Nutrition 34: 2831–2838.

Rolland-Cachera MF, Brambilla P, Manzoni P, Akrout M, Sironi S, Del Maschio A, Chiumello G. (1997). Body composition assessed on the basis of arm circumference and triceps skinfold thickness: a new index validated in children by magnetic resonance imaging. American Journal of Clinical Nutrition 65: 1709–1713.

Ryan AS, Martinez GA, Baumgartner RN, Roche AF, Guo S, Chumlea WC, Kuczmarski RJ. (1990). Median skinfold thickness distributions and fat-wave patterns in Mexican-American children from the Hispanic Health and Nutrition Examination Survey (HHANES 1982–1984). American Journal of Clinical Nutrition 51: 925S–935S.

Sangi H, Mueller WH. (1991). Which measures of body fat distribution is best for epidemiologic research among adolescents? American Journal of Epidemiology 133: 870–883.

Scherf J, Franklin BA, Lucas CP, Stevenson D, Rubenfire M. (1986). Validity of skinfold thickness measures of formerly obese adults. American Journal of Clinical Nutrition 43: 128–135.

Shakir A, Morley D. (1974). Measuring malnutrition. Lancet 1(7860): 758–759.

Siervogel RM, Roche AF, Himes JH, Chumlea WC, McCammon R. (1982). Subcutaneous fat distribution in males and females from 1 to 39 years of age. American Journal of Clinical Nutrition 36: 162–171.

Sinning WE. (1978). Anthropometric estimation of body density, fat and lean body mass in women gymnasts. Medicine and Science in Sports and Exercise 10: 243–249.

Siri WB. (1956). The gross composition of the body. In: Lawrence JH, Tobias CA (eds.) Advances in Biological and Medical Physics. Volume 4. Academic Press, New York, pp. 239–280.

Siri WE. (1961). Body composition from fluid space and density. In: Brozek J, Hanschel A (eds.) Techniques for Measuring Body Composition. National Academy of Sciences, Washington, DC, pp. 223–244.

Slaughter MH, Lohman TG, Boileau RA, Horswill CA, Stillman RJ, Van Loan MD, Bembden DA. (1988). Skinfold equations for estimation of body fatness in children and youth. Human Biology 60: 709–723.

Sloan AW. (1967). Estimation of body fat in young men. Journal of Applied Physiology 23: 23–29.

Sloan AW, Burt JJ, Blyth CS. (1962). Estimation of body fat in young women. Journal of Applied Physiology 17: 967–970.

Spurr GB, Barac-Nieto M, Lotero H, Dahners HW. (1981). Comparisons of body fat estimated from total body water and skinfold thicknesses of undernourished men. American Journal of Clinical Nutrition 34: 1944–1953.

Tanner JM, Whitehouse RH, Cameron N, Marshall W, Healy MJR, Goldstein H. (1983). The Assessment of Skeletal Maturity and Prediction of Adult Height (TW2 Method). 2nd ed. Academic Press, London.

Taylor RW, Jones IE, Williams S, Goulding A. (2000). Evaluation of waist circumference, waist-to-hip ratio, and the conicity index as screening tools for high trunk fat mass, as measured by dual-energy X-ray absorptiometry, in children aged 3–19 y. American Journal of Clinical Nutrition 72: 490–495.

Trowbridge FL, Hiner CD, Robertson AD. (1982). Arm muscle indicators and creatinine excretion in children. American Journal of Clinical Nutrition 36: 691–696.

Ulijaszek SJ, Kerr DA. (1999). Anthropometric measurement error and the assessment of nutritional status. British Journal of Nutrition 82: 165–177.

van der Kooy KVD, Seidell JC. (1993). Techniques for the measurement of visceral fat: a practical guide. International Journal of Obesity and Related Metabolic Disorders 17: 187–196.

Visser M, van den Heuvel E, Deurenberg P. (1994). Prediction equations for the estimation of body composition in the elderly using anthropometric data. British Journal of Nutrition 71: 823–833.

Wagner DR, Heyward VH. (2000). Measures of body composition in blacks and whites: a comparative review. American Journal of Clinical Nutrition 71: 1392–1402.

Werdein EJ, Kyle LH. (1960). Estimation of the constancy of density of the fat-free body. Journal of Clinical Investigation 39: 626–629.

WHO (World Health Organization). (1995). Physical Status: The Use and Interpretation of Anthropometry. Report of a WHO Expert Committee. Technical Report Series No. 854. World Health Organization, Geneva.

WHO (World Health Organization). (2000). Obesity: Preventing and Managing the Global Epidemic. Report on a WHO Consultation. Technical Report Series No. 894. World Health Organization, Geneva.

WHO (World Health Organization), International Association for the Study of Obesity, International Obesity Task Force. (2000). The Asia-Pacific perspective: redefining obesity and its treatment. Health Communications Australia, Sydney.

Wilmore JH, Brown CH. (1974). Physiological profiles of women distance runners. Medicine and Science in Sports and Exercise 6: 178–181.

Wong WW, Stuff JE, Butte NF, O'Brian Smith E, Ellis KJ. (2000). Estimating body fat in African American and white adolescent girls: a comparison of skinfold-thickness equations with a 4-compartment criterion model. American Journal of Clinical Nutrition 72: 348–354.

Yao M, Roberts SB, Ma G, Pan H, McCrory MA. (2002). Field methods for body composition assessment are valid in healthy Chinese adults. Journal of Nutrition 12: 310–317.

Zerfas AJ. (1985). Checking Continuous Measures: Manual for Anthropometry. Division of Epidemiology, School of Public Health, University of California, Los Angeles.

Zhu SK, Wang ZW, Hershka S, Heo M, Faith MS, Heymsfield SB. (2002). Waist circumference and obesity-associated risk factors among whites in the third National Health and Nutrition Examination Survey: clinical action thresholds. American Journal of Clinical Nutrition 76: 743–749.

Zillikens MC, Conway JM. (1990). Anthropometry in blacks: applicability of generalized skinfold equations and differences in fat patterning between blacks and whites. American Journal of Clinical Nutrition 52: 45–51.

12

Anthropometric reference data

Anthropometric reference data comes from local or international sources. Local reference data should be compiled from measurements made on well-nourished, healthy individuals, selected from a local elite group; the group should be ethnically and genetically representative of the population to be investigated. Such data may be preferred where ethnic and genetic factors influencing growth potential predominate, or where it is felt that international reference data, derived from populations with needlessly high energy intakes, are inappropriate.

International reference data are preferred when ethnic and genetic differences are considered less important than the influences of nutrition, infection, parasitic disease, and environmental and economic factors (Habicht et al., 1974; Graitcer and Gentry, 1981). Stephenson et al. (1983) showed that during the first 5 y of life, there is little difference between the growth curves for members of elite groups in less developed countries and those for infants and children of similar age in the industrialized nations.

In 2000, the U.S. Centers for Disease Control and Prevention (CDC) published updated growth charts for children designed to overcome some of the limitations and technical defects of the National Center for Health Statistics (NCHS) 1977 growth data. These new CDC 2000 growth charts now extend to 20 years of age and include body mass index (BMI) percentiles for 2–20 y to aid the diagnosis of overweight and underweight. In the United States, these CDC 2000 charts are the recommended anthropometric reference (Kuczmarski et al. 2000a)

The World Health Organization (WHO, 1995) recommended the development of a new international growth reference for infants and children from birth to 5 y. This growth reference is based on a sample from diverse geographic sites around the world, whose caregivers have complied with WHO feeding recommendations. This new growth reference is planned for release in 2005. A new growth reference is also needed for older children and adolescents. In the interim, WHO continues to recommend the use of the NCHS/WHO 1977 growth reference for children and adolescents, despite its known limitations.

For adults, when no local reference data are available, as is the case in many low-income countries, WHO continues to recommend the use of NCHS/WHO values for height at 18 y as the reference, and not the new CDC 2000 growth charts (WHO, 1995).

For defining overweight and obesity, WHO favors the provisional use of internationally derived age-specific BMI percentile cutoffs for children and adolescents equivalent to the WHO BMI definitions for adults who are overweight (BMI $\geqslant 25$) or obese (BMI $\geqslant 30$), until better reference data become available. WHO has also adopted BMI cutoff points defined by FAO for classifying adults with chronic energy deficiency.

For body composition indices, use of local reference data is preferred in view of the marked racial differences that exist in body proportions, as well as in both the amount and distribution of subcutaneous fat. In practice, however, comprehensive local sets of data for body composition indices are limited.

In the absence of any local reference data for body composition indices, WHO (1995) provisionally recommends the continued use of the NCHS 1977 values derived from the National Health and Nutrition Examination Survey (NHANES) I and NHANES II as reference data for children and younger adults. This recommendation meets the requirement for all anthropometric variables to be derived from the same reference population. However, when interpreting indices of body composition, the potential effect of marked racial differences should always be kept in mind.

WHO (1995) does not recommend the use of 1977 NCHS reference data for the elderly but, instead, has urged countries to compile local data. In the interim, WHO recommends that NHANES III data for persons $\geqslant 60$ y should be used for comparison.

At present, reference data are generally classified by age, sex, and (sometimes) race. Classification by additional variables (such as number of siblings in a family and/or maturity level) may increase the sensitivity and specificity of the data for identifying individuals or groups at risk. This approach has not been extensively investigated, although WHO (1995) now provides guidelines for adjusting comparisons of anthropometric indices of adolescents for maturational status (Section 12.7).

Reference data facilitate international comparisons of anthropometric indices across the populations and enable the proportion of the individuals with abnormal indices to be determined, relative to the reference population. Such comparisons enable the extent and severity of malnutrition in the study group to be estimated. In surveillance studies, reference data allow the evaluation of trends over time, as well as the effectiveness of intervention programs. Reference data can also be used in clinical settings to monitor growth of individuals and to identify those at risk for under- or overnutrition (screening), and

to assess their response to treatment. Valid anthropometric reference data sets have the properties listed in Box 12.1.

12.1 Fetal growth reference data

Fetal growth during the first 6 mo appears to be independent of sex, race, and exposure to common growth-promoting and growth-inhibiting environmental influences. As a result, most published early-gestation reference curves for fetal growth are similar. It is not until later gestation that differences in the existing fetal growth curves become evident. For example, at about 30 wk, female fetuses are smaller on average than male fetuses.

At 34–36 wk gestation, African American infants are larger than Caucasian infants, although the pattern is reversed thereafter (IOM, 1990). These racial differences are small and are likely to be genetically determined. Therefore, the WHO Expert Committee recommended the use of a single, sex-specific international reference for fetal growth (de Onis and Habicht, 1996). Use of a single reference also facilitates regional and international comparisons. Of the 11 fetal growth reference data sets considered by WHO, the data from California of Williams et al. (1982) was chosen (Figure 12.1) based on the criteria listed in Box 12.2.

A secular trend, that is a trend toward earlier maturity and increased height at all ages over generations, must not confound the data.

A random, nationally representative sample must have been drawn to generate the reference data.

The reference data must have external validity and thus be valid for groups other than the sampled population.

No cross-sectional discrepancy must be apparent. On trial, the proportion below any particular reference centile must be consistently within the expected limits.

There must be no longitudinal discrepancy. On trial, there must be a consistent fit to the growth curves with increasing age.

Box 12.1: Properties of valid reference data sets.

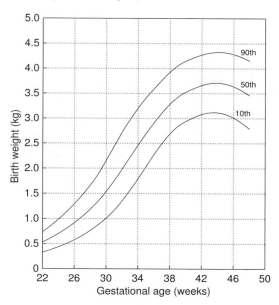

Figure 12.1: 10th, 50th, and 90th percentiles of birth weight for singleton Californian Caucasian boys. Drawn from numerical data of Williams et al., (1982). Fetal growth and perinatal viability in California. Obstetrics and Gynecology 59(5): 624–632.

Birthweight interval (g)	n	Weight gain	
		(g/d)	(g/kg/d)
501–600	53	15.27	13.99
601–700	128	16.81	13.46
701–800	155	18.60	13.96
801–900	139	20.06	14.46
901–1000	184	21.04	14.63
1001–1100	163	22.83	15.22
1101–1200	171	24.73	15.98
1201–1300	187	26.34	16.28
1301–1400	200	27.15	16.17
1401–1500	203	27.77	16.00

Table 12.1: Weight gain by birth-weight interval for very low birth-weight infants. Data from Ehrenkranz et al., Pediatrics 104: 280–289, 1999.

12.2 Growth reference data for preterm infants

Differences in weight, length, and head circumference between preterm and full-term infants are well recognized. The time period over which these differences extend varies with the growth measurement. Differences are significant until 18 mo for head circumference, until 24 mo for weight-for-age, and up to 3.5 y for length/height-for-age.

Multiracial;

Gestational age given in completed weeks.

Large sample size at the lower end of the gestational age distribution.

Separate curves for singleton boys and girls and for multiple births.

Comparable with many other candidate curves.

Neonatal mortality data provided in relation to birth weight and gestational age.

Box 12.2: Desired properties of fetal growth reference data sets.

Postnatal growth curves suitable for clinical settings and research have been constructed for very low birth-weight (VLBW) infants with birth weights between 501 g and 1500 g. The curves are based on infants (n = 1660) admitted to 12 U.S. National Institute of Child Health and Human Development Neonatal Research Network Centers from August 1994 to 1995. Characteristics of the infants are given in Ehrenrkanz et al. (1999).

Measurements (except weight) were taken twice using standardized techniques. Body weight was recorded daily for a minimum of 14 d or until birth weight was regained, and then weekly thereafter using digital electronic scales (to the nearest 10 g). Weekly measurements were made for recumbent length, head circumference, and mid-upper-arm circumference (MUAC) using a special length board for recumbent length and fiber measurement tapes for both head and arm circumferences. Estimates of gestational age were based on last menstrual period, standard obstetrical observations, and ultasonography.

Weight gain by 100-g birth-weight intervals is shown in Table 12.1. The data are based on all the available anthropometric measurements from all infants, irrespective of their nutritional status or clinical course. Gains in length (cm/wk), head circumference (cm/wk), and MUAC (cm/wk) are less dependent on birth weight (Ehrenrkanz et al. 1999).

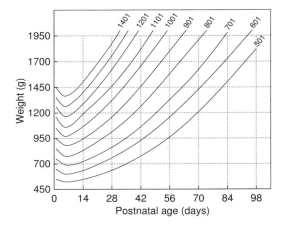

Figure 12.2: Body weight versus postnatal age for very low birth-weight infants, stratified by 100 g birth-weight intervals. From Ehrenkranz et al., Pediatrics 104: 280–289, 1999.

Ehrenkranz et al. (1999) also present additional postnatal growth curves for VLBW infants; these are listed below:

- Average weekly length versus postnatal age in weeks for infants stratified by 100-g birth-weight intervals
- Average weekly head circumference versus postnatal age in weeks for infants stratified by 100-g birth-weight intervals
- Average weekly MUAC versus postnatal age in weeks for infants stratified by 100-g birth-weight intervals
- Growth curves of infants with major morbidities and of reference infants without major morbidities plotted by postnatal age in days
- Growth curves of small-for-gestational age infants and of appropriate-for-gestational age infants plotted by postnatal age in days; the infants are stratified by 100-g birth-weight intervals
- Average body weight versus postmenstrual age in weeks for all study infants with gestational ages 24–25, 26–27, and 28–29 wk; the reference intrauterine growth curves were plotted using the smoothed 10th and 50th percentile birth-weight data reported by Alexander et al. (1996)

These growth curves for VLBW infants

should not be taken as optimal but, instead, should be used to better understand postnatal growth, to identify infants developing illnesses that affect growth, and to design future research studies.

The data shown in Figure 12.2 only extend to about 100 days uncorrected postnatal age or until a body weight of 2000 g is reached. This can be a limitation in clinical practice and public health settings. Hence, to assess the growth of VLBW infants for a longer period, the growth charts compiled by the U.S. Infant Health and Development Program (IHDP) should be used (Casey et al., 1990, 1991; Guo et al., 1996). These charts are based on a relatively large sample ($n = 867$) of VLBW infants from across the United States. They are adjusted for gestational age at birth to account for prematurity, and can be used for low birth-weight (LBW) infants from an age corrected for gestation of 40 wk to 36 mo. However, the data were collected in 1985 and, hence, may not reflect current medical and nutritional care practices.

The IHDP reference includes tables and charts by sex of means, standard deviations (SDs), and selected percentiles (10th, 25th, 50th, 75th, 90th) for length-for-age, weight-for-age, weight-for-length, head circumference-for-length, and head circumference-for-age for two groups of preterm infants: LBW (1501–2500 g) and VLBW ($<$ 1500 g) (Casey et al., 1990, 1991; Guo et al., 1996, 1997). The data are from a combination of small for gestational age (SGA) and appropriate for gestational age (AGA) infants. The head circumference data were expressed in relation to length as well as age, because the former are independent of gestational age, and this is an advantage when gestational ages are not available (Roche et al., 1997).

The measurements were taken on 428 boys and 439 girls on admission, then at 40 wk postconceptional age, and longitudinally at 4, 8, 12, 18, 24, 30, and 36 mo of gestation-corrected age using standardized, appropriate techniques. Gestational age of the infants was assessed within 48 h of birth using the physical criteria of Ballard et al. (1979).

Sherry et al. (2003) recommend the use

of the IHDP reference for comparison of the growth of a VLBW infant with those of other VLBW infants, but for a comparison with non-VLBW infants, then the CDC 2000 growth charts (Section 12.4) should be used.

12.3 Head circumference reference data

Several new sets of head circumference reference curves have been published since 1995. They include the updated CDC 2000 percentile charts (Kuczmarski et al., 2000b), percentile charts from the Euro-Growth study (van't Hof et al., 2000), and the UK90 growth study (Freeman et al., 1995). The upcoming WHO multicenter growth reference for young children will also have head circumference data, as described in Section 12.4.2.

The new CDC 2000 percentile curves for the head circumference of boys from birth to 36 mo are shown in Figure 12.3. A larger version of the data and the reference curves for girls are presented in the Appendix (A12.7 and A12.8). The measurements were taken

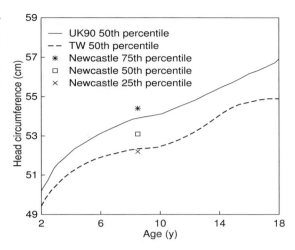

Figure 12.4: Tanner and Whitehouse (TW) and UK90 head circumference 50th percentiles (male data only shown) compared to survey data from Newcastle, 221 boys aged 8.5 y. Data from Wright et al., Archives of Disease in Childhood 86: 11–14, 2002, with permission of the BMJ Publishing Group.

on the same children who provided the length and weight data (Kuczmarski et al., 2000b).

Figure 12.4 presents the 50th percentile curve for head circumference of boys aged 2–18 y from the UK90 data, and compares it with the 50th percentile derived from the earlier Tanner and Whitehouse data (Wright et al., 2002). There is a striking differences between the two curves, both in the shape during puberty and in percentile values. Indeed, the UK90 reference is on average 1–2 percentile spaces (>1 SD) higher, the largest discrepancy occurring at ages 18–20 y. Moreover, neither reference shows an acceptable fit with recent data from a survey in Newcastle in the United Kingdom (Figure 12.4).

In view of these discrepancies, the UK90 reference for head circumference, like the Tanner and Whitehouse reference, is probably not sufficiently robust to correctly diagnose abnormalities of head size after 2 y or for monitoring head growth after the onset of puberty. Nevertheless, it can be used for monitoring head circumference prior to puberty, as long as the same reference is used consistently, and some degree of caution is exercised (Wright et al., 2002). In future, a new robust U.K reference for head circumference for children should be constructed.

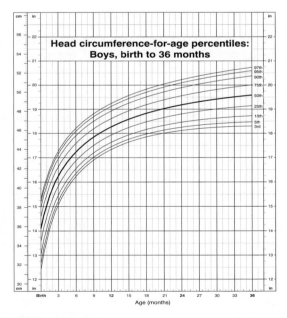

Figure 12.3: Reference data for head circumference-for-age for U.S. boys aged 0–36 mo. From Kuczmarski et al. (2000a).

12.4 Distance growth reference data for infants and children

Growth curves are compiled using data from normal healthy infants and children. They can be developed using two approaches — descriptive and prescriptive. The descriptive approach is more often adopted; it uses a representative sample of normal healthy children to generate a "reference," which describes how children actually grow. In the prescriptive approach, children are selected to include only those who are well nourished and healthy and who adhere to established feeding and health care recommendations. Such data generate a growth "standard," which describes how children should grow.

Most of the growth reference data noted in the following sections are descriptive, with the notable exception of the WHO international growth reference for infants and young children currently in preparation, and the CDC 2000 reference data for weight and BMI (Section 12.4.4). The new WHO reference (Section 12.4.2) aims to represent the best standard possible for optimal growth for all children younger than 5 y.

The term "distance growth" encompasses both stature and weight measurements compiled from cross-sectional sampling — measurements taken once on children of varying ages, preferably on a nationally representative sample. Distance growth reference data allows comparison of stature and weight attained by an individual up to the time of observation (Tanner et al., 1966).

Cross-sectional reference data are suitable for use during the surveillance and screening of population groups studied during cross-sectional surveys. Such reference data can additionally be used to identify individual preadolescent children with unusually low or high values for stature or weight (i.e., screening) and who may be nutritionally at risk.

12.4.1 NCHS/WHO growth reference data

Two WHO publications present percentiles for weight and height, recalculated from the NCHS data, for use as an international reference (WHO, 1978, 1983). The values listed in these two booklets differ and are not identical with the NCHS percentiles.

The "Growth Chart for International Use in Maternal and Child Health Care" (WHO, 1978) presents percentiles (3rd, 50th, and 97th) and the values for $-3\,SD$ and $-4\,SD$, for weight-for-age and stature-for-age (but not weight-for-stature) for male and females from 0–5 y at 1-mo intervals.

Measuring Change in Nutritional Status (WHO, 1983) gives more extensive percentile tables for males and females from 0–36 mo and 2–18 y. Percentile values included are 3rd, 5th, 10th, 20th, 30th, 40th, 50th, 60th, 70th, 80th, 90th, 95th, and 97th for weight-for-age, stature-for-age, and weight-for-stature (for prepubertal children). The median and ± 1, 2, and 3 SD are also given (see abbreviated example, Table 12.2); details of their derivations are given in Dibley et al. (1987). A computer program (EPIINFO) is available from the CDC for calculating anthropometric growth indices from the NCHS/ WHO reference data. The program is in the public domain; information is available at

http://www.cdc.gov/epiinfo/

The U.S. NCHS data, on which the NCHS/ WHO percentile curves are based, are mainly derived from large, nationally representative probability samples. The data consist of accurate measurements made on children from birth to 18 y and are mainly cross-sectional: they are not suitable for the monitoring of individuals during puberty.

The NCHS data are derived from several sources. The values for weight, length, and weight-for-length from birth to 36 mo are taken from longitudinal data collected by the Fels Research Institute, Yellow Springs, Ohio, between 1960 and 1975. The measurements were conducted on 720 Caucasian, predominantly middle-class, infants and children at 3-mo intervals. Nude body weight and recumbent length without shoes were recorded. The majority of the infants were fed proprietary formula-based products (DuRant and Linder, 1981).

Age (mo)	Percentiles							Standard deviations (SD)						
	3rd	10th	20th	50th	80th	90th	97th	-3 SD	-2 SD	-1 SD	Med.	+1 SD	+2 SD	+3 SD
0	2.5	2.7	2.9	3.3	3.7	3.9	4.2	2.0	2.4	2.9	3.3	3.8	4.3	4.8
6	6.0	6.6	7.0	7.8	8.7	9.1	9.7	4.9	5.9	6.9	7.8	8.8	9.8	10.8
12	8.2	8.8	9.3	10.2	11.1	11.6	12.2	7.1	8.1	9.1	10.2	11.3	12.4	13.5
18	9.3	10.0	10.5	11.5	12.5	13.0	13.8	7.9	9.1	10.3	11.5	12.7	13.9	15.2
24	10.1	10.9	11.5	12.6	13.7	14.2	15.0	8.6	9.9	11.3	12.6	13.9	15.2	16.5
30	10.9	11.8	12.4	13.7	14.8	15.4	16.2	9.3	10.8	12.2	13.7	15.0	16.4	17.7
36	11.8	12.7	13.4	14.7	15.9	16.6	17.5	10.0	11.6	13.1	14.7	16.2	17.7	19.1

Table 12.2: Weight (kg) by age of boys from birth to 36 mo. Abstracted with permission from a more complete table of data in WHO (1983).

The data for children aged 2–18 y were compiled by NCHS from three sources: values collected during the Health Examination Survey (HES) Cycle I (1963–1965) for ages 6–11 y; HES Cycle II (1966–1970) for ages 12–17 y; and the first National Health and Nutrition Examination Survey (NHANES I) (1971–1974) for ages 2–17 y.

Because the NCHS/WHO percentiles are recalculated from the U.S. NCHS reference growth data for children, they have the same limitations as detailed later in Section 12.4.4. During early childhood, one of the most severe limitations is the length-height disjuncture at 24 mo which makes it difficult to track the growth of individual children or populations throughout the first 5 y of life. As well, in population studies in low-income countries, weight-for-height cannot be calculated for children less than approximately 2 mo of age (minimum height 49 cm) or above approximately 9 y for girls and 11 y for boys (Gorstein et al., 1994) because of the minimum and maximum height limitations. Because of the marked differences in the age of onset of puberty among populations, authors of the WHO (1983) tables do not recommend using these growth reference data for comparing the nutritional status of groups of children >10 y.

12.4.2 WHO multicenter growth reference data for infants and children

A new anthropometric growth reference is being compiled by WHO for young children from birth to 5 y, as a result of concerns about the limitations of the current NCHS/WHO growth reference (Section 12.5). WHO anticipates that this new growth reference will become available in 2005. The new reference will be especially useful for monitoring growth of children during the first 5 y of life, as discussed earlier. The technical and biological limitations with the earlier NCHS/WHO growth reference are of particular concern when the growth charts are interpreted as generating a "standard," which represents how young children should grow, rather than as a "reference," describing how children do grow. Such a practice has had negative implications, especially when the NCHS/WHO curves have been used to assess the growth patterns of healthy breastfed infants. For example, a sustained Z-score of 0 during the entire 12-mo period is to be expected for breastfed infants when their growth pattern is compared to that of an ideal reference. Instead, in practice, when compared to the NCHS/WHO reference, breastfed infants typically gain more weight than expected between birth and 6–7 mo, but less weight from 7–12 mo of age, as shown in Figure 12.5 (Garza and de Onis, 1999). Observed negative deviations in growth patterns of healthy breastfed infants relative to those reflected in the NCHS/WHO reference, may lead to the premature introduction of complementary feeding (Dewey, 1998).

As a result of these concerns, WHO initiated a multicenter growth reference study for children aged up to 5 y involving more than seven diverse geographic sites. The study combined a longitudinal design from birth to 24 mo with a cross-sectional study of children aged 18–71 mo from the same site (de Onis et al., 2004).

WHO adopted a prescriptive approach for the development of this new international growth reference for young children, unlike the descriptive approach used for the revised 2000 CDC growth charts. Hence, the result will be growth charts that approximate a standard (Garza and de Onis, 1999). In order to achieve this goal, a set of individual eligibility criteria were developed. These included term singleton infants with non-smoking mothers, a health status that did not constrain growth, and mothers who were willing to follow current WHO feeding recommendations (de Onis et al., 2004).

To assess the compliance with the WHO feeding recommendations, a detailed assessment of feeding practices was completed for each home visit. Further, the mothers received breastfeeding support to comply with the WHO feeding recommendations. Infants of mothers who were not complying to WHO feeding recommendations were excluded. Additional exclusion criteria were serious illness, voluntary exclusion and children becoming more than 2 y old.

In the longitudinal study, growth measurements (weight, length, and head circumference) were taken on each cohort at birth, and at 2, 4, 6, and 8 wk, and then monthly until

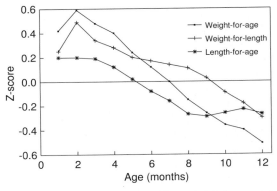

Figure 12.5: Mean Z-scores of breastfed infants aged 1–12 months (n = 226) relative to the NCHS/WHO reference (horizontal line at Z-Score of 0.0). Data from Garza and de Onis, American Journal of Clinical Nutrition 70: 169S–172S, 1999 © Am J Clin Nutr. American Society for Clinical Nutrition.

their first birthday, after which they were measured bimonthly until 2 y of age. Body composition measurements (arm circumference, and triceps and subscapular skinfolds) were also taken with the growth measurements.

For the cross-sectional study, children aged 18–71 mo were categorized into 3-mo groupings. Eligibility criteria were the same as those used for the longitudinal study, with the exception that compliance to the current WHO feeding recommendations was not an inclusion criteria. Nevertheless, information on past and current feeding practices was also obtained. For each age group (18 in total), 70 children were required, resulting in a total of 1260 children per center. To allow for refusals, 1400 children per center were recruited. Measurements included weight, standing height, head and arm circumferences, and triceps and subscapular skinfolds. Children aged 18–30 mo also had their supine length measured to obtain a precise estimate of the length/height disjunction.

12.4.3 European growth reference data

In 1988, the European Union started a multi-center, longitudinal Euro-Growth study to record the growth of contemporary European children presumed to be fed according to prevailing feeding recommendations. A longitudinal study design was selected in part to investigate associations between growth and diet and lifestyle. Healthy term infants with gestational ages between 37 and 44 wk without signs of intrauterine growth retardation and who did not meet the other exclusion criteria were enrolled before 30 days of age (van't Hof and Haschke, 2000a). In total, the cohort consisted of 2245 subjects (1154 boys and 1091 girls) from 22 study centers in 12 European countries.

Measurements were recorded using standardized methodology at monthly intervals from birth to 6 mo, and then at 3-mo intervals until 12 mo, after which measurements were taken at 18, 24, 30, and 36 mo. Details of the reported parental weight and height, education level, socioeconomic and demographic status, and characteristics of the infants at enrollment were also recorded. Ten sites also performed measurements of standing height ($n = 2423$), as well as recumbent length.

From the data, sex- and age-specific percentile curves (3rd, 5th, 10th, 25th, 50th, 75th, 95th, and 97th) were constructed as tables (for raw percentiles) and charts (for smoothed percentiles) for recumbent length, weight, mid-upper arm, thigh, and calf circumferences (Haschke and van't Hof, 2000a). The methods of Wright and Royston (1997) were used. A standing height reference was not constructed.

Influences of parental height, size at birth, birth order, breastfeeding, and time of introduction of solids on subsequent Z-scores for length and weight were also investigated (Haschke and van't Hof, 2000b). In addition, comparisons were made between these new Euro-Growth references for length and weight, and both the NCHS/WHO reference and the WHO interim reference for breastfed infants (WHO, 1994).

12.4.4 U.S. CDC 2000 growth reference data

The 1977 NCHS growth charts have now been revised by the CDC following concerns about the Fels data set. The concerns were:

- The 1977 NCHS growth reference was made from two unrelated sets of curves. Data for children < 3 y were derived from a small select sample ($n = 720$) from Ohio (Fels Research Institute) with restricted genetic, geographic, and socioeconomic backgrounds, whereas the NCHS charts for children and young adults 2–20 y were derived from nationally representative data.
- For the FELS data, recumbent length was measured, but for the NCHS subjects, information on standing height was collected from children aged 2–18 y. For any child, the length measurement is always greater than the height measurement. This has resulted in a length-height disjunction at 24 mo, as noted earlier, that has made it

difficult to track the growth of individual children or of populations throughout the first 5 y of life. This effect is highlighted in Figure 12.6.

- Observations for the Fels growth curves were only recorded at 3-mo intervals from 3 to 12 mo of age. Reference data are needed at 1-mo intervals during infancy.
- Fels data were collected from 1929 to 1975. Distributions of current birth weights are not comparable to earlier birth weights;
- Accuracy of the recumbent length measurements in the Fels data has been questioned.
- Infants in the Fels data set were predominantly formula-fed. Hence their size and growth patterns do not represent growth patterns of combined breast- and formula-fed infants.
- Ability to assess size and growth at extremes beyond the 5th and 95th percentiles is limited.
- No reference data on weight-for-stature for adolescents is available.
- No reference data beyond 17 y is available.
- Curve-fitting procedures used to smooth the data are outdated.

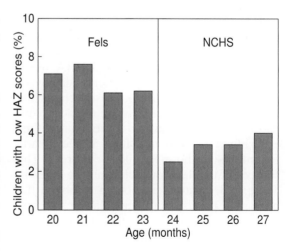

Figure 12.6: Change in the prevalence of low height-for-age for low-income U.S. children, illustrating the effect of the 24-mo disjunction resulting from using the Fels length-based curves for children younger than 2 y of age and the NCHS height-based curves for older children. Data from de Onis and Habicht, American Journal of Clinical Nutrition 64: 650–658, 1996 © Am J Clin Nutr. American Society for Clinical Nutrition.

Chart	Age or height range	Primary data sources[a]	Supplemental data sources
Weight-for-age	Birth to 36 mo	National Surveys 3–5[b]	National birth certificate data from United States Vital Statistics[b]
Length-for-age	Birth to 36 mo	National Surveys 3–5[b,c]	Birth certificate data from Wisconsin and Missouri State Vital Statistics[b,d] CDC Pediatric Nutrition Surveillance System data for birth to 5 mo
Head circum- ference-for-age	Birth to 36 mo	National Surveys 3–5[b]	Fels Longitudinal Study data[b]
Weight-for-length	45–103 cm	National Surveys 3–5[b,e]	Birth certificate data from Wisconsin and Missouri State Vital Statistics[b]
Weight-for-stature	77–121 cm	National Surveys 3–5[e]	None
Weight-for-age	24–240 mo	National Surveys 1–5[e]	None
Stature-for-age	24–240 mo	National Surveys 1–5	None
BMI-for-age	24–240 mo	National Surveys 1–5[e]	None

Table 12.3: U.S. growth charts and data sources. [a]Primary data sources National Survey 1 = NHES II, Survey 2 = NHES III, Survey 3 = NHANES I, Survey 4 = NHANES II, Survey 5 = NHANES III. [b]Excludes birth weight ⩽ 1500 g. [c]Excludes data from NHANES III for ages < 3.5 mo. [d]Wisconsin and Missouri were the only states with available data from birth certificates. [e]Excludes data from NHANES III for ages > 72 mo. From Kuczmarski et al. (2000a).

The revised CDC 2000 growth charts have been compiled by the NCHS through the CDC, in collaboration with the Division of Nutrition and Physical Activity at the National Center for Chronic Disease Prevention and Health Promotion (Kuczmarski et al., 2000a). The revised growth charts are based primarily on physical measurements taken during HES Cycle II and III and NHANES I, II, III, although some supplemental data were also used. Hence, in the revised charts the Fels longitudinal data set were replaced with nationally representative survey data, thus ensuring a smooth transition in the charts for infants to those for older children. The sources of the data for each chart are given in Table 12.3. Data were pooled to obtain the necessary precision for calculating the percentile distributions. For the growth charts, age was truncated to the nearest full month. For example 1.0–1.9 mo was truncated to 1 mo, 11.0–11.9 mo to 11 mo; and so on.

When creating the revised growth charts, two data sets were excluded: growth data for VLBW infants (< 1500 g), whose growth differs from that of normal birth-weight infants, and weight data for children > 6 y who par-

ticipated in the NHANES III survey. The latter data were excluded from both the revised weight and BMI growth charts because the inclusion of these data shifted the upper percentile curves. The exclusion of these selected data resulted in a modified growth reference that is not a purely descriptive growth reference because it does not contain representative national data for all variables.

The newly revised reference data are presented as smoothed percentile curves for nine percentiles (3rd, 5th, 10th, 25th, 50th, 75th, 90th, 95th, and 97th) for each age group (i.e., 0–36 mo and 2–20 y). The complete set of CDC percentile curves are included in the Appendix (A12.1 – A12.6, A12.9 – A12.14). Two examples of percentile charts for weight-for-age (boys, birth to 36 mo) and stature-for-age (girls, 2–20 y) are shown here (Figures 12.7 and 12.8). The charts, tabular data points of the smoothed percentiles, and least median squares (LMS) parameters by age and sex are also available at

http://www.cdc.gov/growthcharts/

The two-stage smoothing used for the CDC 2000 charts was a modified LMS estimation

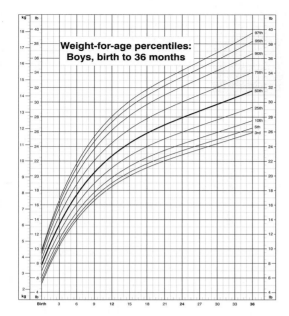

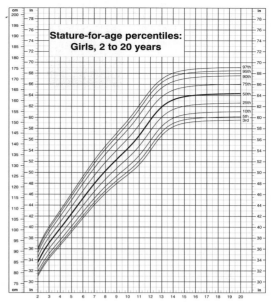

Figure 12.7: CDC 2000 growth chart. Weight-for-age percentiles: boys, birth to 36 mo. From Kuczmarski et al. (2000a).

Figure 12.8: CDC 2000 growth chart. Stature-for-age percentiles: girls, 2 to 20 y. From Kuczmarski et al. (2000a).

procedure (Cole, 1990); in the second stage, Z-scores that match the smoother percentile curves were generated. For the smoothing procedure, data were grouped by single months of age from 1 to 11 mo, and then by 3-mo intervals from 12 to 23 mo, and by 6-mo intervals from 24 mo to 19 y. Data for weight-for-length and weight-for-stature were grouped by 2-cm intervals. The 85th percentile was also included in the weight-for-stature and BMI-for-age charts. The 85th percentile for BMI has been recommended as a cutoff point to identify U.S. children and adolescents at risk for overweight (Himes and Dietz, 1994).

Table 12.4 compares the NCHS 1977 and the more recent CDC 2000 charts. Now the weight-for-stature charts have a broader range (77–121 cm for both boys and girls), and the revised charts for children and adolescents extend to age 20 y. Further, all the revised charts now include the 3rd and 97th percentiles. Comparison of the NCHS 1977 and the revised CDC 2000 growth charts reveals some discrepancies in the percentile lines, especially in the charts for infants.

1977 NCHS growth charts	CDC 2000 growth charts
Weight-for-age	
Birth to 36 mo	Birth to 36 mo
2–18 y	2–20 y
Length-for-age	
Birth to 36 mo	Birth to 36 mo
Weight-for-length	
Birth to 36 mo	Birth to 36 mo
Boys (49–103 cm)	Boys (45–103 cm)
Girls (49–101 cm)	Girls (45–103 cm)
Head circumference-for-age	
Birth to 36 mo	Birth to 36 mo
Stature-for-age	
2–18 y	2–20 y
Weight-for-stature[a]	
(Prepubescent)	
Boys (90–145 cm)	Boys (77–121 cm)
Girls (90–137 cm)	Girls (77–121 cm)
BMI-for-age	
Not available	2–20 y

Table 12.4: Comparison of U.S. NCHS 1977 and CDC 2000 growth charts. [a]The 1977 weight-for-stature charts are not applicable to any child showing the earliest signs of pubescence. The comparable CDC 2000 charts have no such restriction. From Kuczmarski et al. (2000a).

A discussion of these differences is available in Kuczmarski et al. (2000b).

In general, the revised weight-for-age and stature-for-age percentiles are quite similar to the 1977 percentiles for both boys and girls 2–14 y, the revised curves for children 14–17 y tend to be less erratic than the 1977 curves, and the revised percentiles beyond 17 y are smoother than the 1977 curves. Users can compute exact percentiles, Z-scores, and BMI values from weight and stature data using EpiInfo 2000 and the CDC 2000 reference (Section 12.4.1) (Kuczmarski et al., 2000a).

12.4.5 U.K. 1990 growth reference data

An expert working party in the United Kingdom, the Growth Reference Review Group, has recommended the use of the new UK90 cross-sectional growth reference data for both screening and surveillance of samples of U.K. children throughout childhood and adolescence (Wright et al., 2002). The new UK90 reference growth charts were first published in 1995 (Freeman et al., 1995) and then were revised in 1997 (Cole et al., 1998). Two later studies confirmed the validity of these data for monitoring the growth of infants, toddlers, and primary school children in the United Kingdom (Savage et al., 1999; Rudolf et al., 2000).

The UK90 reference data were compiled from several sources described in detail by Freeman et al. (1995) and by Prescott-Clarke and Primatesta (1996), and outlined briefly below. Only measurements of Caucasian subjects were included because the number of non-Caucasian subjects was too small to produce separate reference data for each ethnic group. Therefore, unlike the CDC 2000, the UK90 reference data are not based on a nationally representative sample. Hence, their external validity (Section 1.4.4) is questionable (Cole et al., 1998). The sources of the UK90 reference data are the following:

- Human Measurements Anthropometry and Growth (HUMAG) Research Group's chil-

dren's growth studies: 0–15.99 y for girls; 0–16.99 y for boys; data for boys > 5 y in 1978; data for girls > 5 y in 1986; data for infants 0–1.99 y in 1987; data for toddlers 2–4.99 y in 1987
- HUMAG adult anthropometric measurement: 16–64.99 y for men in 1984 and 16–69.99 y for women in 1984
- The National Study of Health and Growth (NSHG): children (mostly Caucasian) aged 4.5–11.99 y in 1990
- Tayside Growth Study: children aged 3, 5, 7, 9, 11, 14 y in 1989–1990, but only children ⩾ 4.5 y were included in the UK90 reference sample
- Department of Health Survey: statures and weights of British adults aged 16–64.99 y in 1980
- Cambridge Infant Growth Study: 252 infants followed to 2 y, in 1984–1988 (Cole et al., 2002)
- Whittington Birth Data Study: hospital-based study of 999 infants ⩾ 32 weeks gestation born in 1987–1988 (Prescott-Clarke and Primatesta, 1996)

Of these sources, all except the Tayside Growth Study, the Cambridge Infant Growth Study, and the Whittington Birth Data Study, were based on representative samples of England, Scotland, and, in most cases, Wales. The primary sources for the UK90 reference data were the HUMAG studies (British Standards Institution, 1990) augmented with data for infants.

Measurements for the UK90 reference data are based on over 25,000 Caucasian children. The measurements (length or height, and weight) were made using appropriate equipment and trained personnel. For children younger than 2 y, length rather than height was measured. Exact decimal age was calculated from the date of birth and the date of the measurement. In all cases, within- and between-observer errors were ⩽ 0.4 cm for stature and ⩽ 0.05 kg for weight.

The data were adjusted statistically, where necessary, to minimize the effects of methodological differences and any secular trend, using the nationally representative National Study of Health and Growth (NSHG) as the baseline. Data were then pooled, and the percentiles fitted using Cole's LMS method (Cole et al., 1998). Cole's technique permits standard deviation scores to be calculated directly from the data. For the published version of the U.K. 1990 reference data, nine percentiles for weight-for-age and height-for-age (but not weight-for-height) were constructed for clinical use: 0.4th, 2nd, 9th, 25th, 50th, 75th, 91st, 98th, and 99.6th; data for the conventional percentiles — 3rd, 10th, 25th, 50th, 75th, 90th, and 97th — are also available (Freeman et al., 1995).

12.4.6 Growth reference data for children with special needs

Children with developmental disorders, mental retardation, and certain genetic disorders often have growth patterns that differ from the reference growth curves. Growth charts are available for children with Down's syndrome, whose growth rate and stature tend to be reduced, derived from 4650 observations on 730 children (Cronk et al., 1988).

In addition, the U.S. Greenwood Genetic Center has developed growth charts for children with other special conditions including Marfan syndrome, achondroplasia, Noonan syndrome, sickle-cell disease, Turner syndrome, and Williams syndrome (Horton et al. 1978; Saul et al., 1988). Caution must always be used with these specialized growth charts as they are generally developed from relatively small homogeneous samples: sometimes nonstandard measurement techniques were used to collect the data. It is often useful to assess the growth of children with special needs using both specialized growth charts and the CDC 2000 or UK90 growth reference data.

12.5 Parent-allowed-for growth reference data

Several investigators have compiled parent-allowed-for growth reference data in an effort to identify nonfamilial short stature (Tanner et al., 1970; Himes et al., 1985; Cole, 2000).

These charts and tables can be used for children from 2 to 9 y. Prior to about 2 y, the height of a child is not closely correlated to parental heights, while beyond 9 y, the adolescent growth spurt complicates the interpretation of height data. These charts can only be used if the biological parents of the child have achieved their full height potential. In such cases, mid-parent height, based on the average of the two parents' height, can be used to adjust for parental size. No differences exist between the relationships of father with son and father with daughter, and mother with daughter and mother with son (Tanner, 1986). In the most recent U.K. parent-allowed-for height chart, an adjustment can also be made for either parent alone or for a sibling aged 2–9 y; this approach is especially useful in a single-parent family.

Parent-allowed-for growth reference charts provide a clinical tool to distinguish the genetic contribution of parental stature from other factors that affect stature (such as malnutrition) or growth disorders (such as growth hormone deficiency and Turner's syndrome). Two of these tools are described below: the U.S. correction factors compiled by Himes et al. (1985), and a new U.K. familial height chart developed by Cole (2000).

12.5.1 U.S. parent-allowed-for growth reference data

Parent-specific adjustments for evaluating the recumbent length and stature of children, together with clinical application and interpretation guidelines, are given in Himes et al. (1985). The method is based on parent–child relationships for 568 midparent–child pairs participating in the Fels longitudinal study and on more than 16,000 serial measurements of recumbent length or stature. Tables of the parent-specific adjustments for recumbent length of boys and girls 0–36 mo and stature 3–18 y are presented. An excerpt is provided in Table 12.5. The adjustments are rounded to the nearest whole cm, and should be added to the child's measured length or stature. When

Age	Child's length or height (cm)	Midparent stature (cm) 150	160	170	180
Birth					
	40.0–43.9	+2	+1	0	−1
	53.0–56.9	+2	+1	0	−1
6 mo					
	62.0–64.9	+3	+1	0	−2
	74.0–76.9	+4	+2	0	−1
12 mo					
	67.0–71.9	+4	+2	−1	−3
	83.0–84.9	+4	+2	0	−2
2 y					
	78.0–82.9	+5	+2	−1	−3
	93.0–96.9	+6	+3	0	−3
3 y					
	86.0–87.9	+7	+3	−1	−5
	98.0–106.9	+8	+4	0	−4
4 y					
	90.0–93.9	+7	+3	−1	−5
	104.0–112.9	+8	+4	0	−4
5 y					
	96.0–103.9	+8	+3	−1	−6
	114.0–122.9	+9	+5	0	−4

Table 12.5: Examples of adjustments to length (or height) of short and tall boys based on average parental height. The steps in calculating parent-specific adjustments for a hypothetical boy aged 12 mo are:
   Son's actual length is 71.1 cm
   Mother's stature is 153.7 cm
   Father's stature is 165.7 cm
   Midparent stature is $(153.7 + 165.7) \div 2 = 159.7$
   Adjustment is +2 cm
   Son's adjusted length is $71.1 + 2.0 = 73.1$ cm
From Himes et al., Pediatrics 75: 304–313, 1985, © with permission.

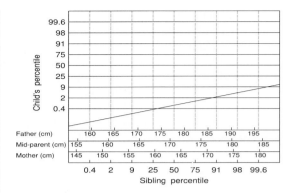

Figure 12.9: A family height chart to adjust for midparent, single parent, or sibling height. The index child and sibling are plotted at height percentiles obtained from a reference chart. Alternatively, the child's percentile is plotted relative to the absolute height of either or both parents. From Cole, Archives of Disease in Childhood 82, 173–176, 2000, with permission of the BMJ Publishing Group.

midparent height is at or close to the norm, the adjustments are zero, but they become larger with increasing disparity between midparent height and the mean.

12.5.2 U.K. familial height chart

Cole (2000) has constructed a novel parent-allowed-for height chart that adjusts for maternal, paternal, midparental, or sibling height based on the UK90 height reference (Section 12.5.1). This chart is shown in Figure 12.9 and is designed specifically for screening and the identification of children suffering from growth failure.

To use the familial height chart, the height percentile of the index child is obtained from the revised UK90 reference growth charts

(Cole et al., 1998). If the child's height falls below the 9th percentile, then more information about the height of the family should be sought. This may include measurement of the height of the child's biological mother or father or of a sibling.

To adjust for sibling height, the height percentile of the index child is plotted against the height percentile of the sibling. To adjust for the height of father or mother alone, the child's percentile is plotted against the height (in cm) of the corresponding parent. When midparent height is used for the adjustment, then the average of the height of the two parents is calculated before plotting the percentile of the index child against the midparent height using the midparent scale.

If the plot for the index child falls below the conditional sloping familially adjusted 0.4th percentile line shown in Figure 12.9, or below the unconditional horizontal 0.4th percentile line, then the child should be referred for follow-up.

12.6 Tempo-conditional growth charts

Misleading assessments for individual adolescent children may result from the use of cross-sectional distance growth data, because of distortions introduced by the adolescent growth spurt. This can occur in children at markedly different ages. This is termed the "phase-difference" effect. For example, some children start their growth spurt at age 10 y or even earlier, whereas for others the onset of the growth spurt may be delayed until age 12 y, or even later. An additional complication is that the timing of the peak weight and peak height velocities do not exactly coincide (Roberts and Dallal, 2001).

To overcome the differences in the timing of the adolescent growth spurt, distance growth charts based on mixed cross-sectional and longitudinal data have been compiled by Tanner and co-workers for both the United States (Tanner and Davies, 1985) and the United Kingdom (Tanner and Buckler, 1997). By using longitudinal growth data at adolescence to define the shape of the curves, and cross-sectional data to obtain the absolute values for the beginning and end of the curves, distance reference data applicable to individual children during adolescence have been constructed. These reference data take into account the phase-difference effect and, therefore, are suitable for the diagnosis and monitoring of *individual* children in clinical settings (Tanner and Whitehouse, 1976). They are termed "tempo-conditional" charts.

12.6.1 U.S. tempo-conditional growth charts

Tanner and Davies (1985) have produced longitudinally based height distance charts for North American male and female children. These tempo-conditional charts, unlike the cross-sectional CDC 2000 reference data, are the appropriate tool for monitoring an individual U.S. child's progress throughout the growth period, including puberty. The prepubertal and adult percentiles for height attained were taken from the earlier NCHS data described in Section 12.3.1, whereas the shape of the curves was taken from a review of longitudinal studies. Selected percentiles (5th, 50th, and 95th) for early and late maturers are also displayed on these growth charts. De-

tails of their method of construction are given in Tanner and Davies (1985). Age standards for puberty stages are also presented.

12.6.2 U.K. tempo-conditional growth charts

The distance growth charts compiled originally by Tanner and co-workers in 1965 were revised in 1976 to emphasize the longitudinal-type percentiles appropriate for individuals, and to deemphasize the curves based on the cross-sectional data (Figure 12.4). The resulting tempo-conditional growth charts allow for whether any given child is an early or a late maturer. In addition, the limits for the ages at which successive stages of pubertal sexual development occur in a normal population were added. These revised tempo-conditional growth charts were known as the "Tanner-Whitehouse 1976 Clinical Standards" (Tanner and Whitehouse, 1976).

These 1976 revised growth charts have now been superseded by a second revision carried out in 1996 by Tanner and Buckler (1997). The most recent revision takes into account the secular trend since the 1960s, and clearly portrays percentiles for both early and late maturers, as well as those who mature at the average time. This has been achieved by including height and weight data for prepubertal and young adults from the recent UK90 growth reference (Freeman et al., 1995), as well as data from a longitudinal study of 198 adolescents that was carried out in Sheffield by Buckler in the 1980s (Buckler, 1990). The range of ages of pubertal events that was used in the 1976 growth chart has also been updated using the recent data of Buckler (1990). The selected percentiles (10th, 50th, and 90th) for early- and late-maturers are clearly displayed on these growth charts. Hence, when assessing the height of any given child, both age and tempo can be jointly taken into account. However, the limitations of the small, non-representative longitudinal data used for these up-dated charts have been emphasized by Cameron (2002).

Figure 12.10, abstracted from the charts of Tanner and Buckler (1997), shows the 50th

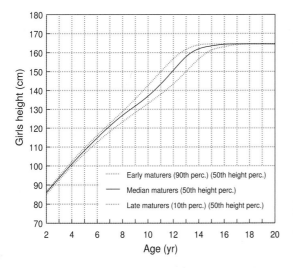

Figure 12.10: Diagrammatic height percentile chart for early-, median-, and late-maturing girls. Adapted from Tanner and Buckler (1997).

height percentiles for girls for early, median, and late maturers. Only the average child, whose growth spurt occurs at the median time, will actually follow the 50th percentile (solid line in Figure 12.10). Children of average height but maturing early will rise above the growth line for median-maturing girls, but later rejoin it. Conversely, late-maturing girls fall below the 50th percentile and later rejoin it. Note that an early-maturing girl — defined as on the 90th developmental percentile — but of median height attains a height of 150 cm at 11 y. This is approximately 2 y earlier than a late-maturing girl of median height on the 10th developmental percentile. The large delay shows the importance of taking into account the phase difference effects when monitoring the growth of individual children during adolescence (Cameron, 2002). Printed versions for clinical use of these revised U.K. growth charts are available from Castlemead Publications, Welwyn Garden City, UK.

12.7 Growth velocity reference data

Growth velocity curves come from longitudinal studies, during which the same child is measured regularly and the growth rate

is calculated for each interval. The curves provide information on the varying rate of growth with age; this rate of growth is generally termed the "growth velocity."

Velocity curves can be used to establish the timing of the adolescent growth spurt, to detect abnormal changes in growth, and to evaluate individuals (rather than populations) in terms of changes in rates of growth and response to therapy. Recent changes in the rates of growth can be identified very much earlier using velocity growth charts rather than attained distance growth charts, because the latter reflect the past history of the child, including the effect of parental size (Tanner, 1976).

Unlike distance curves, a child's percentile placement on the velocity growth curve may change markedly during growth, particularly during adolescence. This arises because velocity growth curves are much more sensitive than distance curves. For example, the range from the 25th to the 75th percentile for stature on the CDC 2000 distance growth charts for 10-y-old boys is approximately 10 cm, compared to an increment range of only 1.5 cm on the velocity growth charts (Roche and Himes, 1980).

A high degree of precision is required for measurements in velocity studies because two measurement errors are included whenever growth increments are calculated. As a result, measurement techniques should be standardized and preferably conducted by the same anthropometrist throughout the study.

During infancy, length increments should be assessed at 1-mo intervals for the first 6 mo and at 2-mo intervals from 6 to 12 mo. Increments measured over 6 mo are the minimum interval that can be used to provide reliable data during adolescence (WHO, 1995). For shorter intervals, the combined errors of two repeated measurements may be too large in relation to the expected mean increments (Marshall, 1971). Seasonal variation in growth may occur. Height velocity, for example, may be faster in the spring than in the fall and winter (Marshall, 1971; Marshall and Swan, 1971).

The following simple formula is used to

calculate velocity:

$$\text{velocity} = (x_2 - x_1)/(t_2 - t_1)$$

where x_2 and x_1 are values of the measurement on two occasions t_2 and t_1. Height velocity is normally expressed as cm/y.

Growth increments during infancy should always be evaluated in relation to gestational age, body size, and weight-for-length at birth; premature and small-for-gestational-age infants tend to have larger increments than term infants. Incremental growth during pubescence should preferably be interpreted in relation to data on maturity levels (e.g., skeletal age, onset of menarche) and the timing of the pubescent growth spurt (WHO, 1995). WHO recommends use of at least two maturational events for each child to assist in the interpretation of anthropometric data during pubescence: for each sex, one marker signals the beginning of the adolescent growth spurt, and another indicates that the peak height velocity and associated changes have passed. The positions of the suggested markers are shown in Figure 12.11; details of the maturational events are also given in the caption.

Currently, no uniform criteria exist for defining growth faltering based on growth velocity data, although in practice, no growth in two consecutive periods is sometimes used (WHO, 1995). Unfortunately, the only available velocity growth charts at the present time are based on small nonrepresentative samples of children measured many years ago; they are discussed below.

12.7.1 U.S. growth velocity reference data

The Fels Research Institute has constructed curves from the longitudinal data recorded between 1929 and 1978 from 818 Caucasian U.S. children. Measurements were recorded on approximately 200 children of each sex, at each increment, using standardized anthropometric techniques six times in the first year (birth and 1, 3, 6, 9, and 12 mo) and then every 6 mo to 18 y. Adjustments were made to the serial data for each child to remove errors

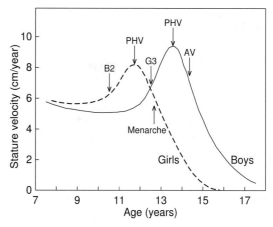

Figure 12.11: Approximate timing of recommended maturational events relative to peak height velocity (PHV) in boys and girls.

B2 = Start of breast development. Identified by examination. Precedes PHV by about 1 y. Indicates adolescent spurt has begun.

Menarche. Determined by questioning. Menstruation usually begins a little more than 1 y after PHV. Indicates that most of the adolescent spurt has been completed.

G3 = Adolescent changes in the penis, characterizing G3. Identified by examination. Precedes PHV by about 1 y. Indicates adolescent spurt has begun.

AV = Attainment of adult voice. Determined by questioning. Usually attained about 1 y after PHV. Indicates that most of the adolescent spurt has been completed. From WHO (1995).

associated with differences in the chronological ages at which examinations were made. No secular or seasonal effects were observed in the data. The charts are similar to those obtained from a representative sample of the U.S. population (Roche and Himes, 1980).

Sex-specific increments were calculated during 6-mo intervals for weight, recumbent length, and head circumference from birth to 3 y, for weight from 2 to 18 y, and for stature from 30 mo to 18 y. Seven percentiles — 3rd, 10th, 25th, 50th, 75th, 90th, and 97th — are presented for each age interval, except below 3.5 years for stature, both graphically (Roche and Himes, 1980) and as reference data tables (Baumgartner et al., 1986). The small sample of young children made it impossible to calculate the extreme percentiles accurately. The percentiles for both stature and weight, but not head circumference and length, are smoothed.

To use the growth velocity charts, the observed increments must be plotted vertically above the age at the *end* of the increment. By using the reference data tables, measurements can be interpreted more precisely, enabling more subtle changes in growth to be detected.

The U.S. infants studied by the Fels Institute tended to have more rapid rates of growth in weight, recumbent length, and head circumference but more rapid decelerations in growth rate over the first 1–2 y, compared with the British infants. Furthermore, the U.S. children had earlier and more pronounced pubescent growth spurts in both stature and weight than the British children had (Baumgartner et al., 1986).

Tanner and Davies (1985) have constructed longitudinal reference data for height velocity for North American children, in which percentiles are given for early-, middle-, and late-maturing children. Fig 12.12 presents a simplified view of these height velocity reference percentiles for boys. Detailed charts for both boys and girls are given in Tanner and Davies (1985). Printed versions for clinical use are available from Castlemead Publications, Welwyn Garden City, UK.

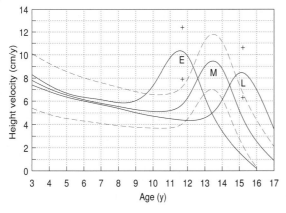

Figure 12.12: Diagrammatic height velocity percentiles for U.S. boys. The 50th percentiles for early- (E), median- (M), and late-maturing (L) boys are shown as solid lines, along with the 3rd and 97th percentiles for the median maturing boys (dashed lines). In addition the positions of the 3rd and 97th percentiles of the peak height velocity for both early- and late-maturing boys are also shown (+). From Tanner and Whitehouse (1976).

12.7.2 U.K. growth velocity reference data

The United Kingdom growth velocity reference data from birth to 11–12 y were compiled from a random sample of about 80 male and 80 female infants born between 1952 and 1954 in central London and followed longitudinally at the Child Study Centre in London. Measurements were made at 3-mo intervals up to age 5.5 y and then annually thereafter. During adolescence, data were based on the 3-mo measurements of 49 boys and 41 girls participating in the Harpenden Growth study and followed throughout the whole of adolescence.

The data are presented as percentile curves for the velocity of growth in both height and weight from birth to maturity (i.e., 0–18 y), centered about the year of maximum or peak height velocity. Data relate to increments calculated over the period of a whole year to eliminate seasonal differences in growth of children (Tanner, 1962). The velocity curves present "individual-type" reference data during adolescence. The latter take into account the phase differences that occur among individuals as a result of variation in the time of onset of the adolescent growth spurt (Figure 12.13). Individual height velocity curves from 10 to 18 y for five boys from the Harpenden Growth Study are shown, each with their peak height velocity at a different age. The dashed line depicts the mean curve, obtained by averaging their values at each age. Such an approach clearly smooths out the adolescent growth spurt (Tanner, 1986). The lower figure shows the same curves plotted according to their peak height velocity, a procedure often referred to as "normalization" for the time of the adolescent growth spurt.

This U.K. Growth velocity reference data has the age scale calibrated in tenths of a year rather than months. Height and weight velocity curves for both boys and girls are available (Tanner and Whitehouse, 1976). Printed versions for clinical use are available from Castlemead Publications, Welwyn Garden City, UK.

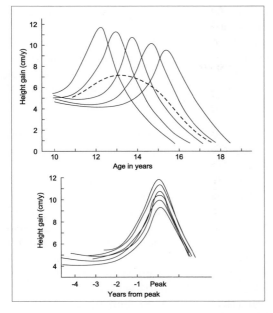

Figure 12.13: The relation between individual and mean velocities during the adolescent spurt. Top: The individual height velocity curves of five boys from the Harpenden Growth Study (solid lines) with the mean curve (dashed) constructed by averaging their values at each age. Bottom: the same curves all plotted according to their peak height velocity. From Tanner et al., *Archives of Disease in Childhood* 41: 454–471, 613–625, 1966, with permission of the authors and of the BMJ publishing group.

12.8 Adult height and weight reference data

Height and weight in adult years have been studied less intensively than during childhood. The interpretation of apparent age-related changes in such data may be confounded by the existence of secular trends in body size over successive generations.

Reference data for height for adults may be used to estimate the degree of stunting during maturation. WHO (1995) indicates that, in the absence of appropriate local reference data, the NCHS/WHO values for height at 18 y should be used for persons aged 18–24 y to be consistent with the reference values recommended for use for children older than 5 y and adolescents (WHO, 1995).

Among adults, weight data are now expressed as weight relative to height. The weight/height ratio of choice for defining both underweight and obesity is the BMI (see Section 10.3). The adult reference data available provide a descriptive reference base for observed weights and do not indicate "desirable" weight (Abraham et al., 1979).

12.8.1 U.S. adult height and weight reference data

Height and weight data for U.S. adults who participated in NHANES III are available. Measurements were taken on 13,645 civilian noninstitutionalized adults from a national probability sample selected for NHANES III (1988–1994) (Kuczmarski et al., 2000a).

Height and weight tables are given in the Appendix (A12.17 to A12.20) for men and women, with mean height values (in cm and kg) for the following age groups: 20–29, 30–39, 40–49, 50–59, 60–69, 70–79, and 80+ y. In addition, the number of persons examined, standard error of the mean, and selected percentiles (5th, 10th, 15th, 25th, 50th, 75th, 85th, 90th, and 95th) for each sex and age group by ethnicity or race are presented. Three ethnic groups are included: Caucasian, African American, and Mexican American. These data are also available on the CDC-NCHS Web site under "Survey Results and Products." The corresponding height and weight tables in inches and pounds are also available.

Kuczmarski et al. (2000b) compiled tables of selected anthropometric reference data for older Americans from the NHANES III data (1988–1994) (Table 12.6). Measurements were from a total of 5700 persons aged ⩾ 60 y and 1861 persons aged 50–59 y. Equal numbers of elderly Caucasian, African American, and Mexican American subjects were sampled. There was no upper age limit, and the oldest group was oversampled (Burt and Harris, 1994).

Data for this sample of older Americans include means and selected percentiles (15th, 50th, 85th) for body weight (and BMI, triceps skinfold, arm muscle circumference) by sex, race or ethnicity, and four age categories (50–59, 60–69, 70–79, 80+ y). Table 12.6 presents the 15th, 50th, and 85th percentiles

Height (in)	n	Weight percentile (lb)		
		15th	50th	85th
Males				
< 65	541	124.5	151.7	174.2
65	283	134.5	157.0	186.2
66	380	142.0	165.5	195.3
67	352	141.9	170.9	194.7
68	377	149.4	176.2	210.6
69	282	154.2	187.4	215.8
70	249	160.7	184.8	223.0
71	235	165.8	200.1	232.6
⩾ 72	150	166.7	199.7	236.5
Females				
< 60	672	101.0	126.1	158.9
60	382	110.2	134.7	169.1
61	451	116.2	140.7	172.6
62	427	117.1	141.6	184.3
63	314	121.4	152.0	186.1
64	272	129.6	156.0	191.7
65	206	130.8	157.5	200.1
66	92	131.0	160.9	198.4
⩾ 67	103	142.5	168.1	206.4

Table 12.6: Weight by height for male and female subjects 60–89 y examined in NHANES III (1988–1994). Data from Kuczmarski et al. (2000b).

for body weight (lb) by height (in) for men and women aged 60 to 89 y. In general, mean body weight was lowest for persons aged 80 y and older, and lower for older Mexican American men and women at each decade than for their African American counterparts.

12.8.2 U.K. adult height and weight reference data

A survey of the heights and weights of a representative sample of the adult population of Great Britain, aged 16 – 64 y, was conducted in 1980. Measurements were conducted in the subjects' homes using standardized methods (Knight, 1984; Rosenbaum et al., 1985). The final sample of 10,021 adults was based on a multistage design with minor biases for age and region. These biases were corrected later by poststratifying the sample at the data-processing stage. No nonresponse bias with respect to height existed, but some underrepresentation of overweight adults may have occurred.

Tables of the mean (± SEM), and median,

for height (cm) and weight (kg) for 10 groups of 4-y age intervals (16–19, 20–24, 25–29, 30–34, 35–39, 40–44, 45–49, 50–54, 55–59, 60–64) for males and females separately are available, together with the number of subjects. These data are also presented by social class, region, and height of parents (for height only). The average height was greatest in age groups 20–24 y for males and 30–34 y for females. For all age groups, height tended to be related to social class.

The distribution for the mean (± SEM) and median weights by sex, in 0.5-kg increments (range ⩽ 45 kg to > 100 kg) for the 10 groups, by social class and region, are also given. Tables of the percentage distribution of weight at each height for all ages, and for five groups of age intervals (16–19, 20–29, 30–39, 40–49, 50–64 years) are also available (Knight, 1984; Rosenbaum et al., 1985). The average weight was greatest in age group 45 – 49 y for males, after which it decreased. For females, the average weight was greatest in age group 55 – 59 y; no decrease with age occurred.

Anthropometric results, including height, weight, and BMI, are also available for 2323 subjects studied in 1986 and 1987 during the Dietary and Nutritional Survey of British Adults (Gregory et al., 1990). These workers noted that the proportion of men classified as overweight or obese increased by about 15% during the 6 y following the 1980 survey, thereby emphasizing the importance of taking into account secular changes when interpreting adult anthropometric measurements.

12.9 Body mass index reference data

Body mass index (wt/ht^2) in adults is a reliable and valid indicator of obesity at the population level (Section 10.3); it correlates with percentage of body fat and is relatively unbiased by height. BMI is used in population studies of adults because measurements of weight and height are easy, quick, relatively noninvasive, and are more precise than skinfold thickness measurements. As an example, BMI tables for men and women, derived from NHANES III, are given in the Appendix (A12.21 and A12.22) for the following age groups: 20–29, 30–39, 40–49, 50–59, 60–69, 70–79 y, and 80+ years. Three ethnic groups are included: Caucasian, African American, and Mexican American.

Appendix A12.21 and A12.22, show that BMI changes very slowly with age in adults, so age-independent cutoffs are used to grade obesity; there is no need for adult reference data for BMI. Details are given in Section 10.3. Separate cutoffs are used to denote underweight in adults (Section 10.3.5).

Use of BMI as an indicator of overweight and obesity in childhood and adolescence is more recent. Unlike adults, in children BMI changes substantially with age, so reference data based on age (and sex) are needed. National BMI-for-age charts and tables are available in several countries, including children in the United Kingdom (Cole et al., 1995), Sweden (Lindgren et al., 1995), Italy (Luciano et al., 1997), Australia (McLennan and Podger, 1998), and the United States (Kuczmarski et al., 2000a). In most of these charts, the BMI distribution was adjusted for skewness using the method of Cole (1990).

WHO (2000) favors an approach proposed by the European Childhood Obesity Group (Poskitt, 1995) to indicate overweight and obesity in childhood and adolescence. This involves the use of internationally derived age-specific BMI percentile cutoffs for children and adolescents that are equivalent to the WHO BMI definitions for adults of overweight (BMI $\geqslant 25$) and obesity (BMI $\geqslant 30$) (Section 12.9.3).

12.9.1 U.S. BMI reference data for children

The CDC 2000 growth charts now include BMI-for-age percentiles for children 2–20 y. As noted in Section 12.4.4, the NHANES III data on weight for U.S children $\geqslant 6$ y were excluded, so that the BMI growth charts are no longer a "true" reference. This strategy was adopted because of the marked increases in weight of children in NHANES III compared with earlier surveys. As a result, underdiag-

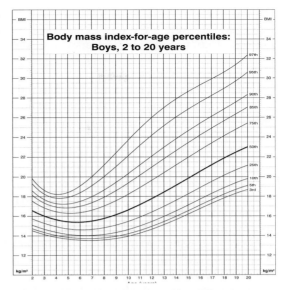

Figure 12.14: CDC growth chart. Body mass index-for-age percentiles: boys, 2 to 20 y. From Kuczmarski et al. (2000a).

nosis of overweight and obesity in children was avoided (Kuczmarski et al., 2000a).

Sex-specific smoothed percentile curves (97th, 95th, 90th, 85th, 75th, 50th, 25th, 10th, 5th, 3rd) have been constructed using the LMS procedure (Cole, 1990); the BMI-for-age percentile chart for boys 2–20 y is shown in Figure 12.14. Larger versions of the percentile chart for both boys and girls are included in the Appendix (A12.15 and A12.16). The 85th percentile was included on the CDC 2000 BMI charts because it is the recommended cutoff for identifying children and adolescents at risk for overweight (Himes and Dietz, 1994). Hence, these BMI-for-age percentiles may be used to identify children and adolescents at the upper end of the distribution who are either at risk for overweight ($\geqslant 85$th and < 95th percentile) or overweight ($\geqslant 95$th percentile) (Himes and Dietz, 1994; Barlow and Dietz, 1998).

12.9.2 U.K. BMI reference data for children

Body mass index reference curves for children from birth to 23 y have been compiled for the U.K. by Cole et al. (1995) and are based on the same large representative sample (i.e., 15,636 boys; 14,899 girls) and the same data as those used for the new UK90 height and weight reference percentile curves (Section 12.4.5). Exact decimal age was calculated from the dates of birth and measurement. Nine percentiles were constructed for clinical use (0.4th, 2nd, 9th, 25th, 50th, 75th, 91st, 98th, 99.6th) using Cole's LMS method and penalized likelihood. The latter permits the calculation of the SD score from BMI, using the equation given in Cole et al. (1995).

The BMI percentile chart for U.K. boys is shown in Figure 12.15. The percentiles are very skewed, with the top percentile channel being over four times as wide as the bottom percentile channel at all ages. The age-related changes observed in median BMI (i.e., 50th percentile) in Figure 12.15 for males are also apparent for females. In contrast, the age of the adiposity rebound — that is, the dip in the BMI — differs between males and females: in boys, it occurs later on the lower than the higher percentiles, by over 3 y, compared with 2 y in girls. After the rebound, the increase in BMI is more rapid in girls than in boys until aged 21.0 y, after which the curves

cross. At this time, the BMI for boys is higher than that for girls. BMI curves are less affected by the timing of the pubertal growth spurt than are height and weight charts.

At the present time, the U.K. BMI reference curves have had only limited use in clinical practice. Children who are unusually thin or fat, and in need of immediate referral, can be identified by the extra 0.4th and 99.6th percentiles shown in Figure 12.15. For infants, such a referral should be done cautiously, unless the pattern is found to persist well into the second year. In older children, care must be taken to avoid classifying the very muscular as obese.

12.9.3 International BMI cutoffs for children for obesity

In adults, the BMI cutoff of 30 kg/m^2 has become recognized internationally as the preferred definition of obesity (WHO, 2000). However, during childhood, BMI changes with age, so that cutoffs related to age are required, as noted earlier. Unfortunately, there has been little agreement on the definitions of obesity during childhood and adolescence.

The European Childhood Obesity Group (Poskitt, 1995) proposed linking the BMI definitions of overweight and obesity in adults to BMI percentiles for children. In 1998 the WHO International Obesity Task Force adopted this approach, and this led to the compilation by Cole et al. (2000) of age-specific BMI values for children equivalent to the BMI definitions of overweight (BMI $\geqslant 25$) and obesity (BMI $\geqslant 30$) in adults. This involved using BMI data from six large nationally representative cross-sectional growth studies to compile an international reference population; the data sets used are listed in Table 12.7.

In each of the six surveys there were more than 10,000 subjects with ages ranging from birth to at least 18 y. For the United States, pooled data were used from four national surveys (i.e., 1963–1980) that predated the period when the prevalence of obesity increased markedly (i.e., NHANES III: 1988–1994).

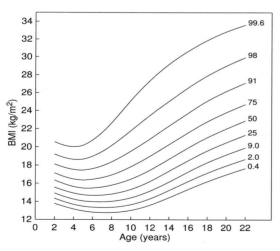

Figure 12.15: Nine percentiles for BMI in British boys, 1990. The percentiles are spaced two-thirds of an SD score apart to emphasize the asymmetric nature of the distribution at any one age. From Cole et al., Archives of Disease in Childhood 73: 25–29, 1995, with permission of the BMJ Publishing Group.

Country	Year	Description	Males Age	*n*	Females Age	*n*
Brazil	1989	Second national anthropometric survey	2–25	15,947	2–25	15,859
Great Britain	1978–93	Data pooled from the national growth surveys	0–23	16,491	0–23	15,731
Hong Kong	1993	National growth survey	0–18	11,797	0–18	12,168
Netherlands	1980	Third nationwide growth survey	0–20	21,521	0–20	20,245
Singapore	1993	School health service survey	6–19	17,356	6–20	16,616
United States	1963–80	Data pooled from four national surveys	2–20	14,764	2–20	14,232

Table 12.7: Six nationally representative datasets of BMI in childhood. From Cole et al., British Medical Journal 320(7244): 1240–1243, 2000, with permission of the BMJ Publishing Group.

For each data set, percentile curves passing through BMI values of 25 (corresponding to overweight) and 30 (corresponding to obesity) at age 18 years were calculated separately for both male and female children. Note that the prevalence of overweight (Table 12.8) and obesity (data not shown) varied greatly among the six countries. Nevertheless, the shape of the percentiles was broadly similar among the six countries, enabling them to be averaged to yield age-specific BMI cutoff points by sex from 2 to 18 y. By definition, these cutoff curves pass through "adult" BMIs of 25 and 30 at age 18 (Table 12.9).

The cutoff points are based purely on a statistical definition of overweight and obesity, and not on adverse health consequences related to obesity in children. Nevertheless, use of these standard cutoff points should allow international comparisons of the prevalence of overweight and obesity in children and adolescents. Further, such an approach ensures consistency with the cutoff points used to identify overweight and obesity in adults. Nevertheless, the validity of using the new approach for identifying cutoffs for children in combination with these new aggregated percentiles requires further confirmation. This is critical for stunted populations in low-income countries: factors other than increased body fat may be responsible for their increased weight-for-height.

Country	Percentile	Z-score	% above cutoff
Males			
Brazil	95.3	1.68	4.7
Great Britain	90.4	1.30	9.6
Hong Kong	88.3	1.19	11.7
Netherlands	94.5	1.60	5.5
Singapore	89.5	1.25	10.5
United States	81.9	0.91	18.1
Females			
Brazil	84.8	1.03	15.2
Great Britain	88.3	1.19	11.7
Hong Kong	90.2	1.29	9.8
Netherlands	93.5	1.52	6.5
Singapore	93.0	1.48	7.0
United States	83.5	0.97	16.5

Table 12.8: Percentiles and Z-scores for overweight corresponding to body mass index of 25 kg/m^2 at age 18 y in six internationally representative data sets. Data from Cole et al., British Medical Journal 320(7244): 1240–1243, 2000, with permission of the BMJ Publishing Group.

12.9.4 Other BMI reference data for children

Several other sets of BMI references exist. Of note are the smoothed BMI-for-age reference percentiles developed by Must et al. (1991). They were recommended by a U.S. Expert Committee for overweight in adolescents (Himes and Dietz, 1994) and were used prior to the publication of the updated CDC 2000 BMI reference. These BMI-for-age percentiles are based on data from NHANES I by year of age from 6 to 19 y. The data meet the criteria recommended by WHO for reference data, and the construction of the smoothed percentile curves employed an appropriate curve-fitting procedure.

BMI-for-age percentiles have also been developed for children in Sweden (Lindgren et al., 1995), Italy (Luciano et al., 1997), and New Zealand (Williams, 2000). BMI percent-

Age (y)	BMI = 25 kg/m²		BMI = 30 kg/m²	
	Males	Females	Males	Females
2.0	18.4	18.0	20.1	20.1
2.5	18.1	17.8	19.8	19.5
3.0	17.9	17.6	19.6	19.4
3.5	17.7	17.4	19.4	19.2
4.0	17.6	17.3	19.3	19.2
4.5	17.5	17.2	19.3	19.1
5.0	17.4	17.2	19.3	19.2
5.5	17.5	17.2	19.5	19.3
6.0	17.6	17.3	19.8	19.7
6.5	17.7	17.5	20.2	20.1
7.0	17.9	17.8	20.6	20.5
7.5	18.2	18.0	21.1	21.0
8.0	18.4	18.4	21.6	21.6
8.5	18.8	18.7	22.2	22.2
9.0	19.1	19.1	22.8	22.8
9.5	19.5	19.5	23.4	23.5
10.0	19.8	19.9	24.0	24.1
10.5	20.2	20.3	24.6	24.8
11.0	20.6	20.7	25.1	25.4
11.5	20.9	21.2	25.6	26.1
12.0	21.2	21.7	26.0	26.7
12.5	21.6	22.1	26.4	27.2
13.0	21.9	22.6	26.8	27.8
13.5	22.3	23.0	27.3	28.2
14.0	22.6	23.3	27.6	28.6
14.5	23.0	23.7	28.0	28.9
15.0	23.3	23.9	28.3	29.1
15.5	23.6	24.2	28.6	29.3
16.0	23.9	24.4	28.9	29.4
16.5	24.2	24.5	28.1	29.6
17.0	24.5	24.7	29.4	29.7
17.5	24.7	24.8	29.7	29.8
18.0	25.0	25.0	30.0	30.0

Table 12.9: International cutoff points for BMI for children for overweight and obesity by sex between 2 and 18 y, defined to pass through BMI = 25 kg/m² and BMI = 30 kg/m² at age 18 y, obtained by averaging data from Brazil, Great Britain, Hong Kong, the Netherlands, Singapore, and the United States. Data from Cole et al., British Medical Journal 320(7244): 1240–1243, 2000, with permission of the BMJ Publishing Group.

iles for ages 0–36 mo were also developed by the Euro-Growth Study Group as part of a longitudinal study of 2145 children at 21 study sites (van't Hof and Haschke, 2000b).

12.10 Waist circumference reference data

Body mass index does not account for the wide variation in the distribution of body fat. Many studies have shown that body fat distribution is a more powerful predictor than is BMI for risk factors and morbidity. In particular, the presence of excess fat in the abdomen is strongly associated with metabolic and cardiovascular disease risk and a variety of chronic diseases (Björntorp, 1993; NIH, 1998). Waist circumference is a better correlate of abdominal fat content than is waist-hip ratio, as noted earlier (Section 11.1.3) (Pouliot et al., 1994; Daniels et al., 2000). Hence, waist circumference is now recommended as the best simple, practical anthropometric measurement for assessing abdominal fat content (NIH, 1998; WHO, 2000); it is unrelated to height (Han et al., 1997).

Nevertheless, caution must be exercised when comparing waist circumference measurements among populations because of discrepancies in the measurement process (Section 11.1.2). There is still no commonly agreed site; some measure at the natural waist, others at the umbilicus level. In some cases, details of the site used have not been provided (Zannolli and Morgese, 1996).

In adults, sex-specific waist circumference cutoffs have been developed by NIH (1998) and WHO (2000) to identify increased risk associated with abdominal fat in adults with a BMI in the range of 25 to 34.9; these are given in Section 11.1.3. The WHO cutoffs were developed from data on waist circumference on a random sample of adults aged 20–59 y from the Netherlands (Han et al., 1995). At present, these cutoffs are applied to all adult ethnic or racial groups, although sex- and ethnic-specific cutoffs are probably warranted.

There is mounting evidence that the use of waist circumference as a surrogate indicator of abdominal fat is not restricted to adults (Goran et al., 1998): relationships between waist circumference and adverse atherogenic lipoprotein profiles have also been observed in children (Flodmark et al., 1994; Freedman et al., 1999).

Comparisons across countries have shown the importance of ethnic-specific and population-specific reference data for waist circumference for children (McCarthy et al.,

2001) and adults (Dowling and Pi-Sunyer, 1993). Populations differ in the level of risk associated with a particular waist circumference.

Several countries have now compiled sex-specific waist circumference reference percentiles; they are described below. Tentatively, the 85th and 95th percentiles for waist circumference are used to classify overweight and obesity, but in the future, cutoff points for waist circumference, similar to those used with BMI percentile curves, may be implemented.

12.10.1 U.S. waist circumference reference data

Waist circumference reference tables for men and women, derived from data collected during NHANES III, are given in the Appendix (A12.24 and A12.25) for the following age groups: 20–29, 30–39, 40–49, 50–59, 60–69, 70–79, and 80+ y. Three ethnic groups are included: Caucasian, African American, and Mexican American. It is noticeable that the age-related variation in the median waist circumference is much larger than for BMI. Nevertheless, age-related cutoffs are probably not warranted for adults; the variation with age may be in part the result of secular changes (Ford et al., 2003).

Waist circumference reference tables for U.S. male and female children from 2 to 19 y, derived, like the tables for adults, from data collected during NHANES III, are shown in Appendix A12.23. These results are more difficult to interpret and use, and age-related cutoff points will need to be established for children.

12.10.2 U.K. waist circumference reference data for children

In the United Kingdom, waist circumference percentile curves have been compiled from a representative sample of children (boys, $n = 3585$; girls, $n = 4770$) 5.0–16.9 y, who participated in surveys by the HUMAG Research Group (McCarthy et al., 2001). All racial groups were included. Waist circum-

Age	n	5th	10th	25th	50th	75th	90th	95th
Boys								
5+	254	46.8	47.7	49.3	51.3	53.5	55.6	57.0
6+	349	47.2	48.2	50.7	52.2	54.6	57.1	58.7
7+	334	47.9	48.9	50.9	53.3	56.1	58.8	60.7
8+	333	48.7	49.9	52.1	54.7	57.8	60.9	62.9
9+	337	49.7	51.0	53.4	56.4	59.7	63.2	65.4
10+	357	50.8	52.3	55.0	58.2	61.9	65.6	67.9
11+	298	51.9	53.6	56.6	60.2	64.1	67.9	70.4
12+	347	53.1	55.0	58.4	62.3	66.4	70.4	72.9
13+	319	54.8	56.9	60.4	64.6	69.0	73.1	75.7
14+	279	56.9	59.2	62.6	67.0	71.6	76.1	78.9
15+	288	59.0	61.1	64.8	69.3	74.2	79.0	82.0
16+	90	61.2	63.3	67.0	71.6	76.7	81.8	85.2
Girls								
5+	401	45.4	46.3	48.1	50.3	52.8	55.4	57.2
6+	400	46.3	47.3	49.2	51.5	54.2	57.0	58.9
7+	376	47.4	48.4	50.3	52.7	55.6	58.7	60.8
8+	413	48.5	49.6	51.5	54.1	57.1	60.4	62.7
9+	395	49.5	50.6	52.7	55.3	58.5	62.0	64.5
10+	364	50.7	51.8	53.9	56.7	60.0	63.6	66.2
11+	357	52.0	53.2	55.4	58.2	61.6	65.4	68.1
12+	375	53.6	54.8	57.1	60.0	63.5	67.3	70.5
13+	390	55.2	56.4	58.7	61.7	65.3	69.1	71.8
14+	404	56.5	57.8	60.2	63.2	66.8	70.6	73.2
15+	433	57.6	58.9	61.3	64.4	67.9	71.7	74.3
16+	462	58.4	59.8	62.2	65.3	68.8	72.6	75.1

Table 12.10: Waist circumference percentiles for U.K. children by age and sex. '5+' means the group of children between 5 y and 5.99 y. Data from McCarthy et al., European Journal of Clinical Nutrition 55: 902–907, 2001 © with permission of the Nature Publishing Group.

ference was measured at the natural waist (i.e., midway between the 10th rib and the top of the iliac crest) (Section 11.1.3). Seven smoothed age- and sex-specific percentile curves (5th, 10th, 25th, 50th, 75th, 90th, 95th) were computed; these are presented in Table 12.10.

Secular trends in waist circumference have been investigated in British youth over the past 10–20 y (McCarthy et al., 2003). This has been done by expressing waist circumference (measured in 1997 during the recent U.K. National Diet and Nutrition Survey of young people aged 4–18 y) (Gregory et al., 2000), as a standard deviation score, using the published reference of McCarthy et al. (2001), discussed above. Standard deviation scores for waist circumference increased in 1997, particularly in females, in whom changes correspond to a shift from the 50th to the 85th percentile for waist circumference. The prevalence of overweight and obesity increased over time, based on arbitrary cutoffs corresponding to the 91st and 98th percentiles (SD scores 1.33 and 2.0), respectively. More than one-third of the females in 1997 were overweight and over one-sixth were obese.

Percentiles for waist circumference have been compiled for children from several other countries, including Cuba (Martinez et al., 1994), Italy (Zannolli and Morgese, 1996), Spain (Moreno et al., 1999), and Cyprus (Savva et al., 2001).

12.11 Triceps and subscapular skinfold reference data

Marked ethnic differences in the amount and distribution of subcutaneous fat — and, to a lesser degree, muscle — occur (Wagner and Heyward, 2000). Native Americans, African Americans, and Polynesians, for example, have more subcutaneous fat deposited on the trunk than on the limbs (i.e., centripetal fat pattern), and this fat tends to be deposited more on the upper than on the lower part of the trunk, compared with Caucasians (Zillikens and Conway, 1990; Malina, 1996). Such a fat pattern is associated with an increased incidence of coronary vascular disease and diabetes (Vague, 1956).

Secular changes have been noted in some industrialized countries for indices of body composition (Wells, 2003), including both triceps and subscapular skinfolds (Moreno et al., 2001). Hence, international reference data for the assessment of indices of body composition should be used with these uncertainties in mind.

WHO (1995) provisionally recommended the use of the NCHS 1977 reference data for subscapular and triceps skinfold thicknesses during childhood and adolescence (Johnson et al.,1981), to ensure that all the anthropometric variables are derived from the same reference population, as well as continuity from one age group to another. In the future, data for mid-upper-arm circumference,

and triceps and subscapular skinfold thickness for young children aged 0–5 y from the WHO multicenter growth reference study will be the recommended international reference (Section 12.4.2).

12.11.1 U.S. triceps and subscapular skinfold reference data

Frisancho (1990) produced race-, sex-, and age-specific percentiles for triceps, subscapular, and sum of triceps and subscapular skinfold thickness for persons aged 1–74 y based on the merged NHANES I (1971–1974) and NHANES II (1976–1980) data. The total sample size for the skinfold measurements was 43,597, with 7,080 African Americans, 35,802 Caucasians, and 716 of other ethnic groups.

These same data have been used to compile age- and sex-specific percentile distributions for triceps and subscapular skinfolds in relation to frame size and height; body composition is known to be influenced by these factors, as well as age and sex (Frisancho, 1984). By using these reference data, investigators can distinguish a large-framed individual from a person who is truly obese, as indicated by excessive body weight and fat tissue. In the former, a large body weight is not associated with excessive fat tissue.

Limited data are now available for triceps and subscapular skinfold percentiles from NHANES III for both children and adults. Reference tables for men and women are included in the Appendix (triceps: A12.27 and A12.28; and subscapular: A12.30 and A12.31). The percentiles are for the following age groups: 20–29, 30–39, 40–49, 50–59, 60–69, 70–79, and 80+ y. Three ethnic groups are included: Caucasian, African American, and Mexican American. Triceps and subscapular skinfold percentiles for U.S. male and female children (2–19 y) are shown in Appendix A12.26 and Appendix A12.29.

In response to a recommendation by WHO (1995) for local contemporary reference data for persons ⩾ 60 y, Kuczmarski et al. (2000a) compiled 15th, 50th, and 85th percentiles for triceps skinfold thickness based on the

Age (y)	n	Mean ± SE	10th	15th	25th	50th	75th	85th	90th
Men									
50–59	813	13.7 ± 0.29	7.5	8.0	9.4	12.6	16.0	18.7	21.8
60–69	1122	14.2 ± 0.25	7.7	8.5	10.1	12.7	17.1	20.2	23.1
70–79	825	13.4 ± 0.28	7.3	7.9	9.0	12.4	16.0	18.8	20.6
80 +	642	12.0 ± 0.28	6.6	7.6	8.7	11.2	13.8	16.2	18.0
Women									
50–59	929	26.7 ± 0.40	16.4	18.3	20.6	26.7	32.1	35.2	37.0
60–69	1090	24.2 ± 0.37	14.5	15.9	18.2	24.1	29.7	32.9	34.9
70–79	902	22.3 ± 0.39	12.5	14.0	16.4	21.8	27.7	30.6	32.1
80 +	705	18.6 ± 0.42	9.3	11.1	13.1	18.1	23.3	26.4	28.9

Table 12.11: Triceps skinfold thickness (mm) percentiles for older men and women examined in NHANES III (1988–1994). Data from Kuczmarski et al. (2000b).

NHANES III results. Data are presented for men and women ($n = 7561$) for each decade commencing at 50 y; persons $\geqslant 80$ y were combined into a single group; percentiles are shown in Table 12.11. As discussed in Section 9.2.2, the apparent age-related changes in triceps skinfold thickness are often difficult to interpret in this age group.

Johnson et al. (1981) generated percentiles for both triceps and subscapular skinfolds for young children and adolescents from the NCHS 1977 data. As noted earlier, these percentiles have been provisionally recommended by WHO (1995) for young children and adolescents. These sex- and age-specific percentiles (5th, 10th, 15th, 25th, 50th, 75th, 85th, 90th, 95th), unlike those of Frisancho (1990), do not include the NHANES II (1971–1974) data. Instead, they are derived from the same sources as those described for the NCHS growth reference in Section 12.4.1. Tables of percentiles based on these data by sex for triceps and subscapular are also available for children 9–18 y in WHO (1995).

12.11.2 U.K. triceps and subscapular skinfold reference data

At present, the only reference data for triceps and subscapular skinfold thickness available for use in the United Kingdom are those of Tanner and Whitehouse; these data were compiled in 1962 (Tanner et al., 1966) and later revised in 1975 (Tanner and Whitehouse, 1975). Smoothed sex-specific percent-

ile distributions (3rd to the 97th) for 1–19 y for triceps and 5–16 y for subscapular are available.

The revised 1975 triceps skinfold Tanner and Whitehouse reference data are based exclusively on U.K. data derived at 1–12 mo on 200 children followed longitudinally in Infant Welfare Clinics, for children 1–5 y from a random sample of West London children, and for 5–19 y from an Inner London Education Authority (ILEA) survey. The latter was also used to construct the subscapular reference data. The ILEA survey consisted of 1000 children of each sex at each year of age (Tanner and Whitehouse, 1975). Davies et al. (1993) have employed the LMS method of Cole (1990) to convert these revised triceps and subscapular skinfold measurements of Tanner and Whitehouse (1975) to standard deviation scores.

Several investigators have examined the adequacy of triceps and subscapular skinfold measurements in U.K. infants and young children, expressed as standard deviation scores relative to the 1975 Tanner-Whitehouse reference data (Paul et al., 1998; Savage et al., 1999; Rudolf et al., 2000). The mean triceps and subscapular skinfold SD scores for a random sample of 127 healthy term infants from the west of Scotland is shown in Figure 12.16 (Savage et al, 1999). These results confirm that the existing 1975 Tanner-Whitehouse reference data for triceps and subscapular skinfold thickness are too high, primarily because of differences in feeding

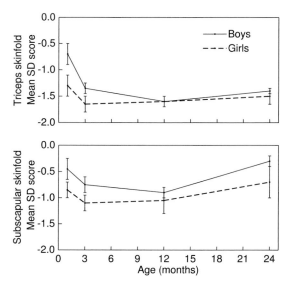

Figure 12.16: Mean triceps and subscapular skinfold SD scores and 95% confidence limits, for a random sample of 127 U.K. infants, relative to Tanner-Whitehouse reference data. From Savage et al., Archives of Disease in Childhood 80: 121–124, 1999, with permission of the BMJ Publishing Group.

practices 30 years ago (Paul et al., 1998), and should no longer be used.

Paul et al. (1998) suggest that smoothed sex-specific percentiles (2nd, 9th, 25th, 50th, 75th, 91st, 98th) for triceps and subscapular for each month from 1 to 24 mo, constructed from the Cambridge infant study, could provide a reference for U.K. infants, especially as these same infants provided the data for the first 2 y of life for the UK90 growth reference.

12.12 Mid-upper-arm circumference reference data

Mid-upper-arm circumference measurements are frequently used to screen for protein-energy malnutrition, when the amount of subcutaneous fat is likely to be small. In such circumstances, mid-upper-arm circumference tends to parallel changes in muscle mass.

WHO (de Onis et al., 1997) have developed age-specific reference data for mid-upper-arm circumference for the correct interpretation of mid-upper-arm circumference and nutritional status, and its relationship

with functional outcomes; details are given in Section 12.14.1. Mid-upper-arm circumference is often used together with triceps skinfold thickness to derive mid-upper-arm fat area or muscle circumference/area. Reference data for these derived parameters are discussed in Sections 12.15 and 12.16.

12.12.1 WHO MUAC reference data by age or height

A WHO Expert Committee has constructed reference data for mid-upper-arm circumference (MUAC) by age using growth data for children 6–59 mo from NHANES I and II. These reference data were compiled because of increasing evidence that MUAC Z-scores that adjust for differences between age and sex are a more useful indicator of nutritional status than is low MUAC determined on the basis of a fixed cutoff value (WHO, 1995). Use of the latter results in wasting being overdiagnosed among younger children and underdiagnosed among older ones (de Onis and Habicht, 1996).

The MUAC reference data were constructed by estimating the mean MUAC for each month of age. This was done by combining MUAC data for the relevant month of each age with data for the 3 mo before and 3 mo after the age. Both the numerical refer-

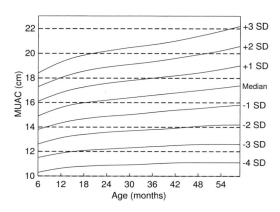

Figure 12.17: Mid-upper-arm circumference (MUAC)-for-age growth reference curves for boys aged 6–59 months. Drawn from full numerical reference data for boys, girls, and sexes combined, given in de Onis et al., Bulletin of World Health Organization 75: 11–18, 1997, with permission.

ence data and sex-specific and sex-combined MUAC-for-age reference growth curves for children 6–59 mo are presented in de Onis et al. (1997). Figure 12.17 provides, as an example, the MUAC-for-age growth reference curve for boys 6–59 mo. Sex- and age-specific differences are evident for the curves for boys and girls < 24 mo.

WHO has also compiled a MUAC-for-height reference for international use based on the same data as that used for the MUAC-for-age reference described above; the methods are described in detail in Mei et al. (1997). Three sets of MUAC-for-height curves were developed, as noted above for the MUAC-for-age reference data, each set with curves representing the median and 1, 2, 3, and 4 SD values above and below the median. Recumbent length was adjusted to standing height when developing the MUAC-for-height reference.

A small disjunction (~ 0.01 cm in MUAC) is exhibited for the recumbent length and standing height at 85 cm. Figure 12.18 shows the MUAC-for-height reference curves for girls and boys of height 65–145 cm as an example. Note that, because of sample size limitations, the reference data only apply to children with a standing height of 65–145 cm.

The WHO Expert Committee recommended that children < 85 cm be measured lying down, but taller children be measured while standing to maintain consistency with the international recommendations (WHO, 1995). The Statistical Analysis System (SAS) code used to calculate the median and upper and lower SD curves for MUAC-for-height is given in Mei et al. (1997), enabling readers to use their own data to calculate exact Z-scores for each child. Details are also provided about the construction and use of the QUAC stick (see Section 13.3.3).

12.12.2 U.S. mid-upper-arm circumference reference data

Both secular and age-related changes in mid-upper-arm circumference percentiles for U.S. men and women have been observed (Bishop et al. 1981). Therefore, earlier U.S. reference data for mid-upper-arm circumference compiled from the Ten-State Nutrition Survey (1968–1970) (Frisancho, 1974) or reference data from the merged NHANES I and II (Frisancho, 1990) should be used with caution.

Mid-upper-arm circumference data from NHANES III are presented in Appendices A12.32 to A12.34. These show means, SDs, and percentile values for arm circumference by age and sex for persons 2–79 y.

Kuczmarski et al. (2000b) compiled a separate reference data set for arm circumference for older Americans from the NHANES III results. Means and percentiles for males and females ≥ 50 y are shown in Table 12.12.

12.13 Mid-upper-arm fat area reference data

Midarm fat area is derived from triceps skinfold thickness and mid-upper-arm circumference measurements. The index, not surprisingly, provides a better estimate of total body fat (i.e., fat weight) than does a single skinfold thickness at the same site. The reference data for mid-upper-arm fat area varies little in children between 1 and 7 y, thus providing an age-independent assessment of total body fat for adequately nourished children of this age group (Gurney and Jelliffe, 1973).

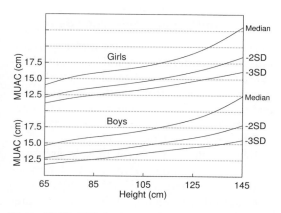

Figure 12.18: Mid-upper-arm circumference (MUAC)-for-height growth reference curves for boys and girls. Drawn from full numerical reference data for boys, girls, and sexes combined, given in Mei et al., Bulletin of World Health Organization 75: 333–341, 1997, with permission.

Age (y)	n	Mean ± SE	10th	15th	25th	50th	75th	85th	90th
Men									
50–59	824	33.7 ± 0.18	29.2	30.0	31.1	33.7	35.6	37.2	37.9
60–69	1126	32.8 ± 0.15	28.4	29.2	30.6	32.7	35.2	36.2	37.0
70–79	832	31.5 ± 0.17	27.5	28.2	29.3	31.3	33.4	35.1	36.1
80+	642	29.5 ± 0.19	25.5	26.2	27.3	29.5	31.5	32.6	33.3
Women									
50–59	970	32.5 ± 0.25	26.6	27.5	28.7	32.0	35.3	37.5	39.2
60–69	1122	31.7 ± 0.21	26.2	26.9	28.3	31.2	34.3	36.5	38.3
70–79	914	30.5 ± 0.23	25.4	26.1	27.4	30.1	33.1	35.1	36.7
80+	712	28.5 ± 0.25	23.0	23.8	25.5	28.4	31.5	33.2	34.0

Table 12.12: Mid-upper-arm circumference percentiles (cm) for older men and women examined in NHANES III (1988–1994). Data from Kuczmarski et al. (2000b).

Secular changes in mid-upper-arm fat area have been demonstrated consistently across many different population groups. Therefore, WHO recommended the use of contemporary reference data, preferably local data, whenever this is possible (de Onis and Habicht, 1996).

12.13.1 U.S. mid-upper-arm fat area reference data

Secular changes in mid-upper-arm fat area have been demonstrated in females, but not in males (Bowen and Custer, 1984). Women from the United States showed a large apparent rise in mid-upper-arm fat area with age between 1962 and 1972. Hence, both age- and sex-specific percentile distributions from contemporary U.S. reference data should be used to evaluate mid-upper-arm fat area values of persons from the United States.

Frisancho (1990) provided age- and sex-specific mid-upper-arm fat-area means, standard deviation, and percentiles (5th, 10th, 15th, 25th, 50th, 75th, 85th, 90th, 95th) for U.S. persons 1–74 y, using the unadjusted data for triceps skinfold and mid-upper-arm circumference described in Sections 12.11.1 and 12.12.2. Data for children were classified into 1-y age groups (e.g., 1.0–1.9), whereas adults aged from 18 to 75 y were grouped into one 7-y age group, and ten 5-y age groups (e.g., 25.0–29.9, 30.0–34.9, 35.0–39.9, etc.). Comparable data are also presented by ethnicity or race.

12.14 Mid-upper-arm muscle-circumference and muscle-area reference data

Secular and age-related trends, and genetic differences, have been described for mid-upper-arm muscle circumference and for arm muscle area indices, so contemporary and locally applicable reference data should be used if possible. Both indices are derived from measurements of the triceps skinfold thickness and mid-upper-arm circumference using the formulae given in Sections 11.2.2 and 11.2.3.

12.14.1 U.S. mid-upper-arm muscle circumference and mid-upper-arm muscle area reference data

Earlier U.S reference data for mid-upper-arm muscle circumference should not be used because of the existence of secular-related changes in mid-upper-arm muscle circumference and mid-upper-arm muscle area in both males and females in the United States (Frisancho, 1974; Bowen and Custer, 1984).

Instead, the use of arm muscle area percentiles (5th through 95th) for U.S. persons based on the merged NHANES I and II data is preferred (Frisancho, 1990). Data are presented by age, sex, and ethnicity or race for persons 1–74 y by height for boys and girls 2–17 y; and by age, sex, and frame size for adults aged 18–74 y. In addition, for Caucasians, arm muscle area percentiles by

Age (y)	n	Mean $\pm$ SE	10th	15th	25th	50th	75th	85th	90th
Men
50–59	811	29.2 $\pm$ 0.15	25.6	26.2	27.4	29.2	31.1	32.1	33.0
60–69	1119	28.3 $\pm$ 0.13	24.9	25.6	26.7	28.4	30.0	30.9	31.4
70–79	824	27.3 $\pm$ 0.14	24.4	24.8	25.6	27.2	28.9	30.0	30.5
80+	639	25.7 $\pm$ 0.16	22.6	23.2	24.0	25.7	27.5	28.2	28.8
Women
50–59	927	23.8 $\pm$ 0.15	20.4	20.9	21.5	23.3	25.4	26.5	27.8
60–69	1090	23.8 $\pm$ 0.12	20.6	21.1	21.0	23.5	25.4	26.6	27.4
70–79	898	23.4 $\pm$ 0.14	20.3	20.8	21.6	23.0	24.8	26.3	27.0
80+	703	22.7 $\pm$ 0.16	19.3	20.0	20.9	22.6	24.5	25.4	26.0

Table 12.13: Arm-muscle circumference percentiles (cm) for older men and women examined in NHANES III (1988–1994). Data from Kuczmarski et al. (2000b).

age, sex, and frame size are also available. In older persons, increased compressibility of fat may result in an overestimation of mid-upper-arm muscle area. The trends in mid-upper-arm muscle area observed in the younger age groups may represent a combined increase in bone diameter and muscle area.

Caution must be used when interpreting estimates of arm muscle area among those who are obese or those with triceps skinfold thickness that exceeds the 85th age- and sex-specific percentiles. In such persons, estimates of arm muscle area by anthropometry are said to overestimate arm muscle area determined by computerized tomography, the degree of overestimation varying directly with the degree of adiposity (Forbes et al., 1988).

At present only arm muscle circumference reference data for Americans $\geqslant 50$ y have been compiled from the NHANES III survey (Kuczmarski et al., 2000b). Mean (SE) and selected percentile values of males and females for four age groups are shown in Table 12.13.

The distributions of the values for mid-upper-arm muscle circumference for adult males and females are similar and change with age. Arm muscle circumference and mid-upper-arm muscle area usually increase up to age 65 y in women and up to middle age in men and then steadily decrease.

Reference percentiles for bone-free mid-upper-arm muscle area, calculated using the equation of Heymsfield et al. (1982) (Section 11.2.3), have been compiled for three categories of frame size for U.S. male and female adults for two age groups, 25–54 y and 55–74 y (Frisancho, 1984). Percentiles ranging from the 5th to the 95th are included.

12.15 Summary

Several sets of fetal growth curves are available; those based on Californian data are recommended for use by WHO. Reference growth data for preterm infants and for children with special needs are also available.

For young children aged 0–5 y, WHO recommends the use of new international growth references that will include both growth and body composition measurements (arm circumference, triceps and subscapular skinfolds). Only those infants whose mothers comply to the current WHO feeding recommendations were included, so that the growth reference approximates a standard. Until this new international growth reference is available, WHO recommends the continued use of the NCHS/WHO reference data. This reference is based on more extensive percentile tables for weight-for-age, stature-for-age, weight-for-stature, and the median and ± 1, 2, 3, and 4 SD, together with new MUAC-for-age and MUAC-for-height percentiles.

New European growth references for children aged 0–3 y have also been compiled, which include sex- and age-specific percentiles (3rd through 97th) for recumbent length, weight, mid-upper arm, thigh, and calf circumferences.

Sources of distance reference growth data include the CDC 2000 (0–3; 2–20 y) for U.S children and the UK90 (23 wk to 20 y) data for U.K. children. Percentiles of weight-for-age, stature-for-age, weight-for-stature (for the U.S. only), head circumference-for-age, and BMI are available for the U.S. and U.K data. The NCHS/WHO reference is still recommended by WHO as the international growth standard for children older than 5 y, until a new reference for this age group is available. This recommendation was made to ensure that all the anthropometric variables are derived from the same reference population. In the absence of local reference data for adults, WHO also suggests that the NCHS/WHO values for height at 18 y should be used for persons aged 18–24 y.

Tempo-conditional, longitudinal-type distance charts, suitable for monitoring growth of individual children, especially during adolescence, are also available for weight-for-age and height-for-age for the United Kingdom and for the United States.

Sources of growth velocity reference data derived from longitudinal data are still limited. Available data are those compiled by the U.S. Fels Institute and by the U.K. London Child Study Centre. These reference data provide information on rate of growth and on weight (for United Kingdom only) and height velocity percentile curves for early and late maturers. Growth velocity reference data are more sensitive to growth abnormalities than are distance growth data, provided accurate and precise measurements are taken.

For adults, WHO, Canada, and the United Kingdom use BMI cutoff points of BMI $\geqslant 25$ and BMI $\geqslant 30$ to define overweight and obesity, respectively, whereas the United States uses these same cutoff points in adults to define risk of overweight and overweight in population studies. For children, WHO recommends the use of internationally derived, age-specific BMI values equivalent to WHO BMI definitions of overweight (BMI = 25) and obesity (BMI = 30) in adults. This

approach was developed and adopted by the European childhood Obesity Group. Both the United States and the United Kingdom use age-specific BMI percentiles compiled from the 2000 CDC and UK90 reference data, respectively, for children and adolescents.

To evaluate the distribution of body fat, waist circumference is now the preferred anthropometric surrogate of abdominal fat, the key variable associated with risk for type 2 diabetes, coronary heart disease, and hypertension. For adults, sex-specific waist circumference cutoff points have been developed by WHO and the NIH, but WHO cautions there is a need to develop sex- and ethnic-specific cutoff points in the future. For children, waist circumference percentiles have been compiled in various countries, with the 85th and 95th percentiles arbitrarily used to define overweight and obesity. In the future, international cutoff points for waist circumference similar to those used for BMI for overweight and obesity may be used for children.

Use of an international reference data set for body composition measurements is not appropriate. When local data are not available, WHO recommends the use of the new international standards for triceps and subscapular skinfolds, and arm circumference for children from 0–5 y, when they are available. For older children, new reference data must be constructed, but in the interim, the NCHS is still recommended by WHO.

Reference data for selected body composition indices are available for the United Kingdom and the United States. However, use of the revised Tanner and Whitehouse reference data for triceps and subscapular skinfolds for U.K. children is no longer appropriate. Instead, smoothed percentiles for triceps and subscapular based on Cambridge infants aged 1–24 mo should be used. For the United States, age-, sex-, and some race-specific reference data, for triceps skinfold, subscapular skinfold, mid-upper-arm circumference, mid-upper-arm muscle circumference and area, and mid-upper-arm fat area are available for persons aged 1–75 years based on NHANES I and NHANES II data, and selected data for persons $\geqslant 50$ y, based on NHANES III.

References

Abraham S, Johnson CL, Najjar MF. (1979). Weight by height and age for adults 18–74 years: United States, 1971–1974. Vital Health Statistics Series 11, No. 208, (PHS 79–1656). Department of Health and Human Services, Hyattsville, MD.

Alexander GR, Himes JH, Kaufman RB, Mor J, Kogan M. (1996). A United States national reference for fetal growth. Obstetrics and Gynecology 87: 163–168.

Ballard JL, Novak KK, Driver M. (1979). A simplified score for assessment of fetal maturation of newly born infants. Journal of Pediatrics 95: 769–774.

Barlow SE, Dietz WH. (1998). Obesity evaluation and treatment: Expert Committee recommendations. Pediatrics 102: E29

Baumgartner RN, Roche AF, Himes JH. (1986). Incremental growth tables: supplementary to previous charts. American Journal of Clinical Nutrition 43: 711–722.

Bishop CW, Bowen PE, Ritchey SJ. (1981). Norms for nutritional assessment of American adults by upper arm anthropometry. American Journal of Clinical Nutrition 34: 230–2539.

Björntorp P. (1993). Visceral obesity: a "civilization syndrome." Obesity Research 1: 206–222.

Bowen PE, Custer PB. (1984). Reference values and age-related trends for arm muscle area, arm fat area, and sum of skinfolds for United States adults. Journal of the American College of Nutrition 3: 357–376.

British Standards Institution. (1990). Body measurements of boys and girls from birth to age 16.9 years, BS 7321. British Standards Institution, London.

Buckler JM. (1990). A Longitudinal Study of Adolescent Growth. Springer-Verlag, London.

Burt VL, Harris T. (1994). The third National Health and Nutrition Examination Survey: contributing data on aging and health. The Gerontologist 34: 486–490.

Cameron N. (2002). British growth charts for height and weight with recommendations concerning their use in auxological assessment. Annals of Human Biology 29: 1–10.

Casey PH, Kraemer HC, Berbaum J et al. (1990). Growth patterns of preterm infants: longitudinal analysis of a large, varied sample. Journal of Pediatrics 117: 298–307.

Casey PH, Kraemer HC, Berbaum J, Yogman MW, Sells JC. (1991). Growth status and growth rates of a varied sample of low birth-weight, preterm infants: a longitudinal cohort from birth to three years of age. Journal of Pediatrics 119: 599–605.

Cole TJ. (1990). The LMS method for constructing normalized growth standards. European Journal of Clinical Nutrition 44: 45–60.

Cole TJ. (2000). A simple chart to identify non-familial short stature. Archives of Disease in Childhood 82: 173–176.

Cole TJ, Freeman JV, Preece MA. (1995). Body mass index reference curves for the U.K., 1990. Archives of Disease in Childhood 73: 25–29.

Cole TJ, Freeman JV, Preece MA. (1998). British 1990 growth reference centiles for weight, height, body mass index, and head circumference fitted by maximum penalized likelihood. Statistics in Medicine 17: 407–429.

Cole TJ, Bellizzi MC, Flegal KM, Dietz WH. (2000). Establishing a standard definition for child overweight and obesity worldwide: international survey. British Medical Journal 320: 1240–1243.

Cole TJ, Paul AA, Whitehead RG. (2002). Weight reference charts for British long-term breastfed infants. Acta Paediatrica 91: 1296–1300.

Cronk CE, Crocker AC, Pueschel SM, Shea AM, Zackai E, Pickens G, Reed RB. (1988). Growth charts for children with Down syndrome: 1 month to 18 years of age. Pediatrics 81: 102–110.

Daniels SR, Khoury PR, Morrison JA. (2000). Utility of different measures of body fat distribution in children and adolescents. American Journal of Epidemiology 152: 1179–1184.

Davies PSW, Dy JME, Cole TJ. (1993). Converting Tanner–Whitehouse reference tricep and subscapular skinfold measurements to standard deviation scores. European Journal of Clinical Nutrition 47: 559–566.

de Onis M, Habicht J-P. (1996). Anthropometric reference data for international use: recommendations from a World Health Organization Expert Committee. American Journal of Clinical Nutrition 64: 650–658.

de Onis M, Yip R, Mei Z. (1997). The development of MUAC-for-age reference data recommended by a WHO Expert Committee. Bulletin of the World Health Organization 75: 11–18.

de Onis M, Garza C, Victora CG, Onyango AW, Frongillo EA, Martinez J. (2004). The WHO Multicentre Growth Reference Study: Planning, study design, and methodology. Food and Nutrition Bulletin 25: S15–S26.

Dewey KG. (1998). Growth characteristics of breast-fed compared to formula-fed infants. Biology of the Neonate 74: 94–105.

Dibley MJ, Goldsby JB, Staehling NW, Trowbridge FL. (1987). Development of normalized curves for the international growth reference: historical and technical considerations. American Journal of Clinical Nutrition 46: 736–748.

Dowling HJ, Pi-Sunyer FX. (1993). Race-dependent health risks of upper body obesity. Diabetes 42: 537–543.

DuRant RH, Linder CW. (1981). An evaluation of five indexes of relative body weight for use with children. Journal of the American Dietetic Association 78: 35–41.

Ehrenkranz RA, Younes N, Lemons JA, Fanaroff AA, Donovan EF, Wright LL, Katsikiotis V, Tyson JE, Oh W, Shankaran S, Bauer C, Korones SB, Stoll BJ, Stevenson DK, Papile LA. (1999). Longitudinal growth of hospitalized very low birth-weight infants. Pediatrics 104: 280–289.

Flodmark CE, Sveger T, Nilsson-Ehle P. (1994). Waist measurement correlates to a potentially atherogenic lipoprotein profile in obese 12–14-year-old children. Acta Paediatrica 83: 941–945.

Forbes GB, Brown MR, Griffiths HJL. (1988). Arm muscle plus bone area: anthropometry and CAT scan compared. American Journal of Clinical Nutrition 47: 929–931.

Ford ES, Mokdad AH, Giles WH. (2003). Trends in waist circumference among U.S. adults. Obesity Research 11: 1223–1231.

Freeman JV, Cole TJ, Chinn S, Jones PRM, White EM, Preece MA. (1995). Cross sectional stature and weight reference curves for the UK, 1990. Archives of Disease in Childhood 73: 17–24.

Freedman DS, Serdula MK, Srinivasan SR, Berenson GS. (1999). Relation of circumferences and skinfold thicknesses to lipid and insulin concentrations in children and adolescents: the Bogalusa Heart Study. American Journal of Clinical Nutrition 69: 308–317.

Frisancho AR. (1974). Triceps skin fold and upper arm muscle size norms for assessment of nutritional status. American Journal of Clinical Nutrition 27: 1052–1058.

Frisancho AR. (1984). New standards of weight and body composition by frame size and height for assessment of nutritional status of adults and the elderly. American Journal of Clinical Nutrition 40: 808–819.

Frisancho AR. (1990). Anthropometric standards for the assessment of growth and nutritional status. University of Michigan Press, Ann Arbor.

Garza C, de Onis M. (1999). A new international growth reference for young children. American Journal of Clinical Nutrition 70: 169S–172S.

Goran MI, Gower BA, Treuth M, Nagy TR. (1998). Prediction of intra-abdominal and subcutaneous abdominal adipose tissue in healthy pre-pubertal children. International Journal of Obesity and Related Metabolic Disorders 22: 549–558.

Gorstein J, Sullivan K, Yip R, de Onis M, Trowbridge F, Fajans P, Clugston G. (1994). Issues in the assessment of nutritional status using anthropometry. Bulletin of the World Health Association 72: 273–283.

Graitcer PL, Gentry EM. (1981). Measuring children: one reference for all. Lancet 2: 297–299.

Gregory J, Foster K, Tyler H, Wiseman M. (1990). The Dietary and Nutritional Survey of British Adults. The Stationery Office, London.

Gregory J, Lowe S, Bates CJ, Prentice A, Jackson LV, Smithers G, Wenlock R, Farron M. (2000). National Diet and Nutrition Survey. Young people aged 4 to 18 years. Volume 1: Report of the diet and nutrition survey. The Stationery Office, London.

Guo SS, Wholihan K, Roche AF, Chumlea WC, Casey PH. (1996). Weight-for-length reference data for preterm, low birth weight infants. Archives of Pediatrics and Adolescent Medicine 150: 964–970.

Guo SS, Roche AF, Chumlea WC, Casey PH, Moore WM. (1997). Growth in weight, recumbent length, and head circumference for preterm low birth weight infants during the first three years of life using gestation-adjusted ages. Early Human Development 47: 305–325.

Gurney JM, Jelliffe DB. (1973). Arm anthropometry in nutritional assessment: nomogram for rapid calculation of muscle circumference and cross-sectional muscle and fat areas. American Journal of Clinical Nutrition 26: 912–915.

Habicht JP, Martorell R, Yarbrough C, Malina RM, Klein RE. (1974). Height and weight standards for preschool children: how relevant are ethnic differences in growth potential? Lancet 1(7858): 611–615.

Han TS, van Leer EM, Seidell JC, Lean ME. (1995). Waist circumference action levels in the identification of cardiovascular risk factors: prevalence study in a random sample. British Medical Journal 311: 1401–1405.

Han TS, Seidell JC, Currall JE, Morrison CE, Deurenberg P, Lean ME. (1997). The influence of height and age on waist circumference as an index of adiposity in adults. International Journal of Obesity and Related Metabolic Disorders 21: 83–89.

Haschke F, van't Hof MA. (2000a). Euro-Growth references for length, weight, and body circumferences. Journal of Pediatric Gastroenterology and Nutrition 31: S14–S38.

Haschke F, van't Hof MA. (2000b). Euro-Growth references for breastfed boys and girls: influence of breast-feeding and solids on growth until 36 months of age. Journal of Pediatric Gastroenterology and Nutrition 31: S60–S71.

Heymsfield SB, McManus C, Smith J, Stevens V, Nixon DW. (1982). Anthropometric measurement of muscle mass: revised equations for calculating bone-free arm muscle area. American Journal of Clinical Nutrition 36: 680–690.

Himes JH, Dietz WH. (1994). Guidelines for overweight in adolescent preventive services: recommendations from an expert committee. American Journal of Clinical Nutrition 59: 307–316.

Himes JH, Roche AF, Thissen D, Moore WM. (1985). Parent-specific adjustments for evaluation of recumbent length and stature of children. Pediatrics 75: 304–313.

Horton WA, Rotter JI, Rimoin DL, Scott CI, Hall JG. (1978). Standard growth curves for achondroplasia. Journal of Pediatrics 3: 435–438.

IOM (Institute of Medicine). (1990). Nutrition during Pregnancy. National Academy Press, Washington, DC.

Johnson CL, Fulwood R, Abraham S, Bryner J. (1981). Basic data on anthropometric measurements and angular measurements of the hip and knee joints for selected age groups 1–74 years of age, United States, 1971–1975. Vital Health Statistics Series 11, No. 219, Department of Health and Human Services, Washington, DC.

Knight I (ed.). (1984). The heights and weights of adults in Great Britain: report of a survey carried out on behalf of the Department of Health and Social Security covering adults aged 16–64 years. Office of Population Censuses and Surveys, Social Survey Division, Her Majesty's Stationery Office, London.

Kuczmarski RJ, Ogden CL, Grummer-Strawn LM, Flegal KM, Guo SS, Wei R, Mei Z, Curtin LR, Roche AF, Johnson CL. (2000a). CDC Growth Charts: United States. Advance Data 314: 1–27.

Kuczmarski KF, Kuczmarski RJ, Najjar M. (2000b). Descriptive anthropometric reference data for older Americans. Journal of the American Dietetic Association 100: 59–66.

Lindgren G, Strandell A, Cole T, Healy M, Tanner J. (1995). Swedish population reference standards for height, weight and body mass index attained at 6 to 16 years (girls) or 19 years (boys). Acta Paediatrica 84: 1019–1028.

Luciano A, Bressan F, Zoppi G. (1997). Body mass index reference curves for children aged 3–19 years from Verona, Italy. European Journal of Clinical Nutrition 51: 6–10.

Malina RM. (1996). Regional body composition: age, sex, and ethnic variation. In: Roche AF, Heymsfield SB, Lohman TG (eds.) Human Body Composition. Human Kinetics, Champaign, IL, pp. 217–255.

Marshall WA. (1971). Evaluation of growth rate in height over periods of less than one year. Archives of Disease in Childhood 46: 414–420.

Marshall WA, Swan AV. (1971). Seasonal variation in growth rates of normal and blind children. Human Biology 43: 502–516.

Martinez E, Devesa M, Bacallao J, Amador M. (1994). Percentiles of the waist-hip ratio in Cuban scholars aged 4.5 to 20.5 years. International Journal of Obesity and Related Metabolic Disorders 18: 557–560.

McCarthy HD, Jarrett KV, Crawley HF. (2001). The development of waist circumference percentiles in British children aged 5.0–16.9 y. European Journal of Clinical Nutrition 55: 902–907.

McCarthy HD, Ellis SM, Cole TJ. (2003). Central overweight and obesity in British youth aged 11–16 years: cross sectional surveys of waist circumference. British Medical Journal 326: 624–627.

McLennan WM, Podger A. (1998). National Nutrition Survey Nutrient Intakes and Physical Measurements. Australia 1995. Australian Bureau of Statistics, Canberra.

Mei Z, Grummer-Strawn LM, de Onis M, Yip R. (1997). The development of a MUAC-for-height reference, including a comparison to other nutritional status screening indicators. Bulletin of the World Health Organization 75: 333–341.

Moreno LA, Fleta J, Mur L, Rodriguez G, Sarria A, Bueno M. (1999). Waist circumference values in Spanish children: gender-related differences. European Journal of Clinical Nutrition 53: 429–433.

Moreno LA, Fleta J, Sarria A, Rodriguez G, Gill C, Bueno M. (2001). Secular changes in body fat patterning in children and adolescents of Zaragoza (Spain), 1980–1995. International Journal of Obesity and Related Metabolic Disorders 25: 1656–1660.

Must A, Dallal GE, Dietz WH. (1991). Reference data for obesity: 85th and 95th percentiles of body mass index (wt/ht^2) and triceps skinfold thickness. American Journal of Clinical Nutrition 53: 839–846. Erratum in: American Journal of Clinical Nutrition 54: 773.

NIH (National Institute of Health). (1998). Clinical guidelines on the identification, evaluation, and treatment of overweight and obesity in adults: the evidence report. Obesity Research 6: 51S–209S.

Paul AA, Cole TJ, Ahmed EA, Whitehead RG. (1998). The need for revised standards for skinfold thickness in infancy. Archives of Disease in Childhood 78: 354–358.

Poskitt EM. (1995). Defining childhood obesity: the relative body mass index (BMI). Acta Paediatrica 84: 961–963.

Pouliot MC, Despres JP, Lemieux S, Moorjani S, Bouchard C, Tremblay A, Nadeau A, Lupien PJ. (1994). Waist circumference and abdominal sagittal diameter: best simple anthropometric indexes of abdominal visceral adipose tissue accumulation and related cardiovascular risk in men and women. American Journal of Cardiology 73: 460–468.

Prescott-Clarke P, Primatesta P (eds.) (1996). Health Survey for England 1996. The Stationery Office, London.

Roberts SB, Dallal GE. (2001). The new childhood growth charts. Nutrition Reviews 59: 31–36.

Roche AF, Himes JH. (1980). Incremental growth charts. American Journal of Clinical Nutrition 33: 2041–2052.

Roche AF, Guo SS, Wholihan K, Casey PH. (1997). Reference data for head circumference-for-length in preterm low-birth-weight infants. Archives of Pediatric Adolescent Medicine 151: 50–57.

Rosenbaum S, Skinner RK, Knight IB, Garrow JS. (1985). A survey of heights and weights of adults in Great Britain, 1980. Annals of Human Biology 12: 115–127.

Rudolf MCJ, Cole TJ, Krom AJ, Sahota P, Walker J. (2000). Growth of primary school children: a validation of the 1990 references and their use in growth monitoring. Archives of Disease in Childhood 83: 298–301.

Saul RA, Stevenson RE, Rogers RC, Skinner SA, Prouty LA, Flannery DB (eds.). (1988). Growth References from Conception to Adulthood. Suppl. 1: Proceedings of the Greeenwood Genetic Center. Jacobs Press, Clinton, SC.

Savage SA, Reilly JJ, Edwards CA, Durnin JVGA. (1999). Adequacy of standards for assessment of growth and nutritional status in infancy and early childhood. Archives of Disease in Childhood 80: 121–124.

Savva SC, Kourides Y, Tornaritis M, Epiphaniou-Savva M, Tafouna P, Kafatos A. (2001). Reference growth curves for Cypriot children 6 to 17 years of age. Obesity Research 9: 754–762.

Sherry B, Mei Z, Grummer-Strawn L, Dietz WH. (2003). Evaluation of and recommendations for growth references for very low birth-weight ($\leqslant 1500$ grams) infants in the United States. Pediatrics 111: 750–758.

Stephenson LS, Latham MC, Jansen AAJ. (1983). A Comparison of Growth Standards: Similarities between NCHS, Harvard, Denver and Privileged African Children and Differences with Kenyan Rural Children. Program in International Nutrition Monograph Series No.12. Cornell University, Ithaca NY.

Tanner JM. (1962). Growth at Adolescence. 2nd ed. Blackwell Scientific, Oxford.

Tanner JM. (1976). Growth as a monitor of nutritional status. Proceedings of the Nutrition Society 35: 315–322.

Tanner JM. (1986). Use and abuse of growth standards. In: Falkner F, Tanner JM (eds.) Human Growth: A Comprehensive Treatise. Volume 3: Methodology, Ecological, Genetic, and Nutritional Effects on Growth. 2nd ed. Plenum Press, New York, pp. 95–109.

Tanner JM, Buckler JMH. (1997). Revision and update of Tanner-Whitehouse clinical longitudinal charts for height and weight. European Journal of Pediatrics 156: 248–249.

Tanner JM, Davies PSW. (1985). Clinical longitudinal standards for height and height velocity for North American children. Journal of Pediatrics 107: 317–329.

Tanner JM, Whitehouse RH. (1975). Revised standards for triceps and subscapular skinfolds in British children. Archives of Disease in Childhood 50: 142–145.

Tanner JM, Whitehouse RH. (1976). Clinical longitudinal standards for height, weight, height velocity, and weight velocity, and the stages of puberty. Archives of Disease in Childhood 51: 170–179.

Tanner JM, Whitehouse RH, Takaishi M. (1966). Standards from birth to maturity for height, weight, height velocity, and weight velocity: British children, 1965. Archives of Disease in Childhood 41: 454–471, 613–625.

Tanner JM, Goldstein H, Whitehouse RH. (1970). Standards for children's height at ages 2–9 years, allowing for height of parents. Archives of Disease in Childhood 45: 755–762.

Vague J. (1956). The degree of masculine differentiation of obesities: a factor determining predisposition to diabetes, atherosclerosis, gout, and uric acid calculous disease. American Journal of Clinical Nutrition 4: 20–34.

van't Hof MA, Haschke F. (2000a). The Euro-Growth study: why, who, and how. Journal of Pediatric Gastroenterology and Nutrition 31: S3–S13.

van't Hof MA, Haschke F. (2000b). Euro-Growth references for body mass index and weight for length. Journal of Pediatric Gastroenterology and Nutrition 2000 31: S48–S59.

van't Hof MA, Haschke F, Darvay S. (2000). Euro-Growth references on increments in length, weight, and head and arm circumference during the first 3 years of life. Journal of Pediatric Gastroenterology and Nutrition 2000 31: S39–S47.

Wagner DR, Heyward VH. (2000). Measures of body composition in blacks and whites: a comparative review. American Journal of Clinical Nutrition 71: 1392–1402.

Wells JC. (2003). Body composition in childhood: effects of normal growth and disease. Proceedings of the Nutrition Society 62: 521–528.

WHO (World Health Organization). (1978). A Growth Chart for International Use in Maternal and Child Health Care. World Health Organization, Geneva.

WHO (World Health Organization). (1983). Measuring Change in Nutritional Status: Guidelines for Assessing the Nutritional Impact of Supplementary Feeding Programmes for Vulnerable Groups. World Health Organization, Geneva.

WHO (World Health Organization). (1994). Working Group on Infant Growth: An Evaluation of Infant Growth. World Health Organization, Geneva.

WHO (World Health Organization). (1995). Physical Status: The Use and Interpretation of Anthropometry. Technical Report Series No. 854. World Health Organization, Geneva.

WHO (World Health Organization). (2000). Obesity: Preventing and Managing the Global Epidemic. Report on a WHO Consultation. Technical Report Series No. 894. World Health Organization, Geneva.

Williams S. (2000). Body mass index reference curves derived from a New Zealand birth cohort. New Zealand Medical Journal 113: 308–311.

Williams RL, Creasy RK, Cunningham GC, Hawes W, Norris FD, Tashiro M. (1982). Fetal growth and perinatal viability in California. Obstetrics and Gynecology 59: 624–632.

Wright CM, Booth IW, Buckler JMH, Cameron N, Cole TJ, Healy MJR, Hulse JA, Preece MA, Reilly JJ, Williams AF. (2002). Growth reference charts for use in the United Kingdom. Archives of Disease in Childhood 86: 11–14.

Wright EM, Royston P. (1997). Simplified estimation of age-specific reference intervals for skewed data. Statistics in Medicine 16: 2785–2803.

Zannolli R, Morgese G. (1996). Waist percentiles: a simple test for atherogenic disease? Acta Paediatrica 85: 1368–1369.

Zillikens MC, Conway JN. (1990). Anthropometry in blacks: applicability of generalized skinfold equations and differences in fat patterning between blacks and whites. American Journal of Clinical Nutrition 52: 45–51.

13

Evaluation of anthropometric indices

Standardized methods of evaluating anthropometric indices are absolutely essential for identifying malnourished individuals in need of treatment and for assessing the nutritional status of population groups. The methods selected will depend on the objectives of the study and the facilities available for data handling.

At the individual level, anthropometric indices can be used to track an individual's pattern of growth over time. They can also be used to identify and classify an individual as "malnourished" or of "normal" nutritional status by comparison with either predetermined reference limits or cutoff points. In some circumstances, individuals may also be classified into risk categories indicative of the severity or type of malnutrition or mortality risk.

In population studies involving nutrition surveys or nutrition surveillance, the data should be presented as frequency distributions of the anthropometric indices. The World Health Organization (WHO) recommends reporting comparison of these distributions with the corresponding NCHS/WHO reference data. For young children aged 0–5 y, the new WHO international growth reference should be used (Section 12.4.2), when it becomes available. Comparisons can also be made with local reference data, when appropriate.

Comparisons with suitable reference data can characterize the nutritional status of the population at baseline in relation to the reference population or highlight changes with successive measurements. As well, the proportion of individuals in the population with indices below or above predetermined reference limits can also be determined. Such prevalence data can be used for assessing the need for, or impact of, an intervention and for comparisons among populations.

In some cases, cutoff points are used that are based on functional impairment or clinical signs of deficiency, and occasionally mortality risk (Section 1.4). Cutoff points may be combined with trigger levels to set the level at which an intervention is initiated (or triggered).

Therefore, to evaluate anthropometric indices at both the individual and population levels, appropriate reference data for each index (discussed in Chapter 12) are required. Various methods of comparing anthropometric indices with the reference data are discussed below, followed by a review of the commonly used systems for identifying and classifying individuals and populations at risk for malnutrition. The uses of anthropometric indices for both individual and population level assessment are also considered.

13.1 Modes of expression of anthropometric indices

For studies of both individuals and populations, the anthropometric indices can be compared to the reference population using percentiles or Z-scores derived from the reference data. In most industrialized countries, percentiles are used, whereas in low-income countries, the use of Z-scores is preferred.

In some circumstances, percentiles and Z-scores cannot be calculated and, instead, the anthropometric indices are expressed in terms of percent-of-median. Percent-of-median, however, provides only limited information on the relative position of the value within the population.

13.1.1 Percentiles

A percentile refers to the position of the measurement value in relation to all the measurements for the reference population, ranked in order of magnitude. Figure 13.1 is a cumulative frequency distribution of the heights of boys aged 13 y, illustrating the use of percentiles. In this figure, a height of 152 cm represents the 50th percentile. This means that 50% of the boys in the reference population have a height at or below this value and 50% at or above this value. Similarly, 10% of the boys have a height at or below the 10th percentile which, in Figure 13.1, falls at 141.8 cm. For data with a Gaussian distribution (e.g., height for age), the 50th percentile corresponds to both the mean and the median; for skewed data (e.g., weight-for-age), the 50th percentile corresponds to the median.

The percentile for an individual of known age and sex can be calculated exactly, if the numerical percentile values are available

for the reference data. Computer programs (e.g., EpiInfo 2002) (Sullivan et al., 1990) are available to calculate exact percentiles based on the NCHS/WHO (Section 12.4.1) or revised CDC 2000 (Section 12.4; Kuczmarski et al., 2000) reference growth curves. Alternatively, the percentile range within which the measurement of an individual falls can be read from graphs or tables of the reference data.

Sometimes, when calculating percentiles, adjustments are made for parental stature, to distinguish between genetic and pathological effects in a child who is unusually short (Section 12.5). The magnitude of the adjustment tends to be greater for older children. An example of adjustments based on midparent height from Himes et al. (1985), is given in Section 12.7.

Adjustments are also important when evaluating the growth percentiles of both low birth weight and preterm infants (i.e., < 38 wk gestation). Specialized growth charts are available for determining the growth percentiles of preterm infants (Section 12.2).

For population studies, the number and percentage of individuals falling within specified percentiles of the reference data can be tabulated or presented graphically to provide an estimate of "relative status," as shown in Figure 13.2. This approach highlights critical features of the distribution of the study population compared to that of the reference population (WHO, 1986).

The percentile reference limits commonly used for designating individuals as "at risk" to malnutrition are either below the 3rd or 5th percentiles or above the 97th or 95th percentiles. The limits chosen depend on the reference data used.

Use of percentiles is recommended for the evaluation of anthropometric measurements from relatively well-nourished populations from industrialized countries, as no errors are introduced if the data have a skewed distribution. Weight-for-age, weight-for-height, and many circumferential and skinfold indices have skewed distributions.

Percentiles are not recommended for evaluating anthropometric indices of individu-

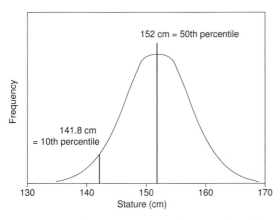

Figure 13.1: Frequency distribution for stature in 13-y-old boys.

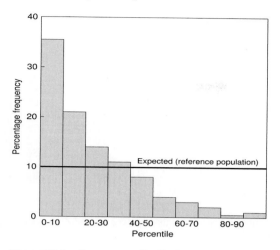

Figure 13.2: Percentage distribution of children by weight/height percentiles. From the 1974 Sahel nutrition studies based on measurements of 798 children. From WHO (1983), with permission.

als or populations from low-income countries if reference data from industrialized countries, such as the NCHS/WHO International Growth Reference (WHO, 1983), are used. In such circumstances, an individual with large deficits in weight and height may have indices below the extreme percentile of the reference distribution (i.e., below 3rd or 5th percentile), making it difficult to characterize the magnitude of the deficit. Likewise, for population studies, many of the population being studied may have indices below the extreme percentile of the reference population, making it difficult to accurately classify large numbers of individuals (Waterlow et al., 1977). Moreover, because data from a population, expressed in terms of percentiles, are often not normally distributed, such populations cannot be correctly described in terms of means and standard deviations of the percentiles.

13.1.2 Z-scores

The World Health Organization recommends the use of Z-scores for evaluating anthropometric data from low-income countries (Gorstein et al., 1994), because Z-scores can be calculated accurately beyond the limits of the original reference data. This is an advantage

in low-income countries because individuals with indices below the extreme percentiles of the reference data can then be classified accurately.

The method measures the deviation of the anthropometric measurement from the reference mean or median in terms of standard deviations or Z-scores. The score is a measure of an individual's value with respect to the distribution of the reference population.

The exact values for the Z-score of an individual can be calculated using selected reference standard deviation values for the NCHS/WHO reference population published by WHO (1983); an example is given in Table 13.1. These reference standard deviations have been calculated by transforming the original NCHS reference data. The specific details of this process are given in Dibley et al. (1987). As the distributions of weight-for-age and weight-for-height are not symmetrical, standard deviations below and above the median differ and hence were calculated separately. In contrast, the distribution for height-for-age is symmetrical, so that a single set of age-specific standard deviations was calculated.

As an example, for a boy 69 cm tall, weighing 7.6 kg (Table 13.1) (i.e., with a weight below the reference population median), the Z-score of the individual corresponds to:

$$\frac{\text{wt of subject} - \text{median reference value of wt-for-ht}}{1 \text{ SD below median reference value of wt-for-ht}}$$

$$\text{Z-score of individual} = \frac{7.6 - 8.5}{8.5 - 7.5} = -0.9$$

These calculations can be carried out using computer programs (e.g., EpiInfo 2002). Alternative reference populations can also be

−3SD	−2SD	−1SD	Median	+1SD	+2SD	+3SD
5.6	6.6	7.5	8.5	9.8	11.1	12.4

Table 13.1: A portion of a table showing weight (kg) for height in a reference population at different SD values. The data are for boys 69 cm in height. Note that 1 SD above the median is not the same relative distance from the median as 1 SD below the median. From WHO (1983), with permission.

used such as CDC 2000 (Kuczmarski et al., 2000).

In population studies, the number and the proportion of individuals within a specified range of Z-scores for each age and sex group can be tabulated or presented graphically to provide an estimate of "relative" status, as shown in Figure 13.3 and as noted previously for percentiles. In addition, the proportion of individuals with anthropometric indices below or above some predetermined reference limits based on Z-scores can also be determined. Such reference limits vary; often scores of below −2 are designated as indicating risk of severe malnutrition, whereas scores above +2 are taken to indicate obesity. The proportion of children in the reference population with a Z-score less than −2 is 2.3%. Clearly, if the proportion in the study population with such low Z-scores is significantly greater than this, then the study population is more severely affected.

An important advantage of using Z-scores for population-based applications is that it is valid to calculate the mean and standard deviation for a group of Z-scores. This allows the nutritional status of the entire population to be described. In addition, because the observed Z-scores from a population are

Below mean		Above mean	
Percentile	Z-score	Percentile	Z-score
5.0	−1.645	55.0	0.126
10.0	−1.282	60.0	0.253
15.0	−1.036	65.0	0.385
20.0	−0.842	70.0	0.524
25.0	−0.675	75.0	0.675
30.0	−0.524	80.0	0.842
35.0	−0.385	85.0	1.036
40.0	−0.253	90.0	1.282
45.0	−0.126	95.0	1.645
50.0	−0.000		

Table 13.2: Equivalents of percentile and Z-scores in a normal distribution.

often normally distributed, statistical analytical procedures that assume normality such as *t*-tests and regression methods can be used (Gorstein et al., 1994).

In some circumstances, however, the mean Z-score will not be useful. For example, in some studies of refugees, the death rate among those most severely malnourished can be high and the lower end of the distribution can be truncated: the mean is hardly affected (Yip and Sharp, 1993). In such cases, a comparison of the distribution of indices of the entire population in relation to the reference population, is more useful (Figure 13.3).

If the distribution of the reference values is normal, percentiles and Z-scores are directly related. As shown in Table 13.2, a Z-score of −1.645 corresponds to an observation on the 5th percentile. Conversely, a value that is at the 85th percentile equates to a Z-score of +1.036. The commonly used −3, −2, and −1 Z-scores are the 0.13th, 2.28th, and 15.8th percentiles, respectively.

An easy way to assess whether the distribution is skewed is to compare the values of the mean and the median. For normal distributions the mean and median will be very similar. As the distribution becomes more skewed, the difference between mean and median increases. Several tests are available for testing normality. Examples include the Kolmogorov-Smirnoff and the Cox tests, of which the latter is generally preferred.

The interpretation of reference limits based

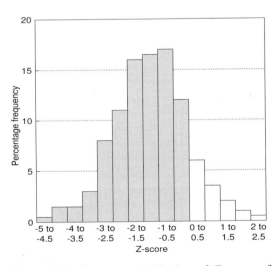

Figure 13.3: Frequency distribution of Z-scores of height-for-age for 1395 children measured during the Sahel nutrition studies and who were 12–23.9 mo. From WHO (1983), with permission.

Characteristic	Z-score	Percentile	Percentage of median
Adherence to reference distribution	Yes	Yes	No
Linear scale permitting summary statistics	Yes	No	Yes
Uniform criteria across all ages and indices	Yes	Yes	No
Useful for detecting changes at extremes of the distributions	Yes	No	Yes

Table 13.3: The characteristics of three anthropometric data-reporting systems. From WHO (1995), with permission.

on percentiles, and Z-scores, is consistent across all ages and indices (Table 13.3). This means that a reference limit of 3rd percentile or –2 Z-scores represents the same degree of malnutrition, irrespective of the anthropometric index used (e.g., weight-for-age or weight-for-height) or the age of the child (Waterlow et al., 1977). Nevertheless, the physiological meaning or consequence of extreme values may differ with age and height.

13.1.3 Percent-of-median

Growth indices can be expressed as percent-of-median value of the reference data when the distribution around the median value is unknown. Percent-of-median is the ratio of a measured anthropometric value (e.g., weight) in the individual, to the median value of the reference data for the same age or height, expressed as a percentage. It is especially useful when the distribution of the reference data has not been normalized, such as the earlier Harvard reference data, and explains why so many of the first classification schemes based on the Harvard reference data (e.g., Gomez and Wellcome classification) used percent-of-median (Gorstein et al., 1994).

Use of percent-of-median does not provide the same information as the Z-score, and the relationship between these two criteria differs

with age and height. Such discrepancies may be especially important if intervention activities are prioritized across populations according to the prevalence of low anthropometric indices. A comparison of selected Z-scores and percent-of-median curves for weight-for-height, height-for-age, and weight-for-age is given in Gorstein et al. (1994).

A further limitation of the percent-of-median is that, unlike percentiles or Z-scores, the interpretation of specific percent-of-median varies across age groups and growth indices. This arises because the calculation of the percent-of-median does not take into account the distribution of the data within the reference set, and particularly the differing widths of the distributions of the weight-for-age, weight-for-height, and height-for-age indices (Waterlow et al., 1977). Indeed, it is this variability that inhibits the universal use of a constant percentage of the reference median (e.g., 70%) across all ages and for all growth indices. For example, 60% of median weight-for-age represents a more severe state of malnutrition for younger than for older children. Moreover, when the index weight-for-height is used, 60% of the median is inappropriate; such a deficit at any age is incompatible with life (Dibley et al., 1987).

The characteristics of the three anthropometric reporting systems—Z-scores, percentiles, and percent-of-median—are compared in Table 13.3. Software can be used to compute percentiles, percent-of-median, and Z-scores for each of the three indices (Fichtner et al., 1989; Sullivan et al., 1990). Of the software available, both the manual and the program for EpiInfo 2002 are in the public domain and may be freely copied, translated, and distributed. Information is available at

http://www.cdc.gov/epiinfo/

13.2 Use of anthropometric indices in clinical settings

Anthropometry in clinical settings has two main applications for individuals: screening for early detection of abnormal changes in growth, and assessing the response of an individual to therapy (WHO, 1995). In both cases, repeated measurements on each child are needed.

13.2.1 Screening to identify abnormal changes in growth

In general, growth measurements in a child should be repeated at 1-mo intervals during the first 6 mo, then every 2–3 mo during later infancy and early childhood, and then every 6–12 mo (Guo et al., 1991). Such serial measurements provide information on the pattern of growth over time. This enables a child with failure to thrive to be identified. Abnormal growth is apparent from the direction of the growth curve: an abnormal height-for-age growth curve is horizontal or, in the case of weight-for-height, moves downwards. The former indicates that the child is not growing, and the latter shows that the child is losing weight.

Figure 13.4 depicts diagrammatically the growth history of a 7-y-old girl who was following a macrobiotic diet, and whose growth, based on stature-for-age, was measured and plotted at least annually on a distance growth chart. Curves for −2 Z-score, the median, and +2 Z-score for the growth reference for stature-for-age are depicted. Growth indices that fall below −2 Z-score or above +2 Z-score are defined as abnormal. In Figure 13.4, the child's height-for-age growth curve fell below the −2 Z-score reference at age 2 y, at which point the curve became nearly horizontal, indicating that the child was growing very, very slowly.

Although changes in a child's growth are apparent on such distance growth charts, abnormal changes in the rate of growth of a child can be detected much earlier when growth velocity charts (Section 12.7), rather than distance growth charts, are used: growth velocity measurements are much more sensitive to recent changes in growth but require careful measurement procedures to be of value.

When a child exhibits deceleration or slow growth of length or height, as shown in the

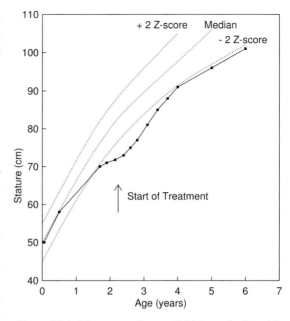

Figure 13.4: Diagrammatic growth history of a 7-y-old girl following a macrobiotic diet.

example given in Figure 13.4, then the child must be evaluated to distinguish between a shifting of linear growth, sometimes termed "rechanneling," constitutional growth delay, and underlying pathology. Any shift in linear growth is determined by genetic influences, and tends to occur within the first 18 mo of life, when the growth of an apparently healthy child may cross one or more Z-score or percentile lines. In contrast, the exact cause of constitutional growth delay is unknown. It occurs later than rechanneling, and is characterized by a temporary delay in skeletal growth and height of a child, and is not accompanied by any other physical abnormalities causing the delay. Alternatively, slow growth can arise from many pathological conditions, such as malnutrition (Figure 13.4), chronic disease (e.g., tuberculosis), non-organic failure to thrive (caused by a severe psychosocial disturbance in the family), or organic disorders. The latter may encompass congenital and acquired disorders, or abnormal function of the endocrine system or metabolism, and gastrointestinal dysfunction (e.g., malabsorption); details are given in WHO (1995).

13.2.2 Assessing response to therapy

Serial measurements are also useful when assessing the response to therapy, as shown in Figure 13.4; again at least two anthropometric measurements are required.

Selection of the indicator of response to the therapy must be made carefully. It must take into account the possible time lag between the start of the intervention and the time when a response is apparent. For example, a wasted infant will respond to a nutrition intervention first by putting on weight and then by "catching" up in linear growth. This will be manifested by an increase in weight-for-length Z-score, followed by an increase in height-for-age Z-score. In the example given in Figure 13.4, the child's stature-for-age growth curve fell below the -2 Z-score reference at 2 y, at which point the curve tended to flatten out, indicating that the child was growing slowly. As a result, the child was enrolled in an intervention program which lasted for 2 y. The catch-up growth in response to therapy is clear, although the child did not approach the -2 Z-score reference until she was age 4 y.

If individuals do not respond to the therapy, then some other medical treatment may be necessary to improve the poor growth, and the earlier therapy should be discontinued.

13.3 Use of anthropometric indices in public health

Anthropometry at the individual level can also be used in the public health setting. However, in public health, it is often not possible to obtain serial measurements. Instead, screening systems are used to identify individuals "at risk" to malnutrition and who may require intervention. Some screening systems are used only in emergency settings, when low-cost portable equipment and the use of trained unskilled personnel are primary considerations. In such circumstances, only one measurement may be taken. All the systems use at least one anthropometric index and one or more reference limits drawn from

appropriate reference data. As an alternative, cutoff points based on functional impairment or clinical signs of deficiency or mortality risk may be used.

An optimal screening system is one in which no misclassification occurs; all the individuals designated as "at risk" are actually malnourished (i.e., there are no false positives; sensitivity is 100%) (Section 1.3). Similarly, those individuals classified as "not at risk" are truly unaffected (i.e., there are no false negatives; specificity is 100%).

In practice, classification schemes are *not* optimal; some misclassification will always occur so that some individuals identified as "at risk" to malnutrition will not be truly malnourished (false positives), and others classified as "not at risk" to malnutrition will in fact be malnourished (false negatives). Unfortunately, specificity and sensitivity data for the anthropometric indices selected are usually not known for the target population. Instead, when selecting a screening system, values for sensitivity and specificity obtained elsewhere are often used and assumed to be appropriate for the target population (Habicht et al., 1979, 1982).

Unfortunately, literature values for sensitivity and specificity are unlikely to apply to the target population when the indices assess an outcome (e.g., low birth weight) which is influenced by several biological factors. For example, low birth weight can be due to both prematurity and intrauterine growth retardation, and its sensitivity as an indicator of neonatal mortality is greater for the former than the latter (WHO, 1995).

A more general way of selecting an optimal screening system is shown in Figure 13.5, which depicts the relationship between the sensitivity and specificity for both height-for-age and weight-for-height in predicting 2-y survival. The position of the Receiver-Operating Characteristic (ROC) curves indicates that, in this case, height-for-age is the better index. Brownie et al. (1986) provide details of statistical methods that can be used to select the best indicator.

In many of the early classification systems, cutoff points were defined as a designated

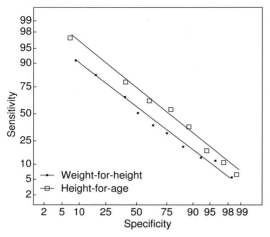

Figure 13.5: Relationship between sensitivity (%) and specificity (%) for height-for-age and weight-for-height in predicting 2-y survival. The Receiver-Operating Characteristic (ROC) Plots have been linearized by the Z-transformation. The linearized height-for-age ROC plot lies above the weight-for-height ROC plot, indicating that the former index generates fewer errors of classification at every level of sensitivity and specificity. From Habicht et al., American Journal of Clinical Nutrition 35: 1241–1245, 1982 © Am J Clin Nutr. American Society for Clinical Nutrition.

percentage of the median of the reference population, for the reason outlined earlier. Now the approach preferred by WHO (1995) is to use reference limits based on Z-scores (WHO, 1995; de Onis et al., 1997; Mei et al., 1997). Examples of screening systems that use this approach, that are based on a single anthropometric index, and that can be used to classify individuals "at risk' to malnutrition are outlined below.

13.3.1 Use of MUAC for children

In the past, mid-upper-arm circumference (MUAC) has been used for screening individual children for targeting interventions if weight and stature measurements are impossible and the precise age of the child is unknown. In such cases, a fixed cutoff point (e.g., 13.5 cm) was used to distinguish normal and malnourished children. Alternatively, a series of cutoff points to classify degrees of malnutrition were defined. Such an approach assumed that MUAC was rela-

tively independent of age for children 1–5 y (Burgess and Burgess, 1969).

More recent studies have questioned this assumption (Ross et al., 1990; Hall et al., 1993; Van den Broeck et al., 1993; Bern and Nathanail, 1995). Data from both affluent and nonaffluent populations show that MUAC is age dependent, resulting in overdiagnosis of wasting among younger children and underdiagnosis among older ones, when a fixed cutoff point is used (de Onis et al., 1997).

Consequently, WHO has developed and now recommend the adoption of MUAC-for-age reference data for children 6–60 mo (Figure 13.6) (Section 12.14.1). The curves show important age-specific differences, as well as significant sex-specific differences for boys and girls < 24 mo.

Several studies have compared the use of a fixed cutoff point with that of MUAC-for-age reference data and noted important sex- and age-related discrepancies. Among Bangladeshi children, use of a fixed cutoff point (i.e., < 12.5 cm) resulted in a markedly higher prevalence of undernutrition among girls than boys aged 12–59 mo, but a much lower prevalence in children aged > 3 y, compared to those for MUAC Z-scores (Hall et al., 1993; Van den Broeck, 1993). In the field, the use of MUAC-for-age reference

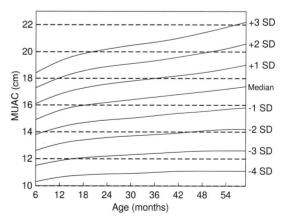

Figure 13.6: Mid-upper-arm circumference (MUAC) for age growth reference curves for boys 6–59 mo. Drawn from full numerical reference data for boys, girls, and sexes combined, given in de Onis et al., Bulletin of the World Health Organization 75: 11–18, 1997, with permission.

Mid-upper-arm circumference			Diagnostic category	BMI		Grade of chronic energy deficiency
Z-score	Men (mm)	Women (mm)		Men	Women	
< -1.0	< 230	< 220	Undernourished	< 17	< 17	3
< -2.0	< 200	< 190	Severe wasting	< 13	< 13	4
< -3.0	< 170	< 160	Extreme wasting	< 10	< 10	5

Table 13.4: A proposed set of mid-upper-arm circumference values for use when screening adults under famine conditions. From Ferro-Luzzi and James, British Journal of Nutrition 75: 3–10, 1996, with permission of the Nutrition Society.

data is no more difficult than using weight-for-height, the conventional index of wasting.

13.3.2 Use of MUAC for adults

The importance of adult malnutrition is becoming increasingly recognized. Both the Food and Agricultural Organization (FAO) and WHO have adopted the body mass index (BMI) to assess adult malnutrition and have defined cutoffs grading the severity of low BMI in adults. However, in emergency situations, measurements of weight and height, required to calculate BMI, are difficult to obtain from severely emaciated individuals who often cannot stand unaided. Therefore, MUAC, a measurement that only requires a tape measure, has been investigated as a substitute for BMI. Significant correlations between measurements of MUAC and BMI have been demonstrated in both normal (James et al., 1994), and severely malnourished adult populations from low-income countries (Collins, 1996). Further, the proportions of the population and the actual individuals identified as malnourished by the two indicators were similar.

Following these investigations, MUAC values corresponding to BMIs of 17, 13, and 10 have been developed for the rapid screening of severely malnourished male and female adults who are in desperate need of supplementary feeding (Ferro-Luzzi and James, 1996). The MUAC cutoff points have been identified from the analyses and extrapolation of anthropometric data based on nine adult surveys from Asia, Africa, and the Pacific. The cutoffs are shown in Table 13.4, together with the corresponding MUAC Z-scores and BMI values.

Note that different cutoffs are used for males and females and to identify malnutrition of varying severity. Severe wasting, grade 4 malnutrition, is identified by a MUAC value equivalent to < -2 Z-score (< 200 mm for men; < 190 mm for women). At this stage, arm fat stores are exhausted, and individuals urgently require food supplements. Wasting is so extreme at grade 5 that there is marked atrophy of both fat and protein stores. This stage is classified by a MUAC value corresponding to < -3 Z-score (i.e., < 170 mm for men; < 160 mm for women). Such individuals will require immediate special feeding regimens to ensure their survival.

Arm circumference during pregnancy has also been investigated as a screening tool for risk of low birth weight and late fetal and infant mortality. Maternal arm circumference is relatively stable during pregnancy, so its measurement is independent of gestational age. Hence, measurement of arm circumference at any time during pregnancy may serve as a useful proxy for prepregnancy weight in situations where these measurements are not available (Krasovec and Anderson, 1991). Ricalde et al. (1998), in a study of 92 pregnant women in São Paulo, Brazil, showed that gestational age, mother's arm circumference, and prepregnancy weight were significant predictors of birth weight.

13.3.3 MUAC-for-height: QUAC stick

The Quaker arm circumference measuring stick (QUAC stick) was developed as a rapid, cheap, and simple screening tool for the nutritional assessment of children. It avoids the use of cumbersome scales and minimizes errors in measuring height (Arnhold, 1969).

The measuring stick is used to compare a child's MUAC with the two reference limits of the MUAC reference data corresponding to the child's height.

The modified QUAC stick developed by WHO uses MUAC-for-height data from the MUAC-for-age reference for children < 5 y (Section 12.14.1) (de Onis et al., 1997; Mei et al., 1997). Three sets of MUAC-for-height curves were developed — one for boys, one for girls, and one for both boys and girls combined. The curves are for children of height 65–145 cm. Recumbent length measurements were adjusted to standing height when the MUAC-for-height reference data were constructed to eliminate any discrepancy caused by differences in the two stature measurements.

Mei et al. (1997) also provide instructions on the construction and use of the modified QUAC stick shown in Figure 13.7 using the new MUAC-for-height reference data. Construction of two sticks, one for the boys and one for girls, is recommended. The WHO-modified QUAC stick consists of a vertical stick, about 150 cm long and 3×3 cm in cross-section. One face is marked from 0 at the bottom up to 145 cm near the top in 0.5 cm increments, as shown in Figure 13.7. On one

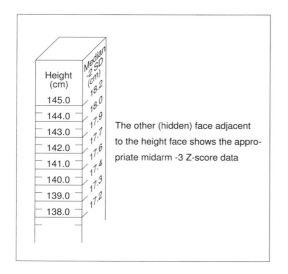

Figure 13.7: The WHO-modified QUAC stick. From Mei et al., Bulletin of the World Health Organization 75: 333–341, 1997, with permission.

adjacent face, the corresponding reference values for the median −2 Z-score of MUAC-for-height are marked; the other face, adjacent to the height measurements, shows the values for median −3 Z-score of the MUAC-for-height.

To use the QUAC stick, it is first placed firmly and upright on a platform against a vertical wall. The child is then asked to stand straight with his or her back against the height measure. Next, the MUAC of the child is measured using the technique described in Section 11.2.1. Then a note is made about whether the value is below that given on the "median −3 Z-score" face at the point on the stick marked by the child's height. If the measurements is below this value, the child is noted as having a severe nutritional deficit; if above and yet still below the appropriate value on the "median −2 Z-score" face, the deficit is recorded as moderate. In this way, all children are identified as having severe, moderate, or no deficit. Note that the method eliminates the necessity of recording both the height and MUAC of the child for subsequent comparison with reference data.

The performance of MUAC-for-height for screening was evaluated using weight-for-age < −2 Z-score as the "gold standard" for identifying malnourished children (Mei et al., 1997). Results indicated that the sensitivity and specificity for MUAC-for-height was better than MUAC based on a fixed cutoff for screening malnourished children 6–59 mo from Sri Lanka, Nepal, Togo, and Malawi.

13.3.4 Weight-for-height wall chart

A wall chart developed by Nabarro and Mc-Nab (1980) is based on weight-for-height and three percentage ranges of the corresponding median weight-for-height of the NCHS reference data. These are 70% − 80%, 80% − 90%, and 90% − 110%. Wasted children are identified as those with a percentage weight-for-height less than 80% of the reference median. The chart has the advantage of visually identifying the extent of wasting in a very simple manner. In addition, during nutritional rehabilitation, a target weight can be readily identified.

The chart is fixed to a smooth wall, and the child is positioned on a level floor against the chart at a point corresponding to the child's weight (Figure 13.8). The top of the child's head will fall into one of three color-coded categories on the chart, equivalent to 70% – 80% (red), 80% – 90% (yellow), and 90% –110% (green) of the expected weight-for-height and representing various degrees of malnutrition. The color should be read off the chart at the point at which the exam-iner's fingers touch the column marked with the child's weight (Figure 13.8).

For small children, two persons may be required to position the child correctly for the measurement. To avoid misclassifying children with edema or ascites (fluid in the abdominal cavity), a brief clinical examina-tion should also be undertaken. The charts

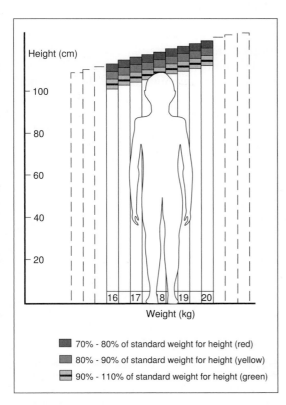

Height (cm)

- 100

- 80

- 60

- 40

- 20

16 17 18 19 20

Weight (kg)

▓ 70% - 80% of standard weight for height (red)
▓ 80% - 90% of standard weight for height (yellow)
▓ 90% - 110% of standard weight for height (green)

Figure 13.8: Weight-for-height wall chart. From Nabarro and McNab, Journal of Tropical Medicine and Hygiene 83: 21–33, 1980, with permission.

can be modified to include different colors, numbers of colors, and alternative reference limits, depending on the resources and needs of the population.

13.3.5 Using combinations of indices for studies of individuals

A combination of two or more anthropo-metric indices can be used to characterize the anthropometric status of an individual in both clinical and public health settings. The growth indices that are generally combined are weight-for-age (for underweight), weight-for-height (for thinness and wasting), and height-for-age (for shortness and stunting); these have been discussed in detail in Sec-tion 10.2. Increasingly, BMI and waist : hip ratio (WHR) or waist circumference are also used as surrogate indicators of obesity and intra-abdominal fat content, respectively (see Sections 10.2.6, 11.1.2, and 11.1.3).

Normally, the growth indices are used in conjunction with the recommended internat-ional (i.e., NCHS/WHO) or local reference data, as noted earlier, to determine "relative" status. BMI, WHR, and waist circumference for adults are generally used with sex-specific cutoffs.

Several important limitations exist when the current NCHS/WHO international growth reference data are used at the individual (and population) level. Of special note is the lim-itation associated with the weight-for-height data. Because of the maximum and minimum height limitations (Section 12.5), weight-for-height cannot be calculated using the NCHS/WHO growth reference curves for some in-fants < 2 mo (minimum height 49 cm), or for girls above about 9 y and boys above 11 y (Table 13.5).

A second limitation is the length-height disjunction at 24 mo in the NCHS/WHO ref-erence growth data (Figure 12.6), discussed in Section 12.4.1. This makes it difficult to estimate height status of a child immedi-ately before and after 24 mo of age, and to track the growth of a child throughout the first 5 y of life. Similar difficulties occur at the population level (Section 13.4). Indeed,

Index	Sex	Age (y) Min.	Age (y) Max.	Height (cm) Min.	Height (cm) Max.
Weight-for-	M	Birth	11.49	49	145
height	F	Birth	9.99	49	137
Weight-for-age	M+F	Birth	17.99	None	None
Height-for-age	M+F	Birth	17.99	None	None

Table 13.5: Age and height limitations for the NCHS/WHO international growth reference curves. There are no weight limitations. From Gorstein et al., Bulletin of the World Health Organization 72: 273–283, 1994, with permission.

the improvement in the age-specific prevalence of low anthropometry that has been observed around the world in children aged ⩾2 y compared to those < 2 y has been attributed, in part, to the disjunction of the NCHS/WHO reference curves (Gorstein et al., 1994).

The NCHS/WHO growth reference data are also not recommended for comparing the nutritional status of a child greater than 10 y because of the marked differences in the age of peak height velocity among populations (Section 12.7) (WHO, 1983).

Ideally, cutoffs for anthropometric indices should be identified on the basis of biological considerations such as an increased risk of mortality or functional impairment, as noted earlier. In practice, however, defining such cutoffs is difficult because the relationship between the indices and mortality or functional impairment cannot be generalized from one region to another. Instead, for the growth indices, statistically derived reference limits are used. For percentiles, these are either below the 3rd or 5th percentiles or above the 95th or 97th percentiles, depending on the reference data. Reference limits used with Z-scores vary; often Z-score of below -2.0 are designated as indicating risk of protein-energy malnutrition, whereas scores above $+2.0$ are taken to indicate risk of obesity.

The use of three growth indices — weight-for-age, weight-for-height, height-for-age — in combination, is especially useful for identifying children at risk of malnutrition and for evaluating a response to an intervention.

Figure 13.9 shows the relation between the classifications of "low," "normal," and "high" for the indices weight-for-age, weight-for-height, and height-for-age using the reference limits at 2 Z-scores above and below the median of the NCHS/WHO reference data; it emphasizes the apparent contradictions that may occur (WHO, 1983).

In this example, for the index height-for-age (horizontal axis), children to the left of -2 Z-score will be classified as short, those to the right of $+2$ Z-score as tall, and those between the two reference limits as normal in height. Likewise, in terms of weight-for-height (indicated on the left vertical axis), children below -2 Z-score are thin and those above $+2$ Z-score obese; those between the two reference limits are normal. The reference limits for weight-for-age run obliquely across those for weight-for-height and height-for-age. Hence, children falling within the lower stippled area have weight-for-age values less than -2 Z-score below the median and are "light," and those within the upper stippled area are "heavy."

The numbered areas shown in Figure 13.9 are different combinations of low, normal,

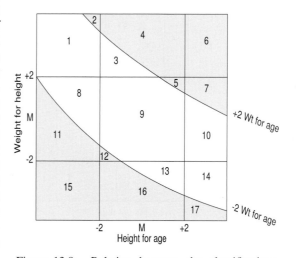

Figure 13.9: Relation between the classifications "low," "normal," and "high" for the indices weight-for-height, height-for-age, and weight-for-age, with reference limits at 2 Z-scores above and below the median. Calculated from the data for 18-mo-old boys in the National Center for Health Statistics (NCHS) reference population. From WHO (1983), with permission.

Nos.	Combination of indices	Nutritional status
16	Low wt/ht + low wt/age + normal ht/age	Currently underfed
17	Low wt/ht + low wt/age + high ht/age	Currently underfed
14	Low wt/ht + normal wt/age + high ht/age	Currently underfed
11	Normal wt/ht + low wt/age + low ht/age	Short, normally nourished
9	Normal wt/ht + normal wt/age + normal ht/age	Normal
7	Normal wt/ht + high wt/age + high ht/age	Tall, normally nourished
1	High wt/ht + normal wt/age + low ht/age	Currently overfed, short
2	High wt/ht + high wt/age + low ht/age	Obese
4	High wt/ht + high wt/age + normal ht/age	Overfed, not necessarily obese

Table 13.6: The results of using various combinations of anthropometric indices and possible interpretations of the results. The numbers in the left hand column are taken from Figure 13.9. From WHO (1983), with permission.

and high for the three indices, examples of which are shown in Table 13.6. From this table it is clear that if low weight-for-age is selected as the index, the children identified will be a mixed group in terms of their nutritional status. Some of the children (e.g., No. 11) will have low weight-for-age as a result of their very short stature, perhaps arising from a history of past malnutrition. In contrast, others (e.g., No. 17) will indeed be currently malnourished with a low weight-for-age and low weight-for-height, even though they have a high height-for-age. These results show the importance of including an index that includes height when screening children for malnutrition.

13.4 Use of anthropometric indices in population studies

Anthropometry has a range of applications at the population level, which have been described in detail by WHO (1995); they are summarized below. Where appropriate, the anthropometric data for children should be presented and analyzed by the age groups recommended by WHO (1983); these are shown in Table 13.7. WHO recommends the use of the NCHS/WHO reference data for all of these applications (Gorstein et al., 1994), until the new WHO international growth standard for children from birth to 5-y is available (Section 12.4.2).

Newborn children, infants and preschool children	0 to < 6 mo 6 to < 12 mo 12 to < 24 mo 24 to < 48 mo 48 to < 72 mo
Primary school children	72 to < 96 mo 96 to < 120 mo

Table 13.7: Suggested age classes or groups for use in the presentation of anthropometric data. Extracted from WHO (1983), with permission.

13.4.1 Targeting interventions

Anthropometry can be used as a screening tool to identify the areas of greatest need (e.g., areas with a high prevalence of stunting or wasting) and, hence, likely to gain the most benefit from any intervention. WHO recognizes the severity of malnutrition in young children < 60 mo for targeting purposes, by classifying the prevalence (as %) of underweight, stunting, and wasting into three levels, as shown in Table 13.8 (Gorstein et al., 1994). This classification is not based on correlations with functional outcomes but reflects a statistical grouping of prevalence levels from different countries (WHO, 1995). Only 2.3% of children in a well-nourished healthy population would be expected to fall below $-2\,Z$-score. This means that even a "low" prevalence of underweight includes communities with up to four times the expected prevalence of the reference popula-

Indicator	Low	% prevalence Medium	High	V.high
Underweight Low wt.-for-age	< 10	10–19.9	20–29.9	⩾ 30
Stunting Low ht.-for-age	< 20	20–29.9	30–39.9	⩾ 40
Wasting Low wt.-for-ht.	< 5	5–9.9	10–14.9	⩾ 15

Table 13.8: Proposed epidemiological criteria for assessing severity of undernutrition in populations of children < 60 mo. Undernutrition is defined as < 2 Z-scores of the median of the reference population. Data from Gorstein et al., Bulletin of the World Health Organization 72: 273–283, 1994, with permission.

tion; at the "medium" level, the prevalence of underweight is up to eight times higher.

Anthropometry can also be used to make decisions about selecting the most appropriate intervention program. For example, in Table 13.9, the prevalence of low anthropometry is compared among four different populations. The results emphasize that for both Côte d'Ivoire and Morocco, the prevalence for both stunting (i.e., height-for-age <–2 Z-score) and wasting (i.e., weight-for-height <–2 Z-score), differs markedly, despite the prevalence of underweight (weight-for-age <–2 Z-score) being similar in both countries. This trend is also apparent for Ethiopia and Burundi. Based on this evaluation of growth indices, intervention activities should first focus on resolving factors associated with wasting in Côte d'Ivoire and

Country and year of survey	Age (mo)	Under-weight	Stunted	Wasted
Côte d'Ivoire (1986)	12–23.9	19.8	19.8	16.5
Morocco (1987)	12–23.9	20.1	31.8	6.4
Ethiopia (1982)	24–35.9	40.2	47.7	12.1
Burundi (1987)	24–35.9	44.9	60.4	3.5

Table 13.9: Comparison of the prevalence of low anthropometry in different populations. Low anthropometry is defined as below –2 Z-scores of the median of the reference population. Data from Gorstein et al., Bulletin of the World Health Organization 72: 273–283, 1994, with permission.

Ethiopia and stunting in Burundi and Morocco (Gorstein et al., 1994).

A high prevalence of wasting often arises as a result of starvation or infectious diseases. In southern Sudan during the 1993 famine, there was a dramatic downward shift of the entire distribution for weight-for-height in relation to the NCHS/WHO reference. In such circumstances, efforts should be made to provide adequate food and to prevent and treat infectious diseases, such as diarrhea and measles (Toole and Waldman, 1990).

In contrast, a high prevalence of stunting is often associated with lower socioeconomic status. Figure 13.10, for example, shows height-for-age Z-scores for Chinese boys in relation the NCHS/WHO reference. This example emphasizes the usefulness of comparing the distribution of anthropometric indices for the entire population, in relation to the reference population, using Z-scores, as well as assessing the prevalence of low anthropometric indices (Table 13.9). Where stunting is prevalent, efforts should be made to increase the availability of food and to improve diet quality. Improvements in hygiene and potable water supplies, as well as the prevention and treatment of infectious diseases, are also important (Gorstein et al., 1994).

When using such a population approach to targeting, then all the children from a high-prevalence group will receive the inter-

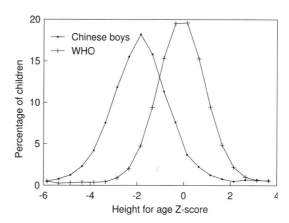

Figure 13.10: Z-score distribution for height-for-age of Chinese boys compared with the NCHS/WHO International reference. From WHO (1995), with permission.

vention, and not just those individuals with anthropometric values below the cutoff, as in the screening approach for individuals.

13.4.2 Assessing response to an intervention

When using anthropometry to evaluate the performance of an intervention at the population level, at least two measurements are required, taken before and after the intervention period. The difference in population mean Z-score of the chosen anthropometric indicator of response is then calculated. Alternatively, the difference in the proportion of the population below the chosen reference limit or cutoff of the indicator is determined. Note that growth velocity data are rarely used in such population studies because, in general, the same children are not examined on both occasions.

The choice of the anthropometric indicator is critical when evaluating the response to an intervention. The choice depends on the type and length of the intervention, the baseline anthropometry, and the study design. The time delay before the indicator can be expected to show evidence of change must also be taken into account. In general, functional indicators are less responsive than biochemical indicators because the latter tend to be more specific measures of nutritional status (Habicht and Pelletier, 1990). The responsiveness of a range of anthropometric and biochemical indicators to supplementary feeding is listed in Habicht et al. (1984).

The relative responsiveness of indicators can be assessed from the ratio d/SD, where d is the expected difference generated by the intervention, and SD is the standard deviation of the measure within the group. Obviously the larger the SD, the less responsive the indicator for a given change. Table 13.10 presents, as an example, the responsiveness of some anthropometric indicators to protein-energy supplementation in children up to 3 y of age. At present, data on the responsiveness of various indicators to different interventions are still limited. More research is needed so

Indicator	Response		
	(d)	SD	d/SD
Attained			
Weight (kg)	0.9	1.3	0.69
Height (cm)	2.3	3.9	0.59
Arm circumference (cm)	0.35	0.9	0.39
Triceps skinfold (mm)	0.15	1.1	0.14
Subscapular skinfold (mm)	0.0	1.1	0.00

Table 13.10: Responsiveness of anthropometric indicators to protein-energy supplementation from birth to 3 y of age. The response is in children who would otherwise have a weight deficit of 4.5 kg at age 3 and who consumed 15% of their energy and 26% of their protein from supplements. From Habicht and Pelletier, Journal of Nutrition 120: 1519–1524, 1990, with permission of The American Society for Nutritional Sciences.

that appropriate indicators for a specific intervention in any given setting can be chosen.

When interpreting the anthropometric data, disjunction in the NCHS/WHO growth reference noted earlier, must also be considered. This disjunction makes it difficult to discriminate between what portion of any apparent improvement in the age-specific prevalence of low anthropometry for children aged < 2 y compared to those aged ⩾ 2 y is attributable to the actual intervention versus the disjunction.

13.4.3 Identifying the determinants and consequences of malnutrition

Anthropometric indices can be used to ascertain both the determinants of malnutrition and its consequences. They are especially useful in extreme and acute situations such as famine, when the causes of very high levels of wasting are severe energy deficits. Such determinants can be confirmed by the rapid response, based on a reduction in the prevalence of low weight-for-height, to re-feeding.

In non-disaster situations, however, the possible causes of low weight-for-height can be more difficult to identify. One approach involves a comparison of wasted and non-wasted children using a cross-sectional or case-control study design. Alternatively, if the prevalence of wasting is low, the use of Z-scores for weight-for-height as a continuous outcome variable is recommended

(WHO, 1995). The same two strategies can also be used to ascertain the determinants of stunting, although the latter is more challenging, because of the long-term and cumulative nature of factors influencing stunting. Instead, intervention studies are best used to identify determinants of stunting, where feasible.

The capacity of an anthropometric indicator to predict the risk of morbidity and mortality has been the subject of much research; it depends on several factors. These include the indicator selected, the specific risk under question, the age of the children, the levels of the anthropometric deficit, and the morbidity and mortality in the study population at baseline. The findings vary according to the study setting. In most non-emergency settings, weight-for-height appears to have the highest predictive value for mortality and is followed by height-for-age, whereas weight-for-age has the poorest predictive value. In contrast, in emergency settings, whether MUAC or weight-for-height performs better at predicting mortality over the short-term is hotly debated (WHO, 1995).

13.4.4 Nutritional surveillance

Nutritional surveillance is defined as:

> the continuous monitoring of the physical status of a population, based on repeated surveys or on data from child health or growth-monitoring programs (WHO, 1995).

A detailed discussion of nutritional surveillance is available in Mason et al. (1984). The indicators of nutritional status used in surveillance may include anthropometric measurements of preschool children, heights (and sometimes also weights) of children at school entry, and the prevalence of low birth weight (i.e., less than 2.5 kg). In addition, infant and child mortality rates, the prevalence of infectious diseases, and certain environmental and socioeconomic data are also used as outcome indicators.

In situations such as famines or refugee crises, the severity of the disaster can be

Classification of severity	Prev. of wasting (% of children < −2 Z-score)	Mean weight-for-height Z-score
Acceptable	< 5	> −0.40
Poor	5–9	−0.40 to −0.69
Serious	10–14	−0.70 to −0.99
Critical	≥ 15	≤ −1.0

Table 13.11: Severity index for malnutrition in emergency situations based on prevalence of wasting and mean weight-for-height Z-score for children under 5 y. From WHO (1995), with permission.

assessed by conducting a rapid survey to estimate the prevalence of low weight-for-height (i.e. < −2 Z-scores) among children younger than 5 y of age. When the prevalence of low weight-for-height exceeds 5% in most preschool populations, with the exception of Southern Asia, then mortality appears to increase. As a result, WHO (1995) has classified the severity of malnutrition in emergency situations based on the prevalence of wasting and the mean weight-for-height Z-score for children younger than 5 y, as shown in Table 13.11.

In the future, MUAC-for-age or MUAC-for-height may be used, particularly in settings where it is difficult to assess the age of the children. More research on the performance of these two indicators in emergency situations is warranted.

13.5 Summary

At the individual level, anthropometry can be used in both clinical and public health settings for screening and assessing response to an intervention. In such cases, the anthropometric index can be compared to the reference population using percentiles or Z-scores derived from the reference data. In industrialized countries, percentiles are generally used, whereas in low-income countries, use of Z-scores is preferred.

In clinical practice, a series of measurements can be performed on an individual, allowing abnormal changes in growth, or a response to an intervention, to be detected. In some cases, stature percentiles of individual children can be adjusted for parental stature, or prematurity.

In public health, serial growth measurements are usually not possible. As an alternative, screening systems are used, to identify individuals at risk for malnutrition. All systems use at least one anthropometric index with its associated reference limit(s) or cut-off point(s) to identify individuals "at risk" to malnutrition, and, in some cases, identify the type and severity of malnutrition. The simplest use a single growth index associated with a single reference limit, based on a Z-score of the reference data. Those developed for field survey use include MUAC-for-age (for children), MUAC (for adults), MUAC-for-height (QUAC stick), and a wall chart showing weight-for-height. The early classification systems based on weight-for-age (as percent-of-median), and the Harvard growth data should no longer be used.

In population studies, the distribution of the anthropometric indices can be evaluated using either percentiles or Z-scores calculated from appropriate reference data. In addition, because the observed Z-scores from a population are generally normally distributed, statistical analytical procedures that assume normality such as t-tests and regression methods can be used. As well, the proportion of individuals with growth indices below predetermined reference limits, based on percentiles (< 3rd or 5th and > 97th, 95th), or Z-scores (< –2 Z-scores or > +2 Z-scores) can also be determined. Use of reference limits based on percentiles and Z-scores is preferred, because unlike percent-of-median, their interpretation is consistent across all ages and growth indices.

Of the anthropometric indices, weight-for-height (for thinness and wasting), height-for-age (for shortness and stunting), weight-for-age (for underweight), and BMI-for-age (for overweight, obesity, and thinness) are used for children. Criteria for assessing severity of undernutrition in population studies of children < 5 y are available, based on < 2 Z-scores for underweight, stunting, and wasting.

References

Arnhold R. (1969). The arm circumference as a public health index of protein-calorie malnutrition of early childhood. The QUAC stick: a field measure used by the Quaker Service team in Nigeria. Journal of Tropical Pediatrics 15: 243–247.

Bern C, Nathanail L. (1995). Is mid-upper-arm circumference a useful tool for screening in emergency settings? Lancet 345: 631–633.

Brownie C, Habicht J-P, Cogill B. (1986). Comparing indicators of health or nutritional status. American Journal of Epidemiology 124: 1031–1044.

Burgess HJL, Burgess AP. (1969). A modified standard for mid upper arm circumference in young children. Journal of Tropical Pediatrics 15: 189–192.

Collins S. (1996). Using middle upper arm circumference to assess severe adult malnutrition during famine. Journal of the American Medical Association 276: 391–395.

de Onis M, Yip R, Mei Z. (1997). The development of MUAC-for-age reference data recommended by a WHO Expert Committee. Bulletin of the World Health Organization 75: 11–18.

Dibley MJ, Goldsby JB, Staehling NW, Trowbridge FL. (1987). Development of normalized curves for the international growth reference: historical and technical considerations. American Journal of Clinical Nutrition 46: 736–748.

Ferro-Luzzi A, James WPT. (1996). Adult malnutrition: simple assessment techniques for use in emergencies. British Journal of Nutrition 75: 3–10.

Fichtner RR, Sullivan KM, Trowbridge FL, Carlson B. (1989). Report of the technical meeting on software for nutritional surveillance. Food and Nutrition Bulletin 11: 57–61.

Gorstein J, Sullivan K, Yip R, de Onis M, Trowbridge F, Fajans P, Clugston G. (1994). Issues in the assessment of nutritional status using anthropometry. Bulletin of the World Health Organization 72: 273–283.

Guo SM, Roche AF, Fomon SJ, Nelson SE, Chumlea WC, Rogers RR, Baumgartner RN, Ziegler EE, Siervogel RM. (1991). Reference data on gains in weight and length during the first two years of life. Journal of Pediatrics 119: 355–362.

Habicht J-P, Pelletier DL. (1990). The importance of context in choosing nutrition indicators. Journal of Nutrition 120: 1519–1524.

Habicht J-P, Yarbrough C, Martorell R. (1979). Anthropometric field methods: criteria for selection. In: Jelliffe DG, Jelliffe EFP (eds.) Human Nutrition. Vol. II: Nutrition and Growth. Plenum Press, New York, pp. 365–387.

Habicht J-P. Meyers LD, Brownie C. (1982). Indicators for identifying and counting the improperly nourished. American Journal of Clinical Nutrition 35: 1241–1254.

Habicht J-P, Mason JB, Tabatabi H. (1984). Basic concepts for the design of evaluation during program implementation. In: Shan DE, Lockwood R,

Scrimshaw NS (eds.) Methods for the Evaluation of the Impact of Food and Nutrition Programmes. United Nations University, Tokyo, Japan.

Hall G, Chowdhury S, Bloem M. (1993). Use of mid-upper-arm circumference Z-scores in nutritional assessment. Lancet 341: 1481.

Himes JH, Roche AF, Thissen D, Moore WM. (1985). Parent-specific adjustments for evaluation of recumbent length and stature of children. Pediatrics 75: 304–314.

James WP, Mascie-Taylor GC, Norgan NG, Bistrian B, Shetty PS, Ferro-Luzzi A. (1994). The value of arm circumference measurements in assessing chronic energy deficiency in Third World adults. European Journal of Clinical Nutrition 48: 883–894.

Krasovec K, Anderson MA. (eds). (1991). Maternal nutrition and pregnancy outcomes: anthropometric assessment. Scientific Publication No. 529. Pan American Health Organization, Washington, DC.

Kuczmarski RJ, Ogden CL, Grummer-Strawn LM, Flegal KM, Guo SS, Wei R, Mei Z, Curtin LR, Roche AF, Johnson CL. (2000a). CDC Growth Charts: United States. Advance Data 314: 1–27.

Mason JB, Habicht J-P, Tabatbai H, Valverde V. (1984). Nutritional Surveillance. World Health Organization, Geneva.

Mei Z, Grummer-Strawn LM, de Onis M, Yip R. (1997). The development of a MUAC-for-height reference, including a comparison to other nutritional status screening indicators. Bulletin of the World Health Organization 75: 333–341.

Nabarro D, McNab S. (1980). A simple new technique for identifying thin children. Journal of Tropical Medicine and Hygiene 83: 21–33.

Ricalde AE, Velasquez-Melendez G, Tanaka AC, de Siqueira AA. (1998). Mid-upper-arm circumference in pregnant women and its relation to birth weight. Revista de Saude Publica 32: 112–117.

Ross DA, Taylor N, Hayes R, McLean M. (1990). Measuring malnutrition in famines: are weight-for-height and arm circumferences interchangeable? International Journal of Epidemiology 19: 636–645.

Sullivan KM, Gorstein J, Dean AM, Fichtner R. (1990). Use and availability of anthropometry software. Food and Nutrition Bulletin 12: 116–119.

Toole MJ, Waldman RJ. (1990). Prevention of excess mortality in refugee and displaced populations in developing countries. Journal of the American Medical Association 263: 3295–3302.

Van den Broeck J, Eeckels R, Vuylsteke J. (1993). Influence of nutritional status on child mortality in rural Zaire. Lancet 341: 1491–1495.

Waterlow JC, Buzina R, Keller W, Lane JM, Nichaman MZ, Tanner JM. (1977). The presentation and use of height and weight data for comparing the nutritional status of groups of children under the age of 10 years. Bulletin of the World Health Organization 55: 489–498.

WHO (World Health Organization). (1983). Measuring Change in Nutritional Status: Guidelines for Assessing the Nutritional Impact of Supplementary Feeding Programmes for Vulnerable Groups. World Health Organization, Geneva.

WHO (World Health Organization). (1986). Use and interpretation of anthropometric indicators of nutritional status. Bulletin of the World Health Organization 64: 929–941.

WHO (World Health Organization). (1995). Physical Status: The Use and Interpretation of Anthropometry. Report of a WHO Expert Committee. WHO Technical Report Series No. 854. World Health Organization, Geneva. 452pp.

Yip R, Sharp TW. (1993). Acute malnutrition and high childhood mortality related to diarrhea. Lessons from the 1991 Kurdish refugee crisis. Journal of the American Medical Association 270: 587–590.

14

Laboratory assessment of body composition

As the human body is a complex unit, it is normal to use a simplified model to represent its composition: two- or four-compartment models are most commonly used. The two-compartment model assumes that the total body mass is composed of two major molecular compartments: body fat and the fat-free mass. The four-compartment model divides the body into four molecular fractions — minerals, water, protein, and fat — all of which can now be determined in vivo. Wang et al. (1995) have formally proposed that the body can be divided not only on a four-compartment molecular basis but also according to parallel elemental, cellular, and functional frameworks. This scheme has become accepted and is shown in Figure 14.1.

Accurate methods for measuring specific components of body composition are necessary to assess the effects of nutritional deprivation and intervention on body composition. Such information is also important to establish the appropriate prognosis and treatment of hospital patients.

Selection of a method to measure body composition depends on the required precision and accuracy, the study objective, cost, convenience to the subject and their health, and equipment and technical expertise needed (Lukaski, 1987). Methods based on the determination of components of body composition indirectly from elemental analysis minimize assumptions related to tissue density, hydration, and structure. This is important because in malnourished individuals and subjects with metabolic disturbances, the relative propor-

tions of the body components may be altered, and losses of protein and fat may occur, often in association with the rapid accumulation of water. Changes such as these invalidate the determination of fat and the fat-free mass in the two-compartment model. Therefore, in such circumstances, the four-compartment model must be used.

It is not possible to validate measurements of body composition with an absolute standard based on results of direct chemical anal-

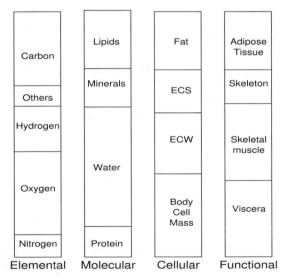

Figure 14.1: Multi compartment models of body composition based on an elemental, molecular, cellular, or functional framework. "Others" includes Ca, P, K, Na, and the trace elements; ECS, extracellular solids; ECW, extracellular water; "viscera" includes all the visceral organs and residua. Compiled from Wang et al. (1992, 1993, 1995).

353

ysis on the same subject. Instead, relative validity is estimated by comparing results with those obtained on the same subject using alternative, indirect methods. The following sections describe the individual procedures used to assess body composition and the assumptions of these methods.

14.1 Chemical analysis of cadavers

Studies of body composition by direct chemical analysis of human cadavers are limited. Most of the cadavers were analyzed between 1945 and 1968 and were adults of varying ages who had died as a result of illness; hence, the values obtained may not be representative of an average healthy adult. Table 14.1 presents data on the contribution of water and protein to the fat-free mass of six adult cadavers, compiled by Garrow (1983). The fat-free tissues of the cadavers were of a relatively constant composition, containing about 72% water and about 20% protein; the potassium content was also relatively constant (about 69 mmol/kg). In contrast, the amount of fat was very variable (data not shown), ranging from 4.3% to 27.9% of body weight in the six cadavers.

14.2 Total body potassium using ^{40}K

Potassium occurs almost exclusively as an intracellular cation, primarily in the muscle and

Sex (y)	Water (g/kg)	Protein (g/kg)	Density (kg/m^3)	Potassium (mmol/kg)
Male (25)	728	195	1120	71.5
Male (35)	775	165	1083	–
Female (42)	733	192	1103	73.0
Male (46)	674	234	1131	66.5
Male (48)	730	206	1099	–
Male (60)	704	238	1104	66.6
Mean	724	205	1106	69.4
SD	34	28	17	3.3

Table 14.1: The contribution of water and protein to the fat-free weights of six adults. From Garrow, Nutrition Abstracts and Reviews 53: 697–708, 1983, with permission.

viscera. Negligible amounts occur in extracellular fluid, bone, and other noncellular sites. Measurement of total body potassium is therefore used as a marker for the body cell mass and also as an index of the fat-free mass in healthy subjects, on the assumption that the fat-free mass has a constant proportion of potassium.

A constant fraction (0.012%) of potassium exists in the body as the isotope ^{40}K (half-life = 1.3×10^9 years). This isotope emits a high-energy γ-ray of 1.46 MeV, allowing the amount of potassium in the body to be estimated by counting with a whole body γ-spectrometer using sodium iodide detectors (Forbes et al., 1961). The isotope occurs in low concentrations so that the background counts from external radiation (cosmic rays and local sources of ionizing radiation) must be minimized. Hence, the whole body counter must be shielded from the background radiation with lead, steel, or concrete shielding. Counting times of at least 15 min are normally required for adults, with proportionately longer times for children and infants. Such times may be a problem for ill patients.

Calibration of the whole body counter must be done carefully because the ^{40}K count detected by the whole body counter is a function of the total body potassium concentration, the geometric configuration of the subject, and internal absorption of the 1.46 MeV by the subject. As a result, the counter must be calibrated to allow for differences in the body build of the subjects. Hansen and Allen (1996) achieved this by using a phantom (also termed a mannequin) containing a known amount of potassium (as KCl solution) and gender-specific correction factors for weight and height. These authors reported CVs of 1.5% for precision and 4.5% for accuracy for measurements on adults. However, the accuracy of the method has not been confirmed by the analysis of human cadavers.

The original factor used for converting the total body potassium content into the fat-free mass (i.e., 69.4 mmol K per kg fat-free mass) was derived from cadaver analysis. However, a single value for all subjects is now known to be inappropriate because the potassium concentration of fat-free tissue tends to decrease with age and is lower in women than in men (Pierson et al., 1974). The potassium concentration of the fat-free mass also appears to increase with muscular development and to decline with obesity (Womersley et al., 1976). However, in obese subjects, some of the decrease may be explained by the lower proportion of muscle in the fat-free mass and by a measurement error resulting from absorption of the γ-rays by adipose tissue. Clearly, if appropriate constants for the potassium concentration of the fat-free mass of muscular, obese, and older individuals are not used, the estimates of fat-free mass derived from ^{40}K measurements will be in error. The latter may be as much as 20%.

Once the fat-free mass is determined, total body fat can be derived indirectly as the difference between total body weight and the fat-free mass, based on a simple two-compartment model. This indirect approach is not recommended, however. Relatively small errors in the fat-free mass generate much larger errors in the much smaller total percentage of body fat when the latter is derived by difference in this way. In particular, this difference method should not be used to derive total body fat for patients with a wasting disease such as cancer (Cohn et al., 1981a), because total body potassium measurements are low in these patients as a result of loss of muscle mass. Hence, in these patients, total body fat derived indirectly as the difference between body weight and the fat-free mass will always be overestimated.

14.3 Total body water using isotope dilution

Body fat contains essentially no water; all the body water is present in the fat-free mass. In healthy adults, the latter contains about 73% water (Kotler et al., 1999).

Total body water can be measured in both healthy and diseased persons using isotope dilution techniques. Deuterium (^{2}H) and tritium (^{3}H) and the stable isotope of oxygen (^{18}O) can be used. Standardized conditions are necessary for the measurement because fluid and food intake and exercise can all affect total body water concentrations. As a result, the samples should be taken in the morning, after an overnight fast, with restriction of fluid intake, and after the bladder has been emptied. A tracer dose of sterile water labeled with an accurately weighed amount of ^{2}H, ^{3}H, or ^{18}O is administered either orally or intravenously to the subject and allowed to equilibrate. No food or water is permitted during equilibration, which may take 2–6 h, depending on the isotope used, the sample form, and the health condition of the patient. Longer equilibration periods are necessary if urine samples are used and for obese patients (Schoeller et al., 1980), or for those with edema, ascites, and shock (McMurrey et al., 1958). Two samples (serum, saliva, urine, or breath) are collected, both prior to the administration of the tracer and at the end of the equilibration period, and total body water is calculated from the dilution observed. Table 14.2 demonstrates that the method is relatively robust and, after equilibration, independent of the different physiological fluids used.

The calculation of total body water is based on the extent to which the isotopic dose is di-

Samples (A) and (B)	Isotope	n	$\dfrac{TBW_A}{TBW_B}$	SD
(A) Saliva at 4 h (B) Serum at 4 h	^{18}O	33	1.006	±0.019
(A) Urine at 6 h (B) Serum at 6 h	^{18}O	11	1.012	±0.027
(A) Urine at 12 h (B) Serum at 12 h	^{18}O	14	1.006	±0.010
(A) Saliva at 3 h (B) Saliva at 4 h	^{18}O	20	0.997	±0.005
(A) Saliva at 3 h (B) Saliva at 4 h	^{2}H	43	0.996	±0.007

Table 14.2: A demonstration of the relatively small variations in total body water, when calculated from isotopic enrichments of different physiological fluids and at different times postdose. From Schoeller et al., 1985 © Ross Laboratories, with permission.

luted by the total body fluid:

$$\text{total body water} = (V \times C) / (C_2 - C_1)$$

where V = volume of dose, C = concentration of administered isotope, C_1 = baseline concentration of isotope in serum/urine/breath, and C_2 = concentration of isotope in serum/urine/breath sample after equilibration. A correction may be necessary for urinary loss of the tracer. Substances or tracers used to measure total body water should:

- Be present only in body water
- Equilibrate rapidly and thoroughly with the body water
- Not be metabolized or excreted
- Be nontoxic in the amounts used
- Not alter normal physiological processes or homeostatic mechanisms

The isotopic tracer chosen and the method used for analysis are interrelated. Tritium (^{3}H) is easy to measure by scintillation counting but involves radiation to the subject, making the technique unsuitable for children and women of childbearing age (Schoeller et al., 1980), and when repeated measurements over a short time period are necessary. The non-radioactive isotope ^{18}O must be measured by mass spectrometry. The stable isotope ^{2}H can be measured by infrared absorption, gas chromatography, or mass spectrometry; details of these methods have been reviewed by Schoeller (1991). The isotope of oxygen (^{18}O) appears to be the tracer of choice, but its use may be limited by the high cost and need for a mass spectrometer for the analysis.

After measuring total body water, the fat-free mass can be estimated:

$$\text{fat-free mass (kg)} = (\text{total body water (kg)}) / 0.732$$

Once the fat-free mass has been determined, total body fat (TBF) and percentage of body fat can be calculated by difference:

$$\text{TBF (kg)} = \text{body weight (kg)} - \text{fat-free mass (kg)}$$
$$\% \text{ body fat} = (\text{TBF (kg)} \times 100) / \text{body weight (kg)}$$

The error associated with the measurement of total body water using these isotopic tracers is typically less than 1 kg. This error equates to an uncertainty of about 10% (about 1.4 kg) in the absolute fat mass of an average adult or 2% in the estimate of percentage of fat. These relatively low errors have resulted in the isotope dilution method becoming the reference or gold-standard method in comparison with other measurement procedures for total body water.

The major limitations of the total body water method for estimating fat-free mass are the assumptions that the fat-free mass of an adult contains a constant percentage of water and that the total body water content is independent of the fat content of the body (Sheng and Huggins, 1979). Chemical analysis of human cadavers has shown that the actual total body water content of the fat-free mass body compartment can vary from 67% to 77% (Table 14.1). These cadavers were not normal healthy subjects, and the degree to which their illnesses may have affected total body water is unknown. Furthermore, the water content of the fat-free tissue has been shown to be relatively higher in obese and pregnant subjects. Consequently, if the usual equation is applied in obese and pregnant individuals, fat-free mass will be overestimated, and body fat will be underestimated. In pregnant women, for example, the estimate of fat mass may be underestimated by as much as 1–2 kg (van Raaij et al., 1988). Special equations have been developed for estimating body fat mass from total body water, which will result in more valid estimates of maternal body fat mass during pregnancy (van Raaij et al., 1988). These equations are shown in Table 14.3. Likewise, for patients with wasting disease, the hydration constant is also increased because of loss of body tissue and the accumulation of extracellular fluid, so the estimate of fat will be too low. Hence, measurement of total body water to estimate total body fat indirectly is not an appropriate method for obese persons and patients with wasting disease; the revised equations of van Raaij et al. (1988) should be used for pregnant women. Details of the limitations of the isotope dilution method for measuring total body water in the field have been summarized by Ellis (2001).

Subject	Equation
Nonpregnant adult female	
	$W_{FM} = W_B - (TBW/0.724)$
No edema or leg edema only	
10 wk gestation	$W_{FM} = W_B - (TBW/0.725)$
20 wk gestation	$W_{FM} = W_B - (TBW/0.732)$
30 wk gestation	$W_{FM} = W_B - (TBW/0.740)$
40 wk gestation	$W_{FM} = W_B - (TBW/0.750)$
Generalized edema	
10 wk gestation	$W_{FM} = W_B - (TBW/0.725)$
20 wk gestation	$W_{FM} = W_B - (TBW/0.734)$
30 wk gestation	$W_{FM} = W_B - (TBW/0.748)$
40 wk gestation	$W_{FM} = W_B - (TBW/0.765)$

Table 14.3: Equations for estimating body fat mass (W_{FM}) during pregnancy from total body water and body weight (W_B). The equations assume that the fraction of water in the fat-free mass is normally 0.724. From van Raaij et al., American Journal of Clinical Nutrition 48: 24–29, 1988 © Am J Clin Nutr. American Society for Clinical Nutrition.

14.4 Other body fluid compartments and isotope dilution

The isotope dilution principle can be used to estimate the volume of various other body fluid compartments, which, in turn, can be used to derive estimates of two components of the fat-free mass (FFM): extracellular mass (ECM) and the body cell mass (BCM). The ECM is defined as the component of the fat-free mass which exists outside the cells. It consists of both fluid (e.g., extracellular fluids, plasma volume) and solid (e.g., skeleton, cartilage, tendons) components which are involved in transport and support and are not metabolically active. The BCM represents the metabolically active, energy-exchanging mass of the body. Measurements of ECM and BCM are especially critical in malnourished patients. Although values for fat-free mass in these patients may remain unchanged, the composition of the fat-free mass is abnormal. Malnutrition results in a reduced body cell mass, concomitant with an expansion of the extracellular mass. These changes are shown in Figure 14.2. Hence, any loss in

body weight in such patients reflects a loss of body fat (Shizgal, 1987).

A dilution technique involving the simultaneous intravenous injection of ^{22}Na and tritiated water has been developed to measure body cell mass, extracellular mass, and body fat (Shizgal, 1985). Body fat is estimated indirectly from total body water, as described in Section 14.3. Body cell mass is derived from total exchangeable potassium (K_e), which, in turn, is determined indirectly from the relationship:

$$K_e = TBW \times R - Na_e$$

where R = the sum of the sodium and potassium content of a sample of whole blood, divided by its water content, and Na_e = total exchangeable sodium (Shizgal et al., 1977). Total exchangeable potassium is not determined directly from ^{42}K because of the short half-life of this isotope (12.5 h). The BCM is then estimated using the following relationship (Moore et al., 1963):

$$BCM (kg) = 0.00833 \times K_e$$

Total exchangeable sodium (Na_e), measured using ^{22}Na, provides a measure of the fluid, but not the solid, component of the extra-

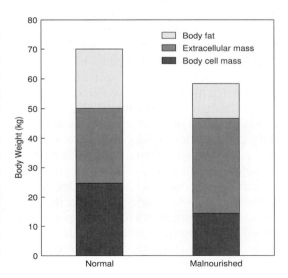

Figure 14.2: The mean body composition of 25 normally nourished healthy volunteers and 75 malnourished patients. From Shizgal, Surgery, Gynecology & Obstetrics 152: 22–26, 1981, with permission.

cellular mass. The total extracellular mass can be calculated, however, from the difference between the FFM (determined via total body water) and the BCM:

$$ECM (kg) = FFM (kg) - BCM (kg)$$

Finally, body fat can be determined as the difference between body weight and the FFM, as discussed earlier. The total radiation exposure from the injected isotopes using this dual isotope procedure is approximately 2.4 mSv (240 mrem) (Shizgal, 1987). This technique can be applied to patients with malnutrition and cancer to evaluate their response to nutritional therapy.

14.5 In vivo activation analysis

A group of related techniques involving in vivo neutron activation analysis (NAA) allow the direct estimation of the amount of a range of chemical elements in the living human body. Most other techniques used in body composition studies, with the exception of whole body counting for potassium, but including bioelectrical impedance and conductance methods, magnetic resonance imaging, computed tomography, and dual-energy X-ray absorptiometry, generate data on tissue density or volume, but not data on the chemical composition. As a result, multi-compartment elemental models based on in vivo NAA have gradually become accepted as reference models for the calibration of the other techniques described here.

Nearly all the major elements present in the body can be analyzed by in vivo NAA, including hydrogen, oxygen, carbon, nitrogen, calcium, phosphorus, sodium, and chlorine. In addition, procedures have been developed to measure in vivo some other specific elements that become concentrated in particular organs in the body. Examples include cadmium, mercury, and iodine. However, the technical difficulties associated with the determination of some of these elements are significant, and at present the method is most commonly used in clinical medicine for the determination of total body calcium (TBCa)

and total body nitrogen (TBN), as discussed below. Even these two elements are only determined in a relatively small number of laboratories worldwide — an indication of the expense involved and technical difficulties associated with the method.

A major negative factor associated with in vivo NAA is that the subject is exposed to radiation. This and the associated risks must always be explained to the subject. At present, the exposure during a session to determine total body nitrogen is about 0.3 mSv. The dose when determining calcium is significantly higher. However, this compares with the natural background radiation from cosmic and other sources of about 3.5 mSv/y.

14.5.1 Total body nitrogen by in vivo NAA

Nitrogen is normally determined by NAA by bombarding the patient, in a supine position, with a low neutron flux from ^{238}PuBe sources or from a cyclotron or neutron generator. During irradiation, a proportion of ^{14}N is converted to an excited state of ^{15}N, which decays almost immediately to its ground state, emitting a "prompt" γ-ray at 10.83 MeV. This activity is counted by an array of sodium iodide detectors in a whole body counter (Figure 14.3). The detected γ-ray counts are proportional to the absolute mass of total body nitrogen (Beddoe and Hill, 1985). Measurement of the nitrogen content of the body gives a measure of total body protein because the mass of nitrogen bears a fixed ratio to the mass of protein (1 g N : 6.25 g protein).

The 10.83 MeV γ-ray is specific to nitrogen and is at an energy which is not affected by interference from other reactions. Extensive shielding, however, is necessary around the sodium iodide detectors to reduce the level of background radiation. Nevertheless, corrections to the γ-spectra must still be made for background counts.

The calibration of the counter is critical and must take into account the height, weight, and adiposity of the subject because of the varying neutron attenuation and internal absorption of the emitted γ-rays. Normally

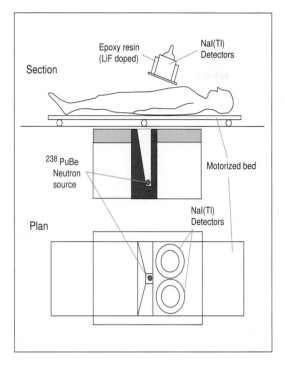

Figure 14.3: In vivo γ-neutron activation. From Cohn et al., 1981b © Ross Laboratories, with permission.

calibration is achieved using phantoms. Vartsky et al. (1979) have described an alternative procedure in which hydrogen is used as an internal standard. Hydrogen is present in almost uniform concentrations in all soft tissues except bone and fat. By obtaining simultaneously an independent measurement of total body hydrogen, the ratio of nitrogen to hydrogen can be calculated. The mass of nitrogen can be derived from the N : H ratio and the known ratio of hydrogen to body weight.

The accuracy of prompt γ-neutron activation for measuring total body nitrogen has been validated by comparing total body nitrogen in two human cadavers with results obtained by direct chemical analysis of nitrogen (Knight et al., 1986). Close agreement between the two techniques was found. This study also confirmed the use of the ratio 6.25 for the relationship between total body protein and total body nitrogen.

Changes in total body protein of hospital patients with diseases such as cancer, renal dysfunction, hypertension, chronic heart disease, rheumatoid arthritis, and anorexia nervosa have been studied using prompt gamma neutron activation (Beddoe and Hill, 1985). Investigators have also used this technique to monitor body composition changes in critically ill patients with severe trauma or sepsis prior to, and following, intravenous feeding (Beddoe and Hill, 1985). The results indicate that substantial losses of body protein may occur in critically ill patients, even when conventionally adequate nutritional support is provided. Further work is required to identify nutritional intervention procedures which minimize loss of body protein.

Prompt γ-neutron activation can also be used to simultaneously measure total body calcium, phosphorus, sodium, and chlorine (Cohn et al., 1984).

14.5.2 Total body calcium by in vivo NAA

The assessment of total body calcium by in vivo neutron activation analysis is discussed in Section 23.1.12 under the assessment of calcium status. The method is based on the conversion of a proportion of the naturally occurring isotope ^{48}Ca in the body to ^{49}Ca (half-life = 8.8 min) by exposing the patient to a low neutron flux. Immediately following irradiation, the patient is transferred to a whole body counter, and the gamma rays emitted by the decay of ^{49}Ca are detected by an array of sodium iodide detectors. The counting geometry is similar to that used for total body potassium, and again care must be taken in positioning the subject and correctly accounting for the varying height, weight, sex, and body mass index of subjects. In particular, for subjects with BMI > 30, the effects of neutron attenuation become significant, necessitating additional corrections or a special calibration (Ma et al., 2000).

14.6 Densitometry

Body density was one of the first measures of body composition to be made (Behnke et al.,

1942). It is relatively easy to measure and is widely used. For these reasons, in the past it has been regarded as the gold-standard method when used to determine body fat, even when the calculation is based on a simple two-component model. However, the calculation makes the assumption that both components, body fat and the fat-free mass, are uniform in density. This is clearly not the case for the fat-free mass. As a result, densitometry is now often combined with other measures, such as isotope dilution or dual-energy X-ray absorptiometry. Three- and four-component models can then used to make an assessment of body fat (Fields and Goran, 2000).

Although hydrostatic weighing was the initial densitometric method described for the determination of body volume, and hence body density, this is now being replaced by two plethysmographic methods that are more acceptable to subjects and in particular, to children (Fields and Goran, 2000). All three methods are described below. A concluding section describes the calculation of body fat from body density (Section 14.6.4).

14.6.1 Hydrostatic weighing

The conventional method of directly measuring whole body density involves weighing the subject and then using Archimedes' principle to determine the volume of the subject. Thus, the subject is weighed first in air and then when completely submerged in water in a large tank. The subject is instructed to squeeze out any air bubbles trapped inside the bathing suit, and to expel as much air as possible from the lungs before immersion. The hydrostatic weight is recorded at the end of the forced expiration. Multiple readings should be taken using a continuous and sensitive recording of underwater mass, the heaviest corresponding to the most complete expiration. This requires a high degree of water confidence and thus the method is not suitable for children younger than 8 y, the elderly, obese, or unhealthy persons.

The body volume is then calculated from the apparent loss of weight in water (i.e., the difference between the weight of the person in air and his or her corresponding weight in water). Once total body mass and body volume have been determined, body density can be readily calculated, on the basis that density is mass per unit volume and the density of water is 1.0 kg/L at 4°C:

$$\text{body density} = \frac{\text{body weight in air (kg)}}{\text{apparent loss in weight (kg)}}$$

Three corrections must be applied:

- Hydrostatic weighing is usually performed in water at 30°C instead of 4°C. At this higher temperature, the density of water is 0.9957 kg/L, and a water temperature correction factor must be applied.
- Air trapped in the lungs also contributes to the amount of water displaced by the subject under water. Residual air in the lungs can be measured while the subject is in the tank. Alternatively, the volume can be estimated using a nitrogen washout, helium dilution, or oxygen dilution (Brodie, 1988). This correction can also be estimated from empirical equations. The residual air volume is then subtracted from the body volume.
- The volume of the air trapped in the gastrointestinal tract also contributes to the total amount of water displaced. This volume is small and is never measured. It is often taken as 100 mL. The within subject variability in gastrointestinal gas volume, however, can be quite large (0 to 500 mL in adults), reducing the precision of the method.

Even when these corrections are carefully applied, considerable uncertainty remains. If the body density is used to calculate the percentage of body fat (see below), these uncertainties become errors in the percentage of body fat. The errors may be systematic rather than random in nature and may be large when the residual air volume is estimated. If the residual air volume is in error by 300 to 500 mL, there will be a corresponding uncertainty in the percentage of body fat from 3% to 5%.

The hydrostatic weighing method can give very reproducible results for body density, provided that the examiners and the subjects are well trained. For example, Durnin and Rahaman (1967) reported a standard deviation of 0.008 kg/L for serial measurements on three subjects over a 1-y period.

14.6.2 Water-displacement plethysmography

The use of a plethysmograph eliminates the necessity for totally immersing the subject in water, a disadvantage with the hydrostatic weighing method (Section 14.6.1). For the measurement, the plethysmograph is zeroed and filled with water (Figure 14.4). The subject is then weighed, and a weight of water equal to the weight of the subject is removed from the plethysmograph. The subject then stands with water up to the neck only, and the head is covered by a clear-plastic dome. The volume of air surrounding the head of the subject, and in the lungs and gut, is then determined by measuring the pressure changes produced by a pump of known stroke volume (Garrow et al., 1979). This allows the total volume of the subject to be determined. The total time for the test, including three measurements on each subject, is about 20 min. The method has been used successfully to measure body density of obese adults (Garrow et al., 1979). Estimates of body fatness obtained compared favorably with those based on total body potassium.

14.6.3 Air-displacement plethysmography

The measurement of body volume has been significantly eased by the development of an air-displacement plethysmograph (Dempster and Aitkens, 1995). This device consists of an ovoid fiberglass structure divided into two sections: a rear reference chamber and a front test chamber containing the seated subject (Figure 14.5). The dividing wall between the two chambers embraces a large diaphragm. This can be made to oscillate under computer control, generating complementary pressure changes in the test and reference chambers which are recorded. These changes and the application of the basic gas laws allows the volume of the test chamber to be calculated. Measurements both with and without seated subjects give information on the total body volume of the subjects.

While they are seated in the test chamber, subjects should wear minimal clothing and

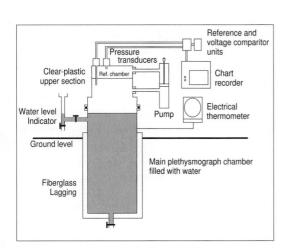

Figure 14.4: Measurement of body density using a plethysmograph. From Garrow et al., British Journal of Nutrition 42: 173–183, 1979, with permission of Cambridge University Press.

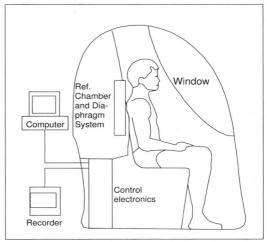

Figure 14.5: Measurement of body volume using an air-displacement plethysmograph. From Dempster and Aitkens, Medicine and Science in Sports and Exercise 27(12): 1692–1697, 1995.

a tightly fitting bathing cap. Measurements over a 1-min period usually suffice, and an average of two separate trials should be used to calculate body volume.

A correction for the average volume of air in the lungs and thorax during normal breathing (V_{TG}) should be applied. This can be measured while the subject is in the test chamber (Dempster and Aitkens, 1995). A predicted estimate of V_{TG} based on age, sex and height can also be used (McCrory et al., 1998).

Nuñez et al. (1999) reported the between-day coefficient of variation for body density for adult subjects 22–33 y and weighing between 52 and 92 kg as 0.0062 kg/L. They also showed no significant difference for the same group of subjects between estimates of body density made using an air-displacement plethysmograph and estimates obtained using conventional hydrostatic weighing. Recently, Utter et al. (2003) showed no significant difference between the two methods in a study of 66 collegiate wrestlers.

14.6.4 Calculation of body fat from body density

The fat content of the body is the most variable component of the body, as noted earlier. It comprises a complex mixture of glycerides, sterols, phospholipids, and glycolipids, some of which are more labile than others. As a result, the average density of fat may change within an individual over time and varies between individuals. Nevertheless, when calculating body fat from body density for normal persons, body fat is assumed to have a relatively constant density, as well as negligible water and potassium contents. Different authors use different values for the density of fat; the Siri equation assumes that the density of fat is about 0.90 kg/L at 37°C (Siri, 1961), and is most widely used as discussed in Section 11.1.5. The percentage of body fat is often calculated from the whole-body density using one of the empirical equations describing the relationship between fat content and body density (Siri, 1961; Brožek et al., 1963). The assumptions on which these

empirical equations are based are outlined in Section 11.1.5 and should be recognized.

Total body fat (TBF) is derived from percentage of body fat by multiplying body weight by percentage of fat:

$$\text{TBF (kg)} = (\text{body weight (kg)} \times \% \text{ body fat}) / 100$$

The fat-free mass (FFM) can then be calculated by subtracting the total body fat from the body weight:

$$\text{FFM (kg)} = \text{body weight (kg)} - \text{total body fat (kg)}$$

Lohman (1981) calculated that the theoretical error in body fat when calculated from densitometric measurements was 3–4%, attributed to variability in the water content of the fat-free mass and in the bone mineral density.

14.7 Total body electrical conductivity

Total body electrical conductivity (TOBEC) is measured by observing the changes induced by placing the subject in an electromagnetic field (Baumgartner, 1996). The extent of the change depends on the overall electrical conductivity of the body and, in particular, on the proportions of the fat-free mass and fat in the body: the lean body mass, comprised largely of electrolyte-containing water, will readily conduct an applied electric current, whereas fat is a poor conductor. Thus with careful calibration, measures of TOBEC can provide an estimate of the lean body mass and total body water.

In the more modern equipment, the subject lies supine on a motorized bed (Figure 14.6) that is passed in a series of steps progressively

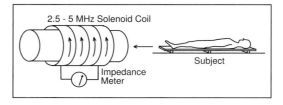

Figure 14.6: Measurement of body composition by total body electrical conductivity. From van Itallie et al., 1985 © Ross Laboratories, with permission.

through a uniform solenoid coil. A 2.5-MHz oscillating radiofrequency current is passed through the coil. This induces an electromagnetic field in the space enclosed by the coil, which, in turn, induces a current in the subject, the magnitude depending on the conductivity of the subject. A second reading is taken when the coil is empty; the difference represents the measurement. The use of Fourier analysis improves the assessment the lean body mass (Van Loan, 1990).

Measurement of TOBEC is simple, safe, and fast and can be used on individuals who cannot be weighed underwater. The instrument, however, is expensive. Disturbances in electrolyte balance, such as edema and dehydration, influence the signal generated. Moreover, the method is relatively insensitive to shifts of fluid or electrolyte between the intracellular and the extracellular compartments and to variations in bone mineralization. Careful consideration must be given to the positioning of the subject and corrections for body geometry and length applied.

Treuth et al. (2001) used a variety of techniques, including TOBEC, to determine body composition in 8-y-old prepubertal girls. The authors concluded that the determinations are highly method dependent and that results from all six methods studied (TOBEC, total body potassium, isotope dilution for total body water, bioelectrical impedance, anthropometry, and dual-energy X-ray absorptiometry) are not interchangeable. The results highlight how TOBEC measurements are evaluated by comparison with other methods. Unfortunately, most of these are also subject to error and bias.

14.8 Bioelectrical impedance

Bioelectrical impedance analysis (BIA) also depends on the differences in electrical conductivity of fat-free mass and fat. The technique measures the impedance of an electrical current (typically 800 µA; 50 KHz), passed between two electrodes, generally located on the right ankle and the right wrist of an individual. The impedance is related to the

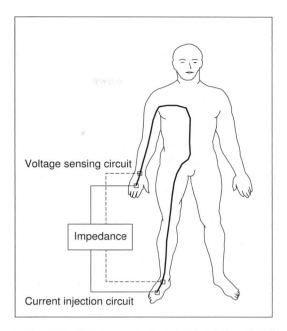

Figure 14.7: Measurement of whole-body bioelectrical impedance, showing diagrammatically the current path through the body and the positioning of the four electrodes.

volume of a conductor (the human body) and the square of the length of the conductor — a distance which is a function of the height of the subject (Figure 14.7). Bioelectical impedance analysis most closely estimates body water, from which fat-free mass is then estimated, on the assumption that the latter contains about 73% water, as described in Section 14.3. Fat mass can then be derived as the difference between body weight and fat-free mass. Details of the principle of BIA is given in Chumlea and Guo (1994).

Standardized procedures must be used to obtain BIA measurements; recommendations are outlined in NIH (1996). Hydration status, recent physical activity, consumption of food or beverages, ambient air and skin temperature, menstrual status, and body position are among the factors that can affect the validity and precision of the measurements. For example, subjects should avoid alcohol and vigorous exercise for 24–48 h before testing, so that body fluids are not perturbed prior to the measurements. The measurements should be taken on subjects approximately 2 h after eating, and within 30 min of voiding, generally with the subjects lying down, with limbs not touching the body.

Variations in the number, type, and positions of the electrodes used may also limit the validity of the BIA measurements. Conventionally, two distal current-inducing electrodes are placed on the dorsal surfaces of a hand and a foot, at the distal metacarpals and metatarsals, respectively. In addition, two voltage-sensing electrodes are placed at the pisiform prominence of a wrist and between the medial and lateral malleoli at an ipislateral (same side) or contralateral (opposite side) ankle. The correct positioning of these electrodes is critical; a 1-cm displacement can result in a 2% change in resistance. A thin layer of electrode gel is applied to each electrode before it is placed on the skin. The resistance component of body impedance between the right wrist and an ankle is then measured to the nearest ohm. The lowest resistance (R) value for an individual is used to calculate conductance (Ht^2/R) and to predict fat-free mass.

Investigators using BIA to estimate total body water, and thus the fat-free mass, have shown that the method is improved by adding an accurate measurement of weight, as well as sex and age, to the basic Ht^2/R parameter. This is not surprising as fat-free mass is a direct function of these parameters: an over- or underestimate of weight or height by 1 kg or 2.5 cm results in an error of 0.2 L and 1.0 L of total body water, respectively.

Numerous prediction equations of varying complexity have been published for the calculation of total body water and fat-free mass from BIA measurements (Baumgartner, 1996), each of which may be useful only for subjects who closely match the reference population on which the original prediction equation was based (NIH, 1996).

To further improve the BIA method, multifrequency measurements can be undertaken (Cornish et al. 1993; Deurenburg et al. 1994), instead of at a single frequency of 50 kHz, as described above. This allows the estimation of both total and extracellular body fluid compartments. Such estimates are es-

pecially useful in certain disease conditions involving disturbances in water distribution (e.g., congestive heart disease, renal disease, and malnutrition) (Van Loan and Mayclin, 1992; Cornish et al., 1993). There is some evidence that multiple-frequency impedance may be more sensitive to physiological variables such as the phase of the menstrual cycle or blood pressure than is single-frequency impedance (Chumlea et al., 1987).

Nevertheless, regardless of whether single or multifrequency observations are made, the prediction equations used to calculate total body water and thus fat-free mass from BIA measures must be validated using a criterion reference method. Of the latter methods, those used most frequently have been total body water by isotope dilution and body density by underwater weighing. In some studies, multicompartment methods have been used. The accuracy of the prediction equations for estimating fat-free mass, fat mass, and relative body fat, in turn, will depend on the assumptions associated with each of the criterion methods; these have been discussed in earlier sections. Further, the user should also confirm the applicability of the validation study to the population under investigation.

Studies to validate the relationship between BIA measures (mainly Ht^2/R, sex, and weight) and fat-free mass derived by a criterion method, have reported prediction errors for young healthy adults of less than 4% (CV). Sources of prediction error include measurement of height, weight, R, the criterion method used, and errors from the prediction equation (Brodie et al., 1998). The performance of the prediction equation also depends on the selection and number of independent variables.

In the future, impedance spectrum analysis derived from multifrequency impedance data, may be increasingly used to distinguish differences in body water and body composition among individuals (Chumlea and Guo, 1994). More validation studies are needed, however, on the elderly, youth, children, neonates, ethnic minority groups, and thin and obese individuals.

Bioelectrical impedance is safe and convenient, and the equipment is portable and relatively inexpensive. A variety of single-frequency, four-electrode BIA devices are commercially available. A smaller number of multifrequency devices are also available. Multifrequency bioelectrical impedance analysis formed part of the National Health and Nutrition Examination Survey (NHANES) III for persons aged ⩾12 y. Impedance measures at 50 frequencies logarithmically spaced from 5 kHz to 1 MHz were used to generate separate estimates of the extracellular (ECF) and intracellular fluid (ICF). Total body water (TBW) can then be calculated as ECF + ICF, and the fat-free mass is assumed to be 73.2% TBW. Data from NHANES III will be used to examine the relationship of body composition based on BIA measures to clinical risk factors such as blood pressure, blood lipids, and glucose tolerance (NIH, 1996).

Recent developments in BIA include the assessment of the composition of specific parts of the body, such as muscle and adipose tissue mass in limbs, and the measurement of skinfold thicknesses; these applications are reviewed by Elia and Ward (1999).

14.9 Computerized tomography

Computerized tomography (CT) is based on the relationship between the degree of attenuation of an X-ray beam and the density of the tissues through which the beam has passed. From this relationship, a two-dimensional radiographic image of the underlying anatomy of the scan area can be constructed.

The CT scanner is made up of two components: a collimated X-ray source and detectors, and a computer that processes the scan data and produces an X-ray image. The subject lies on a movable platform within the scanner gantry. The designated area to be scanned is a plane through the middle of the central aperture of the gantry and parallel to the gantry. The X-ray beam is made to rotate around the subject, generating a cross-sectional "slice" through the patient. As the X-rays pass through the tissue, the beam undergoes attenuation, the intensity of which is

recorded and stored in the scanner computer. The latter then processes the stored information by using a series of complex algorithms to reconstruct cross-sectional images (Figure 14.8). The images consist of a matrix of picture elements, or pixels, each about 1 mm × 1 mm, arranged in rows and columns. The pixels vary in their degree of shading according to the magnitude of the X-ray beam attenuation, which, in turn, depends on the physical density of the scanned tissues. Tissues with a greater density cause a greater absorption of X-ray energy and, consequently, a higher attenuation value. The demarcation between tissues of differing density can be very good. The degree of pixel shading is scaled as the CT number, a measure of attenuation relative to that of water. Examples of the CT numbers and densities (D) are fat, CT = 70, D = 0.91 g/cc; muscle, CT = 20, D = 1.05 g/cc; liver, CT = 25, D = 1.06 g/cc; and water, CT = 0, D = 1.0 g/cc.

The cross-sectional area of each of the tissues can be determined using specialized computer programs. The volume of tissues and organs (such as liver, kidney, and spleen) can also be assessed. When no sharp boundaries exist between structures, the pixels can be plotted as histograms to help separate the fat-free and fat tissues. As the volume of each

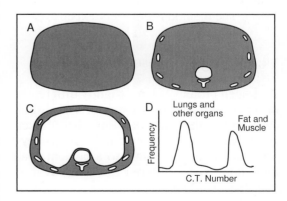

Figure 14.8: Body composition from a computerized tomography scan at the thorax level, showing three images resulting from different computer processings of the same scan. A: The air/skin interface. B: Major skeletal elements. C: Adjusted to show the interface between the lungs and other organs and the surrounding muscle and fat. D: Histogram of the pixel density from scan C.

pixel is known, the volume of the fat-free and fat tissue can then be calculated from the number of pixels forming each slice and the number of slices.

The method has several uses. It can be used to assess changes in the visceral organ mass in undernutrition and obesity, to measure regional muscle mass, to assess the distribution of subcutaneous versus internal fat, and to establish bone density in osteopenia (Heymsfield et al., 1987). For example, Mitsiopoulos et al. (1998) studied the validity of CT to provide regional estimates of both skeletal muscle and adipose tissue embedded within muscle (interstitial adipose tissue) and surrounding muscle (subcutaneous adipose tissue) in cadavers by comparison with measurements performed by magnetic resonance imaging (MRI) and cadaver analysis. Good agreement between CT results for estimates of appendicular skeletal muscle and interstitial and subcutaneous adipose tissue and those measured by magnetic resonance imaging was reported, providing support for the use of CT and MRI as reference methods in vivo.

Computerized tomography, however, involves exposure to ionizing radiation and is not recommended for pregnant women or children, for routine whole-body scans, or for multiple scans on the same person (Lukaski, 1987). The method is also very expensive.

14.10 Magnetic resonance imaging

Hydrogen protons behave slightly differently in adipose versus lean tissues. The differences are in the relaxation time that it takes for the nuclei to release the radio-frequency-induced energy and return to a random configuration. These differences can be used to map the distribution of adipose versus lean tissue in the body (Ross, 1995).

The imaging process involves placing the subject in a very strong magnetic field. Some of the nuclei in the body attempt to align themselves relative to the applied field. The effect is particularly marked for ^1H protons. Only a small fraction of the protons become

aligned, but they are sufficiently numerous for the effect to be detectable when the field is removed or altered. It is then that the differences between the lean and adipose tissue become apparent.

Magnetic resonance imaging (MRI) equipment has been developed that uses the differences in the nuclei relaxation times. Commonly, MRI generates cross-sectional abdominal images, showing the distribution of the lean and adipose tissues. These scans are similar to the images generated by computerized tomography but are based on completely different physical principals. In older equipment, scanning times of 10 min were necessary, but in more modern equipment, this has been reduced to under 2 min.

The principal advantages of MRI versus CT or dual-energy X-ray absorptiometry is that no ionizing radiation is involved. Consequently, unlike CT, whole-body scans, or multiple scans on the same person can be performed. However, the equipment is bulky and expensive and most commonly used to validate other anthropometric measures in which a limited number of high-quality criterion observations are required (Sohlström et al., 1993; Chan et al., 1998; Thomas et al., 1998; Stewart et al., 2003).

14.11 Dual energy X-ray absorptiometry

Dual-energy X-ray absorptiometry (DXA) is now the primary technique for the assessment of the bone mineral content of the axial skeleton; it is described in detail in Section 23.1.8. However, DXA is also used for determining the relative proportions of the fat-free mass, body fat, and bone in subjects by whole body scanning. This application is considered here.

Modern DXA scanners use a dual-energy X-ray source that generates X-rays at 40 KeV and 70–100 KeV; these pass through the subject (Figure 14.9). The relative absorption at these two energies is measured to give two estimates of body composition along the beam path using a two-compartment model. In bone-free regions of the body, the attenuation

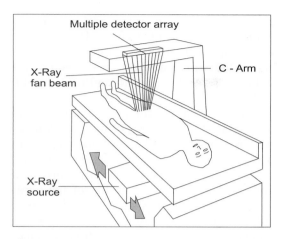

Figure 14.9: Dual-energy X-ray scanner with multiple detector array and X-ray fan beam.

provides an estimate of the relative proportions of fat and lean tissues. In the other regions, the attenuation provides a measure of the proportions of bone and soft tissues. To provide estimates of the overall relative proportions of the three components — the fat-free mass, body fat, and bone — the assumption is made that the soft tissue overlaying bone has the same fat to muscle ratio as that in immediately adjacent non-bone regions. In a typical whole-body scan, as much as 45% of the scanned region contains bone. Thus for nearly half the body, the proportion of body fat is derived from lean-to-fat measurements made elsewhere on the subject.

The computing algorithms used to partition the soft tissue between the body fat and the fat-free mass are critically important in assessing body composition and have been shown to vary significantly with the manufacturer of the equipment (Tothill et al., 2001). Such algorithms should take into account the different fat distributions in males and females and also the differences generated by overall increases in adiposity.

Notwithstanding the uncertainties outlined above, DXA clearly has an important role in body composition assessment. Fan-beam technologies, replacing earlier pencil-beam techniques, are resulting in much shorter scan times (3 min), lower X-ray doses (< 10 μSv compared to 0.3 mSv for total body nitrogen

by NAA), and improved geometrical resolution. These new-generation DXA instruments also have a high precision and with careful calibration can lead to accurate results (Tothill et al., 2001).

Several investigators have tried to establish the absolute accuracy of gross measurements of body composition in vivo performed using DXA. Many of these studies have examined correlations between measurements made by DXA on pig cadavers and subsequent direct chemical analysis; results have been mixed (Jebb, 1997). Visser et al. (1999) describe a validation study on 58 men and women aged 70–79 y, with a body mass index of 17.5–39.8 kg/m^2. A four-compartment body composition model was used as the criterion method for determining the fat-free mass, and the results were compared with determinations using fan-beam DXA. Calculation of the fat-free mass using the four-compartment model required the determination of body density (underwater weighing), total body water (isotope dilution), total body bone mineral mass (DXA), and body weight. A short summary of the results for fat-free mass is presented in Table 14.4 and a graph of the differences (Bland and Altman, 1986) between the methods is shown in Figure 14.10. The study shows that the method has high precision and validity, although there is bias in the DXA results for fat-free mass which are, on average, approximately 1.8 kg higher. Likewise, total body mass by DXA was also 1.1% higher than body weight, suggesting that good agreement on mean fat mass was also achieved. Nevertheless, considerable

	4C model	DXA	Diff.	R^2
M (n = 30)	61.4 ± 6.8	63.4 ± 6.8	1.8 ± 1.7	0.94
W (n = 28)	41.1 ± 5.3	43.0 ± 6.0	1.9 ± 1.5	0.95

Table 14.4: Validation of the dual-energy X-ray absorptiometry technique for measuring the fat-free mass against a four-compartment (4C) model on elderly men (M) and women (W). Data in kg showing the mean (± SD) for the 4C and DXA methods, and the difference (Diff.). R^2 is the explained variance. Data from Visser et al., Journal of Applied Physiology 87: 1513–1520, 1999, with permission.

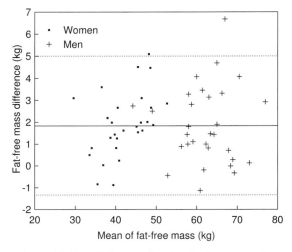

Figure 14.10: Difference in the fat-free mass determined by DXA and a four-compartment model on elderly men and women. Solid line, mean difference; dashed lines, limits of agreement ($\pm 2\,SD$). Data from Visser et al., Journal of Applied Physiology 87: 1513–1520, 1999, with permission.

differences exist between measurements of soft tissue and total body bone made by fan-beam DXA scanners, emphasizing the need for and value of cross-calibration (Tothill et al., 2001).

14.12 Ultrasound

In the ultrasound technique, high-frequency sound waves from an ultrasound source/meter penetrate the skin surface and pass through the adipose tissue until they reach the muscle tissue. At the adipose–muscle tissue interface, a proportion of the sound waves are reflected back as echoes that return to the ultrasound meter.

To use this technique, the measurement site is marked with a water-soluble transmission gel that provides acoustic contact without depression of the dermal surface. The high-resolution ultrasound source/meter is then placed so that the ultrasonic beam is perpendicular to the tissue interfaces at the marked site. A transducer receives the echoes and translates them into depth readings viewed on an oscilloscope screen. Subcutaneous fat thicknesses of 100 mm or more can be meas-

ured, and density interfaces can be detected with an accuracy of 1 mm. The tissue is not compressed, thereby eliminating errors associated with variations in the compressibility of skinfolds (Fanelli and Kuczmarski, 1984).

The ultrasound technique can also be used to measure the thickness of muscle tissue as well as subcutaneous fat, enabling changes in body composition of hospital patients receiving nutritional support to be monitored. In general, studies of the validity of the ultrasound method suggest it provides a reasonable estimate of adipose tissue thickness in humans, compared to total electrical conductivity and skinfold caliper techniques (Fanelli and Kuczmarski, 1984). For obese persons, ultrasound may be superior to skinfold caliper techniques for measuring subcutaneous fat (Kuczmarski et al., 1987). Nevertheless, large studies involving subjects with wide ranges in body fatness should be undertaken before the validity of this technique can be firmly established.

14.13 Summary

The characteristics of the various procedures used to assess body composition are summarized in Tables 14.5 (non-scanning techniques) and Table 14.6 (scanning techniques). Comments on these methods are also given. Selection of any method depends on the objectives of the study, and on the cost, convenience, equipment and technical expertise available, the health of the subject, and the precision and accuracy required. Methods with the lowest cost are often the most imprecise. Methods based on the two-compartment model (i.e., body fat and fat-free mass) include total body water and total body potassium, densitometry, total body electrical conductivity, and bioelectrical impedance. Such methods are not suitable for patients with chronic nutritional deprivation, because in such cases, the basic assumptions of the two-compartment model are invalid. In these patients, techniques using the four-compartment model (i.e., water, protein, minerals,

Method and procedures	Comments
Total body potassium (TBK) TBK is measured by counting radiation from naturally occurring ^{40}K in a whole body counter. FFM is derived from the assumption that average potassium concentration of FFM is constant.	Required equipment is expensive. Obese and elderly subjects have lower potassium concentrations, leading to overestimates of total body fat.
Total body water (TBW) A tracer dose of water, labeled with ^3H, ^2H, or ^{18}O, is given orally or intravenously and then equilibrated. The concentration of isotope is measured in serum, urine, saliva, or breath (for ^{18}O). TBW is calculated from dilution observed.	Involves radiation to the subject if ^3H is used. Water content of fat-free tissue is increased during obesity, pregnancy, and wasting disease, leading to an underestimate of fat.
Neutron activation analysis Radioactive isotopes of N, P, Na, Cl, Ca are created by irradiating the subject. The radioactivity of the element is measured using a whole body counter.	Expensive. Subjects are exposed to radioactivity. Elements are not uniformly activated, and thus sensitivity varies.
Densitometry Body density is derived from measurements of body mass and body volume. The latter is calculated from: (*a*) the apparent loss of weight when the body is totally submerged in water, or (*b*) air-displacement or water-displacement plethysmography. Corrections may be required for water temperature, and the volume of air trapped in the gastrointestinal tract, and residual lung volume.	Total submersion methods require a high degree of cooperation from the subjects and are not suitable for young children, the elderly or sick patients, who should be measured using air-displacement plethysmography. Relatively expensive.
Total body electrical conductivity (TOBEC) Subject lies supine in a solenoid coil through which a 5 MHz current is passed. The latter induces a current in the subject. The conductivity value of the subject is obtained by subtracting the background value when the coil is empty. Conductivity value is proportional to body electrolyte content and, hence, reflects the amount of fat-free tissue.	Edema, ascites, dehydration, and electrolyte balance will alter conductivity and interfere with reading. The extent to which variation in body shape and size affects readings is not yet known. Variations in bone mass may affect readings. Expensive method.
Ultrasound High-frequency sound waves from a combined ultrasound source and meter pass through adipose tissue to the adipose–muscle tissue interface. At the interface, some sound waves are reflected back as echoes, which are translated into depth readings via a transducer.	Validity of technique for subjects with wide range of body fatness unknown. Technique does not provide the same degree of structure resolution that is possible with CT, MRI or DXA.
Bioelectrical impedance (BEI) The impedance to a weak electrical current passed between the right ankle and right wrist of a subject in supine position is measured. Impedance is related to the volume of a conductor (human body) and the square of the length of the conductor — a function of the height of the subject. Multifrequency measurement allow estimation of both total and extracellular compartments	Edema, ascites, and dehydration will alter the resistance measurements and invalidate single frequency measurements. Multifrequency methods allow assessment of body fluid compartment volume changes during clinical interventions and physical activity studies.

Table 14.5: Summary of non-scanning laboratory techniques used to measure body composition.

Method and procedures	Comments
Computerized tomography (CT) Method measures attenuation of X-rays as they pass through tissues, the degree of attenuation being related to differences in physical density of the tissues. An image is reconstructed from the matrix of picture elements (pixels), which vary in their shading.	Exposure to ionizing radiation limits use of CT for whole body scans, multiple scans in same person, and scans of pregnant women or children. Expensive equipment is not readily available. The CT does not provide information on chemical composition of the structures.
Magnetic resonance imaging (MRI) Imaging involves placing a subject in a very strong magnetic field and observing the relative differences in behavior of ^{1}H protons in lean and adipose tissue. Commonly used to generate cross-sectional abdominal images showing fat distribution.	Unlike CT or DXA, no ionizing radiation is involved. However the equipment is bulky and expensive.
Dual energy X-ray absorptiometry (DXA) Primary technique for assessment of the bone mineral content of the axial skeleton. Also used for body fat measurements. Utilizes the attenuation of a dual energy X-ray beam, often during whole-body scanning. New fan-beam technologies replacing earlier pencil-beam techniques lead to lower X-ray doses and improved spatial resolution.	High precision method, but results are calibration dependent and differences between different equipment manufacturers can be significant. Cross-calibration using densitometry and isotope dilution methods on specific subject groups may be helpful.

Table 14.6: Summary of scanning laboratory techniques used to measure body composition.

and fat) are more appropriate. These techniques include neutron activation analysis for protein and minerals and isotope dilution for total body water. Body fat can be calculated by subtracting the protein, minerals, and water from body weight. Three scanning techniques (computerized tomography, magnetic resonance imaging, and dual energy X-ray absorptiometry) can be used to assess the relative proportions of the fat-free mass, body fat, and bone mineral content.

References

Baumgartner RN. (1996). Electrical impedance and total body electrical conductivity. In: Roche AF, Heymsfield SB, and Lohman TG (eds.) Human Body Composition. Human Kinetics, Champaign, IL.

Beddoe AH, Hill GL. (1985). Clinical measurement of body composition using in vivo neutron activation analysis. Journal of Parenteral and Enteral Nutrition 9: 504–520.

Behnke AR, Feen BG, Welham WC. (1942). The specific gravity of healthy men: body weight and volume as an index of obesity. Journal of the American Medical Association 118: 495–498.

Bland JM, Altman DG. (1986). Statistical methods for assessing agreement between two methods of clinical measurement. Lancet 1(8476): 307–310.

Brodie DA. (1988). Techniques of measurement of body composition: Part I and Part II. Sports Medicine 5: 11–40, 74–98.

Brodie DA, Moscrip V, Hutcheon R. (1998). Body composition measurement: a review of hydrodensitomety, anthropometry, and impedance methods. Nutrition 14: 296–310.

Brožek JF, Grande F, Anderson JT, Keys A. (1963). Densitometric analysis of body composition: revision of some quantitative assumptions. Annals of the New York Academy of Sciences 110: 113–140.

Chan YL, Leung SS, Lam WW, Peng XH, Metreweli C. (1998). Body fat estimation in children by magnetic resonance imaging, bioelectrical impedance, skinfold and body mass index: a pilot study. Journal of Paediatrics and Child Health 34: 22–28.

Chumlea WC, Guo SS. (1994). Bioelectrical impedance and body composition: present status and future directions. Nutrition Reviews 52: 123–131.

Chumlea WC, Roche AF, Guo S, Woynarowska B. (1987). The influence of phsyiologic variables and oral contraceptives on bioelectrical impedance. Human Biology 59: 257–270.

Cohn SH, Ellis KJ, Vartsky D, Sawitsky A, Gartenhaus W, Yasumura S, Vaswani AN. (1981a). Comparison of methods of estimating body fat in normal subjects and cancer patients. American Journal of Clinical Nutrition 34: 2839–2847.

Cohn SH, Satwitsky A, Vartsky D, Yasumura S, Zanzi I,

Ellis KJ. (1981b). Body composition as measured by in vivo neutron activation analysis. In: Nutritional Assessment: Present Status, Future Directions and Prospects. Report of the Second Ross Conference on Medical Research. Ross Laboratories, Columbus, OH, pp. 99–102.

Cohn SH, Vaswani AN, Yasumura S, Yuen K, Ellis KJ. (1984). Improved models for determination of body fat by in vivo neutron activation. American Journal of Clinical Nutrition 40: 255–259.

Cornish BH, Thomas BJ, Ward LC. (1993). Improved prediction of extracellar and total body water using impedance loci generated by multiple frequency bioelectrical impedance analysis. Physics in Medicine and Biology 38: 337–346.

Dempster P, Aitkens S. (1995). A new air displacement method for the determination of human body composition. Medicine and Science in Sports and Exercise 27: 1692–1697.

Deurenberg P, Broekhoff C, Andreoli A, Delorenzo A. (1994). The use of multi-frequency impedance in assessing changes in body water compartments. Age and Nutrition 5: 142–145.

Durnin JVGA, Rahaman MM. (1967). The assessment of the amount of fat in the human body from measurements of skinfold thickness. British Journal of Nutrition 21: 681–689.

Elia M, Ward LC. (1999). New techniques in nutritional assessment: body composition methods. Proceedings of the Nutrition Society 58: 33–38.

Ellis KJ. (2001). Selected body composition methods can be used in field studies. Journal of Nutrition 131: 1589S–1595S.

Fanelli MT, Kuczmarski RJ. (1984). Ultrasound as an approach to assessing body composition. American Journal of Clinical Nutrition 39: 703–709.

Fields DA, Goran MI. (2000). Body composition techniques and the four-compartment model in children. Journal of Applied Physiology 89: 613–620.

Forbes GB, Gallup J, Hursh JB. (1961). Estimation of total body fat from potassium-40 content. Science 133: 101–102.

Garrow JS. (1983). Indices of adiposity. Nutrition Abstracts and Reviews 53: 697–708.

Garrow JS, Stalley S, Diethelm R, Pittet PH, Hesp R, Halliday D. (1979). A new method for measuring the body density of obese adults. British Journal of Nutrition 42: 173–183.

Hansen RD, Allen BJ. (1996). Calibration of a total body potassium monitor with an anthropomorphic phantom. Physics in Medicine and Biology 41: 2447–2462.

Heymsfield SB, Rolandelli R, Casper K, Settle RG, Koruda M. (1987). Application of electromagnetic and sound waves in nutritional assessment. Journal of Parenteral and Enteral Nutrition 11: 64S–69S.

Jebb SA. (1997). Measurement of soft tissue composition by dual energy X-ray absorptiometry. British Journal of Nutrition 77: 151–163.

Knight GS, Beddoe AH, Streat SJ, Hill GL. (1986). Body composition of two human cadavers by neutron activation and chemical analysis. American Journal of Physiology 250: E179–E185.

Kotler DP, Thea DM, Heo M, Allison DB, Engleson ES, Wang J, Pierson RN Jr, St.Louis M, Keusch GT. (1999). Relative influence of sex, race, environment, and HIV infection on body composition in adults. American Journal of Clinical Nutrition 69: 432–439.

Kuczmarski RJ, Fanelli MT, Koch GG. (1987). Ultrasonic assessment of body composition in obese adults: overcoming the limitations of the skinfold caliper. American Journal of Clinical Nutrition 45: 717–724.

Lohman TG. (1981). Skinfolds and body density and their relation to body fatness: a review. Human Biology 53: 181–225.

Lukaski HC. (1987). Methods for the assessment of human body composition: traditional and new. American Journal of Clinical Nutrition 46: 537–556.

Ma R, Stamatelatos IE, Yasumura S. (2000) Calibration of the Brookhaven National Laboratory delayed gamma-neutron activation facility to measure total body calcium. Annals of the New York Academy of Sciences 904: 148–151.

McCrory MA, Mole PA, Gomez TD, Dewey KG, Bernauer EM. (1998). Body composition by air-displacement plethysmography by using predicted and measured thoracic gas volumes. Journal of Applied Physiology 84: 1475–1479.

McMurrey JD, Boling EA, Davis JM, Parker HV, Magnus IC, Ball MR, Moore FD. (1958). Body composition: simultaneous determination of several aspects by the dilution principle. Metabolism 7: 651–667.

Mitsiopoulos N, Baumgartner RN, Heymsfiled SB, Lyons W, Gallagher D, Ross R. (1998). Cadaver validation of skeletal muscle measurement by magnetic resonance imaging and computerized tomography. Journal of Applied Physiology 85: 115–122.

Moore FD, Olesen KH, McMurrey JD, Parker HV, Ball MR, Boyden CM (eds.). (1963). The Body Cell Mass and Its Supporting Environment: Body Composition in Health and Disease. W.B. Saunders, Philadelphia.

NIH (National Institutes of Health). (1996). Bioelectrical impedance analysis in body composition measurement: NIH Technology Assessment Conference statement. American Journal of Clinical Nutrition 64: 524S–532S.

Nuñez C, Kovera AJ, Pietrobelli A, Heshka S, Horlick M, Kehayias J, Wang Z, Heymsfield SB. (1999). Body composition in children and adults by air displacement plethysmography. European Journal of Clinical Nutrition 53: 382–387.

Pierson RN Jr, Lin DHY, Phillips RA. (1974). Total-body potassium in health: effects of age, sex, height, and fat. American Journal of Physiology 226: 206–212.

Ross R. (1995). Magnetic resonance imaging provides new insights into the characterization of adipose and lean tissue distribution. Canadian Journal of Physiology and Pharmacology 74: 778–785

Schoeller DA. (1991). Isotope dilution methods. In: Bjorntorp P, Brodoff BN (eds.) Obesity. Lippincott, New York, pp. 80–88.

Schoeller DA, van Santen E, Peterson DW, Dietz W, Jaspan J, Klein PD. (1980). Total body water measurement in humans with ^{18}O and ^2H labeled water. American Journal of Clinical Nutrition 33: 2686–2693.

Schoeller DA, Kushner RF, Taylor P, Dietz WH, Bandini L. (1985). Measurement of total body water: isotope dilution technique. In: Roche AF (ed.) Body-Composition Assessments in Youth and Adults. Sixth Ross Conference on Medical Research. Ross Laboratories, Columbus, OH, pp. 24–28.

Sheng HP, Huggins RA. (1979). A review of body composition studies with emphasis on total body water and fat. American Journal of Clinical Nutrition 32: 630–647.

Shizgal HM. (1981). The effect of malnutrition on body composition. Surgery, Gynecology and Obstetrics 152: 22–26.

Shizgal HM. (1985). Body composition of patients with malnutrition and cancer: summary of methods of assessment. Cancer 55: 250–253.

Shizgal HM. (1987). Nutritional assessment with body composition measurements. Journal of Parenteral and Enteral Nutrition 11: 42S–47S.

Shizgal HM, Spanier AH, Humes J, Wood CD. (1977). Indirect measurement of total exchangeable potassium. American Journal of Physiology 233: F253–F259.

Siri WE. (1961). Body composition from fluid spaces and density: analysis of methods. In: Brozek J, Hanschel A (eds.) Techniques for Measuring Body Composition. National Academy of Sciences, National Research Council, Washington DC., pp. 223–244.

Sohlström A, Wahlund LO, Forsum E. (1993). Adipose tissue distribution as assessed by magnetic resonance imaging and total body fat by magnetic resonance imaging, underwater weighing, and body-water dilution in healthy women. American Journal of Clinical Nutrition 58: 830–838.

Stewart KJ, DeRegis JR, Turner KL, Bacher A, Sung J, Hees PS, Shapiro EP, Tayback M, Ouyang P. (2003). Usefulness of anthropometrics and dual-energy X-ray absorptiometry for estimating abdominal obesity measured by magnetic resonance imaging in older men and women. Journal of Cardiopulmonary Rehabilitation 23: 109–114.

Thomas EL, Saeed N, Hajnal JV, Brynes A, Goldstone AP, Frost G, Bell JD. (1998). Magnetic resonance imaging of total body fat. Journal of Applied Physiology 85: 1778–1785.

Tothill P, Hannan WJ, Wilkinson S. (2001). Comparisons between a pencil beam and two fan beam dual energy X-ray absorptiometers used for measuring total body bone and soft tissue. British Journal of Radiology 74: 166–176.

Treuth MS, Butte NF, Wong WW, Ellis KJ. (2001). Body composition in prepubertal girls: comparison of six methods. International Journal of Obesity and Related Metabolic Disorders 25: 1352–1359.

Utter AC, Gross FL, Swan PD, Harris GS, Robertson RJ, Trone GA. (2003). Evaluation of air displacement for assessing body composition of collegiate wrestlers. Medicine and Science in Sports and Exercise 35: 500–505.

van Itallie TB , Segal KR, Yang M-V, Funk RC. (1985). Clinical assessment of body fat content in adults: potential role of electrical impedance methods. In: Roche AF (ed.) Body-Composition Assessments in Youth and Adults. Report of the Sixth Ross Conference on Medical Research. Ross Laboratories, Columbus, OH, pp. 5–8.

Van Loan MD. (1990). Assessment of fat-free mass in teen-agers; use of TOBEC methodology. American Journal of Clinical Nutrition 52: 586–590.

Van Loan MD, Mayclin PL. (1992). Use of multi-frequency bioelectrical impedance analysis for the estimation of extracellular fluid. European Journal of Clinical Nutrition 46: 117–124.

van Raaij JM, Peek ME, Vermaat-Miedema SH, Schonk CM, Hautvast JG. (1988). New equations for estimating body fat mass in pregnancy from body density or total body water. American Journal of Clinical Nutrition 48: 24–29.

Vartsky D, Prestwich WV, Thomas BJ, Dabek JT, Chettle DR, Fremlin JH, Stammers K. (1979). The use of body hydrogen as an internal standard in the measurement of nitrogen in vivo by prompt neutron capture gamma-ray analysis. Journal of Radioanalytical Chemistry 48: 243–252.

Visser M, Fuerst T, Lang T, Salamone L, Harris TB. (1999). Validity of fan-beam dual-energy X-ray absorptiometry for measuring fat-free mass and leg muscle mass. Journal of Applied Physiology 87: 1513–1520.

Wang ZM, Pierson RN Jr, Heymsfield SB. (1992). The five-level model: a new approach to organizing body-composition research. American Journal of Clinical Nutrition 56: 19–28.

Wang ZM, Ma R, Pierson RN Jr, Heymsfield SB. (1993). Five-level model: reconstruction of body weight at atomic, molecular, cellular, and tissue-system levels from neutron activation analysis. Basic Life Sciences 60: 125–128.

Wang ZM, Heshka S, Pierson RN Jr, Heymsfield SB. (1995). Systematic organization of body-composition methodology: an overview with emphasis on component-based methods. American Journal of Clinical Nutrition 61: 457–465.

Womersley J, Durnin JVGA, Boddy K, Mahaffy M. (1976). Influence of muscular development, obesity, and age on the fat-free mass of adults. Journal of Applied Physiology 41: 223–229.

15

Laboratory assessment

Laboratory assessment is used primarily to detect subclinical deficiency states, but also to confirm a clinical diagnosis. It has become increasingly important with the growing emphasis on preventive medicine, as it provides an objective means of assessing nutritional status, independent of emotional and other subjective factors. The procedures can supplement other methods of nutritional assessment — for example, dietary, clinical, and anthropometric assessment — enabling specific nutritional problems to be more readily identified.

Both static and functional tests can be used in laboratory assessment. Static biochemical tests measure either a nutrient in biological fluids or tissues, or the urinary excretion rate of the nutrient or its metabolites. Theoretically, the test selected should reflect either the total body content of the nutrient or the size of the tissue store that is most sensitive to depletion. In practice, such tests are not available for many nutrients. Further, even if levels of the nutrient or metabolite in the biological tissue or fluid are "low," they may not necessarily reflect the presence of a pathological lesion. Alternatively, their significance to health may be unknown.

Functional tests aim to measure the extent of the functional consequences of a specific nutrient deficiency and, hence, have greater biological significance than the static tests. The tests can be subdivided into two groups: functional biochemical and functional physiological or behavioral tests. Details are given in Section 15.2.

Functional biochemical tests should measure changes associated with the first limiting biochemical system which, in turn, affects health and well-being. Again, for many nutrients, the first limiting biochemical system is often unknown, or inaccessible, or it cannot be measured (Strain, 1999). Unfortunately, static and functional tests are often affected by biological and technical factors other than depleted body stores of the nutrient, which may confound the interpretation of the result. These factors are listed in Box 15.1.

The effects of these factors on specific nutrients are discussed more fully in the following chapters. Their influence (if any) on each test should be established before

---

Method-related limitations: accuracy, precision, sensitivity, specificity, and predictive value of the test

Sampling difficulties, including possible sample contamination and hemolysis

Subject-related factors: age, sex, ethnicity, race, genetic predisposition to disease, physiological state, hormonal status, supplement use, physical activity level, lifestyle, environment, recent dietary intake

Health-related factors: inherited or acquired diseases, infection, inflammation, stress, medication use, unusual weight loss

Biological factors: homeostatic regulation, diurnal and/or circadian variation, nutrient interactions

---

Box 15.1: Technical, biological, and other factors which may confound the interpretation of static and functional tests.

carrying out the tests because often these confounding effects can be minimized or eliminated. For example, in nutrition surveys, the effects of diurnal variation on the concentration of nutrients such as zinc and iron in plasma can be eliminated by collecting the blood samples on all subjects at a standardized time of the day. When factors such as age, sex, race, and physiological state influence the laboratory tests, the observations can be classified according to these variables. The influence of drugs, hormonal status, physical activity, weight loss, and presence of disease conditions on laboratory tests can also be considered if the appropriate questions are included in the survey questionnaire.

During the early stage of an infectious illness or after trauma, certain systemic and clinical changes occur that are referred to as the "acute-phase response." During this reaction, circulating levels of certain nutrients — for example, zinc, iron, and copper — in the blood are altered, due to a redistribution in body compartments rather than to deficiency or excess. The acute phase response can be detected by measurement of elevated levels of several plasma proteins. Of these, C-reactive protein (CRP), α-1-glycoprotein, and α-1-anti-chymotrypsin are most often measured (ICSH, 1988; Doyle et al., 1999).

In general, a combination of laboratory tests should be used, rather than a single test for each nutrient; several concordant abnormal values are more reliable than a single aberrant value in diagnosing a deficiency state. Tables 15.1 and 15.2 summarize the biochemical tests recommended for the assessment of the essential nutrients. This chapter outlines the principles and procedures of static and functional laboratory tests, as well as the factors that affect their choice; subsequent chapters assess the application of these tests to individual nutrients.

15.1 Nutrients in biological fluids and tissues

Static biochemical tests measure either (*a*) a nutrient in biological fluids or tissues or (*b*) the urinary excretion rate of a nutrient or its metabolite. The biopsy material most frequently used for static biochemical tests is whole blood or some fraction of blood. Other body fluids and tissues, less widely used, include urine, saliva, breast milk, semen, amniotic fluid, hair, toenails, skin, and buccal mucosa. Four stages are involved in the analysis of these biopsy materials: sampling, storage, preparation, and analysis. Care must be taken to ensure that the appropriate safety precautions are taken at each stage. Contamination is also a major problem for trace elements, and must be controlled at each stage of their analyses, especially when the expected analyte levels are at or below concentrations of 1×10^{-9} g.

Ideally, as discussed above, the nutrient content of the biopsy material should reflect the level of the nutrient in the tissue most sensitive to a deficiency, and any reduction in nutrient content should reflect the presence of a metabolic lesion. In some cases, however, the level of the nutrient in the biological fluid or tissue may appear adequate, but a deficiency state still arises. This may be because a metabolic defect prevents the utilization of the nutrient.

15.1.1 Blood

Samples of blood are readily accessible, relatively noninvasive, and generally easily analyzed. They must be collected and handled under controlled, standardized conditions to ensure accurate and precise analytical results. Factors such as fasting, fluctuations resulting from diurnal variation and meal consumption, hydration status, use of oral contraceptive agents or hormone replacement therapy, medications, infection, inflammation, and stress may all confound interpretation of results (Pilch and Senti, 1984a; Smith et al., 1985).

Plasma and serum carry newly absorbed nutrients and those being transported to the tissues and thus tend to reflect recent dietary intake. Therefore, plasma and serum nutrient levels provide an acute, rather than long-term, biomarker of nutrient status. The effect of recent dietary intake on plasma and

Nutrient	Test	Analytical method
Calcium	Serum ionized calcium	Ion-specific electrodes
Phosphorus	Serum phosphorus	Colorimetry using molybdenum blue
Magnesium	Serum magnesium	AAS
	Serum ionized magnesium	Ion- specific electrodes
Copper	Erythrocyte superoxide dismutase	Spectrophotometric assay or ELISA
Iodine	Urinary iodine	Acid digestion, followed by spectrophotometric assay using the Sandell-Kolthoff reaction
	TSH (for neonates)	ELISA with dried blood spots or serum
Iron	Serum ferritin	ELISA (in absence of infection)
	Hemoglobin	Cyanmethemoglobin method. Hemocue in field studies
	Serum transferrin receptor	ELISA
Selenium	Plasma selenium	AAS with Zeeman background correction or hydride generation AAS
	Plasma GSHPx-3	ELISA: only useful if Se intakes are habitually low
Zinc	Serum/plasma zinc	Flame AAS (in absence of infection)
	Hair zinc	Measure by NAA or AAS in children with low height percentiles and/or hypogeusia

Table 15.1: Recommended biochemical tests for minerals and trace elements. AAS: atomic absorption spectrometry; ELISA, enzyme-linked immunosorbent assays; TSH, thyroid stimulating hormone; GSHPx-3, glutathione peroxidase; NAA, neutron activation analysis.

serum nutrient concentrations can be reduced by collecting fasting blood samples.

Nutrient concentrations in both plasma and serum may be near normal, even when there is evidence of functional impairment because serum concentrations of some nutrients (e.g., calcium and zinc) are strongly homeostatically regulated (Ruz et al., 1991). In such cases, alternative biochemical markers may be needed.

The risk of contamination during sample collection, storage, preparation, and analysis is a particular problem in trace element analysis of blood. Trace elements are present in low concentrations in blood but are ubiquitous in the environment (Iyengar et al., 1998). Details of strategies to reduce the risk of adventitious sources of trace-element contamination are given in the introduction to Chapter 24. In addition, for certain vitamins such as folate, suitable antioxidants must be added to samples to stabilize the vitamin during collection and storage (Section 22.1.2).

Additional confounding factors in the analysis of trace elements in blood are venous occlusion, hemolysis, use of an inappropriate anticoagulant, collection-separation time, and element losses produced by adsorption on the container surfaces or by volatilization during storage (Tamura et al., 1994; Veillon and Patterson, 1999).

Serum is often preferred for trace element analysis because, unlike plasma, risk of adventitious contamination from anticoagulants is avoided, as well as the tendency to form an insoluble protein precipitate during freezing. Nevertheless, serum is more prone than plasma to both contamination from platelets and hemolysis.

15.1.2 Erythrocytes

The nutrient content of erythrocytes reflects chronic nutrient status because the lifespan of these cells is quite long ($\sim$120 d). An additional advantage is that nutrient concen-

Nutrient	Test	Analytical method
Vitamin A	Liver retinol stores	HPLC
	Modified relative dose response	Serum retinol and dehydroretinol via HPLC 4–6 h after oral dose of 3,4-didehydroretinol acetate (100 μg/kg)
Vitamin D	Serum 25-hydroxyvitamin D	Separation of serum 25(OH)-D by HPLC, followed by a competitive binding assay or RIA
Vitamin E	Ratio of serum tocopherol: serum cholesterol	Reverse phase HPLC with a high sensitivity fluorescence detector
Thiamin	Erythrocyte activity of transketolase with and without added thiamin pyrophosphate	Semi-automated spectrophotometry using glyceraldehyde as an internal standard
	Erythrocyte thiamin pyrophosphate	Reversed-phase HPLC and fluorescence detection
Riboflavin	Erythrocyte activity of glutathione reductase with and without added prosthetic group flavin adenine dinucleotide	Enzyme-coupled kinetic assay whereby glutathione reductase activity is measured spectrophotometrically via oxidation of NADP to $NADP^+$
Niacin	NAD : NADP ratio in erythrocytes	HPLC
Pyridoxine	Plasma pyridoxal-5′-phosphate	Cation-exchange HPLC with fluorescence detection
Vitamin C	Serum or leukocyte ascorbic acid	HPLC with electrochemical detection
Folate	Erythrocyte and serum folate Serum homocysteine	Microbiological assay using *L. casei* (NCIB 10463) Reversed-phase HPLC with fluorescence detection
Vitamin B_{12}	Serum vitamin B_{12} Serum MMA	Radioimmunoassay Mass spectrometry
Protein	Serum transthyretin	Radialimmunodiffusion or nephelometry

Table 15.2: Recommended biochemical tests for the fat- and water-soluble vitamins and protein. NADP, nicotinamide adenine dinucleotide phosphate; NAD, nicotinamide adenine dinucleotide; ELISA, enzyme-linked immunosorbent assays; HPLC, high-performance liquid chromatography; RIA, radioimmunoassay; MMA, methylmalonic acid.

trations in erythrocytes are not subject to the transient variations that can affect plasma.

The anticoagulant used for the collection of erythrocytes must be chosen with care to ensure that it does not induce any leakage of ions from the red blood cells. At present, the best choice is heparin (Vitoux et al., 1999).

The separation, washing, and analysis of erythrocytes is technically difficult and must be carried out with care. For example, the centrifugation speed must be high enough to remove the extracellular water but low enough to avoid hemolysis. Care must be taken to carefully discard the buffy coat containing the leukocytes and platelets, because these cells may contain higher concentrations of the nutrient than the erythrocytes.

After separation, the packed erythrocytes must be washed three times with isotonic saline to remove the trapped plasma, and then homogenized. The latter step is critical because during centrifugation the erythrocytes become density stratified, with younger lighter cells at the top and denser older cells at the bottom.

There is no standard method for expressing the nutrient content of erythrocytes, and each of the methods used has limitations. They include nutrient per liter of packed cells, per number of cells, per g of hemoglobin, or per g of dry material (Vitoux et al.,1999).

Erythrocytes can also be used for the assay of a variety of enzyme systems, especially those depending on B-vitamin-derived cofactors. In such cases, the total concentrations of vitamin-derived cofactors in the erythrocytes, or the extent of stimulation of specific enzymes by their vitamin-containing coenzymes, is determined (Sections 20.1.1, 20.2.1, and 21.1). Some of these tests are sensitive to marginal deficiency states and accurately reflect body stores of the vitamin.

15.1.3 Leukocytes

Leukocytes or some specific cell types such as lymphocytes, monocytes, and neutrophils can be used to monitor medium- to long-term changes in nutritional status because they have a lifespan which is slightly shorter than do erythrocytes. As a result, nutrient concentrations in these cell types reflect the onset of a nutrient deficiency state more quickly than do erythrocytes.

Density centrifugation with Ficoll-Hypaque gradients using commercially available solutions are often used to separate leukocytes or other specific cell types (Field, 1996; Bauer, 1999). Newer techniques to separate and classify specific cell types include partition chromatography (Shibusawa, 1999), counterflow centrifugal elutriation, and flow cytometry (Ito and Shinomiya, 2001). Techniques such as these enable the leukocytes or specific cell types to be isolated in a highly purified viable form without introducing contamination from reagents or from residual platelets or erythrocytes.

Nevertheless, several other technical difficulties may arise when isolating leukocytes or other cell types for biochemical tests. For example, the nutrient content of the cell types varies with the age and size of the cells. In some circumstances (i.e., during surgery or acute infection), there is a temporary influx of new granulocytes, which alters the normal balance between the cell types in the blood and thus may confound the results. Certain illnesses alter the size and protein content of some cell types, and this may also lead to difficulties in the interpretation of their nutrient content (Martin et al., 1993).

When centrifugal force is used for washing and isolating the cell types, it must be standardized; otherwise the precision of the assay may be poor (Peretz et al., 1991). Indeed, coefficients of variation as large as 25% have been reported for elemental concentrations in leukocytes (Martin et al., 1993), although the variation can be markedly reduced when rigorous methods are employed to separate the cells. Because relatively large blood samples are required for harvesting the leukocytes or cell types, the use of these assays is restricted to adults.

Again, as noted for erythrocytes, no standard method exists for expressing the content or concentration of nutrients in cells such as leukocytes. Methods that are used include nutrient per unit mass of protein, nutrient concentration per cell, nutrient concentration per dry weight of cells, and nutrient per unit of DNA (Elin, 1987).

15.1.4 Breast milk

Concentrations of certain nutrients secreted in breast milk — notably vitamins A, B_6, and B_{12}, as well as thiamin, riboflavin, iodine and selenium — can reflect levels in the maternal diet and body stores. Studies have shown that in regions where deficiencies of vitamin A (Underwood, 1994), selenium (Funk et al., 1990), and iodine (Delange, 1985) are endemic, concentrations of these micronutrients in breast milk are low. There are, however, few reported population studies of the concentration of the B-vitamins in breast milk.

In some settings, it is more feasible to collect breast milk samples rather than blood samples. Nevertheless, sampling, extraction, handling, and storage of the breast milk samples must be carried out carefully to obtain accurate information on the nutrient concentrations of breast milk. To avoid sampling colostrum and transitional milk, which often have very high nutrient concentrations, mature breast milk samples should be taken at least 21 d postpartum, when the concentration of most nutrients has stabilized. Ideally, complete 24-h breast milk samples from both breasts should be collected because the concentration of some nutrients (e.g., retinol)

Indicator (month post-partum)	Vitamin A group [n]	Placebo group [n]	Standardized difference
Breast milk vit.A (µg/g fat) in casual samples (3 mo)	2.05 ± 0.44 [36]	1.70 ± 0.47 [37]	0.76
Breast milk vit.A (µmol/L) in casual samples (3 mo)	0.12 ± 0.70 [36]	−0.18 ± 0.48 [37]	0.50
Maternal serum retinol (µmol/L) (3 mo)	1.45 ± 0.47 [34]	1.33 ± 0.42 [35]	0.27
Breast milk vit.A (µmol/L) in full samples (3 mo)	−0.33 ± 0.74 [33]	−0.45 ± 0.53 [35]	0.19
Breast milk vit.A (µg/g fat) in full samples (3 mo)	1.87 ± 0.51 [33]	1.82 ± 0.45 [35]	0.10

Table 15.3: Response to postpartum vitamin A supplementation measured by maternal and infant indicators. The values shown are means ± SD. A natural log transformation was used in all cases to improve normality except for the serum retinol data. The means and SDs of the transformed values are presented. [n], number of samples. Data from Rice et al., American Journal of Clinical Nutrition 71: 799–806, 2000 © Am J Clin Nutr. American Society for Clinical Nutrition.

varies during a feed (Section 18.1.5). In community-based studies, however, this is often not feasible. As a result, alternative breast milk sampling protocols have been developed, the choice depending on the study objectives and the nutrient of interest. To date, only breast milk vitamin A concentrations have been extensively used to provide information about the vitamin A status of both the mother and the breastfed infant (Stoltzfus and Underwood, 1995).

For the assessment of breast milk vitamin A at the individual level, the recommended practice is to collect into a dark glass bottle on ice, the entire milk content of one breast that has not been used to feed an infant for at least 2 h; details are given in Section 18.1.5. This procedure is necessary because the fat content of breast milk, and thus the content of fat-soluble vitamin A, increases from the beginning to the end of a single feed.

If a full-breast milk sample cannot be obtained, then an aliquot (8–10 mL) can be collected before the infant starts suckling, by using either a breast pump or manual self-expression (Section 18.1.5) (Rice et al., 2000).

For population-based studies, WHO (1996) suggests collecting random samples of breast milk throughout the day and at varying times following the last feed (i.e., casual samples) in an effort to ensure that the variation in milk fat is randomly sampled. When random sampling is not achievable, the fat-soluble nutrients should be expressed relative to fat concentrations, using the procedure described in Section 18.1.5.

Before shipping to the laboratory, the complete breast milk sample from each subject should be warmed to room temperature and homogenized by swirling gently, and then an aliquot of the precise volume needed for analysis can be withdrawn. This aliquot is then frozen at −20°C in an amber or yellow polypropylene tube with an airtight cap, preferably in a freezer without a frost-freeze cycle, until it is analyzed. This strategy of homogenization reduces subsequent problems with attaining uniform mixing after prolonged storage in a freezer (Stoltzfus and Underwood, 1995).

Table 15.3 compares the performance of breast milk indicators in detecting a response to postpartum vitamin A supplementation in lactating Bangladeshi women (Rice et al., 2000). The most responsive breast milk indicator in this study was the vitamin A content per gram of fat in casual breast milk samples, based on the absolute values of the standardized differences. For more details, see Section 18.1.5.

The analytical methods for breast milk samples must be chosen carefully. Reagents used must be free of adventitious sources of contamination; bound forms of some of the vitamins (e.g., folate, pantothenic acid and vitamin D) must be released prior to extraction and analysis; and, for microbiological assays, a test organism must be selected that can utilize the nutrient under the conditions of the assay. Finally, because certain nonspecific blocking factors present in breast milk interfere with solid-phase immunoassay procedures, the latter must be selected with care.

15.1.5 Saliva

Several studies have investigated the use of saliva as a biopsy fluid for the assessment of nutritional status. It is readily available so that multiple collections can be made. Collection procedures, unlike those for blood, are non-invasive and can readily be undertaken in the field or in the home.

Saliva is a safer diagnostic specimen than blood; infections from HIV and hepatitis are less of a danger because of the low concentrations of antigens in saliva (Hofman, 2001). Saliva specimens can be collected and stored at room temperature, and then mailed to the laboratory without refrigeration. However, before collecting saliva samples, several factors must be considered; these are summarized in Box 15.2.

Collection of saliva can be accomplished by expectorating saliva directly into tubes or small paper cups, with or without any additional stimulation. Subjects may be requested to rinse their mouth with distilled water, prior to the collection. In some cases, cotton balls or absorbent pads are used to collect saliva. These are then immersed in a preservative which stabilizes the specimen for several weeks. A disadvantage of this method is that it may contribute interfering

substances to the extract and is therefore not suitable for certain analytes.

Alternatively, devices can be placed in the mouth to collect a filtered saliva specimen. These include a small membrane sack that filters out bacteria and enzymes (Saliva Sac; Pacific Biometrics, Seattle, Washington) (Schramm and Smith, 1991), or a tiny plastic tube that contains cyclodextrin to bind the analyte. The latter device, termed the "Oral Diffusion Sink" (ODS), is available from the Saliva Testing and Reference Laboratory, Seattle, Washington (Wade and Haegle, 1991). The ODS device can be suspended in the mouth using dental floss, while the subject is sleeping or performing most of their normal activities, with the exception of eating and drinking. In this way, the content of the analyte in the saliva represents an average for the entire collection time period.

Steroid and other nonpeptide hormones (e.g., thyroxine, testosterone), some therapeutic and other drugs, and antibodies to various bacterial and viral diseases can also be measured in saliva. For example, determinations of salivary IgA and IgG can be used to screen for the presence of infections (Punthuprapasa et al., 2001).

The concentrations of some micronutrients (e.g., zinc) in saliva have also been investigated. However, interpreting the results is still difficult: suitable certified reference materials and interpretive values for normal individuals are limited.

15.1.6 Sweat

Collection of sweat, like saliva, is also non-invasive and can be performed in the field or in the home. Several collection methods for sweat have been used: some are designed to collect whole body sweat, whereas others collect sweat from a specific region of the body, often using some form of enclosing bag or capsule.

Shirreffs and Maughan (1997) have developed a method for collecting whole body sweat involving the subject exercising in a plastic-lined enclosure. The method does not interfere with the normal sweating pro-

---

Is resting or stimulated saliva required? Stimulated saliva can be collected using sugar-free gum.

What volume of saliva is required for the assay?

Is special pretreatment and storage of the saliva required?

What is the health status of the subjects in relation to medications and/or diseases causing a dry mouth?

Will a quantitative or qualitative assay be performed?

Box 15.2: Factors to be considered when collecting saliva samples.

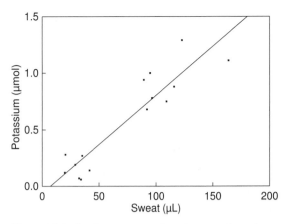

Figure 15.1: Total sweat potassium from patches worn by five healthy subjects vs. total volume of sweat collected. Data from Sarno et al., Clinical Chemistry 45: 1501–1509, 1999, with permission of the AACC.

cess and overcomes difficulties caused by variations in the composition of sweat from different parts of the body. The method cannot be used for treadmill exercise but can be used for subjects exercising on a cycle ergometer.

A method designed to collect sweat from a specific region of the body involves using a nonocclusive skin patch known as the Osteopatch. It consists of a transparent, hypoallergenic, gas-permeable membrane with a cellulose fiber absorbent pad. The patch can be applied to the abdomen or lower back for 5 d. During the collection period, the nonvolatile components of sweat are deposited on the absorbent pad, whereas the volatile components evaporate through the semipermeable membrane.

Sweat volume can be assessed via measurement of potassium by flame atomic emission or ion-selective electrode techniques. Potassium concentrations in sweat are relatively independent of sweat rate (Figure 15.1) and thus the potassium content of the collection pad is a measure of sweat volume. The Osteopatch method was used for sample collection when studying collagen cross-link molecules such as deoxypyridinoline in sweat (Section 23.1.5) (Sarno et al., 1999).

Differences in the composition of human sweat have been linked, in part, to discrepancies in collection methods. Errors may

be caused by contamination, incomplete collection, or real differences induced by the collection procedure.

15.1.7 Adipose tissue

Adipose tissue is becoming an increasingly popular biopsy material for use in population studies. It may be a better biomarker of the long-term intake of fat-soluble nutrients, such as certain fatty acids or vitamin E, than concentrations in the blood (Beynen and Katan, 1985; Parker, 1989; El-Sohemy et al., 2002). The latter change more rapidly and reflect the short-term fluctuations in intake (Kohlmeier and Kohlmeier, 1995; Hunter, 1998).

Simple, rapid sampling methods have been devised for collecting subcutaneous adipose-tissue biopsies, generally from the upper buttock (El-Sohemy et al., 2002), although other sites have also been investigated (Schafer and Overvad, 1990; Zhang et al., 1997). Use of adipose tissue for the assessment of long-term fatty acid and vitamin E status is discussed in Sections 7.3.7 and 18.3.5, respectively.

15.1.8 Liver and bone

Iron and calcium are stored primarily in the body in the liver and bones, respectively. Sampling these sites is too invasive for population studies: they are only sampled in research or clinical settings. Dual photon absorptiometry (DXA) is now used to determine total bone mineral content (Section 23.1.8).

15.1.9 Hair

Scalp hair can be used as a biopsy material for screening populations at risk for certain trace element deficiencies (e.g., zinc, selenium) and to assess excessive exposure to heavy metals (e.g., mercury, arsenic). Detailed reviews are available (IAEA, 1993, 1994). In some circumstances, hair trace element content has been used to provide a retrospective, chronic measure of trace element status during the period of hair growth. Caution must be used when interpreting results for hair mineral analysis from com-

Higher concentrations of trace elements are found in hair, relative to blood or urine, making analysis easier; results for the ultra-trace elements such as chromium and manganese are more consistent.

Concentrations are more stable and hair trace element levels are not subject to the rapid fluctuations associated with diet, diurnal variation, and so on.

No trauma is involved in the collection of hair samples.

No special preservatives are needed, and samples can be stored in plastic bags at room temperature without deterioration.

Box 15.3: Some of the advantages of hair as a biopsy material.

mercial laboratories because results can be unreliable (Seidel et al., 2001).

Analysis of trace element levels in hair has several advantages compared to that of blood or urine; these are summarized in Box 15.3. Nevertheless, a major limitation of the use of scalp hair is its susceptibility to exogenous contamination. Hopps (1977) noted that sweat from the eccrine sweat glands may contaminate the hair with elements derived from body tissues. Other exogenous materials that may modify the trace element composition of hair include air, water, soap, shampoo, lacquers, dyes, and medications. Selenium in antidandruff shampoos, for example, significantly increases hair selenium content, and the selenium cannot be removed by standardized hair-washing procedures (Davies, 1982) (Section 25.2.7). For other trace elements, results from hair-washing procedures have been equivocal. Some (Hilderbrand and White, 1974), but not all (Gibson and Gibson, 1984), investigators have observed marked changes in hair trace element concentrations after hair cosmetic treatments. The relative importance of these sources remains uncertain, and standardized procedures for hair sampling and washing prior to analysis are essential.

The currently recommended hair sampling method is to use the proximal 1.5–2.0 cm of hair, cut from the suboccipital portion of the scalp. This procedure, involving the sampling of recently grown hair, minimizes the effects

of abrasion of the hair shaft and exogenous contamination (Hambidge, 1982).

Several different washing procedures have been investigated, including the use of non-ionic or ionic detergents, followed by rinsing in distilled, deionized water to remove absorbed detergent (Harrison et al., 1969; Petering et al., 1971; Salmela et al., 1981; Kumpulainen et al., 1982). Various organic solvents such as hexane-methanol, acetone (Hambidge et al., 1972a; Salmela et al., 1981; Kumpulainen et al., 1982), and ether (Petering et al., 1971) have also been recommended, either alone or in combination with a detergent. A metal-chelating agent, ethylenediaminetetraacetate (EDTA), has also been included in some hair-washing procedures (Hammer et al., 1971), especially those designed to remove adsorbed zinc and copper. However, use of EDTA is not generally recommended because of the risk of removing endogenous minerals from the hair shaft.

Additional confounding factors that may affect trace element concentrations in hair include hair color, age, sex, pregnancy, smoking, the presence of certain disease states, season, and rate of hair growth (Hambidge et al., 1972b; Creason et al., 1975; McKenzie, 1978; Hambidge, 1982; Taylor, 1986; Laitinen et al., 1988; Gibson et al., 1983; Bertazzo et al., 1996; Perrone et al., 1996). Relationships between hair color and trace element content have been inconsistent. Creason et al. (1975) reported that only the iron content was related to hair color in adults, whereas other investigators have noted higher manganese concentrations in dark versus blond scalp hair samples, and higher iron, nickel, copper, and zinc in red hair compared to brown (Sky-Peck and Joseph, 1983).

Some investigators suggest that the rate of hair growth influences hair trace element concentrations. Scalp hair grows at about 1 cm/mo, but in some cases of severe protein-energy malnutrition (Erten et al., 1978) and the zinc deficiency state acrodermatitis enteropathica (Hambidge et al., 1977), growth of the hair is impaired. In such cases, hair zinc concentrations may be normal or even high. No significant differences, however, were observed in the trace element concentrations of scalp and pubic hair samples (De Antonio et al., 1982), despite marked differences in the rate of hair growth at the two anatomical sites (Hopps, 1977). These results suggest that the relative rate of hair growth is not a significant factor in controlling hair trace element levels.

In summary, more data on other tissues from the same individuals are urgently required to interpret the significance of hair trace element concentrations. Hair is certainly a very useful indicator of the body burden of heavy metals such as lead, mercury, cadmium and arsenic. It is also valuable in the case of selenium, chromium, and zinc. Data for other elements such as iron, calcium, magnesium, and copper should be interpreted cautiously (Seidel et al., 2001).

15.1.10 Fingernails and toenails

Nails have been investigated as biopsy materials for trace element analysis (Bank et al., 1981; van Noord et al., 1987). Like hair, nails are also easy to sample and store but grow more slowly than hair at rates ranging from 0.025 mm/d for toenails to 0.1 mm/d for fingernails. Nails are formed by proliferating cells in the germinal layer of the nail matrix, which are converted during growth into horny lamellae.

The elemental composition of nails is influenced by age, sex, geographical location, and possibly by disease states (e.g., cystic fibrosis, Wilson's disease, Alzheimer's disease, and arthritis) (Takagi et al., 1988; Vance et al., 1988). Environmental contamination could be a potential problem limiting the use of nails as a biopsy material for trace element analysis. Bank et al. (1981) recommend cleaning fingernails with a scrubbing brush and a mild detergent, followed by mechanical scraping to remove any remaining soft tissue, before clipping. Nails should then be washed in aqueous detergents rather than organic solvents and dried under vacuum prior to analysis.

The elemental composition of toenails can be used as a long-term biomarker of nutri-

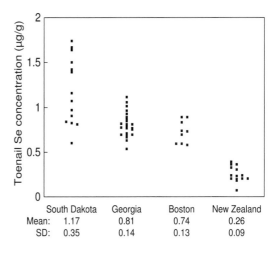

	South Dakota	Georgia	Boston	New Zealand
Mean:	1.17	0.81	0.74	0.26
SD:	0.35	0.14	0.13	0.09

Figure 15.2: Toenail selenium concentrations in a high-selenium area (South Dakota), Georgia, and Boston, compared with a low-selenium area (New Zealand). From Morris et al., Biological Trace Element Research 5: 529–537, 1983 with permission.

tional status for some elements, notably selenium. Selenium concentrations in toenails correlate with geographic differences in selenium exposure (Figure 15.2) (Morris et al., 1983; Hunter et al., 1990). At the individual level, concentrations of selenium in toenails correlate with those in habitual diets, serum, and whole blood (Swanson et al., 1990).

More studies comparing the trace element composition of toenails with corresponding concentrations in other body tissues and fluids, as well as habitual dietary intakes, are needed before any definite recommendations on the use of toenails can be made.

15.1.11 Buccal mucosal cells

Buccal mucosal cells have been investigated as a biopsy sample for assessing α-tocopherol status (Kaempf et al., 1994) (Section 18.3.5) and dietary lipid status (McMurchie et al., 1984) (Section 7.3.7), but interpretive criteria to assess these results are not available. These cells have also been explored as an indicator of folate status (Johnson et al., 1997), although smoking is a major confounder as a localized folate deficiency is generated in tissues exposed to cigarette smoke (Piyathilake et al., 1992). Buccal mucosal cells are also increasingly used in epidemiological studies that involve DNA (Potischman, 2003).

Buccal mucosal cells can be sampled easily and noninvasively by gentle scraping with a spatula. Cells must be washed with isotonic saline prior to sonication and analysis. Contamination of buccal cells with food is a major problem, however, and has prompted research into new methods for the collection of buccal mucosal cells.

15.1.12 Urinary excretion rate of the nutrient or its metabolite

Urine specimens can be used for the biochemical assessment of some trace elements (e.g., chromium, iodine, selenium), protein, the water-soluble B-complex vitamins, and vitamin C, if renal function is normal. Urine cannot be used to assess the status of vitamins A, D, E, and K, as metabolites are not excreted in proportion to the amount of these vitamins consumed, absorbed, and metabolized.

Urinary excretion assessment methods almost always reflect recent dietary intake or the *acute* status, rather than the chronic nutritional status. The methods depend on the existence of a renal conservation mechanism that reduces the urinary excretion of the nutrient and metabolite when their body stores are depleted.

For some of the water-soluble vitamins (e.g., thiamin, riboflavin, and vitamin C), the amount excreted depends on both the nutrient saturation of tissues and the dietary intake. Further, it tends to reflect intake when intakes of the vitamins are moderate to high relative to the requirements, but less so when intakes are habitually low. In other circumstances, such as infections, after trauma, and use of antibiotics or medications, and in conditions that produce negative balance, increases in urinary excretion may occur despite depletion of body nutrient stores. For example, drugs with chelating abilities, alcoholism, and liver disease can increase urinary zinc excretion, even in the presence of zinc deficiency.

For measurement of a nutrient or a corresponding metabolite in urine, it is essential to collect a clean, properly preserved urine sample, preferably over a complete 24-h period (Solomons, 1985). For unstable nutrients (e.g., vitamin C), urine requires acidification and cold storage to prevent degradation.

To monitor the completeness of any 24-h urine collection, urinary creatinine excretion is often measured (Section 7.3.4). This approach assumes that daily urinary creatinine excretion is constant for a given individual, the amount being related to muscle mass. In fact, this excretion can be highly variable within an individual (Waterlow, 1986; Webster and Garrow, 1985). Estimates of the within-subject coefficient of variation for creatinine excretion in sequential daily urine collections range from 1% to 36% (Jackson, 1966; Webster and Garrow, 1985). Hence, creatinine determinations may only detect gross errors in 24-h urine collections (Bingham and Cummings, 1985).

British investigators have used an alternative marker, para-aminobenzoic acid (PABA), to assess completeness of urine collections (Bingham and Cummings, 1983). Possible explanations, for low PABA recovery values, besides the undercollection of urine samples, are summarized in Box 15.4. This substance is taken in tablet form with meals — one tablet of 80 mg PABA three times per day. It is harmless, easy to measure, and rapidly and completely excreted in urine. Studies have shown that any urine collection containing less than 85% of the administered dose is probably incomplete (Bingham and Cummings, 1983), suggesting that PABA is a useful marker for monitoring the completeness of urine collection. The incomplete nature of

---

Failure to take all three tablets

Taking tablets late in the evening with a large meal that reduces gastric emptying time and uptake in the intestine

Impaired renal function

Errors in preparation of urine aliquots

Analytical errors

Box 15.4: Possible reasons for the undercollection of 24-h urine samples.

urine collections with a mean PABA recovery of ⩽ 79% is emphasized in Figure 15.3.

A method has been devised for adjusting urinary concentrations of nitrogen, sodium, and potassium, in cases where the recovery of PABA is between 50% and 80%. It is based on the linear relationship of the PABA recovery and the amount of analytes in the urine, as shown in Figure 15.4, and allows the use of incomplete 24-h urine collections. However, this adjustment method is not recommended in cases where PABA recovery is below 50%.

Twenty-four-hour urine samples can be difficult to collect in noninstitutionalized population groups. Instead, first-voided fasting morning urine specimens are often used as they are less affected by recent dietary intake. Such specimens were used in the U.K. National Diet and Nutrition Survey of young people aged 4–18 y (Gregory et al., 2001). Special Bori-Vial vials containing a small amount of boric acid as a preservative can be used for the collection of first-voided fasting samples. Alternatively, it may only be feasible to collect nonfasting casual urine samples. Such spot urine samples are not recommended for studies at the individual

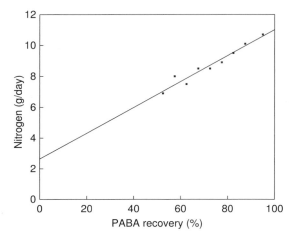

Figure 15.4: The relationship between PABA recovery (%) and the nitrogen output in urine (g/d). The PABA recovery values have been classified into 5% intervals from 50% to 90% and one interval between 90% and 110%. The number of subjects in each interval is 10 or more. Total $n = 312$, $r^2 = 0.9752$. Data from Johansson et al., Public Health Nutrition 2: 587–591, 1999, with permission of the Nutrition Society.

level, because concentrations of nutrients and metabolites in such samples are affected by liquid consumption, recent dietary intake, physical activity, and so on.

When first-voided fasting or casual urine specimens are collected, urinary excretion is sometimes expressed as a ratio of the nutrient to urinary creatinine to correct for both diurnal variation and fluctuations in urine volume. This mode of expression is not recommended, however, by WHO/UNICEF/ICCIDD (1994) for urinary iodine. Instead, they recommend collecting casual samples and expressing the results in terms of μg/L.

15.2 Functional tests

Functional laboratory tests can be classified into two main groups: functional biochemical tests and functional physiological or behavioral tests. They measure the extent of the functional consequences of a specific nutrient deficiency and, hence, have greater biological significance than the static laboratory tests, as noted earlier.

Functional biochemical tests may involve the measurement of an abnormal metabolic

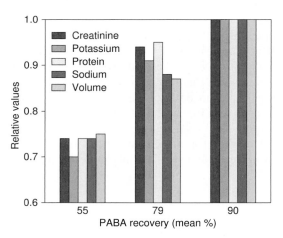

Figure 15.3: The relationship of urinary PABA recovery and urinary creatinine, potassium, protein (derived from nitrogen), sodium, and volume in three groups of patients with median PABA recovery of 55% ($n = 28$), 79% ($n = 24$), and 90% ($n = 21$). The urinary variables are expressed in relative terms in relation to the highest PABA recovery group, which is set to 1.0. Data from Johansson et al., Public Health Nutrition 1: 199–206, 1998, with permission of the Nutrition Society.

product in blood or urine samples arising from a deficiency of a nutrient-dependent enzyme. For some nutrients, reduction in the activity of enzymes that require a nutrient as a coenzyme or prosthetic group can also be measured. Alternatively, changes in blood components related to intake of a nutrient can be determined, as well as load or tolerance tests conducted on subjects in vivo. Sometimes, tissues or cells are isolated and maintained under physiological conditions for tests of in vivo functions. Tests related to host defense and immunocompetence are the most widely used of this type. For some of the nutrients (e.g., niacin), functional biochemical tests are not available.

In research settings, stable isotope techniques are now used to measure the size of the body pool(s) of a nutrient (e.g., the vitamin A content of the liver) (Section 18.1.2), and for kinetic modeling to assess the integrated whole-body response to changes in nutrient status (e.g., protein, copper, zinc). The latter approach is especially useful for detecting subtle changes that may not be responsive to static indices (King et al., 2000). Figure 15.5 shows a marked reduction in the endogenous fecal excretion of zinc over a 6-mo period on

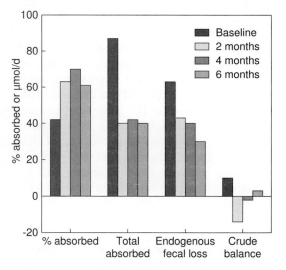

Figure 15.5: Changes in intestinal zinc absorption and endogenous loss over 6 mo while on a low-zinc intake of 63 μmol/d (4.1 mg/d). From King et al., Journal of Nutrition 130: 1360S–1366S, 2000, with permission of The American Society for Nutritional Sciences.

a low-zinc diet. Such a reduction can only be quantified with isotopic techniques. New molecular techniques are also increasingly used in research to measure, for example, mRNA for proteins (e.g., metallothionein), the expression of which is regulated by metal ions such as zinc (Hirschi et al., 2001).

Some important examples of functional tests include the following:

- Abnormal metabolic products in blood or urine arising from reduced activity of a nutrient-dependent enzyme. Such products may include the urinary excretion of xanthurenic acid, formiminoglutamic acid (FIGLU), and methylmalonic acid as a test of vitamin B_6, folate, and vitamin B_{12} deficiency, respectively.
- Changes in blood components (e.g., whole blood hemoglobin for iron assessment) or changes in enzyme activities that depend on a given nutrient (e.g., erythrocyte glutathione reductase activity for riboflavin; erythrocyte transketolase activity for thiamin).
- In vitro tests of in vivo functions (e.g., lymphocyte proliferation for protein-energy, zinc, and iron; deoxyuridine (dU) suppression test for vitamin B_{12} and folate).
- Load and tolerance tests and induced responses in vivo. Examples include the histidine load test for folate, the tryptophan load test for vitamin B_6, and zinc and manganese tolerance tests. Delayed-type hypersensitivity is a well-known example of a test based on an induced response in vivo and is often used to identify protein-energy malnutrition.
- Spontaneous in vivo responses (e.g., dark adaptation and taste acuity for vitamin A; muscle function for protein-energy malnutrition).
- Growth or developmental responses (e.g., sexual maturation for zinc; growth velocity for protein-energy, zinc, etc.; cognitive performance for iron, iodine, zinc, and vitamin B_{12}).

Most functional physiological and behavioral tests are less invasive, often easier to perform, and more directly related to disease mechanisms or health status than are functional tests. However, functional physiological or behavioral tests may not be very specific.

15.2.1 Abnormal metabolic products in blood or urine

Many of the vitamins and minerals act as coenzymes or prosthetic groups for enzyme systems. During deficiency, the activities of these enzymes may be reduced, resulting in the accumulation of abnormal metabolic products in the blood or urine. Hence, measurement of these abnormal metabolic products may provide a sensitive and specific biomarker of nutrient deficiency.

In vitamin B_6 deficiency, for example, the activity of kynureninase in the tryptophan-niacin pathway is reduced because pyridoxal phosphate is a coenzyme for kynureninase. This leads to increased formation and excretion of xanthurenic and other tryptophan metabolites, including both kynurenic acid and 3-hydroxy-kynurenine. Usually, urinary xanthurenic acid is determined because it is easily measured.

Another example is the increase in total plasma homocysteine concentration that is seen in folate and vitamin B_{12} deficiency. Normally, the metabolism of homocysteine follows two pathways, one of which is favored in the postprandial state, and another, the remethylation pathway, that is favored under fasting conditions. The latter pathway requires vitamin B_{12} as a coenzyme and folate as a cosubstrate or methyl donor (Section 22.1.5) (Carmel, 2000). Therefore, in folate or vitamin B_{12} deficiency, homocysteine accumulates, and concentrations in plasma increase. Elevated circulating homocysteine concentrations are now known to have an adverse effect on health. For example, they have been associated with an increased risk of occlusive vascular disease (Refsum et al., 1998).

15.2.2 Reduction in activity of enzymes

Methods that involve measuring a change in the activity of enzymes which require a specific nutrient as a coenzyme or prosthetic group are preferred because they are generally the most sensitive and specific (Bates et al., 1997). Often the enzyme is associated with a specific metabolic defect and associated nutrient deficiency (e.g., lysyl oxidase for copper, aspartate aminotransferase for vitamin B_6, glutathione reductase for riboflavin, transketolase for thiamin).

The activity of the enzyme is sometimes measured with and without the addition of saturating amounts of the coenzyme added in vitro. The in vitro stimulation of the enzyme by the coenzyme indicates the degree of unsaturation of the enzyme, and therefore a measure of deficiency. Such tests, often termed "enzyme stimulation tests," are used for vitamin B_6, riboflavin, and thiamin and employ the activities of aminotransferases, glutathione reductase, and transketolase, respectively.

The tissue selected for the enzyme assay should be particularly sensitive to the pathological lesion. Erythrocytes are often chosen for enzyme stimulation tests because they contain a variety of enzyme systems that depend on B-vitamin-derived cofactors. The tests also appear to be sensitive to marginal deficiencies and provide an accurate reflection of body stores for thiamin, riboflavin, and vitamin B_6.

Unfortunately, for many nutrients, such pathologically sensitive tissues are either inaccessible or unknown. Ideally, the assay selected should (*a*) reflect the amount of the nutrient available to the body, (*b*) respond rapidly to changes in supply of the nutrient, and (*c*) relate to the pathology of deficiency or excess. Measurement of the copper-containing enzyme lysyl oxidase is an example of an assay that fulfills these criteria. Connective tissue defects occur during the early stages of the copper deficiency syndrome. These defects can be attributed to the depressed activity of lysyl oxidase inhibiting cross-linking of collagen and elastin.

Many nutrients have more than one functional role, so that the activities of several enzymes may be affected during the development of a deficiency, thereby providing additional information on the severity of the deficiency state. For example, in the case of copper, platelet cytochrome c oxidase (Section 24.2.4) is more sensitive to deficiency than plasma ceruloplasmin (Section 24.2.2), the activity of which is only reduced in more severe deficiency states (L'Abbé and Fischer, 1984; Milne and Johnson, 1993).

15.2.3 Changes in blood components

Instead of measuring the activity of an enzyme, changes in blood components that are related to the intake of a nutrient can be measured. A well-known example is the measurement of hemoglobin concentrations in whole blood for iron deficiency anemia; iron is an essential component of the hemoglobin molecule (Section 17.1). Other examples include the determination of the three transport proteins transferrin, transthyretin, and retinol-binding protein, as indicators of iron, iodine, and vitamin A status, respectively. The specific factors affecting the binding of transthyretin to thyroxine and of retinol-binding protein to retinol remain uncertain (de Pee and Dary, 2002).

15.2.4 In vitro tests of in vivo functions

Tissue samples or cells can be removed from test subjects and isolated and maintained under physiological conditions. Attempts can then be made to replicate in vitro a corresponding in vivo function. Tests related to host-defense and immunocompetence are probably the most widely used assays of this type. They appear to provide a useful, functional, and quantitative index of nutritional status.

The immune system has two lymphoid components. These are thymus-dependent T-lymphocytes arising in the thymus and also B-lymphocytes originating in the bone marrow. The former are the main effectors of cell-mediated immunity, whereas B-lymphocytes are responsible for humoral immunity. During protein-energy malnutrition, both the proportion and the absolute number of T-cells in the peripheral blood may be reduced (Chan-

dra, 1974). An in vitro test has been developed to measure the total number of T-lymphocytes. Details of this test are given in Section 16.5.2.

Lymphocyte proliferation assays are also examples of tests of this type. They are functional measures of cell-mediated immunity, assessed by the in vitro responses of lymphocytes to selected mitogens. Again, peripheral T-lymphocytes are isolated from blood and incubated in vitro with selected mitogens (Field, 1996). Details are summarized in Section 16.5.3.

Other in vitro tests include the erythrocyte hemolysis test and the dU suppression test. In the former, the rate of hemolysis of erythrocytes is measured; the rate correlates inversely with serum tocopherol levels (Section 18.3.6). Unfortunately, this test is not very specific, as other nutrients, such as selenium, influence the rate of erythrocyte hemolysis.

The dU suppression test is used to diagnose deficiencies of vitamin B_{12} or folic acid in the absence of morphological changes in the blood (Section 22.2.2). In this test, bone marrow cells are preincubated with and without dU. Deoxyuridine suppresses the ability of the bone marrow cells to incorporate the subsequently added radioactive thymidine (^{3}H-thymidine) into DNA. This suppression is subnormal in patients with vitamin B_{12} or folate deficiency (Herbert et al., 1973). Peripheral blood lymphocytes and whole blood can also be used for the dU suppression test.

15.2.5 Induced responses, load and tolerance tests in vivo

Functional tests conducted on the subject in vivo include many well-established load and tolerance tests (Solomons and Allen, 1983). Such tests are used for individuals with a suspected deficiency of a nutrient; they are not suitable for survey studies.

Load tests are used to assess deficiencies of water-soluble vitamins (e.g., tryptophan load test for pyridoxine, histidine load test for folic acid, vitamin C load test), and certain minerals (e.g., magnesium, zinc, and selenium)

(Caddell et al., 1975; Robberecht and Deelstra, 1984; Fickel et al., 1986; Bates et al., 1997).

In a load test, the baseline urinary excretion of the nutrient or metabolite (Robberecht and Deelstra, 1984) is first determined on a timed preload urine collection. Then a loading dose of the nutrient or an associated compound is administered orally, intramuscularly, or intravenously. After the load, a timed sample of the urine is collected, and the excretion level of the nutrient or a metabolite is determined. The net retention of the nutrient is calculated by comparing the basal excretion data with net excretion after the load. In a deficiency state, when tissues are not saturated with the nutrient, excretion of the nutrient or a metabolite will be low because net retention is high.

Tolerance tests, sometimes referred to as plasma appearance tests, are also conducted on the subject in vivo. In these tests, the concentration of the nutrient is measured both in fasting plasma and in plasma after an oral pharmacological dose of the nutrient (e.g., zinc or manganese). The response is enhanced in cases of nutrient depletion because intestinal absorption of the nutrient is assumed to increase in a nutrient deficiency state (Fickel et al., 1986). Use of pharmacological doses limits the usefulness of these tests because such large doses may be handled differently by the gastrointestinal tract than are physiological levels of the nutrient.

Examples of other functional in vivo load tests that involve physiological doses include the relative dose–response test for vitamin A (Section 18.1.6) and, for chromium, changes in an oral glucose tolerance test after chromium supplementation (Section 24.1.7).

A well known example of a test based on an induced response in vivo is delayed-type hypersensitivity (DTH). This test is a direct functional measure of cell-mediated immunity and is used in hospitals and community settings. It involves injecting a battery of specific antigens intradermally in the forearm and noting the induced response at selected time intervals. This test, like the in vitro test of immune function described in Section 15.2.4, is not specific enough to detect individual nutrient deficiencies (Bates et al., 1979; Twomey et al., 1982). Details are given in Section 16.5.4.

15.2.6 Spontaneous in vivo responses

The first functional tests to use a spontaneous physiological response in vivo involved dark adaptation and capillary fragility. A deficit in dark adaptation, resulting in night blindness, was first described in association with vitamin A deficiency.

The classical method of assessing night blindness is formal dark adaptometry. This method is very time-consuming. It has been superseded by a new, interactive, rapid dark adaptation test (RDAT), results of which correlate well with those of the classical method. The RDAT, however, is not appropriate for young children, as noted in Section 18.1.9. Consequently, a new test has been developed, the pupillary and visual threshold test, which can be used with individuals of all ages (Congdon and West, 2002); details are given in Section 18.1.10.

Capillary fragility has been used as a functional test of vitamin C deficiency since 1913 (Hess, 1913) because frank petechial hemorrhages occur in overt vitamin C deficiency. The test, however, is not very specific to vitamin C deficiency states (Section 19.7); static biochemical tests are preferred to assess the status of vitamin C.

Abnormalities in taste function are sometimes associated with suboptimal zinc status in children and adults (Hambidge et al., 1972b; Gibson et al., 1989; Ruz et al., 1991), as well as in some disease states in which secondary zinc deficiency may occur (e.g., cystic fibrosis, Crohn's disease, celiac sprue, and chronic renal disease) (Watson et al., 1983; Henkin, 1984). A few studies have also demonstrated the recovery of taste function with repletion of body zinc stores (Henkin et al., 1975). Taste acuity can be assessed by using the forced drop method which measures both the detection and recognition thresholds (Buzina et al., 1980; Henkin, 1984), or by measuring the recognition thresholds only

(Desor and Maller, 1975; Bartoshuk, 1978) (Section 24.3.13). In some studies, an electrogustometer, which measures taste threshold by an electric current, has been used (Grant et al., 1987). Many other factors affect taste function, and taste acuity alone should not be used to measure zinc status.

Some other tests based on spontaneous physiological responses in vivo include the assessment of the contraction-relaxation characteristics and endurance of skeletal muscle (Section 16.4.1). The reduction in protein stores and muscle catabolism which occurs during protein-energy malnutrition can alter muscle contractility, relaxation rate, and endurance, and may provide a sensitive index of protein status (Russell and Jeejeebhoy, 1983).

Handgrip strength, measured using a dynamometer, assesses upper extremity muscle strength. The latter has been used to measure nutritional status in hospital patients (Klidjian et al., 1982) and the elderly (Chilima and Ismail, 2001).

15.2.7 Growth responses

Growth indices are not specific for any particular nutrient and are preferably used in association with other more specific laboratory indices. Growth velocity, for example, has frequently been used as a functional index of nutritional status of infants and young children and is discussed in Chapter 10. It can be assessed via measurements of changes in recumbent length for children < 2 y and changes in height for older children. Alternatively, measurements of knee height can be used to provide a more sensitive measure of growth velocity (Section 10.1.6) (Cronk et al., 1989).

15.2.8 Developmental responses

The assessment of cognitive function requires rigorous methodology. Even with careful methodology, a relationship between cognitive function and nutrient deficiency can only be established by (*a*) documenting clinically important differences in cognitive function between deficient subjects and healthy controls, and (*b*) demonstrating improvement in cognitive function after an intervention. The subjects should be matched, and the design should preferably involve a double-blind randomized intervention trial (Lozoff and Brittenham, 1986).

Several measurement scales of cognitive function have been used in studies related to iron (Grantham-McGregor and Ani, 2001) and, more recently, zinc deficiency (Sandstead et al., 1998; Castillo-Duran et al., 2001).

In infancy, the Bayley Scales of Infant Development are often used (Black and Matula, 1999). These scales are well standardized and include three components: Mental Scale, Motor Scale, and Infant Behavior Record (BSID-II: The Psychological Corporation). Several other tests of mental functioning have been used during infancy. For example, the Fagan Test of Infant Intelligence was used in a large trial in which Chilean infants supplemented with iron between 6 and 12 mo ($n = 1123$) were compared to a no-added-iron group ($n = 534$) (Lozoff et al., 2003).

In older school children, IQ-test performance (Seshadri et al., 1982; Palti et al., 1983) has been used as a measure of cognitive function in relation to iron deficiency. The Raven's Progressive Matrices and Vocabulary Scales have also been used in school children and adults to assess performance-type abilities (Raven et al., 1986). The test measures the ability to organize perceptual detail, to reason by analogy, and to make comparisons.

Raven's Progressive Matrices were used in a study of Kenyan school children designed to test whether animal source foods have a key role in the optimal cognitive development of children (Whaley et al., 2003). Results are shown in Figure 15.6. Post-hoc analyses showed that children who received a supplement with meat had significantly greater gains on the Raven's Progressive Matrices than all other groups.

A computer-administered Cognition-Psychomotor Assessment System has also been used to assess neuropsychologic performance in both school children and adults (Sandstead et al., 1998; Penland, 2000).

In the elderly, the Mini-Mental State Ex-

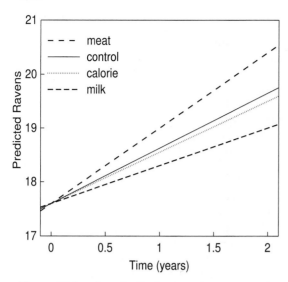

Figure 15.6: Longitudinal regression curves for Raven's scores across five time points, indicating improved cognition in some Kenyan children under four different dietary regimes. Data from Whaley et al., Journal of Nutrition 133: 3965S–3971S, 2003, with permission of The American Society for Nutritional Sciences.

amination (MMSE) is often used in general practice as a screening measure of cognitive impairment (Valente et al., 1992). Italian investigators observed that elevated plasma homocysteine concentrations had an independent, graded association with concurrent cognitive impairment as measured with the MMSE in some healthy elderly community dwellers (Ravaglia et al., 2003).

	Cu (mg/d)		Fe (mg/d)	
	< 1.0	> 2.0	< 5	> 15
Evening bedtime	352*	364	320*	349
Latency to sleep onset	18*	16	11*	9
Night-time awakenings	0.60*	0.51	0.71*	0.59
Total sleep time	358*	346	396*	370
Sleep quality	1.91*	1.97	1.99	1.96

Table 15.4: Effects of dietary copper and iron intakes on the self-reported sleep patterns of women. * Significantly different ($p < 0.05$) than corresponding value for the same mineral. Data from Lukaski and Penland, Journal of Nutrition 126: 2354S–2364S, 1996, with permission of The American Society for Nutritional Sciences.

15.2.9 Sleep behavior

Dietary iron and copper intakes of adults may influence sleep behavior. Women residing in a metabolic unit consumed diets containing varying levels of iron and copper. They completed a sleep behavior inventory immediately upon awakening each morning (Lukaski and Penland, 1996). Results indicated that when receiving low copper diets (i.e., < 1.0 mg/d), women had earlier bedtimes, significantly longer latency to sleep, and longer sleep time, but they felt significantly less rested upon awakening than when they consumed a diet adequate in copper (i.e., > 2.0 mg/d). A comparable finding was noted when women received low dietary intakes of iron, as shown in Table 15.4. These results suggest that sleep quantity may increase during times of illness and stress, although sleep quality may decrease.

15.3 Characteristics of laboratory tests

The objectives of any nutritional assessment system will normally dictate the number and characteristics of the associated laboratory tests. These should be selected with care. Laboratory tests vary in precision, accuracy, analytical specificity, analytical sensitivity, validity, and predictive value. Some of these terms are discussed in Section 1.6. Because almost all techniques are subject to both random and systematic measurement errors, personnel should use calibrated equipment, and be trained to use standardized and validated techniques that are monitored continuously by appropriate quality-control procedures.

15.3.1 Precision

Repeated measurements on a single sample or individual can be used to assess the precision of the laboratory test. The coefficient of variation (CV), as determined by the ratio of the standard deviation to the mean of the replicates ($SD/\bar{x}$), is the best quantitative measure of the precision. Ideally, the CV should be calculated for samples at the bottom, middle, and top of the reference concentration range for the test, as determined on apparently healthy individuals. These same samples serve as quality controls.

Typically, the quality-control samples used to calculate the CV are pooled samples from donors similar to the study participants. It is important that to the analyst, these quality-control samples should appear identical to the samples from the study participants. This means that the same type of vial, label, volume, and so on should be used.

Quality-control samples should be inserted blind into each batch of samples from the study participants. Both the within-run CV and between-run CV should be calculated on these quality-control samples. The former is calculated from the values for the quality-control samples analyzed within the same batch. The between-run CV is normally calculated from the values for the quality-control samples analyzed on different days (Blanck et al., 2003).

The precision of the measurement is a function of the random measurement errors that occur during the actual analytical process, and, in some cases, the within-subject biological variation that occurs naturally over time. As noted earlier (Section 1.4.5), the relative importance of these two sources of uncertainty varies with the measurement. For some measurements (e.g., serum iron), the within-subject biological variation is quite large: coefficients of variation may exceed 30% and be greater than analytical variation. Details of the within-subject, day-to-day variation for other biochemical measurements of iron status are given in Section 17.5.1.

The level of precision attainable for any particular measurement depends on the procedure, whereas the precision required is a function of the study objectives. Some investigators have stipulated that, ideally, the analytical CV for an assay used in epidemiological studies should not exceed 5% (Hunter, 1998). In practice, this level of precision is very difficult to achieve for many assays. Even if precision is acceptable, the method may not be accurate as shown in Figure 15.7.

15.3.2 Analytical accuracy

The difference between the reported and the true amount of the nutrient/metabolite present in the sample is a measure of the analytical accuracy of the laboratory test (Figure 15.7).

Several strategies can be used to ensure that analytical methods are accurate. For methods involving direct analysis of nutrients in tissues or fluids, a recovery test is generally performed. This involves the addition of known amounts of nutrient to the sample. These spiked samples are then analyzed together with unspiked aliquots to assess whether the analytical value accounts for close to 100% of the added nutrient.

As an additional test for accuracy, aliquots of a reference material, similar to the sample and certified for the nutrient of interest, should be included routinely with each batch of specimens (Section 4.4.3). If possible, several reference materials, with values spanning the range observed in the study samples, should be analyzed (Blanck et al., 2003). Such a practice will document the accuracy achieved.

Certified reference materials can be obtained from the U.S. National Institute of Standards and Technology (NIST), the U.S. Centers for Disease Control and Prevention (CDC) (for serum vitamin A and C), the International Atomic Energy Authority (IAEA) in Vienna, the Community Bureau of Reference of the Commission of the European Communities (BCR) in Belgium, and the U.K.

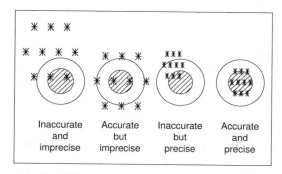

Figure 15.7: Differences between precision and accuracy. From Pi-Sunyer and Woo, 1984 © with permission of Aspen Publishers, Inc.

National Institute of Biological Standards and Controls. A reference material for erythrocyte enzymes for vitamin B_6, riboflavin, and thiamin is also available from the Wolfson Research Laboratory, Birmingham, England. Reference materials for serum ferritin (Reagent 80/578, ICSH, 1984) are available from the U.K. National Institute of Biological Standards and Controls and for human hair (CRM #397) and serum proteins (CRM #470) from the Community Bureau of Reference of the Commission of the European Communities (BCR) in Belgium. Details of the suppliers of these reference materials are given in Appendix A4.1.

If suitable reference materials are not available, aliquots from a single homogeneous pooled test sample should be analyzed by several independent laboratories using different methods. Programs are available which compare the performance of different laboratories in relation to specific analytical methods. Some examples include the programs operated by NIST, IAEA, and the Toxicology Centre in Quebec, Canada.

Important differences distinguish assays undertaken by a hospital clinical laboratory from those completed during a survey or research study. Clinical laboratories often focus on values for the assay that are outside the normal range, whereas in nutrition surveys such as National Health and Nutrition Examination Survey (NHANES) III, and research studies, the emphasis is often on concentrations that fall within the normal range. This latter emphasis requires an even more rigorous level of internal quality control in the laboratory (Potischman, 2003).

Where possible, it is preferable for all specimens to be analyzed in a single batch to reduce between-assay variability. This is not always feasible: in such cases an appropriate number of controls should be included in each batch of samples. Box 15.5 highlights the quality-control procedures adopted in NHANES III to ensure analytical accuracy (Gunter and McQuillan, 1990).

Most clinical chemistry laboratories are required to belong to a certified quality assurance program. The U.S. CDC operates a

National Health Performance Standards Program (NPHPSP) designed to improve the quality of public health practice and performance of public health systems, particularly statewide assessments; details are available from:

http://www.phppo.cdc.gov/nphpsp/index.asp

15.3.3 Analytical sensitivity

Unfortunately, the term "sensitivity" is used in nutritional assessment methodology in two different ways (Section 1.4.10). To clarify the distinction, the term "analytical sensitivity" should always be used in relation to an analytical method. For any analytical method, the smallest concentration that can be distinguished from the blank is termed the "analytical sensitivity" or the "minimum detection limit." The blank should have the same matrix as the test sample and, therefore, usually contains all the reagents but none of the added analyte. Recognition of the analytical sensitivity of a biochemical test is particularly important when the nutrient is present in low concentrations (e.g., the ultra-trace elements Cr, Mn, and Ni).

In practical terms, the minimum detection

Bench quality-control pools for each analyte, at multiple concentration levels

Blind quality-control pools for each analyte, low-normal and high-normal levels

Random reanalysis of 5% of specimens for each method

Split-duplicates from one original specimen submitted from the mobile examination center

Re-collection from sample participants during a stand to provide two time points for comparison of values

External proficiency testing for many analytes, such as the College of American Pathologists, New York State, CDC-Wisconsin programs

Box 15.5: Laboratory quality-control systems used in the National Health and Nutrition Examination Survey III. From Gunter and McQuillan, Journal of Nutrition 120: 1451–1454, 1990, with permission of the American Society for Nutritional Sciences.

limit or the analytical sensitivity is best defined as three times the standard deviation (SD) of the measurement at the blank value (Wolf, 1982). To calculate the SD of the blank value, 20 replicate measurements are generally recommended. Routine work should not include making measurements close to the detection limit and should normally involve analyzing the nutrient of interest at levels at least five times greater than the detection limit. Measured values at or below the detection limit should not be reported (Wolf, 1982).

15.3.4 Analytical specificity

The ability of an analytical method to measure exclusively the substance of interest is a characteristic referred to as the "analytical specificity." Methods that are nonspecific generate false-positive results because of interferences. For example, in NHANES II, the radioassay used gave falsely elevated results for vitamin B_{12}. This arose because the porcine intrinsic factor (IF) antibody source initially used reacted both with vitamin B_{12} and nonspecific cobalamins present in serum. As a result, erroneously high concentrations were reported and the samples had to be reanalyzed using a modified method based on purified human IF, specific for vitamin B_{12} (Gunter and McQuillan, 1990).

Strategies exist to enhance analytical specificity (and sensitivity). Examples include the use of dry ashing or wet digestion to remove organic material prior to the analysis of minerals and trace elements.

15.3.5 Validity

The definition of validity which is given in Section 1.4.4 indicates that a laboratory test can be considered valid if it correctly reflects the nutritional parameter of interest. As an example, if the laboratory test selected reflects recent dietary intake, but the study objective is to assess the total body store of a nutrient, the test is said to be invalid. In NHANES I, thiamin and riboflavin were analyzed on casual urine samples because it was not practical to collect 24-h urine specimens. However, results were not indicative of body stores of thiamin or riboflavin, so these tests were not included in NHANES II or NHANES III (Gunter and McQuillan, 1990).

Unfortunately, the action of certain drugs, hormones, infection, or stress on enzyme activity and nutrient metabolism may alter nutrient status and thus affect the validity of a laboratory test. For example, the acute-phase response observed during the early stages of an infectious illness may cause changes in certain nutrient levels in the blood (e.g., plasma zinc may fall), which do not reflect alterations in the nutrient status per se, but indicate a redistribution of the nutrient mediated by the release of cytokines (Singh et al., 1991). Other disease processes may alter the nutrient status as a result of impaired absorption, excretion, transport, or conversion to the active metabolite and thus confound the validity of the laboratory test. Some of these diseases are hereditary, but others are acquired. Some examples of disease processes that affect nutrient status and, in turn, laboratory tests are shown in Table 15.5.

15.3.6 Predictive value

The predictive value describes the ability of a laboratory test, when used with an associated cutoff, to predict correctly the presence or absence of a nutrient deficiency or disease. Sensitivity, specificity, and prevalence of the nutrient deficiency or disease affect the predictive value of a laboratory test. Of the three, prevalence has the most influence on the predictive value of a laboratory test, as discussed in Section 1.4.13.

15.4 Evaluation of laboratory indices

Laboratory indices and the related indicators, are evaluated using the techniques described in Section 1.5. Evaluation at both the population and individual level, normally requires comparison with reference values obtained

Disease	Nutrient indices that may be altered (usually lowered)
Pernicious anemia	Vitamin B_{12} (secondary effect on folate)
Vitamin-responsive metabolic errors	Usually B-vitamins (e.g., vitamins B_{12}, B_6, riboflavin, biotin, folate)
Tropical sprue	Vitamins B_{12} and folate (local deficiencies); protein
Steatorrhea	Fat-soluble vitamins, lipid levels, energy
Abetalipoproteinemia	Vitamin E
Thyroid abnormality	Riboflavin, iodine, selenium, lipid levels, energy
Diabetes	Possibly vitamin C, zinc, chromium, and several other nutrients; lipid levels
Infections, inflammation, acute phase reaction	Zinc, copper, iron, vitamin C, vitamin A, lipids, protein, energy
Measles, upper respiratory tract infections, diarrheal disease	Especially vitamin A, lipid levels, protein
Renal disease	Increased retention or increased loss of many circulating nutrients, lipid levels, protein
Cystic fibrosis	Especially vitamin A, lipid levels, protein
Various cancers	Lowering of vitamin indices
Acute myocardial infarction	Lipid levels affected for about 3 mo
Malaria, hemolytic disease, hookworm, etc	Iron, vitamin A, lipid
Huntington's chorea	Energy
Acrodermatitis enteropathica; various bowel, pancreatic, and liver diseases	Zinc, lipid levels, protein
Hormone imbalances	Minerals, corticoids, parathyroid hormone, thyrocalcitonin (effects on the alkali metals and calcium), lipid levels affected by oral contraceptive agents and estrogen therapy

Table 15.5: Examples of some disease states that may confound the validity of laboratory tests. From Bates et al., (1997). Biochemical markers of nutrient status. In: Margetts BM, Nelson M (eds.) Design Concepts in Nutritional Epidemiology, 2nd ed. With permission of Oxford University Press.

from a reference sample group. The distribution of these reference values forms the reference distribution, from which reference limits can be derived, as shown in Table 1.9.

Alternatively, the laboratory indices are compared with cutoff points based on values from subjects with clinical or functional manifestations of deficiency or excess. Note that statistically defined "reference limits" are technically not the same as clinically or functionally defined "cutoffs", and the two terms should not be used interchangeably.

15.4.1 Reference distribution and reference limits

Theoretically, the reference distribution is derived from a reference sample group of healthy persons, free from conditions known to affect the status of the nutrient under study.

Hotz et al. (2003) used this approach to define new lower reference limits (i.e., 2.5th percentile values) for serum zinc, by age, sex, fasting status, and time of blood collection. These lower reference limits were based on a reanalysis of the NHANES II results for serum zinc, excluding data for subjects with conditions known to significantly affect serum zinc concentrations. Hence, the reference distribution used was based on a healthy reference sample group (Section 24.3.1).

In NHANES II and NHANES III, the range of normal values for some of the biochemical tests for iron status were also derived from a healthy reference sample (Pilch and Senti, 1984b; Looker et al., 1997). Participants with conditions known to affect iron status, such as pregnant women and those who had been pregnant in the preceding year; persons with white blood cell count $< 3.4 \times 10^9$/L or $>11.5 \times 10^9$/L, protoporphyrin $> 70 \, \mu$g/dL red blood cells, transferrin saturation $< 16\%$, or with a mean corpuscular volume < 80.0 or > 96.0 fL, were excluded. Table 15.6 shows the percentiles for hemoglobin and transferrin saturation for male subjects (all races) aged 20–64 y, drawn from the NHANES II healthy reference sample (Pilch and Senti, 1984b).

"Normal values" in both NHANES II and NHANES III for children 1–14 y were defined as: $>$10th percentile for hemoglobin, > 5th percentile for mean cell volume, and < 90th percentile for erythrocyte protoporphyrin. Because of its greater biological variability, corresponding normal values for transferrin saturation were $>$10th percentile in NHANES II but $>$12th percentile in NHANES III (Looker et al., 1995).

A healthy reference sample group was not compiled from the NHANES II biochemical data for serum zinc published by Pilch and Senti (1984a) (Section 24.5.1), or for the serum vitamin A (Pilch, 1985) (Section 18.1.1), serum folate or red blood cell folate values (Senti and Pilch, 1985) (Sections 22.1.2 and 22.1.3). Further, none of the biochemical data generated from NHANES III, with the exception of iron, have been treated in this way (Looker et al., 1997). Similarly, biochemical data for healthy reference populations were not compiled for the New Zealand national nutrition surveys (Russell et al., 1999; Parnell et al., 2003), or for the U.K. Diet and Nutrition surveys (Gregory et al., 1990, 1995, 2000; Finch et al., 1998).

Because specially selected reference samples are rarely defined, the reference distribution for a laboratory test is often based on a nationally representative, apparently healthy group assumed to be disease-free (Gardner and Scott, 1980). The central part of the reference distribution is chosen to represent the reference interval, often termed the "reference range" or "range of normal." Generally, the latter is defined as the range around an average value, with the 2.5th percentile value corresponding to the lower reference limit and the upper 2.5th percentile value to the upper reference limit (Section 1.5.2). Such reference limits are often race-, age-, and sex-specific, depending on the laboratory test.

The lower and upper 2.5th or 5th percentile values (by age and sex) have been reported for many of the laboratory tests used in the U.K. Diet and Nutrition Surveys (Gregory et al., 1990, 1995, 2000; Finch et al., 1998). Using such data, the number and percentage of the individuals with observed values falling within these designated percentiles can be calculated. Unfortunately, no data are available from national nutrition surveys for the distribution of reference values for physiological functional indices of nu-

Age (y)	Hemoglobin percentiles (g/dL)						
	5	10	25	50	75	90	95
Males							
20–44	13.7	14.0	14.6	15.3	15.9	16.5	16.8
45–64	13.5	13.8	14.4	15.1	15.8	16.4	16.8
Age (y)	Transferrin saturation percentiles (%)						
	5	10	25	50	75	90	95
Males							
20–44	16.6	18.4	23.3	29.1	35.9	43.7	48.5
45–64	15.2	17.6	21.8	27.8	34.2	39.7	44.4

Table 15.6: Selected percentiles for hemoglobin (g/L) and transferrin saturation (%) for male subjects (all races) 20 — 64 y. Percentiles are for the NHANES II "reference population." Abstracted from comprehensive tables which include additional information on the SD, SEM, and the number of subjects studied in each age range. From Pilch and Senti (1984b). These results can be compared with those for the NHANES III general population (Appendix A17.1 [hemoglobin] and A17.2 [serum transferrin saturation]).

tritional status (e.g., relative dose–response for vitamin A). Such tests are not feasible in large-scale nutrition surveys. Some notable exceptions are the indices of body size and body composition (Chapter 12). Consequently, physiological functional indices are often evaluated by monitoring their improvement serially, during a nutrition intervention program (Solomons, 1985). Alternatively, the observed values may be compared with cutoff points, described below.

15.4.2 Cutoff points

A cutoff point for a specific laboratory test is generally based on data from subjects with either clinical or functional manifestations of a nutrient deficiency. In national nutrition surveys in industrialized countries, nutrient deficiencies (with the exception of iron) are rarely observed in the general population and tests measuring physiological or behavioral functions have not been performed. As a result, the cutoff points employed are generally based on ranges associated with clinical signs, or impairment in a biochemical or physiological function, as reported in the clinical literature (Pilch, 1985). Sometimes, multiple laboratory tests are used to aid in the choice of a biologically relevant cutoff point (van den Berg, 1994).

Cutoff points, like reference limits, are often age, race, or sex specific, depending on the laboratory test. For biochemical tests, cutoff points must also take into account the precision of the assay. Poor precision leads to overlap of individuals with low or deficient values with those having normal values and thus to misclassification of individuals, as shown in Figure 1.4. This affects the sensitivity and specificity of the test. The International Vitamin A Consultative Group (IVACG), for example, now recommends the use of HPLC for measuring serum retinol concentrations because this is the best method for detecting concentrations $< 0.70\,\mu mol/L$ with adequate precision (de Pee and Dary, 2002).

In earlier nutrition surveys, multiple cutoff points were used to define several levels

of nutritional status. The Interdepartmental Committee on Nutrition for National Defense (ICNND) (1963) chose four levels, designated as deficient, low, acceptable, and high. However, this multiple level approach has largely been abandoned in favor of a simpler approach, usually involving only one cutoff. The IVACG has now adopted only one cutoff (i.e., $< 0.70\,\mu mol/L$) to determine whether vitamin A deficiency is a public health problem among preschool age children (de Pee and Dary, 2002).

It is emphasized again that cutoff points can never separate the "deficient" and the "adequately nourished" without some misclassification occurring. There will always be some overlap between persons who actually have the deficiency and those falsely identified (i.e., false positives) (Figure 1.4). This arises because the physiological normal levels defined by a laboratory test vary among persons, depending on their individual nutrient requirements. As well, for many tests there is a high within-subject variance, as noted earlier, which influences both the sensitivity and the specificity of the test, and on the population prevalence estimates. These estimates can be more correctly determined if the effect of within-subject variation is taken into account. This can only be done by obtaining repeated measurements for each individual or at least on a subsample of the subjects. The number of repeated measurements required depends on the ratio of the within-subject variation to the between subject variation for the laboratory test and population concerned (Tangney et al., 1987) (See analogous discussion of adjustments to dietary intake estimates in Sections 3.3.4 and 6.2.)

The specificity of the laboratory diagnosis can be enhanced by combining measures, as discussed earlier. The presence of two or more abnormal values can be taken as indicative of deficiency, often improving the specificity of the diagnosis. This approach has been used in several national nutrition surveys (e.g., United States and New Zealand) to define iron deficiency (Looker et al., 1997; Russell et al., 1999; Parnell et al., 2003). Use of multiple indices to aid in the diagnoses of specific nutrient deficiency states is also described, where appropriate, in the following chapters. Ten of these chapters include details of the laboratory tests for those nutrients for which primary nutritional deficiency states in humans, have been described. Clinical assessment and the nutritional assessment of hospital patients are discussed in Chapters 26 and 27 respectively.

References

Bank HL, Robson J, Bigelow JB, Morrison J, Spell LH, Kantor R. (1981). Preparation of fingernails for trace element analysis. Clinica Chimica Acta 116: 179–190.

Bartoshuk LM. (1978). The psychophysics of taste. American Journal of Clinical Nutrition 31: 1068–1077.

Bates CJ, Thurnham DI, Bingham SA, Margetts BM, Nelson M. (1997). Biochemical markers of nutrient status. In: Margetts BM, Nelson M (eds.) Design Concepts in Nutritional Epidemiology, 2nd ed. Oxford University Press, Oxford, pp. 170–240.

Bates SE, Suen JY, Tranum BL. (1979). Immunological skin testing and interpretation: a plea for uniformity. Cancer 43: 2306–2314.

Bauer J. (1999). Advances in cell separation: recent developments in counterflow centrifugal elutriation and continuous flow cell separation. Journal of Chromatography B, Biomedical Sciences Applications 722: 55–69.

Bertazzo A, Costa C, Biasiolo M, Allegri G, Cirrincione G, Presti G. (1996). Determination of copper and zinc levels in human hair: influence of sex, age, and hair pigmentation. Biological Trace Element Research 52: 37–53.

Beynen AC, Katan MB. (1985). Rapid sampling and long-term storage of subcutaneous adipose-tissue biopsies for determination of fatty acid composition. American Journal of Clinical Nutrition 42: 317–322.

Bingham S, Cummings JH. (1983). The use of 4-aminobenzoic acid as a marker to validate the completeness of 24-h urine collections in man. Clinical Science 64: 629–635.

Bingham S, Cummings JH. (1985). The use of creatinine output as a check on the completeness of 24-hour urine collections. Human Nutrition: Clinical Nutrition 39C: 343–353.

Black MM, Matula K. (1999). Essentials of Bayley Scales of Infant Development II Assessment. John Wiley & Sons, New York.

Blanck HM, Bowman BA, Cooper GR, Myers GL, Miller DT. (2003). Laboratory issues: use of nutritional biomarkers. Journal of Nutrition 133: 888S–894S.

Buzina R, Jusic M, Sapunar J, Milanovic N. (1980). Zinc nutrition and taste acuity in school children with impaired growth. American Journal of Clinical Nutrition 33: 2262–2267.

Caddell JL, Saier FL, Thomason CA. (1975). Parenteral magnesium load tests in postpartum American women. American Journal of Clinical Nutrition 28: 1099–1104.

Carmel R. (2000). Current concepts in cobalamin deficiency. Annual Review of Medicine 51: 357–375.

Castillo-Duran C, Perales CG, Hertrampf ED, Marin V, Rivera FA, Icaza G. (2001). Effect of zinc supplementation on development and growth of Chilean infants. Journal of Pediatrics 138: 229–235.

Chandra RK. (1974). Rosette-forming T lymphocytes and cell-mediated immunity in malnutrition. British Medical Journal 3:(5931) 608–609.

Chilima DM, Ismail SJ. (2001). Nutrition and handgrip strength of older adults in rural Malawi. Public Health Nutrition 4: 11–17.

Congdon NG, West KP. (2002). Physiologic indicators of vitamin A status. Journal of Nutrition 132: 2889S–2894S.

Creason JP, Hinners TA, Bumgarner JE, Pinkerton C. (1975). Trace elements in hair, as related to exposure in metropolitan New York. Clinical Chemistry 21: 603–612.

Cronk CE, Stallings VA, Spender QW, Ross JL, Widdoes HD. (1989). Measurement of short-term growth with a new knee height measuring device. American Journl of Human Biology 1: 421–428.

Davies TS. (1982). Hair analysis and selenium shampoos. Lancet 2:(8304) 935.

DeAntonio SM, Katz SA, Scheiner DM, Wood JD. (1982). Anatomically-related variations in trace-metal concentrations in hair. Clinical Chemistry 28: 2411–2413.

Delange F. (1985). Physiopathology of iodine nutrition. In: Chandra RD (ed.) Trace Elements in Nutrition in Children. Nestle Nutrition Workshop Series Vol 8. Raven Press, New York, pp. 291–299.

de Pee S, Dary O. (2002). Biochemical indicators of vitamin A deficiency: serum retinol and serum retinol binding protein. Journal of Nutrition 132: 2895S–2901S.

Desor JA, Mallor O. (1975). Taste correlates of disease states: cystic fibrosis. Journal of Pediatrics 87: 93–96.

Doyle W, Crawley H, Robert H, Bates CJ. (1999). Iron deficiency in older people: interactions between food and nutrient intakes with biochemical measures of iron; further analysis of the National Diet and Nutrition Survey of people aged 65 years and over. European Journal of Clinical Nutrition 53: 552–559.

Elin RJ. (1987). Status of the mononuclear blood cell magnesium assay. Journal of the American College of Nutrition 6: 105–107.

El-Sohemy A, Baylin A, Kabagambe E, Ascherio A, Spiegelman D, Campos H. (2002). Individual carotenoid concentrations in adipose tissue and plasma as biomarkers of dietary intake. American Journal of Clinical Nutrition 76: 172–179.

Erten J, Arcasoy A, Cavdar AO, Cin S. (1978). Hair zinc levels in healthy and malnourished children. American Journal of Clinical Nutrition 31: 1172–1174.

Fickel JJ, Freeland-Graves JH, Roby MJ. (1986). Zinc tolerance tests in zinc deficient and zinc supplemented diets. American Journal of Clinical Nutrition 43: 47–58.

Field CJ. (1996). Using immunological techniques to determine the effect of nutrition on T-cell function. Canadian Journal of Physiology and Pharmacology 74: 769–777.

Finch S, Doyle W, Lowe C, Bates CJ, Prentice A, Smithers G, Clarke PC. (1998). National Diet and Nutrition Survey: People Aged 65 Years or Older. Volume 1: Report of the Diet and Nutrition Survey. The Stationery Office, London.

Funk MA, Hamlin L, Picciano MF, Prentice A, Milner JA. (1990). Milk selenium of rural African women: influence of maternal nutrition, parity, and length of lactation. American Journal of Clinical Nutrition 51: 220–224.

Gardner MD, Scott R. (1980). Age- and sex-related reference ranges for eight plasma constituents derived from randomly selected adults in a Scottish new town. Journal of Clinical Pathology 33: 380–385.

Gibson RS, Gibson IL. (1984). The interpretation of human hair trace element concentrations. Science of the Total Environment 39: 93–101.

Gibson RS, Anderson BM, Scythes CA, (1983). Regional differences in hair zinc concentrations: a possible effect of water hardness. American Journal of Clinical Nutrition 37: 37–42.

Gibson RS, Vanderkooy PD, MacDonald AC, Goldman A, Ryan BA, Berry M. (1989). A growth limiting mild zinc deficiency syndrome in some Southern Ontario boys with low height percentiles. American Journal of Clinical Nutrition 49: 1266–1273.

Grant R, Ferguson MM, Strang R, Turner JW, Bone I. (1987). Evoked taste thresholds in a normal population and the application of electrogustometry to trigeminal nerve disease. Journal of Neurology Neurosurgery and Psychiatry 50: 12–21.

Grantham-McGregor S, Ani C. (2001). A review of studies on the effect of iron deficiency on cognitive development in children. Journal of Nutrition 131: 649S–668S.

Gregory J, Foster K, Tyler H, Wiseman M. (1990). The Dietary and Nutritional Survey of British Adults. Her Majesty's Stationery Office, London.

Gregory JR, Collins DL, Davies PSW, Hughes JM, Clarke PC. (1995). National Diet and Nutrition Survey: Children Aged One-and-a-Half to Four-and-a-Half Years. Volume 1: Report of the Diet and Nutrition Survey. Her Majesty's Stationery Office, London.

Gregory JR, Lowe S, Bates CJ, Prentice A, Jackson LV, Smithers G, Wenlock R, Farron M. (2000). National

Diet and Nutrition Survey: Young People Aged 4 to 18 Years. Volume 1: Report of the Diet and Nutrition Survey. The Stationery Office, London.

Gunter EW, McQuillan G. (1990). Quality control in planning and operating the laboratory component for the Third National Health and Nutrition Examination Survey. Journal of Nutrition 120: 1451–1454.

Hambidge KM. (1982). Hair analyses: worthless for vitamins, limited for minerals. American Journal of Clinical Nutrition 36: 943–949.

Hambidge KM, Franklin ML, Jacobs MA. (1972a). Hair chromium concentration: effect of sample washing and external environment. American Journal of Clinical Nutrition 25: 384–389.

Hambidge KM, Hambidge C, Jacobs M, Baum JD. (1972b). Low levels of zinc in hair, anorexia, poor growth, and hypogeusia in children. Pediatric Research 6: 868–874.

Hambidge KM, Walravens PA, Neldner KH. (1977). The role of zinc in the pathogenesis and treatment of acrodermatitis enteropathica. In: Brewer GJ, Prasad AS (eds.) Zinc Metabolism: Current Aspects in Health and Disease. Alan R. Liss, New York, pp. 329–340.

Hammer DI, Finklea JF, Hendricks RH, Shy CM, Horton RJ. (1971). Hair trace metal levels and environmental exposure. American Journal of Epidemiology 93: 84–92.

Harrison WW, Yurachek JP, Benson CA. (1969). The determination of trace elements in human hair by atomic absorption spectroscopy. Clinica Chimica Acta 23: 83–91.

Henkin RI. (1984). Review: zinc in taste function. Biological Trace Element Research 6: 263–280.

Henkin RI, Patten BM, Re PK, Bronzert DA. (1975). A syndrome of acute zinc loss: cerebellar dysfunction, mental changes, anorexia, and taste and smell dysfunction. Archives of Neurology 32: 745–751.

Herbert V, Tisman G, Le-Teng-Go, Brenner L. (1973). The dU suppression test using ^{125}I-UdR to define biochemical megaloblastosis. British Journal of Haematology 24: 713–723.

Hess AF. (1913). The involvement of the blood and blood vessels in infantile scurvy. Proceedings of the Society for Experimental Biology and Medicine 11: 130–132.

Hilderbrand DC, White DH. (1974). Trace-element analysis in hair: an evaluation. Clinical Chemistry 20: 148–151.

Hirschi KD, Kreps JA, Hirrschi KK. (2001). Molecular approaches to studying nutrient metabolism and function: an array of possibilities. Journal of Nutrition 131: 1605S–1609S.

Hofman LF. (2001). Human saliva as a diagnostic specimen. Journal of Nutrition 131: 1621S–1625S.

Hopps HC. (1977). The biologic bases for using hair and nail for analyses of trace elements. Science of the Total Environment 7: 71–89.

Hotz C, Peerson JM, Brown KH. (2003). Suggested lower cutoffs of serum zinc concentrations for assessing zinc status: reanalysis of the second National Health and Nutrition Examination Survey data (1976–1980). American Journal of Clinical Nutrition 78: 756–764.

Hunter D. (1998). Biochemical indicators of dietary intake. In: Willett W (ed.) Nutritional Epidemiology. 2nd ed. Oxford University Press, New York, pp. 174–243.

Hunter DJ, Morris JS, Chute CG, Kushner E, Colditz GA, Stampfer MJ, Speizer FE, Willett WC. (1990). Predictors of selenium concentration in human toenails. American Journal of Epidemiology 132: 114– 122.

IAEA (International Atomic Energy Authority). (1993). The Significance of Hair Mineral Analysis as a Means for Assessing Internal Body Burdens of Environmental Pollutants. NAHRES-18. IAEA, Vienna.

IAEA (International Atomic Energy Authority). (1994). Application of Hair as an Indicator for Trace Element Exposure in Man: A Review. NAHRES-22. IAEA, Vienna.

ICNND (Interdepartmental Committee on Nutrition for National Defense). (1963). Manual for Nutrition Surveys, 2nd ed. National Institutes of Health, Bethesda, MD.

ICSH (International Committee for Standardization in Haematology). (1988). Expert Panel on Blood Rheology: guidelines on selection of laboratory tests for monitoring the acute phase response. Journal of Clinical Pathology 41: 1203–1212.

ICSH (International Committee for Standardization in Haematology). (1984). Preparation, characterization, and storage of human ferritin for use as a standard for the assay of serum ferritin. Clinical and Laboratory Haematology 6: 177–191.

Ito Y, Shinomiya K. (2001). A new continuous-flow cell separation method based on cell density: principle, apparatus, and preliminary application to separation of human buffy coat. Journal of Clinical Apheresis 16: 186–191.

Iyengar GV, Subramamian KS, Woittiez JRW. (1998). Element analysis of biological samples: principles and practice. CRC Press, Boca Raton, FL.

Jackson S. (1966). Creatinine in urine as an index of urinary excretion rate. Health Physics 12: 843–850.

Johansson G, Akesson A, Berglund M, Nermell B, Vahter M. (1998). Validation with biochemical markers for food intake of a dietary assessment method used by Swedish women with three different dietary preferences. Public Health Nutrition 1: 199–206.

Johansson G, Bingham S, Vahter M. (1999). A method to compensate for incomplete 24-hour urine collections in nutritional epidemiology studies. Public Health Nutrition 2: 587–591.

Johansson L, Solvoll K, Bjømeboe GE, Drevon CA. (1998). Under- and overreporting of energy intake related to weight status and lifestyle in a nationwide sample. American Journal of Clinical Nutrition 68: 266–274.

Johnson EJ, Qin J, Krinsky NI, Russell RM. (1997). β-Carotene isomers in human serum, breast milk and buccal mucosa cells after continuous oral doses of all-*trans*- and 9-*cis*-β-carotene. Journal of Nutrition 127: 1993–1999.

Kaempf DE, Miki M, Ogihara T, Okamoto R, Konishi K, Mino M. (1994). Assessment of vitamin E nutritional status in neonates, infants and children on the basis of alpha-tocopherol levels in blood components and buccal mucosal cells. International Journal of Vitamin and Nutrition Research 64: 185–191.

King JC, Shames DM, Woodhouse LR. (2000). Zinc homeostasis in humans. Journal of Nutrition 130: 1360S–1366S.

Klidjian AM, Archer TJ, Foster KJ, Karran SJ. (1982). Detection of dangerous malnutrition. Journal of Parenteral and Enteral Nutrition 6: 119–121.

Kohlmeier L, Kohlmeier M. (1995). Adipose tissue as a medium for epidemiologic exposure assessment. Environmental Health Perspectives 103(suppl. 3): 99–106.

Kumpulainen J, Salmela A, Vuori E, Lehto J. (1982). Effects of various washing procedures on the chromium content of human scalp hair. Analytica Chimica Acta 138: 361–364.

L'Abbé MR, Fischer PW. (1984). The effects of high dietary zinc and copper deficiency on the activity of copper-requiring metalloenzymes in the growing rat. Journal of Nutrition 114: 813–822.

Laitinen R, Vuori E, Åkerblom HK. (1988). Hair zinc and copper: relationship to hair type and serum concentrations in children and adolescents. Biological Trace Element Research 16: 227–237.

Looker AC, Gunter EW, Johnson CL. (1995). Methods to assess iron status in various NHANES surveys. Nutrition Reviews 53: 246–254.

Looker AC, Dallman PR, Carroll MD, Gunter EW, Johnson CL. (1997). Prevalence of iron deficiency in the United States. Journal of of the American Medical Association 277: 973–976.

Lozoff B, Brittenham GM. (1986). Behavioral aspects of iron deficiency. Progress in Hematology 14: 23–53.

Lozoff B, De Andraca I, Castillo M, Smith JB, Pino P. (2003). Behavioral and developmental effects of preventing iron-deficiency anemia in healthy full-term infants. Pediatrics 112: 846–854.

Lukaski HC, Penland JG. (1996). Functional changes appropriate for determining mineral element requirements. Journal of Nutrition 126: 2354S–2364S.

Martin BJ, Lyon TDB, Walker W, Fell GS. (1993). Mononuclear blood cell magnesium in older subjects: evaluation of its use in clinical practice. Annals of Clinical Biochemistry 30: 23–27.

McKenzie JM. (1978). Alteration of the zinc and copper concentration of hair. American Journal of Clinical Nutrition 31: 470–476.

McMurchie EJ, Potter JD, Rohan TE, Hertzel BS (1984). Human cheek cells: a noninvasive method for determining tissue lipid profiles in dietary and nutritional studies. Nutrition Reports International 29: 519–526.

Milne DB, Johnson PE. (1993). Assessment of copper status: effect of age and gender on reference ranges in healthy adults. Clinical Chemistry 39: 883–887.

Morris JS, Stampfer MJ, Willett W. (1983). Dietary selenium in humans: toenails as an indicator. Biological Trace Element Research 5: 529–537.

Palti H, Pevsner B, Adler B. (1983). Does anemia in infancy affect achievement on developmental and intelligence tests? Human Biology 55: 189–194.

Parker RS. (1989). Carotenoids in human blood and tissues. Journal of Nutrition 119: 101–104.

Parnell W, Scragg R, Wilson N, Schaaf D, Fitzgerald E. (2003). NZ Food NZ Children: Key Results of the 2002 National Children's Nutrition Survey. Ministry of Health, Wellington.

Penland JG. (2000). Behavioural data and methodology issues in studies of zinc nutrition in humans. Journal of Nutrition 130: 361S–364S.

Peretz A, Neve J, Jeghers O, Leclercq N, Praet J-P, Vertongen F, Famaey J-P. (1991). Interest of zinc determination in leucocyte fractions for the assessment of marginal zinc status. Clinica Chimica Acta 203: 35–46.

Perrone L, Moro R, Caroli M, Di Toro R, Gialanella G. (1996). Trace elements in hair of healthy children sampled by age and sex. Biological Trace Element Research 51: 71–76.

Petering HG, Yeager DW, Witherup SO. (1971). Trace metal content of hair. I: Zinc and copper content of human hair in relation to age and sex. Archives of Environmental Health 23: 202–207.

Pilch SM (ed). (1985). Assessment of the Vitamin A Nutritional Status of the U.S. Population Based on Data Collected in the Second National Health and Nutrition Examination Survey, 1976–1980. Life Sciences Research Office, Federation of the American Societies for Experimental Biology, Bethesda, MD.

Pilch SM, Senti FR (eds). (1984a). Assessment of the Zinc Nutritional Status of the U.S. Population Based on Data Collected in the Second National Health and Nutrition Examination Survey, 1976–1980. Life Sciences Research Office, Federation of the American Societies for Experimental Biology, Bethesda, MD.

Pilch SM, Senti FR (eds). (1984b). Assessment of the Iron Nutritional Status of the U.S. Population Based on Data Collected in the Second National Health and Nutrition Examination Survey, 1976–1980. Life Sciences Research Office, Federation of the American Societies for Experimental Biology, Bethesda, MD.

Pi-Sunyer FX, Woo R. (1984). Laboratory assessment of nutritional status. In: Simko MD, Cowell C, Gilbride JA (eds.) Nutrition Assessment: A Comprehensive Guide for Planning Intervention. Aspen Systems Corporation, Rockville, MD, pp. 139–174.

Piyathilake CJ, Hine RJ, Dasanayake AP, Richards EW, Freeberg LE, Vaughn WH, Krumdieck CL. (1992). Effect of smoking on folate levels in buccal mucosal cells. International Journal of Cancer 52: 566–569.

Potischman N. (2003). Biologic and methodologic issues for nutritional biomarkers. Journal of Nutrition 133: 875S–880S.

Punthuprapasa P, Thammaplerd N, Chularerk U, Charoenlarp K, Bhaibulaya M. (2001). Diagnosis of intestinal amebiasis by salivary IgA antibody detection. Southeast Asian Journal of Tropical Medicine and Public Health 32(Suppl. 2): 159–164.

Ravaglia G, Forti P, Maioli F, Muscari A, Sacchetti L, Arnone G, Nativio V, Talerico T, Mariani E. (2003). Homocysteine and cognitive function in healthy elderly community dwellers in Italy. American Journal of Clinical Nutrition 77: 668–673.

Raven JC, Court JH, Raven J. (1986). Manual for Raven's Progressive Matrices and Vocabulary Scales. Raven JC Ltd, KK Lewis and Co Ltd., London.

Refsum H, Ueland PM, Nygärd O, Vollset SE. (1998). Homocysteine and cardiovascular disease. Annual Review of Medicine 49: 31–62.

Rice AL, Stoltzfus RJ, de Franciso A, Kjolhede CL. (2000). Evaluation of serum retinol, the modified-relative-dose-response ratio, and breast milk vitamin A as indicators of response to postpartum maternal vitamin A supplementation. American Journal of Clinical Nutrition 71: 799–806.

Robberecht HJ, Deelstra HA. (1984). Review: selenium in human urine — concentration levels and medical implications. Clinica Chimica Acta 136: 107–120.

Russell D, Parnell W, Wilson N, Faed J, Ferguson E, Herbison P, Horwath C, Nye T, Walker R, Wilson B. (1999). NZ Food: NZ People. Key results of the 1997 National Nutrition Survey. Ministry of Health, Wellington, New Zealand.

Russell DM, Jeejeebhoy KN. (1983). The assessment of the functional consequences of malnutrition. Nutrition Abstracts and Reviews 53: 863–877.

Ruz M, Cavan KR, Bettger WJ, Thompson L, Berry M, Gibson RS. (1991). Development of a dietary model for the study of mild zinc deficiency in humans and evidence of some biochemical and functional indices of zinc status. American Journal of Clinical Nutrition 53: 1295–1303.

Salmela S, Vuori E, Kilpio JO. (1981). The effect of washing procedures on trace element content of human hair. Analytica Chimica Acta 125: 131–137.

Sandstead HH, Penland JG, Alcock NW, Dayal HH, Chen XC, Li JS, Zhao F, Yang JJ. (1998). Effects of repletion with zinc and other micronutrients on neuropsychologic performance and growth of Chinese children. American Journal of Clinical Nutrition 68: 470S–475S.

Sarno M, Powell H, Tjersland G, Schoendorfer D, Harris H, Adams K, Ogata P, Warnick GR. (1999). A collection method and high-sensitivity enzyme immunoassay for sweat pyridinoline and deoxypyridinoline cross-links. Clinical Chemistry 45: 1501–1509.

Schafer L, Overvad K. (1990). Subcutaneous adipose-tissue fatty acids and vitamin E in humans: relation to diet and sampling site. American Journal of Clinical Nutrition 52: 486–490.

Schramm W, Smith RH. (1991). An ultrafiltrate of saliva collected in situ as a biological sample for diagnostic evaluation. Clinical Chemistry 37: 114–115.

Seidel S, Kreutzer R, Smith D, McNeel S, Gilliss D. (2001). Assessment of commercial laboratories performing hair mineral analysis. Journal of the American Medical Association 285: 67–72.

Senti FR, Pilch SM. (1985). Assessment of the Folate Nutritional Status of the U.S. Population Based on the Data Collected in the Second National Health and Nutrition Examination Survey, 1976–1980. Life Sciences Research Office, Federation of American Societies for Experimental Biology, Bethesda, MD.

Seshadri S, Hirode K, Naik P, Malhotra S. (1982). Behavioural responses of young anaemic Indian children to iron-folic acid supplements. British Journal of Nutrition 48: 233–240.

Shibusawa Y. (1999). Surface affinity chromatography of human peripheral blood cells. Journal of Chromatography B Biomedical Science Applications 722: 71–88.

Shirreffs SM, Maughan RJ. (1997). Whole body sweat collection in humans: an improved method with preliminary data on electrolyte content. Journal of Applied Physiology 82: 336–341.

Singh A, Smoak BL, Patterson KY, LeMay LG, Veillon C, Deuster PA. (1991). Biochemical indices of selected trace minerals in men: effect of stress. American Journal of Clinical Nutrition 53: 126–131.

Sky-Peck HH, Joseph BJ. (1983). The 'use' and 'misuse' of human hair in trace metal analysis. In: Brown SS, Savory J (eds.) Chemical Toxicology and Clinical Chemistry of Metals. Academic Press, London, pp. 159–163.

Smith JC, Holbrook JT, Danford DE. (1985). Analysis and evaluation of zinc and copper in human plasma and serum. Journal of the American College of Nutrition 4: 627–638.

Solomons NW. (1985). Assessment of nutritional status: functional indicators of pediatric nutriture. Pediatric Clinics of North America 32: 319–334.

Solomons NW, Allen LH. (1983). The functional assessment of nutritional status: principles, practice, and potential. Nutrition Reviews 41: 33–50.

Stoltzfus RJ, Underwood BA. (1995). Breastmilk vitamin A as an indicator to assess vitamin A status of women and infants. WHO Bulletin 73: 703–711.

Strain JJ. (1999). Optimal nutrition: an overview. Proceedings of the Nutrition Society 58: 395–396.

Swanson CA, Longnecker MP, Veillon C, Howe M, Levander OA, Taylor PR, McAdam PA, Brown CC, Stampfer MJ, Willett WC. (1990). Selenium intake, age, gender, and smoking in relation to indices of selenium status of adults residing in a seleniferous area. American Journal of Clinical Nutrition 52: 858–862.

Takagi Y, Matsuda S, Imai S, Ohmori Y, Masuda T,

Vinson JA, Mehra MC, Puri BK, Kaniewski A. (1988). Survey of trace elements in human nails: an international comparison. Bulletin of Environmental Contamination and Toxicology 41: 690–695.

Tamura T, Johnston KE, Freeberg LE, Perkins LL, Goldenberg RL. (1994). Refrigeration of blood samples prior to separation is essential for the accurate determination of plasma or serum zinc concentrations. Biological Trace Element Research 41: 165–173.

Tangney CC, Shekelle RB, Raynor W, Gale M, Betz EP. (1987). Intra- and interindividual variation in measurements of beta-carotene, retinol, and tocopherols in diet and plasma. American Journal of Clinical Nutrition 45: 764–769.

Taylor A. (1986). Usefulness of measurements of trace elements in hair. Annals of Clinical Biochemistry 23: 364–378.

Twomey P, Ziegler D, Rombeau J. (1982). Utility of skin testing in nutritional assessment: a critical review. Journal of Parenteral and Enteral Nutrition 6: 50–58.

Underwood BA. (1994). Maternal vitamin A status and its importance in infancy and early childhood. American Journal of Clinical Nutrition 59: 517S–522S

Valente C, Maione P, Lippi A et al. (1992). Validation of the Mini Mental State Examination (MMSE) as a screening instrument for dementia in an Italian Population. Giornale di Gerontologia 40: 161–165.

Vance DE, Ehmann WD, Markesbery WR. (1988). Trace element imbalances in hair and nails of Alzheimer's disease patients. Neurotoxicology 9: 197–208.

van den Berg H. (1994). Functional vitamin status assessment. Bibliotheca Nutritio et Dieta 51: 142–149.

van Noord PAH, Collette HJA, Maas MJ, de Waard F. (1987). Selenium levels in nails of premenopausal breast cancer patients assessed prediagnostically in a cohort-nested case-referent study among women screened in the DOM project. International Journal of Epidemiology 16: 318–322.

Veillon C, Patterson KY. (1999). Analytical issues in nutritional chromium research. Journal of Trace Elements in Experimental Medicine 12: 99–109.

Vitoux D, Arnaud J, Chappuis P. (1999). Are copper, zinc and selenium in erythrocytes valuable biological indexes of nutrition and pathology? Journal of Trace Elements in Medicine and Biology 13: 113–128.

Wade SE, Haegle AD. (1991). Differential measurement of cortisol and cortisone in human saliva by HPLC with UV detection. Journal of Liquid Chromatography 14: 1813–1827.

Waterlow JC. (1986). Observations on the variability of creatinine excretion. Human Nutrition: Clinical Nutrition 40: 125–129.

Watson AR, Stuart A, Wells FE, Houston IB, Addison GM. (1983). Zinc supplementation and its effects on taste acuity in children with chronic renal failure. Human Nutrition: Clinical Nutrition 37: 219–225.

Webster J, Garrow JS. (1985). Creatinine excretion over 24 hours as a measure of body composition or of completeness of urine collection. Human Nutrition: Clinical Nutrition 39: 101–106.

Whaley SE, Sigman M, Neumann C, Bwibo N, Guthrie D, Weiss RE, Alber S, Murphy S. (2003). The impact of dietary intervention on the cognitive development of Kenyan school children. Journal of Nutrition 133: 3965S–3971S.

WHO (World Health Organization). (1996). Indicators for assessing vitamin A deficiency and their application in monitoring and evaluating intervention programmes. WHO/NUT/941. World Health Organization, Geneva.

WHO / UNICEF / ICCIDD. (World Health Organization / United Nations Children's Fund / International Council for the Control of Iodine Deficiency).(1994). Indicators for assessing iodine deficiency disorders and their control through salt iodization. World Health Organization, Geneva.

Wolf WR. (1982). Trace element analysis in food. In: Prasad AR (ed.) Clinical, Biochemical and Nutritional Aspects of Trace Elements. Alan R. Liss, New York, pp. 427–446.

Zhang S, Tang G, Russell RM, Mayzal KA, Stampfer MJ, Willett WC, Hunter DJ. (1997). Measurements of retinoids and carotenoids in breast adipose tissue and a comparison of concentrations in breast cancer cases and control subjects. American Journal of Clinical Nutrition 66: 626–320.

16

Assessment of protein status

The body of the adult 70 kg reference man contains about 11 kg of protein (i.e., 16%) which is widely distributed throughout the different tissues of the body, as shown in Table 16.1. Most of the body protein is present in the skeletal muscle (about 43%) and in the smaller visceral protein pool. Visceral protein is made up of serum proteins, erythrocytes, granulocytes, and lymphocytes, as well as the solid tissue organs such as the liver, kidneys, pancreas, and heart. The skeletal muscle protein (termed somatic protein) and the visceral protein pool together comprise the metabolically available protein known as the "body cell mass" (Section 14.4).

The other major protein components of the body are found in the extracellular connective tissue and constitute the noncellular structural proteins of the cartilaginous, fibrous, and skeletal tissues. Such noncellular structural proteins are not readily exchangeable with other body pools of protein. Hence, although alterations may occur in both the somatic and visceral protein components during protein malnutrition and disease, much of the protein in the extracellular connective tissue cannot be mobilized to counteract these changes (Phinney, 1981).

The data in Table 16.1 are for an adult; the distribution of protein among the organs such as the brain, lung, heart, and bone varies with developmental age so that the neonate has proportionately less muscle and much more brain and visceral tissue than an adult.

Functions of protein

Protein is important in the diet as a source of amino acids, which are required for the synthesis of body protein and other important nitrogen-containing compounds. The latter include creatine, nucleotides and nucleic acids, polypeptide hormones (e.g., insulin, thyroid hormones, growth hormone, and glucagon), and some neurotransmitters and other nonpolypeptide hormones; some further examples are given in Table 16.2.

Amino acids consumed in excess of the amounts needed for the formation of nitrogenous compounds are not stored but are degraded; the nitrogen is excreted in the urine as urea, and the keto acids left after removal of the amino groups are either used directly as sources of energy or are converted to carbohydrate or fat. Nitrogen is also lost in feces, sweat, and other body secretions and in sloughed skin, hair, and nails. Therefore, a continuous supply of amino acids must be obtained from the diet to replace these losses, even after growth has ceased.

	g/kg
Muscle	22
Skeleton	20
Viscera and skin	18
Extracellular	17
Fat	6

Table 16.1: The protein content of adult body tissues, calculated from Forbes et al., Journal of Biological Chemistry 203: 359–366, 1953 © The American Society for Biological Chemists, Inc., with permission.

Alanine	Glucogenic precursor; N-carrier from peripheral tissues to liver for N-excretion
Aspartate	Urea biosynthesis; glucogenic precursor; pyrimidine precursor
Cysteine	Precursor of taurine (used in bile acid conjugation and for other functions); reducing agent, also part of glutathione (important in the defense against oxygen radicals)
Glutamate	Intermediate in amino acid interconversions; precursor of proline, ornithine, arginine, polyamines, neurotransmitter α-aminobuyric acid (GABA); NH_3 source
Glutamine	Amino group donor to many nonamino acid reactions; N-carrier (crosses membranes more easily than glutamate); NH_3 source
Glycine	Precursor in purine biosynthesis and for glutathione and creatine; neurotransmitter
Histidine	Precursor of histamine; donates to 1-C pool
Lysine	For cross-linking proteins (as in collagen); precursor of carnitine biosynthesis (used in fatty acid transport)
Methionine	Methyl group donor for many synthetic processes; cysteine precursor
Phenylalanine	Precursor of tyrosine; and via tyrosine, precursor of catecholamines, dihydroxyphenyl-alanine, melanin, thyroxine
Serine	Constituent of phospholipids; precursor of sphingolipids; precursor of ethanolamine and choline
Tryptophan	Precursor of serotonin; precursor of nicotinamide (B-vitamin)
Tyrosine	See phenylalanine

Table 16.2: Functions of amino acids other than for protein synthesis and energy production. From Linder (1991), with permission of the author.

Absorption and metabolism of protein and amino acids

Proteins in the diet are hydrolyzed in the gastrointestinal tract by a series of proteolytic enzymes. The end products of protein digestion — free amino acids and small peptides — are taken up by mucosal cells of the small intestine by an energy-requiring process involving several carrier systems. Trace amounts of whole proteins are also absorbed through the intestinal mucosa and can enter the blood stream.

Upon entering the portal blood, the free amino acids are taken up by the liver and other organs and metabolized along three possible pathways. These are: (*a*) incorporation into tissue proteins, (*b*) catabolism by degradation pathways that involve deamination or transamination and, (*c*) synthesis of new nitrogen-containing compounds such as purine bases, creatine, and epinephrine, as well as nonessential amino acids. About one

third of the amino acids entering the liver from the portal blood are used for protein synthesis, energy metabolism, or gluconeogenesis. Skeletal muscle is the main site of metabolism of the branched-chain amino acids (leucine, isoleucine, and valine). For further details see Crim and Munro (1994) and IOM (2002).

There are 20 amino acids required for protein synthesis, of which 8 are essential (sometimes termed indispensable) for adults and must be provided preformed in the diet. These are lysine, methionine, phenylalanine, threonine, tryptophan, leucine, isoleucine, and valine. The remainder are either nonessential (dispensable), because they can be formed in the body from carbon and nitrogen precursors, or conditionally essential (conditionally indispensable). The term conditionally essential recognizes that under certain physiological circumstances (e.g., neonates) the ability to synthesize some of these amino acids endogenously relative to the demand is limited. Conditionally essential amino acids may include tyrosine, glycine, serine, arginine, glutamine, asparagine, proline, and histidine, depending on the physiological circumstance.

The amount of protein synthesized daily depends on the requirements for growth, the manufacture of digestive and other enzymes, and the repair of body tissues. Even in healthy adults, proteins and other nitrogenous compounds are being continuously degraded and resynthesized in the body. This process is termed "protein turnover" and varies with age, physiological status, and level of protein intake.

In healthy adults, the rate of protein synthesis is balanced by an equal amount of protein degradation, so that the amount of body protein remains approximately constant over long periods of time. During growth, however, protein synthesis exceeds protein degradation so there is a net deposition of protein. When protein intake is inadequate or diets are limiting in certain essential amino acids, then there is a shift in this balance so that rates of synthesis of some body proteins decrease while protein degradation continues in an effort to provide an endogenous source of those amino acids most in need. Conversely, when amino acids are consumed in excess of the amounts actually needed, the excess are not stored but are degraded, as noted earlier.

Protein deficiency in humans

There are no dispensable protein stores in humans, and therefore loss of body protein results in the loss of essential structural elements as well as impaired function.

Initially, during short-term changes in dietary intake, the main loss of protein occurs from the visceral protein pool (de Blaauw et al., 1996). In chronic deficiency states, however, the largest single contributor to protein loss is the skeletal muscle (Hansen et al., 2000).

Loss of muscle mass (and adipose tissue) characterizes the marasmic form of protein-energy malnutrition. This is the form most frequently encountered in low-income countries, and it is known as nutritional marasmus. It generally results from a prolonged reduction of food intake. Marasmus may also occur in more affluent countries in hospital patients with chronic illnesses such as cancer, or from the prolonged use of clear fluid diets and hypocaloric intravenous infusions of 5% dextrose (Naber et al., 1997; Corish and Kennedy, 2000).

Kwashiorkor, a second form of protein-energy malnutrition, occurs in children from certain regions of low-income countries. In these countries, kwashiorkor is often precipitated by a series of infections or aflatoxin exposure in concert with a diet with a low protein content relative to energy (Fuhrman et al., 2004). This condition may also occur in adult hospital patients in more affluent countries, where it is termed "adult kwashiorkor" (Hill, 1992). Kwashiorkor tends to arise from an inadequate intake of dietary protein accompanied by acute protein losses and metabolic reactions induced by the stresses associated with hypermetabolism (e.g., trauma or sepsis) (Jeejeebhoy, 1981).

Unlike marasmus, kwashiorkor does not result in any depletion of skeletal muscle protein; instead, the visceral protein pool is depleted and edema occurs. In hospitalized patients "marasmic-kwashiorkor" is most commonly observed, and is characterized by wasting of muscle and fat with hypoalbuminemia (Hill, 1992). Marasmic kwashiorkor also occurs in children in low-income countries where protein-energy malnutrition is endemic. For further details about these two forms of protein-energy malnutrition see Waterlow (1992).

Food sources and dietary intakes

In many affluent countries, foods of animal origin are the major source of protein in the diets of adults, with the proportion from the meat and dairy groups varying with age and region (USDA, 1983; Gregory et al., 1990; Subar et al., 1998; Russell et al., 1999). Nevertheless, cereal grains can supply up to 23% of the total protein intake in these diets

(Gregory et al., 1990) compared with more than 50% in some low-income countries such as Malawi (Ferguson et al., 1993).

The adequacy of dietary protein depends on quality as well as quantity; methods for estimating the protein quality of diets are given in Section 4.8.8. In western countries, the amino acid pattern of mixed diets meets the requirement levels for most age groups. Even vegetarian diets are likely to meet the requirement levels as long as they contain complementary mixtures of plant proteins (IOM, 2000). In low-income countries, some concerns have been raised about the adequacy of protein intakes, especially among children with low energy intakes. Beaton et al. (1992) concluded, however, that protein intake was unlikely to a primary limiting factor for the growth of toddlers in Egypt, Kenya, and Mexico.

In low-income countries, it is often useful to express the protein content of the staple foods as the proportion of the energy in the foods provided by protein. Using this approach foods such as cassava, plantains, sweet potatoes, and taros are classified as examples of poor sources of protein (in relation to their energy), whereas potatoes, unrefined maize, rice, and sorghum are classified as adequate, and groundnuts, beans, and peas, cow's milk (skimmed), soybean, and dried fish as good.

Effects of high intakes

In most western countries, habitual intakes of protein are substantially above the recommended intakes. Based on current evidence, high protein diets do not appear to improve protein nutriture and physical performance. Whether such high protein intakes are harmful is debatable. Metges and Barth (2000) have summarized the undesirable metabolic effects of high dietary protein intakes in adults, based on existing experimental and epidemiological evidence. There is some evidence that a high intake of protein may increase the risk of diabetes (Kitagawa et al., 1998; Wolever et al., 1997), renal cell cancer (Chow et al., 1994), and prostate can-

cer (Vlajinac et al., 1997). Additional adverse health effects on bone health, immune competence, and body protein synthesis have also been reported, although some of these effects are very controversial (Section 23.1). At present, the U.S. Food and Nutrition Board have not set a Tolerable Upper Intake Level for protein for adults. Metges and Barth (2000) caution that protein intakes should not be increased above 2g/kg per day, a level also recommended by the International Dietary Energy Consultancy Group (Durnin et al., 1999).

Indices of protein status

Whole body protein can be estimated from the measurement of total body nitrogen described in Section 14.5.1. Alternatively, changes in total body protein nutriture can be monitored indirectly, using anthropometric indices such as mid-upper-arm muscle area (Section 11.2.3), which provides an estimate of changes in skeletal muscle, a major component of body protein (Table 16.1). The skeletal muscle mass can be estimated using bioelectrical impedance (Section 14.8), computerized tomography (Section 14.9), magnetic resonance imaging (Section 14.10) and by dual energy X-ray absorptiometry (Section 14.11).

Biochemical measurements can also be used to estimate skeletal muscle protein. Examples include urinary creatinine (Section 16.1.1) or 3-methylhistidine (Section 16.1.2). Concentrations of specific proteins in serum (e.g., albumin, transferrin, and transthyretin) are often used to evaluate visceral protein status (Section 16.2). Levels are reduced in kwashiorkor but not in the marasmic form of protein-energy malnutrition. Protein-energy malnutrition also leads to metabolic changes, some of which (e.g., nitrogen balance) are used to monitor the effectiveness of nutritional support in hospital patients, and is discussed in Section 16.3.3.

The measurements discussed above do not necessarily provide information on functional status. Consequently, they are often performed in combination with selected physiological functional indices, such as tests of muscle and immune function; examples are given in Sections 16.4 and 16.5.

16.1 Assessment of somatic protein status

The metabolism of protein and amino acids in skeletal muscle is profoundly affected by inadequate intakes of dietary nitrogen, energy, and some specific essential amino acids. This can lead to a reduction in the size and metabolic status of muscle protein. These changes can be monitored by the measurement of creatinine and 3-methylhistidine in urine, as described below.

16.1.1 Urinary creatinine excretion

Urinary creatinine is derived from the catabolism of creatine phosphate, a metabolite present mainly in muscle. The measurement of urinary creatinine thus provides an estimate of the creatine pool. If the creatine content of muscle is assumed to be constant, urinary creatinine is also an index of muscle mass. This assumption has been confirmed in animal studies by the chemical analysis of muscle mass and the use of labeled creatine (Meador et al., 1968). In humans, the assumption is supported by a highly significant linear relationship between muscle mass and creatinine excretion (Cheek, 1968).

Some investigators suggest that each gram of creatinine excreted in a 24-h urine sample represents a constant weight of about 18–20 kg of fat-free muscle (Cheek et al., 1966; Cheek, 1968; Heymsfield et al., 1983). Others consider it is inappropriate to use a constant ratio of creatinine per kg of fat-free muscle in a population, unless factors such as age, gender, maturity, physical training, and metabolic state are considered (Boileau et al., 1972; Forbes and Bruining, 1976).

When estimating the muscle mass from urinary creatinine, it is assumed that (*a*) most creatine (i.e., 98%) is in the skeletal muscle, (*b*) the diet is creatine-free, (*c*) the total creatine pool and the average concentration

Diurnal and day-to-day variations within an individual occur, which are independent of diet and physical activity. These normally range from 4% to 8%, although larger variations ranging from 8.7% to 34.4% have been noted for obese subjects (Webster and Garrow, 1985). Use of several consecutive 24-h urine samples eliminates some of this variation (Waterlow, 1986).

Strenuous exercise increases urinary creatinine excretion by 5%–10% (Srivastava et al., 1957). The mechanism inducing such changes is unknown.

Emotional stress affects the variability but not the absolute amount of creatinine excretion. The cause is unknown.

Dietary intakes of creatine and creatinine from meat or supplements increase urinary creatinine excretion. Dietary protein also has a small effect on urinary creatinine excretion because it is the main source of the two dietary amino acid precursors of creatine — arginine and glycine.

Menstruation affects creatinine excretion. It increases by 5%–10% late in the second half of the menstrual cycle, decreasing just before and during menstrual flow (Smith, 1942).

Age influences creatinine excretion, a decline occurring with increasing age. This effect is attributed to a probable progressive decrease in lean body mass in absolute terms, a decrease in the proportion of muscle in lean body mass, especially in men, and a probable lower meat intake in older subjects (Walser, 1987).

Infection, fever, and trauma result in an apparent increase in urinary creatinine excretion because noncreatinine chromogens interfere with the analysis (Walser, 1987).

Chronic renal failure results in decreased excretion of creatinine. The decrease is not related to depletion in muscle mass but to a recycling of creatinine to creatine, to intestinal degradation of creatinine to products other than creatine, and to a decreased urine volume (Mitch et al., 1980). Hence, the use of urinary creatinine to estimate muscle mass or lean body mass in patients with chronic renal failure is invalid.

Box 16.1: Factors affecting daily creatinine excretion. Adapted from Heymsfield et al., American Journal of Clinical Nutrition 37: 478–494, 1983 © Am J Clin Nutr. American Society for Clinical Nutrition.

of creatine per kg of muscle remain constant, (*d*) creatine is converted to creatinine at a constant daily rate nonenzymatically and irreversibly, and (*e*) creatinine undergoes a constant rate of renal excretion (Heymsfield et al., 1983). Unfortunately, these assumptions are not all true. Box 16.1 details some of the factors that are known to affect daily creatinine excretion and limit the validity of urinary creatinine as an index of muscle mass.

In general, the longer the collection period for the urinary creatinine determination, the more precise the prediction of muscle mass and, hence, lean body mass. In practice, three consecutive 24-h urine collections are generally used. Some investigators recommend placing subjects on a constant, low-creatine, meat-free diet containing 60–80 g protein/d to stabilize the creatinine excretion, prior to the collection of the urine samples. However, because the half-life of the creatine pool is long (approximately 43 d), it takes many weeks to eliminate the creatine contribution, and, consequently, this approach is impractical in the clinical setting. Instead, meat should be eliminated from the diet only during the collection of the 24-h urine samples (Walser, 1987).

Several methods are used to express urinary creatinine excretion:

- Urinary creatinine excretion (mg) / 24-h
- Daily urinary creatinine excretion (mg) per cm body height
- Creatinine height index (CHI) as %:

$$= \frac{\text{measured 24-h urinary creatinine} \times 100\%}{\text{ideal 24-h urinary creatinine for height}}$$

- CHI as a percent deficit

$$\text{percent deficit} = 100 - \text{CHI (\%)}$$

where a mild deficit is 5–15%, a moderate deficit is 15–30%, and a severe deficit is > 30%

Creatinine excretion expressed in terms of height is the preferred mode of expression as it is unaffected by variations in adipose tissue and fluid imbalances (e.g., edema). Moreover, knowledge of the exact age of the child is not required. Figure 16.1 presents the relationship between urinary creatinine excretion and height for children. The relationship can be used to estimate the "ideal" 24-h urinary creatinine, and, with the measured 24-h urinary creatinine, a child's CHI.

For the calculation of adult CHI values, the ideal 24-h urinary creatinine excretion

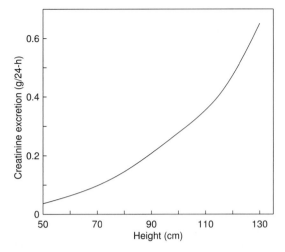

Figure 16.1: Relationship between urinary creatinine excretion (g/24-h) and height (cm) for children. Redrawn from Sauberlich (1999).

for height has been derived from a population of 30 healthy young adults receiving a creatine-free diet (Bistrian et al., 1975; Bistrian, 1977). However, these ideal values are not appropriate for the elderly, as a 20% decline in creatinine excretion, expressed as mg/cm body height, occurs from age 65–74 y (Driver and McAlvey, 1980). Consequently, use of standard adult reference data is likely to overestimate protein depletion in elderly patients.

Age-corrected creatinine excretion rates (Imbembo and Walser, 1984) have been derived from linear regression equations for predicting creatinine excretion, expressed as mg/kg per day, in relation to age, with "ideal" weights for height derived from the 1983 tables of the Metropolitan Life Insurance Company. The resulting tables of Imbembo and Walser (1984) can be used to determine an age-corrected CHI in subjects consuming self-selected diets, until observations of age-corrected creatinine excretion in a large series of healthy men and women of varying age are available.

A CHI of 60%–80% of the standard has been suggested as representing a moderate deficit in body muscle mass, whereas < 60% indicates a severe deficit (Blackburn et al., 1977). These interpretive values for the creatinine height index, however, should be used with caution because they have not been validated and may be insensitive. For example, if the CHI for a patient is initially at the upper end of the normal range, significant muscle mass will have been lost before detection by measuring CHI.

The CHI is most frequently used to assess the degree of depletion of muscle mass in children with the marasmic form of protein-energy malnutrition. In such subjects, there will be a decrease in CHI as a result of loss of lean body mass to maintain serum protein levels. The CHI can also be used to monitor the effects of long-term nutritional intervention on repletion of lean body mass in hospital patients. It is not sensitive to weekly changes in lean body mass and so should be used over longer periods. The CHI is also useful for patients for whom measurements of weight or skinfolds are unobtainable or inaccurate (e.g., in patients with severe edema, marked obesity, or pendulous skinfolds). Studies have revealed that the CHI is not useful for predicting morbidity and mortality (Mullen et al., 1979a).

One of the major difficulties in estimating urinary creatinine excretion is ensuring that 24-h urine collections are complete. Forbes and Bruining (1976) stressed that an error as small as 15 min in a collection period represents an error of 1% in the determination of 24-h urinary creatinine excretion.

Measurement of urinary creatinine

Urinary creatinine is usually assayed by the Jaffé reaction (Cook, 1975), using precise automated methods (Boileau et al., 1972). Acetoacetate in the urine interferes with this method, so urinary CHI is an unsuitable index for insulinopenic (type 1) diabetic patients who excrete large amounts of this metabolite (Bleiler and Schedl, 1962).

16.1.2 Excretion of 3-methylhistidine

Measurements of the amino acid 3-methyl-histidine (3-MH) in urine can theoretically be used to assess the size and turnover of the skeletal muscle protein mass. This amino acid is present almost exclusively in the actin of all skeletal muscle fibers and the myosin of white fibers. It is formed by the methylation of histidine residues after the synthesis of actin and myosin. When the proteins actin and myosin are catabolized, 3-MH is released and is not reused for protein synthesis; instead, it is excreted quantitatively into the urine without further metabolism. Therefore, if muscle protein synthesis and catabolism in adults are in balance, 3-MH excretion should reflect muscle mass.

Several investigators have attempted to validate the relationship between muscle mass and 3-MH excretion in adults fed meat-free diets (Lukaski et al., 1981). Results confirm that skeletal muscle mass, estimated from a mathematical model based on the measured ratio of total body potassium to total body nitrogen, is related to the endogenous urinary 3-MH excretion.

Urinary 3-MH excretion may be useful for monitoring the effectiveness of nutritional support; the latter should result in a reduction in muscle protein breakdown, indicated by a decrease in urinary 3-MH excretion. Whether output of 3-MH can be used to predict morbidity and mortality has not been extensively investigated.

There are several limitations to the use of 3-MH (Box 16.2) for assessing the size and turnover of the skeletal protein mass. These must be considered when interpreting 3-MH excretion. Unfortunately, data on excretion of 3-MH in a variety of populations are limited, so that interpretive criteria have not been established.

Measurement of 3-methylhistidine

Complete 24-h urine collections are essential for the measurement of 3-MH and should be collected over three consecutive 24-h periods. Several precise methods are available for the analysis of 3-MH in urine. Some involve the use of ion-exchange chromatography (Vielma et al., 1981; Robert and Serog, 1984). Others use high-performance liquid chromatography (Teerlink and de Boer, 1989).

A meat-free diet should be consumed by the subjects for at least 3 d prior to urine collection to eliminate 3-MH from dietary sources, in addition dietary protein intakes should be held constant (Wassertheil-Smollers et al., 1990). After such a period, mean daily 3-MH excretion is relatively constant, with a coefficient of variation of 4.5% (Lukaski et al., 1981).

Other sources contribute to the endogenous urinary 3-MH. Not all comes from skeletal muscle; some is derived from cardiac and smooth muscle (Afting et al., 1981).

Other excretionary forms also occur. About 5% of urinary 3-MH in adults is excreted in the N-acetyl form (Long et al., 1975). This is not normally analyzed.

Age also affects 3-MH excretion when expressed per kg body weight. Excretion is higher in the neonate than in the mature adult (Munro and Young, 1978), and it declines further in the elderly, presumably because of their decreasing muscle mass.

Catabolic states such as fever, starvation, trauma, and infection generally increase muscle turnover and alter the relationship between muscle mass and the excretion of 3-MH, thus confounding the interpretation of the measured level of 3-MH excretion.

Chronic renal failure results in a prolonged period of adaptation to a meat-free diet and reduced 3-MH excretion (Gutierrez et al., 1992).

Box 16.2: Factors affecting daily 3-methylhistidine (3-MH) excretion.

16.2 Assessment of visceral protein status

Visceral protein status is frequently assessed by the measurement of one or more of the serum proteins. The main site of synthesis for most of these is the liver, one of the first organs to be affected by a restricted intake of dietary protein. In such circumstances, the limited supply of protein substrate impairs the synthesis of plasma proteins, resulting in a relatively early decline in serum protein concentrations.

Many non-nutritional factors influence the concentration of serum proteins (Box 16.3) and reduce their specificity and sensitivity. Indeed, reductions in the serum proteins arising from infection and inflammation occur so frequently in critically ill hospital patients that many investigators recommend including a measurement of an acute-phase reactant, such as C-reactive protein, and using serum proteins *only* during convalescence. In such patients, serum proteins may be indicators of morbidity and those most at risk of developing malnutrition (Fuhrman et al., 2004).

During convalescence, serum protein concentrations probably correlate with total body protein, although their rate of change may not be related to the relative change in body protein (Grant, 1986). At this time, serum proteins with short half-lives provide an index of the effectiveness of nutritional therapy (Carpentier et al., 1982).

Serum proteins useful for measuring short-term changes in protein status have a small body pool, a rapid rate of synthesis, a major proportion present within the vascular space, a fairly constant catabolic rate that responds specifically to protein-energy deprivation but is not affected by extraneous factors, and a very short biological half-life.

The half-lives, body pool size, and factors that influence the individual serum proteins most commonly used to measure protein status are shown in Table 16.3.

Inadequate protein intake resulting from low dietary intakes, anorexia, unbalanced diets, hypocaloric intravenous infusions

Altered metabolism generated by trauma, stress, sepsis, and hypoxia

Specific deficiency of plasma proteins caused by protein-losing enteropathy and liver disease

Reduced protein synthesis resulting from inadequate energy intake, electrolyte deficiency, trace element deficiencies (e.g., iron and zinc), vitamin A deficiency

Pregnancy-induced changes in the amount and distribution of body fluids

Capillary permeability changes

Drugs (e.g., oral contraceptive agents)

Strenuous exercise

Box 16.3: Factors affecting serum protein concentrations. Adapted from Jeejeebhoy, British Medical Bulletin 37: 11–17, 1981, with permission of Oxford University Press.

Protein	Half-life	Body pool size (g/kg body weight)	Clinical use	Influencing factors
Albumin	18–20 d	3–5	Severe malnutrition	Hydration status; renal and liver disease; trauma, surgery, sepsis; edema; dietary protein; burns; zinc status; hypothyroidism; protein-losing enteropathy
Retinol-binding protein	12 h	0.0002	Acute depletion	Chronic renal failure; liver diseases; cystic fibrosis; hyperthyroidism; vitamin A and zinc status; dietary protein
Fibronectin	15 h	?		Trauma, infection, stress; burns
Somatomedin C	2 h	?		Hypothyroidism; estrogen; renal and liver disease; autoimmune diseases
Transferrin	8–9 d	< 0.1	Limited — chronic deficiency	Pregnancy; acute hepatitis; infection; oral contraceptives; end-stage hepatic disease, neoplastic disease; high-dose antibiotic therapy; iron status, dietary protein
Transthyretin	2 d	0.010		Stress; hyperthyroidism; active chronic inflammatory disease; acute phase response; steroid administration; dietary protein

Table 16.3: Serum proteins mainly of hepatic origin. Adapted from Logan and Hildebrandt (2003).

16.2.1 Total serum protein

Earlier national nutrition surveys used total serum protein as an index of visceral protein status (Health and Welfare Canada, 1973). It is easily measured but is a rather insensitive index of protein status. For example, the total serum protein concentration is maintained initially within normal limits, despite restricted protein intake, and is only significantly depleted when clinical signs of protein malnutrition are apparent. The observed decline results largely from a marked decrease in the serum albumin concentrations, which represent 50%–60% of total serum protein.

In severely ill hospital patients, blood products such as albumin are sometimes given, which affect the concentration of total serum protein. Furthermore, many other factors influence the concentration of total serum protein and, hence, compromise the specificity and sensitivity of this index. Consequently, this index is rarely used today.

16.2.2 Serum albumin

There is a relatively large body pool of albumin (from 3 to 5 g/kg body weight), of which

> 50% is present outside the vascular space. Serum albumin concentrations only reflect changes occurring within the intravascular space and not the total visceral protein pool. Because albumin has a large pool size and a long half-life (14–20 d), serum albumin is not very sensitive to short-term changes in protein status (Table 16.3). Even during chronic malnutrition, when the hepatic synthesis of albumin is reduced, concentrations in serum may be maintained by a compensatory reduction in albumin catabolism, along with redistribution of extravascular albumin to the intravascular space.

Serum albumin levels are influenced by a variety of other conditioning factors, some of which are noted in Table 16.3. Low serum albumin levels (hypoalbuminemia) may be generated in some gastrointestinal diseases (e.g., ulcerative colitis and Crohn's disease) and renal diseases by loss of protein, in liver disease and hypothyroidism by reduced protein synthesis, in congestive heart failure by increases in plasma volume, and in pregnancy by hemodilution. Infection and zinc depletion are also associated with reductions in serum albumin levels (Taylor et al., 1949; Wahlqvist et al., 1981).

In the presence of traumatic injury or with ongoing stress, a shift of albumin from the intravascular to the extravascular space results in a transient fall in serum albumin, whereas in semistarvation, the opposite effect occurs. As a result, serum albumin concentrations are artificially elevated in semistarvation (James and Hay, 1968). Hyperalbuminemia may also occur in patients with dehydration, as a result of a diminished plasma volume. Parenteral administration of albumin in some patients may mask such changes in serum albumin levels and confound its use as an index of protein status.

Age also influences serum albumin, with concentrations rising until the second or third decade of life and then declining thereafter, especially in the elderly. This trend in the elderly is probably associated with a decreased rate of albumin synthesis, which responds slowly to increases in protein intake. In adults, gender also affects serum albumin levels, with males tending to have higher values than females, the maximum difference occurring at 25 y (Ritchie et al., 1999a).

In low-income countries, serum albumin concentrations may be used to identify malnourished children who may be susceptible to edema, because hypoalbuminemia is a major contributory factor in the development of this condition (Whitehead et al., 1971). In such cases, a deficit in weight-for-age is not apparent (Table 16.4), and therefore an alternative index for identifying marginal kwashiorkor is essential. In contrast, in marasmus, there is no change in serum albumin concentration but deficits in weight-for-age are severe. In the more affluent countries, however, serum albumin is not useful for screening patients for protein-energy malnutrition. Potter and Luxton (1999) reported that 50% of patients with protein-energy malnutrition had normal serum albumin concentrations. Even elderly women receiving a diet low in protein but adequate in calories showed no change in plasma albumin concentration, despite losses of lean body mass and muscle function (Castenada et al., 1995).

The use of serum albumin concentrations as a prognostic index for the development of postoperative complications has been extensively studied. The results are inconsistent. Mullen et al. (1979b) reported that serum albumin levels < 30 g/L were associated with a complication rate two and half times greater than that of patients with levels > 30 g/L. In contrast, Ryan and Taft (1980) found no relationship between plasma albumin levels and complication rate after major abdominal surgery. Further, the use of serum albumin for evaluating the nutritional status of postoperative patients appears questionable (Erstad et al., 1994).

The prognostic potential of serum albumin for survival in the elderly has also been investigated. Decreased serum albumin values (< 35 g/L) appear to be a risk factor for mortality in elderly persons living at home (Lesourd et al., 1996) and in institutions (Sullivan and Walls, 1995).

Interpretive criteria and measurement of serum albumin

Ritchie et al. (1999a) have derived selected percentiles stratified by age and gender for serum albumin from a cohort of over 124,000 Caucasians in the northeastern United States. Individuals with evidence of inflammation (i.e., C-reactive protein $\geqslant 10$ mg/L) were excluded. These percentiles are presented in Table 16.5. Measurements were standardized against the Certified Reference Material (CRM) 470-RPPHS (Whicher et al., 1994)

Group	Serum albumin ($\overline{x} \pm$ SEM)	Weight for age ($\overline{x} \pm$ SEM)
Children with early signs of edema ($n = 33$)	25.9 ± 0.9	76 ± 2
Children with no signs of edema ($n = 65$)	32.6 ± 0.5	79 ± 3
Significance of difference	$p < 0.001$	NS

Table 16.4: Comparison of serum albumin levels (g/L) and weights-for-age (as percentage of Tanner and Whitehouse reference median) in two groups of Ugandan children. From Whitehead et al., Lancet 2(7719): 287–289, 1971, with permission.

Age (y)	2.5th	50th	97.5th
Males			
1.0	35.9	43.1	51.9
4.0	36.6	44.0	52.9
7.0	36.9	44.3	53.3
10.0	37.1	44.6	53.8
14.0	37.7	45.3	54.5
18.0	38.1	45.9	55.1
20.0	38.2	45.9	55.2
30.0	37.9	45.5	54.8
40.0	37.0	44.6	53.6
50.0	36.1	43.6	52.3
60.0	35.2	42.3	50.9
70.0	34.3	41.2	49.6
80.0	33.4	40.2	48.3
Females			
1.0	36.1	43.5	52.2
4.0	36.9	44.3	53.3
7.0	37.2	44.7	53.7
10.0	37.3	44.9	54.0
14.0	36.6	44.0	52.9
18.0	36.3	43.7	52.5
20.0	35.0	43.6	52.4
30.0	35.0	43.3	52.0
40.0	35.6	42.8	51.4
50.0	35.1	42.1	50.7
60.0	34.4	41.4	49.7
70.0	33.7	40.6	48.8
80.0	33.0	39.7	47.8

Table 16.5: Reference medians and selected percentiles for serum albumin (g/L), stratified by age and gender. Data from Ritchie et al., Journal of Clinical Laboratory Analysis 143: 273–279, 1999 © Wiley-Liss, Inc., with permission.

and analyzed using a statistical approach outlined in Ritchie et al. (1999b).

CRM 470-RPPHS (Whicher et al., 1994) is available from the International Federation of Clinical Chemists, the Community Bureau of Reference in Brussels, and from the College of American Pathologists in the United States (Baudner et al., 1994). It should be used to check the accuracy of all methods used to determine serum albumin.

Serum albumin is assayed in most clinical laboratories using an automated dye-binding method with bromocresol green (McPherson and Everard, 1972). Other methods include standard electrophoresis and immunonephelometry. Values for serum albumin depend on the analytical method used. Hence, these differences should be considered when interpreting serum albumin levels.

16.2.3 Serum transferrin

Transferrin is a serum β-globulin protein, synthesized primarily in the liver, but unlike albumin, it is located almost totally intravascularly. Transferrin serves as the iron transport protein, each molecule of transferrin binding with two molecules of iron. Normally, in well-nourished persons, from 30% to 40% of the transferrin is used for iron transport. Transferrin is also bacteriostatic: it binds with free iron and prevents the growth of gram-negative bacteria, which need iron for growth.

Transferrin has a shorter half-life (8–19 d, Table 16.3) and a much smaller body pool (< 0.1 g/kg body weight) than albumin and therefore responds more rapidly to changes in protein status. Nevertheless, the range of serum transferrin concentrations reported among individuals with subclinical, marginal, or moderate malnutrition is wide, limiting its usefulness (Roza et al., 1984).

Unfortunately, serum transferrin concentrations, like serum albumin concentrations, are affected by many factors, including liver, gastrointestinal, and renal diseases; congestive heart failure; neoplastic disease; and inflammation. Concentrations also fall when the requirements for iron transport are reduced by decreased iron absorption (e.g., in conditions of chronic infection, iron overload, and pernicious anemia). Conversely, iron deficiency leads to increased transferrin synthesis in response to increased iron absorption, leading to elevated serum transferrin levels. These higher levels also occur in pregnancy, during estrogen therapy, and during acute hepatitis (Spiekerman, 1993).

In concomitant iron deficiency and protein-energy malnutrition, a decrease in transferrin concentrations may be masked by an increase caused by iron deficiency (Table 16.6). In cases of severe kwashiorkor, however, when liver function is impaired, there may be no concomitant increase in transferrin synthesis in the liver, even when iron deficiency exists. Hence, in general, serum transferrin is not an appropriate index of protein status where both iron-deficiency anemia and chronic protein-

	Group I (mean ± SE)	Group II (mean ± SE)
Age (mo)	32.8 ± 2.3	27.6 ± 2.5
Weight-for-height.(%)	90.6 ± 1.6	91.4 ± 1.9
Height-for-age (%)	93.8 ± 0.6	91.0 ± 0.9
Serum iron (μmol/L)	11.7 ± 1.1	7.8 ± 1.0
Transferrin (g/L)	3.51 ± 0.1	3.91 ± 0.2
% Transferrin sat.	15.8 ± 1.5	9.8 ± 1.3
Transthyretin (g/L)	0.125 ± 0.006	0.097 ± 0.007

Table 16.6: Biochemical and other comparative data for two groups of children from North Cameroon, grouped according to their blood hemoglobin concentrations (Group I: > 100 g/L; Group II: < 80 g/L). Group differences are significant ($p < 0.05$), except for age and weight-for-height. From Delpeuch et al., British Journal of Nutrition 43: 375–379, 1980, with permission of the authors and the Nutrition Society.

energy malnutrition are widespread. Instead, alternative serum proteins should be selected.

Serum transferrin is also not appropriate as a marker of protein status when patients are given high concentrations of antibiotics and fungicides. Unlike serum albumin and transthyretin, concentrations of serum transferrin fall rapidly during tetracycline therapy, as shown in Figure 16.2.

Studies on the value of serum transferrin to predict morbidity and mortality in hospital patients have produced conflicting results. Some suggest that the concentration of serum transferrin, either individually or as part of a multiparameter index, is one of the strongest

Age (y)	2.5th	50th	97.5th
Males			
1.0	1.86	2.65	3.77
4.0	1.89	2.69	3.83
7.0	1.90	2.71	3.86
10.0	1.91	2.72	3.88
14.0	1.89	2.70	3.84
18.0	1.79	2.55	3.64
20.0	1.77	2.52	3.60
30.0	1.76	2.51	3.58
40.0	1.78	2.53	3.61
50.0	1.77	2.53	3.60
60.0	1.74	2.49	3.54
70.0	1.70	2.42	3.44
80.0	1.63	2.33	3.31
Females			
1.0	1.80	2.57	3.66
4.0	1.80	2.56	3.65
7.0	1.83	2.61	3.72
10.0	1.92	2.74	3.91
14.0	1.91	2.72	3.88
18.0	1.88	2.68	3.82
20.0	1.87	2.66	3.79
30.0	1.83	2.61	3.72
40.0	1.82	2.60	3.71
50.0	1.82	2.59	3.69
60.0	1.80	2.57	3.66
70.0	1.77	2.53	3.60
80.0	1.73	2.47	3.52

Table 16.7: Reference medians and selected percentiles for serum transferrin (g/L), stratified by age and gender. Data from Ritchie et al., Journal of Clinical Laboratory Analysis 143: 273–279, 1999.

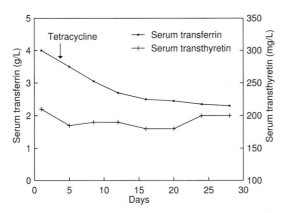

Figure 16.2: Serial levels of serum transthyretin and serum transferrin following tetracycline therapy. Data from Spiekerman, Clinics in Laboratory Medicine 13: 353–369, 1993.

predictors of morbidity and mortality in hospital patients (Mullen et al., 1979a; Rainey-Macdonald et al., 1983), and in children with cystic fibrosis (Ramsey et al., 1992). Other investigators, however, have not confirmed these findings (Ryan and Taft, 1980).

Interpretive criteria

Ritchie et al. (1999b) have also derived selected percentiles for serum transferrin by age and gender. The percentiles, based on the same Caucasian cohort as that used for serum albumin, are given in Table 16.7. Again, serum transferrin values rise until the second decade of life and then decrease thereafter, as described for serum albumin. Above 10 y,

Parameter	Protein deficit		
	None	Mild	Severe
Transferrin (g/L)	> 2.0	1.5–2.0	< 1.0
Retinol-binding protein (g/L)	0.026–0.076	—	—
Transthyretin (g/L)	0.16–0.40	0.11–0.16	< 0.11

Table 16.8: Interpretive guidelines for serum transferrin, retinol-binding protein, and transthyretin. Compiled from Grant et al. (1981) and Logan and Hildebrandt (2003).

transferrin values become increasingly higher among females than males (7% at 20 y).

Guidelines for the interpretation of serum transferrin concentrations in relation to the protein deficit are shown in Table 16.8.

Measurement of serum transferrin

Serum transferrin concentrations can be assayed by a radial immunodiffusion technique using commercial kits. The test sera and controls, together with three standards, are placed in the wells, after which the plates are left at room temperature for about 3 d. During this time, the sera and standards diffuse through the plate, forming a ring around each well. The diameter of each ring is then measured with either a jewelers' eyepiece (using a micrometer) or an electronic radial immunodiffusion plate reader. The concentrations of transferrin in the test sera are determined from a calibration line derived from the three standards.

Although the radial immunodiffusion technique is quite easy, it is expensive and time consuming and not routinely performed in most clinical laboratories. The technique is also vulnerable to between-examiner error so that it is preferable for one examiner to take all the measurements (de Pee and Dary, 2002).

Leonberg et al. (1987) have developed an accurate and precise assay for plasma transferrin, based on an antigen-antibody reaction using a commercially available transferrin antibody. The method requires only 15 μL of plasma and is rapid (60–90 min), sensitive, and easily performed. All assay methods

for serum transthyretin should be checked against CRM 470-RPPHS (Whicher et al., 1994) as noted for serum albumin.

16.2.4 Serum retinol-binding protein

Retinol-binding protein (RBP) is the carrier protein for retinol, with a single binding site for one molecule of retinol. The resultant complex of retinol-binding protein + retinol is the smallest of the circulatory serum proteins. The complex normally travels together with one molecule of plasma transthyretin to form a trimolecular complex of retinol, retinol-binding protein, and transthyretin. In this way, loss of RBP during filtration at the kidney glomerulus is prevented.

The half-life of RBP is approximately 12 h (Table 16.3), and the body pool is quite small (0.0002 g/kg body weight). As a result, serum RBP concentrations fall rapidly in response to protein and, to a lesser extent, energy deprivation and then respond quickly to dietary treatment (Shetty et al., 1979). For example, low levels were observed in obese subjects following a low-protein diet, with and without energy restriction (Table 16.9) (Shetty et al., 1979), and also in children with marasmus, kwashiorkor, and marasmic kwashiorkor (Smith et al., 1975). Later, more-detailed studies of children with both vitamin A deficiency and protein-energy malnutrition showed that RBP synthesis is, in fact, less affected in marasmus than in kwashiorkor (Large et al., 1980).

Unfortunately, like other serum transport proteins, the specificity of RBP as an index of protein status is low. Some of the factors affecting concentrations of RBP are similar to those described earlier for serum albumin and serum transferrin. For example, concentrations generally fall in liver diseases such as cirrhosis and hepatitis, as a result of interference with the storage and synthesis of RBP in the liver. Likewise, serum RBP concentrations are reduced in acute catabolic states, postsurgery, and hyperthyroidism.

A fall in serum RBP levels is also observed during deficiencies of vitamin A and zinc, in response to a reduced demand for the

Energy intake	Daily protein intake (g)			
	80	60	40	20
	Plasma-transthyretin (mean $\pm$ SEM mg/L)			
High-energy diet				
Day 10	298 ± 14	298 ± 5^{a}	290 ± 40	240 ± 32
Low-energy diet				
Day 6	280 ± 18	166 ± 14	208 ± 32	153 ± 12
Day 12	208 ± 43	199 ± 14	167 ± 20	147 ± 34
Day 24	193 ± 19	169 ± 27	150 ± 10	127 ± 29
Refeeding (Day 4)	—	240 ± 53	—	—
	Plasma-RBP (mean $\pm$ SEM mg/L)			
High-energy diet				
Day 10	57 ± 5	69 ± 2^{a}	54 ± 5	37 ± 4
Low-energy diet				
Day 6	51 ± 3	53 ± 3	35 ± 6	—
Day 12	54 ± 3	44 ± 5	33 ± 9	29 ± 11
Day 24	36 ± 5	36 ± 1	34 ± 9	33 ± 5
Refeeding (Day 4)	—	72 ± 9	—	—

Table 16.9: Changes in plasma transthyretin and retinol-binding protein on energy and/or protein restriction with four obese adults in each treatment group. [a]Observation from day 7. From Shetty et al., Lancet 2(8136): 230–232, 1979, with permission.

vitamin A transport protein. The reduction in demand for RBP occurs because deficiencies of both vitamin A and zinc inhibit the mobilization of RBP from the liver (Christian and West, 1998). Following vitamin A and/or zinc supplementation, serum RBP levels rise.

Decreased levels of serum RBP have been noted in cases of cystic fibrosis, possibly associated with a defect at the molecular level or the release of retinol-binding complex from the liver (Smith et al., 1975). A reduction in RBP, unlike serum transferrin, is not associated with iron-deficiency anemia.

In chronic renal failure, there is decreased catabolism of RBP by the kidney. As a result, the half-life of RBP is increased and serum concentrations become elevated. In contrast, concentrations of albumin and transthyretin in the serum become only slightly higher. These changes limit the usefulness of the absolute values of serum RBP for patients with renal failure, although monitoring the rate of change in response to nutritional therapy may still be helpful (Spiekerman, 1993). Oral contraceptive agents are also known to increase serum RBP concentrations (Beetham et al., 1985).

Interpretive criteria

There are no well-established guidelines for the interpretation of serum RBP concentrations. Normal levels for serum RBP are low ($0.026 - 0.076$ g/L; mean 0.051 ± 0.025 g/L), making it difficult to measure RBP precisely. Hence, a sensitive method should be used.

Measurement of retinol-binding protein

Serum retinol-binding protein, like serum transferrin, is most commonly measured by radial immunodiffusion methods using commercial kits, as described above for serum transferrin. The method is easy and requires little equipment, but the sensitivity for RBP is limited. More sensitive techniques include nephelometry (Hallworth et al., 1984), but the equipment needed is expensive.

An enzyme-linked immunosorbent assay (ELISA) has also been developed. In this technique, an enzyme is attached to an antibody that changes the color of a substrate, the intensity of the color change depending on the amount of RBP bound. Commercial ELISA kits are available, facilitating the determination of serum RBP concentration in 10 μL samples.

Sensitive radioimunoassays have also been developed for RBP in serum, plasma, and urine; these assays involve labeling radio-active antibodies, and a purified protein is used as a calibrant (Beetham et al., 1985). In the future, it may be possible to measure RBP concentrations in whole blood preserved on filter paper using an enzyme immunoassay method. All assays must be calibrated against CRM 470-RPPHS (Whicher et al., 1994) prior to use.

Parameter	Pre-TPN	Week 1	Week 2	End of TPN
RBP	38	74*	87*	87*
Transthyretin	56	64*	65*	66*
Transferrin	46	38	35	65*
Albumin	30	28	17	38

Table 16.10: Plasma protein concentrations during total parenteral nutrition (TPN). Values are percentages of patients ($n = 68$) who have normal concentrations of the proteins. $*p < 0.05$ vs. pre-TPN by chi-square. From Winkler et al., Journal of the American Dietetic Association 89: 684–687, 1989 © with permission of the American Dietetic Association.

16.2.5 Serum transthyretin

Transthyretin, known also as prealbumin or thyroxine-binding prealbumin, serves as a transport protein for thyroxine, and as a carrier protein for RBP (Section 16.2.4). It has a longer half-life (i.e., 2 d) (Table 16.3) and a slightly larger body pool (0.010 g/kg body weight), compared to RBP, although the sensitivities of these two serum proteins to protein deprivation and treatment are similar. Transthyretin has a high content of the amino acid tryptophan and a high proportion of essential to nonessential amino acids. Thus it can be used as an indicator of the availability of essential amino acids in the body (Spieker-man, 1993).

Serum transthyretin can be used in hospital settings as a screening tool to identify patients at risk for protein-energy malnutrition; more details are given in Section 27.1. Potter and Luxton (1999) examined the results of using transthyretin as a routine diagnostic test for protein-energy malnutrition in emergency room admissions. They emphasized that transthyretin was a more sensitive indicator of protein-energy malnutrition than was serum albumin and was significantly associated with length of hospital stay.

Serum transthyretin responds rapidly to the short-term effects of nutritional therapy. As a result, serum transthyretin is also used to monitor the progress of patients receiving total parenteral nutrition postoperatively and during the transition from total parenteral nutrition to oral or enteral feeding (Win-

kler et al., 1989). Table 16.10 shows results for plasma RBP, transthyretin, transferrin, and albumin in 68 patients receiving total parenteral nutrition (TPN). Improvements in serum transthyretin and RBP occurred within the first week of TPN and persisted throughout its duration, whereas there was no improvement in transferrin until the end of the therapy. In contrast, there were no significant differences in mean serum albumin levels between the pre- and post-TPN levels (Winkler et al., 1989).

Other investigators have also reported a rapid rise in serum transthyretin levels in patients who improve clinically, in contrast to the much longer time required to show an increase in serum albumin. Indeed, Bernstein et al. (1995) reported weekly increases in serum transthyretin of 40–50 mg/L in response to adequate nutritional support and suggested that a response of less than 20 mg/L in a week is indicative of either inadequate nutritional support or a failure to respond to the treatment.

Deficiencies of vitamin A, zinc, and iron do not affect the levels of transthyretin, unlike those of RBP and transferrin, as noted previously. In contrast, the presence of other conditions — such as gastrointestinal diseases, hepatic and kidney diseases, surgical trauma, stress, inflammation, and infection — leads to modifications in the metabolism of transthyretin and reduces its specificity as an index of protein status. Nevertheless, hepatic disease does not affect transthyretin as early or to the same extent as the other serum proteins, particularly RBP. Further, although serum transthyretin is moderately elevated in renal disease due to decreased catabolism by the kidney, nonetheless, in patients with stable renal failure, the direction of change in transthyretin concentration rather than the actual value can be used to monitor the adequacy of nutritional therapy (Winkler et al., 1989).

The response of serum transthyretin concentrations to dietary protein intake has also been investigated. Shetty et al. (1979), reported that serum transthyretin concentrations did not respond to a short-term (10-d) protein restriction if energy intake was maintained, but levels fell markedly when both energy and, to a lesser extent, protein intakes were restricted (Table 16.9). Ramsey et al. (1992) suggested that because of its very short half-life, serum transthyretin probably reflects acute protein intake rather than risk of protein malnutrition, which occurs over about 7 to 10 d. Nevertheless, Ogunshina and Hussain (1980) noted an inverse relationship of plasma transthyretin concentrations to the severity of malnutrition as assessed by the anthropometric classification of Waterlow (1972) (Figure 16.3; Section 13.2.5).

Age (y)	2.5th	50th	97.5th
Males			
1.0	0.12	0.18	0.26
4.0	0.12	0.18	0.27
7.0	0.13	0.18	0.27
10.0	0.15	0.22	0.32
14.0	0.18	0.26	0.37
18.0	0.19	0.28	0.41
20.0	0.20	0.29	0.42
30.0	0.21	0.30	0.44
40.0	0.21	0.31	0.45
50.0	0.21	0.30	0.44
60.0	0.20	0.29	0.43
70.0	0.19	0.28	0.41
80.0	0.19	0.27	0.40
Females			
1.0	0.12	0.18	0.26
4.0	0.13	0.18	0.27
7.0	0.13	0.19	0.28
10.0	0.15	0.23	0.33
14.0	0.17	0.25	0.36
18.0	0.18	0.26	0.37
20.0	0.18	0.26	0.38
30.0	0.18	0.26	0.38
40.0	0.18	0.26	0.39
50.0	0.18	0.27	0.39
60.0	0.18	0.27	0.39
70.0	0.18	0.27	0.39
80.0	0.18	0.26	0.39

Table 16.11: Reference medians and selected percentiles for serum transthyretin (g/L), stratified by age and gender. Data from Ritchie et al., Journal of Clinical Laboratory Analysis 143: 273–279, 1999 © Wiley-Liss Inc., with permission.

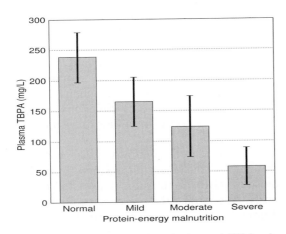

Figure 16.3: Plasma transthyretin (mean ± SE) levels in children classified as normal or with mild, moderate, and severe protein-energy malnutrition according to the Waterlow classification of protein-energy malnutrition. From Ogunshina and Hussain, American Journal of Clinical Nutrition 33: 794–800, 1980 © Am J Clin Nutr. American Society for Clinical Nutrition.

Certain medications can influence serum transthyretin levels. Levels rise with anti-inflammatory medications including some over-the-counter products (Ingelbleek and Young, 1994). They are also altered by endogenous estrogen (e.g., during pregnancy) (Haram et al., 1983) or the use of estrogen-containing preparations (e.g., oral contraceptive agents, estrogen replacement therapy).

Transthyretin values vary according to age and sex (Ritchie et al., 1999b). Values rise until the second or third decade of life and then decrease thereafter (Table 16.11). Males have higher values than females during mid-life, this difference being highest at about age 40 y (i.e., 16%).

Interpretive criteria

Interpretive values for adults based on nephelometry and the extent of the protein deficit are given in Table 16.8. Nutritional risk is high when serum transthyretin concentrations fall below 0.11 g/L, whereas poor outcome is predicted when a level < 0.50 g/L is observed (Logan and Hildebrandt, 2003).

Table 16.11 presents selected percentiles for serum transthyretin by age and gender, derived from the same Caucasian cohort used for both serum albumin and serum transferrin (Ritchie et al., 1999b).

Measurement of serum transthyretin

Serum levels of transthyretin are four to five times higher than those of RBP and thus are easier to measure. Radial immunodiffusion techniques can also be used to determine transthyretin using commercial assay kits, as described for transferrin and RBP. Other more sensitive and precise immunoassay techniques include nephelometry and turbimetry, both of which can operate on large automated chemistry analyzers.

16.2.6 Insulin-like growth factor I

Insulin-like growth factors are growth-hormone-dependent serum growth factors which are produced mainly in the liver. They have a pro-insulin-like structure and broad anabolic properties. The insulin-like growth factor I (IGF-I), sometimes referred to as somatomedin-C, circulates bound to carrier proteins and has a half-life of 12–15 h (Thissen et al., 1994).

In studies of children suffering chronic undernutrition, decreased concentrations of circulating IGF-I in the serum occur, which respond rapidly to dietary treatment (Smith et al., 1981). When acutely malnourished patients received nutritional support for 3–16 d, IGF-I levels increased from initial levels, although no significant changes in serum albumin, transferrin, RBP, or transthyretin concentrations occurred (Unterman et al., 1985). These results suggest that serum IGF-I may be more sensitive to acute changes in protein status than are the other serum proteins. Further, serum IGF-I levels are not subject to diurnal variation and are not influenced by stress, sleep, or exercise, although levels are decreased in patients with hypothyroidism and with estrogen administration. In patients with liver disease, kidney failure, and several autoimmune diseases, serum IGF-I levels are very variable, unless the carrier protein is completely removed by the acid chromatography extraction method, as noted below.

More studies are necessary to establish the sensitivity and specificity of IGF-I measurements as an index of malnutrition before it can be used as a routine biochemical marker of protein status and as a marker for the response to nutritional therapy.

Measurement of insulin-like growth factor I

IGF-I can be assayed using commercially available radioimmunoassay kits, provided a gamma counter is available. Quality controls are provided with the assay kits. Other immunoassays including immunoradiometric assays, enzyme-linked immunosorbent assays (ELISAs), and immunofunctional assays are also used. A number of different commercial kits are now available (Popii and Bauman, 2004).

Prior to the assay of IGF-I, any interfering binding proteins must be removed from the sample by an extraction procedure. Either acid-gel chromatography or acid-ethanol extraction is the most frequently used method. Of these, acid-gel chromatography is more difficult technically, but it is preferred because it removes 98% of the binding protein with a recovery of IGF-I of approximately 75%.

Either serum or plasma specimens can be used for the assay, but they must be separated as soon as possible after collection. Serum must be frozen promptly after separation to avoid falsely high values (Isley et al., 1990). Samples can be frozen at −20°C, but repeated freezing and thawing must be avoided.

16.2.7 Plasma alkaline ribonuclease activity and fibronectin

The activity of plasma alkaline ribonuclease (EC 3.1.4.2.2) has been investigated as a measure of protein status. Enzyme activity is reportedly increased in infants and children with protein malnutrition but returns to normal within 2–4 wk after rehabilitation (Scott et al., 1984). The measurement may be especially useful for monitoring the response of malnourished patients to nutrition interventions. A method for measuring alkaline ribonuclease activity in serum has been developed by Scott (1979).

Young et al. (1990) suggest that concentrations of fibronectin may also have potential as an index of protein status, and this warrants further study. Fibronectin is a glycoprotein which, unlike other serum proteins discussed above, is not synthesized exclusively by the liver but also by the endothelial cells, peritoneal macrophages, and fibroblasts. It has a half-life of about 15 h. Fibronectin serves numerous physiological functions, including cell–matrix interactions, and the binding of macrophages and fibroblasts. In protein malnutrition, levels of fibronectin are reduced, but they return to normal rapidly after nutritional rehabilitation (Buonpane et al., 1989). Fibronectin, like the other serum proteins shown in Table 16.3, also responds to certain non-nutritional factors, including infection, trauma, and burns, but again returns to normal on recovery. Special precautions must be taken when collecting serum samples for the assay of fibronectin. Analysis can be performed by competitive enzyme immunoassay (Ylatupa et al., 1993).

16.3 Metabolic changes as indices of protein status

Several striking changes in metabolism can develop in response to a reduced or inadequate supply of dietary protein or of some specific indispensable amino acids; the changes have been reviewed by Young and Marchini (1990). Of these, changes in free amino acid profiles in plasma have been described in children with frank kwashiorkor that are much more pronounced than those for children with the marasmic form of protein-energy malnutrition. Such changes have been linked to the hyperinsulinemia that occurs in kwashiorkor, which, in turn, results in characteristic alterations in serum amino acid concentrations via its effect on muscle protein synthesis (Coward and Lunn, 1981). Other metabolic changes, such as reduced urinary hydroxyproline excretion and increased urinary nitrogen excretion, occur in both the kwashiorkor and the marasmic forms of protein-energy malnutrition, and these changes are used as less-specific indices of protein-energy malnutrition.

16.3.1 Plasma amino acid ratio

Concentrations of free amino acids in plasma have been extensively studied in children with marasmus and frank kwashiorkor. Earlier work suggested that the serum amino acid profile of children with frank kwashiorkor was markedly abnormal (Coward and Lunn, 1981). Concentrations of nonessential amino acids (NEAA) — such as alanine, glycine, serine, and proline — were elevated, whereas those for the essential (indispensable) amino acids (EAA) were lowered, resulting in a high NEAA to EAA ratio. Such changes in serum amino acid profiles were much less pronounced in marasmic children.

Based on apparent differences in serum amino acid profiles, Whitehead and Dean (1964) developed a simplified technique for use in the field to determine serum amino acid ratios using one-dimensional paper chromatography and a fingerprick blood sample. The method was devised in an effort to distinguish between subclinical kwashiorkor and marasmus. Unfortunately, plasma NEAA:EAA ratios didn't show a consistent response in relation to the type or severity of protein-energy malnutrition. Saunders et al. (1967) reported that the amino acid profile reflected the dietary protein intake immediately prior to the test and plasma amino acid profiles are no longer used to assess protein status.

16.3.2 Urinary 3-hydroxyproline excretion

Urinary 3-hydroxyproline, principally in the peptide form, is an excretory product derived from the soluble and insoluble collagens of both soft and calcified tissues. In malnourished children with impaired growth resulting from kwashiorkor, marasmus, or marasmic kwashiorkor, urinary 3-hydroxyproline excretion levels are significantly lower than those in age-matched, well-nourished controls. In adults, levels of 3-hydroxyproline in the urine can be used as a marker of bone resorption and, hence, can help diagnose certain metabolic bone diseases and connective tissue or endocrine disorders. A variety of extraneous factors influence urinary 3-hydroxyproline excretion. These are outlined in Box 16.4

Interpretive criteria

The marked changes in hydroxyproline excretion with age and sex necessitate the use

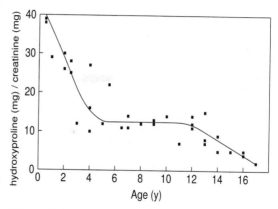

Figure 16.4: The hydroxyproline : creatinine ratio of normal individuals from 6 mo to 17 y. From Allison et al., Clinica Chimica Acta 14: 729–734, 1966.

of age- and sex-specific interpretive reference data. Investigators have therefore developed alternative methods for evaluating urinary hydroxyproline excretion levels which are independent of age. Excretion can be expressed as the hydroxyproline:creatinine ratio. This ratio corrects at least partially for differences in adult body size:

$$\frac{\text{hydroxyproline (mg) per 24 h}}{\text{creatinine (mg) per 24 h}}$$

As a result, ratios in adults are independent of age and are similar in males and females. For children, however, the ratio changes rapidly with age as shown in Figure 16.4: hydroxyproline decreases with age, while creatinine excretion increases.

As an alternative, hydroxyproline excretion can be expressed as the hydroxyproline index. Whitehead (1965) developed this index as an age-independent interpretive criteria for use with children, which additionally attempts to take body weight into account:

hydroxyproline index =

$$\frac{\text{mg hydroxyproline per mL urine}}{\text{mg creatinine per mL urine}} \times \text{kg body weight}$$

In normal children, between 1 and 6 y, the hydroxyproline index is relatively constant and

---

Age-related changes in urinary 3-hydroxyproline excretion are related to differences in growth velocity: excretion rises rapidly during periods of fast growth. Hence, the highest excretion is apparent during the adolescent growth period (11–16 y), after which there is a gradual reduction in hydroxyproline excretion.

Gender influences urinary 3-hydroxyproline excretion. Males, for example, have greater amounts of soft and calcified tissue and excrete larger amounts of hydroxyproline than females.

Infection influences urinary 3-hydroxyproline excretion and complicates the interpretation of the results.

Intake of collagen or gelatin increases urinary 3-hydroxyproline excretion.

Disease states involving disturbances in collagen metabolism such as rheumatoid arthritis are associated with elevated hydroxyproline excretion.

Parasitic infections such as hookworm and malarial infestations increase urinary 3-hydroxyproline excretion. .

Box 16.4: Factors affecting urinary 3-hyroxyproline excretion.

	Less than acceptable		Acceptable (low risk)
	Deficient (high risk)	Low (medium risk)	
Hydroxyproline index (3 mo to 10 y of age)	< 1.0	1.0–2.0	> 2.0
Creatinine height index (3 mo to 17 y of age)	< 0.5	0.5–0.9	> 0.9
Urea nitrogen : creatinine ratio	< 6.0	6.0–12.0	> 12.0

Table 16.12: Guidelines for the interpretation of urinary hydroxyproline index, creatinine height index, and urinary urea nitrogen:creatinine ratios. From Sauberlich (1999).

is approximately 3.0. In malnourished children, however, the hydroxyproline index is low, irrespective of the type of malnutrition, and statistically related to the extent of the weight deficit (Whitehead, 1965). Interpretive guidelines for the hydroxyproline index are shown in Table 16.12 (Sauberlich, 1999).

Measurement of hydroxyproline in urine

The use of 24-h urine specimens is preferred, but it is not practical for children. Instead, early morning fasting samples can be collected, thereby minimizing the effects of the dietary ingestion of hydroxyproline. Prockop and Udenfriend (1960), LeRoy (1967), and Dabev and Struck (1971) have all described methods for the analysis of hydroxyproline in urine. The method of Prockop and Udenfriend (1960) requires that the urine samples are first hydrolyzed, then decolorized and neutralized prior to oxidation to pyrrole. Pyrrole is estimated colorimetrically after coupling with ρ-dimethylaminobenzaldehyde.

16.3.3 Nitrogen balance

Nitrogen balance is a measure of the net status of protein metabolism. It provides no information on the size of the protein stores or about nutritional status. Nitrogen balance is most useful when used to monitor changes arising from nutritional therapy.

The nitrogen balance method is based on the assumption that nearly all of total body nitrogen is incorporated into protein. As protein contains 16% nitrogen:

$$\text{nitrogen (g)} = \text{protein (g)} / 6.25$$

In healthy adults with adequate energy and nutrient intakes, nitrogen losses are dependent mostly on the amounts and proportions of essential amino acids in the diet and on the total nitrogen intake. When nitrogen intakes are adequate to replace the endogenous nitrogen losses and for the growth of hair and nails, the subject is said to be in nitrogen balance. In such conditions, a correlation between daily nitrogen intake and daily nitrogen excretion can be expected. The expression for nitrogen balance is

$$\text{N balance} = I - (U - \text{Ue}) + (F - \text{Fe}) + S$$

where I = nitrogen intake (protein / 6.25), U = total urinary nitrogen, Ue = endogenous urinary nitrogen, F = nitrogen voided in feces (as unabsorbed protein), Fe = endogenous fecal nitrogen losses, and S = dermal nitrogen losses.

Nitrogen intake is generally estimated from the protein intake. For mixed diets, approximately 16% of the protein intake can be assumed to be nitrogen. For parenteral solutions containing free amino acids, specific conversion factors can be used to calculate the nitrogen content exactly. Alternatively, nitrogen intakes can be determined accurately by analyzing the nitrogen content of the diets or parenteral/enteral formulas using the micro-Kjeldahl technique.

When the nitrogen intake exceeds nitrogen output, subjects are in positive balance. This occurs during growth, late pregnancy, athletic training, and recovery from illness. In contrast, when nitrogen output exceeds nitrogen intake, subjects are in negative nitrogen balance. A negative nitrogen balance of 1 g/d is equivalent to a reduction in total body protein of 6.25 g/d. If the negative balance persists, the resultant protein depletion may have adverse effects on all organ systems.

Several factors may precipitate a negative nitrogen balance. They include inadequate protein or energy intakes, an imbalance in the NEAA : EAA ratio, conditions of accelerated protein catabolism (e.g., trauma, sepsis, infection, and burns), and excessive loss of nitrogen arising from fistulas or excessive diarrhea. The range of nitrogen balance values observed in hospital patients can vary from +4 to –20 g of nitrogen per day.

About 90%–95% of daily nitrogen losses are excreted in the urine, the remainder being lost through the skin and stools. Small losses through nasal secretions, menstrual fluid, semen, and nail and hair cuttings also occur. As a result, measurements of urinary nitrogen excretion and nitrogen intake over a defined period of time can be used to estimate the state of nitrogen balance.

Note that nitrogen balance results tend to be biased toward a positive balance. This bias arises because intakes tend to be overestimated as a result of unconsumed food, whereas excretion tends to be underestimated because of unmeasured nitrogen losses. Some of the sources of error and limitations associated with nitrogen balance studies are listed in Box 16.5. These must be kept in mind when interpreting nitrogen balance results (Kopple, 1987).

Expensive and time consuming. Most balance studies require substantial resources and significant amounts of time of the patient and staff.

Losses of foods that adhere to dishware, cooking, and eating utensils may lead to an overestimate of intake.

Losses of feces or urine on toilet paper and in stool and urine containers lead to an underestimate of output.

Unmeasured losses from skin (including exfoliated cells, sweat, hair and nail growth), flatus respiration, toothbrushing, menstrual fluid, semen, and blood sampling lead to an underestimate of output. Some of these unmeasured outputs are not constant and can vary with intake of nitrogen, the degree of sweating, and disease state.

Difficulty in precise collections of fistula or wound drainage, or, in incontinent individuals, of urine or stool, leads to errors in measurement of output.

Nitrogenous compounds (e.g., nitrate) are not measured by standard techniques, and this may introduce errors in the estimation of the intake and excretion.

Errors in the balance may be significant, as this is usually calculated as the small difference between two much larger numbers (intake and output). Hence, small percentage errors in these latter measurements can lead to large errors in the calculated balance.

Cumulative balance measurements (e.g. calculation of the total positive or negative balance over the entire period of study) are particularly likely to be erroneous.

The fate of the compounds ingested, their intermediary metabolism, and the tissue or cellular sources of the nitrogen outputs are not defined by the balance technique.

Box 16.5: Limitations and sources of error in nitrogen balance studies.

16.3.4 Estimated nitrogen balance and apparent net protein utilization

Total urinary nitrogen levels are rarely measured in routine hospital clinical laboratories because the conventional Kjeldahl technique is time consuming and laborious. Instead, urinary urea nitrogen is more frequently determined and can be used to replace the estimation of total urinary nitrogen in some circumstances. This is possible because in individuals who are consuming a normal mixed Western diet, and are in overall nitrogen balance, $> 80\% – 90\%$ of the total nitrogen in the urine is normally excreted as urea (Bingham et al., 1988). Moreover, the excretion of the nonurea nitrogen components (e.g., creatinine nitrogen 6.4%, ammonia nitrogen 7.4%, uric acid nitrogen 2%–3%, and other minor nitrogenous compounds 1%–2%) remains fairly stable in such conditions (Allison and Bird, 1977).

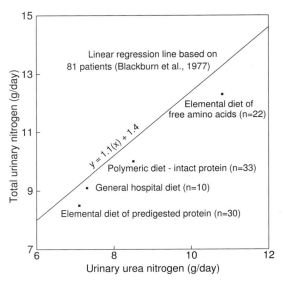

Figure 16.5: The relationship of total urinary nitrogen to urinary urea nitrogen for 81subjects and four groups of hospital patients. From Blackburn et al., Journal of Parenteral and Enteral Nutrition 1: 11–22, 1977 ⓒ American Society for Parenteral and Enteral Nutrition. From Allison and Bird (1977). Elimination of nitrogen from the body. In: Munro HN, Allison JB (eds.) Mammalian Protein Metabolism, Volume 1. American Medical Association ⓒ Academic Press, with permission.

Figure 16.5 depicts the relationship between measured total urinary nitrogen and measured urinary urea nitrogen observed in 81 patients for 564 study days and with a variety of clinical and nutritional conditions. The difference between the total nitrogen and the urea nitrogen in the urine averaged 1.8 g/d (range 0–5.8 g/d) with a standard deviation of 0.9 g/d (Blackburn et al., 1977; MacKenzie et al., 1985). On the basis of these results, an estimate of 2 g of nitrogen per day is commonly used for the nonurea nitrogen components of the urine.

The estimated nitrogen balance can be calculated from the urinary urea nitrogen using the following equation:

$$\frac{\text{protein intake (g)}}{6.25} - (\text{urinary urea N (g)} + 2 + 2)$$

In this equation, two correction factors are included: 2 g for dermal and fecal losses of nitrogen which occur but which are not meas-

ured; and 2 g for the nonurea nitrogen components of the urine (e.g., ammonia, uric acid, and creatinine), which are also not measured (MacKenzie et al., 1985).

Several factors can affect the validity of urinary urea nitrogen as a measure of nitrogen balance. The most important of these relate to the amount and quality of the protein intake. A low protein intake results in a decrease in urinary nitrogen excretion and the urea nitrogen accounts for a decreasing percentage of total urinary nitrogen (e.g., 61–70%) (Allison and Bird, 1977) (Figure 16.6). In such circumstances, urinary urea nitrogen is no longer a valid index of total urinary nitrogen excretion, and total urinary nitrogen must be determined. As well, nitrogen losses in skin may also be reduced. Calloway et al. (1971) estimated skin nitrogen losses as 3 mg/kg body weight per day on a protein-free diet formula, compared to 5 mg/kg body weight per day on a normal mixed diet.

Dietary protein of low biological value can result in ureagenesis or the increased excretion of urea. Ureagenesis, which also occurs when parenteral or enteral solutions contain-

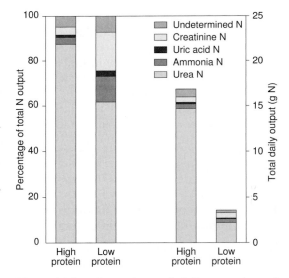

Figure 16.6:   Comparison of daily excretion of nitrogen-containing compounds for subjects on high- and low-protein diets. From Allison and Bird (1977). Elimination of nitrogen from the body. In: Munro HN, Allison JB (eds.) Mammalian Protein Metabolism, Volume 1. American Medical Association, ⓒ Academic Press, with permission.

Box 16.6:

Severe energy restriction or starvation increases the production of renal ammonia to such an extent that the nonurea nitrogen correction factor of 2 g is no longer adequate (Winterer et al., 1980).

Certain disease states and burns may result in alterations in the unmeasured nitrogen losses from the integument, sweat, exfoliated skin, and growing hair and nails compared to levels for normal healthy subjects (Kopple, 1987).

Malabsorption syndromes may increase fecal losses of nitrogen, resulting in levels as high as 3.5 g/d (41%). Therefore, for patients with malabsorption, fecal nitrogen should be measured on a timed stool specimen.

Metabolic acidosis and alkalosis result in increases and decreases in urinary ammonia levels, respectively.

Free-amino-acid formula feedings decrease fecal nitrogen losses to levels as low as 0.2 g/day.

Environmental conditions in which the ambient temperature is high may induce increased nitrogen losses through sweat.

Nitrogen retention diseases such as renal or hepatic failure also invalidate the equation.

Box 16.6: Factors affecting the validity of urinary urea nitrogen as a measure of nitrogen balance.

ing certain amino acids (e.g., arginine and glutamine) are administered, invalidates urinary urea nitrogen as an index of total urinary nitrogen.

Other factors affecting the validity urinary urea nitrogen as an index of total urinary nitrogen are shown in Box 16.6. In cases where the nitrogen balance has clearly been influenced by nitrogen-retention diseases such as renal or hepatic failure, then the nitrogen balance must be adjusted for changes in body urea nitrogen (BUN), using the following equations:

adjusted N balance = measured N balance
$$- \text{change in body urea nitrogen (BUN)}$$

$$\text{change in BUN (g)} = [(\text{SUN}_f - \text{SUN}_i) \times \text{BW}_i \times 0.6]$$
$$+ [(\text{BW}_f - \text{BW}_i) \times \text{SUN}_f \times 1.0]$$

where BW = body weight (kg), SUN = serum urea nitrogen (g/L), and the suffixes i and f indicate the initial and final values of the

measurement (Harvey et al., 1980). In this equation, the fraction of the body weight that is water is assumed to be 0.6. Unfortunately, although this fraction varies depending on the age and condition of the patient, no simple corrections are available. For example, in lean patients or those with edema, the fraction (i.e., 0.6) is too low, whereas in obese or very young persons, the fraction is too high (Kopple, 1987).

Once the nitrogen intake and urinary urea nitrogen excretion have been determined, an estimate of the apparent net protein utilization can be calculated as:

$$\frac{P}{6.25} - \frac{(\text{UUN} + 2 - \text{NL}) \times 6.25}{P}$$

where P = protein intake (g), UUN = urinary urea nitrogen (g), and NL = obligatory nitrogen loss (approximately 0.1 g for each kg of ideal body weight) (Blackburn et al., 1977).

Measurement of urinary urea nitrogen

Nitrogen balance in hospital patients is best determined by using at least three consecutive, complete 24-h urine collections, because the within-subject variation for urinary nitrogen excretion can be large. The collection of the urine should be made after an equilibrium period, to allow for readjustment to a new, steady-state level of nitrogen balance. The length of the readjustment period required depends on the relative change in protein intake but it would be expected to be at least a few days (Meakins and Jackson, 1994). Care must be taken to avoid spills, discards, and inadvertent omissions of urine during collection, because these lead to a positive error in the nitrogen balance.

In community surveys, a simplified system has been devised to collect 24-h urine samples, which is both easily transported and readily cleaned (Mann, 1988). Using this system, subjects can collect an accurate aliquot of each urine sample voided during a 24-h period, in a container which can later be mailed to the laboratory.

Urea nitrogen in the urine can be assessed by the enzymatic method of Searcy et al. (1965) using an auto-analyzer.

16.3.5 Urea nitrogen : creatinine ratios

Estimations of nitrogen balance are seldom made in field surveys because 24-h urine collections are usually impractical. As an alternative, first-voided, fasting urine specimens are sometimes used for determining urinary urea nitrogen : creatinine ratios. Urea, as discussed above, is the largest source of urinary nitrogen and is synthesized in the liver by the Krebs-Henseleit cycle. Urinary urea nitrogen : creatinine ratios have been proposed for evaluating dietary protein intakes. Several early studies have shown a relationship between the level of protein intake and the ratio (Simmons, 1972; Allison and Bird, 1977).

Creatinine excretion is measured in an attempt to take into account variations in urine volume, on the assumption that excretion of creatinine is relatively constant over a 24-h period. Nevertheless, many factors affect the urinary creatinine excretion (Section 16.1.1) and thus severely limit the use of this ratio as an index of the protein intake of individuals. If this ratio is used to compare the adequacy of dietary protein intakes of groups, the time of day for urine collection should be standardized—preferably by using the next urine sample after the first-voided, morning, fasting sample. Such samples will minimize the effect of diuresis on urea output. If possible, dietary data should also be collected to provide confirmatory information on the intake of dietary protein.

Several extraneous factors can influence urinary urea nitrogen : creatinine ratios. The specific factors affecting urinary creatinine have been discussed in Section 16.1.1. Conditions such as trauma, sepsis, infections, burns, fistulas, and diarrhea all increase the level of urinary nitrogen excretion and, hence, in turn, the excretion of urea. Urea excretion is also influenced by the presence of urinary tract infections, which reduce the glomerular filtration rate.

Interpretive criteria

Interpretive criteria that can be used for urinary urea nitrogen : creatinine ratios are shown in Table 16.12. These are very tentative because of the uncertain effects of age. Note that the ratio is primarily a measure of recent dietary protein intake and not a measure of protein nutriture of an individual (Simmons, 1972).

16.4 Muscle function tests

Muscle wasting characterizes the marasmic form of protein-energy malnutrition. Significant changes in muscle function, such as muscle contractility, relaxation rate, and endurance induced by electrical stimulation, may precede body composition changes and, as a result, are used to detect functional impairment at the subclinical level (Lopes et al., 1982). Muscle function can also be assessed by voluntary handgrip and by pulmonary function testing. In critically ill patients, changes in muscle function may alter respiratory function and precipitate respiratory failure. Tests of muscle function by electrical stimulation of the adductor pollicis muscle and by voluntary handgrip are discussed below.

16.4.1 Skeletal muscle function after electrical stimulation

Muscle function tests usually measure the function of the adductor pollicis muscle after electrical stimulation of the ulnar nerve. The changes in the adductor pollicis muscle appear to be representative of muscle function as a whole.

For the test, the right arm and hand are placed in an arm support with an integral fixation device. The ulnar nerve at the wrist is then electrically stimulated with a square wave impulse of 50–100 µs duration, of between 80 and 120 volts, and at frequencies increasing from 10 to 100 Hz. The force produced by the adductor pollicis muscle is measured using a force transducer, and the

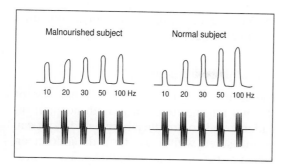

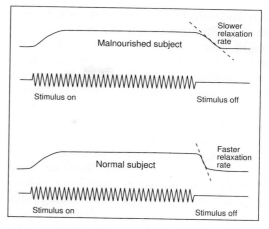

Figure 16.7: Comparison of the force of contraction with electrical stimulation at 10, 20, 30, 50, and 100 Hz in a malnourished and a normal subject. The typical malnourished patient shows an increased force at 10 Hz (expressed as the percentage of the force at 100 Hz) compared with a normal subject. The lower tracing shows diagrammatically the surface EMG, demonstrating constant nerve stimulation. From Russell and Jeejeebhoy, Nutrition Abstracts and Reviews 53: 863–877, 1983, with permission.

Figure 16.8: Comparison of the force of contraction (and EMG recording) at 30 Hz in typical malnourished and normal subjects. The maximal relaxation rate is calculated from the gradient of the initial phase of relaxation (dotted line) and is slower in the malnourished subject. From Russell and Jeejeebhoy, Nutrition Abstracts and Reviews 53: 863–877, 1983, with permission.

electromyograms (EMG) of the adductor pollicis muscle are recorded.

Supramaximal nerve stimulation during the study is ensured by placing surface electrodes over the adductor pollicis muscle and on the tip of the index finger (Edwards et al., 1977). The force generated depends on the frequency of stimulation and on whether the muscle is fresh or fatigued. In malnourished patients, tetany occurs at a lower stimulation frequency. There is also a loss of force at high-frequency stimulation so that the force at 10 Hz (expressed as a percentage of the force at 100 Hz) is increased. This procedure can also be used to measure muscle relaxation rate and muscle endurance (Lopes et al., 1982).

The method has been investigated using both animal models and human studies of nutritional deprivation and refeeding. In patients with clinical and biochemical features of severe nutritional depletion, three abnormalities of muscle function have been noted, all of which can be reversed by refeeding. These include (*a*) altered force-frequency pattern with an increased force at 10 Hz stimulation when expressed as a percentage of the maximal force (Figure 16.7), (*b*) lower maximal relaxation rate, expressed as percentage of force loss per 10 ms (Figure 16.8); and (*c*)

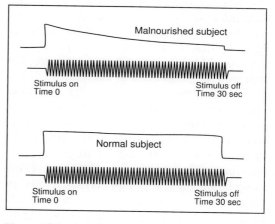

Figure 16.9: Comparison of the force of contraction (and EMG recording) at 20 Hz stimulation for 30 s, in typical malnourished and normal subjects. The malnourished subject shows significant muscle fatigue. From Russell and Jeejeebhoy, Nutrition Abstracts and Reviews 53: 863–877, with permission.

increased muscle fatigability (Figure 16.9). These abnormalities have also been reported in obese patients during a period of fasting and were restored to normal within 2 wk of refeeding.

In contrast, no significant changes in the anthropometric measures of body composition and selected biochemical indices (e.g. serum albumin, serum transferrin, creatinine height index, and total body nitrogen and potassium) were observed in the group of obese subjects noted above, during fasting and refeeding (Russell et al., 1983a). Similar results were also reported in patients with primary anorexia nervosa (Russell et al., 1983b).

The results discussed above suggest that changes in skeletal muscle function may be more sensitive to nutritional deprivation and repletion than are other nutritional assessment indices. Nevertheless, the changes that occur after 5 d of total starvation are still too small to detect short-term nutritional depletion (Lennmarken et al., 1986). Moreover, when both body composition (assessed by multiple-isotope dilution, Section 14.4) and skeletal muscle function were simultaneously evaluated in some malnourished and normally nourished patients, no significant correlations were noted between the two measurements (Shizgal et al., 1986). Further, in critically ill and septic patients, contraction/relaxation properties of the adductor pollicis muscle did not reflect proteolysis (measured by in vivo neutron activation), but appeared to reflect cellular energetics.

Skeletal muscle function after electrical stimulation has also been assessed using large muscle groups, e.g., the knee extensors (Hanning et al., 1993; Cupisti et al., 2004). In such cases values should be normalized for limb cross-sectional area. However, when using larger muscle groups, issues related to specificity and sensitivity, noted for the adductor pollicis muscle (e.g., training effects), may be even more pronounced. Application of this technique to ill patients was limited by poor acceptance and neuromuscular blockade (Finn et al., 1996).

Unfortunately, despite the indications that muscle function tests are useful for identifying patients at increased risk for medical complications, their use has been rather limited. The technology needs to become more widely available, so that additional data can be generated, before it is incorporated into clinical practice. It is still not known whether restoring muscle function with nu-

tritional support improves clinical outcome (Klein et al., 1997).

16.4.2 Handgrip strength

Handgrip strength is often used as a test of skeletal muscle function in both hospital in-patients and community-based studies. It can be measured with a handgrip dynamometer, which tests grip strength to 90 kg. The instrument can be adjusted for hand size. Subjects are asked to perform a maximal contraction for a few seconds, generally with the non-dominant hand. This is repeated 3–4 times, and the highest value achieved is recorded (Fleeman et al. 1983).

Age-related changes in handgrip strength have been observed; performance in older persons is consistently lower than that of their younger counterparts (Beckett et al., 1996; Chilima and Ismail, 2001; Pieterse et al., 2002). This trend has been attributed to the decline in both muscle mass and muscle strength that occurs with age, as well as to a decrease in physical activity (Bassey and Harries, 1993). Arthritis may also have a role (Bohannon, 1987).

Men appear to have a higher handgrip strength than women (Chilima and Ismail, 2001). This sex-related difference cannot be explained exclusively by differences in muscle mass or pain. Pieterse et al. (2002), for example, showed that men had a significantly higher strength per cm^2 arm muscle area than women.

Occupation is also a factor in handgrip strength. Persons engaged in heavy agricultural work have reportedly greater handgrip strength than urban-dwellers. Psychological factors, such as motivation and anxiety, may also play a role and confound the interpretation of the results (Lennmarken et al., 1986).

Table 16.13 summarizes handgrip strength results in four community studies, and highlights the age and sex-related relationships noted above.

In community studies of older adults, a poor handgrip strength has been related to poor nutritional status, based on low body mass index (BMI), in both low-income (Chil-

Country (*n*)	Sex	Age (y)	Handgrip kg (SD)
Malawi rural[a] (284)	Male	55–59	32.3 (5.5)
		60–69	29.0 (6.1)
		≥70	25.9 (5.2)
	Female	55–59	22.9 (4.0)
		50–69	21.7 (4.9)
		≥70	19.7 (3.2)
Thailand rural[b] (244–280)	Male	60–69	31.4 (7.8)
		70–79	25.0 (6.3)
	Female	60–69	22.6 (4.7)
		70–79	19.7 (4.5)
India urban[c] (1097)	Male	50–64	23.7 (6.5)
		≥65	20.8 (6.5)
	Female	50–64	13.4 (4.5)
		≥65	11.1 (4.2)
U.K. community[d] (1023)	Male	>65	34.8 (10.5)
	Female	>65	20.0 (6.8)

Table 16.13: Mean handgrip strength in four populations. Data from: [a]Chilima (1998); [b]Varakamin et al. (1998); [c]Manandhar (1999); [d]Finch et al. (1998).

ima and Ismail, 2001; Pieterse et al., 2002) and more affluent countries (Galanos et al., 1994). Pieterse et al. (2002) noted that in some U.K. elderly, higher handgrip strength was associated with much higher BMI values.

In some hospitalized patients, handgrip has been shown to be better than weight loss and plasma proteins as a predictor of postoperative complications and mortality (Klidjian et al., 1980; Windsor and Hill 1988). Nevertheless, to obtain a reliable assessment of nutritional status or postoperative risk using handgrip, appropriate age- and sex-specific data may be required. Moreover, the effects of medication (e.g., opiates, sedatives) and disease on handgrip strength need to be evaluated (Guo et al., 1996; Corish and Kennedy, 2000).

Interpretive criteria

Bassey and Harries (1993) have compiled normal values for handgrip strength in 920 men and women aged >65 y. Age- and sex-specific lower limits of acceptable grip strength have also been compiled by Webb et al. (1989). In some studies, a population-specific cutoff based on the lowest 25th percentile value has been used as an indicator of impaired handgrip strength (Pieterse et al., 2002).

Handgrip strength was measured in the U.K. National Diet and Nutrition Survey of people aged 65 y and over. Tables of the mean, median, and lower and upper 2.5th percentiles were compiled (Finch et al., 1998).

16.5 Immunological tests

The immune system is part of the host's defense against destructive forces from outside the body (i.e., bacteria, viruses, and parasites) or those from within, such as malignant and autoreactive cells (Field, 1996). Conventionally, the immune system is divided into two branches: the cell-mediated arm of the immune system in which $CD8^+$ thymus-dependent lymphocytes (T-cells) affect destruction of virus-infected cells, bacteria, and some malignant cells, and a humoral component in which B lymphocytes (B-cells) produce antibodies (IgM, -A, -D, -E) in response to specific antigens. Antigens are defined as any substance that can induce the production of antibodies.

Both arms of the immune system are under the control of $CD4^+$ T-cells which have a role in activating the immune response. T-cells acquire immune specificity in the thymus during early life. B-cells originate in bone mucous and peripheral lymphoid tissues, and make up 20–30% of peripheral blood lymphocytes.

Consistent changes in immunological responses have been observed during protein-energy malnutrition, and they have been reversed with nutritional repletion (Delafuente, 1991). As a result, measurements of immunocompetence have been used as a functional index of nutritional status in hospital patients since the 1970s (Bistrain et al., 1975).

Many other factors influence the immune response in the absence of protein-energy malnutrition. These include certain micronutrient deficiencies, infections, illnesses, major burns, medications, general anesthesia and surgery, as well as emotional and physical stress. The immune response is also involved in the pathophysiology of many diet-related chronic diseases (e.g., cardiovascular disease, insulin-dependent diabetes mellitus, and cancer) (Romagnani, 1994). Hence, to correctly interpret the results of immunological measurements in hospital and community-based studies, the results should always be interpreted in conjunction with other laboratory tests for specific micronutrient deficiencies. In addition, information on nutritional intake, concurrent illness, exposure to infectious agents, duration of the deficit, and genetic factors is also required. Results of some of the early observational studies are difficult to interpret because the influence of these confounding factors has not always been taken into account.

Nearly all aspects of the immune system can be impaired by nutritional deficiencies; details are reviewed by Delafuente (1991) and Alexander (1995). In general, humoral immunity is said to be less affected by protein-energy malnutrition than cell-mediated immunity (Stiehm, 1980).

Therefore, no single test can measure the adequacy of the immune response. For practical and ethical reasons, the most frequently sampled immune cells in human nutrition studies are those from the peripheral blood (Field, 1996). Hence tests involving peripheral blood lymphocytes are summarized here; for further details see Paxton et al. (1995).

	Cells /mm^3	Normal range (cells/mm^3)	Total white cells (%)
Total WBCs	9000	4000–11,000	
Granulocytes			
Neutrophils	5400	3000–6000	50–70
Eosinophils	275	150–300	1–4
Basophils	35	0–100	0.4
Lymphocytes	2750	1500–4000	20–40
Monocytes	540	300–600	2–8

Table 16.14: Classes of leukocytes in the peripheral blood of the average adult. Conversion factor to SI units $(10^9/L) = \times 0.001$. WBC, white blood cell count.

16.5.1 Lymphocyte count

Lymphocytes are the most frequently sampled immune cells in human nutrition studies (Field, 1996). They are small cells that circulate between blood and lymphoid tissues, and are derived from hematopoietic stem cells in the bone marrow. Lymphocytes are the primary cells of the acquired immune system, and comprise 20%–40% of the total white blood cells (WBCs) (leukocytes) (Table 16.14).

The total lymphocyte count in the peripheral circulation is usually monitored routinely in hospital patients in industrialized countries (Hendricks et al., 1995). A decrease in total lymphocytes ($< 0.9 \times 10^9/L$) is characteristic of severe protein energy malnutrition. Even in mildly undernourished elderly (Group B), the total lymphocyte count is often reduced compared with data for both healthy elderly and young adults (Table 16.15) (Lesourd, 1995).

The total lymphocyte count is a variable included in two preoperative screening systems that can be used to assess nutritional risk — the Likelihood of Malnutrition Index (Coats et al., 1993) and the Instant Nutritional Assessment (Seltzer et al., 1979). However, many other factors can affect the absolute lymphocyte count, notably stress, sepsis, acute and chronic infections, uremia, neoplasia, and the use of steroids. Hence, the specificity and sensitivity of this test is low.

The relationship of total lymphocyte count to patient prognosis has not been extensively investigated, although Riesco (1970) noted a link between depressed total lymphocyte count in cancer patients and prognosis. Suchner et al. (1996) showed that lymphocyte concentrations decreased after gastrointestinal surgery but rose during enteral nutrition. The levels of lymphocytes (and leukocytes, neutrophils, and monocytes) also decreased in adult obese subjects fed a very low-energy diet (Field et al., 1991).

Measurement of lymphocyte count

The lymphocyte count is derived from the percentage of lymphocytes multiplied by the

	Group A	Group B	Group C
Total absolute lymphocyte count	1940 ± 630	1460 ± 450	2157 ± 611
Proliferation (cpm).			
Phytohemagglutin A (1.0 µg/10⁶ cells)	$66,000 \pm 44,000$	$55,000 \pm 37,000$	$139,000 \pm 45,000$
Phytohemagglutin A. (0.25 µg/10⁶ cells)	$34,000 \pm 21,500$	$17,000 \pm 17,500$	$64,000 \pm 38,000$
DCH measured by multitest CMI (in females)			
Positive responses / 7	4.1 ± 2.3	1.3 ± 0.7	4.3 ± 2.1
Score in mm	18.3 ± 6.2	3.1 ± 1.7	17.4 ± 5.2

Table 16.15: Absolute lymphocyte counts, lymphocyte proliferation, and delayed cutaneous hypersensitivity (DCH) in healthy populations. Group A, healthy elderly subjects with a mean age 78.7 y who met the SENIEUR protocol for "optimally aged" (Ligthart et al., 1984); Group B, mildly undernourished elderly (mean age 79.4 y) with a serum albumin of 30–35 g/L; Group C, younger healthy adults 20–50 y. Data from Lesourd, Nutrition Reviews 53: S86–S94, 1995, with permission of the International Life Sciences Institute.

WBC and divided by 100:

$$\text{total lymphocyte count} = \frac{\text{lymphocytes (\%)} \times \text{WBC}}{100}$$

In clinical laboratories, the total white cell count and lymphocyte count are usually determined automatically using an electronic particle counter (e.g., Coulter Counter, Coulter Electronics Inc., Hialeah, FL.). These counters discriminate cells on the basis of the induced resistance as they pass through an electrical potential (Field, 1996).

In healthy subjects, the average lymphocyte count in peripheral blood is generally above 2.75×10^9/L. In malnutrition, the blood lymphocyte count is reduced. A level of $0.9 - 1.5 \times 10^9$/L indicates moderate depletion, whereas $< 0.9 \times 10^9$/L represents severe depletion (Blackburn et al., 1977). Obviously, the total lymphocyte count does not provide information on which specific lymphocyte subpopulation is responsible for the lowered count.

16.5.2 Thymus-dependent lymphocytes

Approximately 75%–80% of the circulating lymphocytes are T-cells. During severe protein-energy malnutrition, both the proportion and absolute number of T-cells in the peripheral blood may be reduced (Keusch, 1990). This low proliferation of T-cells has been attributed in part to alterations in monokine metabolism, particularly decreased activity of interleukin-1 (IL-1) (Hoffman-Goetz and Kluger, 1979a, 1979b; Bhaskaram and Sivakumar, 1986). In most cases, these changes can be rapidly reversed with nutritional therapy. Hence, sequential measurements of T-cell numbers can provide an index of the effect of a nutrition intervention and monitor nutritional recovery in malnourished patients.

Measurement of T-cells is now performed by flow cytometry. When a simple four-parameter flow cytometer is used, cells must be in a single-cell suspension for analysis. This can be achieved by density-gradient centrifugation on Ficoll-Hypaque using commercially available solutions, or by "whole blood lysis" (Janossy and Amlot, 1987). In the whole blood lysis procedure, the major cellular elements of the blood (lymphocytes, monocytes, granulocytes) can be discriminated. A bitmap gate can be drawn around the lymphocytes, excluding most other cell types, so that further analysis is restricted to lymphoid cells. Lymphocytes are stained with fluorescent-labeled monoclonal antibodies (mAbs) prior to analysis on a flow cytometer. This instrument is capable of analyzing single cells as they pass through an orifice at high velocity. Cells larger and smaller than lymphocytes can be "gated" out electronically so that the analysis concentrates solely on lymphocytes. The flow cytometer measures the properties of light scattering by the cells and the emission of light from fluorescent-labeled mAbs bound to the surface of the cell; details are given in Field (1996). Blood for flow cytometry should be collected in heparinized tubes, preferably in the morning (Nicholson et al., 1993).

16.5.3 Lymphocyte proliferation assays

Lymphocyte proliferation assays measure the functional capability of lymphocytes to respond to antigenic or mitogenic stimulation. Hence, the assays are a more direct test of immunocompetence than a total lymphocyte count. Indeed, they are the most frequently used in vitro method to assess the cell-mediated response to a nutrition intervention. Investigators report a decrease in the response to mitogens in both children and adults with protein-energy malnutrition (Miller, 1978; McMurray, 1984). Decreases in cell-mediated responses occur early in the development of protein-energy malnutrition, so that the lymphocyte proliferation is said to represent a sensitive measure of nutritional status.

For the assay, peripheral lymphocytes are harvested from blood and incubated in vitro with mitogens, which stimulate carbohydrate receptors on the lymphocyte surfaces, thereby causing division. In cases of immune dysfunction, decreases in the mitogen-induced proliferation occur. Mitogens commonly used include concanavalin A (Con A) and phytohemagglutinin (PHA), which primarily stimulate the division of T-lymphocytes, and the thymus-dependent B-lymphocyte mitogen, pokeweed mitogen (PWM).

Table 16.15 compares PHA-stimulated lymphocyte proliferation for three population groups. Note that the lymphocyte proliferation was much lower in the healthy elderly than the healthy young controls, unlike the results for total lymphocyte count, and that these differences were more pronounced in the undernourished elderly (Lesourd, 1995). Hence, these results emphasize that both aging per se and decreased nutritional status influence the immune response during aging.

Measurement of lymphocyte proliferation

To measure lymphocyte proliferation, lymphocytes are first purified from heparinized peripheral whole blood by density-gradient centrifugation on Ficoll-Hypaque gradients using commercially available solutions. Cells are then incubated in 96-well microtiter plates in a complete culture media supplemented with 5%–10% heat-inactivated serum. Either autologous (collected from the subject), pooled standard human sera, or fetal calf serum can be selected. Cells are incubated with and without mitogens for a defined period (usually 48 h), after which DNA synthesis is measured by pulse labeling the cultures in each well with a radioactive precursor (usually tritiated thymidine). The incorporation of tritiated thymidine into the newly synthesized chromosomal DNA reflects the rate of cell proliferation. As an alternative, either nonradioactive assays (which employ fluorescent dyes that are incorporated into DNA) or dyes that measure oxidative respiration can be used (Lowell, 2001). The cells are harvested onto glass filters using a multiwell automated cell harvester.

Controversy exists over the way to express the results from proliferative assays. They can be expressed as either the amount of thymidine incorporated or the response by stimulated cells relative to unstimulated cells. The results must be interpreted with caution: technical variations, such as culture time and the dose response, and difficulties in the assays can influence the results. Lymphocyte proliferation assays should always be performed with normal healthy controls as well as the test subjects, and the responses of the cells of the controls should not vary by more than 15% between tests.

16.5.4 Delayed cutaneous hypersensitivity

Delayed cutaneous hypersensitivity (DCH) response is a direct functional measure of cell-mediated immunity in vivo. Suppression of cell-mediated immunity signals a failure of multiple components of the host-defense system (Twomey et al., 1982).

When healthy persons are reexposed to recall antigens intradermally, the T-cells respond by proliferation and then by the release of soluble mediators of inflammation.

This produces an induration (hardening) and erythema (redness). These skin reactions are often reduced in malnourished persons with marasmus or kwashiorkor and in those with nutrient deficiencies such as vitamin A, zinc, iron, and pyridoxine, but the reactions are reversed after nutritional rehabilitation. Because several diseases and drugs also influence DCH, it is a poor measure of malnutrition in sick patients.

Several investigators have studied the use of DCH testing in assessing risk of morbidity and mortality in hospital patients. Anergy, or loss of cutaneous hypersensitivity to skin testing, has been associated with poor clinical outcomes. In general, anergic hospitalized patients have an increased risk for complications after surgery (Mullen et al., 1979b), such as sepsis and death (Meakins et al., 1977; Christou et al., 1995), compared with patients with normal responses to skin test antigens. Indeed, DCH was selected as one of the four indices in the prognostic nutritional index developed by Mullen and associates (Mullen et al., 1979a) (Section 26.2). The DCH response does not appear to be useful, however, for assessing the effectiveness of nutrition intervention involving total parenteral nutrition (Law et al., 1973).

Measurement of DCH

To measure DCH, a battery of specific antigens are injected intradermally in the forearm and the area of induration measured at one or two selected times subsequently. The recall skin test antigens commonly used are purified protein derivative (PPD), mumps, Tricophyton, *Candida albicans*, and dinitrochlorobenzene (DNCB).

The time course chosen for interpreting the DCH test is an important consideration. Usually, the area of induration is measured 24 h and 48 h after the antigen injection. However, some individuals being tested for the first time may develop reactions more slowly, so that 72 h may be needed (Sokal, 1975), whereas in some others who have undergone repeated testing, accelerated reactions may occur. As a result, multiple readings should

---

Infections — sepsis as a result of viral, bacterial, and granulomatous infections can suppress normal DCH.

Metabolic disorders — uremia, cirrhosis, hepatitis, inflammatory bowel diseases, and sarcoidosis suppress normal DCH.

Malignant diseases — most solid tumors, leukemias, lymphomas, chemotherapy, and radiotherapy impair DCH.

Medications — corticosteroids, immunosuppressants, cimetidine, coumarin, warfarin, and possibly aspirin may influence DCH.

Surgery and anesthesia — can alter DCH.

Patient factors — age, race, geographic location, prior exposure to antigen, circadian rhythm, and psychological state may all affect DCH.

Box 16.7: Non-nutritional factors affecting the delayed cutaneous hypersensitivity (DCH) response.

---

be taken and the largest reading used. If only one reading can be taken, the peak reaction is most likely to occur at 48 h.

Many non-nutritional factors affect skin test reactivity (Box 16.7), as noted earlier and, hence, reduce the specificity and sensitivity of the test (Twomey et al., 1982). Some of the effects of the technical factors can be minimized if standard procedures are adopted. The technical factors include reader variability, dilution of the antigens used, the time course of interpretation, and the "booster effect" of repeated antigen administration. The booster effect is particularly significant when DCH is tested serially and applied at the same site each time. In such cases, the responses will be enhanced. Box 16.8 summarizes the recommendation by Bates et al. (1979) for standardization of DCH testing procedures.

A cell mediated immunity (CMI) test kit for measuring DCH has been developed by the Institute Merieux (Lyons, France) (Kniker et al., 1979). This kit eliminates some of the methodological problems associated with the traditional skin testing method. It consists of a sterile, disposable plastic multipuncture applicator consisting of eight test heads preloaded with standardized doses of

Use **uniform dilutions** for the antigens.

Use **uniform measurement techniques** such as the ballpoint pen technique of Sokal (1975). In this method, a ballpoint pen is placed on the skin 1 – 2 cm away from the margin of the skin reaction and is moved slowly toward the center. When resistance at the edge of induration is reached, the pen is lifted, and the procedure is repeated from the opposite side. The distance between the opposite lines is the diameter of induration.

Record erythema (redness) and induration.

Use a **uniform interpretation method** such as a modification of the gradual scale of Sokal (1975). In this method both the size of the erythema and induration is noted: 1+, erythema ≥ 10 mm without induration or induration 1 – 5 mm; 2+, induration 6 – 10 mm; 3+, induration 11 – 20 mm; 4+, induration > 20 mm.

Box 16.8: Recommendations for the standardization of delayed cutaneous hypersensitivity testing. From Bates et al., Cancer 43: 2306–2314, 1979.

seven antigens (tuberculin, tetanus toxoid, diphtheria toxoid, *Streptococcus, Candida, Tricophyton,* and *Proteus*) in glycerin solution and a glycerin control. Use of seven antigens reduces the number of false negatives and increases the sensitivity of the test. Results for DCH measured by the multitest CMI in three groups of female patients are presented in Table 16.15. Note that the DCH responses in the healthy elderly group (A) were comparable to those of the young adult control group (C) (Lesourd, 1995).

16.5.5 Cytokine production

Cytokines are soluble peptide/glycoprotein mediators of immunity that are secreted by activated immune cells lining the liver and spleen. They influence cells involved in the immune and inflammatory responses. These nonantibody proteins act at the local level on other immune cells, as well as systemically. Cytokines are considered to be accessory molecules that transmit immune messages. The most extensively characterized cytokine is interleukin-1 (IL-1), which has numerous biological activities in cell-mediated and humoral immunity, as well as nonspecific immunity. Interleukin-1 enhances lym-

phocyte proliferation and stimulates helper T cells to produce interleukin-2 (IL-2), and thus is directly related to the availability of IL-2 (Whicher and Evans, 1990). Interleukin-1 is involved in the induction of fever, slow wave sleep, bone resorption, and muscle proteolysis.

In children with severe edematous protein-energy malnutrition, whether as a cause or a consequence, there are alterations in cytokine metabolism, particularly decreased activity of IL-1, which, in turn, may contribute to the low proliferation of T-cells in severe malnutrition (Hoffman-Goetz and Kluger, 1979a, 1978b; Bhaskaram and Sivakumar, 1986).

Interleukin-1 has a half-life of 2–4 h and has a small body pool. Hence, it has the potential to be a sensitive marker of nutritional status, although it is not specific to protein-energy malnutrition; IL-1 production can also be reduced in severe and moderate deficiencies of iron (Helyar and Sherman, 1987) and copper (Lukasewycz and Prohaska, 1990). Romagnani (1994) summarizes the role of cytokines in various disease states.

Measurement of cytokines

Currently, assays of cytokine responses are used primarily in research studies because of their high cost (Spiekerman, 1993). Immunoassays are generally used because they are simpler and less time consuming than bioassays, and they do not require any specialized equipment. They detect both biologically active and inactive cytokines, whereas bioassays measure only biologically active cytokine. Measurement of most cytokines can now be made using enzyme-linked-immunosorbent assay (ELISA) procedures with commercial kits. Results vary according to the kit used (Ledur et al., 1995).

Mire-Sluis et al. (1995) have highlighted several factors that influence the quality and validity of the data generated by these commercial kits. At present, results from immunoassay kits are best used to compare treatments within studies rather than between studies. Commercially available standards produced by the Lymphokine Standardization Committee of the International Union of Immunological Societies should be used with all assay methods (Wadhwa et al., 1999). In the future, flow cytometry methods may be used in nutrition studies to measure cytokines (Hoefakker et al., 1995).

16.5.6 Other methods

Many laboratories now test for the level of individual complement proteins, particularly C3. This protein acts as an acute phase reactant and, in well-nourished persons, serum C3 levels rise in response to infection. In malnourished individuals, serum C3 is generally low and decreases further with infection.

Serum C3 can be quantified using a variety of methods, particularly rate nephelometry. Alternatively, ELISA methods are also available. For the analysis of C3, serum must be separated immediately after the blood has clotted at room temperature, and the serum must be stored at $-70°C$ or lower prior to testing. During storage, C3 spontaneously converts to C3c, which has a smaller molecular size than native C3. Hence, an important source of error in the assay of C3 and other complement proteins is poor sample handling. Details of the assay methods are given in Parslow et al. (2001).

Other acute-phase plasma proteins that are often measured include C-reactive protein (CRP), α_1-acid glycoprotein, α_1-antichymotrypsin, and α_2-macroglobulin; details are given in Section 17.6.1. When there is evidence of an acute-phase response (e.g., increased CRP), decreased concentrations of plasma proteins such as albumin, transferrin, retinol-binding protein, and transthyretin cannot be assumed to reflect protein malnutrition (Box 16.3) (Fleck, 1989; Gabay et al., 1999).

16.6 Summary

Laboratory indices of protein status measure (*1*) somatic protein status, (*2*) visceral protein status, (*3*) metabolic changes, (*4*) muscle function, and (*5*) immune function.

Indices of somatic protein status include

urinary excretion of creatinine (frequently expressed as the creatinine height index) and 3-methylhistidine. The former is used to assess the degree of depletion of muscle mass in marasmic patients, as well as the degree of repletion, after long-term nutrition intervention, provided that accurately timed 72-h urine collections are made. Urinary excretion of 3-methylhistidine appears to be promising as a marker of muscle protein except in conditions of severe sepsis and major physical trauma, although it has not been widely used.

To assess the visceral protein status, concentrations of one or more serum proteins are measured. Of the most widely used proteins — albumin, transferrin, retinol-binding protein, and transthyretin — transferrin and albumin are most frequently used in hospital assessment protocols. They are not necessarily the most appropriate, particularly for monitoring short-term changes in protein status. They show a relatively slow response, which, like most serum proteins, may be complicated by the effects of such confounding factors as stress, sepsis, and hydration, thereby severely limiting their use for critically ill patients. As a result, serum albumin and transferrin are more usefully applied for monitoring long-term changes during convalescence.

To monitor short-term changes in visceral protein status during convalescence, serum transthyretin should be used. It has a smaller total body pool, a shorter half-life, and a relatively higher specificity than serum albumin and transferrin have. In the future, studies may include measurement of serum insulin-like growth factor I; it is said to be more sensitive to acute changes in protein status than are the other serum proteins.

Some metabolic changes that occur in protein-energy malnutrition are sometimes used as indices of protein status, although none of them differentiate between kwashiorkor and marasmus. Early studies in children have used the hydroxyproline index as an index of impaired growth arising from protein-energy malnutrition. For hospital patients, urinary urea nitrogen excretion on at least three 24-h urine samples, in association with nitrogen intake data, can provide an estimate of nitrogen balance. The latter is a particularly useful indicator for monitoring the nutritional status of hospital patients during the course of therapy. In field surveys, 24-h urine collections are impractical. Instead, the urinary urea nitrogen : creatinine ratio on casual urine samples can be calculated to assess the adequacy of protein intake.

Functional indices of protein status include muscle function, handgrip strength, and immunological tests. Muscle function tests measure changes in muscle contractility, relaxation rate, and endurance in malnourished patients.

Tests of immunocompetence may be used as functional indices of protein status, although their specificity and sensitivity are low. Many aspects of the immune system can be impaired by nutritional deficiencies, and no single test can measure the adequacy of the immune response. Hence, multiple immunological tests are needed. These may include total lymphocyte count, measurement of thymus-dependent lymphocytes and lymphocyte proliferation, delayed cutaneous hypersensitivity, and measurement of cytokines such as interleukin-1. The latter enhances lymphocyte proliferation and stimulates the helper T-cells to produce interleukin-2.

References

Afting EG, Bernhardt W, Janzen RW, Rothig H. (1981). Quantitative importance of non-skeletal muscle N tau-methylhistidine and creatinine in human urine. Biochemical Journal 200: 449–452.

Alexander JW. (1995). Specific nutrients and the immune response. Nutrition 11: 229–232.

Allison JB, Bird JWC. (1977). Elimination of nitrogen from the body. In: Munro HN, Allison JB (eds.) Mammalian Protein Metabolism. Volume 1. American Medical Association, Chicago, pp. 141–146.

Allison DJ, Walker A, Smith QT. (1966). Urinary hydroxyproline:creatinine ratio of normal humans at various ages. Clinica Chimica Acta 14: 729–734.

Bassey EJ, Harries UJ. (1993). Normal values for handgrip strength in 920 men and women aged over 65 y, and longitudinal changes over 4 y in 620 survivors. Clinical Science 84: 331–337.

Baudner S, Haupt H, Hubner R. (1994). Manufacture and characterization of a new reference preparation for 14 plasma proteins/CRM 470 = RPPHS lot 5. Journal of Clinical Laboratory Analysis 8: 177–190.

Bates SE, Suen JY, Tranum BL. (1979). Immunological skin testing and interpretation: a plea for uniformity. Cancer 43: 2306–2314.

Beaton GH, Calloway DH, Murphy S. (1992). Estimated protein intakes of toddlers: predictive prevalence of inadequate intakes in village populations in Egypt, Kenya, and Mexico. American Journal of Clinical Nutrition 55: 902–911.

Beckett LA, Brock DB, Lemke JH, Mendes de Leon C, Guralnik JM, Fillenbaum GG, Branch LG, Wetle T, Evans DA. (1996). Analysis of change in self-reported physical function among older persons in four population studies. American Journal of Epidemiology 143: 766–778.

Beetham R, Dawnay A, Landon J, Cattell WR. (1985). A radioimmunoassay for retinol-binding protein in serum and urine. Clinical Chemistry 31: 1364–1367.

Bernstein LH, Bachman TE, Meguid M, Arment M, Baumgartner T, Kinosian B, Martindale R, Spilekerman M. (1995). Measurement of visceral protein status in assessing protein and energy malnutrition: standard of care. Nutrition 11: 169–171.

Bhaskaram P, Sivakumar B. (1986) Interleukin-1 in malnutrition. Archives of Disease in Childhood 61: 182–185.

Bingham SA, Williams R, Cole TJ, Price CP, Cummings JH. (1988). Reference values for analytes of 24-h urine collections known to be complete. Annals of Clinical Chemistry 25: 610–619.

Bistrian BR. (1977). Nutritional assessment and therapy of protein-calorie malnutrition in the hospital. Journal of the American Dietetic Association 71: 393–397.

Bistrian BR, Blackburn GL, Sherman M, Scrimshaw N. (1975). Therapeutic index of nutritional depletion in hospitalized patients. Surgery, Gynecology and Obstetrics 141: 512–516.

Blackburn GL, Bistrian BR, Maini BS, Schlamm HT, Smith MF. (1977). Nutritional and metabolic assessment of the hospitalized patient. Journal of Parenteral and Enteral Nutrition 1: 11–22.

Bleiler RE, Schedl HP. (1962). Creatinine excretion: variability and relationship to diet and body size. Journal of Laboratory and Clinical Medicine 59: 945–955.

Boileau RB, Horstman DH, Buskirk ER, Mendez J. (1972). The usefulness of urinary creatinine excretion in estimating body composition. Medicine and Science in Sports and Exercise 4: 85–90.

Bohannon RW. (1987). The clinical measurement of strength. Clinical Rehabilitation 1: 5–16.

Buonpane EA, Brown RO, Boucher BA, Fabian TC, Luther RW. (1989). Use of fibronectin and somatomedin-C as nutritional markers in the enteral nutritional support of traumatized patients. Critical Care Medicine 17: 126–132.

Calloway DH, Odell ACF, Margen S. (1971). Sweat

and miscellaneous nitrogen losses in human balance studies. Journal of Nutrition 101: 775–786.

Carpentier YA, Barthel J, Bruyns J. (1982). Plasma protein concentration in nutritional assessment. Proceedings of the Nutrition Society 41: 405–417.

Castanada C, Charnley JM, Evans WJ, Crim MC. (1995). Elderly women accommodate to a low protein diet with losses of body cell mass, muscle function, and immune response. American Journal of Clinical Nutrition 62: 30–39.

Chandra RK. (1981). Immunodeficiency in undernutrition and overnutrition. Nutrition Reviews 39: 225–231.

Chandra RK. (1991). Immunocompetence is a sensitive and functional barometer of nutritional status. Acta Paediatrica Scandinavica Supplement 374: 129–132.

Cheek DB. (1968). Human Growth: Body Composition, Cell Growth, Energy, and Intelligence. Lea & Febiger, Philadelphia.

Cheek DB, Brasel JA, Elliot D, Scott R. (1966). Muscle cell size and number in normal children and in dwarfs (pituitary, cretins, and primordial) before and after treatment. Bulletin of Johns Hopkins Hospital 119: 46–62.

Chilima DM. (1998). Nutritional status and functional ability of older people in rural Malawi. PhD thesis, London School of Hygiene and Tropical Medicine.

Chilima DM, Ismail SJ. (2001). Nutrition and handgrip strength of older adults in rural Malawi. Public Health Nutrition 4: 11–17.

Chow WH, Gridley G, McLaughlin JK, Mandel JS, Wacholder S, Blot WJ, Niwa S, Fraumeni JF Jr. (1994). Protein intake and risk of renal cell cancer. Journal of the National Cancer Institute. 86: 1131–1139.

Christian P, West KP Jr. (1998). Interactions between zinc and vitamin A: an update. American Journal of Clinical Nutrition 68: 435S–441S.

Christou NV, Meakins JL, Gordon J, Yee J, Hassanzahraee M, Nohr CW, Shizgal HM, Maclean LD. (1995). The delayed hypersensitivity response and host resistance in surgical patients: 20 years later. Annals of Surgery 222: 534–548.

Coats KG, Morgan SL, Bartolucci AA, Weinsier RL. (1993). Hospital-associated malnutrition: a reevaluation 12 years later. Journal of the American Dietetic Association 93: 27–33.

Cook JGH. (1975). Factors influencing the assay of creatinine. Annals of Clinical Biochemistry 12: 219–232.

Corish CA, Kennedy NP. (2000). Protein-energy undernutrition in hospital in-patients. British Journal of Nutrition 83: 575–591.

Coward WA, Lunn PG. (1981). The biochemistry and physiology of kwashiorkor and marasmus. British Medical Bulletin 37: 19–24.

Crim MC, Munro HN. (1994). Proteins and amino acids. In: Shils ME, Olson JA, Shike M (eds.) Modern Nutrition in Health and Disease. Volume 1. 8th ed. Lea & Febiger, Philadelphia. pp. 3–35.

Cupisti A, Licitra R, Chisari C, Stampacchia G, D'Alessandro C, Galetta F, Rossi B, Barsotti G. (2004). Skeletal muscle and nutritional assessment in chronic renal failure patients on a protein-restricted diet. Journal of Internal Medicine 255: 115–124.

Dabev D, Struck H. (1971). Microliter determination of free hydroxyproline in blood serum. Biochemical Medicine 5: 17–21.

de Blaauw I, Deutz NE, Von Meyenfeldt MF. (1996). In vivo amino acid metabolism of gut and liver during short and prolonged starvation. American Journal of Physiology 270: G298–G306.

Delafuente JC. (1991). Nutrients and the immune response. Rheumatic Diseases Clinics of North America 17: 203–212.

Delpeuch F, Cornu A, Chevalier P. (1980). The effect of iron-deficiency anaemia on two indices of nutritional status, prealbumin and transferrin. British Journal of Nutrition 43: 375–379.

de Pee S, Dary O. (2002). Biochemical indicators of vitamin A deficiency: serum retinol and serum retinol binding protein. Journal of Nutrition 132: 2895S–2901S.

Driver AG, McAlvey MT. (1980). Creatinine height index as a function of age. American Journal of Clinical Nutrition 33: 2057.

Durnin JV, Garlick P, Jackson AA, Schurch B, Shetty PS, Waterlow JC. (1999). Report of the IDECG Working Group on lower limits of energy and protein and upper limits of protein intakes. International Dietary Energy Consultative Group. European Journal of Clinical Nutrition 53(Suppl.1): S174–S176.

Edwards RH, Young A, Hosking GP, Jones DA. (1977). Human skeletal muscle function: description of tests and normal values. Clinical Science and Molecular Medicine 52: 283–290.

Erstad BL, Campbell DJ, Rollins CJ, Rappaport WD. (1994). Albumin and prealbumin concentrations in patients receiving postoperative parenteral nutrition. Pharmacotherapy 14: 458–462.

Ferguson EL, Gibson RS, Opare-Obisaw C, Osei-Opare F, Lamba C, Ounpuu S. (1993). Seasonal food consumption patterns and dietary diversity of rural preschool Ghanaian and Malawian children. Ecology of Food and Nutrition 29: 219–234.

Field CJ. (1996). Using immunological techniques to determine the effect of nutrition on T-cell function. Canadian Journal of Physiology and Pharmacology 74: 769–777.

Field CJ, Gougeon R, Marliss EB. (1991). Changes in circulating leukocytes and mitogen responses during very low energy all-protein reducing diets. American Journal of Clinical Nutrition 54: 123–129.

Finch S, Doyle W, Lowe C, Bates CJ, Prentice A, Smithers G, Clarke PC. (1998). National Diet and Nutrition Survey: People Aged 65 Years and Over. Report of the Diet and Nutrition Survey. The Stationery Office, London.

Finn PJ, Plank LD, Clark MA, Connolly AB, Hill GL. (1996). Assessment of involuntary muscle function in patients after critical injury or severe sepsis. Journal of Parenteral and Enteral Nutrition 20: 332–337.

Fleck A. (1989). Clinical and nutritional aspects of changes in acute-phase proteins during inflammation. Proceedings of the Nutrition Society 48: 347–354.

Fleeman C, Rodgers L, Miller B, Wright RA. (1983). The use of a dynamometer in nutritional assessment. Journal of the American College of Nutrition 4: 397–400.

Forbes GB, Bruining GJ. (1976). Urinary creatinine excretion and lean body mass. American Journal of Clinical Nutrition 29: 1359–1366.

Forbes RM, Cooper AR, Mitchell HH. (1953). Composition of adult human body as determined by chemical analysis. Journal of Biological Chemistry 203: 359–366.

Fuhrman MP, Charney P, Mueller CM. (2004). Hepatic proteins and nutrition assessment. Journal of the American Dietetic Association 104: 1258–1264.

Galanos AN, Pieper CF, Cornoni-Huntley JC, Bales CW, Fillenbaum GG. (1994). Nutrition and function: is there a relationship between body mass index and the functional capabilities of community-dwelling elderly? Journal of American Geriatrics Society 42: 368–373.

Gabay C, Kushner I. (1999). Acute-phase proteins and other systemic responses to inflammation. New England Journal of Medicine 340: 448–454.

Grant JP. (1986). Nutritional assessment in clinical practice. Nutrition in Clinical Practice 1: 3–11.

Grant JP, Custer PB, Thurlow J. (1981). Current techniques of nutritional assessment. Surgical Clinics of North America 61: 437–463.

Gregory J, Foster K, Tyler H, Wiseman M. (1990). The Dietary and Nutritional Survey of British Adults. The Stationery Office, London.

Gutierrez A, Alvestrand A, Qureshi GA, Bergstrom J. (1992). Influence of a meat-free diet on the urinary excretion of 3-methylhistidine and creatinine in chronic renal failure. Journal of Internal Medicine 232: 129–132.

Guo CB, Zhang W, Ma DQ, Zhang KH, Huang JQ. (1996). Hand grip strength: an indicator of nutritional state and the mix of postoperative complications in patients with oral and maxillofacial cancers. British Journal of Oral Maxillofacial Surgery 34: 325–327.

Hallworth MJ, Calvin J, Price CP. (1984). Determination of retinol-binding protein in serum by kinetic immunonephelometry with polyethylene glycol pretreatment. Annals of Clinical Biochemistry 21: 484–487.

Hanning RM, Blimkie CJ, Bar-Or O, Lands LC, Moss LA, Wilson WM. (1993). Relationships among nutritional status and skeletal and respiratory function in cystic fibrosis: does early dietary supplementation make a difference. American Journal of Clinical Nutrition 57: 580–587.

Hansen RD, Raja C, Allen BJ. (2000). Total body

protein in chronic diseases and in aging. Annals of the New York Academy of Sciences 904: 345–352.

Haram K, Augensen K, Elsayed S. (1983). Serum protein in normal pregnancy with special reference to acute-phase reactants. British Journal of Obstetrics and Gynecology 90: 139–145.

Harvey KB, Blumenkrantz MJ, Levine SE, Blackburn GL. (1980). Nutritional assessment and treatment of chronic renal failure. American Journal of Clinical Nutrition 33: 1586–1597.

Health and Welfare Canada. (1973). Nutrition Canada National Survey. Health and Welfare, Ottawa.

Helyar L, Sherman AR. (1987). Iron deficiency and interleukin 1 production by rat leukocytes. American Journal of Clinical Nutrition 46: 346–452.

Hendricks KM, Duggan C, Gallagher L, Carlin AC, Richardson DS, Collier SB, Simpson W, Lo C. (1995). Malnutrition in hospitalized pediatric patients: current prevalence. Archives of pediatrics & adolescent medicine 149: 1118–1122.

Heymsfield SB, Arteaga C, McManus CB, Smith J, Moffitt S. (1983). Measurement of muscle mass in humans: validity of the 24-hour urinary creatinine method. American Journal of Clinical Nutrition 37: 478–494.

Hill GL. (1992). Body composition research: implications for the practice of clinical nutrition. Journal of Parenteral and Enteral Nutrition 16: 197–218.

Hoffman-Goetz L, Kluger MJ. (1979). Protein deprivation: its effect on fever and plasma iron during bacterial infection in rabbits. Journal of Physiology 295: 419–430.

Hoffman-Goetz L, Kluger MJ. (1979). Protein deficiency: its effect on body temperature in health and disease states. American Journal of Clinical Nutrition 32: 1423–1427.

Hoffman-Goetz L, McFarlane D, Bistrain BR, Blackburn GL. (1981). Febrile and plasma iron responses of rabbits injected with endogenous pyrogen from malnourished patients. American Journal of Clinical Nutrition 34: 1109–1116.

Hunt SV. (1987). Preparation of lymphocytes and accessory cells. In: Klaus GGB (ed.) Lymphocytes: A Practical Approach. IRL Press, Washington, DC, pp. 1–34.

Imbembo AL, Walser M. (1984). Nutritional assessment. In: Walser M, Imbembo AL, Margolis S, Elfert GA (eds.) Nutritional Management: The John Hopkins Handbook. W.B. Saunders, Philadelphia, pp. 9–30.

Ingelbleek Y, Young V. (1994). Transthyretin (prealbumin) in health and disease: nutritional implications. Annual Review of Nutrition 14: 495–533.

IOM (Institute of Medicine). (2002). Dietary Reference Intakes for Energy, Carbohydrate, Fiber, Fat, Fatty Acids, Cholesterol, Protein, and Amino Acids (Macronutrients). National Academy Press, Washington, DC.

Isley WL, Lyman B, Pemberton LB. (1990). Somatomedin-C as a nutritional marker in traumatized patients. Critical Care Medicine 18: 795–796.

Jacob RA, Sandstead HH, Solomons NW, Rieger C, Rothberg R. (1978). Zinc status and vitamin A transport in cystic fibrosis. American Journal of Clinical Nutrition 31: 638–644.

James WP, Hay AM. (1968). Albumin metabolism: effect of the nutritional state and the dietary protein intake. Journal of Clinical Investigation 47: 1958–1972.

Janossy G, Amlot P. (1987). Immunofluorescence and immunohistochemistry. In: Klaus GGB (ed.) Lymphocytes: A Practical Approach. IRL Press, Washington, DC. pp. 67–108.

Jeejeebhoy KN. (1981). Protein nutrition in clinical practice. British Medical Bulletin 37: 11–17.

Keusch GT. (1990). Malnutrition, infection and immune function. In: Suskind RM, Lewinter-Suskind L. (eds.) The Malnourished Child. Nestlé Nutrition Workshop Series Vol. 19. Raven Press, New York, pp. 37–59.

Kitagawa T, Owada M, Urakami T, Yamauchi K.(1998). Increased incidence of non-insulin dependent diabetes mellitus among Japanese school-children correlates with an increased intake of animal protein and fat. Clinical Pediatrics 37: 111–115.

Klein S, Kinney J, Jeejeebhoy K, Alpers D, Hellerstein M, Mirray M, Twomey P. (1997). Nutrition support in clinical practice: review of published data and recommendations for future research directions. American Journal of Clinical Nutrition 66: 683–706.

Klidjian AM, Foster KJ, Kammerling RM, Cooper A, Karran SJ. (1980). Relation of anthropometric and dynamometric variables to serious postoperative complications. British Medical Journal 281: 899–901.

Kniker WT, Anderson CT, Roumiantzeff M. (1979). The multi-test system: a standardized approach to evaluation of delayed hypersensitivity and cell-mediated immunity. Annals of Allergy 43: 73–79.

Kopple JD. (1987). Uses and limitations of the balance technique. Journal of Parenteral and Enteral Nutrition 11: 79S–85S.

Large S, Neal G, Glover J, Thanangkul O, Olson RE. (1980). The early changes in retinol-binding protein and prealbumin concentrations in plasma of protein-energy malnourished children after treatment with retinol and an improved diet. British Journal of Nutrition 43: 393–402.

Law DK, Dudrick SJ, Abdou NI. (1973). Immunocompetence of patients with protein-calorie malnutrition: the effects of nutritional repletion. Annals of Internal Medicine 79: 545–550.

Ledur A, Fitting C, David B, Hamberger C, Cavaillon J. (1995). Variable estimates of cytokine levels produced by commercial ELISA kits: results using international cytokine standards. Journal of Immunological Methods 186: 171–179.

Lennmarken C, Sandstedt S, Schenck HV, Larsson J. (1986). The effect of starvation on skeletal muscle function in man. Clinical Nutrition 5: 99–103.

Leonberg BL, Crosby LO, Buzby GP. (1987). A rapid, accurate, precise assay for determination of plasma transferrin. Journal of Parenteral and Enteral Nutrition 11: 74–76.

LeRoy EC. (1967). The technique and significance of hydroxyproline measurement in man. Advances in Clinical Chemistry 10: 213–253.

Lesourd B. (1995). Protein undernutrition as the major cause of decreased immune function in the elderly: clinical and functional implications. Nutrition Reviews 53: S86–S94.

Lesourd B, Decarli B, Dirren H. (1996). Longitudinal changes in iron and protein status of elderly Europeans. SENECA investigators. European Journal of Clinical Nutrition 50: S16–S24.

Ligthart GJ, Corberand JX, Fournier C, Galanaud P, Hijmans W, Kennes B, Muller-Hermelink HK, Steinmann GG. (1984). Admission criteria for immunogerontological studies in man: the SENIEUR protocol. Mechanisms of Ageing and Development 28: 47–55.

Linder MC (ed.) (1991). Nutritional Biochemistry and Metabolism with Clinical Applications. 2nd ed. Appelton & Lange, Norwalk, CT.

Logan S, Hildebrandt LA. (2003). The use of prealbumin to enhance nutrition-intervention screening and monitoring of the malnourished patient. Nutrition Today 38: 134–138.

Long CL, Haverberg LN, Young VR, Kinney JM, Munro HN, Geiger JW. (1975). Metabolism of 3-methylhistidine in man. Metabolism 24: 929–935.

Lopes J, Russell DM, Whitwell J, Jeejeebhoy KN. (1982). Skeletal muscle function in malnutrition. American Journal of Clinical Nutrition 36: 602–610.

Lowell C. (2001). Clinical laboratory methods for detection of cellular immunity. In: Parslow TG, Stites DP, Terr AI, Imboden JB (eds.) Medical Immunology. 10th ed. McGraw-Hill, New York, pp. 234–249.

Lukasewycz OA, Prohaska JR. (1990). The immune response in copper deficiency. Annals of the New York Academy of Sciences 587: 147–159.

Lukaski HC, Mendez J, Buskirk ER, Cohn SH. (1981). Relationship between endogenous 3-methylhistidine excretion and body composition. American Journal of Physiology 240: E302–E307.

MacKenzie TA, Clark NG, Bistrian BR, Flatt JP, Hallowell EM, Blackburn GL. (1985). A simple method for estimating nitrogen balance in hospitalized patients: a review and supporting data for a previously proposed technique. Journal of the American College of Nutrition 4: 575–581.

Manandhar MC. (1999). Undernutrition and impaired functional ability amongst elderly slum dwellers in Mumbai, India. PhD thesis, London School of Hygiene and Tropical Medicine.

Mann GV. (1988). A simplified system for collecting 24-hour urine samples. Journal of the American College of Nutrition 7: 141–145.

Mason DW, Penhale WJ, Sedgwick JD. (1987). Preparation of lymphocyte subpopulation. In: Klaus GGB (ed.) Lymphocytes: A Practical Approach. IRL Press, Washington, DC, pp. 35–54.

McMurray DN. (1984). Cell-mediated immunity in nutritional deficiency. Progress in Food and Nutrition Science 8: 193–228.

McPherson IG, Everard DW. (1972). Serum albumin estimation: modification of the bromocresol green method. Clinica Chimica Acta 37: 117–121.

Meador CK, Kreisberg RA, Friday JP, Bowdoin B, Coan P, Armstrong J, Hazelrig JB. (1968). Muscle mass determination by isotopic dilution of creatine-^{14}C. Metabolism 17: 1104–1108.

Meakins JL, Pietsch JB, Bubernick O, Kelly R, Rode H, Gordon J, MacLean LD. (1977). Delayed hypersensitivity: Indicator of acquired failure of host defenses in sepsis and trauma. Annals of Surgery 186: 241–250.

Meakins TS, Jackson AA. (1996). Salvage of exogenous urea nitrogen enhances nitrogen balance in normal men consuming marginally inadequate protein diets. Clinical Science 90: 215–225.

Metges CC, Barth CA. (2000). Metabolic consequences of a high dietary-protein intake in adulthood: assesment of the available evidence. Journal of Nutrition 130: 886–889.

Miller CL. (1978). Immunological assays as measurements of nutritional status: a review. Journal of Parenteral and Enteral Nutrition 2: 554–566.

Mire-Sluis AR, Gaines-Das R, Thorpe R. (1995). Immunoassays for detecting cytokines: what are they really measuring? Journal of Immunological Methods 186: 157–160.

Mitch WE, Collier VU, Walser M. (1980). Creatinine metabolism in chronic renal failure. Clinical Science 58: 327–335.

Mullen JL, Buzby GP, Waldman MT, Gertner MH, Hobbs CL, Rosato EF. (1979a). Prediction of operative morbidity and mortality by preoperative nutritional assessment. Surgical Forum 30: 80–82.

Mullen JL, Gertner MH, Buzby GP, Goodhart GL, Rosato EF. (1979b). Implications of malnutrition in the surgical patient. Archives of Surgery 114: 121–125.

Munro HN, Young VR. (1978). Urinary excretion of N gamma-methylhistidine (3-methylhistidine): a tool to study metabolic responses in relation to nutrient and hormonal status in health and disease in man. American Journal of Clinical Nutrition 31: 1608–1614.

Naber THJ, Schermer T, de Bree A, Nusteling K, Eggink L, Kruimel JW, Bakkeren J, van Heereveld H, Katan MB. (1997). Prevalence of malnutrition in nonsurgical hospitalized patients and its association with disease complications. American Journal of Clinical Nutrition 66: 1232–1239.

Nicholson JK, Jones BM, Hubbard M. (1993). CD4 T-lymphocyte determinations on whole blood specimens using a single-tube three color assay. Cytometry 14: 685–689.

Ogunshina SO, Hussain MA. (1980). Plasma thyroxine-binding prealbumin as an index of mild protein-energy malnutrition in Nigerian children. American Journal of Clinical Nutrition 33: 794–800.

Parnell W, Scragg R, Wilson N, Schaaf D, Fitzgerald E. (2003). NZ Food NZ Children: Key Results of the 2002 National Children's Nutrition Survey. Ministry of Health, Wellington.

Parslow TG, Stites DP, Terr AI, Imboden JB (eds.) (2001). Medical Immunology. 10th ed. McGraw-Hill, New York.

Paxton H, Cunningham-Rundles S, O'Gorman MRG. (1995). Laboratory evaluation of the cellular immune system. In: Henry JB (ed.) Clinical Diagnosis and Management by Laboratory Methods. WB Saunders, New York, pp. 877–912.

Phinney SD. (1981). The assessment of protein nutrition in the hospitalized patient. Clinics in Laboratory Medicine 1: 767–774.

Pieterse S, Manandhar M, Ismail S. (2002). The association between nutritional status and handgrip strength in older Rwandan refugees. European Journal of Clinical Nutrition 56: 933–939.

Popii V, Baumann G. (2004). Laboratory measurement of growth hormone. Clinica Chimica Acta 350: 1–16.

Potter MA, Luxton G. (1999). Prealbumin measurement as a screening tool for protein calorie malnutrition in emergency hospital admissions: a pilot study. Clinical and Investigative Medicine 22: 44–52.

Prockop DJ, Udenfriend S. (1960). A specific method for the analysis of hydroxyproline in tissues and urine. Analytical Biochemistry 1: 228–239.

Rainey-Macdonald CG, Holliday RL, Wells GA, Donner AP. (1983). Validity of a two-variable nutritional index for use in selecting candidates for nutritional support. Journal of Parenteral and Enteral Nutrition 7: 15–20.

Ramsey BW, Farrell PM, Pencharz P. (1992). Nutritional assessment and management in cystic fibrosis: a consensus report: The Consensus Committee. American Journal of Clinical Nutrition 55: 108–116.

Riesco A. (1970). Five-year cancer cure: relation to total amount of peripheral lymphocytes and neutrophils. Cancer 25: 135–140.

Ritchie RF, Palomaki GE, Neveux LM, Navolotskaia O. (1999a). Reference distributions for the negative acute-phase serum proteins, albumin, transferrin and transthyretin: a comparison of a large cohort to the world's literature. Journal of Clinical Laboratory Analysis 13: 280–286.

Ritchie RF, Palomaki GE, Neveux LM, Navolotskaia O, Ledue TB, Craig WY. (1999b). Reference distributions for the negative acute-phase serum proteins, albumin, transferrin and transthyretin: a practical, simple and clinically relevant approach in a large cohort. Journal of Clinical Laboratory Analysis 13: 273–279.

Robert JC, Serog P. (1984). Determination of 3 methyl-L-histidine in human urine by ion exchange high performance liquid chromatography: applications to patients in postoperative surgical care. Clinica Chimica Acta 142: 161–181.

Romagnani S. (1994). Lymphokine production by human T cells in disease states. Annual Review of Immunology 12: 227–257.

Roza AM, Tuitt D, Shizgal HM. (1984). Transferrin: a poor measure of nutritional status. Journal of Parenteral and Enteral Nutrition 8: 523–528.

Russell DM, Jeejeebhoy KN. (1983). The assessment of the functional consequences of malnutrition. Nutrition Abstracts and Reviews 53: 863–877.

Russell DM, Leiter LA, Whitwell J, Marliss EB, Jeejeebhoy KN. (1983a). Skeletal muscle function during hypocaloric diets and fasting: a comparison with standard nutritional assessment parameters. American Journal of Clinical Nutrition 37: 133–138.

Russell DM, Prendergast PJ, Darby PL, Garfinkel PE, Whitwell J, Jeejeebhoy KN. (1983b). A comparison between muscle function and body composition in anorexia nervosa: the effect of refeeding. American Journal of Clinical Nutrition 38: 229–237.

Russell D, Parnell W, Wilson N, Faed J, Ferguson E, Herbison P, Horwath C, Nye T, Walker R, Wilson B. (1999). NZ Food, NZ People: Key Results of the 1997 National Nutrition Survey. Ministry of Health, Wellington, New Zealand.

Ryan JA, Taft DA. (1980). Preoperative nutritional assessment does not predict morbidity and mortality in abdominal operations. Surgical Forum 31: 96–98.

Sauberlich HE. (1999). Laboratory Tests for the Assessment of Nutritional Status. CRC Press, Cleveland, OH.

Saunders SJ, Truswell AS, Barbezat GO, Wittman W, Hansen JDL. (1967). Plasma free amino acid pattern in protein-calorie malnutrition: reappraisal of its diagnostic value. Lancet 2(7520): 795–797.

Schlesinger L, Olbaum A, Grez L, Stekel A. (1977). Cell-mediated immune studies in marasmic children from Chile: delayed hypersensitivity, lymphocyte transformation, and interferon production. In: Suskind RM (ed.) Malnutrition and the Immune Response. Raven Press, New York, pp. 91–98.

Scott PH. (1979). A method for the determination of alkaline ribonuclease (EC 3.1.4.22) activity in human serum. Analytical Biochemistry 100: 233–239.

Scott PH, Berger HM, Wharton BA. (1984). A critical assessment of plasma alkaline ribonuclease as an indicator of protein nutritional status in infancy. Annals of Clinical Biochemistry 21: 357–362.

Searcy RL, Simms NM, Foreman JA, Bergquist LM. (1965). A study of the specificity of the Berthelot colour reaction. Clinica Chimica Acta 12: 170–175.

Seltzer MH, Bastidas JA, Cooper DM, Engler P, Slocum B, Fletcher HS. (1979). Instant nutritional assessment. Journal of Parenteral and Enteral Nutrition 3: 157–159.

Shetty PS, Watrasiewicz KE, Jung RT, James WPT. (1979). Rapid-turnover transport proteins: an index of subclinical protein-energy malnutrition. Lancet 2(8136): 230–232.

Shizgal HM, Vasilevsky CA, Gardiner PF, Wang WZ, Tuitt DA, Brabant GV. (1986). Nutritional assessment and skeletal muscle function. American Journal of Clinical Nutrition 44: 761–771.

Simmons WK. (1972). Urinary urea nitrogen-creatinine ratio as an indicator of recent protein intake in field studies. American Journal of Clinical Nutrition 25: 539–542.

Smith OW. (1942). Creatinine excretion in women: data collected in the course of urinalysis for female sex hormones. Journal of Clinical Endocrinology 2: 1–12.

Smith FR, Suskind R, Thanangkul O, Leitzmann C, Goodman DS, Olson RE. (1975). Plasma vitamin A, retinol-binding protein and prealbumin concentrations in protein- calorie malnutrition. III. Response to varying dietary treatments. American Journal of Clinical Nutrition 28: 732–738.

Smith IF, Latham MC, Azubuike JA, Butler WR, Phillips LS, Pond WG, Enwonwu CO. (1981). Blood plasma levels of cortisol, insulin, growth hormone and somatomedin in children with marasmus, kwashiorkor, and intermediate forms of protein-energy malnutrition. Proceedings of the Society for Experimental Biology and Medicine 167: 607–611.

Sokal JE. (1975). Measurement of delayed skin-test responses. New England Journal of Medicine 293: 501–502.

Spiekerman AM. (1993). Proteins used in nutritional assessment. Clinics in Laboratory Medicine 13: 353–369.

Srivastava SS, Mani KV, Soni CM, Bhati J. (1957). Effect of muscular exercises on urinary excretion of creatine and creatinine. Indian Journal of Medical Research 55: 953–960.

Stiehm ER. (1980). Humoral immunity in malnutrition. Federation Proceedings 39: 3093–3097.

Subar AF, Krebs-Smith SM, Cook A, Kahle LL. (1998). Dietary sources of nutrients among US adults, 1989 to 1991. Journal of the American Dietetics Association 98: 537–547.

Suchner U, Senftleben U, Eckart T, Scholz M, Beck K, Murr R, Enzenbach R, Peter K. (1996). Enteral versus parenteral nutrition: effects on gastrointestinal function and metabolism. Nutrition 12: 13–22.

Sullivan DH, Walls RC. (1995). The risk of life-threatening complications in a select population of geriatric patients: the impact of nutritional status. Journal of the American College of Nutrition 14: 29–36.

Taylor HL, Mickelsen O, Keys A. (1949). Effects of induced malaria, acute starvation and semistarvation on the electrophoretic diagram of the serum proteins of normal young men. Journal of Clinical Investigation 28: 273–281.

Teerlink T, de Boer E. (1989). Determination of 3-methylhistidine in urine by high-performance liquid chromatography using pre-column derivatization with 9-fluorenylmethyl chloroformate. Journal of Chromatography 491: 418–423.

Thissen JP, Ketelslegers JM, Underwood LE. (1994). Nutritional regulation of the insulin-like growth factors. Endocrine Research 15: 80–101.

Twomey P, Ziegler D, Rombeau J. (1982). Utility of skin testing in nutritional assessment: a critical review. Journal of Parenteral and Enteral Nutrition 6: 50–58.

Unterman TG, Vazquez RM, Slas AJ, Martyn PA, Phillips LS. (1985). Nutrition and somatomedin. XIII: Usefulness of somatomedin-C in nutritional assessment. American Journal of Medicine 78: 228–234.

USDA (United States Department of Agriculture) (1983). Nationwide Food Consumption Survey 1977–1978. Report No. 1-1. Consumer Nutrition Division, Human Nutrition Information Service, U.S. Department of Agriculture, Hyattsville, MD.

Varakamin C, Henry J, Golden M, Tontisirin K. (1998). Body composition and muscular strength in an elderly Thai population. Proceedings of the Nutrition Society 57: 64A.

Vielma H, Mendez J, Druckenmiller M, Lukaski H. (1981). A practical and reliable method for determination of urinary 3-methylhistidine. Journal of Biochemistry and Biophysics Methods 5: 75–82.

Vlajinac HD, Marinkovic JM, Ilic MD, Kocev NI. (1997). Diet and prostate cancer: a case control study. European Journal of Cancer 33: 101–107.

Wadhwa M, Mire-Sluis A, Thorpe R. (1999). Standardization and calibration of cytokine immunoassays. Revue de l'ACOMEN (Action Concertée en Medicine Nucléaire) 5: 276–284.

Wahlqvist ML, Flint DM, Prinsley DM, Dryden PA. (1981). Effect of zinc supplementation on serum albumin and folic acid concentrations in a group of hypo-albuminaemic and hypozincaemic aged persons. In: Howard AN, Baird I M (eds.) Recent Advances in Clinical Nutrition. Volume 1. John Libbey, London, pp. 83–84.

Walser M. (1987). Creatinine excretion as a measure of protein nutrition in adults of varying age. Journal of Parenteral and Enteral Nutrition 11: 73S–78S.

Wassertheil-Smollers S, Langford HG, Yamori Y, Blaufox MD, Oberman A, Davis B, Nara Y, Wylie-Rosett J, Zimbaldi N. (1990) Estimation of protein intake: comparison of dietary assessment and urinary excretion. Journal of Cardiovascular Pharmacology 1658: S28–S31.

Waterlow JC. (1972). Classification and definition of protein-calorie malnutrition. British Medical Journal 3: 566–569.

Waterlow JC. (1986). Observations on the variability of creatinine excretion. Human Nutrition: Clinical Nutrition 40C: 125–129.

Waterlow JC. (1992) (ed.) Protein-Energy Malnutrition. Edward Arnold, London.

Webb AR, Newman LA, Taylor M, Keogh JB. (1989). Handgrip dynamometry as a predictor of postoperative complications: reappraisal using age standardized grip strengths. Journal of Parenteral and Enteral Nutrition 13: 30–33.

Webster J, Garrow JS. (1985). Creatinine excretion over 24 hours as a measure of body composition or of completeness of urine collection. Human Nutrition: Clinical Nutrition 39C: 101–106.

Whicher JT, Evans SW. (1990). Cytokines in disease. Clinical Chemistry 36: 1269–1281.

Whicher JT, Ritchie RF, Johnson AM, Baudner S, Biemvenu J, Blirup-Jensen S, Carlsrom A, Dati F, Ward AM, Svendsen PJ. (1994). New international reference preparation for protein in human serum (RPPHS). Clinical Chemistry 40: 934–938.

Whitehead RG. (1965). Hydroxyproline creatinine ratio as an index of nutritional status and rate of growth. Lancet 2(7412): 567–570.

Whitehead RG. (1967). Biochemical tests in differential diagnosis of protein and calorie deficiencies. Archives of Disease in Childhood 42: 479–484.

Whitehead RG, Dean RFA. (1964). Serum amino acids in kwashiorkor. I: Relationship to clinical conditions. American Journal of Clinical Nutrition 14: 313–319.

Whitehead JDL, Frood JDL, Poskitt EME. (1971). Value of serum-albumin measurements in nutritional surveys: a reappraisal. Lancet 2(7719): 287–289.

Windsor JA, Hill GL. (1988). Weight loss with physiologic impairment: a basic indicator of surgical risk. Annals of Surgery 207: 290–296.

Winkler MF, Gerrior SA, Pomp A, Albina JE. (1989). Use of retinol-binding protein and prealbumin as indicators of the response to nutrition therapy. Journal of the American Dietetic Association 89: 684–687.

Winterer J, Bistrian BR, Bilmazes C, Blackburn GL, Young VR. (1980). Whole body protein turnover studied with 15N-glycine, and muscle protein breakdown in mildly obese subjects during a protein-sparing diet and a brief total fast. Metabolism 29: 575–581.

Wolever TM, Hamad S, Gittelsohn J, Gao J, Hanley AJ, Harris SB, Zinman B. (1997). Low dietary fiber and high protein intakes associated with newly diagnosed diabetes in a remote aboriginal community. American Journal of Clinical Nutrition 66: 1470–1471.

Ylatupa S, Partanen P, Haglund C, Virtanen I. (1993). Competitive enzyme immunoassay for quantification of the cellular form of fibronectin (EDAcFN) in blood samples. Journal of Immunological Methods 163: 41–47.

Young VR, Marchini JS. (1990). Mechanisms and nutritional significance of metabolic responses to altered intakes of protein and amino acids, with reference to nutritional adaptation in humans. American Journal of Clinical Nutrition 51: 270–289.

Young VR, Marchini JS, Cortiella J. (1990). Assessment of protein nutritional status. Journal of Nutrition 120: 1496–1502.

17

Assessment of iron status

The assessment of the iron status of the population is critical: iron deficiency is the most frequently occurring micronutrient deficiency in low-income and industrialized countries.

Functions of iron

The human body contains about 2.5 to 4 g of elemental iron. Of this, about 70% is present in the hemoglobin, the oxygen-carrying pigment of the red blood cells that plays a critical role in transferring oxygen from lung to tissues. Hemoglobin is made up of four heme subunits, each with a polypeptide chain of globin attached. Each molecule of heme consists of a protoporphyrin IX molecule with one iron atom. In addition, about 4% of body iron is present in myoglobin, the oxygen-binding storage protein found in muscle. The structure of myoglobin is similar to hemoglobin, except that it contains only one heme unit and one globin chain.

Trace amounts of iron are also associated with electron transport and several enzymes. Examples include the heme-containing cytochromes that serve as electron carriers within the cell, iron-sulfur proteins (flavoproteins, heme-flavoproteins) that are required for the first reaction in the electron transport chain, and hydrogen peroxidases (e.g., catalase and peroxidase). The cytochrome P450 family of enzymes also contain heme and are located in microsomal membranes of liver cells and intestinal mucosal cells. Key functions of cytochrome P450 involve detoxification of foreign substances in the liver, and synthesis of steroid hormones and bile acids (Yip and Dallman, 1996; Beard et al., 1996).

In addition to these functional forms, as much as 25% of total body iron is present as storage iron, found primarily in the liver. Smaller amounts occur in the reticulo-endothelial cells of the bone marrow and spleen; and in the muscle tissues. Of the storage iron, approximately two-thirds consists of ferritin, the soluble fraction of the nonheme iron stores. Small quantities of ferritin can be synthesized in all cells of the body, even those with no special iron storage function. Ferritin also appears in small concentrations in the serum but is not involved in iron transport. The remainder of storage iron is insoluble hemosiderin (Yip and Dallman, 1996).

Stored iron serves as a reservoir to supply cellular needs, mainly hemoglobin production, and is especially important in the third trimester of pregnancy. The size of the storage component is most strongly influenced by age, sex, body size, and either the magnitude of iron losses or the presence of diseases of iron overload (Brittenham et al., 1981).

Iron transport is carried out by the transport protein transferrin. The latter delivers iron to the tissues by means of cell membrane receptors specific for transferrin (Section 17.8). About 20–30 mg of iron cycles through the transport component each day.

Absorption and metabolism of iron

Three main factors in the body operate to maintain iron balance and prevent iron deficiency and iron overload. These are: (a) intake, (b) storage, and (c) loss of iron. The interrelationship of these factors has now been described mathematically, so that the amount of storage iron can be predicted as long as iron losses and bioavailability of iron are known (Hallberg et al., 1998).

Intake of iron is determined by the quantity and bioavailability of iron in the diet and the capacity to absorb iron. The amount of dietary iron absorbed is determined by the nutritional needs of the individual and by factors influencing the bioavailability of the ingested iron (Miret et al., 2003).

The two different forms of dietary iron, heme and nonheme, are absorbed by separate mechanisms. Heme iron is derived from the hemoglobin and myoglobin in meat, and is absorbed readily as the intact moiety. Nonheme iron is found primarily in plant-based foods, meat, and iron-fortified foods, and is absorbed from the common nonheme pool within the gut. The absorption of nonheme iron is affected by the simultaneous ingestion of many other dietary components; some inhibit and others enhance nonheme iron absorption.

Inhibitors of nonheme iron absorption include phytate and polyphenols, as well as certain vegetable proteins (e.g., soybean protein). Calcium inhibits both nonheme and heme iron absorption, although the precise mechanism is unclear. In contrast, vitamin C, other organic acids, and animal tissues (meat, fish, and poultry) enhance nonheme iron absorption (Hallberg and Hulthen, 2000). Details are given in Section 4. 8 and IOM (2001).

The amount of iron in the stores varies widely, depending on sex and iron status. The iron bound to ferritin is more readily mobilized than iron bound to hemosiderin. In cases of chronic iron deficiency, iron stores in the bone marrow, spleen, and liver are depleted first, after which tissue iron deficiency occurs. In contrast, when iron balance is positive, iron stores gradually increase. In general, depletion of iron stores alone does not have any adverse functional consequences, although there are some exceptions (Beard et al., 1996).

Total daily iron losses are small and occur mainly in the feces (0.6 mg/d), although very small amounts are also lost in desquamated skin cells and sweat (0.2 to 0.3 mg/d), and in urine ($<$ 1 mg/d). In premenopausal women, total iron losses are larger (about 1.3 mg/d) because of the additional loss of iron in menstrual blood. On average, menstrual blood loss is 30 to 40 mL per cycle or 0.4 to 0.5 mg iron per day, although in some women it is much greater (Yip and Dallman, 1996).

Most of the iron in erythrocytes is recycled for hemoglobin synthesis at the end of their functional lifetime (i.e., on average 120 d). At this time, the erythrocytes are degraded by the macrophages of the reticular endothelium, and the iron is rereleased in the form of iron bound to transferrin or ferritin. This process is termed iron turnover; each day 0.66% of the total iron content of the body is recycled in this way. For more details on the functions, absorption, and metabolism of iron see Fairbanks (1994), Hallberg (2001), and Miret et al. (2003).

Deficiency of iron in humans

Iron deficiency is particularly prevalent in infants, young children, and pregnant women. It may arise from inadequate intakes of dietary iron, poor absorption, excessive losses, or a combination of these factors. In normal circumstances, only a small amount of iron is lost each day, with the exception of menstrual losses in premenopausal women.

Overt physical manifestations of iron deficiency include anemia, angular stomatitis, glossitis, dysphagia, hypochlorhydria, and koilonychia (spoon nails). Behavioral disturbances such as pica, characterized by the abnormal consumption of nonfood items such as dirt (geophagia) and ice (pagophagia), can also occur. Other less-specific physiological manifestations that are associated with iron deficiency include fatigue, anorexia, tiredness, impaired exercise or work performance, developmental delay, and cognitive impairment. These functional consequences of iron deficiency are most likely to occur when the iron deficiency is accompanied by a measurable decrease in hemoglobin concentration (IOM, 2001). Whether adverse pregnancy outcomes such as preterm delivery and higher maternal mortality are associated with iron deficiency is still uncertain (Allen, 1997).

Food sources and dietary intakes

High iron foods include liver, kidney, mussels, and red meat. Foods with a medium iron content include chicken, processed meat, fish, and legumes (non-heme iron only). Milk and milk products are poor sources of dietary iron (USDA, 2003). Flesh foods are especially important because of their high content of bioavailable heme iron, and their enhancing effect on nonheme iron absorption (Hallberg and Rossander, 1984).

In many industrialized countries, cereal products fortified or enriched with iron, provide the highest proportion of dietary iron, followed by meat, poultry, and fish, and then vegetables and fruits (Gregory et al., 1990; McLennan and Podger, 1998; Russell et al., 1999). The bioavailability of iron in these mixed diets probably ranges from 15% to 18%, provided they contain ample quantities of flesh foods and ascorbic acid. In low-income countries, the proportion of heme iron in the diet is generally much lower, so that absorption of dietary iron is probably only about 5%–10% (FAO/WHO, 1988).

Effects of high intakes of iron

Cases of acute iron toxicity have been reported, mainly among children who accidentally ingest medicinal iron supplements (IOM, 2001). More common are adverse gastrointestinal effects following the administration of high doses of iron supplements, especially when they are taken without food (Brock et al., 1985). A reduction in zinc absorption has also been associated with high intakes of iron supplements given in the fasting state (Sandström et al., 1985), but not when the iron is given as a fortificant in food (Davidsson et al., 1995).

Some people are at risk from iron overload as a consequence of hereditary hemochromatosis, injections of therapeutic iron, multiple blood transfusions, or at least in part from excessive intakes of dietary iron (e.g., some Bantu in South Africa) (Andrews, 1999).

The U.S. Food and Nutrition Board has set the Tolerable Upper Intake Level (UL) for iron for adults, including pregnant and lactating women $\geqslant 19$ y, at 45 mg/d, whereas the level for infants and children 1–18 y is 40 mg/d (IOM, 2001).

Development of iron-deficiency anemia

Three stages in the development of iron-deficiency anemia can be recognized and are best characterized by the use of multiple indices (Section 17.9). The three stages are the following:

Iron depletion, the first stage, is characterized by a progressive reduction in the amount of storage iron in the liver. At this stage, the supply of iron to the functional compartment is not compromised so levels of transport iron and hemoglobin are normal. However, the progressive depletion of iron stores will be reflected by a fall in serum ferritin concentrations.

Iron-deficient erythropoiesis, the second stage, is characterized by the exhaustion of iron stores and is also referred to as "iron deficiency without anemia." At this stage the iron supply to the erythropoietic cells is progressively reduced and decreases in transferrin saturation occur (Section 17.5). At the same time, there are increases in serum transferrin receptor (Section 17.8) and erythrocyte protoporphyrin concentrations (Section 17.7). Hemoglobin levels may decline slightly at this stage, although they usually remain within the normal range.

Iron-deficiency anemia, the third and final stage of iron deficiency, is characterized by the exhaustion of iron stores, declining levels of circulating iron, and presence of frank microcytic, hypochromic anemia. The main feature of this stage is a reduction in the concentration of hemoglobin in the red blood cells, arising from the restriction of iron supply to the bone marrow. Decreases in the hematocrit and red cell indices also occur (Sections 17.2 and 17.3). Examination of a stained blood film allows confirmation of the presence of hypochromia and microcytosis.

The different measures of iron status are each discussed in the remainder of this chapter, starting with those used in the diagnosis of anemia — hemoglobin and hematocrit.

17.1 Hemoglobin

Iron is an essential component of the hemoglobin molecule, the oxygen-carrying pigment of red blood cells. Each hemoglobin molecule is a conjugate of a protein (globin) and four molecules of heme. Measurement of the concentration of hemoglobin in whole blood is probably the most widely used test for iron-deficiency anemia. It is important to note that some misclassification will always arise because the range of hemoglobin values for normal nonanemic persons overlap with values for persons with iron-deficiency. This means that hemoglobin should not be used as the only measure of iron status in individuals. Indeed it can only be used as the sole indicator of iron-deficiency anemia in populations under very specific circumstances (Section 17.1.3). The use of hemoglobin as a measure of iron status has other, more specific, limitations, as discussed below.

17.1.1 Factors affecting hemoglobin concentrations

Biological variation in hemoglobin concentrations are significant. Hemoglobin values tend to be lower in the evening than in the morning, by amounts of up to 10 g/L. Day-to-day variation is low (Table 17.10).

Age and sex are important determinants, particularly for younger subjects: median hemoglobin values rise during the first 10 years of childhood, with a further increase at puberty (Table 17.1). Sex differences in hemoglobin

are apparent at 6 mo of age, with boys having significantly lower hemoglobin concentrations than girls. Such discrepancies appear to be greater in infants with a birth weight < 3500 g (Domellöf et al., 2002a). By the second decade of life, however, females have lower values that change very little after 12 y of age. Hemoglobin levels of males during adolescence are strongly influenced by testosterone and thus by the age of sexual maturation. In young adults, the hemoglobin concentration for men is on average about 20 g/L higher than for women. These sex-related differences diminish gradually with increasing age.

Race is known to influence hemoglobin concentrations. Individuals of African descent have hemoglobin values 5–10 g/L lower than Caucasians, irrespective of age, income, or iron deficiency. It is likely that a genetic factor is involved. As a result, race-specific cutoffs for diagnosing anemia in persons of African descent may be necessary (Johnson-Spear and Yip, 1994). WHO/UNICEF/UNU (2001) recommends moving the hemoglobin cutoffs downward by 10 g/L for individuals of African descent, irrespective of age. In contrast, the Caucasian cutoffs for anemia seem to be appropriate for persons in Thailand (Charoenlarp and Polpothi, 1987) and Indo-

Age (y)	Females	Males
1–2	122.0 (7.34)	
3–5	124.4 (7.57)	
6–11	130.9 (7.92)	
12–15	134.3 (9.27)	142.4 (10.0)
16–19	133.7 (8.21)	152.9 (10.03)
20–49	134.8 (9.12)	153.0 (9.68)
50–69	136.5 (9.82)	150.1 (10.64)
⩾70	135.6 (10.68)	145.3 (12.87)

Table 17.1: Mean (SD) hemoglobin concentrations (g/L) by age and sex. Data from National Health and Nutrition Examination Survey III (1988–1994). Individuals of all races with abnormal or missing values for transferrin saturation, erythrocyte protoporphyrin, serum ferritin, or mean cell volume were excluded. From Looker et al., Journal of the American Medical Association 277: 973–976, 1997.

nesia (Khusun et al., 1999), after excluding subjects with abnormal hemoglobin types.

Pregnancy results in an expansion of both plasma volume and the red cell mass. The greater expansion is of plasma volume so hemoglobin becomes diluted. As a result, there is a fall in hemoglobin concentration. This is most evident near the end of the second trimester of pregnancy, after which, during the third trimester, hemoglobin concentrations gradually rise (Section 17.1.2).

Higher altitudes generate an adaptive response in the body to both the lower partial pressure of oxygen and the reduced oxygen saturation of blood (Hurtado et al., 1945). This becomes significant at elevations above 1000 m, with usual hematocrit and hemoglobin concentrations increasing gradually with altitude. Consequently, a series of adjustments for altitude for hemoglobin cutoffs have been published by the Centers for Disease Control and Prevention (CDC, 1989) (Section 17.1.2).

Iron-deficiency anemia develops only during the third stage of iron deficiency, when iron stores are exhausted and the supply of iron to the tissues is compromised. Hemoglobin is therefore an insensitive measure of iron deficiency as the concentrations only fall during this late stage. In addition, considerable overlap exists in the hemoglobin values of normal nonanemic and iron-deficient individuals (Figure 1.4), further decreasing the sensitivity of this measure.

Certain other micronutrient deficiencies are associated with anemia and, by definition, with low hemoglobin concentrations. These include deficiencies of vitamin A, B_6, and B_{12}, and riboflavin, folic acid, and copper (van den Broek and Letsky, 2000); details of the role of vitamins in the etiology of anemia are given in Fishman et al. (2000).

Parasitic infections such as with the malarial protozoan *Plasmodium falciparum* cause low hemoglobin concentrations by rupturing

Age (y)	Hemoglobin cutoff value (g/L) Males and females	Males	Females
NHANES III (from Looker et al., 1997)			
1–2	< 110	—	—
3–5	< 112	—	—
6–11	< 118	—	—
12–15	—	< 126	< 119
16–19	—	< 136	< 120
20–49	—	< 137	< 120
50–69	—	< 133	< 120
≥ 70	—	< 124	< 118
INACG/WHO/UNICEF			
0.5–5	< 110	—	—
5–11	< 115	—	—
12–13	< 120	—	—
Men	—	< 130	—
Pregnant women	—	—	< 110
Nonpregnant women	—	—	< 120

Table 17.2: Two different sets of hemoglobin cutoffs used to define anemia. The INACG/WHO/UNICEF cutoffs are for individuals living at sea level and are from Stoltzfus and Dreyfuss (1998).

erythrocytes and suppressing the production of new erythrocytes. Helminths (such as hookworms) and flukes (e.g., schistosomes) may also cause low hemoglobin values as a result of loss of blood and thus iron (Stoltzfus et al., 2000; Nestel and Davidsson, 2002).

Certain disease states can affect hemoglobin concentrations, significantly reducing the specificity of the measure. Low hemoglobin values arise in chronic infections and inflammation, chronic disease states including HIV-AIDS, hemorrhage, protein-energy malnutrition, hemoglobinopathies, and other states in which there is overhydration or acute plasma volume expansion. In contrast, hemoglobin values are elevated in polycythemia and hemoconcentration caused by dehydration.

Cigarette smoking is associated with higher concentrations of hemoglobin (3–7 g/L) in adults. This is attributed to a reduction in the oxygen-carrying capacity of the blood arising from the carbon monoxide induced increase in carboxyhemoglobin levels.

17.1.2 Interpretive criteria

In the United States hemoglobin values are often compared with data from the distribution of hemoglobin from a healthy, nonpregnant reference sample studied during the National Health and Nutrition Examination Survey (NHANES) III, 1988–1991. The reference sample consisted of individuals of all races, but excluded pregnant women and those with a higher risk of iron deficiency based on an abnormal value or missing value for 3 of the 4 tests (free erythrocyte protoporphyrin, transferrin saturation, serum ferritin, and mean cell volume (MCV) (Looker et al. (1997). The hemoglobin "cutoff values" were calculated as the mean of the reference sample minus 1.645 SD, giving values corresponding to the 5th percentile, shown in Table 17.2.

Although often termed hemoglobin "cutoff values," the values from Looker et al. (1997) in Table 17.2 are more appropriately called "reference limits" for hemoglobin: they are not based directly on observed clinical or functional impairment (Section 15.4). Implicit in the use of a 5th percentile reference limit derived from the distribution of hemoglobin values for a healthy reference sample is the concept that most individuals with hemoglobin concentrations below the limit/cutoff will be at risk of having suboptimal hemoglobin concentrations (i.e., the hemoglobin would increase in response to iron supplementation). However some misclassification will always occur (Figure 1.4).

Cutoff values for hemoglobin for identifying anemia during infancy were not defined by Looker et al. (1997). The commonly used cutoff at 6–12 mo of age is < 110 g/L, a level used by INACG/WHO/UNICEF (Table 17.2) and by CDC (1998). This value was extrapolated from older age groups and may not be appropriate for infants (Emond et al., 1996). Domellöf et al. (2002b) have defined cutoffs for hemoglobin for infants, based on iron-replete, breastfed infants. These are < 105 g/L for infants at 4 and 6 mo of age and < 100 g/L at 9 mo of age.

The criteria used by the CDC (1989) to

Stage of pregnancy (trimester)	Hemoglobin (g/L)
First	−10
Second	−15
Third	−10
Trimester unknown	−10

Table 17.3: Hemoglobin adjustment for pregnancy in women living at sea level. From Nestel (2002).

identify anemia in pregnant women during trimesters 1, 2, and 3, respectively, are 110, 105, and 110 g/L. The International Nutritional Anemia Consultative Group (INACG) recommend trimester-specific adjustments and a generic value for use when the trimester is unknown; these are shown in Table 17.3 (Nestel, 2002). In contrast, the earlier recommendations by INACG/WHO/UNICEF use one cutoff of 110 g/L throughout pregnancy (Stoltzfus and Dreyfuss, 1998).

Adjustments for altitude and smoking have also been compiled by the CDC (1989), as noted earlier. These adjustments have been adopted by INACG (Nestel, 2002), and are shown in Table 17.4 and Table 17.5. They can either be added to the cutoff values shown in Table 17.2 or subtracted from the measured hemoglobin values. When applying the altitude adjustments, the altitude at which the blood sample is taken should be rounded up or down to the nearest 500 m. The CDC adjustments for altitude can also be used for pregnant women (Nestel, 2002). Note that

Altitude (m)	Hemoglobin (g/L)
< 1000	0
1000	+1
1500	+4
2000	+7
2500	+12
3000	+18
3500	+26
4000	+34
4500	+44
5000	+55
5500	+67

Table 17.4: Hemoglobin adjustment for altitude; adjustments for altitudes above 3000 m are extrapolated. From Nestel (2002).

Amount smoked	Hemoglobin (g/L)
0.5–1 pack/d	+3
1–2 packs/d	+5
> 2 packs/d	+7
All smokers	+3

Table 17.5: Hemoglobin adjustment for smokers. From Nestel (2002).

the adjustments for smoking, altitude, race, and pregnancy are additive.

Tables of mean and selected percentiles for hemoglobin by age and sex for *all* persons except breastfeeding infants and children in the NHANES III population are included in Appendix A17.1 (IOM, 2001). Potentially iron-deficient subjects were not excluded when generating this compilation.

The U.K. national surveys present data for hemoglobin (Gregory et al., 1990, 1995, 2000; Finch et al., 1998). Mean, median, and lower and upper 2.5 percentiles by age and sex are presented. Again, potentially iron-deficient subjects are not specifically excluded. The New Zealand national surveys for persons 15 y and over (Russell et al., 1999) and children 5–14 y (Parnell et al., 2003) also present mean hemoglobin concentration by age, sex, and race or ethnicity.

17.1.3 Using hemoglobin distribution to assess population iron status

Hemoglobin distribution can be used in large-scale field studies to assess the iron status of a population (Yip et al., 1996). This simplified approach is designed to assess the prevalence and etiology of anemia, based solely on hemoglobin, and is especially useful when it is not feasible to use multiple biochemical tests for iron status because of cost or operational constraints. It is also useful in developing countries where factors other than inadequate intakes of dietary iron, such as parasitic infections and hemoglobinopathies, often affect red cell production and thus interfere with the interpretation of iron status measures.

The hemoglobin distribution approach in-

volves comparing the hemoglobin distribution curves for men, women, and children of the study population, with optimal hemoglobin distributions derived from a healthy reference sample. These have been compiled from NHANES II (Pilch and Senti, 1984) and NHANES III (Looker et al., 1997) populations by excluding subjects with biochemical evidence of iron deficiency, as noted earlier. Figure 17.1 depicts the hemoglobin distributions for the NHANES II reference samples. These distributions can be used as a standard for comparison with the hemoglobin distributions from other surveys.

If anemia is prevalent in the population then the distribution will be shifted to the left. The distribution approach can also indicate when inadequate dietary intake of iron is the main factor causing iron deficiency in a population. In this case the hemoglobin distributions for children and women are disproportionately affected. Both subgroups have significantly lower median hemoglobin values when compared with their respective reference distributions, whereas the median of the distribution for adult men is virtually unaffected. For example, comparison of the hemoglobin distributions for both school-

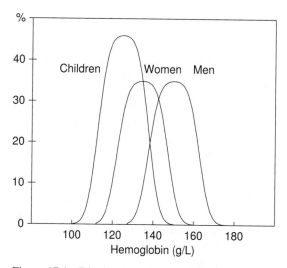

Figure 17.1: Distribution of hemoglobin in children aged 1–5 y and in women and men aged 18–44 y. Data from NHANES II after exclusion of subjects with abnormal values for indicators of iron status. From Yip et al. (1996).

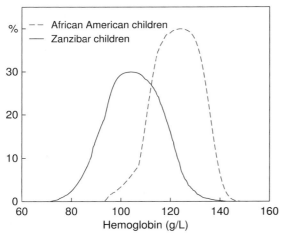

Figure 17.2: Distribution of hemoglobin in a reference population of African American children with no biochemical signs of iron deficiency and school-age children from Zanzibar. From Yip et al. (1996).

aged children (Figure 17.2) and men from Zanzibar with the corresponding U.S. reference sample for African Americans shows a marked shift of hemoglobin concentrations. In Zanzibar, the decreased hemoglobin levels were related to gastrointestinal blood loss as a result of hookworm infection rather than inadequate dietary iron intake.

17.1.4 Measurement of hemoglobin

Hemoglobin is best determined using venous blood, anticoagulated with EDTA. Alternatively, capillary blood from heel-, ear-, or fingerpricks, collected in heparinized capillary tubes, can be used. Hemoglobin concentrations determined using capillary blood are less precise than are the corresponding measurements on venous blood, primarily because interstitial fluid may dilute capillary samples (Burger and Pierre-Louis, 2003).

The cyanmethemoglobin method, which is recommended by the International Committee for Standardization in Hematology (ICSH, 1987), is the most reliable, provided that the blood specimen has been accurately diluted. Incorrect dilution of the sample is one of the main sources of error in this method (Pilch and Senti, 1984). The method involves converting all of the usually encountered forms of hemoglobin (oxyhemoglobin, methemoglobin, and carboxyhemoglobin) to cyanmethemoglobin. The analysis is then normally performed with a spectrophotometer. The coefficients of both analytical and biological variation for hemoglobin by the cyanmethemoglobin method using venous blood are often less than 4% (Worwood, 1996). A WHO international standard is available to assess the accuracy of the assay (ICSH, 1987). Hemoglobin can also be determined in this way from blood spots collected in the field on filter paper discs; levels remain unchanged during storage for 1 mo (Feraudi and Mejia, 1987).

Alternatively, hemoglobin can be measured electronically on an automated counter (e.g., Coulter counter system) using EDTA-anticoagulated blood.

A portable hemoglobin photometer can be used for population assessment in remote field settings. The "HemoCue" is battery operated and uses a dry reagent (sodium azide) in a microcuvette for direct blood collection and measurement. The accuracy and precision of hemoglobin values based on the HemoCue are comparable to those obtained using the cyanmethemoglobin method, provided standardized procedures for the sample collection and analysis are followed (Von Schenck et al., 1986). Details of standardization procedures to enhance the accuracy and reliability of hemoglobin concentrations measured by the HemoCue are given in Burger and Pierre-Louis (2003).

17.2 Hematocrit

The hematocrit is defined as the volume fraction of packed red cells, sometimes termed the "packed cell volume" (PCV). In iron deficiency, the hematocrit falls after hemoglobin formation has become impaired. As a result, in early cases of moderate iron deficiency, a marginally low hemoglobin value may be associated with a nearly normal hematocrit (Graitcer et al., 1981). Only in more severe iron-deficiency anemia are both hemoglobin and hematocrit reduced. Limitations

Box 17.1:

> **Poor sensitivity,** with hematocrit falling only in the third stage of iron deficiency
>
> **Poor specificity,** as hematocrit is affected by the same factors that influence hemoglobin
>
> **Poor precision,** particularly when capillary blood samples are used
>
> **Values that are age and sex dependent** (Figure 17.3), with similar trends to those described for hemoglobin (Table 17.1)

Box 17.1: Limitations of the hematocrit determination.

Age (y) or group	Hematocrit cutoff
0.5–5	< 0.33
5–11	< 0.34
12–13	< 0.36
Men	< 0.39
Nonpregnant women	< 0.36
Pregnant women	< 0.33

Table 17.6: Hematocrit cutoffs used to define anemia. From Stoltzfus and Dreyfuss (1998).

of the hematocrit determination are shown in Box 17.1.

Hematocrit, like hemoglobin, is usually determined on EDTA-anticoagulated blood from a venipuncture or capillary blood. The measurement is relatively easy, rapid, and often used in screening for iron-deficiency anemia, although the technical errors for the measurement of hematocrit are greater than for hemoglobin. Measurement errors may result from:

- Poorly packed iron-deficient cells, resulting in spuriously elevated values
- Improper mixing of blood caused by intermittent blood flow from the puncture site
- Excessive anticoagulant in the collection tube (e.g., if collection tube is not filled with blood)
- Dilution of blood by an alcohol solution because the finger was not dried before it was punctured
- Elevated white blood cell counts, leading to a poorly defined boundary between erythrocytes and plasma in the hematocrit tube

17.2.1 Interpretive criteria

The cutoff values for hematocrit, compiled by INACG / WHO / UNICEF, are presented in Table 17.6 (Stoltzfus and Dreyfuss, 1998).

The U.K. national surveys (Gregory et al., 1990, 1995, 2000; Finch et al., 1998) present the mean, median, and lower and upper 2.5 or 5th percentiles for hematocrit. Again, potentially iron-deficient subjects are not specifically excluded.

17.2.2 Measurement of hematocrit

Hematocrit can be measured manually by centrifuging a minute amount of blood in a heparinized capillary tube until the red cells have been reduced to a constant packed cell volume. The hematocrit is calculated by comparing the height of the column of packed red cells with the height of the entire column of red cells and plasma.

Alternatively, hematocrit can be measured electronically using an automated counter. It is noteworthy that when hematocrit is determined manually as described above, values are about 1% lower than those generated electronically from automated counters (Fairbanks, 1980; Looker et al., 1995).

17.3 Red cell indices

Red cell indices are derived from measurements of hemoglobin, hematocrit, and red blood cell count. They are used to define cell size and the concentration of hemoglobin within the cell so that different types of anemia can be diagnosed. Their accuracy,

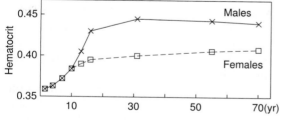

Figure 17.3: Median values for hematocrit by age and sex. From Yip et al., American Journal of Clinical Nutrition 39: 427–436, 1984 © Am J Clin Nutr. American Society for Clinical Nutrition.

Red cell index	Iron-deficiency anemia (microcytic hypochromic)	Macrocytic anemia (macrocytic)	Anemia of chronic inflammation (normocytic normochromic)
MCV	Low	High	Normal
MCH	Low	High	Normal
MCHC	Low	Normal	Normal

Table 17.7: Expected changes in red cell indices during iron-deficiency anemia, macrocytic anemia, and anemia of chronic inflammation. MCV, mean cell volume; MCH, mean cell hemoglobin; MCHC, mean cell hemoglobin concentration. From Wintrobe et al. (1981).

precision, and use have increased with the growing availability of automated electronic cell-counting instruments. Fresh samples of whole anticoagulated blood are required. Values for red cell indices from automated counters are slightly higher than those determined manually (Fairbanks, 1980).

If subnormal values for the red cell indices are noted in the absence of thalassemia trait, anemia of inflammatory disease, and other known causal conditions, additional measures of iron status are recommended to confirm the diagnosis of iron deficiency. The confirmatory tests commonly used are serum iron and total iron-binding capacity, serum ferritin, erythrocyte protoporphyrin, and more recently, serum transferrin receptor. These tests are discussed in Sections 17.5 to 17.8.

Table 17.7 summarizes the expected changes in the more important red cell indices during iron-deficiency anemia, macrocytic anemia resulting from vitamin B_{12} or folic acid deficiency, and anemia of chronic inflammation (also known as anemia of chronic disease). The anemia of chronic inflammation (e.g., due to rheumatic fever, Crohn's disease, or ulcerative colitis) results from a defect in iron recycling. There appears to be a defect in the release of iron from macrophages, or the transfer of iron from the reticulo-endothelial cells to plasma transferrin, or both. The anemia is generally mild, and can be normochromic and normocytic or slightly hypochromic and microcytic (Andrews, 1999). Changes in red cell indices during vitamin B_{12} and folic acid deficiency

are described in more detail in Section 22.1.1. In iron-deficiency anemia, the fall in hemoglobin is followed by a fall in mean cell volume, then mean cell hemoglobin, and finally mean cell hemoglobin concentration.

17.3.1 Mean cell volume

Mean cell volume or mean corpuscular volume (MCV) is a measure of the average size of the red blood cells expressed in femtoliters (fL). Cells may be abnormally large (macrocytosis), as in vitamin B_{12} or folic acid deficiency, or abnormally small (microcytosis), as in iron and vitamin B_6 deficiency. Mean cell volume is best determined directly with an electronic counter as results obtained in this way are highly reproducible. If an electronic counter is not available, mean cell volume can be calculated from the hematocrit and the red blood cell count determined manually (Wintrobe et al., 1981):

$$\text{MCV (fL)} = \frac{\text{hematocrit (volume fraction)}}{\text{red blood cell count } (10^{12}/\text{L})}$$

Mean cell volume is less affected by sampling errors in skin puncture capillary blood samples than hemoglobin, because red cell size is unaffected if the sample is diluted by the interstitial fluid.

A low MCV value only occurs when iron deficiency is severe. It is a relatively specific index for iron-deficiency anemia, provided that the anemias of chronic inflammation, certain hemoglobinopathies, and lead poisoning are excluded. In macrocytic anemias associated with vitamin B_{12} or folate deficiency, MCV values are high (Table 17.7). Spuriously high values for MCV may be apparent when determined electronically as a consequence of hyperglycemia or hypernatremia.

The MCV increases progressively from 6 mo of age to early adulthood (Yip et al., 1984). Differences according to sex are small; MCV is slightly higher in young adult females than in males. Individuals of African descent have lower MCV values than do Caucasians. Such differences are said to have a genetic basis, as described for hemoglobin (Section 17.1).

Cutoff values for MCV used during the NHANES III survey were slightly higher than those used for NHANES II, and correspond to the 5th percentiles of the NHANES III reference sample. The cutoffs are given in Table 17.8 and include values for children in four age groups. Values greater than 98 fL indicate macrocytosis.

Percentile distributions for MCV levels by race, sex, and age, for all persons 1–74 y in the NHANES II population, are available, and for the NHANES II "reference population" for all races as described for hemoglobin in Section 17.1.2 (Pilch and Senti, 1984). At present, comparable data are not available for NHANES III.

Age- and sex-specific data for MCV are available for the U.K. national surveys (Gregory et al., 1990, 1995, 2000; Finch et al., 1998). Mean, median, and lower and upper 2.5 or 5th percentiles are presented. In these data, potentially iron-deficient subjects are not specifically excluded.

Age (y)	Mean cell volume (fL)
1–3	< 77
3–5	< 79
6–11	< 80
11–14	< 82
15–74	< 85

Table 17.8: Cutoff points used to identify abnormal values of MCV in data from NHANES III phase I, 1988–1991. From Dallman et al. (1996).

17.3.2 Mean cell hemoglobin

Mean cell hemoglobin (MCH) is the mean hemoglobin content of individual red blood cells. It is derived from the ratio of hemoglobin to the red blood cell count:

$$\text{MCH (pg)} = \frac{\text{hemoglobin (g/L)}}{\text{red blood cell count } (10^{12}/L)}$$

The MCH changes progressively from infancy to adulthood, when values range from 27 to 32 pg. The changes in iron-deficiency anemia are similar to those for MCV; MCH is low in iron-deficiency anemia but high in the macrocytic anemias of both vitamin B_{12} and folate deficiency (Table 17.7). In the latter, the red blood cells are laden with hemoglobin but are reduced in number. In severe iron deficiency, the relative fall in MCH is greater than the corresponding fall in MCV (Dallman, 1977).

Age- and sex-specific data for MCH are available for the U.K. national surveys (Gregory et al., 1990, 1995, 2000; Finch et al., 1998). Mean, median, and lower and upper 2.5 or 5th percentiles are given. Potentially iron-deficient subjects are not excluded.

17.3.3 Mean cell hemoglobin concentration

If both the hemoglobin concentration and the hematocrit are known, the concentration of hemoglobin in the red blood cells can be determined. This is known as the mean cell hemoglobin concentration (MCHC) and is calculated as:

$$\text{MCHC (g/L)} = \frac{\text{hemoglobin (g/L)}}{\text{hematocrit (vol. fraction}}$$

The MCHC is normally determined with an electronic counter, although manual determinations are possible. After the first few months of life, MCHC is less affected by age than any other red cell index (Matoth et al., 1971). Nevertheless, this index is the least useful of the red cell indices because it is last to fall during iron deficiency.

Mean cell hemoglobin concentrations are low in iron-deficiency anemia but normal in the macrocytic anemia of vitamin B_{12} and folic acid deficiency, and in the anemia of chronic disease (Table 17.7). Values in normal adults range from 320 to 360 g/L. Values of < 300 g/L indicate hypochromia and are associated with advanced iron deficiency.

Age- and sex-specific data for MCHC are available for the U.K. national surveys (Gregory et al., 1990, 1995, 2000; Finch et al., 1998). The mean, median, and lower and upper 2.5 or 5th percentiles are presented. Potentially iron-deficient subjects are not specifically excluded.

17.4　Red cell distribution width

Red cell distribution width (RDW) is a measure of the variation in red cell size (i.e., anisocytosis). It is normally expressed as the coefficient of variation of the mean cell volume:

RDW (%) = (SD of MCV (fL) $\times$ 100%) / MCV (fL)

The RDW can be determined routinely as part of a complete blood count on many automated electronic counters. Some counters output only the standard deviation as the measure of RDW.

Red cell distribution width increases in iron-deficiency anemia and was included as a marker of iron status in the NHANES III survey (Looker et al., 1995). A single cutoff for RDW of 14% was used in NHANES III. Using this, 65% of women of African descent aged 20–49 y with an elevated RDW were also iron deficient based on the ferritin model (Section 17.6); 36% were anemic. In contrast, only 6% with a normal RDW showed similar signs of iron deficiency, and only 5% were anemic. For children 1–2 y, the sensitivity of this cutoff was significantly worse, suggesting that different cutoffs are needed for children and adults.

Bessman et al. (1983) classified anemic disorders based on a combination of a low, normal, and high MCV and two categories of RDW — normal ($< 15.1\%$) and high (indicating anisocytosis). The anemias identified in this way are listed in Table 17.9.

Clearly, a high RDW is not specific for iron deficiency. High values also occur in folate or vitamin B_{12} deficiency and when iron and folate, or iron and vitamin B_{12} deficiencies coexist. Also, in some hemoglobinopathies (e.g. in S β-thalassemia and SS and SC hemoglobinopathy) RDW is elevated (Table 17.9). However, iron-deficiency anemia results in a greater increase in RDW than does the microcytic anemia of the hemoglobinopathy S β-thalassemia (Bessman and Feinstein, 1979). Hence, RDW may be useful for differentiating between these two conditions. In contrast, in the anemia of inflammatory disease, RDW is normal.

Some of the U.K. national surveys (Gregory et al., 1990, 2000) include data on red cell distribution width. Mean, median, and lower and upper 2.5 percentiles by age and sex are presented. The New Zealand National Children's Nutrition Survey also provide data on red cell distribution width by age, sex, race or ethnicity, and the prevalence of elevated values (defined as $> 14\%$) (Parnell et al., 2003).

17.5　Serum iron, TIBC, and transferrin saturation

Three interrelated variables, serum iron, total iron-binding capacity (TIBC), and transferrin saturation are very useful for differentiating between nutritional iron deficiency and anemia arising from chronic infections, inflammation, or chronic neoplastic diseases. Nutritional iron deficiency is characterized by a low serum iron, elevated TIBC and, thus, low transferrin saturation, whereas in chronic infections, inflammation, or chronic neoplastic diseases, both serum iron and TIBC are low, so transferrin saturation tends towards the low end of the normal range.

Almost all iron in the serum is bound to the iron transport protein transferrin. In the fasting state, serum iron levels reflect iron in transit from the reticulo-endothelial system to the bone marrow. Each molecule of transferrin (MW $\approx$ 80kDa) can be bound to one or two atoms of iron, although usually

	Normal RDW	High RDW
Low MCV	Chronic disease Heterogeneous thalassemia	Iron deficiency Red cell fragmentation Hemoglobin H and S β-thalassemia

Normal MCV	Normal healthy subjects
	Chronic disease
	  (including chronic liver disease)
	Hemorrhage
	Chemotherapy
	Chronic myelocytic leukemia
	Transfusion
	Nonanemic hemoglobinopathy
	  (e.g., AS, AC)
	Chronic lymphocytic leukemia
	Hereditary spherocytosis
		Early iron or folate deficiency
		Anemic hemoglobinopathy (e.g., SS, SC)
		Myelofibrosis
		Sideroblastic anemia

High MCV	Aplastic anemia Preleukemia	Folate or vitamin B_{12} deficiency Immune hemolytic anemia Cold agglutinins Chronic lymphocytic leukemia (high count)

Table 17.9: Classification of anemias based on a normal reference range for MCV of 79–101 fL and two categories for RDW: normal ($< 15.1\%$) and high. From Bessman et al., 1983 © American Society of Clinical Pathologists, with permission.

only about one third of the binding sites are occupied.

The TIBC is the sum of all unfilled iron-binding sites on transferrin, and is measured as the total quantity of iron (μmol/L) that saturates all of the iron-binding sites on transferrin after the addition of exogenous iron to serum. Hence, TIBC is closely related to the concentration of transferrin. The TIBC of serum rises once the iron stores are depleted because of an increase in transferrin synthesis in response to increased iron absorption. This increase in TIBC occurs before there is any evidence of an inadequate supply of iron to erythropoetic tissue.

Serum iron and TIBC are usually determined at the same time, and the transferrin saturation is then calculated, as shown below. Transferrin saturation measures the iron supply to the erythroid bone marrow: as the iron supply decreases, the serum iron concentration falls and the saturation of transferrin decreases.

$$\text{transferrin sat. } (\%) = \frac{\text{serum iron } (\mu\text{mol/L})}{\text{TIBC } (\mu\text{mol/L})} \times 100\%$$

Levels $< 16\%$ saturation indicate that the rate of delivery of iron is insufficient to maintain normal hemoglobin synthesis. However, low transferrin saturation levels are not specific for iron deficiency, as discussed below.

17.5.1 Factors influencing serum iron, TIBC, and transferrin saturation

Biological variation for serum iron may be quite large: coefficients of variation may exceed 30% — mainly as a result of variation in the release of iron from the reticulo-endothelial system to the plasma among individuals (Worwood, 1996, 1997). In general, serum iron values tend to be elevated in the morning, decreasing in the afternoon and evening. As a result, measurements of serum iron should be determined on fasting morning blood samples. In this way, the effects of both recent dietary intake and diurnal variation are minimized.

TIBC is less subject to biological variation — especially diurnal effects — than is serum iron, but it is more susceptible to analytical errors. Table 17.10 compares the overall variability of serum iron, hemoglobin, and serum ferritin as indicated by within-subject,

Reference	Hemoglobin	Serum ferritin	Serum iron
Dawkins et al. (1979)	—	15 (M, F)	—
Gallagher et al. (1989)	1.6 (F)	15 (F)	—
Statland and Winkel (1977)	—	—	29 (F)
Statland et al. (1976)	—	—	27 (F)
Statland et al. (1978)	3 (M, F)	—	—
Pilon et al. (1981)	—	15 (M, F)	29 (M, F)
Romslo and Talstad (1988)	—	13 (M, F)	33 (M, F)
Borel et al. (1991a)	4 (M, F)	14 (M)	27 (M)
Borel et al. (1991)	4 (F)	26 (F)	28 (F)

Table 17.10: Within-subject, day-to-day coefficient of variation (CV%) for hemoglobin, serum ferritin, and serum iron for healthy subjects. M, male; F, female.

day-to-day variation for healthy subjects. The results for serum iron have obvious implications for its use at the population and individual levels. They highlight the importance of using multiple indices of iron status to provide a more valid assessment of iron status than any single measurement (Section 17.9).

In NHANES III, the large diurnal variation for serum iron is reflected in the results for transferrin saturation shown in Figure 17.4.

Age-related changes in serum iron and, to a lesser extent, TIBC are marked. Serum iron levels rise during childhood, whereas TIBC falls (Figure 17.5). Values for both measures are highest in young adults, and decline steadily with advancing age (Yip et al., 1984).

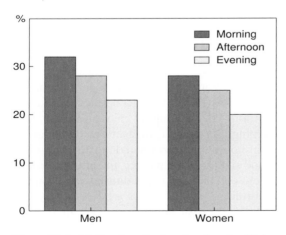

Figure 17.4: Median transferrin saturation (as %) by time of blood collection, Caucasian reference sample 20–49 y, NHANES III phase 1. From Looker et al., Nutrition Reviews 53: 246–254, 1995, with permission of the International Life Sciences Institute.

Sex has only a small effect on serum iron and TIBC levels. In NHANES II, there was a tendency for serum iron levels to be higher in males than females after the middle of the second decade of life (Figure 17.5) (Pilch and Senti, 1984). In NHANES III, the median transferrin saturation was 26% to 30% for men and 21% to 24% for women (Appendix A17.2).

Oral contraceptive agents result in elevated levels of TIBC similar to those observed in iron deficiency (Pilch and Senti, 1984).

Iron deficiency leads to a fall in serum iron levels and a rise in serum transferrin and, thus, a rise in TIBC. Consequently, transferrin saturation is low. These changes appear during the second stage of iron deficiency, after iron stores are depleted. Hence, transferrin saturation is a more sensitive index of iron status than the red cell indices discussed in Section 17.3. It is also more consistently useful for diagnosing iron deficiency than either serum iron or total TIBC alone: a low transferrin saturation in association with an elevated TIBC is specific for iron deficiency.

Iron overload results in an elevated body iron store and, thus, a high serum iron level, leading to a low TIBC and an elevated transferrin saturation level. In NHANES III, a transferrin saturation > 70% was used as a criterion for detecting iron overload in adults (Looker et al., 1997). Iron overload occurs in conditions such as hereditary hemochromatosis, hemolytic anemia, chronic liver disease,

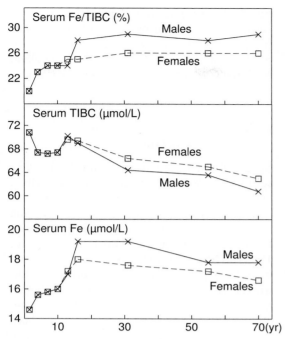

Figure 17.5: Median values for serum Fe/total iron-binding capacity (TIBC) (%), serum TIBC (μmol/L), and serum iron (μmol/L), by age and sex. From Yip et al., American Journal of Clinical Nutrition 39: 427–436, 1984 © Am J Clin Nutr. American Society for Clinical Nutrition.

and long-term transfusion therapy (Andrews, 1999). Hemochromatosis is one of the most common genetic diseases in populations of Northern European origin. In these countries, approximately 50 per 10,000 will be affected by the condition (Hansen et al., 2001).

Chronic disease states, infection, inflammatory conditions, and chronic neoplastic diseases typically produce both low serum iron and low TIBC and, hence, a transferrin saturation that tends toward the low end of the normal range. These trends are the result of defects in the release of iron from the reticulo-endothelial cells and the subsequent transport of iron from these stores by transferrin. Together, these defects result in a shortage of iron in the bone marrow, despite adequate or even slightly increased iron stores. As the iron stores are adequate, the body does not respond to the fall in serum iron by increasing absorption of iron from the diet. Consequently, transferrin synthesis is not increased, and levels of TIBC are low. Hence, the determination of TIBC allows one to distinguish between the low transferrin saturation associated with the anemia of chronic disease and that of true iron deficiency.

Decreased erythropoiesis is often associated with vitamin B_{12} or folic acid deficiency, as well as with the action of certain drugs and toxins. In these circumstances, serum iron levels are normal or slightly above normal because of decreased utilization of iron for hemoglobin synthesis; levels of TIBC are often normal or low. Consequently, transferrin saturation may be high.

Increased erythropoiesis can occur after recovery from bone marrow depression, in response to vitamin B_{12} and folate therapy, in hemolysis, and sometimes in polycythemia. In such cases, the serum iron concentration may fall below normal limits, whereas the TIBC is often high-normal or even high, a trend comparable to that observed in iron deficiency. As a result, some additional alternative measures of iron status (e.g., serum ferritin) should be used to distinguish between iron deficiency and increased erythropoiesis.

17.5.2 Interpretive criteria

In adults, a transferrin saturation below about 16% will be associated with iron-deficient erythropoiesis, if the subjects with infection and inflammation are excluded (Beard et al., 1996). Cutoff points are not as clearly defined for infants and children, because age-related differences in serum iron (but not TIBC) occur. This results in corresponding changes in the normal levels of transferrin saturation (Dallman et al., 1996). The extent of these changes is still uncertain.

Looker et al. (1997) suggested using cut-off values ranging from $< 10\%$ to $< 14\%$ for transferrin saturation in children 1–15 y, and $< 15\%$ for adults $\geqslant 16$ y when assessing the prevalence of iron deficiency in the NHANES III survey, as shown in Table 17.14.

The cutoffs of Looker et al. (1997) for transferrin saturation are slightly lower than those used earlier in NHANES II (Pilch and Senti, 1984) and approximate the 12th percentile. Lower cutoffs were used because of a change in the methodology for the measurement of serum iron in NHANES III (see below) and the fact that more blood samples were drawn late in the day, when serum iron values are normally lower.

Transferrin saturation values $> 70\%$ were used as a criterion for detecting iron overload in adult males and females in both the NHANES II and III surveys, in combination with elevated serum ferritin levels (Section 17.6). In some studies, a lower cutoff value for transferrin saturation for screening for iron overload in women (i.e., $> 50\%$) has been used (Hallberg, 1995).

Tables of mean and selected percentiles by age and sex, for percentage of transferrin saturation, derived from all the persons in the NHANES III survey, with the exception of breastfeeding infants and children, are given in Appendix A17.2 (IOM, 2001). A diagrammatic summary of this information is shown in Figure 17.6.

The U.K. National Diet and Nutrition Survey of young people aged 4 to 18 y (Gregory et al., 2000), and that of people aged 65 y and older (Finch et al., 1998) present data on the mean, median, and lower and upper 2.5 percentile values for percentage of transferrin saturation, as well as for plasma iron and TIBC. Tables of the mean percentage

transferrin saturation by age, sex, race or ethnicity, and the prevalence of low values (i.e., $< 12\%$ if aged 5 y and $< 14\%$ if aged 6–15 y), are also given for the New Zealand National Children's Nutrition Survey (Parnell et al., 2003).

17.5.3 Measurement of serum iron and TIBC

Several methods are available for the assay of serum iron, some of which can be performed using a clinical chemistry autoanalyzer. Colorimetric procedures frequently use ferrozine as the chromogen to react with Fe(II) to form a violet complex (Giovanniello et al., 1968). Other chromogens that can be used include bathophenanthroline sulfonate and tripyridyltriazine (Zak et al., 1980). Alternatively, serum iron can be assayed by atomic absorption spectrophotometry. Often there are large discrepancies between serum iron concentrations assayed by different methods (Tietz et al., 1996), particularly at the lower end of the range where the diagnosis of iron deficiency is important (Worwood, 1996).

The assay of TIBC involves saturating the transferrin iron-binding capacity with excess iron, and then removing the excess unbound iron with magnesium carbonate, charcoal, or an iron exchange resin. The transferrin-bound iron in solution is then measured (ICSH, 1978). Uncertainties in this assay include variations in the type and amount of magnesium carbonate used to remove unbound iron, and in the concentration of the saturating-iron solution (Pilch and Senti, 1984). In 1990, the ICSH published revised recommendations for this assay (ICSH, 1990).

A more sensitive method for determining the total iron-binding capacity of serum is now available that can be readily applied to serum which is turbid, moderately jaundiced, or even slightly hemolyzed (Ramsay, 1997).

Potential sources of error in the measurement of both serum iron and TIBC include contamination by exogenous iron, interference by lipids and bilirubin in the spectrometric methods, and a copper interference with colorimetric assays (Tietz et al., 1996).

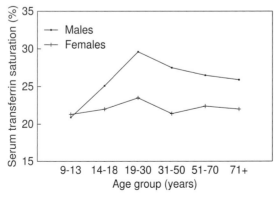

Figure 17.6: NHANES III median serum transferrin saturation by sex/age category. Data from IOM (2001).

To overcome the copper interference, the assay employing ferrozine, used for serum iron and TIBC in NHANES III, was improved by the addition of 1% thiourea (Looker et al., 1997). This led to lower serum iron values (by about 1.6 µmol/L) in this survey than those for NHANES II, with a much larger discrepancy at low concentrations than at higher ones (Looker et al., 1995).

Quality-control sera, with certified values for serum iron and TIBC and covering a wide range, should be included with each assay. A reference material for serum iron has been prepared by the ICSH Expert Panel on Iron (ICSH, 1978). Iron-free water should also be used. In the future, an immunological method that determines serum transferrin directly may be the method of choice. Correlation between the chemical and immunological methods appears high (Huebers et al., 1987). At present, however, there is no agreed recommended method and no international reference standard. Indeed, measurements of iron transport are now often omitted from nutrition surveys because of the large volume of serum sample required, cumbersome analytical methods, and their poor sensitivity and specificity for iron deficiency; their greatest value is in distinguishing between the anemia of inflammatory disease and that of true iron deficiency (Cook, 1999).

17.6 Serum ferritin

Ferritin was first identified in human serum by Addison et al. (1972). Its function in the serum is unknown. Ferritin appears to enter the serum by secretions from the reticuloendothelial system (Cook and Skikne, 1982). In most healthy individuals and those with uncomplicated iron deficiency, the concentration of serum or plasma ferritin parallels the total amount of storage iron (Cook et al., 1974). Once iron stores become exhausted, however, serum ferritin concentrations no longer reflect the *severity* of the iron-deficiency state. Serum ferritin is the only measure of iron status that can reflect a deficient, excess, or normal iron status.

Stainable bone marrow stores correlate positively with serum ferritin levels.

Iron removal by phlebotomy produces a fall in serum ferritin levels, the decline paralleling changes in liver iron stores as measured by liver biopsy.

Iron therapy and repeated blood transfusions generate a positive response in serum ferritin levels.

Box 17.2: Evidence for the quantitative relationship between serum ferritin and storage iron.

Evidence for the quantitative relationship between serum ferritin and storage iron is shown in Box 17.2.

Translation of serum ferritin values into the size of the iron stores should be made cautiously, in view of the limited knowledge of this relationship and the confounding factors that influence serum ferritin concentrations. There is also considerable between-subject variation in the relationship between serum ferritin and tissue iron. In normal healthy subjects with serum ferritin concentrations from 20 to 300 µg/L, a serum ferritin concentration of 1 µg/L is said to be equivalent to approximately 10 mg of storage iron (Cook, 1999).

17.6.1 Factors affecting serum ferritin

Biological variation in serum ferritin levels is less marked than for serum iron. The overall within-subject day-to-day coefficient of variation for serum ferritin in healthy subjects over a period of weeks is about 15%, compared with approximately 30% for serum iron (Table 17.10): the diurnal variation appears to be minimal. Analytical variation for the serum ferritin assay is greater than for serum iron (Worwood, 1996, 1997).

Age-related changes in serum ferritin concentrations are relatively marked and differ according to sex. At birth, concentrations are high, as iron stores in the liver are abundant. During the first 2 mo, serum ferritin levels rise further, as iron is released from the fetal red cells and the rate of erythropoiesis is slow. Serum ferritin concentrations

Age group (y)	Males	Females
1–3		22.9
4–8		28.7
9–13	32.9	30.6
14–18	46.7	27.0
19–30	112.5	36.0
31–50	155.9	39.9
51–70	154.5	89.4
⩾71	137.1	95.3
Pregnant	–	28.0
Lactating	–	32.9

Table 17.11: Changes in serum ferritin concentrations (μg/L) with age. The NHANES III data are abstracted from IOM (2001) and are the median values and representative of all races. Breast-feeding infants and children were excluded.

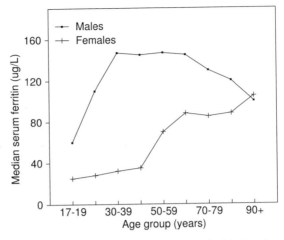

Figure 17.7: NHANES III mean serum ferritin data by decade of age for women and men. From Zacharski et al., American Heart Journal 140: 98–104, 2000.

then fall throughout later infancy (Domellöf et al., 2002b).

During adolescence, trends in serum ferritin concentrations differ according to sex. Levels in males rise sharply and then reach a maximum between 30 and 39 y. After this, levels remain constant until about 70 y, when they decline. In females, serum ferritin levels remain relatively low until menopause, after which they rise steeply (Table 17.11 and Figure 17.7) (Zacharski et al., 2000; IOM, 2001).

Sex differences in serum ferritin concentrations exist. Among infants, males have lower values than females at 4, 6, and 9 mo, and these values are not responsive to iron supplementation (Domellöf et al., 2002a). As a result, there may be a need to develop sex-specific cutoffs for serum ferritin in infancy. During adolescence, females have lower values than males, a trend that persists throughout adulthood (Table 17.11, Figure 17.7) (Zacharski et al., 2000; IOM, 2001).

Race is known to influence serum ferritin concentrations. In NHANES III, adult male African Americans had higher serum ferritin values than Caucasians and Hispanics of comparable age for each decade of life. In the adult females, serum ferritin levels were only higher in the African Americans

after menopause. Overall, serum ferritin values were approximately 7%–8% greater for the African Americans than for the Caucasians throughout the second half of life. Such differences are unlikely to be associated with increased intakes of dietary iron but, instead, may be due to genetic factors (Zacharski et al., 2000).

Iron deficiency leads to lower iron stores: serum ferritin values fall progressively as the stores decline, before the characteristic changes in serum iron and TIBC. In conditions of frank iron-deficiency anemia, when classic microcytic hypochromic anemia occurs, serum ferritin levels are very low or zero, reflecting the exhaustion of storage iron. It is important to note that a low concentration of serum ferritin is characteristic *only* of iron deficiency (Dallman et al., 1980).

Iron overload results in a rise in body iron stores, an associated increase in ferritin synthesis, and, hence, a rise in serum ferritin. A measure of serum ferritin provides information similar to that for serum iron and TIBC in conditions of iron overload and is used alongside transferrin saturation in the diagnosis of iron overload. Cutoff values for serum ferritin indicative of iron overload in adults used

Age group (y)	Males	Females
20–44	> 200	> 150
45–64	> 300	> 200
65–74	> 400	> 300

Table 17.12: Cutoff values for serum ferritin (μg/L) indicative of iron overload in adults. From Pilch and Senti (1984).

in NHANES II and NHANES III are given in Table 17.12.

Acute and chronic infections, inflammatory diseases, certain neoplastic diseases, and liver disorders elevate serum ferritin because ferritin is an acute-phase protein. These disorders can lead an increased rate of ferritin synthesis in the reticulo-endothelial system, which is reflected by an elevated concentration of ferritin in the serum. Hence, serum ferritin is inappropriate as an indicator of iron status where infection and inflammation are widespread and coexist with iron deficiency because values may be within the normal range despite the presence of iron deficiency (Brown, 1998). In such cases, an alternative measure of iron status, preferably serum transferrin receptor (Section 17.8), should be used.

Acute-phase proteins are often used in surveys as markers for infection or inflammation that induce elevated serum ferritin concentrations. For example, in NHANES III (Looker et al., 1997) and the New Zealand national surveys (Russell et al., 1999; Parnell et al., 2003), C-reactive protein was used. The latter is a good measure of acute infection or inflammation but is less appropriate when these conditions are chronic, as is common in the elderly (Looker et al., 1997). In older persons, both serum α_1-glycoprotein (ICSH, 1988) and α_1-antichymotrypsin are more suitable measures (ICSH, 1988) as they remain elevated longer than C-reactive protein (Thompson et al., 1992). Of the two, serum α_1-antichymotrypsin was used in the U.K. surveys of young people aged 4 to 18 y (Gregory et al., 2000) and people $\geqslant 65$ y

(Doyle et al., 1999). The normal upper limit of α_1-antichymotrypsin for adults is 0.65 g/L.

Decreased erythropoiesis may be associated with a deficiency of specific nutrients such as vitamin B_{12} and folic acid, and with certain drugs and toxins. This results in a decreased utilization of iron for hemoglobin synthesis, and, hence, serum ferritin levels may be normal or slightly above normal.

Increased erythropoiesis leads to a decline in storage iron as it is used for hemoglobin synthesis. As a result, serum ferritin levels also decline.

Acute and chronic liver disease may lead to abnormally high serum ferritin concentrations (Table 17.13), probably resulting from the release of ferritin from damaged liver cells. Liver damage may also interfere with the clearance of ferritin from the circulation (Worwood, 1997). Such damage is one of the factors contributing to the elevated serum ferritin concentrations that are observed in children with protein-energy malnutrition. These elevated serum ferritin levels do not reflect a high intracellular concentration of ferritin.

Leukemia and Hodgkin's disease also result in raised serum ferritin concentrations. In leukemia, these may be associated with (*a*) increased deposition of iron in cells of the reticulo-endothelial system; (*b*) circulating leukemic cells containing high levels of ferritin; or (*c*) increased release of ferritin

	Age (y)	Sexes combined
Iron deficiency anemia	3–14	< 10
	15–74	< 12
Idiopathic hemochromatosis	Adults	1000–10,000
Liver disease	Adults	400–3000+
Inflammation	Adults	10–1650
Acute infections	Children	100–510

Table 17.13: Serum ferritin (μg/L) concentrations associated with specific disease states. Adapted from Wormwood, CRC Critical Reviews in Clinical Laboratory Sciences 10: 171–204, 1979.

from damaged cells, as in liver disease. In Hodgkin's disease, the increased ferritin in the serum possibly comes from the lymphocytes (Worwood, 1979).

Other factors such as high alcohol consumption (Leggett et al., 1990; Osler et al., 1998), elevated plasma glucose concentrations (Tuomainen et al., 1997; IOM, 2001), and high body mass index (IOM, 2001) have been associated with elevated serum ferritin concentrations in epidemiological studies.

17.6.2 Interpretive criteria

Controversy exists over the most appropriate cutoffs for serum ferritin concentration to indicate totally depleted iron stores. In NHANES III the cutoff value used for serum ferritin was $< 10\,\mu g/L$ for children 1–5 y and a value of $< 12\,\mu g/L$ for all older subjects (Looker et al., 1997) (Table 17.14). Hallberg et al. (1993) have proposed a cutoff of $< 16\,\mu g/L$ to indicate totally depleted iron stores in adults. There is some evidence that a higher cutoff for serum ferritin may be necessary to diagnose iron depletion in the elderly (Guyatt et at., 1990; Fleming and Wood, 1996).

Lower cutoffs for infants have been proposed by Domellöf et al. (2002b). The cutoffs are based on serum ferritin concentrations at –2 SD for iron-replete infants (Table 17.15).

Elevated serum ferritin values are useful for diagnosing iron overload disorders. The cutoff values for serum ferritin indicative of

	4 mo	6 mo	9 mo
Hemoglobin (g/L)	< 105	< 105	< 100
MCV (fL)	< 73	< 71	< 71
ZnPP (μmol/mol heme)	> 75	> 75	> 90
Ferritin (μg/L)	< 20	< 9	< 5
TfR (mg/L)	> 11	> 11	> 11

Table 17.15: Suggested –2 SD cutoff values for iron status variables for infants at 4, 6, and 9 mo, based on iron-replete, breastfed infants. MCV, mean cell volume (data from Swedish infants); ZnPP, zinc protoporphyrin; TfR, transferrin receptor. From Domellöf et al., Journal of Nutrition 132: 3680–3686, 2002, with permission of The American Society for Nutritional Sciences.

iron overload in adults, used in NHANES II and III in conjunction with a transferrin saturation $> 70\%$, are shown in Table 17.12 (Pilch and Senti, 1984). To be sure, these high serum ferritin levels are not specific to iron overload disorders, as they also occur in liver disease, neoplasms (e.g., leukemia), inflammatory disease, and decreased erythropoiesis, as discussed above. If these conditions coexist with iron deficiency, individuals may be incorrectly diagnosed as iron replete based on serum ferritin alone.

Tables of mean and selected percentiles for serum ferritin by age and sex for children and adults in the NHANES III are given in Appendix A17.3. (Note that only breast-feeding infants and children were excluded). Serum ferritin concentrations were markedly higher in NHANES III than in NHANES II, in both children and adults (Dallman et al., 1996). This probably reflects increasing iron stores in the U.S. population as a whole rather than methodological difference in serum ferritin assays between the two surveys (Looker et al., 1995).

Mean, median, and lower and upper 2.5 or 5th percentiles for serum ferritin by age and sex are also presented in the U.K. national surveys (Gregory et al., 1990, 1995, 2000; Finch et al., 1998). Mean serum ferritin values by age, sex, and race or ethnicity for persons aged 15 y and older (Russell et al., 1999), and children aged 5 to 14 y are given in the New Zealand National Nutrition Survey

Age group (y)	Transferrin saturation (%)	Serum ferritin (μg/L)	Erythrocyte protoporphyrin μmol/L RBCs
1–2	< 10	< 10	> 1.42[a]
3–5	< 12	< 10	> 1.24[b]
6–11	< 14	< 12	> 1.24
12–15	< 14	< 12	> 1.24
$\geqslant 16$	< 15	< 12	> 1.24

Table 17.14: Cutoff points used for identifying abnormal values of iron status measures in the analysis of the NHANES III data. [a] 80 μg/dL red blood cells (RBCs). [b] 70 μg/dL RBCs. From Looker et al., Journal of the American Medical Association 277: 973–976, 1997.

and the National Children's Nutrition Survey, respectively (Parnell et al., 2003).

17.6.3 Measurement of serum ferritin

Serum ferritin is often determined with a two-site immunoradiometric assay (IRMA) (Miles et al., 1974). This procedure was used for NHANES II, the Hispanic Health and Nutrition Examination Survey (HANES), for NHANES III, and in the recent U.K. national surveys. Venipuncture or capillary blood samples can be used (Segall et al., 1979), although within- and between-sample variation tends to be larger with capillary than venous specimens (Pootrakul et al., 1983). Because the assay requires a gamma counter and a trained technician, it is a relatively expensive procedure. The within- and between-assay analytical coefficients of variation for serum ferritin analyzed from venous blood using IRMA are approximately 3% and 7%, respectively (Dallman, 1984).

Sensitive, enzyme-linked immunosorbent assays (ELISA) with colorimetric fluorescent or chemiluminescent endpoints are increasingly being used (Cook, 1999). These ELISA methods eliminate the need for gamma counters and require only a few μL of serum or plasma, which can be obtained from a single microhematocrit tube (Lu et al., 1987). Comparable results for the IRMA and ELISA methods have been reported (Flowers et al., 1986). Nevertheless, differences among kits may be marked particularly at low values, and can alter the apparent prevalence of iron deficiency (Hallberg, 1995).

Dried-serum spot (DSS) samples can also be used (Ahluwalia et al., 2002). This is a major advantage for field studies because the serum can be pipetted directly onto filter paper, and the spots can be air-dried and placed in airtight plastic bags for storage at room temperature for 2 wk; use of a desiccant is not required. Before analysis, the DSS must be digested for 6 h with cellulase from *Trichoderma reesei*.

A ferritin reference material was used in NHANES III and is available from the National Institute for Biological Standards and Controls, London (reagent 80/578; ICSH, 1984). Use of this international reference preparation of ferritin as a calibration check is encouraged.

Either serum or plasma can be used for ferritin assays. Samples may be stored refrigerated at 2–8°C for at least 5 d. For longer storage of up to 6 mo, samples should be frozen at –20°C. Repeated thawing and freezing should be avoided.

17.7 Zinc protoporphyrin and free erythrocyte protoporphyrin

There is some confusion in the literature because protoporphyrin is reported as both zinc protoporphyrin (ZnPP) and total metal-free erythrocyte protoporphyrin (FEP). Indeed, in many of the earlier studies these two terms were used interchangeably. This arose, in part, because in the early analytical procedures, ZnPP was unknowingly converted to FEP during analysis.

Zinc protoporphyrin is a product of disordered heme biosynthesis. If the supply of iron is adequate, heme is synthesized by the incorporation of iron into protoporphyrin IX by ferrochetalase. However, when there is insufficient iron for this reaction to occur, zinc is substituted for iron, forming ZnPP instead of heme. The ZnPP then accumulates within the iron-deprived circulating erythrocytes, where it can be measured in samples of whole blood.

Zinc protoporphyrin remains in the erythrocytes for the duration of their lifespan. Therefore, an increased ZnPP concentration in the blood indicates that the majority of the erythrocytes matured at a time when the iron supply was suboptimal.

The preferred mode of expression for ZnPP is a ratio based on μmol of ZnPP per mol of heme (NCCLS, 1996). Use of the ratio minimizes the effect of dilution that results from changes in plasma volume: ZnPP, RBCs, hemoglobin, and heme are diluted equally. This avoids the misinterpretation of laboratory results that may arise, for example, from plasma-volume changes in pregnancy.

As the zinc-for-iron substitution occurs

mainly in the bone marrow, the ZnPP:heme ratio in erythrocytes reflects the iron status at this site (McLaren et al., 1975). The ratio is a sensitive and relatively specific index of iron status, and is used specifically to detect an undersupply of iron to developing erythrocytes. Factors affecting ZnPP and FEP concentrations are discussed below. Table 17.16 provides an interpretation of the ZnPP:heme ratio in the diagnosis of iron disorders.

17.7.1 Factors affecting ZnPP and FEP

Age-related trends and sex differences in levels of ZnPP or FEP after about 3 y are small, although mean values in females >12 y are slightly higher than in men.

Iron deficiency of increasing severity produces progressively elevated concentrations of both ZnPP and FEP. A ZnPP:heme ratio of 40–60 μmol/mol heme is associated with iron-deficient erythropoiesis, and values of >80 μmol/mol heme with iron-deficiency anemia. When FEP is measured, levels range from 1.47 to 8.09 μmol/L RBC.

Chronic disease states such as infection, inflammation, and some neoplastic diseases are associated with elevated levels of ZnPP or FEP as a result of low iron levels in the bone marrow (Section 17.5.1). Hence, measurements of ZnPP or FEP do not distinguish between the anemia of iron deficiency and the anemia of chronic disease.

Lead toxicity can result in elevated concentrations of ZnPP and FEP because lead impairs the delivery of iron to, or its utilization in, mature erythrocytes. In NHANES II, FEP values were elevated in children 1–4 y with high blood lead values. Levels were lower in NHANES III, following the introduction of lead-free petrol (Looker et al., 1997).

17.7.2 Interpretive criteria

Table 17.15 presents suggested 2 SD cutoff values for ZnPP:heme ratios for infants aged

4, 6, and 9 mo compiled by Domellöf et al. (2002). In children and adults, ZnPP:heme ratios of 60–80 μmol/mol heme are sometimes associated with iron-deficient erythropoiesis, and values of >80 μmol/mol heme with iron-deficiency anemia (Labbé et al., 1999).

In the 1997 New Zealand National Nutrition Survey for persons aged ≥15 y, a cutoff value for ZnPP:heme ratio of >60 μmol/mol heme (in combination with a serum ferritin <12 μg/L) was used to indicate iron-deficient erythropoiesis. The mean and SEM for the ZnPP:heme ratio by age, sex, and race or ethnicity are also presented for this survey (Russell et al., 1999). The ratios of ZnPP:heme were assayed by hematofluorometry.

In both NHANES II and NHANES III, an acid-extraction method was used to measure total metal-free protoporphyrin (FEP) in whole blood (see below), which was then expressed as the ratio of μmoles of FEP per liter of RBCs:

$$FEP = \frac{\text{protoporphyrin in whole blood (μmol/L)}}{\text{hematocrit (vol. fraction)}}$$

The cutoffs used for FEP in NHANES III for children and adults approximate the 95th percentile of the NHANES III reference sample (Looker et al., 1997). They are shown in Table 17.14. A lower cutoff value for FEP was used for children 3–5 y in NHANES III than NHANES II because of the correspondingly lower FEP levels, following the introduction of lead-free petrol (Looker et al., 1997).

Tables of means and selected percentiles, by race, sex, and age are available for FEP for all persons in NHANES II and for the reference sample only (Pilch and Senti, 1984).

17.7.3 Measurement of ZnPP and FEP

The easiest, cheapest and fastest method for measuring ZnPP is by hematofluorometry, and a hematofluorometer has been designed for field use to measure the ratio of ZnPP to heme in a thin film of whole blood (NCCLS, 1996). Currently no automated method is available.

Lab results	Interpretation	Recommendations
Low ZnPP : heme ($< 60\,\mu$mol/mol)	Adequate systemic iron supply; no further deficiency work-up needed	Iron stores can be determined using serum ferritin concentration. If ZnPP : heme is $< 40\,\mu$mol/mol, consider testing for iron overload using either serum ferritin concentration or percentage transferrin saturation.
Medium ZnPP : heme ($60\text{–}80\,\mu$mol/mol)	Possible nonreplete iron status; consider inadequate diet, blood loss, anemia of chronic disease, and other causes	Hemoglobin or hematocrit values may indicate a state of iron depletion. If clinically indicated, measure serum ferritin to differentiate between low iron stores and block of iron release arising from inflammation. Identify the inflammation using C-reactive protein.
High ZnPP : heme ($> 80\,\mu$mol/mol) and low ferritin ($< 20\,\mu$g/L)	Indication of iron-deficient erythropoiesis attributable to low marrow iron supply, possibly related to depleted iron stores	Iron supplementation indicated once abnormal blood loss, anemia of chronic disease, or chronic lead exposure has been ruled out. Monitor therapy with decrease in ZnPP : heme or increase in reticulocyte count.
High ZnPP : heme ($> 80\,\mu$mol/mol) and high ferritin ($> 200\,\mu$g/L)	Severe inflammatory block, anemia of chronic disease, other causes of impaired iron utilization.	Treat causes of impaired iron utilization. Effectiveness of iron supplementation is limited. Consider severe chronic lead poisoning

Table 17.16: Interpretation of the ratio of ZnPP : heme in the diagnosis of iron disorders. From Labbé et al., Clinical Chemistry 45: 146–148, 1999, with permission of the AACC.

Complete oxygenation of the hemoglobin is required when using the hematofluorometric method, as incomplete oxygenation produces falsely low values because of a shift in hemoglobin absorption. To ensure complete oxygenation and dissolution of red cell aggregates, the blood film must be mixed vigorously using a disposable plastic pipet tip. Wooden applicator sticks should not be used for mixing as they may contain fluorescent by-products. Successive observations should be within 10%.

Several other limitations of the hematofluorometric method may lead to falsely elevated values, including the effect of some interfering substances such as bilirubin, certain drugs, and high riboflavin concentrations in plasma. Several strategies exist to eliminate these interferences, such as washing the erythrocytes free of plasma (Hastka et al., 1992); the strategies are discussed in detail in Labbé et al. (1999).

Artificial calibration slides are normally provided with the equipment to check the stability of the hematofluorometer. In addition, the method should be checked against quality-control samples in which ZnPP has been measured by a second method, which also measures the fluorescence and is readily standardized (NCCLS, 1996); details are given in Labbé et al. (1999). Persons planning to set up a ZnPP test may wish to contact the New York State Department of Health Protoporphyrin Proficiency Testing Program.

The method used for the analysis of erythrocyte protoporphyrin in NHANES II and NHANES III (Looker et al., 1997) yielded values for total metal-free protoporphyrin. It involved the extraction of both ZnPP and free protoporphyrin from anticoagulated whole blood with an ethyl acetate and acetic acid solvent, then back-extraction into dilute hydrochloric acid, followed by measurement of total metal-free protoporphyrin by fluorimetry (Gunter et al., 1989; NCCLS, 1996). The between-assay CV is are lower for ZnPP analyzed via the hematofluorometer than for FEP by the extraction method.

17.8 Serum transferrin receptor

Transferrin receptor (TfR) is an iron-related protein that regulates the uptake of transferrin iron into all body cells (Baynes et al., 1994). The surfaces of the cells express TfRs in proportion to their requirement for iron. A soluble form of TfR circulates in human serum; its concentration is proportional to the total body mass of cellular transferrin receptors (Cook, 1999).

Levels of TfRs circulating in the serum are a sensitive indicator of the degree of tissue iron deficiency. In mild iron deficiency, when iron availability to tissues is compromised because iron stores are depleted, TfR expression by cells increases, allowing the cells to compete more effectively for transferrin-bound iron. As a result, serum TfR levels increase in proportion to the functional iron deficit (Gimferrer et al., 1997). For example, in elderly women with iron deficiency, but not necessarily anemia, plasma TfR levels were 1.3 times the levels in iron-sufficient controls (Ahluwalia et al., 1995). In contrast in those with microcytic, hypochromic anemia, serum TfR levels were 5.8 times that of the controls (Gimferrer et al., 1997).

One of the main advantages of using serum TfR is that, unlike serum ferritin, concentrations are not significantly affected by the anemia of chronic disease. Consequently, serum TfR concentrations can be used to help distinguish individuals with anemia of chronic disease from those with iron-deficiency anemia — a distinction that used to require a bone marrow examination for stainable iron. Figure 17.8 shows that for patients with coexisting iron deficiency and anemia of chronic disease, serum TfR levels are elevated and comparable to those for patients with only iron-deficiency anemia. This finding is particularly important because the diagnosis of iron deficiency in individuals with concurrent anemia of chronic disease has been especially difficult in the past (Ahluwalia, 1998).

In humans, the majority of TfR (75%–80%) is derived from the erythroid bone marrow; therefore, any change in erythropoiesis

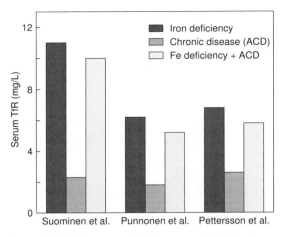

Figure 17.8: Serum transferrin receptor levels in iron-deficiency anemia, anemia of chronic disease (ACD), and ACD plus iron deficiency. From Ahluwalia, Nutrition Reviews 56: 133-141, 1998, with permission of the International Life Sciences Institute.

(e.g., as a result of vitamin B_{12} or folate deficiency), will, in turn, affect serum TfR concentrations. For this reason, conditions that alter erythrocyte production may confound the interpretation of serum TfR values for iron status assessment.

17.8.1 Factors affecting serum TfR

Biological variation for serum TfR concentrations is low. Cooper and Zlotkin (1996) determined the total day-to-day within-subject coefficient of variation (CV) for a group of healthy men ($n = 10$) and women ($n = 11$) aged 19–46 y, based on measurements on 10 nonconsecutive days over a 4-wk period. Biological variation for serum TfR in this study was 12.5%, compared with 8.9% (Ahluwalia et al. 1993) and 12.7% (Lammi-Keefe et al., 1996) in other population groups.

Age-related changes in serum TfR occur. Levels in neonates and infants are comparable but higher than adult levels (Choi et al., 1999; Olivares et al., 2000; Domellöf et al., 2002b), perhaps partly as a result of a higher erythropoietic activity per unit of body weight during infancy. Other mechanisms may also be involved. Further, there is more overlap of serum TfR values between iron-deficient and iron-replete infants than in corresponding adults. This may result from the higher variability in the erythroid mass in healthy infants (Olivares et al., 2000).

Limited data are available to define age-related trends in serum TfR levels during childhood and adolescence. Choi et al. (1999) noted that mean serum TfR values decreased gradually from infancy through childhood but were still higher than adult levels. For adolescents, values were higher at 14–16 y than at 17–19 y, when values reached adult levels. Virtanen et al. (1999) also reported higher serum TfR levels in children than in adults, as well as higher levels in infants than in prepubertal boys. Such differences were said to be a response to physiologically low iron stores. Studies in the elderly are limited, but some results suggest that both the levels and the magnitude of the response of serum TfR to iron deficiency may be lower in this age group (Ahluwalia et al., 1995).

Sex-related differences in serum TfR exist. During early infancy, values may be higher for males than for females, perhaps as a result of sex differences in fetal iron accretion (Domellöf et al., 2002a), although such differences have not been consistently reported in older infants (9–15 mo) (Yeung and Zlotkin, 1997). In contrast, in both children and adults, sex-related differences in serum TfR concentrations are small (Raya et al., 2001; Worwood, 2002).

Race may influence serum TfR concentrations. African Americans have been reported to have values that were 9% higher than those for Caucasians, Asians, and Hispanics. Such race-related differences may be attributed to the well-established but unexplained lower hemoglobin concentration known to occur among persons of African descent (Allen et al., 1998).

Tissue iron deficiency leads to increases in serum TfR, as noted earlier. Even after iron stores are totally depleted, serum TfR concentrations continue to increase in proportion to the increasing tissue iron deficit,

as hemoglobin concentrations fall (Skikne et al., 1990). This trend has been observed in neonates (Rusia et al., 1996), infants (Olivares et al., 2000), pregnant women (Carriaga et al., 1991), and adults (Skikne et al., 1990). Whether serum TfR concentrations change before the iron stores become totally depleted (i.e., serum ferritin $< 12\,\mu g/L$) is more controversial (Skikne et al., 1990; Zhu et al., 1998).

Increased erythropoiesis, as noted earlier, is associated with elevated serum TfR. Numerous other conditions, some of which are listed in Table 17.17, result in increased erythroid proliferation.

Decreased erythropoiesis associated with chronic renal disease and aplastic anemia leads to a fall in serum TfR concentrations (Beard et al., 1996; Ahluwalia, 1998). Fortunately, these conditions can usually be identified by other laboratory tests, such as serum ferritin, which is normal in hematologic dis-

TfR	Condition
Increased	Increased erythroid proliferation: – Autoimmune hemolytic anemia – Hereditary spherocytosis – Beta thalassemia/HbE – Hemoglobin H disease – Sickle cell anemia – Polycythemia vera – Vitamin B_{12} deficiency – Folic acid deficiency Decreased tissue iron stores: – Iron-deficiency anemia
Normal to increased	Idiopathic myelofibrosis Myelodysplastic syndrome Chronic lymphocytic leukemia
Normal	Hemochromatosis Acute and chronic myeloid leukemia Most lymphoid malignancies Solid tumors Anemia of chronic disease
Decreased	Chronic renal failure Aplastic anemia Post bone-marrow transplantation

Table 17.17: Serum transferrin receptor concentration changes in human disease. From Worwood, Annals of Clinical Biochemistry 39: 221–230, 2002.

orders with decreased erythropoiesis (Section 17.6).

High altitudes may also result in higher serum TfR concentrations, as a consequence of the increase in the total body erythroid mass (Allen et al., 1998).

Cigarette smoking (10 per day) has been linked to a significant decrease in serum TfR concentration in males and females (Raya et al., 2001).

Nutrient deficiencies, such as folic acid deficiency and vitamin B_{12} deficiency, are also associated with defective but elevated erythropoiesis. As a result, individuals with the later stages of vitamin B_{12} deficiency have elevated TfR levels associated with megaloblastic anemia (Carmel and Skikne, 1992; Remacha et al., 1997). In such cases, use of serum TfR measurement alone would yield a false-positive diagnosis for iron deficiency.

Acute malaria may result in reduced levels of serum TfR (Williams et al., 1999; Beesley et al., 2000). This means that in areas where both iron deficiency and clinical episodes of malaria occur, the reliability of serum TfR as an indicator of iron status is uncertain.

Pregnancy and the resulting hemodilution do not appear to decrease serum TfR concentrations. Serum TfR may thus be a reliable indicator of iron deficiency during pregnancy. Carriaga et al. (1991) observed elevated serum TfR concentrations in the third trimester of pregnancy, but only in pregnant women with depleted iron stores as defined by low serum ferritin concentrations.

Nevertheless, questions still remain about the effect of changes in erythropoiesis in early pregnancy on serum TfR levels; such changes may mask iron deficiency at this time (Åkesson et al., 1998). Choi et al. (2000) observed that increases in serum TfR appeared to relate to increased erythropoiesis rather than iron depletion. Also, van den Broek et al. (1998) reported that serum TfR did not enhance the sensitivity and specificity for the

determination of iron-deficiency anemia in pregnant women from Malawi where anemia and chronic disease are very prevalent. In a study of Jamaican pregnant women, however, serum TfR readily distinguished those who received an iron supplement from the women who did not (Simmons et al., 1993).

Oral contraceptive agents and hormone replacement therapy, as well as anti-inflammatory and anti-hypertensive drugs do not affect serum TfR concentrations (Raya et al., 2001).

Other factors such as severe protein-energy malnutrition may alter serum TfR levels, perhaps because of the impact of the severe malnutrition on the bone marrow. Erythropoiesis may be reduced, leading to a fall in serum TfR levels; this effect warrants further investigation (Kuvibidila et al., 1996).

17.8.2 Interpretive criteria

Defining normal values for TfR in healthy subjects is difficult because TfR values and the units of expression vary with the assay; even different kits based on the ELISA technique are associated with different "normal" ranges. In addition, at present, there is no international standard for TfR. This makes comparison of results across studies difficult (Worwood, 2002).

Currently, the recommended approach to interpret serum TfR values is to examine their direction and magnitude of change in relation to the severity of iron deficiency, rather than the absolute levels. In general, the correlation among different TfR assays is good, and their ability to identify iron deficiency is similar, provided the cutoff values for the particular assay used are applied.

Only limited data are available to define serum TfR levels by age and sex. No serum TfR data have been reported for NHANES III or for the UK national surveys. Choi et al. (1999) have compiled a set of reference data based on 849 apparently healthy nonanemic subjects ranging in age from neonates (birth weight $\geqslant 2500\,g$) to adults 23–62 y, as shown in Table 17.18. Those with a history of

	Age	Mean ± SD (mg/L)	95% CI (mg/L)
Neonates	0–5 min	4.95 ± 1.24	2.21–6.74
Children			
Infants	4–24 mo	4.51 ± 1.12	2.15–6.31
Young children	3–7 y	3.02 ± 0.76	1.47–4.24
Adolescents			
Middle school	14–16 y	2.86 ± 0.74	1.35–4.19
High school	17–19 y	2.09 ± 0.55	1.18–3.23
Adults	23–62 y	2.13 ± 0.51	1.22–3.31

Table 17.18: Serum transferrin concentrations in various apparently healthy nonanemic populations. Data for neonates from cord blood. 95% confidence intervals (CI) calculated using non-parametric methods. Data from Choi et al., Clinical Chemistry 45: 1562–1563, 1999, with permission of the AACC.

blood transfusions, major surgery, recent infections, or disease were excluded. Subjects were nonanemic (i.e., hemoglobin ≥ 110 g/L) with no evidence of iron deficiency. Serum TfR levels were measured using an ELISA kit (Orion Diagnostica, Espoo, Finland).

Reference percentiles for serum TfR for persons aged from 3 y to ≥ 60 y, assayed using an automated nephelometer and the N Latex sTfR assay (Dade-Behring, Marburg, Germany), are given in Table 17.19.

Some investigators have advocated the use of the ratio of serum TfR to serum ferritin to assess iron status (Skikne et al., 1990) on the

Age in years (n)	5%	50%	75%	90%	95%
Males					
3–10 (64)	1.28	1.58	1.70	1.78	1.84
11–20 (68)	1.05	1.42	1.67	1.90	2.10
21–40 (87)	0.83	1.16	1.31	1.50	1.59
41–60 (110)	0.87	1.14	1.31	1.50	1.60
> 60 (106)	0.79	1.15	1.32	1.46	1.59
Females					
3–10 (64)	1.23	1.63	1.75	1.98	2.05
11–20 (56)	0.93	1.33	1.50	1.70	1.79
21–40 (79)	0.91	1.17	1.32	1.46	1.48
41–60 (108)	0.84	1.15	1.35	1.47	1.56
> 60 (102)	0.92	1.26	1.42	1.59	1.69

Table 17.19: Reference percentiles for serum transferrin receptor concentrations (mg/L) in males and females. From Raya et al., Clinical Chemistry and Laboratory Medicine 39: 1162–1168, 2001.

basis that serum ferritin reflects the amount of storage iron, whereas serum TfR reflects tissue iron need. Use of this ratio to assess iron stores in epidemiological studies and to evaluate the efficacy of fortification trials appears promising, but more research is needed (Cook et al., 2003).

17.8.3 Measurement of serum TfR

Several methods are used to determine serum TfR concentrations. Originally a two-site immunoradiometric assay and commercially available monoclonal antibodies were used (Kohgo et al., 1986). Subsequently, ELISA and monoclonal antibodies (Flowers et al., 1989) or polyclonal antibodies (Huebers et al., 1990) have been used. Commercial kits that use ELISA techniques are also available, but they are expensive and still require standardization (Cook, 1999).

In the United States, several ELISA commercial kits have been approved for use by the Food and Drug Administration (FDA): these use only a few µL of serum. However, major differences have been reported in values for serum TfR concentrations with different assay systems (Wians et al., 2001), including those approved by the U.S. FDA. Nevertheless, the analytical and clinical performance of the three approved commercial kits are similar (Åkesson et al., 1999; Wians et al., 2001). An international TfR certified reference material is urgently required to enable different laboratories to calibrate their own assays, facilitating comparisons across countries. Recommendations on the assay protocol by the ICSH are also needed. In the future, assays on whole-blood spots dried on filter paper may be possible (Cook et al., 1998).

Serum is the preferred matrix although some assays can use EDTA-heparin or citrate plasma. Both venous and capillary blood samples can be used; biological and analytical variation for serum TfR are lower than for serum ferritin (Table 17.10) (Cooper and Zlotkin, 1996).

Serum samples should be stored for no longer than 2 d at room temperature, 7 d at

2–8°C, 1–6 mo at –20°C, and 1 y at –70°C. Repeated freezing and thawing is not recommended. Moderate hemolysis does not confound the results.

17.9 Multiple indices

The use of several different measures of iron status simultaneously provides a more valid assessment of iron status than any single measurement because the misclassification that can occur due to overlapping normal and abnormal values for a single measure is minimized. Moreover, multiple measures differentiate the severity of iron deficiency more readily. A combination of three tests of iron status are frequently used, with abnormal values for at least two of the three tests indicating iron deficiency. At present, there is no consensus on the best definition of iron deficiency when based on multiple measures.

In NHANES II and NHANES III (Pilch and Senti, 1984; Dallman et al., 1996; Looker et al., 1997), two models were used to assess the relative prevalence of impaired iron status and anemia in selected groups of the U.S. population: one model involved ferritin, and one used MCV (Figure 17.9). In the ferritin model, serum ferritin, transferrin saturation, and FEP were included, whereas the MCV model was based on MCV, transferrin saturation, and FEP. In NHANES III, individuals with iron deficiency, based on at least two of three abnormal values in the ferritin model, concurrent with low hemoglobin concentrations, were considered to have iron-deficiency anemia (Looker et al., 1997). It is noteworthy that neither model can provide a definitive diagnosis of iron deficiency because none of the measures (with the exception of serum ferritin) distinguishes between changes resulting from iron deficiency and those arising from infection or inflammation. The cutoff values used in the NHANES III survey are presented in Table 17.14.

The inclusion of serum TfR as one of the laboratory criteria is recommended because of its ability to distinguish the anemia of chronic disease from iron-deficiency anemia,

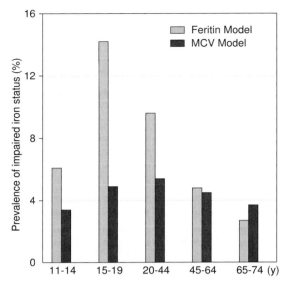

Figure 17.9: Prevalence of impaired iron status in subjects of varying ages estimated using the ferritin model and the MCV model: NHANES II, 1976–1980. From Pilch and Senti (1984).

even in the presence of chronic infection or inflammation (Figure 17.8). Hence, in future surveys, a combination of serum TfR, serum ferritin, and hemoglobin measurements may be used to describe the iron status of a population: serum ferritin levels reflect the decline and eventually the exhaustion of body iron stores; serum TfR reflects the degree of deficiency in functional iron after the stores have been depleted, even in the presence of the anemia of chronic disease; hemoglobin measures the presence of anemia. This combination may be especially useful because it provides diagnostic information over a wide spectrum of iron status, ranging from replete iron stores to overt iron deficiency anemia.

17.10 Summary

Table 17.20 summarizes the changes in biochemical measures of iron status that occur during each of the three phases in the development of iron-deficiency anemia. The first phase is a decrease in iron stores, reflected by a decline in serum or plasma ferritin concentrations. The second phase, iron-deficient erythropoiesis, is characterized by exhausted

	Iron overload	Normal	Iron depletion	Iron-deficient erythro-poiesis	Iron-deficiency anemia
TIBC (µg/dL)	< 300	330 ± 30	360	390	410
Serum ferritin (µg/L)	> 300	100 ± 60	20	10	< 10
Iron absorption (%)	> 15	5–10	10–15	10–20	10–20
Serum iron (µg/dL)	> 175	115 ± 50	115	< 60	< 40
Transferrin saturation (%)	> 60	35 ± 15	30	< 15	< 15
Serum transferrin receptor (mg/L)[a]	Low	Normal	Normal	High	High
FEP µg/dL RBC)	30	30	30	> 70	> 70
Erythrocytes	Normal	Normal	Normal	Normal	Microcytic/ Hypochromic

Table 17.20: Sequential stages in the development of iron deficiency and iron overload. TIBC, total iron-binding capacity; [a]Serum transferrin receptor values vary with the assay; FEP, free erythrocyte protoporphyrin. To convert µg iron to SI units (nmol) multiply by 17.9. From Herbert, American Journal of Clinical Nutrition 46: 387–402, 1987 © Am. J. Clin. Nutr. American Society for Clinical Nutrition.

iron stores, reflected by a further decline in serum ferritin to $< 12\mu g/L$, at which time serum TfR levels increase. At about the same time, serum iron concentrations fall to $< 11\mu mol/L$, which is associated with an elevation in TIBC, and a corresponding fall in percentage of transferrin saturation to $< 15\%$. Erythrocyte free protoporphyrin or the ZnPP : heme ratio, however, changes after the increase in serum TfR, rising to $1.24\,\mu mol/L$ RBCs or to $> 60 - 80\,\mu mol/mol$ heme, respectively, because the supply of iron is no longer adequate for heme synthesis. At this second stage, the hemoglobin remains within the normal range. In the third and final stage of iron deficiency, frank microcytic, hypochromic anemia occurs, when decreases in both the hemoglobin concentration and the hematocrit occur, resulting in a low MCHC. The presence of hypochromic microcytosis can be confirmed at this stage using a stained blood film.

Table 17.20 also presents the changes in the iron status measures that occur during iron overload. As elevated serum ferritin concentrations also occur during chronic inflammatory conditions, measurements of serum iron and total iron-binding capacity are the preferred screening tests for iron overload.

To provide the best assessment of iron status, several measures should be used at the same time. The presence of two or more abnormal values generally indicates impaired iron status. At present there is no consensus on the best combination to use. The selection of the most appropriate combination depends on the health of the individual(s) and on the study objectives. Diagnosis of iron deficiency is difficult in the presence of other conditions that confound the interpretation of laboratory results. For example, the diagnosis may be obscured by the coexistence of chronic inflammation, unless serum TfR is determined.

The prevalence of low iron status will vary according to the combination of measures selected. When serum ferritin is included, prevalence values will always be higher, because serum ferritin is the most sensitive measure of the early depletion of body iron stores.

References

Addison GM, Beamish MR, Hayles CN, Hodgkins M, Jacobs A, Llewellyn P. (1972). An immunoradiometric assay for ferritin in the serum of normal subjects and patients with iron deficiency and iron overload. Journal of Clinical Pathology 25: 326–329.

Ahluwalia N. (1998). Diagnostic utility of serum transferrin receptors measurement in assessing iron status. Nutrition Reviews 56: 133–141.

Ahluwalia N, Lammi-Keefe CJ, Haley NR, Beard JL. (1993). Day-to-day variation in iron-status indexes is similar for most measures in elderly women with and without rheumatoid arthritis. Journal of the American Dietetics Association 96: 247–251.

Ahluwalia N, Lammi-Keefe CJ, Bendel RB, Morse EE, Beard JL, Haley NR. (1995). Iron deficiency and anemia of chronic disease in elderly women: a discriminant-analysis approach for differentiation. American Journal of Clinical Nutrition 61: 590–596.

Ahluwalia N, de Silva A, Atukorala S, Weaver V, Molls R. (2002). Ferritin concentrations in dried serum spots from capillary and venous blood in children in Sri Lanka: a validation study. American Journal of Clinical Nutrition 75: 289–294.

Åkesson A, Bjellerup P, Berglund M, Bremme K, Vahter M. (1998). Serum transferrin receptor: a specific marker of iron deficiency in pregnancy. American Journal of Clinical Nutrition 68: 1241–1246.

Åkesson A, Bjellerup P, Vahter M. (1999). Evaluation of kits for measurement of soluble transferrin receptor. Scandinavian Journal of Clinical Laboratory Investigation 59: 77–81.

Allen J, Backstrom KR, Cooper JA, Cooper MC, Detwiler TC, Essex DW, Fritz RP, Means RT, Meier PB, Pearlman SR, Roitman-Johnson B, Seligman PA. (1998). Measurement of soluble transferrin receptor in serum of healthy adults. Clinical Chemistry 44: 35–39.

Allen LH. (1997). Pregnancy and iron deficiency: unresolved issues. Nutrition Reviews 51: 49–52.

Andrews NC. (1999). Disorders of iron metabolism. New England Journal of Medicine 341: 1986–1995.

Baynes RD, Skikne BS, Cook JD. (1994). Circulating transferrin receptors and assessment of iron status. Journal of Nutritional Biochemistry 5: 322–330.

Beard JL, Dawson H, Piñero DJ. (1996). Iron metabolism: a comprehensive review. Nutrition Reviews 54: 295–317.

Beesley R, Filteau S, Tomkins A, Doherty T. Ayles H, Reid A et al. (2000). Impact of acute malaria on plasma concentrations of transferrin receptors. Transactions of the Royal Society of Tropical Medicine and Hygiene 94: 295–289.

Bessman JD, Feinstein DI. (1979). Quantitative anisocytosis as a discriminant between iron deficiency and thalassemia minor. Blood 53: 288–293.

Bessman JD, Gilmer PR Jr, Gardner FH. (1983). Improved classification of anemias by MCV and RDW. American Journal of Clinical Pathology 80: 322–326.

Borel MJ, Smith SM, Derr J, Beard JL. (1991). Day-to-day variation in iron status indices in healthy men and women. American Journal of Clinical Nutrition 54: 729–735.

Bothwell TH, Seftel H, Jacobs P, Torrance JD, Baum-slag N. (1964). Iron overload in Bantu subjects: studies on the availability of iron in Bantu beer. American Journal of Clinical Nutrition 14: 47–51.

Brittenham GM, Danish EH, Harris JW. (1981). Assessment of bone marrow and body iron stores: old techniques and new technologies. Seminars in Hematology 18: 194–221.

Brock C, Curry H, Hanna C, Knipfer M, Taylor L. (1985). Adverse effects of iron supplementation: a comparative trial of wax-matrix iron preparation and conventional ferrous sulfate tablets. Clinical Therapy 7: 568–573.

Brown KH. (1998). Effect of infections on plasma Zn concentrations and implications for zinc status assessment in low-income countries. American Journal of Clinical Nutrition 68: 425S–429S.

Burger S, Pierre-Louis J. (2003). A Procedure to Estimate the Accuracy and Reliability of HemoCue™ Measurements of Survey Workers. International Life Sciences Institute, Washington, DC.

Carmel R, Skikne BS. (1992). Serum transferrin receptor in the megaloblastic anemia of cobalamin deficiency. European Journal of Haematology 49: 246–250.

Carriaga MT, Skikne BS, Finley B, Cutler B, Cook JD. (1991). Serum transferrin receptor for the detection of iron deficiency in pregnancy. American Journal of Clinical Nutrition 54: 1077–1081.

CDC (Centers for Disease Control and Prevention). (1989). Criteria for anemia in children and childbearing-aged women. Morbidity and Mortality Weekly Report 38: 400–404.

CDC (Centers for Disease Control and Prevention). (1998). Recommendations to prevent and control iron deficiency in the United States. Morbidity and Mortality Weekly Report 47: 1–36.

Charoenlarp P, Polpothi T. (1987). The distribution of haemoglobin concentration in healthy Thai children. Southeast Asian Journal of Tropical Medicine and Public Health 18: 567–568.

Choi JW, Pai SH, Im MW, Kim SK. (1999). Change in transferrin receptor concentrations with age. Clinical Chemistry 45: 1562–1563.

Choi JW, Im MW, Pai SH. (2000). Serum transferrin receptor concentrations during normal pregnancy. Clinical Chemistry 46: 725–727.

COMA (Committee on Medical Aspects of Food Policy). (1991). Dietary Reference Values for Food Energy and Nutrients for the United Kingdom: Report of the Panel on Dietary Reference Values. Report on Health and Social Subjects No. 46. Her Majesty's Stationery Office, London.

Cook JD. (1999). Defining optimal body iron. Proceedings of the Nutrition Society 58: 489–495.

Cook JD, Skikne BS. (1982). Serum ferritin: a possible model for the assessment of nutrient stores. American Journal of Clinical Nutrition 35: 1180–1185.

Cook JD, Lipschitz DA, Miles LEM, Finch CA. (1974). Serum ferritin as a measure of iron stores in normal subjects. American Journal of Clinical Nutrition 27: 681–687.

Cook JD, Flowers CH, Skikne BS. (1998). An assessment of dried blood spot technology for identifying iron deficiency. Blood 92: 1807–1813.

Cook JD, Flowers CH, Skikne BS. (2003). The quantitative assessment of body iron. Blood 101: 3359–3364.

Cooper MJ, Zlotkin SH. (1996). Day-to-day variation of transferrin receptor and ferritin in healthy men and women. American Journal of Clinical Nutrition 64: 738–742.

Dallman PR. (1977). New approaches to screening for iron deficiency. Journal of Pediatrics 90: 678–681.

Dallman PR. (1984). Diagnosis of anemia and iron deficiency: analytic and biological variations of laboratory tests. American Journal of Clinical Nutrition 39: 937–941.

Dallman PR, Siimes MA, Stekel A. (1980). Iron deficiency in infancy and childhood. American Journal of Clinical Nutrition 33: 86–118.

Dallman PR, Looker AC, Johnson CL, Carroll M. (1996). Influence of age on laboratory criteria for the diagnosis of iron deficiency anaemia and iron deficiency in infants and children. In: Hallberg L, Asp N-G (eds.) Iron Nutrition in Health and Disease. John Libbey and Co, London, pp. 65–74.

Davidsson L, Almgren A, Sandström B, Hurrell RF. (1995). Zinc absorption in adult humans: The effect of iron fortification. British Journal of Nutrition 74: 417–425.

Dawkins S, Cavill I, Ricketts C, Worwood M. (1979). Variability of serum ferritin concentrations in normal subjects. Clinical Laboratory Haematology 1: 41–46.

Domellöf M, Lönnerdal B, Dewey KG, Cohen RJ, Rivera IL, Hernell O. (2002a). Sex differences in iron status during infancy. Pediatrics 110: 545–552.

Domellöf M, Dewey KG, Lönnerdal B, Cohen RJ, Hernell O. (2002b). The diagnostic criteria for iron deficiency in infants should be reevaluated. Journal of Nutrition 132: 3680–3686.

Doyle W, Crawley H, Robert H, Bates CJ. J. (1999). Iron deficiency in older people: interactions between food and nutrient intakes with biochemical measures of iron; further analysis of the National Diet and Nutrition Survey of people aged 65 years and over. European Journal of Clinical Nutrition 53: 552–559.

Emond AM, Hawkins N, Pennock C, Golding J. (1996). Haemoglobin and ferritin concentrations in infants at 8 months of age. Archives of Disease in Childhood 74: 36–39.

Fairbanks VG. (1980). Nonequivalence of automated and manual hematocrit and erythrocyte indices. American Journal of Clinical Pathology 73: 55–62.

Fairbanks VF. (1994). Iron in medicine and nutrition. In: Shils M, Olson JA, Shike M (eds.) Modern Nutrition in Health and Disease. 8th ed. Volume 1. Lea & Febiger, Philadelphia, pp. 185–213.

FAO/WHO (Food & Agriculture Organization / World Health Organization). (1988). Requirements of Vitamin A, Iron, Folate, and Vitamin B_{12}. FAO Food and Nutrition Series No. 23. FAO, Rome.

Feraudi M, Mejia LA. (1987). Development and evaluation of a simplified method to collect blood samples to determine hemoglobin and hematocrit using chromatographic paper discs. American Journal of Clinical Nutrition 45: 790–796.

Finch S, Doyle W, Lowe C, Bates CJ, Prentice A, Smithers G, Clarke PC. (1998). National Diet and Nutrition Survey: People aged 65 Years or Older. Volume 1: Report of the Diet and Nutrition Survey. The Stationery Office, London.

Fishman SM, Christian P, West KJ Jr. (2000). The role of vitamins in the prevention and control of anaemia. Public Health Nutrition 3: 125–150.

Fleming D, Wood RJ. (1996). Plasma transferrin receptor helps to predict iron deficiency in the anemia of chronic disease. Nutrition Reviews 53: 167–175.

Flowers CH, Kuizon M, Beard JL, Skikne BS, Covell AM, Cook JD. (1986). A serum ferritin assay for prevalence studies of iron deficiency. American Journal of Hematology 23: 141–151.

Flowers CH, Skikne BS, Covell AM, Cook JD. (1989). The clinical measurement of serum transferrin receptor. Journal of Laboratory and Clinical Medicine 114: 368–377.

Gallagher SK, Johnson LK, Milne DB. (1989). Short-term and long-term variability of indices related to nutritional status. I: Ca, Cu, Fe, Mg and Zn. Clinical Chemistry 35: 369–373.

Gimferrer E, Ubeda J, Royo MT, Marigo GJ, Marco N, Fernandez N, Oliver A, Padros R, Gich I. (1997). Serum transferrin receptor levels in different stages of iron deficiency. Blood 90: 1332–1334.

Giovanniello TJ, DiBenedetto G, Palmer DW, Peters T Jr. (1968). Fully- and semi-automated methods for the determination of serum iron and total iron-binding capacity. Journal of Laboratory and Clinical Medicine 71: 874–883.

Graitcer PL, Goldsby JB, Nichaman MZ. (1981). Hemglobins and hematocrits: are they equally sensitive in detecting anemias? American Journal of Clinical Nutrition 34: 61–64.

Gregory J, Foster K, Tyler H, Wiseman M. (1990). The Dietary and Nutritional Survey of British Adults. Her Majesty's Stationery Office, London.

Gregory JR, Colllins DL, Davies PSW, Hughes JM, Clarke PC. (1995). National Diet and Nutrition Survey: Children Aged One-and-a-Half to Four-and-a-Half Years. Volume 1: Report of the Diet and Nutrition Survey. Her Majesty's Stationery Office, London.

Gregory J, Lowe S, Bates CJ, Prentice A, Jackson LV, Smithers G, Wenlock R, Farron M. (2000). National Diet and Nutrition Survey: Young People Aged 4 to 18 Years. Volume 1: Report of the Diet and Nutrition Survey. The Stationery Office, London.

Gunter EW, Turner WE, Huff DL. (1989). Investigation of protoporphyrin IX standard materials used in acid-extraction methods, and a proposed correction for the millimolar absorptivity of protoporphyrin IX. Clinical Chemistry 35: 1601–1608.

Guyatt GH, Patterson C, Ali M, Singer J, Levine M,

Turpie I, Meyer R. (1990). Diagnosis of iron-deficiency anemia in the elderly. American Journal of Medicine 88: 205–209.

Hallberg L. (1995). Results of surveys to assess iron status in Europe. Nutrition Reviews 53: 314–322.

Hallberg L. (2001). Perspectives on nutritional iron deficiency. Annual Review of Nutrition 21: 1–21.

Hallberg L, Hulthen L. (2000). Prediction of dietary iron absorption: an algorithm for calculating absorption and bioavailability of dietary iron. American Journal of Clinical Nutrition 71: 1147–1160. Erratum in: American Journal of Clinical Nutrition 72: 1242, American Journal of Clinical Nutrition 74: 274.

Hallberg L, Rossander L. (1984). Improvement of iron nutrition in developing countries: comparison of adding meat, soy protein, ascorbic acid, citric acid and ferrous sulphate on iron absorption from a simple Latin American-type of meal. American Journal of Clinical Nutrition 39: 577–583.

Hallberg L, Bengtsson C, Lapidus L, Lindstedt G, Lundberg PA, Hultén L. (1993). Screening for iron deficiency: an analysis based on bone marrow examinations and serum ferritin determinations in a population sample of women. British Journal of Haematology 85: 787–798.

Hallberg L, Hulthén L, Garby L. (1998). Iron stores in man in relation to diet and iron requirements. European Journal of Clinical Nutrition 52: 623–631.

Hansen EH, Imperatore G, Burke W. (2001). HFE Gene and Hereditary hemochromatosis: a huGE review. American Journal of Epidemiology 154: 193–206.

Hastka J, Lasserre JJ, Schwarzbeck A, Strauch M, Hehlmann R. (1992). Washing erythrocytes to remove interferents in measurements of zinc protoporphyrin by front-face hematofluorometry. Clinical Chemistry 38: 2184–2189.

Herbert V. (1987). Nutrition science as a continually unfolding story: the folate and vitamin B_{12} paradigm. American Journal of Clinical Nutrition 46: 387–402.

Huebers HA, Eng MJ, Josephson BM, Ekpoom N, Rettmer RL, Labbe RF, Pootrakul I, Finch CA. (1987). Plasma iron and transferrin iron-binding capacity evaluated by colorimetric and immunoprecipitation methods. Clinical Chemistry 33: 273–277.

Huebers HA, Beguin Y, Pootrakul P, Einspahr D, Finch CA. (1990). Intact transferrin receptors in human plasma and their relation to erythropoiesis. Blood 75: 102–107.

Hurtado A, Merino C, Delgado E. (1945). Influence of anoxemia on the hemopoietic activity. Archives of Internal Medicine 75: 284–323.

ICSH (International Committee for Standardization in Haematology). (1978). Recommendations for measurement of serum iron in human blood. British Journal of Haematology 38: 291–294.

ICSH (International Committee for Standardization in Haematology). (1984). Preparation, characterization, and storage of human ferritin for use as a standard for the assay of serum ferritin. Clinical and Laboratory Haematology 6: 177–191.

ICSH (International Committee for Standardization in Haematology). (1987). Recommendations for reference method for haemoglobinometry in human blood and specifications for international haemoglobin-cyanide reference preparation (3rd edition) Clinical and Laboratory Haematology 9: 73–79.

ICSH (International Committee for Standardization in Haematology). (1988). Expert Panel on Blood Rheology: guidelines on selection of laboratory tests for monitoring the acute phase response. Journal of Clinical Pathology 41: 1203–1212.

ICSH (International Committee for Standardization in Haematology) (1990). Revised recommendations for measurement of serum iron in human blood. British Journal of Haematology 38: 291–294.

IOM (Institute of Medicine). (2001). Dietary Reference Intakes for Vitamin A, Vitamin K, Arsenic, Boron, Chromium, Copper, Iodine, Iron, Manganese, Molybdenum, Nickel, Silicon, Vanadium, and Zinc. National Academy Press, Washington, DC.

Johnson-Spear MA, Yip R. (1994). Hemoglobin difference between black and white women with comparable iron status: justification for race-specific anemia criteria. American Journal of Clinical Nutrition 60: 117–121.

Khusun H, Yip R, Schultink W, Dillon DHS. (1999). World Health Organization hemoglobin cutoff points for the detection of anemia are valid for an Indonesian population. Journal of Nutrition 129: 1669–1674.

Kohgo Y, Nishisato T, Kondo H, Tsushima N, Niitsu Y, Urushizaki I. (1986). Circulating transferrin receptor in human serum. British Journal of Haematology 64: 277–281.

Kuvibidila S, Warrier RP, Ode D, Yu L. (1996). Serum transferrin receptor concentrations in women with mild malnutrition. American Journal of Clinical Nutrition 63: 596–601.

Labbé RF, Dewanji A, McLaughlin K. (1999).Observations on the zinc protoporphyrin/heme ratio in whole blood. Clinical Chemistry 45: 146–148.

Lammi-Keefe CJ, Lickteig ES, Ahluwalia N, Haley NR. (1996). Day-to-day variation in iron status indexes is similar for most measures in elderly women with and without rheumatoid arthritis. Journal of the American Dietetic Association 96: 247–251.

Leggett BA, Brown NN, Bryant SJ, Duplock L, Powell LW, Halliday JW. (1990). Factors affecting the concentrations of ferritin in serum in a healthy Australian population. Clinical Chemistry 36: 1350–1355.

Looker AC, Gunter EW, Johnson CL. (1995). Methods to assess iron status in various NHANES surveys. Nutrition Reviews 53: 246–254.

Looker AC, Dallman PR, Carroll MD, Gunter EW, Johnson CL. (1997). Prevalence of iron deficiency in the United States. Journal of the American Medical Association 277: 973–976.

Lu Y, Lynch SR, Cook JD, Madan N, Bayer WL.

(1987). Use of capillary blood for the evaluation of iron status. American Journal of Hematology 24: 365–374.

Matoth Y, Zaizov R, Varsoni I. (1971). Postnatal changes in some red cell parameters. Acta Paediatrica Scandinavica 60: 317–323.

McLaren GD, Carpenter JT Jr, Nino HV. (1975). Erythrocyte protoporphyrin in the detection of iron deficiency. Clinical Chemistry 21: 1121–1127.

McLennan W, Podger A. (1998). National Nutrition Survey: Nutrient Intakes and Physical Measurements. Australian Bureau of Statistics, Canberra.

Miles LEM, Lipschitz DA, Bieber CP, Cook JD. (1974). Measurement of serum ferritin by a 2-site immunoradiometric assay. Annals of Biochemistry 61: 209–224.

Miret S, Simpson RJ, McKie AT. (2003). Physiology and molecular biology of dietary iron absorption. Annual Review of Nutrition 23: 283–301.

Nestel P. (2002). Adjusting Hemoglobin Values in Program Surveys. International Nutritional Anemia Consultative Group, International Life Sciences Institute, Washington, DC.

Nestel P, Davidsson L. (2002). Anemia, Iron Deficiency, and Iron Deficiency Anemia. International Nutritional Anemia Consultative Group, International Life Sciences Institute, Washington, DC.

NCCLS (National Committee on Clinical Laboratory Standards). (1996). Erythrocyte Protoporphyrin Testing: Approved Guideline. C42-A. NCCLS. Villanova, PA.

Olivares M, Walter T, Cook JD, Hertrampf E, Pizarro F. (2000). Usefulness of serum transferrin receptor and serum ferritin in diagnosis of iron deficiency in infancy. American Journal of Clinical Nutrition 72: 1191–1195.

Osler M, Milman N, Heitmann BL. (1998). Dietary and non-dietary factors associated with iron status in a cohort of Danish adults followed for six years. European Journal of Clinical Nutrition 52: 459–463.

Parnell W, Scragg R, Wilson N, Schaaf D, Fitzgerald E. (2003). NZ Food, NZ Children: Key Results of the 2002 National Childrens Nutrition Survey. Ministry of Health, Wellington, New Zealand.

Pilch SM, Senti FR (eds.) (1984). Assessment of the Iron Nutritional Status of the U.S. Population Based on Data Collected in the Second National Health and Nutrition Examination Survey, 1976–1980. Life Sciences Research Office, Federation of the American Societies for Experimental Biology, Bethesda, MD.

Pilon VA, Howanitz PJ, Howanitz JH, Domres N. (1981). Day-to-day variation in serum ferritin concentrations in healthy subjects. Clinical Chemistry 27: 78–82.

Pootrakul P, Skikne BS, Cook JD. (1983). The use of capillary blood for measurements of circulating ferritin. American Journal of Clinical Nutrition 37: 307–310.

Ramsay WNM. (1997). The determination of the total iron-binding capacity of serum. Clinica Chimica Acta 259: 25–30.

Raper NR, Rosenthal JC, Woteki CE. (1984). Estimates of available iron in diets of individuals 1 year old and older in the Nationwide Food Consumption Survey. Journal of the American Dietetic Association 84: 783–787.

Raya G, Henny J, Steinmatz J, Herbeth B, Siest G. (2001). Soluble transferrin receptor (sTfR): biological variations and reference limits. Clinical Chemistry and Laboratory Medicine 39: 1162–1168.

Remacha AF, Bellido M, Garcia-Die F, Marco N, Ubeda J, Gimferrer E. (1997). Serum erythropoietin and erythroid activity in vitamin B_{12} deficiency. Haematologica 82: 67–68.

Romslo I, Talstad I. (1988). Day-to-day variations in serum iron, serum iron-binding capacity, serum ferritin and erythrocyte protopophyrin concentrations in anaemic subjects. European Journal of Haematology 40: 79–82.

Rusia U, Flowers C, Madan N, Agarwal N, Sood SK, Sikka M. (1996). Serum transferrin receptor levels in the evaluation of iron deficiency in the neonate. Acta Paediatrica Japonica 38: 455–459.

Russell D, Parnell W, Wilson N, Faed J, Ferguson E, Herbison P, Horwath C, Nye T, Walker R, Wilson B. (1999). NZ Food, NZ People: Key Results of the 1997 National Nutrition Survey. Ministry of Health, Wellington, New Zealand.

Sandström B, Davidsson L, Cederblad A, Lönnerdal B. (1985). Oral iron, dietary ligands and zinc absorption. Journal of Nutrition 115: 411–414.

Segall ML, Heese HV, Dempster WS. (1979). Estimation of serum ferritin in blood obtained by heelstick. Journal of Pediatrics 95: 65–67.

Simmons WK, Cook JD, Bingham KC, Thomas M, Jackson J, Jackson M, Ahluwalia N, Kahn SG, Patterson AW. (1993). Evaluation of a gastric delivery system for iron supplementation in pregnancy. American Journal of Clinical Nutrition 58: 622–626.

Skikne BS, Flowers CH, Cook JD. (1990). Serum transferrin receptor: a quantitative measure of tissue iron deficiency. Blood 75: 1870–1876.

Statland BE, Winkel P. (1977). Relationship of day-to-day variation of serum iron concentrations to iron-binding capacity in healthy young women. American Journal of Clinical Pathology 67: 84–90.

Statland BE, Winkel P, Bokieland H. (1976). Variation of serum iron concentration in young healthy men: within-day and day-to-day changes. Clinical Biochemistry 9: 26–29.

Statland BE, Winkel P, Harris SC, Burdsall MJ, Saunders AM. (1978). Evaluation of biologic sources of variation of leukocyte counts and other hematologic quantities using very precise automated analyzers. American Journal of Clinical Pathology 69: 48–54.

Stoltzfus RJ, Dreyfuss ML. (1998). Guidelines for the Use of Iron Supplements to Prevent and Treat Iron Deficiency Anemia: International Nutritional

Anemia Consultative Group (INACG), World Health Organization (WHO), United Nations Children's Fund (UNICEF). International Life Sciences Institute Press, Washington, DC.

Stoltzfus RJ, Chwaya HM, Montresor A, Albonico M, Savioli L, Tielsch JM. (2000). Malaria, hookworms and recent fever are related to anemia and iron status indicators in 0-to 5-y old Zanzibari children and these relationships change with age. Journal of Nutrition 130: 1724–1733.

Thompson D, Milford-Ward A, Whicher JT. (1992). The value of acute phase protein measurements in clinical practice. Annals of Clinical Biochemistry 29: 123–131.

Tietz NW, Rinker AD, Morrison SR. (1996). When is a serum iron really a serum iron? A follow-up study on the status of iron measurements in serum. Clinical Chemistry 42: 109–111.

Tuomainen T, Nyyssonen K, Salonen R, Tervahauta A, Korpela H, Lakka T, Kaplan GA, Salonen J. (1997). Body iron stores are associated with serum insulin and blood glucose concentrations. Population study in 1,013 eastern Finnish men. Diabetes Care 20: 426–428.

USDA (U.S. Department of Agriculture). (2003). USDA National Nutrient Database for Standard Reference. Release 16. Nutrient Data Laboratory (http://www.nal.usda.gov/fnic/foodcomp/)

van den Broek NR, Letsky EA. (2000). Etiology of anemia in pregnancy in south Malawi. American Journal of Clinical Nutrition 247S–256S.

van den Broek NR, Letsky EA, White SA, Shenkin A. (1998). Iron status in pregnant women: which measurements are valid? British Journal of Haematology 103: 817–824.

Virtanen MA, Viinikka LU, Virtanen MKG, Svahn JC, Anttila RM, Krusius T, Cook JD, Axelsson IEM, Räihä NCR, Siimes MA. (1999). Higher concentrations of serum transferrin receptor in children than in adults. American Journal of Clinical Nutrition 69: 256–260.

von Schenck H, Falkensson M, Lundberg B. (1986). Evaluation of "HemoCue," a new device for determining hemoglobin. Clinical Chemistry 332: 526–529.

WHO/UNICEF/UNU (World Health Organization / United Nations Childrens Fund / United Nations University) (2001). Iron deficiency anaemia, assessment, prevention and control: a guide for programme managers. WHO/NHD/01.3. World Health Organization, Geneva.

Wians FH Jr, Urban JE, Kroft SH, Keffer JH. (2001). Soluble transferrin receptor (sTfR) concentration quantified using two sTfR kits: analytical and clinical performance characteristics. Clinica Chimica Acta 303: 75–81.

Williams TN, Maitland K, Rees DC, Peto TEA, Bowden DK, Weatherall DJ, Clegg JB. (1999). Reduced soluble transferrin receptor concentrations in acute malaria in Vanuatu. American Journal of Tropical Medicine and Hygiene

Wintrobe MM, Lee GR, Boggs DR, Bithell TC, Foerster J, Athens JW, Lukens JN (eds.) (1981). Clinical Hematology. 8th ed. Lea & Febiger, Philadelphia.

Worwood M. (1979). Serum ferritin. CRC Critical Reviews in Clinical Laboratory Sciences 10: 171–204.

Worwood M. (1996). The importance of standardization of methodology for determination of iron status. In: Hallberg L, Asp N-G (eds.) Iron Nutrition in Health and Disease. John Libbey and Co, London, pp. 75–79.

Worwood M. (1997). The laboratory assessment of iron status — an update. Clinica Chimica Acta 259: 3–23.

Worwood M. (2002). Serum transferrin receptor assays and their application. Annals of Clinical Biochemistry 39: 221–230.

Yeung GS, Zlotkin SH. (1997). Percentile estimates for transferrin receptors in normal infants 9–15 mo of age. American Journal of Clinical Nutrition 66: 342–346.

Yip R, Dallman PR. (1996). Iron. In: Ziegler EE, Filer LJ (eds.) Present Knowledge in Nutrition. 7th ed. International Life Sciences Institute Press, Washington, DC. pp. 277–292.

Yip R, Johnson C, Dallman PR. (1984). Age-related changes in laboratory values used in the diagnosis of anemia and iron deficiency. American Journal of Clinical Nutrition 39: 427–436.

Yip R, Stoltzfus RJ, Simmons WK. (1996). Assessment of the prevalence and the nature of iron deficiency for populations: the utility of comparing haemoglobin distributions. In: Hallberg L, Asp N-G (eds.) Iron Nutrition in Health and Disease. John Libbey and Co, London. pp. 31–48.

Zacharski LR, Ornstein DL, Woloshin S, Schwartz LM. (2000). Association of age, sex, and race with body iron stores in adults: analysis of NHANES III data. American Heart Journal 140: 98–104.

Zak B, Baginski ES, Epstein E. (1980). Modern iron ligands useful for the measurement of serum iron. Annals of Clinical and Laboratory Science 10: 276–289.

Zhu YI, Haas JD. (1998). Response of serum transferrin receptor to iron supplementation in iron-depleted, nonanemic women. American Journal of Clinical Nutrition 67: 271–275.

18

Assessment of the status of vitamins A, D, and E

The three vitamins A, D, and E are similar, with a structure based on the isoprene unit: [–CH$_2$–C(CH$_3$)=CH–CH$_2$)–]. They are all fat-soluble vitamins. Vitamin A and E can be stored in the body, mainly in the liver and adipose tissue, respectively. In contrast, very little vitamin D is stored, but it is readily synthesized by the action of ultraviolet light on a precursor of vitamin D present in the skin.

Generally, deficiencies of vitamin A, D, and E develop more slowly than those for the water-soluble vitamins; secondary deficiencies may occur in patients with malabsorption syndromes and other disease states and in association with certain drug therapies.

Vitamin A has physiological functions related to vision, bone growth, differentiation of epithelial tissues, embryonic development, and immune function. Vitamin D, following hydroxylation to a biologically active form, is involved in calcium metabolism, whereas vitamin E acts as a nonspecific lipid antioxidant.

Major food sources of vitamins A and D include liver and fish liver oils; precursors of vitamin A also occur in plants and oils as pro-vitamin A carotenoids. Vegetable and seed oils are important sources of vitamin E.

The status of vitamins A, D, and E is generally assessed by measurement of the vitamins and/or their metabolites in serum. High-performance liquid chromatography (HPLC) is the preferred method of analysis. Urinary excretion of metabolites is not used because their concentrations do not reflect the status of these fat-soluble vitamins. Several functional physiological tests are also available for assessing vitamin A and E status, some of which have been modified for use in field studies. Comparable tests for vitamin D are not currently available.

Vitamin K, another fat-soluble vitamin, is not considered in this chapter because a primary nutritional deficiency is very rare. Some newborn infants may be at risk because vitamin K is poorly transported across the placenta. However, in most western countries, infants routinely receive vitamin K either intramuscularly or orally within 6 h of birth (IOM, 2002). Vitamin K functions as a coenzyme in the synthesis of the active form of several proteins involved in blood coagulation and bone metabolism. Phylloquinone, the major form of vitamin K in the diet in western countries, is widely distributed in plant and animal tissues and is synthesized by the microbiological flora of the normal gut. Deficiency of vitamin K may be secondary to some disease states (e.g., biliary obstruction, liver disease, and malabsorption syndromes). Broad-spectrum antibiotics which destroy the intestinal flora, or anticoagulant drugs, may also produce secondary vitamin K deficiency. New HPLC techniques can be used for the direct determination of plasma or serum phylloquinone. More often, functional tests, such as the prothrombin time or the assessment of the plasma procoagulant factor VII activity, are used to assess vitamin K status, but neither of these tests responds to changes in vitamin K intakes in healthy subjects (Bach et al., 1996).

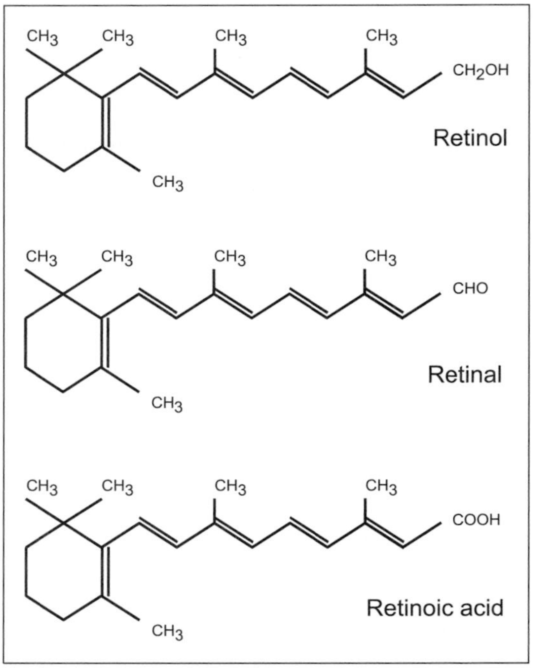

Figure 18.1: The various forms of vitamin A: retinol, retinal, and retinoic acid.

18.1 Vitamin A

Vitamin A is a generic term for all retinoids that qualitatively exhibit the biological activity of all-*trans* retinol. The various biologically active forms of vitamin A are shown in Figure 18.1. Certain carotenoids have provitamin A activity. Of these, β-carotene is the most biologically active and the most widely distributed in plant products.

Functions of vitamin A

Vitamin A has a clearly defined role in vision: when retinal tissue is deprived of vitamin A, rod and cone function is impaired. However, only the biochemical role of the 11-*cis* retinaldehyde form of vitamin A, in the visual process in rod cells, has been studied in detail. Vitamin A is also required for the integrity of epithelial cells throughout the body, via the regulatory action of retinoic acid at the level of the gene. In addition, retinoic acid has an important role in embryonic development, as well as in the maintenance of

immune function. Both cell-mediated immunity and systemic and mucosal humoral immunity are affected. A review by Gerster (1997) outlines the various functions of vitamin A

Vitamin A deficiency in humans

Early signs of vitamin A deficiency in humans include growth failure, loss of appetite, and impaired immune response with lowered resistance to infection. Night blindness develops when liver reserves of vitamin A are nearly exhausted. Later, ocular lesions such as conjunctival xerosis, Bitot's spots, keratomalacia, and xerophthalmia may occur.

Xerophthalmia and vitamin A deficiency blindness are endemic in many parts of southern and eastern Asia, parts of Latin America, and in many countries in Africa and the Middle East. The International Vitamin A Consultative Group (IVACG) have recently defined vitamin A deficiency disorders as

> any health and physiological consequences attributable to vitamin A deficiency, irrespective of whether there is any clinical evidence of deficiency.

Hence, the definition includes both clinical manifestations — xerophthalmia, anemia, growth retardation, increased infectious morbidity and mortality — as well as the following functional consequences: impaired iron mobilization, disturbed cellular differentiation, and depressed immune response (Sommer and Davidson, 2002).

Severe deficiencies of certain other nutrients may also simulate vitamin A deficiency. Examples include zinc (Christian and West, 1998) and protein-energy malnutrition (Russell et al., 1983); details are given in Section 18.1.1.

Vitamin A deficiency may occur secondary to some disease states, including cystic fibrosis, severe intestinal and liver diseases, and some severe defects in lipid absorption (e.g., cholestasis). In developed countries, the prevalence of frank nutritional deficiency of vitamin A is low. In the most recent U.S. National Health and Nutrition Examination Survey (NHANES III), for example, the prevalence of low serum retinol concentrations ($< 0.70\,\mu mol/L$) was less than 2% in all age, sex, race or ethnic strata, although from 17% to 34% of the children had serum retinol levels $<1.05\,\mu mol/L$, indicative of potentially suboptimal vitamin A status (Ballew et al., 2001a). These findings are of concern because serum retinol concentrations may be related to cancer risk (Willett et al., 1984; Reichman et al., 1990; Nagata et al., 1999).

Food sources and dietary intakes

Preformed vitamin A is found only in foods of animal origin: fish-liver oils, liver, butterfat, and egg yolk are major sources. Muscle meats are poor sources of preformed vitamin A, and nuts, grains, and vegetable oils have none.

Provitamin A carotenoids are found in both plant and animal products, but in low-income countries the main food sources are yellow- and orange-colored fruits (West, 2000) and dark-green leafy vegetables. Red palm oil, and certain indigenous plants such as palm fruits (buriti) in Latin America, and the fruit termed "gac" in Vietnam, are unusually rich sources of provitamin A carotenoids (FAO/WHO, 2002).

Provitamin A carotenoids, when derived from ripe yellow- and orange-colored fruits and cooked yellow tubers (e.g., sweet potatoes), appear to be more efficiently converted to retinol than when derived from dark green leafy vegetables, as noted previously (Sections 4.4.5 and 4.8.8) (IOM, 2001; West et al., 2002). Processing methods and the food matrix also affect the bioavailability of provitamin A carotenoids (Torronen et al., 1996; Rock et al., 1998; van het Hof et al., 1998).

In more affluent countries such as Canada, the United States, and the United Kingdom, the major sources of preformed vitamin A in the diet are liver and milk and milk products, followed by fish in the United States and Canada (IOM, 2001), and fat spreads (e.g., fortified margarine) in the United Kingdom (Gregory et al., 1990). The major contributors of provitamin A carotenoids are generally vegetables (Gregory et al., 1990; Chug-Ahuja et al., 1993).

Currently there is lack of consensus on the most appropriate conversion factors to use for calculating the amount of vitamin A activity in foods (Section 4.4.5). The U.S. Food and Nutrition Board and the IVACG have concluded that the bioavailability of provitamin A β-carotene from plant sources is only half of that previously assumed (IOM, 2002; IVACG, 2002). Vitamin A intakes calculated from current food composition data are likely to be overestimated if the lower bioconversion factors for provitamin A carotenoids have been used.

Effects of high intakes

Suggestions that vitamin A and its carotenoid precursors are cancer-preventive agents have led to increased consumption of large doses of vitamin A. This is a serious health hazard, particularly during pregnancy: hypervitaminosis A has been associated with birth defects (Rothman et al., 1995; Azais-Braesco and Pascal, 2000). Clinical manifestations of vitamin A toxicity include a pseudobrain tumor, skeletal pain, desquamating dermatitis, and hepatic inflammation (Frame et al., 1974; Russell, 2000). Concomitant consumption of ethanol appears to enhance the toxicity of vitamin A (Leo and Lieber, 1999).

A U.S. Tolerable Upper Intake Level (UL) has not been set for β-carotene or carotenoids (IOM, 2000), although β-carotene supplements are not advised for the general population. For preformed vitamin A, the U.S. UL varies according to life-stage group, ranging from 600 μg/d for infants to 2,800 μg/d for adolescents. For nonpregnant, pregnant, and lactating women, the UL is 3000 μg/d (IOM, 2001).

The U.S. UL is not applicable to vitamin A-deficient populations who should receive vitamin A prophylactically. In such cases, the IVACG (Sommer and Davidson, 2002) endorses the following recommendations for routine high-dose vitamin A supplementation in developing countries. For infants 0–5 mo, 150,000 International Units (IU) as three doses of 50,000 IU with at least 1-mo interval between doses, whereas for infants 6–11 mo, 100,000 IU should be given as a single dose every 4–6 mo. Children aged 12 mo and older should receive 200,000 IU as a single dose every 4–6 mo. IVACG (2002) also recommends that postpartum women should receive 400,000 IU as two doses of 200,000 IU at least 1 d apart, as soon as possible after delivery and not more than 6 wk later, or 10,000 IU daily or 25,000 IU weekly during the first 6 mo after delivery.

Indices of vitamin A status

Most of the vitamin A in the body is stored in the form of retinyl ester in the liver. Therefore, a measure of liver vitamin A stores is the best index of vitamin A nutriture. Indeed, the conventional definition of vitamin A deficiency is when liver stores of retinol are below 0.07 µmol/g (Sommer and Davidson, 2002). Unfortunately, however, vitamin A is not uniformly distributed in the liver (Olson et al., 1979), and liver biopsies are impractical in population studies. Instead, total serum vitamin A, or more recently, serum retinol concentrations are more often determined. However, the serum or plasma contains only about 1% of the total body reserve of vitamin A, and concentrations do not reflect body stores until they are severely depleted or excessively high. Consequently, it is best to use other biochemical and physiological functional tests of vitamin A status in combination with serum retinol levels. In the future, the validity of these tests will probably be assessed through estimates of total body vitamin A stores derived from stable isotope dilution methods. Details of tests currently used are given in WHO (1996) and are discussed briefly in the following sections.

18.1.1 Serum retinol

Vitamin A in the serum circulates largely in the form of a 1:1 complex of retinol and retinol-binding protein (RBP); the remainder is in the form of retinyl ester (approximately

8%) and very small amounts of retinoic acid and other metabolites (Olson, 1984). Until recently, total serum vitamin A, rather than retinol, was assayed. Results for the two assays are comparable for levels <1.2 µmol/L (Driskell et al., 1982). At higher concentrations, the discrepancy between the assays is greater, with total serum vitamin A about 0.14 µmol/L higher than serum retinol.

Serum retinol levels reflect the vitamin A status only when liver vitamin A stores are severely depleted (<0.07 µmol/g liver) or excessively high (>1.05 µmol/g liver) (Figure 18.2). When liver vitamin A concentrations are between these limits, serum retinol concentrations are homeostatically controlled and levels remain relatively constant and do not reflect total body reserves of vitamin A (Olson, 1984). Hence, it is not surprising that in populations from developed countries, such as the United States, where the liver vitamin A concentrations are generally within these limits, positive relationships between serum retinol concentrations and usual intakes of vitamin A are rare (Hallfrisch et al., 1994; Nierenberg et al., 1997).

Functional impairment has been seen in malnourished children with extremely low serum vitamin A values. For example, results in India (Pirie and Anbunathan, 1981)

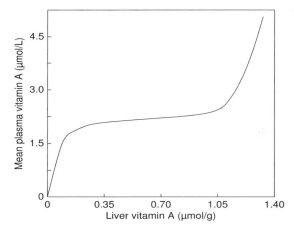

Figure 18.2: Hypothetical relationship between mean plasma vitamin A levels and liver vitamin A concentrations. From: Olson, Journal of the National Cancer Institute 73: 1439–1444, 1984, with permission of Oxford University Press.

	n	Percent with serum Vit A		
		<0.35 μmol/L	0.35–0.69 μmol/L	⩾0.7 μmol/L
Normal children	252	8	37	55
Night-blindness or Bitot's spots	325	30	55	15
Corneal xerophthalmia	98	75	24	1

Table 18.1: Serum vitamin A levels (μmol/L) in a sample of Indonesian children with and without ocular lesions. Compiled from Sommer et al., American Journal of Clinical Nutrition 33: 887–891, 1980 © Am J Clin Nutr. American Society for Clinical Nutrition.

and Indonesia (Sommer, 1982) showed that at least 75% of the children with corneal xerophthalmia had serum vitamin A levels < 0.35 μmol/L. In contrast, in a sample of 252 clinically normal Indonesian children, only 8% had serum vitamin A at this low level (Table 18.1).

A cutoff for serum vitamin A levels of < 0.70 μmol/L is a less specific measure of vitamin A deficiency; its ability to predict a deficiency of the vitamin varies widely by region, probably depending on the presence and severity of other risk factors such as infection. For example, in Sri Lanka, serum vitamin A levels < 0.70 μmol/L were found in only 28% of children ($n = 29$) with clinical signs of vitamin A deficiency (Bitot's spots, corneal scars, or blindness) and in 5% of the children without positive eye findings (Brink et al., 1979). In Indonesia, 85% of children < 6 y ($n = 325$) with either night blindness or Bitot's spots had serum vitamin A levels < 0.70 μmol/L (Sommer et al., 1980). In contrast, 28% of the children with eye findings and 48% of the children without eye findings had serum vitamin A concentrations > 1.05 μmol/L. Additional tests may therefore be required to confirm vitamin A depletion at the individual level when a cutoff of < 0.70 μmol/L is used. At a population level, however, a cutoff of < 0.70 μmol/L can be used to indicate whether vitamin A deficiency is likely to be public health problem.

Factors affecting serum retinol concentrations

Age, sex, and race influence levels, as indicated by the NHANES II and NHANES III results (Pilch, 1985; Stephensen and Gildengorin, 2000; Ballew et al., 2001a). African American children and adolescents had lower serum retinol levels than Caucasians (Ballew et al., 2001a; Neuhouser et al. 2001). In the U.K. National Diet and Nutrition Survey of young people, mean values increased with increasing age in both boys and girls (Gregory et al., 2000). In the U.K. Survey of British Adults, mean values were highest for males and females aged 50–64 y (Gregory et al., 1990). Age-specific criteria should always be used when interpreting serum retinol concentrations.

Low fat diets (i.e., < 5 to 10 g daily) impair the absorption of provitamin A carotenoids (Jayarajan et al., 1980), and over the longer term lower plasma retinol concentrations. In contrast, the ingestion of meals containing relatively large amounts of either dietary or supplemental vitamin A during the previous 4 h does not alter serum retinol concentrations in children or adults (Mejia and Arroyave, 1983; Mejia et al., 1984). Consequently, the collection of fasting blood samples is not necessary for serum retinol determinations.

Other nutrient deficiencies can affect serum retinol concentrations. Protein-energy malnutrition decreases liver apo-retinol binding protein (RBP) production because of a limited supply of protein substrate (Russell et al., 1983). Consequently, hepatic release of vitamin A is impaired, resulting in decreased serum retinol levels, despite the presence of adequate vitamin A stores in the liver. Zinc deficiency decreases serum retinol levels via its role in the hepatic synthesis or secretion of RBP, again even in the presence of adequate liver vitamin A stores (Christian and West, 1998).

Disease may significantly alter serum retinol levels. Chronic renal disease increases serum

Vit. A μmol/L	Age 3–11 y	Age 12–17 y	Age 18–74 y
< 0.35	Vitamin A status is very likely to improve with increased consumption of vitamin A. Impairment of function is likely.		
< 0.70	Vitamin A status is likely to improve with increased consumption of vitamin A	Vitamin A status is likely to improve with increased consumption of vitamin A; some individuals might exhibit impairment of function.	Vitamin A status is likely to improve with increased consumption of vitamin A; impairment of function is likely.
0.70–1.05	Vitamin A status of some subjects may improve with increased consumption of vitamin A. Improvement is most likely in those with values 0.70–0.95 μmol/L.	Vitamin A status may improve with increased consumption of vitamin A. Improvement is more likely in those with values 0.70–0.95 μmol/L.	Vitamin A status may improve with increased consumption of vitamin A. Some individuals may exhibit impairment of function.

Table 18.2: Cutoff points recommended by the NHANES II committee for interpreting low serum total vitamin A concentrations in three age categories. Vitamin A status refers to serum and tissue levels of the nutrient. Impairment of function may include impaired dark adaptation, night blindness, and ocular lesions. From Pilch (1985).

retinol concentrations by reducing catabolism of vitamin A and its carriers. In contrast, liver disease decreases serum retinol levels, probably as a result of a combination of decreased synthesis and secretion of RBP. Cystic fibrosis is also associated with decreased levels of circulating retinol and RBP, probably because of a defect in the transport of vitamin A from the hepatic stores to the periphery.

Infections including HIV (Kafwembe et al., 2001), measles (Thurnham., 1997), and parasitic infections (e.g., malaria and *Ascaris lumbricoides*) are associated with low serum retinol levels, in some cases because of malabsorption of vitamin A (Sivakumar and Reddy, 1972, 1975). Infections may also cause low serum retinol as a result of transient decreases in the concentrations of acute-phase proteins, RBP, and transthyretin, even in the presence of adequate liver vitamin A stores. In NHANES III, inflammation, indicated by a serum C-reactive protein concentration above 10 mg/L, was associated with lower serum retinol concentrations. This, in turn, led to misclassification of vitamin A status (Stephensen and Gildengorin, 2000). The confounding effect of the acute-phase response on serum retinol was not evaluated

in earlier NHANES investigations. Clearly, it is important to include a measure of this response to interpret serum retinol concentrations correctly.

Estrogens, either endogenous or those used in contraceptive agents or hormone replacement therapy, increase serum retinol and RBP apparently as a result of increased mobilization of vitamin A from the liver.

Interpretive criteria

Age-specific cutoff points for serum retinol concentrations developed for NHANES II are shown in Table 18.2 (Pilch, 1985). These same cutoffs were used for the interpretation of the serum vitamin A values in the Hispanic Health and Nutrition Examination Survey (HHANES) and in NHANES III (Ballew et al., 2001a). In the latter survey, the prevalence of serum retinol < 0.70 μmol/L was very low for all age and sex groups. However, the prevalence of potentially suboptimal concentrations of serum retinol, defined as < 1.05 μmol/L, was high among certain minority groups of children. Racial and ethnic differences were significant, even after controlling for confounding factors; non-Hispanic African American and Mexican American children were more at risk than were non-Hispanic Caucasian children.

The U.S. serum retinol cutoff points used for NHANES III are based on their relationship with functional indices of vitamin A deficiency, such as impaired dark adaptation, night blindness, ocular lesions, and possibly impaired immune function and on the serum vitamin A distributions from the earlier NHANES investigations (Pilch, 1985). It is not known if these cutoffs are appropriate for other countries.

Both WHO (1996) and IVACG (de Pee and Dary, 2002) chose a single cutoff for serum retinol concentrations of < 0.70 μmol/L as indicative of a low vitamin A status for children 6–71 mo. This cutoff should not be applied to infants < 6 mo but is otherwise considered to be independent of age and is applied irrespective of the prevalence of infection in a particular population.

WHO (1996) has also proposed that prevalence levels of serum retinol concentrations < 0.70 μmol/L be used to indicate the possible presence of a public health problem. These define whether vitamin A is either a mild (2% to <10% prevalence), moderate (10% to < 20% prevalence), or severe (>20% prevalence) public health problem. In contrast, IVACG recommend only one level (i.e., ⩾15% prevalence) as indicating a likely public health problem (de Pee and Dary, 2002; Sommer and Davidson, 2002).

Data for mean and selected percentiles for serum retinol concentrations classified by age, sex, and race or ethnicity for NHANES III are presented in Ballew et al. (2001a) and IOM (2001). A subset of this information is shown in Appendix A18.1. Serum retinol concentrations were also determined in the U.K. national surveys (Gregory et al., 1990, 1995, 2000; Finch et al., 1998). Mean, median, and lower and upper 2.5th or 5th percentiles by age and sex are given.

Measurement of serum retinol

Special precautions must be taken in the preparation and storage of serum samples for vitamin A and retinol. Serum should be centrifuged soon after the blood is drawn, where possible, and hemolysis and exposure to bright light should be avoided. If separation is not possible within a short time period, then the blood sample should be stored in an icebox at ice temperature (Mejia and Arroyave, 1983). If serum is to be stored for prolonged periods of time prior to analysis, it should be quickly frozen in temperature-resistant tubes, and then flushed with argon or oxygen-free nitrogen. The tubes should be closed tightly with a screw top, and only a small gas space should be left within the tube. Tubes should be stored, together with a reference serum sample, in the dark at temperatures below −70°C (Olson, 1984). Thawing and refreezing should be kept to a minimum.

Several methods are available for the analysis of total serum vitamin A or retinol. Only high-performance liquid chromatography can distinguish retinol from the retinyl esters. All the other methods measure total serum vitamin A and generally give comparable results, provided that conditions of collection, storage, and analysis are clearly controlled.

A standard reference material (SRM 968: Fat-Soluble Vitamins in Human Serum) is available from the National Institute of Standards and Technology (NIST) (Gaithersburg, MD) which is certified for both retinol and retinyl palmitate (Appendix A4.1). The within-subject daily CV for serum retinol for subjects following their normal dietary pattern was 11.3% (Gallagher et al., 1992).

High-performance liquid chromatography

(HPLC) is the method of choice for the separation and analysis of serum retinol because it has the required precision at low concentrations (de Pee and Dary, 2002). It is also specific and easy to use (WHO, 1996). Usually 100–200 μL of serum or plasma are required for analysis. Either reverse- (Bieri et al., 1979; Furr et al., 1984) or normal-phase (Bankson et al., 1986) HPLC is used. The former technique is preferred for serum and was used in NHANES III (Ballew et al., 2001a).

All interfering compounds, such as retinyl

esters and phytofluene, can be separated from retinol using HPLC. Moreover, hemolysis does not affect serum retinol concentrations measured by HPLC (Marinovic et al., 1997).

Fluorometric methods based on the direct measurement of fluorescence of the retinol-binding complex are used for measuring total serum vitamin A. They are highly sensitive and simple, and critical timing is not necessary. Nevertheless, other highly fluorescent substances, particularly phytofluene and phytoene, interfere but can be removed by column chromatography. Alternatively, a correction factor can be used (Thompson et al., 1971). Severe but not moderate hemolysis may also be a confounding factor which could lead to serum vitamin A concentrations being underestimated (Marinovic et al., 1997).

A portable fluorometer optimized for vitamin A fluorescence that operates from a direct current power supply (battery, automobile cigarette lighter, or AC/DC power supply) has been developed for field use. It weighs less than 6 kg, has no moving parts and uses a cuvet-shaped fluorescent calibration block. Use of this instrument eliminates the necessity for the transport and storage of samples, and can generate immediate results provided a portable centrifuge is also available. It also reduces the cost of serum retinol analyses (Craft, 2001).

Dried blood spots (DBS) can be used for the measurement of retinol (Erhardt et al., 2002a). Positive correlations have been recorded between retinol concentrations in dried blood spots and conventional plasma samples (Figure 18.3, Craft et al., 2000). Blood should be collected from a fingerprick onto filter paper (Schleicher and Schuell 903 specimen collection paper), dried for 3 h in the dark, and stored with a desiccant in the dark in bags and at room temperature (i.e., up to 25°C) before analysis. Storage under humid conditions causes loss of retinol in DBS and should be avoided.

Extraction of the DBS retinol can be followed by analysis using normal-phase HPLC with a highly sensitive detector. To reduce

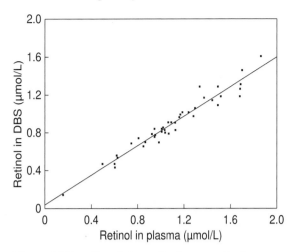

Figure 18.3: Correlation of plasma retinol concentrations with dried blood spot (DBS) retinol concentrations ($n = 46$). DBS retinol was measured after at least 1 wk of storage at room temperature. Data from Erhardt et al., Journal of Nutrition 132: 318–321, 2002, with permission of the American Society for Nutritional Sciences.

the variability of the method, it is recommended that the individual volume of the spots be taken into account by measuring their sodium content by flame photometry or by weighing the blood spots before extraction. The method has been used on blood spot samples from India, Nepal, Nicaragua, Indonesia, and Guatemala.

18.1.2 Serum retinol-binding protein

Retinol-binding protein (RBP) is a specific vitamin A transport protein. It is called holo-RBP when it is bound to retinol; the portion without retinol is called apo-RBP. If the liver becomes depleted in retinol, as occurs in the late stages of vitamin A deficiency, RBP accumulates in the liver as apo-RBP, and levels of both serum retinol and RBP decline.

Retinol binding protein has a single high-affinity binding site for a molecule of retinol. The resultant complex of RBP + retinol, together with one molecule of plasma transthyretin, form a trimolecular complex. Thus, the molar ratio of retinol to RBP in circulation is about one to one. Concentrations of serum RBP may thus be used as a surrogate measure for serum retinol. The assay of RBP is particularly useful in populations where resources and technical support are limited: sample collection and the analytical procedures are easier and cheaper than for serum retinol, and the analysis can be performed on serum from a fingerprick blood sample.

Several studies have confirmed the positive correlation of serum retinol and serum RBP (Solomons et al., 1990; Almekinder et al., 2000; Hix et al., 2004). In a study in the Republic of the Marshall Islands of children who were deficient in vitamin A, Gamble et al. (2001) showed significant correlations between serum retinol and serum RBP ($r = 0.94$) across all retinol concentrations. Severe vitamin A deficiency (serum retinol $< 0.35\,\mu mol/L$) was predicted with a 96% sensitivity and 91% specificity using serum RBP $\leqslant 0.48\,\mu mol/L$ as the cutoff, and more moderate vitamin A deficiency (serum retinol $<0.70\,\mu mol/L$) with 87% sensitivity and 98% specificity using a serum RBP cutoff of $\leqslant 0.70\,\mu mol/L$. Hence, the measurement of serum RBP concentrations appeared to be a practical alternative to using serum retinol in this population. Similar findings were noted for pregnant women in Malawi (Almekinder et al., 2000).

Nevertheless, a variety of factors may influence the binding of RBP to retinol. These include the presence and magnitude of the acute-phase response, protein-energy malnutrition, liver disease, and chronic renal failure. To overcome these confounding effects, use of the ratio of serum RBP : transthyretin (TTR) has been proposed (Rosales and Ross, 1998; Rosales et al., 2002). Transthyretin is unaffected by vitamin A status but, like RBP and serum retinol, decreases in infection and trauma. Hence, theoretically, the ratio of RBP : TTR should decline during vitamin A deficiency but not during an acute-phase response, thus enabling these two conditions to be distinguished. Indeed, Rosales et al. (2002) suggest that a cutoff value of $\leqslant 0.36$ for RBP : TTR is indicative of marginal vitamin A deficiency. However, use of this ratio has been questioned (Filteau et al., 2000), and more research on the use of the RBP : TTR ratio is warranted.

Interpretive criteria for RBP

There is no consensus on a cutoff value for RBP equivalent to a serum retinol concentration of $< 0.70\,\mu mol/L$ (de Pee and Dary, 2002). More research on the relationship of serum RBP and serum retinol concentrations in populations with a range of serum retinol concentrations is required before such a cutoff can be defined. In the interim, investigators are advised to first establish the relationship between serum retinol and serum RBP in a subsample of the population under study before using serum RBP as a surrogate for serum retinol levels. This is especially important during pregnancy, when both the transport and the metabolism of RBP are altered (Sapin et al., 2000).

Measurement of RBP

Retinol-binding protein, unlike serum retinol, is not photosensitive and is less temperature sensitive and more stable during refrigeration — all attributes that facilitate its use in field surveys.

The RBP assay can be performed using a specific and sensitive radioimmunoassay procedure in which the RBP is bound to radioactively labeled antibodies. This method has a lower limit of detection of 0.5 nmol/L (Blaner, 1990; Rosales, 1998). Alternatively, a new rapid quantitative enzyme immunoassay (EIA) can be used that has an average intra- and interassay variability of 6.7% and 8.0%, respectively (Hix et al., 2004). Tests indicate that this new RBP EIA correlates well with serum retinol measured by HPLC. The commercial radial immunodiffusion kits are simple to use and require the minimum of equipment, but are vulnerable to inter-examiner error. Positive correlations between serum RBP measured by radial immuno-diffusion and EIA have been reported (Hix et al., 2004). Nephelometry can also be used to measure serum RBP but the equipment needed is expensive (Malvy et al., 1993).

An EIA method is also being developed to measure RBP in dried blood spots. The kit contains three calibrants over the deficient to normal range for RBP. In the future, it may become feasible to measure RBP directly in a drop of whole blood using a portable fluorometer in the field (Craft, 2001).

18.1.3 Serum retinyl ester

In normal healthy persons, retinyl esters constitute less than 5% of the total vitamin A content of fasting serum samples. However, when the capacity of the liver to store vitamin A is exceeded — for example, after the chronic ingestion of excessive amounts of vitamin A (hypervitaminosis A), or in liver disease — vitamin A is released into the circulation as retinyl esters, and then elevated concentrations of serum retinyl esters are observed. For example, in three patients with hypervitaminosis A, retinyl esters made up 67%, 65%, and 33% of the total vitamin A present in the plasma (Smith and Goodman, 1976).

A cutoff point of retinyl esters >10% of total vitamin A is said to reflect potential hypervitaminosis. Ballew et al. (2001b) studied the validity of this cutoff by examining the distribution of concentrations of serum retinyl esters in samples from NHANES III. They noted that 37% of the sample of adults aged ≥18 y had serum retinyl ester concentrations above the cutoff point, but they were unable to find any associations between serum retinyl ester concentrations and five biochemical indices of liver dysfunction.

Fasting blood samples are essential for serum retinyl ester measurements as concentrations rise transiently after the ingestion of a vitamin A–rich meal or of vitamin A supplements. Measurement of retinyl ester concentrations in serum is best performed using normal-phase HPLC, when the low levels in fasting serum can be measured concurrently with serum retinol concentrations.

18.1.4 Serum carotenoids

Approximately 50 carotenoids show provitamin A activity and provide about 50% of the total vitamin A intake in the United States, as well as larger percentages in Asia, Africa, and parts of South America. In those countries where dietary carotenoids from plants are the major source of vitamin A and where dietary patterns are relatively constant, serum carotenoids may serve as a useful secondary index of vitamin A intake. For populations receiving most of their vitamin A from animal sources, serum carotenoid concentrations provide no information on vitamin A status.

Major components of serum carotenoids are β-carotene, lycopene, and some hydroxylated carotenoids. Serum carotenoids are of increasing interest because of their possible antioxidant properties and their relationship to the risk of certain cancers, cardiovascular disease, macular degeneration, and the onset of cataracts (Omenn et al., 1996).

Unfortunately, several non-nutritional factors are known to influence serum carotenoid concentrations, including age, sex, alcohol intake, physiological state, body mass index, and season (Brady et al., 1996; Neuhouser et al., 2001). Smoking may also modify the relationship of dietary β-carotene and serum β-carotene levels (Järvinen et al., 1993).

Serum carotenoids were measured following NHANES III (Appendix A18.2). Ford (2000) and Ford et al. (2002) measured serum concentrations of α-carotene, β-cryptoxanthin, lutein, zeaxanthin, and lycopene in samples from NHANES III and presented data for the mean and selected percentiles by age, sex, and race or ethnicity. Serum carotenoid concentrations were not uniformly distributed among the population groups. Children, adolescents, and adults of African descent had the highest total carotenoid concentrations whereas overweight children, Caucasian adolescents, and adults had the lowest.

Plasma β-carotene, α-cryptoxanthin, lycopene, and lutein results are available for the U.K. national surveys (Gregory et al., 1990, 1995, 2000; Finch et al., 1998). Mean, median, and lower and upper 2.5th or 5th percentiles by age and sex are presented.

Carotenoids can be both separated and measured by HPLC combined with ultraviolet/visual detection (Sowell et al., 1994). Care must be taken to store frozen serum samples for carotenoid analysis at −70°C or −80°C to avoid decay. A standard reference material for β-carotene can be obtained from NIST (Gaithersburg, MD). The within-subject daily CV for serum β-carotene for subjects following their normal dietary pattern is 7.2% (Gallagher et al., 1992).

18.1.5 Breast milk retinol

Breast milk retinol concentrations can indicate when the maternal vitamin A status is suboptimal, as lactating women then secrete breast milk with a reduced content of retinol. This usually reflects inadequacies in both maternal dietary intake and body stores of vitamin A. Breast milk retinol concentrations can also be used as an indirect indicator of the vitamin A status of breastfed infants (Stoltzfus and Underwood, 1995).

Most of the vitamin A in breast milk is in the form of retinyl palmitate in the milk fat. Concentrations are very high in colostrum and transitional breast milk (days 7–21 postpartum). After about day 21, the concentration stabilizes, so that breast milk samples taken after the first month postpartum are the most useful. The concentration of retinol in breast milk always varies over the course of a feed: the lowest concentration is in the first milk expressed from a full breast because the fat content is highest at the end of a feed. Hence, preferably all the milk from a full breast that has not been used to feed an infant for at least 2 h should be collected.

Stoltzfus et al. (1993) used full breast milk samples to investigate the effect of high-dose vitamin A supplementation on the vitamin A status of mothers and their infants in Indonesia. At 1–8 mo postpartum, the breast milk retinol concentrations of the supplemented mothers were significantly higher than in the placebo group (Figure 18.4).

In practice, collecting the entire contents of one breast is often difficult to achieve. Instead, a standardized collection procedure can be used to assess vitamin A status at the individual level. This involves collecting a small sample of breast milk (8–10 mL) from a full breast before the infant starts suckling, either by manual self-expression or by

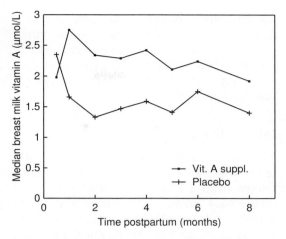

Figure 18.4: Retinol concentrations (μmol/L) in breast milk at baseline and during the subsequent 8 mo in supplement and placebo groups. Data from Stoltzfus et al., Journal of Nutrition 123: 666–675, 1993, with permission of the American Society for Nutritional Sciences.

using a breast pump (Stoltzfus and Underwood, 1995).

For population assessment, casual breast milk samples can be taken randomly throughout the day and at varying times after the infants were last fed. This will ensure that the variation in milk fat is randomly sampled. However, if random sampling is not possible, then the breast milk retinol concentrations can be expressed in terms of the fat content (Table 15.3) (WHO, 1996). In a study of rural women from Bangladesh, Rice et al. (2000) noted that breast milk vitamin A concentrations expressed per gram of milk fat were a particularly responsive indicator of vitamin A status.

There are two circumstances when it may be preferable to express breast milk retinol concentrations per unit volume rather than per gram of fat. First, when a field survey includes mothers with a wide range in the stage of lactation, there will be a large standard deviation around the mean retinol concentrations because of the marked variation in milk retinol concentration from early to late lactation. This large variation may be masked by expressing the retinol concentration in terms of fat content. Secondly, in studies in which both the β-carotene and the fat content of breast milk are increased as a result of a vitamin A intervention, retinol concentrations expressed per unit volume will provide a better measure of the response than when expressed in terms of the fat content (de Pee et al., 1997).

Interpretive criteria

The average retinol content of breast milk from vitamin A–sufficient lactating women ranges from 1.7 to 2.5 μmol/L; values are often <1.4 μmol/L for vitamin A–deficient mothers. The cutoff value defined by WHO (1996) at which both mother and breastfed infant are likely to be at risk of vitamin A deficiency is <1.05 μmol/L retinol. This equates to ⩽ 8 μg/g milk fat.

WHO (1996) has also defined two population prevalence levels that are indicative of a public health problem. When 10% to <25% of the sample population of mothers have breast milk retinol concentrations <1.05 μmol/L, then the public health problem for vitamin A deficiency is classified as moderate; when the prevalence is ⩾25%, the problem is severe.

Measurement of breast milk retinol

After collecting breast milk samples, they must be placed immediately in an insulated ice box for transport from the field to the base laboratory. If the analysis cannot be completed immediately, samples may be frozen at below –20°C. Care must be taken to ensure that the thawed samples are thoroughly mixed before aliquots are removed for analysis into amber or yellow polypropylene tubes with airtight caps. Analysis of retinol in breast milk can be performed by HPLC, after saponifying the breast milk samples.

The fat content of breast milk can be determined in the field by using the creamatocrit method. This involves collecting a sample (about 75 μL) of well-mixed breast milk into a hematocrit capillary tube, which is then sealed at one end. The tubes are then spun in a hematocrit centrifuge, after which the length of the cream layer is measured. The amount of fat is then determined by comparison with a standard curve of fat concentrations compiled using a standard lipid assay (Ferris and Jensen, 1984).

18.1.6 Relative dose response

The relative dose response (RDR) test can be used to estimate the liver stores of vitamin A and thereby identify individuals with marginal vitamin A deficiency. The test is based on the observation that during vitamin A deficiency, when liver stores are diminished, RBP accumulates in the liver as apo-RBP. Following the administration of a test dose of vitamin A, some of the vitamin A binds to the excess apo-RBP in the liver. It is then released as holo-RBP (i.e., RBP bound to retinol) into the circulation (Loerch et al., 1979). Consequently, in vitamin A–depleted individuals, there is a rapid and sustained increase in serum retinol after a small oral dose of vitamin A, whereas in individuals with normal liver vitamin A stores, this rise in serum retinol is either very small or does not occur.

The validity of the RDR test as an index of body stores of vitamin A has been studied by comparing vitamin A concentrations in liver biopsy samples with corresponding RDR test results for otherwise healthy surgical patients (Amédée-Manesme et al., 1984, 1987). Of the 12 surgical patients, the two with the lowest liver vitamin A concentrations had the highest RDR values (Figure 18.5). Following supplementation with vitamin A, RDR values fell to <5%. Patients with liver vitamin A concentrations ranging from 0.2 to 1.5 μmol/g had RDR values from 0% to 12% (Amédée-Manesme et al., 1984).

In a study of Brazilian children from low-income families, all the children with serum retinol concentrations <0.70 μmol/L had elevated RDR values. Moreover, 86% of the children with serum retinol concentrations of 0.74–1.02 μmol/L, and 26% with serum retinol concentrations of 1.05–1.40 μmol/L also had elevated RDR values (Flores et al., 1984) (Table 18.3). After supplementation with vitamin A, all the elevated RDR values reverted to normal. These results indicate

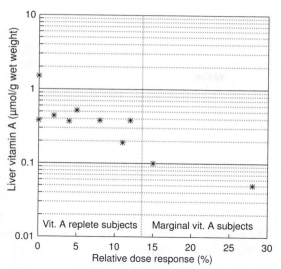

Figure 18.5: Liver vitamin A concentration from biopsies compared with corresponding RDR test results in a group of adult American surgical patients. From Amédée-Manesme et al., American Journal of Clinical Nutrition 39: 898–902, 1984 © Am J Clin Nutr. American Society for Clinical Nutrition.

that the RDR is a more sensitive index of marginal vitamin A status than using serum vitamin A levels <0.70 µmol/L, but it does not distinguish among different levels of adequate vitamin A reserves (Solomons et al., 1990).

Other factors associated with low RDR values include malabsorption, infection, liver disease, severe protein-energy malnutrition, and zinc deficiency. Such factors reduce the sensitivity and the specificity of the RDR test (Mobarhan et al., 1981; Russell et al.,

Serum retinol (µmol/L)	%	No. tested
≤ 0.70	100	12
0.71–1.04	86	21
1.05–1.39	26	19
> 1.40	3	39
Total tested		91

Table 18.3: Percentage of children with a positive RDR test classified by serum retinol levels. From Flores et al., American Journal of Clinical Nutrition 40: 1281–1289, 1984 © Am J Clin Nutr. American Society for Clinical Nutrition.

1983; Campos et al., 1987). For example, when an oral dose of vitamin A was given to patients with varying degrees of liver dysfunction and protein-energy malnutrition, no correlation was observed between the vitamin A content of liver biopsies and the RDR test result (Mobarhan et al., 1981; Russell et al., 1983). These results were attributed to malabsorption of the oral dose because when an intravenous injection of retinyl palmitate was given to children with liver disease, the RDR test proved to be a reliable and sensitive index of vitamin A status (Amédée-Manesme et al., 1987).

Protein deficiency interferes with the RDR test by decreasing liver synthesis of the rapid turnover apo-RBP, while zinc deficiency interferes with the liver synthesis or secretion of RBP (Christian and West, 1998). A further limitation of the RDR test is low precision, which may lead to serious errors in classifying subjects with vitamin A deficiency, especially in populations where the prevalence is moderate (Solomons et al., 1990).

Interpretive criteria for the RDR test

Vitamin A–replete subjects have RDR values ranging from zero to 14%. Relative dose response values > 20% are generally considered indicative of inadequate hepatic stores of vitamin A and marginal vitamin A status (WHO, 1996). When > 20% to < 30% of the sample population show abnormal RDR values (i.e., > 20%), then a public health problem of moderate importance may be assumed. When the prevalence is ≥ 30%, the public health problem is severe (WHO, 1996).

Measurement of relative dose response

Two blood samples are needed for the RDR test. A baseline fasting blood sample is taken immediately before the administration of a small oral dose (450 µg for children; about 600 µg for adults) of vitamin A (as retinyl acetate or retinol palmitate). Next, a high-fat snack that contains minimal vitamin A is consumed to ensure absorption of vitamin A. The second blood sample is then taken 5 h later. The RDR (%) is calculated as:

$$\frac{\text{plasma retinol at 5 h} - \text{plasma retinol at 0 h}}{\text{plasma retinol at 5 h}} \times 100\%$$

Concentrations of serum retinol for the RDR test should be measured by reverse-phase HPLC because this method has the required precision at low concentrations. Even a small analytical error can alter the RDR value significantly, especially when serum retinol concentrations are low.

18.1.7 Modified relative dose response

The modified relative dose response (MRDR) test requires only one blood sample, avoiding the necessity of taking a second sample. This modified test has been used to assess the vitamin A status in children and in pregnant and lactating women (Tanumihardjo et al., 1990, 1994, 1995, 1996).

For the test, a small oral dose of vitamin A is administered, usually 3,4-didehydroretinyl acetate (DRA). Often this is followed by a high-fat, low-vitamin A snack to facilitate the absorption of the DRA. The latter combines with the RBP in the same way as retinol but, unlike retinol, is not normally found in human plasma except when high levels of freshwater fish are consumed. The DRA is hydrolyzed in the gastrointestinal tract to 3,4-didehydroretinol (DR), absorbed, and re-esterified, mainly with palmitic acid in the intestinal mucosal cells (Tanumihardjo et al., 1995). The serum concentrations of DR and retinol (R) in the single blood sample are measured by HPLC. The molar ratio of [DR]:[R] in the blood sample is a measure of the response.

Interpretive criteria for the MRDR

Ratios > 0.060 are considered indicative of marginal vitamin A status (subclinical deficiency), whereas those < 0.030 are satisfactory (Tanumihardjo et al., 1996). The WHO (1996) criteria for a moderate public health problem are a prevalence of MRDR ratios $\geqslant 0.060$ of between 20% and 30%. If the prevalence is $> 30\%$, the public health problem is severe.

Unfortunately, the MRDR test is subject to the same limitations as the RDR test. Within-subject variation in the ratio can be large, because the analysis of DR is difficult and variations in absorption occur (de Pee et al., 1997; Olson and Tanumihardjo, 1998). A further limitation is that DRA is not yet commercially available and presently must be synthesized in the laboratory.

Measurement of the MRDR

The recommended doses of DRA for use in the field are 3.0 µmol for preschool children (< 6 y), 7.0 µmol for preadolescent children (6–12 y), and 8.8 µmol for teenagers and adults (> 12 y) (Tanumihardjo et al., 1996). The acceptable time between administering the oral DRA dose and obtaining a single blood sample (about 0.5–2 ml) is reportedly 4–7 h. To enhance the stability of the DRA dose, it should be dissolved in corn oil and stored in amber vials inside a cooler on ice in the field, or at $-20°C$ to $-70°C$ for longer-term storage. The blood sample should also be stored on ice in a light-protected cooler after collection, prior to separation of the serum. Analyses of DR and retinol (R) concentrations in the serum should be performed by HPLC. The molar ratio of [DR]:[R] is then calculated.

18.1.8 Subjective assessment of night blindness

Night blindness, or the inability to see after dusk or at night, is frequently reported among young children and women of reproductive age in developing countries with moderate to severe vitamin A deficiency (Escoute et al., 1991; Christian et al., 1998a). It is the most common ocular manifestation of vitamin A deficiency and is often described by specific terms in countries or cultures where the prevalence is high. For example, in some cultures it is known as "chicken eyes" or "chicken blindness" (Christian, 2002a). Poor dark adaptation resulting in night blindness arises when there is reduced production in the rods of the visual pigment rhodopsin, or opsin protein bound to the retinal form of vitamin A.

To assess the prevalence of night blindness, the local term for night blindness must first be identified through focus group discussion (Dawson et al., 1993) and its reliability field tested. Next, a night blindness history is elicited via interviews. Care should always be taken during this stage to exclude those individuals whose night blindness results from other causes, such as the rare hereditary eye disease retinitis pigmentosa.

Some studies of children > 2 y have been based on interviews to elicit any history of night blindness. In general, reliable data on night blindness cannot be determined for children < 2 y in this way because they are not able to move around freely after dusk and bump into objects. In studies of children > 2 y, WHO (1996) recommends the use of specific questions to increase the specificity and reduce misclassification of self-reported night blindness. Sommer et al. (1980) reported that 85% of Indonesian preschool children with reported night blindness had low serum vitamin A levels (i.e., < 0.70 µmol/L). This strong association between night blindness and serum retinol levels is shown in Table 18.4. This also shows similar positive findings for a second clinical sign of vitamin A deficiency — Bitot's spots with conjunctival xerosis.

Determination of the prevalence of night blindness is now recommended as a simple and easy tool to assess vitamin A deficiency in women of reproductive age. When using maternal night blindness in this way, only women with a previous pregnancy that ended in a live birth in the past 3 y should be included (Christian, 2002a). Significant associations between maternal night blindness and low serum and breast milk retinol concentrations, as well as functional indices such as abnormal conjunctival impression cytology (Section 18.1.11) and impaired dark adaptation (Section 18.1.9), have been reported among pregnant Nepalese women, as shown in Table 18.5.

Clinical status	n	Mean (µmol/L)
Night blindness reported; no conjunctival xerosis or Bitot's Spots	174	0.49
Controls	161	0.62
No night blindness; conjunctival xerosis and Bitot's Spots present	51	0.47
Controls	45	0.60
Night blindness reported; with conjunctival xerosis and Bitot's Spots	79	0.42
Controls	76	0.64

Table 18.4: Mean serum vitamin A level in Indonesian preschool children by clinical indicators of vitamin A status: night blindness and conjuctival xerosis with Bitot's spots. Data from Sommer et al., American Journal of Clinical Nutrition 33: 887–891, 1980 © Am J Clin Nutr. American Society for Clinical Nutrition.

In a large population-based control study in Nepal, women with night blindness were also less likely to consume dietary sources of vitamin A (Christian et al., 1998a). In a randomized placebo-controlled supplementation trial in Nepal, women in the placebo group with night blindness during pregnancy had a mortality rate four times higher than did women without night blindness. This mortality level was reduced by 68% after weekly vitamin A supplementation (Christian et al., 1998b).

Interpretive criteria

The cutoff recommended by IVACG at which vitamin A deficiency is considered a significant public health problem within a community is when the prevalence of maternal night blindness is 5% or greater (Christian, 2002a). This cutoff value was chosen by IVACG to take into account the misclassification that may occur (i.e., false positives) among women who report problems with daytime vision (i.e., daytime blindness). Efforts should be made during surveys to ex-

Vitamin A status indicators	Night blind N	Night blind n (%)	Not night blind N	Not night blind n (%)	OR	95% CI
Serum retinol < 0.7 µmol/L	85	44 (51.0)	90	19 (21.1)	4.0	2.2–7.4
Serum retinol <1.05 µmol/L	85	65 (76.5)	90	50 (55.5)	2.5	1.4–4.6
CIC abnormal	85	24 (28.2)	90	11 (12.2)	2.8	1.3–6.1
Dark adaptation abnormal	94	67 (71.2)	98	42 (43.8)	3.3	1.8–6.0
Breast milk vitamin A <1.05 µmol/L	94	56 (59.6)	97	41 (42.3)	2.0	1.1–3.6

Table 18.5: Association of night blindness with other indicators of vitamin A deficiency in pregnant women in Nepal. *N*, sample size; n, number of subjects below cutoff; OR, odds ratio; CI, confidence interval; CIC, conjunctival impression cytology. From Christian, Journal of Nutrition 132: 2884S–2888S, 2002, with permission of the American Society for Nutritional Sciences.

clude those women whose night blindness is likely due to daytime blindness.

WHO (1996) have proposed cutoffs for the prevalence of night blindness for children 24–71 mo. Three recommended cutoffs for the prevalence of night blindness to define a public health problem and its level of importance (i.e., mild, moderate, or severe) are given; these are shown in Table 18.6, together with the minimum sample sizes required. However, the large minimum sample sizes required together with the increasing use of vitamin A supplements among young children in most developing countries preclude the use of these WHO cutoffs for children. Instead, in most developing countries, the assessment of nightblindness in women of reproductive age is probably more useful.

18.1.9 Rapid dark adaptation test

Before night blindness develops, disturbances in dark adaptation occur. These can be detected by specially designed noninvasive tests

		Min. sample	
	Prevalence	20%	50%
Mild	<1%	—	—
Moderate	≥1% to < 5%	4706	753
Severe	≥5%	1825	292

Table 18.6: Prevalence of night blindness in children 24–71 mo, and the minimum sample sizes for identifying a mild, moderate, or severe vitamin A deficiency public health problem with a relative precision of 20% and 50% at the 95% confidence level. From WHO (1996).

(Congdon et al., 1995). The conventional laboratory-based, formal dark adaptometry test is a tedious and time-consuming procedure. Instead, a rapid dark adaptation test (RDAT), suitable for field conditions, has been developed. This is based on the measurements of the timing of the Purkinje shift (Thornton, 1977), in which the peak wavelength sensitivity of the retina shifts from the red toward the blue end of the visual spectrum during the transition from photopic or cone-mediated day vision to scotopic or rod-mediated night vision. This shift causes the intensity of blue light to appear brighter than that of red light under scotopic lighting conditions.

The rapid dark adaptation test requires a light-proof room, a light source, a dark, nonreflective work surface, a standard X-ray view box, and sets of red, blue, and white discs; details are given in Vinton and Russell (1981).

Measurements for the RDAT are undertaken during the first few minutes of dark adaptation. This is a major disadvantage because the measurements rely mainly on the cones or light vision cells in the retina instead of the rods or dark vision cones. As a result, the test is not very sensitive to the early signs of vitamin A deficiency (Favaro et al., 1986; Kemp et al., 1988). An additional disadvantage is that the RDAT is not appropriate for preschool children, who are too young to perform the test accurately. This is unfortunate because preschool children are the group most at risk for vitamin A deficiency. False positives may also occur and between-examiner variability may produce inconsistencies in the results.

Age influences dark adaptation and hence must be taken into account when determining the normal range of the rapid test adaptation times for healthy reference populations (Vinton and Russell, 1981).

18.1.10 Pupillary and visual threshold test

A scotopic (dim light vision) device has been developed to assess the responsiveness and sensitivity of the pupil to light as an indication of an individual's dark adaptation threshold. The test measures the threshold of light at which pupillary contraction occurs under dark adapted conditions (Congdon et al., 1995).

Unlike the RDAT, the pupillary and visual threshold test can be conducted in the field on individuals of all ages, including preschool children, who cannot be tested by the RDAT. The test requires minimal cooperation from the subjects and takes about 20 min per subject. A darkened facility is required for this test. A portable tent has been developed and tests devised to ensure that the darkness in the testing area is adequate (Sanchez et al., 1997). If a darkened facility is not available, then night-time testing may be more practical.

The apparatus consists of two handheld illuminators, each having a yellow-green, light-emitting diode light source (dominant wavelength = 572 nm) with 12 intensity settings. Each illuminator is designed to fit entirely over one eye and to illuminate the entire retina. One of the illuminators is designed to measure light of "low intensity" (illumination range −8.75 to −3.00 log cd/m^2) and the other "high intensity" (illumination range −4.16 to 0.44 log cd/m^2).

Before testing, participants are subjected to a camera-flash "partial bleach" of the full retina, which involves placing the subjects in a dark room and exposing them to a camera flash reflected through a foil-lined cone, after which they are allowed 10 min of dark adaptation. The visual threshold is measured first by placing the low-intensity illuminator over the subject's left eye. The light

intensity is then incremented over 11 intensity settings (roughly a 4-log unit range) at 10-s intervals until a pupillary response (i.e., quick contraction of the pupil on presenting the stimulus) is seen in the uncovered right eye on two successive trials. The uncovered right eye is observed with an obliquely mounted red LED light source (dominant wave-length = 626 nm), which preserves dark adaptation in both the subjects and the observer. Next, the pupillary threshold is measured, as described above, using the high intensity illuminator; further details are given in Congdon et al. (1995, 2000) and Christian et al. (2001). All tests should be performed using standardized procedures and well-trained examiners, as discussed in Christian et al. (2001).

The stimulus for the visual or the pupillary threshold is defined as the lowest level at which the subject can correctly distinguish stimulus from nonstimulus on three successive trials. High pupillary and visual scores reflect a pupillary response achieved at a greater light intensity, and indicate poorer dark adaptability (Congdon et al., 1995).

Additional studies are needed to establish whether testing for both pupillary and visual thresholds is necessary, because the latter requires less training and standardization of personnel. In some studies on young children aged 1 to 2 y, only pupillary testing has been performed because complete visual testing on such young children is not always possible (Congdon et al., 1995).

The pupillary and visual threshold tests have been validated as an index of vitamin A status using controlled vitamin A supplementation trials on children and pregnant women (Congdon et al., 1995, 2000; Congdon and West, 2002). Significant improvements in dark adaptation as assessed by visual and/or pupillary testing were reported in those subjects supplemented with vitamin A but not with a placebo. Moreover, dark adaptation scores, measured by visual and/or pupillary testing, correlate well with serum retinol, as shown in Figure 18.6, and with RDR (Congdon et al., 1995, 2000; Sanchez et al., 1997).

Nevertheless, there are limitations assoc-

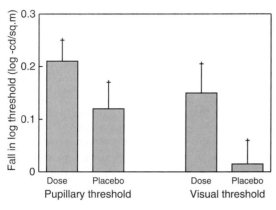

Figure 18.6: Change in mean dark-adaptation thresholds for 235 preschool Indonesian children given 105 μmol vitamin A or placebo. Decline is significant in children receiving vitamin A for both pupillary ($p < 0.0001$) and visual ($p < 0.01$) testing, but not significant for children receiving placebo. Data from Congdon et al., American Journal of Clinical Nutrition 61: 1076-1082, 1995 © Am J Clin Nutr. American Society for Clinical Nutrition.

iated with the pupillary and visual threshold tests. For example, some investigators have shown overlapping values for deficient and nondeficient population groups, so that scotopic threshold testing may be more suitable for population assessment than for individuals. Further, the time required to administer the test is about 20 min per subject, so it is probably not feasible to test large numbers of individuals. Sanchez et al. (1997) suggest that for populations at high risk for vitamin A deficiency, as few as six subjects may be sufficient to show that the group mean thresholds differ significantly from normal. In populations with mild vitamin A deficiency, testing about 100 subjects is probably adequate (Sanchez et al., 1997).

Another limitation is that recovery of the normal pupillary response after dosing with vitamin A supplements takes about 4–6 wk. One must wait at least this long before retesting treated individuals. Finally, the period required to train examiners to recognize the pupillary response is 1–3 d.

The IVACG has proposed two cutoff values to indicate whether vitamin A deficiency is a problem or not in an area, based on a mean pupillary dark adaptation score for a population. Scores worse than the cutoff of $-1.11 \log cd/m^2$ are said to indicate vitamin A deficiency, whereas scores better than the normal cutoff of $-1.24 \log cd/m^2$ should indicate that a population is normal, or that an intervention has successfully improved vitamin A status (Congdon and West, 2002). The population mean should be calculated for this test, rather than the proportion falling below a specific value, as has been stipulated for the other tests of vitamin A nutriture. This approach is recommended because in populations with marginal vitamin A status, the small proportion of subjects with abnormal values for the test could potentially markedly increase the sample size required for testing.

18.1.11 Conjunctival impression cytology with transfer

Conjunctival impression cytology (CIC) can detect some of the early physiological changes characteristic of vitamin A deficiency. Such changes include both the progressive loss of goblet cells in the conjunctiva and the appearance of enlarged, partially keratinized, epithelial cells (Wittepenn et al., 1986; Natadisastra et al., 1988). The original (CIC) test has been modified for ease of use in developing countries and is now referred to as impression cytology with transfer (ICT).

The ICT test involves gently applying a strip (25×5 mm) or disc of cellulose acetate filter paper (Keenum et al., 1990) to the inferior temporal bulbar conjunctiva for 2–3 s (Wittepenn et al., 1986). The filter paper is then peeled off gently, and the cells adhering to the filter paper are immediately transferred to a clean glass slide through finger pressure. The slide is then placed for 20 min into a jar containing a fixative stain solution of alcohol, carbol-fuchsin, and alcian blue. After staining and water washing, the slide is examined with a microscope. Nuclei and cytoplasm of epithelial cells and nuclei of goblet cells are stained pink by acid fuchsin, whereas the acid mucous substance is stained blue with alcian blue.

The test is usually painless, although if a layer of cells is pulled off with the filter paper, a pricking sensation may be felt. As a result, the test is sometimes difficult to perform on young children (Carlier et al., 1992). In some studies, 0.5% proparacaine has been applied to each eye (Natadisastra et al., 1988).

Normal results are characterized by small epithelial cells with distinct borders and the presence of goblet cells or mucin spots with nuclei. Abnormal ICT results, indicative of suboptimal vitamin A status, are suggested by the appearance of enlarged, separated or keratinized epithelial cells and the progressive disappearance of goblet cells and mucin droplets. These changes lead to a lowered resistance to invasion by potentially pathogenic organisms.

Several investigators have examined the validity of this test as a measure of vitamin A status by comparison with other indices of vitamin A status (e.g., serum retinol or RDR) (Natadisastra et al., 1987, 1988; Reddy et al., 1989; Escoute et al., 1991; Resnikoff et al., 1992; Rahman et al., 1995). Results have been inconsistent and dependent in part on the severity of the vitamin A deficiency state (Table 18.7) and on which measures are used. Ocular infections may confound the interpretation (Carlier et al., 1992). In general, good agreement of ICT results with serum retinol has been reported for cases of clinical vitamin A deficiency (e.g., xerophthalmia) (Natadisastra et al., 1987; Reddy et al., 1989) but not subclinical (Gadomski et al., 1989; Rahman et al., 1995). These findings suggest that ICT may not be helpful in indicating subclinical vitamin A deficiency. Indeed, the relatively low sensitivity and specificity of the ICT emphasize the need to combine this test with other indicators of vitamin A status, preferably one that measures acute status such as serum retinol, dietary intake, or MRDR (WHO, 1996).

The validity of the test has also been examined in relation to vitamin A supplementation. Again, the responses have been variable, ranging from a 100% response in a study in Thai school-aged children (Udomkesmalee et al., 1992) to only 46% in undernourished Sengalese preschool children (Carlier et al., 1992). Several factors may influence such responses, including the level and frequency of the supplemental dose, the duration of the study, the possible existence of zinc and folic acid deficiencies, other nutritional disorders, intercurrent disease states (e.g., ocular infection), and environmental factors (Congdon and West, 2002). Hence, the use of ICT to evaluate the influence of vitamin A intervention programs is uncertain.

Interpretive criteria for CIT test

The WHO (1996) has proposed the following abnormal ICT prevalence cutoffs to define a public health problem and its level of importance: < 20% (mild); ≥ 20% to < 40% (moderate); ≥ 40% (severe) (Table 18.8). They caution the need to combine this test with other indicators of vitamin A status to determine the existence of an important public health problem. IVACG suggests that a prevalence of ≥ 20% abnormal results is indicative of a public health problem (Congdon and West, 2002).

Interpretation of ICT specimens requires extensive training because of the progressive nature of the changes: several interim stages may coexist. In addition, there is often considerable variation within and between microscopic fields and between the eyes of the subject. This often leads to large between-observer errors and, hence, discrepancies in the classification of the ICT results. A standard set of reference slides must be used to aid the interpretation of ICT specimens.

Classification of the results is based on the relative numbers of goblet cells, mucin droplets, and character of epithelial cells. Four classes are used: normal (N), marginal

Serum (μmol/L)	Sensitivity	Specificity
< 0.35	75	48
< 0.70	62	63
<1.05	59	100

Table 18.7: Comparison of the sensitivity and specificity of impression cytology at different cutoffs for serum retinol. Data from WHO (1996).

Indicator (cutoff)	Prevalence below cutoffs to define a public health problem and its level of importance		
	Mild	Moderate	Severe
Night blindness present	> 0 to <1%	⩾ 1% to 5%	⩾ 5%
Serum retinol ⩽ 0.70 µmol/L	⩾ 2% to <10%	⩾ 10% to < 20%	⩾ 20%
Breast milk retinol ⩽ 1.05 µmol/L			
or ⩽ 0.028 µmol/g (⩽ 8µg/g) milk fat	<10%	⩾ 10% to < 25%	⩾ 25%
RDR ⩾ 20%	< 20%	⩾ 20% to < 30%	⩾ 30%
MRDR ratio ⩾ 0.06	< 20%	⩾ 20% to < 30%	⩾ 30%
CIC/ICT abnormal at 24–71 mo of age	< 20%	⩾ 20% to < 40%	⩾ 40%

Table 18.8: Indicators of subclinical vitamin A deficiency in children 6–71 mo of age and their use in detecting a public health problem. The prevalence in a population of at least two of the above indicators of vitamin A status, at levels below the cutoff, indicates a public health problem. RDR, relative dose response; MRDR, modified relative dose response; CIC, conjunctival impression cytology; ICT, impression cytology with transfer. From WHO (1996).

normal (M+), marginal deficient (M−), and deficient (D) (Carlier et al., 1992). Generally, subjects with M+, M−, and D are regarded as having an abnormal ICT.

18.1.12 Stable isotope methods and total body stores of vitamin A

An isotope dilution procedure is the only method that provides a quantitative measure of the hepatic stores of vitamin A. It involves the administration of an oral dose of tetra-deuterated vitamin A. The isotopic dose is allowed to equilibrate with the vitamin A pool in the body. Then a blood sample is taken, and the ratio of the deuterated to the non-deuterated compound in serum is measured by mass spectrometry. The amount of total body stores of vitamin A is related to the extent of dilution of the labeled tracer and is calculated using the model of Furr et al. (1989).

The isotope dilution method has been validated in adult surgical patients in the United States and Bangladesh by measuring liver vitamin A biopsy samples (Furr et al., 1989; Haskell et al., 1997). For example, in ten U.S. surgical patients, the correlation coefficient between calculated and measured liver vitamin A concentrations was 0.88.

The length of time required for the isotopic dose to equilibrate with the vitamin A pool in the body varies according to the age and total body vitamin A stores of the study group. Equilibration periods after the test dose ranging from 11 to 26 d have generally been used (Furr et al., 1989; Haskell et al., 1998; Ribaya-Mercado et al., 1999), although Tang et al. (2002) suggest that 3 d may suffice. A shorter equilibration time facilitates the use of this isotope-dilution method in field settings.

The isotope dilution method is expensive, and the isolation and analysis of retinol by mass spectrometry is complex. Although some uncertainties still exist with the validity of this quantitative technique (Olson, 1997, 1999), estimates of total body vitamin A stores derived from stable isotope dilution are likely to be used increasingly in the future.

18.1.13 Multiple indices

Vitamin A deficiency disorders are not defined with any certainty using a single measure of vitamin A status. WHO (1996) has recommended a combination of biochemical, functional, and clinical indicators for children aged 6–71 mo; the indicators are given in Table 18.8, together with the corresponding cutoff values used in population assessment. Some caution is needed when applying these cutoffs to individuals because of the influence of the many confounding factors. Table 18.8 also provides information on the population prevalence levels of each indicator for defining a mild, moderate, or severe public health problem in relation to vitamin A.

According to WHO (1996) a public health problem exists when a population has at least two biological indicators with a prevalence above the level corresponding to a deficiency, or one biological indicator of deficiency supported by a composite of at least four demographic and ecological risk factors, two of which must be nutrition- and diet-related. Details of these demographic and ecological risk factors are given in WHO (1996); their cutoff values are still somewhat arbitrary and additional field testing and experience is needed.

IVACG has recently proposed a revised list of criteria for evaluating vitamin A programs and have set the minimal prevalence levels above which vitamin A deficiency is considered to be a public health problem. Only one biochemical criterion has been specified by IVACG. Further, IVACG recommends that any one of the prevalence criteria listed in Table 18.9 can be used to indicate significant vitamin A deficiency within a defined population. This was done in an effort to simplify assessment and elicit prompt action by policy makers (Sommer and Davidson, 2002).

IVACG also recommends the use of the under-five mortality rate, as a surrogate indicator for assessing the likelihood of vitamin A deficiency within a country or specific population group. They suggest that countries with under-five mortality rates $> 50/1000$ live births are likely to have a problem, whereas those with rates from 20 to $50/1000$ live births may have a problem, and further investigation is warranted (Schultink, 2002).

The selection of the most appropriate combination of criteria depends on the purpose of the study, the expected range of vitamin A status for the study group, and the resources available.

18.2 Vitamin D

Vitamin D (calciferol) is a generic term for a group of related fat-soluble substances, including vitamin D_2 (ergocalciferol), vitamin D_3 (cholecalciferol) (Figure 18.7), and their metabolites. Vitamin D_2 is derived from the yeast and plant sterol, ergosterol, and is the form widely used in pharmaceutical

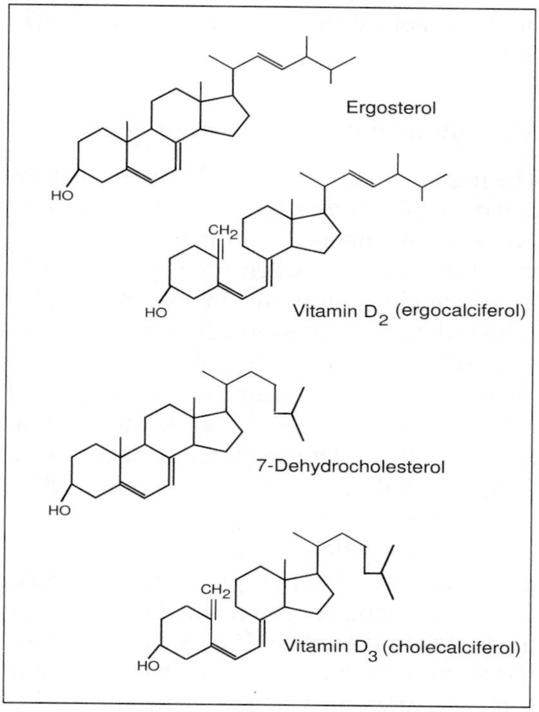

Criteria	Prevalence (%)
Clinical	
Children 2–5 y	
Night blindness	> 1.0
Bitot's spots	> 0.5
Corneal xerosis	> 0.01
Corneal ulcers	> 0.01
Corneal scars	> 0.05
Women of childbearing age	
Night blindness	
during recent pregnancy	> 5.0
Biochemical	
Serum retinol $< 0.70\,\mu mol/L$	> 15

Table 18.9: IVACG 2001 prevalence criteria indicating significant vitamin A deficiency within a defined population. From Sommer and Davidson, Journal of Nutrition 132: 2845S–2850S, 2002, with permission of The American Society for Nutritional Sciences.

Figure 18.7: The structure of the various forms of vitamin D and the major metabolites.

preparations. Vitamin D_3 originates from the action of sunlight or ultraviolet light on its precursor sterol, 7-dehydrocholesterol, which is present in the skin, or from dietary sources. The latter include some fish liver oils, the flesh of fatty fish, and organ meats. Some foods are also fortified with vitamin D (e.g., milk, cereals, margerine) depending on the country (Lips et al., 1996).

Functions of vitamin D

The principal role of vitamin D is to ensure adequate intestinal absorption of calcium and phosphorus and to regulate bone mineralization. Vitamin D also has a critical role in a number of cellular functions in tissues other than bone, notably modulators of the immune response and the regulation of cell differentiation, proliferation, and apoptosis (Omdahl et al., 2002). It is these immuno-modulatory and cell-differentiating properties that have led to the use of vitamin D derivatives in the treatment of psoriasis and other skin disorders (FAO/WHO, 2002). For further details of these noncalcemic functions see Holick (2003).

Absorption and metabolism of vitamin D

The requirement for vitamin D can be met by dietary intake and/or by skin synthesis. The synthesis of vitamin D_3 in the skin involves two stages: the photochemical transformation of 7-dehydrocholesterol to previtamin D_3, followed by thermal isomerization of the previtamin to vitamin D_3. Variables influencing the formation of previtamin D_3 in the skin include skin pigmentation and the intensity of the solar ultraviolet light (Holick et al., 1981; Clemens et al., 1982; Matsuoka et al., 1991; Goswami et al., 2000).

The major metabolic steps involved in the metabolism of vitamin D_2 are similar to those for the metabolism of vitamin D_3, although the latter is more active. Hence, in the following discussion, the term vitamin D without a subscript refers to either or both vitamin D_2 and vitamin D_3 and its metabolites.

Vitamin D enters the circulation from the

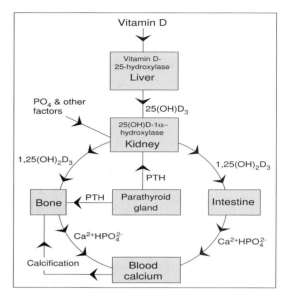

Figure 18.8: Metabolism of vitamin D_3 to $25(OH)D_3$ and $1,25(OH)_2D_3$. Once formed, the latter carries out the biological functions of vitamin D, acting on the intestine and the bone. Parathyroid hormone (PTH) promotes the synthesis of $1,25(OH)_2D_3$, which, in turn, stimulates intestinal calcium transport and bone calcium mobilization and regulates the synthesis of PTH by negative feedback. Adapted from Holick, Kidney International 32: 912–929, 1987.

skin or from the lymph via the thoracic duct, bound to a specific vitamin D–binding protein. Vitamin D is transported to the liver, where it is hydroxylated to 25-hydroxyvitamin D ($25(OH)D$ [calcidiol]), the major circulating form of vitamin D (Figure 18.8). The $25(OH)D$ formed is then converted in the kidney by an enzyme ($25(OH)D$-1-α-hydroxylase) to produce two dihydroxylated metabolites. These are $1,25(OH)_2D$ (calcitriol), the biologically active form, and $24R,25(OH)_2D$, a less active metabolite.

The production of $1,25(OH)_2D$ in the kidney is homeostatically controlled, mainly by the action of parathyroid hormone in response to serum calcium and phosphorus levels. A decrease in serum calcium prompts an increase in parathyroid hormone secretion from the parathyroid gland that acts to mobilize calcium stores from the bone. Parathyroid hormone also promotes the synthesis of $1,25(OH)_2D$ in the kidney which, in turn, stimulates the mobilization of calcium from the bone and intestine (Figure 18.8). It is now known that 1,25(OH)$_2$D can also be locally produced by activated macrophages, some lymphoma cells, and cultured skin and bone cells (Holick, 1996).

Both 25(OH)D and 1,25(OH)$_2$D circulate in plasma. The former reflects the sum of vitamin D from dietary intake and sunlight exposure, whereas plasma 1,25(OH)$_2$D concentrations reflect the immediate physiological need and are under homeostatic control. Concentrations of 1,25(OH)$_2$D in plasma are about 0.1% of those of 25(OH)D. In vitamin D deficiency, serum 1,25(OH)$_2$D levels may be normal or even elevated, as a result of increased renal production of 1,25(OH)$_2$D in response to the rise in serum parathyroid levels (Holick, 2003). In contrast, serum 25(OH)D concentrations remain low until a reserve accumulates. As a result, serum 25(OH)D concentrations reflect medium- to long-term vitamin D availability from both dietary and endogenous sources.

Vitamin D deficiency in humans

Persons who are housebound or living in institutions depend primarily on dietary sources of vitamin D (Lester et al., 1980; McKenna et al., 1985; Gibson et al., 1986). Free-living subjects meet their requirement largely from the synthesis of vitamin D$_3$ by the action of ultraviolet light on 7-dehydrocholesterol in the skin (Fraser, 1983). Thus the elderly (Dattani et al., 1984; McKenna et al., 1985) or subjects living in northern latitudes (Lester et al., 1980) may be particularly vulnerable to vitamin D deficiency. Cultural dress habits may also reduce skin exposure to sunlight.

The influence of the regular use of sunscreen on serum 25(OH)D levels is unclear (Moloney et al., 2002). Over 2 y, use of a clinically prescribed sunscreen (sun protection factor 15) caused only a minor decrease in 25(OH)D levels, which did not induce an increment in bone biological markers (Farrerons et al., 1998). Nevertheless, excessive use of sunscreen may limit cutaneous synthesis of vitamin D.

Severe vitamin D deficiency in adults can produce osteomalacia, a condition characterized by a failure in the mineralization of the organic matrix of bone. This results in weak bones, diffuse skeletal bone tenderness, proximal muscle weakness, and an increased frequency of fractures. Such disturbances are associated with serum 25(OH)D concentrations below 7.5 nmol/L (Haddad and Stamp, 1974). After treatment with vitamin D supplements, serum 25(OH)D values rise and radiological lesions heal (Preece et al., 1975).

Some adult patients with chronic renal failure, gastrectomy, intestinal malabsorption and steatorrhea arising from celiac disease, inflammatory bowel disease, pancreatic insufficiency, or massive bowel resection may also develop osteomalacia.

Some functional disturbances have even been described in adults with serum 25(OH)D concentrations which are low but still above 7.5 nmol/L. These include secondary hyperparathyroidism, an increased bone turnover, and reduced bone mass (Chan et al., 1992; Nieves et al., 1994; van der Wielen et al., 1995; Chapuy et al., 1997). In the elderly, suboptimal vitamin D status may also be responsible for decreased absorption of calcium, a factor associated with a lowering of the bone mineral content during postmenopausal aging (Heaney et al., 1978).

In infants and children, severe vitamin D deficiency may result in rickets, in which abnormal softness of the skull (craniotabes) occurs. This may be accompanied by enlargement of the epiphyses of the long bones and of the costochondral junction (rachitic rosary). Bow legs and knock knees may arise from these bone deformities. Rickets, arising from primary vitamin D deficiency, is now rare in children from industrialized countries because of widespread vitamin D supplementation of some dairy products. Cases have been described among Asian immigrant children living in the United Kingdom and also among African American children (Welch et al., 2000).

Rickets can also arise in association with certain metabolic defects including vitamin D–resistant rickets (familial hypophos-

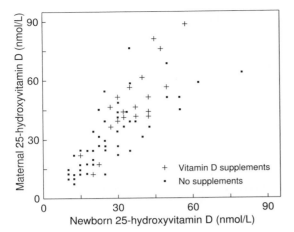

Figure 18.9: Correlation between maternal and newborn serum 25-hydroxyvitamin D concentrations. Results from vitamin D supplemented mothers and their neonates are represented by filled circles. Data from Zeghoud et al., American Journal of Clinical Nutrition 65: 771–778, 1997 © Am J Clin Nutr. American Society for Clinical Nutrition.

phatemia) and also in children with malabsorption syndromes.

Breast-fed infants may be especially vulnerable to low vitamin D status during early infancy if their mothers enter pregnancy with a low vitamin D status. Zeghoud et al. (1997) noted a strong positive correlation ($r = 0.80$; $p < 0.0001$) between maternal and neonatal 25(OH)D levels in 80 normal healthy French neonates and their mothers studied at the end of winter. Moreover, the effect of vitamin D supplementation on maternal and neonatal concentrations was marked (Figure 18.9.). A low vitamin D status may be a particular concern for African American women and their infants: nearly one-third enter pregnancy with low serum 25(OH)D concentrations (< 37.5 nmol/L) (Nesby-O'Dell et al., 2002). Cases of nutritional rickets have been reported in African American breast-fed infants (Kreiter et al., 2000).

Epidemiological studies suggest that vitamin D deficiency may be associated with an increased risk of specific types of cancers (Garland et al., 1990; Schwartz and Hulka, 1990). Epidemiological data also indicate a suboptimal vitamin D status in some chronic diseases, including tuberculosis, rheumatoid arthritis, inflammatory bowel disease, and multiple sclerosis, as well as in hypertension (Zittermann, 2003). More studies are needed to confirm these associations.

Food sources and dietary intakes

Natural food sources rich in vitamin D are restricted to fatty fish and organ meats. In some countries — for example, the United States, Canada, France, and Australia — fluid milk is fortified with vitamin D. In the United Kingdom and Europe, low amounts of vitamin D are added to some breakfast cereals, margarine and fat spreads, vegetable oils, breakfast beverages, and breads (Lips et al., 1996).

Data on vitamin D intakes from national nutrition surveys are sparse. No data are available from the New Zealand or Australian national nutrition surveys (McLennan and Podger, 1998; Russell et al., 1999; Parnell et al., 2003). Likewise, data on vitamin D intakes were not calculated for NHANES III, in part because of the variable vitamin D content of fortified foods (Chen et al., 1993). Estimates have been derived based on food consumption data only from NHANES II; intakes for young women ranged from 0 to 49 µg per day, with a median intake of 2.9 µg per day (Murphy and Calloway, 1986). The U.K national surveys present intakes for vitamin D from food sources and supplements; mean, median, and the lower and upper 2.5th or 5th percentiles by age and sex are given (Gregory et al., 1990; 1995, 2000; Finch et al., 1998). For U.K. adults, median intakes of vitamin D from all sources were 3.0 µg for men and 2.3 µg for women. Major food sources were fats and spreads (30%), cereal products (24%), and fish and fish dishes (22%) (Gregory et al., 1990).

Effects of high intakes of vitamin D

Self-dosing with excessive amounts of vitamin D supplements has been described, but considerable individual variation exists in the dose required to induce vitamin D toxicity (Parfitt et al., 1982). There are no reports of vitamin D intoxication arising from the consumption of conventional, unfortified foods (Chesney, 1989). Cases have arisen, however, from accidental excessive overfortification of milk with vitamin D_3 (Blank et al., 1995). Clinical signs of vitamin D toxicity include hypertension, hypercalcemia, and extraosseous calcification (Blum et al., 1977; Parfitt and Kleerekoper, 1980).

The U.S. Tolerable Upper Intake Level (UL) for vitamin D for infants is 25 µg/d, whereas for children aged >1 y and adults, it is 50 µg/d (IOM, 1997). However, evidence for the threshold of 25 µg/d for infants is limited, and controversy exists about the UL for children and adults.

Indices of vitamin D status

Historically, vitamin D status was assessed indirectly by measuring alkaline phosphatase activity, as well as calcium and phosphorus concentrations in serum — all very nonspecific indices. Methods are now available for the direct measurement of vitamin D metabolites in serum, and these are described below. If possible, these measurements should be performed in conjunction with an assay of serum parathyroid hormone and some functional assessment of skeletal health. In adults, this assessment may include measurement of bone mineral content or bone mineral density.

18.2.1 Serum 25-hydroxyvitamin D

Of the circulating metabolites of vitamin D, 25-hydroxyvitamin D (25(OH)D) is the most abundant and has the longest half-life of all the vitamin D derivatives. Concentrations of 25(OH)D in serum are also the most useful measure of vitamin D status in humans, as they reflect the total supply of vitamin D from both cutaneous synthesis and dietary intake of either vitamin D_2 or vitamin D_3 (Holick, 1996). Moreover, they can be used to define vitamin D deficiency, insufficiency, hypovitaminosis, sufficiency, and toxicity (IOM, 1997). Concentrations in healthy adults vary from 20 to 130 nmol/L, depending in part on exposure to solar ultraviolet light.

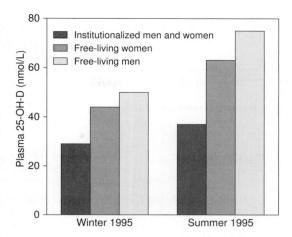

Figure 18.10: Comparison of mean plasma 25(OH)D levels by season for free-living elderly men and women and participants in institutions. Data from Finch et al. (1998).

Factors affecting serum 25(OH)D

Seasonal effects on serum vitamin D status are marked. The highest serum 25(OH)D levels occur in the late summer, and the lowest are in the late winter. This trend parallels the seasonal change in solar ultraviolet light in temperate regions. For example, Dattani et al. (1984) reported that serum 25(OH)D levels of men and women ≥ 65 y were significantly higher in the summer than in the winter, and they correlated with exposure to sunlight as measured by a "sunshine score."

In the U.K. national survey of people ≥ 65 y (Finch et al., 1998), mean plasma 25(OH)D concentrations were also significantly higher in free-living participants surveyed in the summer (July–September) than in the winter (Figure 18.10). Similar findings have been reported by others (McKenna, 1992; Need et al., 1993; Jacques et al., 1997).

Place of work and residence can affect the serum vitamin D status. Outdoor workers from Dundee, Scotland, exposed to increased levels of solar ultraviolet light, had significantly higher levels of serum 25(OH)D at all seasons compared to the indoor workers consuming similar diets (Devgun et al., 1981). Similarly, Finch et al. (1998) noted that in the summer, 6% of a free-living group

	Males		Females	
	Without Vit. D supplements	With Vit. D supplements	Without Vit. D supplements	With Vit. D supplements
25(OH)D (nmol/L)	33.0 ± 16.3 (37)	38.5 ± 12.0 (22)	26.3 ± 13.3 (45)	30.3 ± 11.8 (29)
Alkaline phosphatase (μmol/L)	94.4 ± 23.1 (37)	76.9 ± 23.7 (23)	95.7 ± 23.6 (49)	90.5 ± 19.6 (29)
Calcium (mmol/L)	2.4 ± 0.1 (37)	2.4 ± 0.1 (24)	2.5 ± 0.1 (49)	2.5 ± 0.1 (29)
Phosphorus (mmol/L)	0.9 ± 0.1 (37)	0.9 ± 0.1 (24)	1.0 ± 0.1 (48)	1.1 ± 0.1 (29)

Table 18.10: Plasma 25(OH)D, alkaline phosphatase, calcium, and phosphorus levels of male and female healthy American elderly subjects in relation to vitamin D supplementation. The number of subjects in each group is shown in parenthesis. Both sex and supplementation effects on the plasma 25(OH)D and alkaline phosphatase levels are significant ($p < 0.05$). From Omdahl et al., American Journal of Clinical Nutrition 36: 1225–1233, 1982 © Am J Clin Nutr. American Society for Clinical Nutrition.

of elderly subjects had plasma 25(OH)D concentrations < 25 nmol/L compared to 35% of a comparable group of institutionalized participants (Figure 18.10).

Vitamin D supplement usage and fortification normally leads to higher 25(OH)D concentrations in serum (Omdahl et al., 1982; van der Wielen et al., 1995; Lehtonen-Veromaa et al., 1999; Calvo and Whiting, 2003). In an American elderly population, for example, higher concentrations were observed in both male and female subjects taking vitamin D supplements compared with levels for unsupplemented subjects (Table 18.10), irrespective of the season (Omdahl et al., 1982). Similarly, African American women aged 15–49 y taking vitamin D supplements during NHANES III also had significantly higher 25(OH)D concentrations compared to levels for unsupplemented subjects (Nesby-O'Dell et al., 2002). Such differences were not observed among comparable Caucasian women. A positive relationship between the intake of vitamin D from fortified milk or supplements and serum 25(OH)D concentrations in Canadian women has also been reported (Vieth et al., 2001).

Age-related changes in the concentrations of serum 25(OH)D can be marked. Newborn infants have serum concentrations that correlate with maternal 25(OH)D concentrations (Figure 18.9), but which are usually lower. Concentrations in preterm infants increase very rapidly after birth (Salle et al., 1983). Serum 25(OH)D levels in children of both sexes decline with increasing age (Gregory et al., 2000). In the U.K. survey of young people, boys aged 11–18 y were most likely to have poor vitamin D status (i.e., < 25 nmol/L) (Gregory et al., 2000). A similar decline with age occurs among adults, attributed, in part, to a more limited exposure to solar radiation. Low dietary intakes of vitamin D, reduced capacity of the skin to produce vitamin D, and impaired intestinal absorption of ingested vitamin D may also be involved (van der Wielen et al., 1995). The age-related decline in skin thickness may be an additional factor (Need et al. 1993).

Sex differences in concentrations of serum 25(OH)D have been noted. Generally, concentrations are lower in females than in males (van der Wielen et al., 1995; Jacques et al., 1997; Finch et al., 1998; Gregory et al., 2000), irrespective of season or vitamin D supplement usage (Table 18.10, Figure 18.10). Reasons for these differences are unclear. In elderly women, absorption of dietary vitamin D may be less or their activity pattern may result in less sunlight exposure (Omdahl et al., 1982).

Race also influences 25(OH)D concentrations in serum, as skin pigmentation affects the cutaneous production of vitamin D_3. For example, serum 25(OH)D concentrations in African and Mexican Americans tend to be lower than in Caucasians. In NHANES III, 42% of African American women had serum concentrations of 25(OH)D $\leq$37.5 nmol/L but only 4.2% of Caucasian females of comparable age had such low levels (Nesby-O'Dell et al., 2002).

Latitude effects are marked. Subjects from lower latitudes, exposed to increased levels of solar ultraviolet light, have higher values when the effects of variation in dietary intake and season are taken into account (Figure 18.11). Conversely, when living at higher latitudes such as on the Antarctic continent, serum 25(OH)D concentrations are usually lower (Oliveri et al., 1994). Indeed, synthesis of vitamin D_3 in the skin is absent during most of the winter months in subjects living above and below latitudes of approximately 40°N and 40°S, respectively (Ladizesky et al., 1995).

Smoking depresses serum 25(OH)D concentrations. This may partly explain the reported increased risk of osteoporosis among smokers. The mechanism is unclear, but the relationship does not appear to result exclusively from additional confounding lifestyle factors (Brot et al., 1999). Smoking, however, was not a determinant of 25(OH)D concentrations in either African American or Caucasian women in NHANES III (Nesby-O'Dell et al., 2002).

Obesity is a significant factor in some population groups, and is associated with a trend towards lower serum 25(OH)D levels (Nesby-O'Dell, 2002). Some investigators attribute this trend to a tendency of vitamin D, whether from cutaneous or dietary sources, to be deposited in adipose tissue, where it is not bioavailable (Wortsman et al., 2000). Others suggest that the vitamin D endocrine system is altered in obesity, with the increased production of 1,25(OH)$_2$D exerting a negative

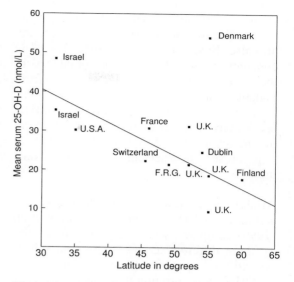

Figure 18.11: Relationship between latitude of country and serum 25(OH)D levels in groups of healthy elderly subjects studied in winter-spring. The regression equation, excluding the Danish results, is $y = 67 - 0.88x$, $r = -0.85$, $p < 0.001$. From McKenna et al., American Journal of Clinical Nutrition 41: 101–109, 1985 © Am J Clin Nutr. American Society for Clinical Nutrition.

feedback control on the hepatic synthesis of 25(OH)D (Bell et al., 1985).

Oral contraceptive use leads to higher concentrations of serum 25(OH)D (e.g., Harris and Dawson-Hughes, 1998; Nesby-O'Dell et al., 2002). Estrogen may alter the relative proportion of free and protein-bound 25(OH)D by increasing the concentrations of vitamin D-binding protein (Kleerekoper et al., 1991).

Anticonvulsant drugs, such as diphenylhydantoin and phenobarbital, if used for a long time, are also associated with low serum 25(OH)D concentrations and the development of rickets or osteomalacia (Hahn et al., 1975). The etiology of these conditions is unclear; they may result from calcium malabsorption caused by suppression of both absorption and metabolism of vitamin D by the drug.

Disease states such as intestinal malabsorption and steatorrhea caused by pancreatic insufficiency, inflammatory bowel disease, celiac disease, or massive bowel resection are also linked to lower serum 25(OH)D concentrations, rickets, and osteomalacia. In these cases, vitamin D depletion arises from malabsorption of dietary vitamin D (Efstathi-adou et al., 1999). Low serum 25(OH)D levels may also occur in diseases affecting the organs involved in vitamin D metabolism (e.g., hepatic disorders and chronic renal failure).

Analytical method has a marked effect on serum 25(OH)D concentrations. Lips et al. (1999) compared serum 25(OH)D measured by three different assays. The competitive protein-binding assay gave a mean serum 25(OH)D concentration that was 80% higher than the level obtained using HPLC, whereas the radioimmunoassay gave intermediate values. In general, the radioimmunoassay methods yield values that are about 30% lower than the competitive protein-binding assay. Hence, a cutoff value of 37.5 nmol/L based on the radioimmunoassay method is said to be comparable to 50 nmol/L when the competitive protein-binding method is used (Calvo and Whiting, 2003).

Interpretive criteria

Although it is now agreed that serum levels of 25(OH)D can be used to define vitamin D deficiency, insufficiency, hypovitaminosis, sufficiency, and toxicity (IOM, 1997), nevertheless, the cutoff values indicative of each stage are still uncertain. At present, two methods based on cutoff points are used to interpret serum 25(OH)D concentrations: a two-stage and a multistage approach.

The two-stage approach is the simplest and uses only two cutoffs to indicate hypovita-minosis D and hypervitaminosis D. In hypo-vitaminosis D, body stores of vitamin D are depleted and parathyroid levels are slightly elevated (although still within the normal range). Hence, low serum 25(OH)D levels associated with elevated parathyroid hormone concentrations are taken to indicate hypovita-

minosis D. However, there is no consensus on the cutoff indicative of hypovitaminosis D. In part, this is because the assay method used affects serum 25(OH)D concentrations, as noted earlier. In addition, age, latitude, race or ethnicity, vitamin D fortification, season, and sunlight exposure influence serum 25(OH)D levels. Hence, results in the literature must be interpreted cautiously.

In NHANES III, hypovitaminosis D was defined by a cutoff of $\leqslant 37.5$ nmol/L for serum 25(OH)D, based on a two-site radio-immunoassay (Nesby-O'Dell et al., 2002). This cutoff was based on studies among older Caucasians in whom parathyroid hormone levels were elevated when serum 25(OH)D concentrations were < 37.5 nmol/L (Webb et al., 1990; Gloth et al., 1995; Norman, 1998; Thomas et al., 1998). This same cutoff, in conjunction with a high parathyroid hormone concentration of > 6.4 pmol/L, has also been used to define vitamin D deficiency in neonates (Table 18.9) (Zeghound et al., 1997).

Others have used different 25(OH)D levels in serum, ranging from 50 to 100 nmol/L, as the cutoff indicative of hypovitaminosis D (Docio et al., 1998; McKenna and Freaney, 1998; Lamberg-Allardt et al., 2001). Nesby-O'Dell et al. (2002) note that the lower limit of the normal range for serum 25(OH)D levels in adults varies from a low of 20 to as high as 37.5 nmol/L. For children, the lower limit of the desirable level may be between 30 and 50 nmol/L, based on the response of serum 1,25(OH)$_2$D and PTH concentrations in Spanish children to supplemental vitamin D (Docio et al., 1998).

Cutoff values indicative of hypervitamin-osis D are also not clearly defined. In all the reported cases of vitamin D toxicity, serum 25(OH)D concentrations exceed 200 nmol/L. Values above 500 nmol/L have been associated with concomitant hypercalcemia, which is clear evidence of vitamin D toxicity (Haddad and Stamp, 1974). Such high levels have been linked to excessive consumption of milk fortified with vitamin D (Jacobus et al.,1992). The U.S. Food and Nutrition Board (IOM, 1997) suggests that serum 25(OH)D concentrations ranging from 400 to 1250 nmol/L have been associated with disturbances indicative of hypervitaminosis D.

The multistage approach recognizes five stages of vitamin D status: vitamin D deficiency, vitamin D insufficiency, hypovitaminosis D, vitamin D sufficiency, and vitamin D toxicity, as shown in Figure 18.12. However, as noted earlier, currently there is no consensus on the serum 25(OH)D cutoff values that should be used to define these stages.

In vitamin D deficiency, there is evidence of severe hyperparathyroidism, calcium malabsorption, and bone diseases such as rickets in infants and osteomalacia in adults. Vitamin D insufficiency is characterized by mild hyperparathyrodism, a reduction in calcium absorption, reduced bone mineral density, and possibly subclinical myopathy; in hypovitaminosis D, in contrast, body stores of vitamin D are low, and the parathyroid hormone levels may be elevated. No disturbances of vitamin D–dependent functions are apparent in vitamin D sufficiency; in vitamin D toxicity, however, increases in absorption of calcium and net bone resorption lead to hypercalcemia (Zitterman, 2003).

Only a few studies have correlated bone diseases such as rickets in infants and osteomalacia in adults with serum 25(OH)D concentrations (Haddad and Stamp, 1974; Preece et al., 1975; Scharla, 1998; Blok et al., 2000). In these studies, serum 25(OH)D concentra-

tions <12.5 nmol/L have been consistently related to disturbances in bone mineralization. Hence, serum 25(OH)D concentrations of <12.5 nmol/L are often used to define vitamin D deficiency.

Cutoff points used to define vitamin D insufficiency, however, are not so well defined, and are highly controversial. Proposed cutoff values have ranged from 12.5–100 nmol/L, depending on the geographic location, analytical method, etc. (IOM, 1997; Malabanan et al., 1998; Need et al., 2000; Vieth et al., 2001; Calvo and Whiting, 2003). These cutoffs have been associated with mild hyperparathyroidism and, in some cases, increased bone turnover and a decreased bone-mass density (Gloth et al., 1995; Ooms et al., 1995; van der Wielen et al., 1995).

Hypovitaminosis D in the multistage approach is defined by the cutoff values for serum 25(OH)D indicative of the same disturbances, noted earlier for hypovitaminosis D in the two-stage approach. Serum 25(OH)D concentrations indicative of vitamin D sufficiency are in the range of 100 to 200 nmol/L, depending on the assay method and the influencing factors noted earlier. Zittermann (2003) suggests that serum 25(OH)D concentrations > 250 nmol/L indicate vitamin D toxicity.

The U.K. national surveys used an alternative approach for the interpretation of serum 25(OH)D levels, analyzed using a radioimmunoassay commercial kit. Mean, median, and lower and upper 2.5 or 5th percentiles are presented by age and sex for children and persons aged 65 y and older, respectively (Gregory et al., 1995, 2000; Finch et al., 1998). Note that in a population, the distribution of 25(OH)D values in serum is often skewed, and log transformations are often performed in the statistical analysis to normalize the data.

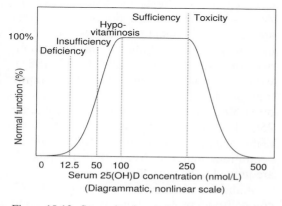

Figure 18.12: Stages in vitamin D status. From Zittermann et al., British Journal of Nutrition 89: 552–572, 2003, with permission of the authors.

Measurement of 25-hydroxyvitamin D

Most clinical assays, with the exception of the HPLC method, do not distinguish between 25(OH)D$_2$ and 25(OH)D$_3$ in serum, and the sum of these two components is therefore usually reported as 25(OH)D. Methods available include competitive protein-binding assays, radioimmunoassays, and HPLC with subsequent direct ultraviolet (UV) detection. In all of these methods, the sterols must first be extracted from the serum with an organic solvent. Recovery of the sterol can only be monitored for the radioimmunoassay methods based on the use of a tritiated tracer.

Only the HPLC method is capable of separating and measuring both $25(OH)D_2$ and $25(OH)D_3$ (Jones, 1978; Aksnes et al., 1992) in a single serum sample (Hummer et al., 1985), but it requires a large sample volume, expensive equipment, and considerable technical expertise. The competitive binding assay uses either mammalian serum or a tissue-binding protein for 25(OH)D. Coefficients of variation for within and between assays are 4%–7% and 7%–10%, respectively (van der Wielen et al., 1995); they tend to be higher in the lower range of measurements (Lips et al., 1999).

Commercial radioimmunoassay (RIA) kits use either tritiated or a radioiodine tracer (^{125}I), and a scintillation or gamma counter, respectively. Of the methods available, a RIA using a radioiodine tracer is now the method of choice for measuring circulating serum 25(OH)D (Hollis, 2000). Care must be taken, however, to ensure that the RIA kit chosen measures both circulating $25(OH)D_2$ and $25(OH)D_3$ equally so that total 25(OH)D in serum is not underestimated. Hollis (2000) recommends the kit manufactured by Dia-Sorin Corporation (Stillwater, MN). Some of the RIA kits allow the assay of both 25(OH)D and $1,25(OH)_2D$ (Hollis et al., 1996).

Performance of all the 25(OH)D assays should be monitored through the Vitamin D External Quality Assessment Scheme (Vieth and Carter, 2001). Serum or plasma samples collected using EDTA or heparin as an anticoagulant can be used for the assays, and samples can be frozen, although repeated freezing and thawing should be avoided.

18.2.2 Serum $1,25(OH)_2D$

$1,25(OH)_2D$ [calcitriol] is the active form of vitamin D. It interacts with its nuclear receptor in the intestine, bone, and kidney to regulate calcium and bone metabolism. $1,25(OH)_2D$ also has several other noncalcemic cellular actions. For further details see Holick (2003).

Measurement of $1,25(OH)_2D$ in serum is not a useful marker of vitamin D status because it has a short half-life (4–6 h) and levels are under stringent homeostatic regulation by a variety of factors at the site of $1,25(OH)_2D$ synthesis in the kidney. Hence, it is not surprising that no seasonal variation in serum $1,25(OH)_2D$ concentrations has been reported (Landin-Wilhelmsen et al., 1995).

Synthesis of $1,25(OH)_2D$ in the kidney is stimulated by low serum concentrations of calcium or phosphorus and is inhibited by excess $1,25(OH)_2D$. In cases of vitamin D sufficiency, a positive relationship exists between serum $1,25(OH)_2D$ and 25(OH)D concentrations (Kinyamu et al., 1997; Need et al., 2000), presumably because 25(OH)D is the substrate for $1,25(OH)_2D$, but in vitamin D deficiency, this relationship is reversed. This occurs because as serum 25(OH)D concentrations fall there is a rise in the concentration of parathyroid hormone (Section 18.2.5) (Need et al., 2000), which increases the renal production of $1,25(OH)_2D$. As a result the circulating concentrations of $1,25(OH)_2D$ often become normal or even elevated. In contrast, serum $1,25(OH)_2D$ levels decrease in renal disease (which affects the hydroxylase enzyme — 25(OH)D-1-α-hydroxylase); levels are very low in anephric patients (i.e., those lacking a functional kidney), and patients on hemodialysis (DeLuca and Schnoes, 1983). Even in normal healthy subjects, concentrations of serum $1,25(OH)_2D$ are very low, often 500–1000 times lower than circulating $25(OH)D_2$ levels, making analysis difficult (Zittermann, 2003). Serum $1,25(OH)_2D$ concentrations ranging from 48 to 100 pmol/L are judged to be normal.

Methods of analysis include HPLC, competitive protein binding assays, and radioimmunoassays using a radioiodine or tritiated tracer.

18.2.3 Serum alkaline phosphatase

Alkaline phosphatase (EC 3.1.1.1) activity in serum can be used as an indirect measure of vitamin D status. Activity increases in osteomalacia in adults and childhood rickets but is generally normal in osteoporosis.

Increases in the activity of alkaline phosphatase are usually proportional to the severity of vitamin D depletion. McKenna et al. (1985) showed that elderly Irish individuals with serum 25(OH)D levels indicative of severe or marginal vitamin D depletion had slightly higher serum alkaline phosphatase activity than those with 25(OH)D levels classified as replete (Figure 18.13). Seasonal changes in serum alkaline phosphatase activity have also been observed in cross-sectional studies of Irish and American elderly persons, levels decreasing with seasonal rises in serum 25(OH)D levels (Omdahl et al., 1982; McKenna et al., 1985).

Serum alkaline phosphatase activity is also affected by sex and age, again in the opposite direction to changes in the levels of serum 25(OH)D. Serum alkaline phosphatase activity is significantly higher in females relative to males (Table 18.10) and in older versus younger adults; activity is also higher in growing children and pregnant women, especially during the third trimester (McKenna, 1992). In the U.K. national survey of young people 4–18 y, mean activity was lowest in the oldest age group (15–18 y), especially among the girls (Gregory et al., 2000).

The activity of serum alkaline phosphatase is also altered by various disease states such as hyperparathyroidism, Paget's disease, secondary bone cancer, and cholestasis (Sauberlich, 1999). Serum alkaline phosphatase activity may decrease in zinc deficiency but, as noted earlier, appears to be close to normal in osteoporosis.

In general, measurement of alkaline phosphatase activity in serum is best used to confirm a clinical diagnosis of vitamin D deficiency, or as a screening tool, but it is not very useful for detecting subclinical vitamin D deficiency.

Interpretive criteria

Serum alkaline phosphatase activity is normally expressed as U/L. The reference range for normal adults is 30–135 U/L (Gregory et al., 2000). Total plasma alkaline phosphatase activity was measured in the recent U.K. national surveys (Gregory et al., 1995, 2000, Finch et al., 1998), with the exception of the survey on pre-school children. Mean, median, and lower and upper 2.5 or 5th percentiles by age and sex are presented.

Measurement of alkaline phosphatase

Several methods are available for the assay of serum alkaline phosphatase; both manual and automated procedures can be used. The method of Bessey et al. (1946) is often used for the assay of alkaline phosphatase in serum or plasma. The activity of serum alkaline phosphatase should be expressed as U/L. The within-subject coefficient of variation for serum alkaline phosphatase activity ranges from 4.6% to 9.2%, depending on the time frame and dietary regimen (Gallagher et al., 1989). Serum and plasma from heparinized blood samples can both be used. The enzyme is reasonably stable in frozen serum or plasma.

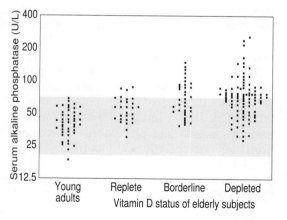

Figure 18.13: Serum alkaline phosphatase values in elderly subjects with serum 25(OH)D concentrations classified as replete, borderline, or depleted. From McKenna et al., American Journal of Clinical Nutrition 41: 101–109, 1985 © Am J Clin Nutr. American Society for Clinical Nutrition.

18.2.4 Serum parathyroid hormone

Parathyroid hormone (PTH) levels in serum or plasma are considered to be a functional index of vitamin D status in the normocalcemic state. In vitamin D deficiency, when calcium absorption is reduced, serum PTH levels rise to induce calcium mobilization from the bone and increase tubular reabsorption of calcium in the kidney. In this way, serum calcium is maintained at a physiologically optimum level. As a result, serum PTH concentrations are inversely related to serum 25(OH)D levels (Meulmeester et al., 1990; Chapuy et al., 1997; Zeghoud et al., 1997; Need et al., 2000; Holick, 2003).

Several researchers have investigated the threshold values for serum 25(OH)D concentrations that induce an increase in serum parathyroid secretion. Reported threshold values have varied: in a study of Australian postmenopausal women the threshold value was 40 nmol/L, as shown in Figure 18.14 (Need et al., 2000), whereas in French adults it was 78 nmol/L (Chapuy et al., 1997). Even small increases in PTH levels may have a negative influence on bone mass and increase the risk of non-vertebral fracture (Chapuy et al., 1997). Hence, a combination of serum PTH and serum 25(OH)D concentrations is often recommended as an indicator of vitamin D status.

Serum PTH levels increase with age (Endres et al., 1987). Season also influences PTH concentrations, as might be expected (Rapuri et al., 2002). Parathyroid hormone can be measured by radioimmunoassay using commercial kits.

18.2.5 Calcium and phosphorus in serum and urine

Many studies of vitamin D status have included the measurement of calcium and phosphorus concentrations in serum or urine. The measurements are most useful if combined with the measurements of serum 25(OH)D and PTH concentrations. In vitamin D deficiency in infants and children, the serum calcium and phosphorus levels are usually re-

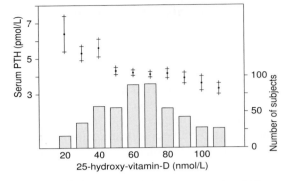

Figure 18.14: Mean (± SEM) serum parathyroid hormone (PTH) concentrations at 10 nmol/L intervals of serum 25(OH)D concentrations in 496 postmenopausal women. Serum PTH (+) is significantly higher in the minority of women with serum 25(OH)D concentrations ≤ 40 nmol/L ($p < 0.001$). Data from Need et al., American Journal of Clinical Nutrition 71: 1577–1581, 2000 © Am J Clin Nutr. American Society for Clinical Nutrition.

duced. For example, significantly lower mean serum calcium concentrations were reported in French neonates with serum 25(OH)D concentrations < 30 nmol/L and elevated PTH concentrations, in comparison with subjects with normal values for these biochemical parameters (Zeghoud et al., 1997). Unlike total serum calcium alone, the existence of such a triad of biochemical disturbances strongly indicates vitamin D deficiency.

Serum calcium is also used to identify possible vitamin D intoxication. In such cases, concentrations of serum 25(OH)D and serum calcium are elevated and provide additional evidence for hypervitaminosis D.

The response of urinary calcium and phosphorus levels to changes in vitamin D status varies, as excretion of these minerals is also affected by dietary intakes. Hence changes in urinary calcium and phosphorus concentrations are not specific for vitamin D status. Details of the measurement of calcium and phosphorus in serum and urine are given in Chapter 23.

18.3 Vitamin E

In the past, vitamin E was the generic term for a group of eight naturally occurring toco-

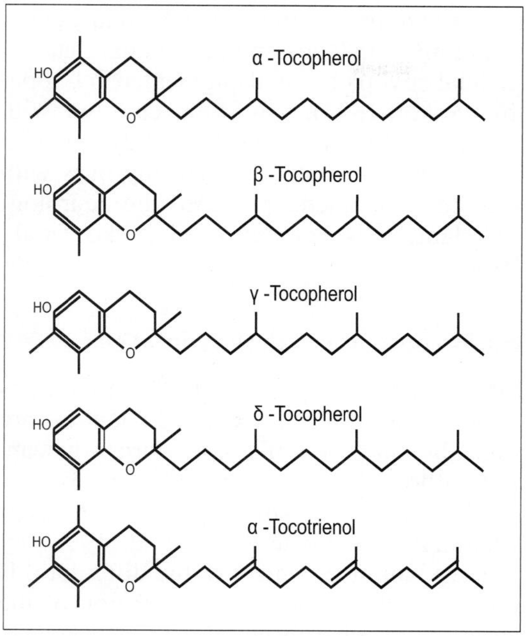

Figure 18.15: The structure of naturally occurring vitamin E compounds. All the tocopherols are in the RRR-form.

pherol and tocotrienol derivatives. The tocotrienols have similar structures to their corresponding tocopherols, but the side chains are unsaturated, as for α-tocotrienol shown in Figure 18.15. It is now known that these various forms of vitamin E are not interconvertible in humans and do not behave in the same way in metabolism. Only the naturally occurring form of α-tocopherol (i.e., RRR-α-tocopherol), and the synthetic forms (RSR-, RRS-, and RSS-) which are commonly used for fortification and in dietary supplements, are presently considered to be active forms of vitamin E. The other forms are equally well absorbed from the diet but their release from the liver into plasma lipoproteins is minimal. For this reason only α-tocopherol is considered when assessing nutrient requirements.

Functions of vitamin E

Vitamin E functions primarily as a lipid antioxidant. It prevents cellular damage by inhibiting the peroxidation of polyunsaturated fatty acids in cell membranes. Vitamin E performs this function by scavenging free radicals formed by the reaction of polyunsaturated fatty acids with oxygen (Sokol, 1996).

Vitamin E may also have other specific functions, besides antioxidant activity. Some investigators suggest that vitamin E may be involved in anti-atherosclerotic mechanisms through the modulation of cellular signaling and transcriptional regulation. Also, vitamin E has been associated with anticarcinogenic properties, through its proposed role in modulating immune function, and in the induction of apoptosis. More research is required to confirm these suggestions. For more details on the biological functions of vitamin E see Brigelius-Flohé et al. (2002).

Absorption and metabolism of vitamin E

The mechanism involved in the absorption of vitamin E is not fully understood. Absorption from the intestine into the mucosal cell depends on pancreatic function, biliary secretion, micelle formation, uptake into enterocytes, and chylomicron secretion. Defects at any stage may lead to impaired absorption. Hence, in diseases where severe and chronic malabsorption of fat exists (e.g., cystic fibrosis, celiac disease, and chronic cholestatic liver disease), the absorption of vitamin E is compromised. A rare genetic disorder, abetalipoproteinemia, involving a defect in chylomicron synthesis, also causes vitamin E malabsorption.

Vitamin E is initially transported in chylomicrons and enters the circulation via the lymphatic system. Chylomicrons are then hydrolyzed by lipoprotein lipase in the systemic circulation, during which some vitamin E may be released to the muscle and adipose tissue or transferred to high-density lipoproteins (HDLs). The vitamin E acquired by HDLs can also be transferred to other circulating lipoproteins, such as low-density lipoproteins (LDLs) and the very low-density lipoproteins (VLDLs) (Traber et al., 1990). However, not all forms of vitamin E are incorporated equally into VLDL in the liver. The RRR-α-tocopherol is preferentially incorporated into VLDL by the action of a binding protein, α-tocoperol-transfer-protein, in the liver. As a result, VLDL secreted from the liver is rich in RRR-α-tocopherol. The other forms of tocopherol (i.e., β, γ, and δ) are excreted in the bile. The VLDLs also accumulate in non-hepatic tissues, especially at sites where free radical protection is greatest.

During the conversion of VLDL to LDL in the circulation, some α-tocopherol remains within the core lipids and thus is incorporated in LDL. Most α-tocopherol then enters the cells of the peripheral tissues within the intact lipoprotein through the LDL receptor pathway. For more details see Farrell and Roberts (1994).

Deficiency of vitamin E

In animals, various vitamin E deficiency syndromes have been identified. These include sterility in male rats, fetal resorption in female rats, muscular dystrophy in rabbits and guinea pigs, encephalomalacia in chicks, and hematological disorders in monkeys. Vitamin E deficiency in animals has also been linked to increased prostaglandin synthesis, platelet aggregation, impaired cell-membrane function, and red cell defects.

In humans, dietary vitamin E deficiency is rare. Indeed, cases of this deficiency in normal persons consuming diets low in vitamin E have never been described. Vitamin E deficiency in humans may be caused by defects in the gene for hepatic α-tocopherol transfer protein (Cavalier et al., 1998), or may be the result of protein-energy malnutrition (Kalra et al., 1998). Alternatively, vitamin E deficiency may be secondary to fat-malabsorption syndromes (Rada and Brewer, 1993). Those most frequently implicated include cystic fibrosis, abetalipoproteinemia, chronic cholestatic liver diseases, celiac disease, and short bowel syndrome.

Premature infants may also be at risk for vitamin E deficiency, induced by transient malabsorption of α-tocopherol and low reserves. In such cases, hemolytic anemia may be observed (Hassan et al., 1966; Oski and Barness, 1967; Johnson et al., 1974).

Peripheral neuropathy is the primary symptom of vitamin E deficiency in humans. Other symptoms include spinocerebellar ataxia, skeletal myopathy, and pigmented retinopathy (Sokol, 1993). In some children with chronic cholestasis, neurological dysfunction has been documented, which improves with vitamin E treatment, provided the neurological damage is not advanced (Sokol et al., 1984).

Foods sources and dietary intakes

Major food sources of vitamin E in the diets of populations in industrialized countries are vegetable and seed oils (e.g., corn, soybean, and safflower oils) and margarine. Hence, low-fat diets may result in reduced intakes of vitamin E (Velthuis-te Wierik et al., 1996).

The vitamin E content of the different oils varies widely, as does the proportion of the different tocopherols (Figure 18.16). Hence, there are marked differences in per capita supply of α-tocopherol among countries, depending in part on the type and quantity of dietary oils used (Bellizzi et al., 1994). Levels range from 8 to 10 mg/capita per day in Iceland and Finland to about 20–25 mg/capita per day in France, Greece, and Spain. In southern Europe, sunflower seed oils, a rich source of α-tocopherol, are often consumed, whereas in northern Europe, soybean oil, a poor source of α-tocopherol (Figure 18.16),

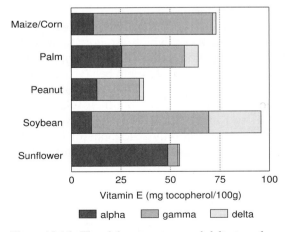

Figure 18.16: The alpha-, gamma-, and delta-tocopherol content of some vegetable oils. From FAO/WHO (2002).

is preferred. Animal products are very poor sources of vitamin E.

The bioavailability of vitamin E in the diet is variable, ranging from 20% to 80% in published studies, and depends on the form of the vitamin E and the amount per meal; absorption decreases at high intakes.

Details of the method used to calculate the vitamin E activity of mixed diets is given in Section 4.3.5. The commercially available synthetic forms of vitamin E consist of an approximately equal mixture of eight stereoisomeric forms of α-tocopherol.

Effect of high intakes of vitamin E

Self-supplementation with vitamin E is increasingly common in many industrialized countries because of an assumed beneficial effect on sexuality, aging, and the prevention of chronic diseases such as cardiovascular disease and cancer. So far, results of several prospective, randomized, placebo-controlled trials have been inconsistent and have failed to confirm a clear benefit of vitamin E on the prevention of chronic disease (Brigelius-Flohé et al., 2002).

Fortunately, excessive doses of vitamin E, unlike vitamins A and D, do not appear to produce deleterious effects (Farrell and Bieri, 1975). The Tolerable Upper Intake (UL) for all adults $\geqslant 19$ y has been set by the U.S. Food and Nutrition Board (IOM, 2000) at 1000 mg/d of any form of supplementary α-tocopherol; recommendations for children and adolescents are given in IOM (2000). The Tolerable Upper Intake Levels for α-tocopherol set by the Scientific Committee on Food for the European Commission are lower. Details are available at:

http://www.europa.eu.int/comm/food/index_en.html

Further research is needed before it can be concluded that long-term self-supplementation with vitamin E is without risk.

Indices of vitamin E status

At present, there are no suitable, practical biomarkers to accurately reflect dietary intakes or body stores of vitamin E. Several alternatives are described below, some of which reflect oxidant stress.

18.3.1 Serum α-tocopherol

Most vitamin E in human serum is in the LDL fractions; more than 90% is in the form of α-tocopherol (Behrens et al., 1982). The concentration of α-tocopherol in serum is the most commonly used biochemical marker of vitamin E status and is technically simple to measure.

In a vitamin E depletion–repletion study, a linear increase in plasma α-tocopherol concentrations with increasing vitamin E intake up to 17 mg/d was reported (Horwitt, 1960). In observational studies, reported correlations between vitamin E intakes and serum α-tocopherol concentrations have been variable. They range from about 0.15 to 0.65, the highest being noted in groups of individuals taking vitamin E supplements (Gregory et al., 1990; Gascón-Vila et al., 1997; Finch et al., 1998).

Concentrations of serum α-tocopherol tend to be lower in persons living in low-income countries, where they are often associated with lower tocopherol intakes. Rahman et al. (1964) reported that 21% of persons living in rural East Pakistan had serum tocopherol levels <11.6 μmol/L. Even in industrialized countries, however, serum α-tocopherol concentrations < 20 μmol/L have been reported. Indeed, in NHANES II, after age standardization, about 28% of the U.S. population had α-tocopherol concentrations lower than 20 μmol/L (Ford and Sowell, 1999). In the U.K. national surveys, 20% of British adults and about 6% of persons aged 65 y and older had low levels (Gregory et al., 1990; Finch et al., 1998).

Factors affecting serum α-tocopherol

Age-related changes in serum tocopherol concentrations may occur (Vandewoude and Vandewoude, 1987). Concentrations increase up to the sixth decade of life, as shown in data from NHANES III and HHANES (Ford and

Age Group	Concentration
NHANES III 1988–1994	
M, 9–13	18.3 ± 0.18
M, 19–30	20.7 ± 0.24
M, 51–70	30.0 ± 0.42
F, 9–13	18.4 ± 0.26
F, 19–30	21.6 ± 0.22
F, 51–70	33.0 ± 0.60
HHANES, 1982–1984	
M+F 6–11	17.1 ± 0.14
M+F 12–19	16.0 ± 0.20
M+F 20–44	22.4 ± 0.42
M+F 45–74	29.2 ± 0.59

Table 18.11: Mean serum tocopherol concentrations (μmol/L ± SEM) for subjects of various ages. Data from NHANES III (IOM, 2000) and HHANES (Sauberlich, 1999). A more complete summary of serum vitamin E data from NHANES III is given in Appendix 18.3.

Sowell, 1999) (Table 18.11). The age-related increase parallels the increase in total serum lipids.

Sex differences are not significant. The concentrations in adult males and females were similar in both NHANES III (Ford and Sowell, 1999), and the U.K. national adult surveys (Gregory et al., 1990; Finch et al., 1998).

Racial differences reported in NHANES III were significant. African Americans had the lowest concentration of α-tocopherol of any racial or ethnic group (Ford and Sowell, 1999), with 41% having a serum α-tocopherol level < 20 μmol/L. A similar trend was reported among adolescents from three U.S. cities (Neuhouser et al., 2001). Reasons for this racial difference in serum α-tocopherol concentrations are unclear.

Vitamin E supplement use increases serum α-tocopherol concentrations but the correlation of the amount ingested and α-tocopherol concentrations in serum is usually weak (Neuhouser et al., 2001). Factors that complicate this relationship include the variable biological activity of the different forms of vitamin E and their incomplete and variable

absorption. In the U.K. adult national survey, where 7-d weighed food records were used, significant but modest correlations between serum α-tocopherol and supplemented diets were found (Gregory et al., 1990; Finch et al., 1998). No significant correlations were noted in NHANES III when intakes were obtained using 24-h dietary recalls (Ford and Sowell, 1999).

Total serum lipid levels often correlate positively with serum concentrations of α-tocopherol because α-tocopherol circulates in the blood mainly with the low-density lipoprotein fraction (Behrens et al., 1982). In NHANES III, serum cholesterol, particularly HDL cholesterol, correlated strongly with serum α-tocopherol concentrations (Ford and Sowell, 1999), consistent with the findings of others (Herbeth et al., 1989).

Smoking appears to impact negatively on serum α-tocopherol concentrations in some (Bolton-Smith et al., 1991; Herbeth et al., 1989) but not all (Ford and Sowell, 1999) studies. The decrease may be linked to the high and sustained load of free radicals that exist in cigarette tar and smoke (Pryor and Stone, 1993), as well as from oxidants produced by activated phagocytes (Duthie et al., 1991). Vitamin E supplementation of smokers does appear to reduce indicators of lipid peroxidation (Morrow et al., 1995; Reilly et al., 1996).

Premature infants have low concentrations of serum α-tocopherol, often ranging from 4.6 to 6.5 μmol/L (Bortolotti et al., 1993). This arises from low reserves and transient malabsorption of α-tocopherol.

Pregnant women with adequate intakes of vitamin E have elevated serum α-tocopherol values, in parallel with an increase in total lipids (Horwitt et al. 1972). There are no reports of vitamin E deficiency during pregnancy, and no evidence that supplementation during pregnancy would prevent deficiency signs appearing in premature infants (IOM, 2000).

Fat-malabsorption syndromes often induce low serum α-tocopherol values, which are associated with early functional signs of vitamin E deficiency such as muscle weakness, ceroid deposition, and decreased erythrocyte survival time in vivo (Farrell et al., 1977). Malabsorption syndromes implicated in children include cystic fibrosis, celiac disease, and chronic cholestatic liver disease (Sokol et al., 1989a). In adults, primary biliary cirrhosis is associated with intestinal malabsorption of vitamin E (Sokol et al., 1989b).

Genetic defects in apolipoprotein B or the hepatic α-tocopherol transfer protein lead to impaired transfer of vitamin E to tissues and, hence, low serum α-tocopherol levels. Neurological symptoms, characteristic of a severe vitamin E deficiency syndrome, develop if supplements of α-tocopherol are not given (Brigelius-Flohé et al., 2002). The symptoms include loss of deep tendon reflexes, cerebellar ataxia, dysarthria, and mental retardation. In some cases, skeletal myopathy and *retinitis pigmentosa* are observed (Sokol, 1993; Gotoda et al., 1995).

Interpretive criteria

Serum α-tocopherol levels of <11.6 µmol/L in adults usually indicate a biochemical deficiency of vitamin E, but not always a clinical deficiency (Sauberlich, 1999). Adults with such low levels often show elevated (> 5%) hemolysis of erythrocytes in the peroxide hemolysis test (Section 18.3.6). Many infants and children have serum tocopherol levels <11.6 µmol/L because of lower lipid concentrations, but no evidence of vitamin E deficiency (Farrell et al., 1978). Hence, the adult cutoff is not appropriate for pediatric populations.

In NHANES III, serum α-tocopherol concentrations < 20 µmol/L were classified as "low" (Ford and Sowell, 1999). This more conservative cutoff was selected because of the apparent increased risk of cardiovascular disease below this concentration (Riemersma et al., 1991; Singh et al., 1995).

Data for mean and selected percentiles for serum vitamin E concentrations (µg/dl) by age and sex, but not by race or ethnicity, for persons from 4 to > 71 y from NHANES III can be found in Appendix 18.3 (Ford and Sowell, 1999). Data on mean, median, and lower and upper 2.5 or 5th percentiles by age and sex for plasma α-tocopherol concentrations and tocopherol : cholesterol ratios are available for the U.K. adult national surveys (Gregory et al., 1990; Finch et al., 1998).

Measurement of serum α-tocopherol

The preferred method for measuring the tocopherols in serum is HPLC. This method can also be used for erythrocytes, platelets, adipose tissue, and buccal mucosal cells. Several HPLC methods are available, involving fluorescence (Epler et al., 1993), electrochemical (Vandewoude et al., 1984), or UV detection (Bortolotti et al., 1993). These techniques are relatively simple, rapid, noninvasive, and suitable for studies of pediatric populations because only small samples (e.g., 100–200 µg plasma) are required (Bieri et al., 1979; Driskell et al., 1982). Most HPLC techniques (e.g., normal-phase HPLC) can analyze α-, β-, and γ-tocopherols separately (Tangney et al., 1979).

The CV for duplicate samples for α-tocopherol via HPLC can be as low as 2% for serum (Schåfer and Overvad, 1990), but the within-subject CV for serum α-tocopherol can be as high as 12.9%, even when the diet is constant (Gallagher et al., 1992).

A certified reference material for α-tocopherol is available from the National Institute of Sciences and Technology (NIST) (Gaitherburg, MD). Special precautions must be taken during both preparation and storage of samples for tocopherol analyses because vitamin E is subject to oxidation. Exposure to bright light, as well as repetitive freezing and thawing should be avoided. Fasting blood samples are preferred to reduce the influence of dietary lipids on serum tocopherol levels. Frozen serum samples are stable for at least 16 mo if stored at −70°C (Driskell et al., 1982).

18.3.2 Serum α-tocopherol: cholesterol ratio

Vitamin E, largely in the form of α-tocopherol, circulates in the blood mainly with the low-density lipoprotein fraction (Behrens et al., 1982). In adults, levels of α-tocopherol in serum are highly correlated with total lipid levels (Horwitt et al., 1972; Vatassery et al., 1983a). As a result, α-tocopherol : lipid ratios have been used to assess vitamin E status.

Blood lipids consist of mainly cholesterol, triglycerides, and phospholipids and α-tocopherol correlates best with the cholesterol fraction. Indeed, in NHANES III, serum cholesterol was one of the strongest predictors of serum α-tocopherol concentrations (Ford and Sowell, 1999). As a result, the α-tocopherol : total cholesterol ratio is now the preferred measure of vitamin E status. Its use prevents the overestimation of vitamin E deficiency in developing countries, where serum lipid levels are often low, and permits comparisons between different age groups within populations (Gregory et al., 1990).

Ratios of α-tocopherol : cholesterol that are > 2.2 μmol α-tocopherol / mmol cholesterol are judged to indicate an adequate vitamin E status; lower ratios have been associated with erythrocyte hemolysis after exposure to oxidizing agents (Department of Health, 1992). In surveys in some more developed countries, few people have α-tocopherol : cholesterol ratios below the cutoff of 2.25 μmol/mmol (Thurnham et al., 1986). In NHANES III, the mean α-tocopherol : cholesterol ratio for adults > 18 y was 5.1 μmol/mmol (Ford and Sowell, 1999). Levels were lower in the U.K. national survey of adults; the mean α-tocopherol : cholesterol ratios for men and women were 4.65 and 4.58 μmol/mmol, respectively. The U.K. surveys provide data on the mean, and selected percentiles by age and sex (Gregory et al., 1990, 1995, 2000; Finch et al., 1998).

18.3.3 Erythrocyte tocopherol

Studies of erythrocyte tocopherol concentrations as a measure of vitamin E status are limited. This is probably because it is technically more difficult to determine tocopherol in the erythrocytes than in the serum. Concentrations of tocopherol in erythrocytes are approximately 20% of those in plasma.

Initial studies in rats suggested that tocopherol levels in erythrocytes and plasma were closely correlated (Poukka and Bieri, 1970). Later work showed marked variation in erythrocyte tocopherol levels in rats fed the same dietary levels of vitamin E, especially at low dosage levels (Lehmann, 1981). There appears to be no justification for using erythrocyte tocopherol as a routine biomarker of vitamin E status in humans.

18.3.4 Platelet tocopherol

Platelets contain significant concentrations of α-tocopherol and small amounts of γ-tocopherol. As a result, the platelet tocopherol content appears to be a promising marker of vitamin E status in humans (Kaempf et al., 1994). Platelet aggregation is inhibited by α-tocopherol, and both deficiencies and excess of α-tocopherol appear to alter platelet function.

A linear relationship between platelet tocopherol and the dosage of DL-α-tocopherol was noted in five human subjects, up to the daily dose of 1800 IU (Vatassery et al., 1983a). These findings were confirmed by Lehmann et al. (1988), who concluded that platelets were more sensitive for measuring dose response than use of plasma, erythrocytes, or lymphocytes. Levels of tocopherol in platelets are independent of serum lipid concentrations. This is an important advantage relative to serum tocopherol concentrations (Table 18.12). Platelet α-, γ-, and total tocopherol concentrations decline significantly with age, but it is not known whether such decreases affect platelet function in the elderly (Vatassery et al., 1983b).

18.3.5 Tissue tocopherol

Analysis of adipose tissue or liver biopsy samples for tocopherol may be a useful index of body stores of vitamin E and thus long-

	Plasma		Platelet	
	α-toc.	γ-toc.	α-toc.	γ-toc.
Total lipid	0.79*	0.60*	0.22	0.15
Cholesterol	0.58*	0.46*	0.27	0.17
Triglyceride	0.78*	0.61*	0.08	0.09

Table 18.12: Correlation coefficients showing the relation of α- and γ-tocopherol in plasma and platelets to total lipid, cholesterol, and triglyceride concentrations in 49 male subjects. * indicates that correlations are statistically significant ($p < 0.001$). From Vatassery et al., American Journal of Clinical Nutrition 37: 1020–1024, 1983 © Am J Clin Nutr. American Society for Clinical Nutrition.

term vitamin E status. For example, adipose tissue with a low vitamin E content was seen in vitamin E–deficient children with chronic cholestasis (Sokol et al., 1983) and adults with a-beta-lipoproteinemia (Kayden et al., 1983). Relationships between dietary intake of α-tocopherol and adipose-tissue tocopherol concentrations have also been noted in healthy adults (Kardinaal et al., 1995; Su et al., 1998), which are independent of the adipose tissue site (Schäfer and Overvad, 1990). During weight reduction, however, this correlation is weakened because weight loss is accompanied by a rise in the adipose tissue tocopherol concentration relative to triglycerides.

Collection of adipose tissue samples for large population studies is still difficult as the method is quite invasive, although rapid methods have now been developed. Biopsy samples are generally collected from the upper buttock (Section 7.3.7) (El-Sohemy et al., 2002).

Buccal mucosal cells have also been investigated as an alternative biopsy sample for assessing α-tocopherol status (Kaempf et al., 1994), although their usefulness is still uncertain (Erhardt et al., 2002b). They can be sampled easily and noninvasively by gentle scraping with a spatula. Cells adhering to the spatula are then suspended and washed three times with isotonic saline prior to sonication and analysis. The preferred mode of expression for the α-tocopherol content of buccal mucosal cells is in terms of μmol per gram of protein (Kaempf et al., 1994).

Interpretive criteria for evaluating α-tocopherol concentrations in biopsy samples from both adipose tissue and buccal mucosal cells are still required.

18.3.6 Erythrocyte hemolysis test

The erythrocyte hemolysis test has been used as a functional index of vitamin E status and is based on the antioxidant properties of vitamin E. The test measures the ability of red cells to resist oxidant damage. The level of hemolysis correlates inversely with serum total tocopherol levels, increasing with vitamin E deficiency (Binder and Spiro, 1967), provided the technique is rigorously standardized. It is easy to perform and requires only a small blood sample.

The test, however, lacks specificity; changes in the status of other nutrients can also influence the rate of erythrocyte hemolysis (Melhorn et al., 1971). In children with cholestasis, the hemolysis test underestimates the level of vitamin E deficiency, as indicated by plasma vitamin E, the vitamin E : lipid ratio, and the formation of malondialdehyde (Section 18.3.7) (Cynamon and Isenberg, 1987).

Freshly prepared samples of erythrocytes must be used for the erythrocyte hemolysis test, making it an impractical method for field studies. Hydrogen peroxide is most commonly used as the hemolyzing agent. Modifications have been made to enhance the sensitivity of this test such as measurement of potassium release (by flame photometry) rather than hemoglobin release. However, this modification did not enhance the reliability of the erythrocyte hemolysis test as a measure of vitamin E status in preterm infants (van Zoeren-Grobben et al., 1998). Details of the test are given in Sauberlich (1999).

18.3.7 Erythrocyte malondialdehyde release in vitro

This functional test is based on quantifying the formation of malondialdehyde generated from the lipid peroxidation of polyunsaturated fatty acids of erythrocytes exposed to hydrogen peroxide in vitro (Cyanamon et al., 1985). Thus the test is a modification of the erythrocyte hemolysis test described above.

Cyanamon and Isenberg (1987) evaluated the erythrocyte malondialdehyde test in a study of 24 children with cholestatic liver disease at risk of vitamin E deficiency and 11 healthy controls. In the children with vitamin E deficiency, mean malondialdehyde formation was 41% compared to < 6% in control children. Nevertheless, the assay is not recommended for the routine assessment of vitamin E status, particularly in marginal vitamin E deficiency. It suffers from most of the limitations noted above for the hydrogen peroxide hemolysis test. Malondialdehyde is generally measured by using thiobarbituric acid–reactive substances, which are not specific for malondialdehyde (Morrissey and Sheehy, 1999). However, analysis of malondialdehyde by HPLC could increase the specificity of this test.

18.3.8 Breath pentane and ethane

Measurements of the concentration of exhaled pentane and ethane, the peroxidation products of linolenic and linoleic acids, respectively, have potential for assessing vitamin E deficiency states in humans. Lemoyne et al. (1987) standardized a technique for collecting and measuring breath pentane. They compared the results with serum vitamin E levels in both vitamin E–deficient and normal adults and found a significant negative correlation between serum vitamin E levels and breath pentane. Moreover, supplementing five normal subjects with vitamin E for 10 days significantly decreased breath pentane concentrations.

Breath ethane has also been measured and shown to be inversely correlated with plasma α-tocopherol concentrations in children and adults with vitamin E deficiency (Refat et al., 1991). Hence, breath pentane and ethane concentrations, as measures of vitamin E status, may help to assess the role of vitamin E in altering the in vivo peroxidation of polyunsaturated fatty acids. However, the effects of other antioxidant systems on this test need further study. More research that includes other indices of vitamin E status for comparison with breath pentane and ethane measurements is necessary before the validity of these functional tests can be firmly established.

18.4 Summary

Vitamin A

Ocular lesions, characteristic of vitamin A deficiency, are endemic in many developing countries. Serum retinol concentrations are the most frequently determined biochemical marker of vitamin A status. They reflect total body reserves of vitamin A when liver vitamin A stores are either severely depleted or excessively high, but not when liver vitamin A concentrations are between these limits. Several confounding factors affect serum retinol concentrations and, hence, limit their specificity and sensitivity as an index of vitamin A status.

Age-specific guidelines for the interpretation of low serum retinol concentrations are available for U.S. persons. Both WHO and IVACG recommend a single cutoff value for serum retinol of < 0.70 µmol/L as being indicative of a low vitamin A status in children 6–71 mo. WHO defines vitamin A deficiency as a public health problem based on the prevalence of serum retinol levels < 0.70 µmol/L; Mild public health problem: 2% to < 10% prevalence; Moderate public health problem: 10% to < 20% prevalence; Severe public health problem $\geqslant$ 20% prevalence. IVACG has proposed only one cutoff as indicative of a public health problem: a prevalence of > 15% of serum retinol concentrations < 0.70 µmol/L. Generally, serum retinol values $\geqslant$ 1.05 µmol/L are indicative of adequate vitamin A status. New biochemical tests include serum retinol-binding protein and the measurement of breast milk retinol concentrations. Elevated serum retinyl ester concentrations in fasting blood samples are used to assess vitamin A toxicity.

The physiological functional tests for vitamin A status include the relative dose response or modified relative dose response, the assessment of night blindness, the rapid dark adaptation test, pupillary and visual threshold tests, and conjunctival impression cytology with transfer. WHO has also proposed cutoff values for these physiological functional tests to define subclinical vitamin A deficiency and the prevalence of unacceptable values that denote a mild, moderate, or severe public health problem. In contrast, IVACG only provide criteria for maternal night blindness and the minimum prevalence for this indicator above which vitamin A deficiency is considered to be a public health problem. IVACG also recommends the use of the under-five mortality rate as surrogate indicator for assessing the likelihood of vitamin A deficiency within a population group.

Newer methods for measuring vitamin A body stores include stable isotope dilution procedures and the determination of serum retinoic acid. The preferred analytical method for total vitamin A, retinol, and retinyl esters in serum is HPLC. Conditions of collection, storage, and analysis of serum samples should be carefully controlled.

Vitamin D

In industrialized countries, suboptimal vitamin D status may occur in persons with inadequate skin exposure to sunlight, and in those living in northern geographical latitudes. The elderly and subjects with dark-skins or a habit of dress that limits exposure to sunlight are especially at risk. Additionally, malabsorption or the prolonged use of certain anticonvulsant drugs may precipitate secondary vitamin D deficiency. Severe vitamin D deficiency may result in rickets in infants and children and osteomalacia in adults. Moderate deficiency has been associated with increased bone turnover, secondary hyperparathyroidism, and decreased bone density in adults. Indiscriminate self-dosing with excessive intakes of vitamin D may produce vitamin D toxicity.

Serum 25(OH)D concentrations are the most useful marker of vitamin D status. They reflect the total supply of vitamin D from both cutaneous synthesis and dietary intake and can be used to define vitamin D deficiency, vitamin D insufficiency, hypovitaminosis D, vitamin D sufficiency, and vitamin D toxicity. Relationships of serum 25(OH)D concentrations and season, place of work, use of fortified foods or vitamin D supplements, latitude, and clinical signs of vitamin D deficiency provide further evidence that serum 25(OH)D is a valid index of vitamin D status.

Interpretive criteria for serum 25(OH)D concentrations are based on cutoffs that are indicative of hypovitaminosis D and hypervitaminosis D or on a multistage approach, with cutoffs for vitamin D deficiency, insufficiency, hypovitaminosis D, vitamin D sufficiency, and toxicity. Most of these cutoffs are controversial and poorly defined. The cutoff value proposed as indicative of vitamin D deficiency is < 12.5 nmol/L; it has been related to clinical signs of vitamin D deficiency. NHANES III defined hypovitaminosis D as a serum 25(OH)D concentration < 37.5 nmol/L, a cutoff also used (with a high parathyroid hormone concentration) to define vitamin D deficiency in neonates. Cutoffs indicative of toxicity vary: > 250 nmol/L has been proposed for the multistage approach. Methods for assaying serum 25(OH)D include HPLC, competitive binding assays, and radioimmunoassays.

Although serum alkaline phosphatase activity has been used as an indirect index of vitamin D status, it is also affected by a variety of other disease states. Hence, its specificity and sensitivity as an index of vitamin D status is poor. Serum PTH levels rise in vitamin D deficiency, so the existence of elevated levels > 6.4 pmol/L in combination with low serum 25(OH)D is a useful indicator of vitamin D status. Serum calcium can be used to identify vitamin D intoxication; in such cases, both serum calcium and serum 25(OH)D are elevated. Urinary excretion levels of calcium and phosphorus are not specific for vitamin D status, and their use as an index of the status of vitamin D is not recommended.

Vitamin E

Various syndromes of vitamin E deficiency have been identified in animals, but in humans dietary deficiency of vitamin E is rare. Nevertheless, signs of vitamin E deficiency have been reported in premature infants, in persons with chronic cholestasis and certain fat malabsorption syndromes.

Serum α-tocopherol is the most frequently used measure of vitamin E status. Concentrations vary according to age, physiological state, method of analysis, and total serum lipid levels. To account for the latter, the ratio of serum α-tocopherol to cholesterol used, with ratios of ⩾ 2.2 μmol/mmol indicating adequate vitamin E status. Erythrocyte tocopherol concentrations are not useful as a marker of vitamin E status. Platelet tocopherol concentrations are independent of serum lipid concentrations, but isolation of platelets is impractical for surveys. New functional tests appear promising, including the measurement of breath pentane and ethane, and possibly erythrocyte malondialdehyde release in vitro. More studies are needed, however, before the validity of these functional tests for assessing marginal vitamin E deficiency states is established.

At the present time, the interpretation of serum tocopherol concentrations is based on the observed relationship with erythrocyte hemolysis, which increases in vitamin E deficiency. Hemolysis in vivo is observed when serum tocopherol levels fall to ⩽ 4.6 μmol/L. Serum concentrations of < 11.6 μmol/L in adults are generally accepted as indicating vitamin E deficiency, but in NHANES III, concentrations < 20.0 μmol/L were considered low.

Although vitamin E levels of liver and adipose tissue provide a measure of tissue stores of vitamin E, adipose tissue biopsies are quite invasive for population studies and are difficult to standardize. The α-tocopherol content of buccal mucosal cells, expressed in terms of μg/g protein, may be a more practical biopsy sample for field studies, but cutoffs need to be defined. Analysis of tocopherol in tissues and blood is best performed by HPLC.

References

Aksnes L. (1992). A simplified high-performance liquid chromatographic method for determination of vitamin D3, 25-hydroxyvitamin D2 and 25-hydroxyvitamin D3 in human serum. Scandinavian Journal of Clinical Laboratory Investigation 52: 177–182.

Almekinder J, Manda W, Soko D, Lan Y, Hoover DR, Semba RD. (2000). Evaluation of plasma retinol-binding protein as a surrogate measure for plasma retinol concentrations. Scandinavian Journal of Clinical Laboratory Investigation 60: 199–204.

Amédée-Manesme O, Anderson D, Olson JA. (1984). Relation of the relative dose response to liver concentrations of vitamin A in generally well nourished surgical patients. American Journal of Clinical Nutrition 39: 898–902.

Amédée-Manesme O, Mourey M, Hanck A, Therasse J. (1987). Vitamin A relative dose response test: validation by intravenous injection in children with liver disease. American Journal of Clinical Nutrition 46: 286–289.

Azais-Braesco V, Pascal G. (2000). Vitamin A in pregnancy: requirements and safety limits. American Journal of Clinical Nutrition 71: 1325S–1333S.

Bach AU, Anderson SA, Foley AL, Williams EC, Suttie JW. (1996). Assessment of vitamin K status in human subjects administered "minidose" warfarin. American Journal of Clinical Nutrition 64: 894–902.

Ballew C, Bowman BA, Sowell AL, Gillespie C. (2001a). Serum retinol distributions in residents of the United States: third National Health and Nutrition Examination Survey, 1988–1994. American Journal of Clinical Nutrition 73: 586–593.

Ballew C, Bowman BA, Russell RM, Sowell AL, Gillespie C. (2001b). Serum retinyl esters are not associated with biochemical markers of liver dysfunction in adult participants in the third National Health and Nutrition Examination Survey (NHANES III), 1988–1994. American Journal of Clinical Nutrition 73: 934–940.

Bankson DD, Russell RM, Sadowski JA. (1986). Determination of retinyl esters and retinol in serum or plasma by normal-phase liquid chromatography: method and applications. Clinical Chemistry 32: 35–40.

Behrens WA, Thompson JN, Madère R. (1982). Distribution of α-tocopherol in human plasma lipoproteins. American Journal of Clinical Nutrition 35: 691–696.

Bell NH, Epstein S, Greene A, Shary J, Oexmann MJ, Shaw S. (1985). Evidence for alteration of the vitamin D–endocrine system in obese subjects. Journal of Clinical Investigation. 76: 370–373.

Bellizzi MC, Franklin MF, Duthie GG, James WPT. (1994). Vitamin E and coronary heart disease: the European paradox. European Journal of Clinical Nutrition 48: 822–831. Erratum in 49: 230.

Bessey OA, Lowry OH, Brock MJ. (1946). Method for rapid determination of alkaline phosphatase with

5 cubic millimeters of serum. Journal of Biological Chemistry 164: 321–329.

Bieri JG, Tolliver TJ, Catignani GL. (1979). Simultaneous determination of α-tocopherol and retinol in plasma or red cells by high pressure liquid chromatography. American Journal of Clinical Nutrition 32: 2143–2149.

Binder HJ, Spiro HM. (1967). Tocopherol deficiency in man. American Journal of Clinical Nutrition 20: 594–603.

Blaner WS. (1990). Radioimmunoassays for retinol-binding protein, cellular retinol-binding protein, and cellular retinoic acid-binding protein. Methods in Enzymology 189: 270–281.

Blank S, Scanlon KS, Sinks TH, Lett S, Falk H. (1995). An outbreak of hypervitaminosis D associated with the overfortification of milk from a home-delivery dairy. American Journal of Public Health 85: 656–659.

Blok BH, Grant CC, McNeil AR, Reid IR. (2000). Characteristics of children with florid vitamin D deficient rickets in the Auckland region in 1998. New Zealand Medical Journal 113: 374–376.

Blum M, Kirsten M, Worth MH Jr. (1977). Reversible hypertension: caused by the hypercalcemia of hyperparathyroidism, vitamin D toxicity, and calcium infusion. Journal of the American Medical Association 237: 262–263.

Bolton-Smith C, Casey CE, Gey KF, Smith WC, Tunstall-Pedoe H. (1991). Antioxidant vitamin intakes assessed using a food-frequency questionnaire: correlation with biochemical status in smokers and nonsmokers. British Journal of Nutrition 65: 337–346.

Bortolotti A, Lucchini G, Barzago MM, Stellari F, Bonati M. (1993). Simultaneous determination of retinol, α-tocopherol and retinyl palmitate in plasma of premature newborns by reversed-phase high-performance liquid chromatography. Journal of Chromatography 617: 313–317.

Brady WE, Mares-Perlman JA, Bowen P, Stacewicz-Sapuntzakis M. (1996). Human serum carotenoid concentrations are related to physiologic and lifestyle factors. Journal of Nutrition 126: 129–137.

Brigelius-Flohé R, Kelly FJ, Salonen JT, Neuzil J, Zingg J-M, Azzi A. (2002). The European perspective on vitamin E: current knowledge and future research. American Journal of Clinical Nutrition 76: 703–716.

Brink EW, Perera WD, Broske SP, Cash RA, Smith JL, Sauberlich HE, Bashor MM. (1979). Vitamin A status of children in Sri Lanka. American Journal of Clinical Nutrition 32: 84–91.

Brot C, Jørgensen NR, Sørensen OH. (1999). The influence of smoking on vitamin D status and calcium metabolism. European Journal of Clinical Nutrition 53: 920–926.

Calvo MS, Whiting SJ. (2003). Prevalence of vitamin D insufficiency in Canada and the United States: importance to health status and efficacy of current food fortification and dietary supplement use. Nutrition Reviews 61: 107–113.

Campos FA, Flores H, Underwood BA. (1987). Effect of an infection on vitamin A status of children as measured by the relative dose response (RDR). American Journal of Clinical Nutrition 46: 91–94.

Carlier C, Coste J, Etchepare M, Amédée-Manesme O. (1992). Conjunctival impression cytology with transfer as a field-applicable indicator of vitamin A status for mass screening. International Journal of Epidemiology 21: 373–380.

Cavalier L, Ouahchi K, Kayden HJ, Di Donato S, Reutenauer L, Mandel J-L, Koenig M. (1998). Ataxia with isolated vitamin E deficiency: Heterogeneity of mutations and phenotypic variability in a large number of families. American Journal of Human Genetics 62: 301–310.

Chan EL, Lau E, Shek CC, MacDonald D, Woo J, Leung PC, Swaminathan R. (1992). Age-related changes in bone density, serum parathyroid hormone, calcium absorption and other indices of bone metabolism in Chinese women. Clinical Endocrinology 36: 375–381.

Chapuy M-C, Preziosio P, Maamer M, Arnaud S, Galan P, Hercberg S, Meunier PJ. (1997). Prevalence of vitamin D insufficiency in an adult normal population. Osteoporosis International 7: 439–443.

Chen TC, Shao A, Heath H 3rd, Holick MF. (1993). An update on the vitamin D content of fortified milk from the United States and Canada. New England Journal of Medicine 329: 1507.

Chesney RW (1989). Vitamin D: can an upper limit be defined? Journal of Nutrition 119: 1825–1828.

Christian P. (2002a). IVACG Statement. Maternal Night Blindness: A New Indicator of Vitamin A Deficiency. International Vitamin A Consultative Group (IVACG), International Life Sciences Institute Research Centre, Washington, DC.

Christian P. (2002b). Recommendations for indicators: night blindness during pregnancy — a simple tool to assess vitamin A deficiency in a population. Journal of Nutrition 132: 2884S–2888S.

Christian P, West KP Jr. (1998). Interactions between zinc and vitamin A: an update. American Journal of Clinical Nutrition 68: 435S–441S.

Christian P, West KP Jr, Khatry SK, Katz J, Shrestha SR, Pradhan EK, LeClerq SC, Pokhrel RP, (1998a). Night blindness of pregnancy in rural Nepal: nutritional and health risks. International Journal of Epidemiology 27: 231–237.

Christian P, West KP Jr, Khatry SK, Katz J, LeClerq S, Pradhan EK, Shresta SR. (1998b). Vitamin A or β-carotene supplementation reduces but does not eliminate maternal night blindness in Nepal. Journal of Nutrition 128: 1458–1463.

Christian P, Khatry SK, Yamini S, Stallings R, LeClerq SC, Shrestha SR, Pradhan EK, West KP Jr. (2001). Zinc supplementation might potentiate the effect of vitamin A in restoring night vision in pregnant Nepalese women. American Journal of Clinical Nutrition 73: 1045–1051.

Chug-Ahuja KJ, Holden JM, Forman MR, Mangels AR, Beecher GR, Lanza E. (1993). The development and application of a carotenoid database for fruits, vegetables and selected multicomponent foods. Journal of the American Dietetics Association 93: 318-323.

Clemens TL, Adams JS, Henderson SL, Holick MF. (1982). Increased skin pigment reduces the capacity of skin to synthesize vitamin D3. Lancet 1(8263): 74–76.

Congdon NG, West KP Jr. (2002). Physiologic indicators of vitamin A status. Journal of Nutrition 132: 2889S–2894S.

Congdon N, Sommer A, Severns M, Humphrey J, Friedman D, Clement L, Wu L-S-F, Natadisastra G. (1995). Pupillary and visual thresholds in young children as an index of population vitamin A status. American Journal of Clinical Nutrition 61: 1076–1082.

Congdon NG, Dreyfuss ML, Christian P, Navitsky RC, Sanchez AM, Wu LS, Khatry SK, Thapa MD, Humphrey J, Hazelwood D, West KP Jr. (2000). Responsiveness of dark-adaptation threshold to vitamin A and β-carotene supplementation in pregnant and lactating women in Nepal. American Journal of Clinical Nutrition 72: 1004–1009.

Craft NE. (2001). Innovative approaches to vitamin A assessment. Journal of Nutrition 131: 1626S–1630S.

Craft NE, Bulux J, Valdez C, Li Y, Solomons NW. (2000). Retinol concentrations in capillary dried blood spots from healthy volunteers: method validation. American Journal of Clinical Nutrition 72: 450–454.

Cynamon HA, Isenberg JN. (1987). Characterization of vitamin E status in cholestatic children by conventional laboratory standards and a new functional assay. Journal of Pediatric Gastroenterology and Nutrition 6: 46–50.

Cynamon HA, Isenberg JN, Nguyen C. (1985). Erythrocyte malondialdehyde release in vitro: a functional measure of vitamin E status. Clinica Chimica Acta 151: 169–176.

Dattani JT, Exton-Smith AN, Stephen JM. (1984). Vitamin D status of the elderly in relation to age and exposure to sunlight. Human Nutrition: Clinical Nutrition 38C: 131–137.

Dawson S, Manderson L, Tallo VS. (1993). A Manual for the Use of Focus Groups: Methods for Social Research in Disease. International Nutrition Foundation for Developing Countries (INFDC), Boston, MA.

DeLuca HF, Schnoes HK. (1983). Vitamin D: recent advances. Annual Review of Biochemistry 52: 411–439.

Department of Health. (1992). The Nutrition of Elderly People. Report on Health and Social Subjects No. 43. Her Majesty's Stationery Office, London.

de Pee S, Dary O. (2002). Biochemical indicators of vitamin A deficiency: serum retinol and serum retinol binding protein. Journal of Nutrition 132: 2895S–2901S.

de Pee S, Yuniar Y, West CE, Muhilal. (1997). Evaluation of biochemical indicators of vitamin A status in breast-feeding and non-breast-feeding Indonesian women. American Journal of Clinical Nutrition 66: 160–167.

Devgun MS, Patterson CR, Johnson BE, Cohen C. (1981). Vitamin D nutrition in relation to season and occupation. American Journal of Clinical Nutrition 34: 1501–1504.

Docio S, Riancho JA, Pérez A, Olmos JM, Amado JA, González-Macías J. (1998). Seasonal deficiency of vitamin D in children: a potential target for osteoporosis-preventing strategies? Journal of Bone Mineral Research 13: 544–548.

Driskell WJ, Neese JW, Bryant CC, Bashor M. (1982). Measurement of vitamin A and vitamin E in human serum by high performance liquid chromatography. Journal of Chromatography 231: 439–444.

Duthie GG, Arthur JR, James WP. (1991). Effects of smoking and vitamin E on blood antioxidant status. American Journal of Clinical Nutrition 53: 1061S–1063S.

Efstathiadou Z, Bitsis S, Tsatsoulis A. (1999) Gastrectomy and osteomalacia: an association not to be forgotten. Hormone Research 52: 295–297.

El-Sohemy A, Baylin A, Kabagambe E, Ascherio A, Spiegelman D, Campos H. (2002). Individual carotenoid concentrations in adipose tissue and plasma as biomarkers of dietary intake. American Journal of Clinical Nutrition 76: 172–179.

Endres DB, Morgan CH, Garry PJ, Omdahl JL. (1987). Age-related changes in serum immunoreactive parathyroid hormone and its biological action in healthy men and women. Journal of Endocrinology and Metabolism 65: 724–731.

Epler KS, Ziegler RG, Craft NE. (1993). Liquid chromatographic method for the determination of carotenoids, retinoids and tocopherols in human serum and in food. Journal of Chromatography 619: 37–48.

Erhardt JG, Craft NE, Heinrich F, Biesalski HK. (2002a). Rapid and simple measurement of retinol in human dried whole blood spots. Journal of Nutrition 132: 318–321.

Erhardt JG, Mack H, Sobeck U, Biesalski HK. (2002b). β-carotene and α-tocopherol concentration and antioxidant status in buccal mucosal cells and plasma after oral supplementation. British Journal of Nutrition 87: 471–475.

Escoute AJ, Chirambo MC, Luzeau R, Amédée-Manesme O. (1991). Assessment of vitamin A deficiency in Republic of Malawi by impression cytology method. International Journal for Vitamin and Nutrition Research 61: 10–16.

FAO/WHO (Food and Agriculture Organization/World Health Organization (2002). Human Vitamin and Mineral Requirements. Report of a Joint FAO/WHO Expert Consultation, Bangkok, Thailand. World Health Organization, Food and Agricultural Organization of the United Nations, Rome.

Farrell PM, Bieri JG. (1975). Megavitamin E supplementation in man. American Journal of Clinical Nutrition 28: 1381–1386.

Farrell PM, Roberts RJ. (1994). Vitamin E. In: Shils ME,

Olson JA, Shike M (eds.) Modern Nutrition in Health and Disease. Volume 1. Lea & Febiger, Philadelphia, pp. 326–341.

Farrell PM, Bieri JG, Fraantoni JF, Wood RE, di Sant'Agnese PA. (1977). The occurrence and effects of human vitamin E deficiency: a study in patients with cystic fibrosis. Journal of Clinical Investigation 6: 233–241.

Farrell PM, Levine SL, Murphy MD, Adams A. (1978). Plasma tocopherol levels and tocopherol-lipid relationships in a normal population of children as compared to healthy adults. American Journal of Clinical Nutrition 31: 1720–1726.

Farrerons J, Barnadas M, Rodriguez J, Renau A, Yoldi B, Lopez-Navidad A, Moragas J. (1998). Clinically prescribed sunscreen (sun protection factor 15) does not decrease serum vitamin D concentration sufficiently either to induce changes in parathyroid function or in metabolic markers. British Journal of Dermatology 139: 422–427.

Favaro RM, de Souza NV, Vannucchi H, Desai ID, de Oliveira JE. (1986). Evaluation of rose bengal staining test and rapid dark-adaptation test for the field assessment of vitamin A status of preschool children in Southern Brazil. American Journal of Clinical Nutrition 43: 940–945.

Ferris AM, Jensen RG. (1984). Lipids in human milk: a review. 1: Sampling, determination, and content. Journal of Pediatric Gastroenterology and Nutrition 3: 108–122.

Filteau SM, Willumsen JF, Sullivan K, Simmank K, Gamble M. (2000). Use of the retinol-binding protein: transthyretin ratio for assessment of vitamin A status during the acute-phase response. British Journal of Nutrition 83: 513–520.

Finch S, Doyle W, Lowe C, Bates CJ, Prentice A, Smithers G, Clarke PC. (1998). National Diet and Nutrition Survey: People Aged 65 Years or Over. Volume 1: Report of the Diet and Nutrition Survey. The Stationery Office, London.

Flores H, Compos F, Araujo CRC, Underwood BA. (1984). Assessment of marginal vitamin A deficiency in Brazilian children using the relative dose response procedure. American Journal of Clinical Nutrition 40: 1281–1289.

Ford ES. (2000). Variations in serum carotenoid concentrations among United States adults by ethnicity and sex. Ethnicity and Disease 10: 208–217.

Ford ES, Sowell A. (1999). Serum α-tocopherol status in the United States population: findings from the Third National Health and Nutrition Examination Survey. American Journal of Epidemiology 1: 290–300.

Ford ES, Gillespie C, Ballew C, Sowell A, Mannino D. (2002). Serum carotenoid concentrations in U.S. children and adolescents. American Journal of Clinical Nutrition 76: 818–827.

Frame B, Jackson CE, Reynolds WA, Umphrey JE. (1974). Hypercalcemia and skeletal effects in chronic hypervitaminosis A. Annals of Internal Medicine 80: 44–48.

Fraser DR. (1983). The physiological economy of vitamin D. Lancet 1(8331): 969–972.

Furr HC, Amédée-Manesme O, Olson JA. (1984). Gradient reversed-phase high-performance liquid chromatographic separation of naturally occurring retinoids. Journal of Chromatography 309: 229–307.

Furr HC, Amédée-Manesme O, Clifford AJ, Bergen HR 3rd, Jones AD, Anderson DP, Olson JA. (1989). Vitamin A concentration in liver determined by isotope dilution assay with tetradeuterated vitamin A and by biopsy in generally healthy adult humans. American Journal of Clinical Nutrition 49: 713–716.

Gadomski AM, Kjolhede CL, Wittpenn J, Bulux J, Rosas AR, Forman MR. (1989). Conjunctival impression cytology (CIC) to detect subclinical vitamin A deficiency: comparison of CIC with biochemical assessments. American Journal of Clinical Nutrition 49: 495–500.

Gallagher SK, Johnson LK, Milne DB. (1989). Short- and long-term variability of indices related to nutritional status. I: Ca, Cu, Fe, Mg, and Zn. Clinical Chemistry 35: 369–373.

Gallagher SK, Johnson LK, Milne DB. (1992). Short- and long-term variability of selected indices related to nutritional status. II: Vitamins, lipids, and protein indices. Clinical Chemistry 38: 1449–1453.

Gamble MV, Ramakrishnan R, Palafox NA, Briand K, Berglund L, Blaner WS. (2001). Retinol binding protein as a surrogate measure for serum retinol: studies in vitamin A–deficient children from the Republic of the Marshall Islands. American Journal of Clinical Nutrition 73: 594–601.

Garland FC, Garland CF, Gorham E, Young JF. (1990). Geographic variation in breast cancer mortality in the United States: a hypothesis involving exposure to solar radiation. Preventive Medicine 19: 614–622.

Gascón-Vila P, Garcia-Closas R, Serra-Majem L, Pastor MC, Ribas L, Ramon JM, Mariné-Font A, Salleras L. (1997). Determinants of the nutritional status of vitamin E in a non-smoking Mediterranean population: analysis of the effect of vitamin E intake, alcohol consumption and body mass index on the serum α-tocopherol concentration. European Journal of Clinical Nutrition 51: 723–728.

Gerster H. (1997). Vitamin A: functions, dietary requirements and safety in humans. International Journal for Vitamin and Nutrition Research 67: 71–90.

Gibson RS, Draper HH, McGirr LG, Nizan P, Martinez OB. (1986). The vitamin D status of a cohort of postmenopausal noninstitutionalized Canadian women. Nutrition Research 6: 1179–1187.

Gloth FM 3rd, Gundberg CM, Hollis BW, Haddad JG, Tobin JD. (1995). Vitamin D deficiency in homebound elderly persons. Journal of the American Medical Association 274: 1683–1686.

Goswami R, Gupta N, Goswami D, Marwaha RK, Tandon N, Kochupillai N. (2000). Prevalence and significance of low 25-hydroxyvitamin D concentrations in healthy subjects in Delhi. American Journal of Clinical Nutrition 72: 472–475.

Gotoda T, Arita M, Arai H, Inoue K, Yokota T, Fukuo Y, Yazaki Y, Yamada N. (1995). Adult-onset spinocerebellar dysfunction caused by a mutation in the gene for alpha-tocopherol-transfer protein. New England Journal of Medicine 333: 1313–1318.

Gregory J, Foster K, Tyler H, Wiseman M. (1990). The Dietary and Nutritional Survey of British Adults. Her Majesty's Stationery Office, London.

Gregory J, Collins DL, Davies PSW, Hughes JM, Clarke PC. (1995). National Diet and Nutrition Survey: Children Aged One-and-a-Half to Four-and-a-Half Years. Volume 1: Report of the Diet and Nutrition Survey. Her Majesty's Stationery Office, London

Gregory J, Lowe S, Bates CJ, Prentice A, Jackson LV, Smithers G, Wenlock R, Farron M. (2000). National Diet and Nutrition Survey: Young People Aged 4 to 18 Years. Volume 1: Report of the Diet and Nutrition Survey. The Stationery Office, London.

Haddad JG, Stamp TCB. (1974). Circulating 25-hydroxyvitamin D in man. American Journal of Medicine 57: 57–62.

Hahn TJ, Hendin BA, Scharp CR, Boisseau VC, Haddad JG. (1975). Serum 25-hydroxy-calciferol levels and bone mass in children on chronic anti-epileptic therapy. New England Journal of Medicine 292: 550–554.

Hallfrisch J, Muller DC, Singh VN. (1994). Vitamin A and E intakes and plasma concentrations of retinol, β-carotene, and α-tocopherol in men and women of the Baltimore Longitudinal Study of Aging. American Journal of Clinical Nutrition 60: 176–182.

Harris SS, Dawson-Hughes B. (1998). The association of oral contraceptive use with plasma 25-hydroxyvitamin D levels. Journal of American College of Nutrition 17: 282–284.

Haskell MJ, Handelman GJ, Peerson JM, Jones AD, Rabbi MA, Awal MA, Wahed MA, Mahalanabis D, Brown KH. (1997). Assessment of vitamin A status by the deuterated-retinol-dilution technique and comparison with hepatic vitamin A concentration in Bangladeshi surgical patients. American Journal of Clinical Nutrition 66: 67–74.

Haskell MJ, Islam MA, Handelman GJ, Peerson JM, Jones AD, Wahed MA, Mahalanabis D, Brown KH. (1998). Plasma kinetics of an oral dose of $^2H_4$retinyl acetate in human subjects with estimated low or high total body stores of vitamin A. American Journal of Clinical Nutrition 68: 90–95.

Hassan H, Hashim SA, Van Itallie TB, Sebrell WH. (1966). Syndrome in premature infants associated with low plasma vitamin E levels and high polyunsaturated fatty acid diet. American Journal of Clinical Nutrition 19: 147–157.

Heaney RP, Recker RR, Saville PD. (1978). Menopausal changes in calcium balance performance. Journal of Laboratory and Clinical Medicine 92: 953–963.

Herbeth B, Chavance M, Musse N, Mejean L, Vern-

hes G. (1989) Dietary intake and other determinants of blood vitamins in an elderly population. European Journal of Clinical Nutrition 43: 175–186.

Hix J, Martinez C, Buchanan I, Morgan J, Tam M, Shankar A. (2004). Development of a rapid enzyme immunoassay for the detection of retinol binding protein. American Journal of Clinical Nutrition 79: 93–98.

Holick MF. (1987). Vitamin D and the kidney. Kidney international 32: 912–929.

Holick MF. (1996). Vitamin D: photobiology, metabolism, mechanism of action, and clinical application. In: Favus MJ (ed.) Primer on the Metabolic Bone Diseases and Disorders of Mineral Metabolism. 3rd ed. Lippincott-Raven, Philadelphia, pp. 74–81.

Holick MF. (2003). Vitamin D: photobiology, metabolism, mechanism of action, and clinical applications. In: Favus MJ (ed.) Primer on the Metabolic Bone Diseases and Disorders of Mineral Metabolism. 5th ed. American Society for Bone and Mineral Research. Washington, DC. pp. 129–137.

Holick MF, MacLaughlin JA, Doppelt SH. (1981). Regulation of cutaneous previtamin D_3 photosynthesis in man: skin pigment is not an essential regulator. Science 211: 590–593.

Hollis BW. (2000). Comparison of commercially available ^{125}I-based RIA methods for the determination of circulating 25-hyroxyvitamin D. Clinical Chemistry 46: 1657–1661.

Hollis BW, Kamerud JQ, Kurkowski A, Beaulieu J, Napoli JL. (1996). Quantification of circulating 1,25-dihydroxyvitamin D by radioimmunoassay with ^{125}I-labeled tracer. Clinical Chemistry 42: 586–592.

Horwitt MK. (1960). Vitamin E and lipid metabolism in man. American Journal of Clinical Nutrition 8: 451–461.

Horwitt MK, Harvey CC, Dahm CH Jr, Searcy MT. (1972). Relationship between tocopherol and serum lipid levels for determination of nutritional adequacy. Annals of New York Academy of Sciences 203: 223–236.

Hummer L, Riis BJ, Christiansen C, Rickers H. (1985). Determination of mono- and dihydroxy-vitamin D metabolites in normal subjects and patients with different calcium metabolic diseases. Scandinavian Journal of Clinical Laboratory Investigation 45: 611–619.

IOM (Institute of Medicine). (1997). Dietary Reference Intakes for Calcium, Phosphorus, Magnesium, Vitamin D, and Fluoride. Food and Nutrition Board, National Academy Press, Washington, DC.

IOM (Institute of Medicine). (2000). Dietary Reference Intakes for Vitamin C, Vitamin E, Selenium, and Carotenoids. Food and Nutrition Board, National Academy Press, Washington, DC.

IOM (Institute of Medicine). (2001). Dietary Reference Intakes for Vitamin A, Vitamin K, Arsenic, Boron, Chromium, Copper, Iodine, Iron, Manganese, Molybdenum, Nickel, Silicon, Vanadium, and

Zinc. Food and Nutrition Board, National Academy Press, Washington, DC.

IVACG (International Vitamin A Consultative Group). (2002). Vitamin A conversion to SI units. International Life Sciences Institute Press, Washington, DC.

Jacobus CH, Holick MF, Shao Q, Chen TC, Holm IA, Kolondney JM, Fuleihan G E-H, Seely EW. (1992). Hypervitaminosis D associated with drinking milk. New England Journal of Medicine 326: 1173–1177.

Jacques PF, Felson DT, Tucker KL, Mahnken B, Wilson PWF, Rosenberg IH, Rush D. (1997). Plasma 25-hydroxyvitamin D and its determinants in an elderly population sample. American Journal of Clinical Nutrition 66: 929–936.

Järvinen R, Knekt P, Seppänen R. Heinonen M, Aaran R-K. (1993). Dietary determinants of serum β-carotene and serum retinol. European Journal of Clinical Nutrition 47: 31–41.

Jayarajan P, Reddy V, Mohanram M. (1980). Effect of dietary fat on absorption of β-carotene from green leafy vegetables in children. Indian Journal of Medical Research 71: 53–56.

Johnson L. Schaffer D, Boggs TR Jr. (1974). The premature infant, vitamin E deficiency and retrolental fibroplasia. American Journal of Clinical Nutrition 27: 1158–1173.

Jones G. (1978). Assay of vitamins D_2 and D_3 and 25-hydroxyvitamins D_2 and D_3 in human plasma by high-performance liquid chromatography. Clinical Chemistry 24: 287–298.

Kaempf DE, Miki M, Ogihara T, Okamoto R, Konishi K, Mino M. (1994). Assessment of vitamin E nutritional status in neonates, infants and children on the basis of α-tocopherol levels in blood components and buccal mucosal cells. International Journal for Vitamin and Nutrition Research 64: 185–191.

Kafwembe EM, Kelly P, Ngalande P. (2001). Vitamin A levels in HIV/AIDS. East African Medical Journal 78: 451–453.

Kalra V, Grover J, Ahuja GK, Rathi S, Khurana DS. (1998). Vitamin E deficiency and associated neurological deficits in children with protein-energy malnutrition. Journal of Tropical Pediatrics 44: 291–295.

Kardinaal AF, van't Veer P, Brants HA, van den Berg H, van Schoohoven J, Hermus RJ. (1995). Relations between antioxidant vitamins in adipose tissue, plasma, and diet. American Journal of Epidemiology 141: 440–450.

Kayden HJ, Hatam LJ, Traber MG. (1983). The measurement of nanograms of tocopherol from needle aspiration biopsies of adipose tissue: normal and abetalipoproteinemic subjects. Journal of Lipid Research 24: 652–656.

Keenum DG, Semba RD, Wirasasmita S, Natadisastra G, Muhilal, West KP Jr., Sommer A. (1990). Assessment of vitamin A status by a disk applicator for conjunctival impression cytology. Archives of Ophthalmology 108: 1436–1441.

Kemp CM, Jacobson SG, Faulkner DJ, Walt R. (1988).

Visual function and rhodopsin levels in humans with vitamin A deficiency. Experimental Eye Research 46: 185–197.

Kinyamu HK, Gallagher JC, Balhorn KE, Petranick KM, Rafferty KA. (1997). Serum vitamin D metabolites and calcium absorption in normal young and elderly free-living women and in women living in nursing homes. American Journal of Clinical Nutrition 65: 790–797.

Kleerekoper M, Brienza RS, Schultz LR, Johnson CC. (1991). Oral contraceptive use may protect against low bone mass. Archives of Internal Medicine 151: 1971–1976.

Kreiter SR, Schwartz RP, Kirkman HN, Charlton PA, Calikoglu AS, Davenport M. (2000). Nutritional rickets in African American breast-fed infants. Journal of Pediatrics 137: 2–6.

Ladizesky M, Lu Z, Oliveri B, San Roman N, Diaz S, Holick MF, Mautalen C. (1995). Solar ultraviolet B radiation and photoproduction of vitamin D_3 in central and southern areas of Argentina. Journal of Bone and Mineral Research 10: 545–549.

Lamberg-Allardt CJE, Outila TA, Kärkkäinen MUM, Rita HJ, Valsta LM. (2001). Vitamin D deficiency and bone health in healthy adults in Finland: could this be a concern in other parts of Europe? Journal of Bone and Mineral Research 16: 2066–2073.

Landin-Wilhelmsen K, Wilhelmsen L, Wilske J, Lappas G, Rosen T, Lindstedt G, Lundberg P-A, Bengtsson B-A. (1995). Sunlight increases serum 25(OH) vitamin D concentrations whereas 1,25(OH)2D3 is unaffected. Results from a general population study Gøteborg, Sweden (the WHO MONICA project). European Journal of Clinical Nutrition 49: 400–407.

Lehmann J. (1981). Comparative sensitivities of tocopherol levels of platelets, red blood cells, and plasma for estimating vitamin E nutritional status in the rat. American Journal of Clinical Nutrition 34: 2104–2110.

Lehmann J, Rao DD, Canary JJ, Judd JT. (1988). Vitamin E and relationships among tocopherols in human plasma, platelets, lymphocytes, and red blood cells. American Journal of Clinical Nutrition 47: 470–474.

Lehtonen-Veromaa M, Möttönen T, Irjala K, Kärkkäinen M, Lamberg-Allardt C, Hakola P, Viikari J. (1999). Vitamin D intake is low and hypovitaminosis D common in healthy 9- to 15-year-old Finnish girls. European Journal of Clinical Nutrition 53: 746–751.

Lemoyne M, van Gossum A, Kurian R, Ostro M, Axler J, Jeejeebhoy KN. (1987). Breath pentane analysis as an index of lipid peroxidation: a functional test of vitamin E status. American Journal of Clinical Nutrition 46: 267–272.

Leo MA, Lieber CS. (1999). Alcohol, vitamin A, and β-carotene: adverse interactions, including hepatotoxicity and carcinogenicity. Clinical Nutrition 69: 1071–1085.

Lester E, Skinner RK, Foo AY, Lund B, Sørenson OH. (1980). Serum 25-hydroxyvitamin D levels and vitamin D intake in healthy young adults in Britain and Denmark. Scandinavian Journal of Clinical and Laboratory Investigation 40: 145–150.

Lips P, Graafmans WC, Ooms ME, Bezemer PD, Bouter LM. (1996). Vitamin D supplementation and fracture incidence in elderly persons: a randomized placebo-controlled clinical trial. Annals of Internal Medicine 124: 400-406.

Lips P, Chapuy MC, Dawson-Hughes B, Pols HAP, Holick MF. (1999). An international comparison of serum 25-hydroxyvitamin D measurements. Osteoporosis 9: 394–397.

Loerch JD, Underwood BA, Lewis KC. (1979). Response of plasma levels of vitamin A to a dose of vitamin A as an indicator of hepatic vitamin A reserves in rats. Journal of Nutrition 109: 778–786.

Malabanan A, Veronikis IE, Holick MF. (1998). Redefining vitamin D insufficiency. Lancet 351: 805–806.

Malvy DJ, Poveda JD, Debruyne M, Burtschy B, Dostalova L, Amédée-Manesme O. (1993). Immunonephelometry and radial immunodiffusion compared for measuring serum retinol-binding protein. European Journal of Clinical Chemistry and Clinical Biochemistry 31: 47–48.

Marinovic AC, May WA, Sowell AL, Khan LK, Huff DL, Bowman BA. (1997). Effect of hemolysis on serum retinol as assessed by direct fluorometry. American Journal of Clinical Nutrition 66: 1160–1164.

Matsuoka LY, Wortsman J, Haddad J, Kolm P, Holis B. (1991). Racial pigmentation and the cutaneous synthesis of vitamin D. Archives of Dermatology 127: 536–538.

McKenna MJ. (1992). Differences in vitamin D status between countries in young adults and the elderly. American Journal of Medicine 93: 69–77.

McKenna MJ, Freaney R. (1998). Secondary hyperparathyroidism in the elderly: means to defining hypovitaminosis D. Osteoporosis International 8(Suppl. 2): S3–S6.

McKenna MJ, Freaney R, Meade A, Muldowney FP. (1985). Hypovitaminosis D and elevated serum alkaline phosphatase in elderly Irish people. American Journal of Clinical Nutrition 41: 101–109.

McLennan W, Podger A. (1998). National Nutrition Survey: Nutrient Intakes and Physical Measurements, Australia, 1995. Australian Bureau of Statistics, Canberra.

Mejia LA, Arroyave G. (1983). Determination of vitamin A in blood: some practical considerations on the time of collection of the specimens and the stability of the vitamin. American Journal of Clinical Nutrition 37: 147–151.

Mejia LA, Pineda O, Noriega JF, Benitez J, Fall G. (1984). Significance of postprandial blood concentrations of retinol, retinol-binding protein, and carotenoids when assessing the vitamin A status of children. American Journal of Clinical Nutrition 39: 62–65.

Melhorn DK, Gross S, Lake GA, Leu JA. (1971). The hydrogen peroxide fragility test and serum tocopherol level in anemias of various etiologies. Blood 37: 438–446.

Meulmeester JF, van den Berg H, Wedel M, Boshuis PG, Hulshof KFAM, Luyken R. (1990). Vitamin D status, parathyroid hormone and sunlight in Turkish, Moroccan and Caucasian children in the Netherlands. European Journal of Clinical Nutrition 44: 461–470.

Mobarhan S, Russell RM, Underwood BA, Wallingford J, Mathieson RD, Al-Midani H. (1981). Evaluation of the relative dose response test for vitamin A nutriture in cirrhotics. American Journal of Clinical Nutrition 34: 2264–2270.

Moloney FJ, Collins S, Murphy GM. (2002). Sunscreens: safety, efficacy and appropriate use. American Journal of Clinical Dermatology 3: 185–191.

Morrissey PA, Sheehy PJA. (1999). Optimal nutrition: vitamin E. Proceedings of the Nutrition Society 58: 459–468.

Morrow JD, Frei B, Longmire AW, Gaziano JM, Lynch SM, Shyr Y, Strauss WE, Oates JA, Roberts LJ 2nd. (1995). Increase in circulating products of lipid peroxidation (F2-isoprostanes) in smokers: smoking as a cause of oxidative damage New England Journal of Medicine 332: 1198–1203.

Murphy SP, Calloway DH. (1996). Nutrient intakes of women in NHANES II, emphasizing trace minerals, fiber, and phytate. Journal of the American Dietetic Association 86: 1366–1372.

Nagata C, Shimizu H, Higashiiwai H, Sugahara N, Morita N, Komatsu S, Hisamichi S. (1999). Serum retinol level and risk of subsequent cervical cancer in cases with cervical dysplasia. Cancer Investigation 17: 253–258.

Natadisastra G, Wittpenn JR, West KP Jr, Muhilal, Sommer A. (1987). Impression cytology for detection of vitamin A deficiency. Archives of Ophthalmology 105: 1224–1228.

Natadisastra G, Wittpenn JR, Muhilal, West K, Mele L, Sommer A. (1988). Impression cytology: a practical index of vitamin A status. American Journal of Clinical Nutrition 48: 695–701.

National Heart, Lung, and Blood Institute. (1996). Morbidity and Mortality: 1996 Chartbook on Cardiovascular, Lung, and Blood Diseases. National Heart, Lung, and Blood Institute, Bethesda, MD.

Need AG, Morris HA, Horowitz M, Nordin C. (1993). Effects of skin thickness, age, body fat, and sunlight on serum 25-hydroxyvitamin D. American Journal of Clinical Nutrition 58: 882–885.

Need AG, Horowitz M, Morris HA, Nordin BEC. (2000). Vitamin D status: effects on parathyroid hormone and 1,25-dihyroxyvitamin D in postmenopausal women. American Journal of Clinical Nutrition 71: 1577–1581.

Nesby-O'Dell S, Scanlon K, Cogswell M, Gillespie C, Hollis BW, Looker AC, Allen C, Dougherty C, Gunter EW, Bowman BA. (2002). Hypovitaminosis D prevalence and determinants among African American and white women of reproductive age:

third National Health and Nutrition Examination Survey, 1988–1994. American Journal of Clinical Nutrition 76: 187–192.

Neuhouser ML, Rock CL, Eldrige AL, Kristal AR, Patterson RE, Cooper DA, Neumark-Sztainer D, Cheskin LJ, Thornquist MD. (2001). Serum concentrations of retinol, α-tocopherol and the carotenoids are influenced by diet, race and obesity in a sample of healthy adolescents. Journal of Nutrition 131: 2184–2191.

Nierenberg DW, Dain BJ, Mott LA, Baron JA, Greenberg ER. (1997). Effects of 4 y of oral supplementation with β-carotene on serum concentrations of retinol, tocopherol, and five carotenoids. American Journal of Clinical Nutrition 66: 315–319.

Nieves J, Cosman F, Herbert J, Shen V, Lindsay R. (1994). High prevalence of vitamin D deficiency and reduced bone mass in multiple sclerosis. Neurology 44: 1687–1692

Norman AW. (1998). Sunlight, season, skin pigmentation, vitamin D and 245-hydroxyvitamin D: integral components of the vitamin D endocrine system. American Journal of Clinical Nutrition 67: 1108–1110.

Oliveri M, Mautalen C, Bustamante L, Gómez García V. (1994). Serum levels of 25-hydroxyvitamin D in a year of residence on the Antarctic continent. European Journal of Clinical Nutrition 48: 397–401.

Olson JA. (1984). Serum levels of vitamin A and carotenoids as reflectors of nutritional status. Journal of the National Cancer Institute 73: 1439–1444.

Olson JA. (1997). Isotope dilution techniques: a wave of the future in human nutrition. American Journal of Clinical Nutrition 66: 186–187.

Olson JA. (1999). Vitamin A assessment by the isotope-dilution technique: good news from Guatemala. American Journal of Clinical Nutrition 69: 177–178.

Olson JA, Tanumihardjo SA. (1998). Evaluation of vitamin A status. American Journal of Clinical Nutrition 67: 148–150.

Olson JA, Gunning D, Tilton R. (1979). The distribution of vitamin A in human liver. American Journal of Clinical Nutrition 32: 2500–2507.

Omdahl JL, Garry PJ, Hunsaker LA, Hunt WC, Goodwin JS. (1982). Nutritional status in a healthy elderly population: vitamin D. American Journal of Clinical Nutrition 36: 1225–1233.

Omdahl JL, Morris HA, May BK. (2002). Hydroxylase enzymes of the vitamin D pathway: expression, function, and regulation. Annual Reviews of Nutrition 22: 139–166.

Omenn GS, Goodman GE, Thomquist MD, Barnes J, Cullen MR, Glass A, Keogh JP, Meyskens FL, Valanis B, Williams JH, Barnhart S, Hammar S. (1996). Effects of a combination of β-carotene and vitamin A on lung cancer and cardiovascular disease. New England Journal of Medicine 334: 1150–1155.

Ooms ME, Lips P, Roos JC, van der Vijgh WJ, Popp-Snijders C, Bezemer PD, Bouter LM. (1995). Vitamin D status and sex hormone binding globulin: determinants of bone turnover and bone mineral density in elderly women. Journal of Bone Mineral Research 10: 1177–1184.

Oski FA, Barness IA. (1967). Vitamin E deficiency: a previously unrecognized cause of hemolytic anemia in the premature infant. Journal of Pediatrics 70: 211–220.

Parfitt AM, Kleerekoper M. (1980). Clinical disorders of calcium, phosphorus and magnesium metabolism. In: Maxwell MH, Kleeman CR (eds.) Clinical Disorders of Fluid and Electrolyte Metabolism. 3rd ed. McGraw-Hill, New York, pp. 947–1151.

Parfitt AM, Gallagher JC, Heaney RP, Johnston CC, Neer R, Whedon GD. (1982). Vitamin D and bone health in the elderly. American Journal of Clinical Nutrition 36: 1014–1031.

Parnell W, Scragg R, Wilson N, Schaaf D, Fitzgerald E. (2003). NZ Food, NZ Children: Key Results of the 2002 National Children's Nutrition Survey. Ministry of Health, Wellington, New Zealand.

Pilch SM. (ed). (1985). Assessment of the Vitamin A Nutritional Status of the U.S. Population Based on Data Collected in the Health and Nutrition Examination Surveys. Life Sciences Research Office, Federation of American Societies for Experimental Biology, Bethesda, MD.

Pirie A, Anbunathan P. (1981). Early serum changes in severely malnourished children with corneal xerophthalmia after injection of water-miscible vitamin A. American Journal of Clinical Nutrition 34: 34–40.

Poukka RKH, Bieri, JG. (1970). Blood alpha-tocopherol: erythrocyte and plasma relationships in vitro and in vivo. Lipids 5: 757–761.

Preece MA, Tomlinson S, Ribot CA, Pietrek J, Korn H, Davies DM, Ford JA, Dunnigan MG, O'Riordan JLH. (1975). Studies of vitamin D deficiency in man. Quarterly Journal of Medicine 44: 575–589.

Pryor WA, Stone K. (1993). Oxidants in cigarette smoke, radicals, hydrogen peroxide, peroxynitrate, and peroxynitrite. Annals of the New York Academy of Sciences 686: 12–27.

Rader DJ, Brewer HB. (1993). Abetalipoproteinemia. New insights into lipoprotein assemby and vitamin E metabolism from a rare genetic disease. Journal of the American Medical Association 270: 865–869.

Rahman MM, Hossain S, Talukdar SA, Ahmad K, Bieri JG. (1964). Serum vitamin E levels in the rural population of East Pakistan. Proceedings of the Society of Experimental Biology and Medicine 117: 133–135.

Rahman MM, Mahalanabis D, Wahed MA, Islam M, Habte D, Khaled MA, Alvarez JO. (1995). Conjunctival impression cytology fails to detect subclinical vitamin A deficiency in young children. Journal of Nutrition 125: 1869–1874.

Rapuri PB, Kinyamu HK, Gallagher JC, Haynatzka V. (2002). Seasonal changes in calciotropic hormones, bone markers, and bone mineral density in elderly women. Journal of Clinical Endocrinology and Metabolism 87: 2024–2032.

Reddy V, Rao V, Arunjyothi, Reddy M. (1989). Conjunctival impression cytology for assessment of vitamin A status. American Journal of Clinical Nutrition 50: 814–817.

Refat M, Moore TJ, Kazui M, Risby TH, Perman JA, Schwarz KB. (1991). Utility of breath ethane as a noninvasive biomarker of vitamin E status in children. Pediatric Research 30: 396–403.

Reichman ME, Hayes RB, Ziegler RG, Schatzkin A, Taylor PR, Kahle LL, Fraumeni JF Jr. (1990). Serum vitamin A and subsequent development of prostate cancer in the first National Health and Nutrition Examination Survey Epidemiologic Follow-up Study. Cancer Research 50: 2311–2315.

Reilly M, Delanty N, Lawson JA, Fitzgerald G. (1996). Modulation of oxidant stress in vivo in chronic cigarette smokers. Circulation 94: 19–25.

Resnikoff S, Luzeau R, Filliard G, Amédée-Manesme O. (1992). Impression cytology with transfer in xeropthalmia and conjunctival diseases. International Opthalmology 16: 445–451.

Ribaya-Mercado JD, Mazariegos M, Tang G, Romero-Abal ME, Mena I, Solomons NW, Russell RM. (1999). Assessment of total body stores of vitamin A in Guatemalan elderly by the deuterated-retinol-dilution method. American Journal of Clinical Nutrition 69: 278–284.

Rice AL, Stoltzfus RJ, de Francisco A, Kjolde CL. (2000). Evaluation of serum retinol, the modified-relative-dose-response ratio, and breast-milk vitamin A as indicators of response to postpartum maternal vitamin A supplementation. American Journal of Clinical Nutrition 71: 799–806.

Riemersma RA, Wood DA, Macintyre CCA, Elton RA, Gey KF, Oliver MF. (1991). Risk of angina pectoris and plasma concentrations of vitamins A, C, and E and carotene. Lancet 337: 1–5.

Rock CL, Lovalvo JL, Emenhiser C, Ruffin MT, Flatt SW, Schwart SJ. (1998). Bioavailability of β-carotene is lower in raw than in processed carrots and spinach in women. Journal of Nutrition 128: 913–916.

Rosales FJ. (1998). Comments on the paper by Willumsen et al. (1997). Journal of Nutrition 128: 782–783.

Rosales FJ, Ross AC. (1998). A low molar ratio of retinol binding protein to transthyretin indicates vitamin A deficiency during inflammation: studies in rats and a posterior analysis of vitamin A-supplemented children with measles. Journal of Nutrition 128: 1681–1687.

Rosales FJ, Chau KK, Haskell MH, Shankar AH. (2002). Determination of a cut-off value for the molar ratio of retinol-binding protein to transthyretin (RBP:TTR) in Bangladeshi patients with low hepatic vitamin A stores. Journal of Nutrition 132: 3687–3692.

Rothman KJ, Moore LL, Singer MR, Nguyen US, Mannino S, Milunsky A. (1995). Teratogenicity of high vitamin A intake. New England Journal of Medicine 333: 1369–1373.

Russell D, Parnell W, Wilson N, Faed J, Ferguson E, Herbison P, Horwath C, Nye T, Walker R, Wilson B. (1999). NZ Food, NZ People: Key Results of the 1997 National Nutrition Survey. Ministry of Health, Wellington, New Zealand.

Russell RM. (2000). The vitamin A spectrum: from deficiency to toxicity. American Journal of Clinical Nutrition 71: 878–884.

Russell RM, Iber FL, Krasinski SD, Miller P. (1983). Protein-energy malnutrition and liver dysfunction limit the usefulness of the relative dose response (RDR) test for predicting vitamin A deficiency. Human Nutrition: Clinical Nutrition 37C: 361–371.

Salle BL, Glorieux FH, Delvin EE, David LS, Meunier G. (1983). Vitamin D metabolism in preterm infants: serial serum calcitriol values during the first four days of life. Acta Paediatrica Scandinavica 72: 203–206.

Sanchez AM, Congdon N, Sommer A, Rahmathullah L, Venkataswamy PG, Chandravathi PS, Clement L. (1997). Pupillary threshold as an index of population vitamin A status among children in India. American Journal of Clinical Nutrition 65: 61–66.

Sapin V, Alexandre MC, Chaïb S, Bournazeau JA, Sauvant P, Borel P, Jacquetin B, Grolier P, Lémery D, Dastugue B, Azaïs-Braesco V. (2000). Effect of vitamin A status at the end of term pregnancy on the saturation of retinol binding protein with retinol. American Journal of Clinical Nutrition 71: 537–548.

Sauberlich H, (1999). Laboratory Tests for the Assessment of Nutritional Status. CRC Press, Cleveland, OH.

Schåfer L, Overvad K. (1990). Subcutaneous adipose-tissue fatty acids and vitamin E in humans: relation to diet and sampling site. American Journal of Clinical Nutrition 52: 486–490.

Scharla SH. (1998). Prevalence of subclinical vitamin D deficiency in different European countries. Osteoporosis International 8(Suppl. 2): S7–S12.

Schwartz GG, Hulka BS. (1990). Is vitamin D deficiency a risk factor for prostate cancer? Anticancer Research 10: 1307–1311.

Schultink W. (2002). Use of under-five mortality rate as an indicator for vitamin A deficiency in a population. Journal of Nutrition 132: 2881S–2883S.

Singh RB, Ghosh S, Niaz MA, Singh R, Beegum R, Chibo H, Shoumin Z, Postiglione A. (1995). Dietary intake, plasma levels of antioxidant vitamins, and oxidative stress in relation to coronary artery disease in elderly subjects. American Journal of Cardiology 76: 1233–1238.

Sivakumar B, Reddy V. (1975). Absorption of labelled vitamin A in children during infection. British Journal of Nutrition 27: 299–304.

Sivakumar B, Reddy V. (1975). Absorption of vitamin A in children with ascariasis. Journal of Tropical Medicine and Hygiene 78: 114–115.

Smith FR, Goodman DS. (1976). Vitamin A transport in human vitamin A toxicity. New England Journal of Medicine 294: 805–808.

Sokol RJ. (1993). Vitamin E deficiency and neurological disorders. In: Pacher L, Fuchs J (eds.) Vitamin E in Health and Disease. Marcel Dekker, New York. pp. 815–849.

Sokol RJ. (1996). Vitamin E. In: Ziegler EE, Filer LJ (ed.) Present Knowledge in Nutrition. 7th ed. International Life Sciences Institute, Washington, DC. pp. 130–136.

Sokol RJ, Heubi JE, Iannaccone ST, Bove KE, Balistreri WF. (1983). Mechanism causing vitamin E deficiency during chronic childhood cholestasis. Gastroenterology 85: 1172–1182.

Sokol RJ, Heubi JE, Iannaccone ST, Bove KE, Balistreri WF. (1984). Vitamin E deficiency with normal serum vitamin E concentrations in children with chronic cholestasis. New England Journal of Medicine 310: 1209–1212.

Sokol RJ, Butler-Simon N, Heubi JE, Iannaccone ST, McClung HJ, Accuso F, Hammond K, Heytman M, Sinatra F, Riely C, et al. (1989a). Vitamin E deficiency neuropathy in children with fat malabsorption: studies in cystic fibrosis and chronic cholestasis. Annals of the New York Academy of Sciences 570: 156–169.

Sokol RJ, Kim YS, Hoofnagle JH, Heubi JE, Jones EA, Balistreri WF. (1989b). Intestinal malabsorption of vitamin E in primary biliary cirrhosis. Gastroenterology 96: 479–486.

Solomons NW, Morrow FD, Vasquez A, Bulux J, Guerrero AM, Russell RM. (1990). Test–retest reproducibility of the relative dose response for vitamin A status in Guatemalan adults: issues of diagnostic sensitivity. Journal of Nutrition 120: 738–744.

Sommer A. (1982). Nutritional Blindness: Xerophthalmia and Keratomalacia. Oxford University Press, New York.

Sommer A, Davidson FR. (2002). Assessment and control of vitamin A deficiency: the Annecy Accords. Journal of Nutrition 132: 2845S–2850S.

Sommer A, Hussaini G, Muhilal, Tarwotjo I, Susanto D, Saroso JS. (1980). History of night blindness: a simple tool for xerophthalmia screening. American Journal of Clinical Nutrition 33: 887–891.

Sowell AL, Huff DL, Yeager PR, Caudill SP, Gunter E. (1994). Simultaneous determination of retinol, α-tocopherol, lutein/zeaxanthin, β-cryptoxanthin, lycopene, α-carotene, *trans*-β-carotene, and four retinyl esters in serum by reversed-phase high-performance liquid chromatography with multi-wavelength detection. Clinical Chemistry 40: 411–416.

Stephensen CB, Gildengorin G. (2000). Serum retinol, the acute-phase response, and the apparent misclassification of vitamin A status in the third National Health and Nutrition Examination Survey. American Journal of Clinical Nutrition 72: 1170–1178.

Stoltzfus RJ, Underwood BA. (1995). Breastmilk vitamin A as an indicator to assess vitmin A status of women and infants. WHO Bulletin 73: 703–711.

Stoltzfus RJ, Haskimi M, Miller KW, Rasmussen KM, Dawiesah S, Habicht JP, Dibley MJ. (1993). High dose vitamin A supplementation of breast-feeding Indonesian mothers: effect on the vitamin A status

of mother and infant. Journal of Nutrition 123: 666–675,

Su LC, Bui M, Kardinaal A, Gomez-Aracena J, Martin-Moreno J, Martin B, Thamm M, Simonsen N, van't Veer P, Kok F, Strain S, Kohlmeier L. (1998). Differences between plasma and adipose tissue biomarkers of carotenoids and tocopherols. Cancer Epidemiology. Biomarkers and Prevention 7: 1043–1048.

Tang G, Qin J, Hao LY, Yin SA, Russell RM. (2002). Use of a short-term isotope-dilution method for determining the vitamin A status of children. American Journal of Clinical Nutrition 76: 413–418.

Tangney CC, Driskell JA, McNair HM. (1979). Separation of vitamin E isomers by high-performance liquid chromatography. Journal of Chromatography 172: 513–515.

Tanumihardjo SA, Muhilal, Yuniar Y, Permaesih D, Sulaiman Z, Karyadi D, Olson JA. (1990). Vitamin A status in preschool-age Indonesian children as assessed by the modified relative dose response assay. American Journal of Clinical Nutrition 52: 1068–1072.

Tanumihardjo SA, Muherdiyantiningsih, Permaesih D, Dahro AM, Muhilal, Karyadi D, Olson JA. (1994). Assessment of the vitamin A status in lactating and nonlactating, nonpregnant Indonesian women by use of the modified relative dose response (MRDR) test. American Journal of Clinical Nutrition 60: 142–147.

Tanumihardjo SA, Suharno D, Permaesih D, Muherdiyantiningsih, Dahro AM, Muhilal, Karyadi D, Olson JA. (1995). Application of the modified relative dose response test to pregnant Indonesian women for assessing vitamin A status. European Journal of Clinical Nutrition 49: 897–903.

Tanumihardjo SA, Cheng JC, Permaesih D, Muherdiyantiningsih, Rustan E, Muhilal, Karyadi D, Olson JA. (1996). Refinement of the modified-relative-dose-response test as a method for assessing vitamin A status in a field setting: experience with Indonesian children. American Journal of Clinical Nutrition 64: 966–971.

Thomas MK, Lloyd-Jones DM, Thadhani RI, Shaw AC, Deraska DJ, Kitch BT, Vamvakas EC, Dick IM, Prince RL, Finkelstein JS. (1998). Hypovitaminosis D in medical inpatients. New England Journal of Medicine 338: 777–783.

Thompson JN, Erdody P, Brien R, Murray TK. (1971). Fluorometric determination of vitamin A in human blood and liver. Biochemical Medicine 5: 67–89.

Thornton SP. (1977). A rapid test for dark adaptation. Annals of Ophthalmology 9: 731–734.

Thurnham DI. (1997). Impact of disease on markers of micronutrient status. Pro Nut Soc 56: 421-431

Thurnham DI, Davies JA, Crump BJ, Situnayake RD, Davis M. (1986). The use of different lipids to express serum tocopherol: lipid ratios for the measurement of vitamin E status. Annals of Clinical Biochemistry 23: 514–520.

Torronen R, Lehmusaho M, Hakkinen S, Hanninen O, Mykkanen H. (1996). Serum β-carotene response to supplementation with raw carrots, carrot juice or purified β-carotene in healthy non-smoking women. Nutrition Research 16: 565–575.

Traber MG, Sokol RJ, Burton GW, Ingold KU, Papas A, Huffaker JE, Kayden HJ. (1990). Impaired ability of patients with familial isolated vitamin E deficiency to incorporate α-tocopherol into lipoproteins secreted by the liver. Journal of Clinical Investigation 85: 397–407.

Udomkesmalee E, Dhanamitta S, Sirisinha S, Charoenkiatkul S, Tuntipopipat S, Banjong O, Rojroongwasinkul N, Kramer TR, Smith JC Jr. (1992). Effect of vitamin A and zinc supplementation on the nutriture of children in Northeast Thailand. American Journal of Clinical Nutrition 56: 50–57.

van der Wielen RPJ, Løwik MRH, van den Berg H, de Groot L, Haller J, Moreiras O, van Staveren WA. (1995). Serum vitamin D concentrations among elderly people in Europe. Lancet 346: 207–210.

Vandewoude M, Claeys M, De Leeuw I. (1984). Determination of alpha-tocopherol in human plasma by high performance liquid chromatography with electrochemical detection. Journal of Chromatography 311: 176–182.

Vandewoude MFJ, Vandewoude MG. (1987). Vitamin E status in a normal population: the influence of age. Journal of the American College of Nutrition 6: 307–311.

van het Hof KM, Gartner C, West CE, Tisburg LB. (1998). Potential of vegetable processing to increase the delivery of carotenoids to man. International Journal of Vitamin Nutrition Research 68: 366–370.

van Zoeren-Grobben D, Jacobs NJM, Houdkamp E, Lindeman JHN, Drejer DF, Berger HM. (1998). Vitamin E status in preterm infants: assessment by plasma and erythrocyte vitamin E–lipid ratios and hemolysis tests. Journal of Pediatric Gastroenterology and Nutrition 26: 73–79.

Vatassery GT, Kezowski AM, Eckfeldt JH. (1983a). Vitamin E concentrations in human blood plasma and platelets. American Journal of Clinical Nutrition 37: 1020–1024.

Vatassery GT, Johnson GJ, Krezowski AM. (1983b). Changes in vitamin E concentrations in human plasma and platelets with age. Journal of the American College of Nutrition 2: 369–375.

Velthuis-te Wierik EJ, van den Berg H, Weststrate JA, van het Hof KH, de Graaf C. (1996). Consumption of reduced-fat products: effects on parameters of antioxidative capacity. European Journal of Clinical Nutrition 50: 214–219.

Vieth R, Carter G. (2001). Difficulties with vitamin D

nutrition research: objective targets of adequacy, and assays of 25-hydroxyvitamin D. European Journal of Clinical Nutrition 55: 221–222.

Vieth R, Cole DE, Hawker GA, Trang HM, Rubin LA. (2001). Wintertime vitamin D insufficiency is common in young Canadian women, and their vitamin D intake does not prevent it. European Journal of Clinical Nutrition 55: 1091–1097.

Vinton NE, Russell RM. (1981). Evaluation of a rapid test of dark adaptation. American Journal of Clinical Nutrition 34: 1961–1966.

Webb AR, Pilbean C, Hanafin N, Holick MF. (1990). An evaluation of the relative contributions of exposure to sunlight and of diet to the circulating concentrations of 25-hydroxyvitamin D in an elderly nursing home population in Boston. American Journal of Clinical Nutrition 51: 1075–1081.

Welch TR, Bergstrom WH, Tsang RC. (2000). Vitamin D–deficient rickets: the reemergence of a once-conquered disease. Journal of Pediatrics 137: 143–145.

West CE. (2000). Meeting requirements for Vitamin A. Nutrition Reviews 58: 341–345.

West CE, Eilander A, van Lieshout M. (2002). Consequences of revised estimates of carotenoid bioefficacy for dietary control of vitamin A in developing countries. Journal of Nutrition 132: 2920S–2926S.

WHO (World Health Organization). (1996). Indicators for assessing vitamin A deficiency and their application in monitoring and evaluating intervention programmes. WHO/NUT/96.10. World Health Organization, Geneva.

Willett WC, Polk BF, Underwood BA, Stampfer MJ, Pressel S, Rosner B, Taylor J, Schneider K, Hames C (1984). Relation of serum vitamins A and E and carotenoids to the risk of cancer. New England Journal of Medicine 310: 430–434.

Wittepenn JR, Tseng SC, Sommer A. (1986). Detection of early xerophthalmia by impression cytology. Archives of Ophthalmology 104: 237–239.

Wortsman J, Matsuoka LY, Chen TC, Lu Z, Holick MF. (2000). Decreased bioavailability of vitamin D in obesity. American Journal of Clinical Nutrition 72: 690–693.

Zeghoud F, Vervel C, Guillozo H, Walrant-Debray O, Boutignon H, Garabédian M. (1997). Subclinical vitamin D deficiency in neonates: definition and response to vitamin D supplements. American Journal of Clinical Nutrition 65: 771–778.

Zittermann A. (2003). Vitamin D in preventive medicine: are we ignoring the evidence? British Journal of Nutrition 89: 552–572.

19

Assessment of vitamin C status

For centuries, the consumption of citrus fruit has been associated with the prevention of the vitamin C deficiency disease scurvy, but it was not until 1932 that the active compound was isolated (King and Waugh, 1932; Svirbely and Szent-Györgyi, 1932). A year later, ascorbic acid was characterized and synthesized. The term "ascorbic acid" is now used to embrace both L-ascorbic acid and dehydroascorbic acid; both have approximately equal vitamin C activity. Ascorbic acid is the enolic form of an α-ketolactone (2,3-didehydro-L-threo-hexano-1,4-lactone), which in solution is then easily oxidized to the diketo form — dehydro-L-ascorbic acid; their structures are shown in Figure 19.1.

Functions of ascorbic acid

Ascorbic acid acts as an electron donor for enzymes in the body involved in several important hydroxylation reactions (Tsao, 1997).

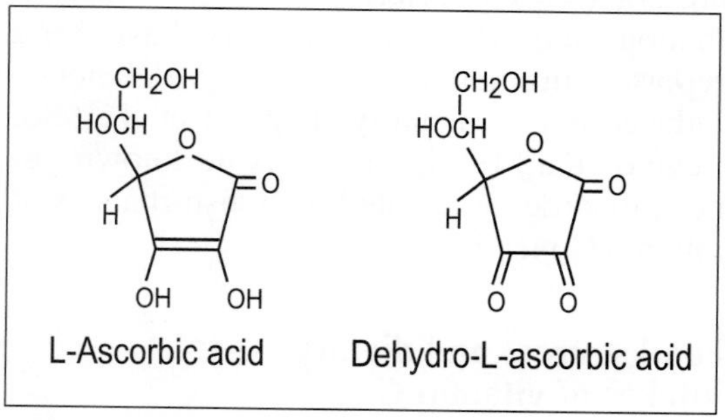

Figure 19.1: Structure of L-ascorbic and dehydroascorbic acid.

Of these, the most notable is hydroxylation of proline and lysine for collagen synthesis, the major connective tissue protein in the body. Ascorbic acid acts in these hydroxylation reactions by reducing the metal sites of prolyl (iron) hydroxylase (EC 1.14.11.2) and lysyl (copper) hydroxylase (EC 1.14.11.4). Reduced activity of these two enzymes leads to the defects in connective tissue that in turn cause the characteristic clinical features of scurvy. They include joint pains, tooth loss, bone and connective tissue disorders, and poor wound healing,

Ascorbic acid is also involved in the hydroxylation of dopamine to noradrenaline, by acting as a cofactor for the copper-containing enzyme dopamine-β-monooxygenase (EC 1.14.17.1). Noradrenaline is a neurotransmitter, and deficient dopamine hydroxylation may be associated with the mood changes, depression, and hypochondria that can occur with scurvy. The early symptoms of scurvy — fatigue, lethargy, and muscle weakness — are related to the role of ascorbic acid as a cofactor for maximal activity of two dioxygenases involved in carnitine biosynthesis. Carnitine is essential for the transport of activated long-chain fatty acids into the mitochondria, where they are converted to energy by way of β-oxidation (Carr and Frei, 1999).

Several other enzymes depend on ascorbic acid as a cofactor, although their role in the development of scurvy is still uncertain. These include enzymes involved in the metabolism of tyrosine and amidation of peptide hormones. Ascorbic acid has also

been implicated in the metabolism of cholesterol to bile acids via the enzyme cholesterol-
7-α-monooxygenase, and in steroids in the
adrenal glands (Carr and Frei, 1999).

Ascorbic acid also has several nonenzy-
matic functions based on its role as a reducing
agent (i.e., antioxidant) and ability to quench
a wide range of intra- and extracellular free
radicals. For example, ascorbic acid enhances
the gastrointestinal absorption of nonheme
iron, through its ability to reduce intraluminal
iron to its more absorbable ferrous form, or
possibly by chelation (Hallberg et al., 1987).
Ascorbic acid also provides important antioxidant protection to plasma lipids and lipid
membranes, to the ocular tissues, and for the
neutralization of phagocyte-derived oxidants.

At high intakes, ascorbic acid has also been
associated with protection against cardiovascular disease, cataracts, and cancer (Block,
1991; Garland, 1991; Gershoff, 1993), and
a variety of immune-related functions (Anderson et al., 1980; Johnston et al., 1992).
Additional research, however, is needed to
establish a causal relationship between ascorbic acid and these degenerative diseases and
immunocompetence. For more details on the
functions of ascorbic acid, see Jacob (1999).

Absorption and metabolism of vitamin C

Ascorbic acid is absorbed in the intestine by
a sodium-dependent active transport mechanism that can become saturated and is dose
dependent (Tsao, 1997). About 70%–90%
of vitamin C is absorbed when daily intakes
range from 30 to 180 mg, but absorption falls
to ⩽ 50% at intakes above 1 g/d (Kallner et al.,
1979). Indeed, the osmotic diarrhea and
intestinal discomfort sometimes experienced
by persons ingesting large doses of vitamin C
is due to the presence of a large amount of
unabsorbed vitamin C.

Regulation of the whole body vitamin C
content is achieved in part by this dose-
dependent intestinal absorption of vitamin C.
Renal action to conserve or excrete unmetabolized vitamin C also plays an important part.
In addition, there is some evidence that homeostatic regulation of vitamin C may operate at

the cellular level (Jacob, 1990). Catabolism
of vitamin C in humans occurs through oxidation of dehydroascorbic acid. However,
with large intakes, most of the vitamin C is
excreted in its unmetabolized form (Olson
and Hodges, 1987).

Deficiency of vitamin C in humans

Clinical manifestations of scurvy — such as
weakness, petechial hemorrhages, gingival
bleeding, ecchymoses and subperiosteal hemorrhage, anemia, and defects in bone development in children — are rare in industrialized countries at present. Nevertheless, mild
ascorbic acid deficiency has been observed
in institutionalized elderly subjects, probably
arising from inadequate intakes of vitamin C
(Newton et al., 1985; VanderJagt et al., 1987;
Monget et al., 1996), although impaired absorption may also be involved (Davies et al.,
1984). Alcoholic patients (Lemoine et al.,
1980) and some Inuit in Canada (Health and
Welfare Canada, 1973) may also be vulnerable to vitamin C deficiency. Infantile scurvy
is rare because breast milk provides adequate
amounts of ascorbic acid and infant formulas
are fortified with sufficient ascorbic acid.

Subclinical vitamin C deficiency may develop secondarily to some disease states such
as liver disease, cancer, gastrointestinal disorders, and rheumatoid disease. Rheumatoid
patients may utilize ascorbic acid at a faster
rate, perhaps as a result of an interaction between aspirin and ascorbic acid (Basu, 1981).

The functional health consequences of both
mild and moderate ascorbic acid deficiency
are not well characterized. Gingival inflammation, fatigue, and irritability have been
reported in moderate vitamin C deficiency
induced experimentally (Leggott et al.,1986;
Levine et al., 1996). There is no known genetic disorder associated with disturbances of
vitamin C metabolism.

Food sources and dietary
intakes of vitamin C

The vitamin C content of foods is highly
variable. Values depend on the growing con-

ditions, season of the year, stage of maturity, location, and storage time prior to consumption (Erdman and Klein, 1982). Exposure to high temperatures, oxidation, or cooking in large amounts of water all reduce the ascorbic acid content of foods.

Major food sources of vitamin C in diets of most developed countries are fresh fruits and fruit juices and some fresh vegetables; they often contribute up to 90% of the vitamin C intake. Citrus fruits and juices are particularly rich sources of vitamin C, whereas meat, fish, eggs, and dairy products are poor sources. Of the vegetables, in the United Kingdom potatoes are the most important single source of vitamin C in the diets of adults (Gregory et al.,1990).

In developing countries, the supply of food sources of vitamin C is often seasonal, so intakes may vary widely. In The Gambia, for example, intakes ranged from zero to 115 mg/d in one community, depending on the seasonal availability of mangos, oranges, and grapefruit (Bates et al., 1994).

The bioavailability of vitamin C from food sources is similar to that of supplements and is not affected by the type of food consumed (Mangels et al., 1993).

Excessive intakes of vitamin C

Therapeutic benefits from the consumption of high doses of ascorbic acid on the common cold have been reported (Pauling, 1971; Hemila and Herman, 1995), but not confirmed by objective, well-controlled studies (Moertel et al., 1985; Herbert, 1995). Nevertheless, such reports have stimulated the consumption of large doses of vitamin C. Indeed, of all the dietary supplements, those for vitamin C are often taken most frequently, especially among the elderly (Jacob et al., 1988).

The toxicity of vitamin C is low; adverse effects have only been reported after very large doses (>3 g/d) (Johnston, 1999). Some possible adverse effects include an increase in the absorption of dietary iron leading to iron overload, diarrhea and other gastrointestinal disturbances, uricosuria, oxaluria, hypoglycemia, and allergic skin reactions (Stein

et al., 1976; Sauberlich, 1981). Reductions in vitamin B_{12} and copper status have also been reported (Rivers, 1987). Current evidence is insufficient to implicate high intakes of ascorbic acid as a risk factor in oxalate stone formation. Nonetheless, individuals with hemochromatosis, glucose-6-phosphate dehydrogenase deficiency, and renal disorders, may be susceptible to adverse effects from excessive intakes of vitamin C (IOM, 2000).

The U.S. Food and Nutrition Board (IOM, 2000) has defined the Tolerable Upper Intake Level (UL) for adults 19 y and older, pregnant and lactating women as 2000 mg per day of vitamin C; ULs for children and adolescents are given in IOM (2000).

Indices of vitamin C status

There are no reliable functional tests of vitamin C status. Instead, static biochemical tests, particularly the measurement of serum or leukocyte ascorbic acid concentrations, are most frequently used to assess vitamin C status. These static biochemical tests are discussed in detail below.

19.1 Serum ascorbic acid

Vitamin C is transported in the serum but is not bound to any protein; almost all is present as ascorbic acid. Serum ascorbic acid concentrations are the most frequently used and practical index of vitamin C status in studies of individuals and populations. Levels are influenced by recent intake of the vitamin, making fasting blood samples essential (Omaye et al., 1979). Such fasting morning samples have the added advantage of being free of erythorbic acid. The latter is an epimer of L-ascorbic acid and is used as a food additive, but it lacks any antiscorbutic activity. It is cleared rapidly from the body.

Serum (or plasma) ascorbic acid levels exhibit a characteristic sigmoidal relationship with intake, as shown in Figure 19.2. In adults, the steepest change is evident at intakes between about 30 and 90 mg/d vita-

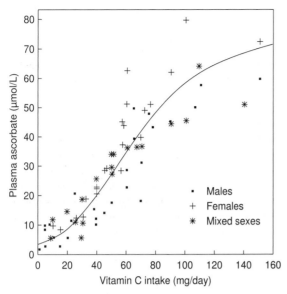

Figure 19.2: The relationship of group mean values of plasma ascorbate and daily vitamin C intake. From Bates et al. (1997), with permission of Oxford University Press.

min C. When intakes are below ~ 20 mg/d, most of the vitamin C enters the tissues, so there is very little available for circulation in the blood. For intakes greater than 60 to 70 mg/d, serum or plasma concentrations tend to plateau at about 75 µmol/L, a level representing the renal threshold (Figure 19.2). When intakes exceed about 200 mg/d, intestinal absorption of vitamin C becomes the limiting factor (Hornig et al., 1980).

Such trends in serum or plasma ascorbic acid concentrations were first noted as early as 1947 in a series of studies conducted on young women who received controlled intakes of ascorbic acid (Dodds and MacLeod, 1947). The trends have since been observed in several later studies, including those of Garry et al. (1982) and Levine et al. (1996).

As a result of this threshold effect with only limited intestinal absorption at intakes > 200 mg/d, and the excess circulating ascorbic acid being excreted in the urine, serum ascorbic acid levels cannot be used to identify persons who are regularly consuming excessive amounts of vitamin C. Hence, it is not surprising that in the National Health and Nu-

trition Examination Survey (NHANES) II, a correlation between serum ascorbic acid and vitamin C intakes was only reported for persons not taking vitamin C supplements (Loria et al., 1998).

Strong correlations of dietary intakes of vitamin C and serum or plasma ascorbic acid concentrations have only been reported when habitual dietary intakes of ascorbic acid are relatively modest (30–80 mg/d) (Bates et al., 1979). In the U.K. survey of preschool children, for example, the intakes of vitamin C, calculated from 7-d weighed records, correlated with plasma ascorbic acid levels in both boys ($n = 369$, $r = 0.43$, $p < 0.01$) and girls ($n = 354$, $r = 0.43$, $p < 0.01$) (Gregory et al., 1995). In some community studies, modest positive correlations between intakes of vegetables or fruits and serum ascorbic acid have also been documented (Drewnowski et al., 1997; Ness et al., 1999).

Persons consuming chronically low intakes of vitamin C probably have serum ascorbic acid concentrations that reflect the ascorbic acid content of the body (Jacob et al., 1987). Indeed, in such circumstances, serum levels are probably as accurate an indicator as concentrations in leukocytes. However, the relationship may be obscured in epidemiological studies by other factors that affect the absorption or metabolic turnover of vitamin C. In NHANES III, for example, only 50% of adult men had serum ascorbic acid concentrations >38 µmol/L, although more than 75% had dietary intakes higher than the estimated average requirement (i.e., 75 mg/d) (IOM, 2000). Such a discrepancy may be due in part to the high proportion of U.S. adult males who smoke or who are exposed to environmental tobacco smoke.

Factors affecting serum ascorbic acid

Cigarette smoking has a marked effect on serum ascorbic acid levels. Many studies report lower serum ascorbic acid levels in smokers (e.g., Weber et al., 1996), as well as in those regularly exposed to environmental cigarette smoke (Figure 19.3) (Tribble et al., 1993).

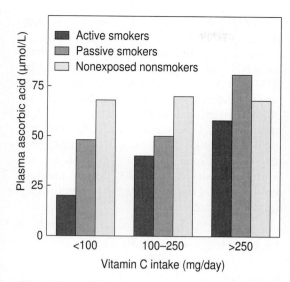

Figure 19.3: The effects of cigarette-smoke exposure on plasma ascorbic acid concentrations in 141 premenopausal women who were active or passive smokers, or nonexposed nonsmokers. Three levels of dietary vitamin C intake are represented in the results. Data from Tribble et al., American Journal of Clinical Nutrition 58: 886–890, 1993 © Am J Clin Nutr. American Society for Clinical Nutrition.

The mechanism controlling the influence of cigarette smoking on serum ascorbic acid levels appears to be related to the higher metabolic turnover of vitamin C in smokers than in nonsmokers (Kallner et al., 1981), which is probably induced by increased oxidative stress from substances in smoke (Lehr et al., 1997). Certainly, studies using isotopically labeled ascorbic acid show an increased metabolic turnover of ascorbic acid in smokers (70.0 ± 20.2 mg/d versus 35.7 ± 9.3 mg/d for nonsmokers), resulting in a 40% greater requirement for vitamin C (IOM, 2000).

Sex influences serum or plasma ascorbic acid concentrations; women have higher serum ascorbic acid levels than men who consume similar intakes of vitamin C. This suggests that there are sex-related physiological differences in the metabolism or retention of vitamin C (Dodds, 1969; Garry et al., 1982; VanderJagt et al., 1987).

Gender differences in serum ascorbic acid levels are not apparent before adolescence.

In NHANES III, higher serum ascorbate concentrations in women than in men were only apparent in those aged >19 y; no gender-related differences were reported in younger age groups (IOM, 2000).

Differences in renal handling of ascorbic acid are probably not responsible for the sex-related differences in serum ascorbic acid concentrations: no differences in measures of renal clearance of ascorbic acid according to sex have been reported (Oreopoulos et al., 1993). Gender differences in lean body mass may be a contributing factor (Blanchard, 1991).

Age-related changes in serum or plasma ascorbic acid concentrations have been reported. The elderly, especially those who are institutionalized or housebound (Cheng et al., 1985), may have lower levels than those of younger persons. This trend has been attributed in part to lower dietary intakes because of problems of poor dentition or subclinical diseases that may influence absorption or renal functioning; many other factors may also have a role (Jacob, 1994). At present, there is no evidence that the elderly have higher vitamin C requirements than those for young adults.

Pregnancy lowers serum ascorbic acid concentrations due to hemodilution, as well as active transfer to the fetus, especially during the last trimester.

Acute or chronic infection lowers serum or plasma ascorbic acid concentrations. For example, Pfitzenmaeyer et al. (1997) showed that plasma ascorbate values were significantly lower in eight hospitalized elderly subjects with acute infection than in healthy control subjects. The relative contribution of diet and stress in such circumstances is uncertain. There is some evidence that urinary excretion of ascorbic acid increases under conditions of acute infection and stress.

Chronic use of aspirin by individuals with inflammatory diseases such as rheumatoid arthritis may result in lower serum ascorbic acid levels because of an interaction between aspirin and ascorbic acid (Basu, 1981).

Oral contraceptive users often have lower serum vitamin C concentrations than non-users (Rivers, 1975). The reasons for these differences are unclear.

19.1.1 Interpretive criteria

Protracted intakes of vitamin C < 20 mg/d cause serum ascorbic acid levels to decline rapidly to 11.4 µmol/L or less (Hodges et al., 1971; Jacob et al., 1987). At such low serum ascorbic acid concentrations, clinical signs of scurvy such as follicular hyperkeratosis, swollen or bleeding gums, petechial hemorrhages, and joint pain occur (Hodges et al., 1969). Therefore, serum or plasma ascorbic acid concentrations < 11.4 µmol/L are taken as indicative of vitamin C deficiency. This cutoff value was also used in NHANES II as indicative of deficiency (Table 19.1) (Loria et al., 1998).

The cutoff values for serum or plasma ascorbic acid concentrations used to define a low vitamin C status are poorly defined. The European FLAIR study used a serum ascorbic acid level <17 µmol/L to indicate partially depleted body reserves of vitamin C (Maiani et al., 1993). NHANES II used a range of values from 11.4 to 22.8 µmol/L to indicate low vitamin C status, and also defined "normal" (22.8–56.8 µmol/L) and "saturated" (>56.8 µmol/L) levels (Loria et al., 1998). Jacob (1994) and Sauberlich (1999) adopted interpretive criteria similar to that

used by NHANES II to define low levels; they also defined two other levels (Table 19.1).

Serum ascorbic acid concentrations from NHANES III (1988–1994) were reported by IOM (2000). Mean and selected percentiles by age and sex are given (Appendix A19.1). Plasma ascorbic acid levels were also determined in the U.K. surveys for children (Gregory et al., 1995, 2000), and people aged 65 y and older (Finch et al., 1998), but not for adults (Gregory et al., 1990). Mean, median, and lower and upper 2.5 or 5th percentiles by age and sex are reported.

19.1.2 Measurement of serum ascorbic acid

Fasting blood samples are required for serum or plasma ascorbic acid analysis. The samples need to be preserved when collected to avoid degradation of the ascorbic acid. Metaphosphoric acid is often used to precipitate the protein and to stabilize the ascorbic acid in samples prior to analysis. Alternatively, trichloracetic acid or dithiothreitol (DTT) can be used; the latter is an effective stabilizing agent over a wide pH range (Okamura, 1980; Margolis and Davis, 1988).

Serum samples for ascorbic acid analysis that have been prepared in this way and frozen at –20°C are stable for several weeks and at –70°C for at least 1 y (Margolis and Duewer, 1996). If the samples cannot be processed immediately, whole blood can be stored for up to 8 h at 4°C in the dark before processing (Galan et al., 1988).

Several methods are available for measuring vitamin C in both the reduced form or as total ascorbic acid. The older assays use 2,6-dichlorophenolindophenol, dipyridil, dinitrophenylhydrazine, or *o*-phenylenedi-amine. These methods have limitations, however. Their sensitivity and specificity is low, and they are often subject to interference by other biological substances and yield falsely high readings at low ascorbic acid concentrations. In some circumstances, inadvertent oxidation of ascorbic acid or hydrolysis of dehydroascorbic acid may occur.

The method of choice for measuring ascor-

Status	Serum (µmol/L)	Mixed leukocytes (nmol/ 10^8 cells)	Mononuclear leukocytes (nmol/ 10^8 cells)
Deficient	< 11.4	< 57	< 114
Low	11.4–23	57–114	114–142
Adequate	> 23	> 114	> 142

Table 19.1: Interpretive criteria for serum and leukocyte ascorbic acid concentrations. From Jacob (1994).

bic acid in serum or plasma samples is high performance liquid chromatography (HPLC); only 50 µL are required for the measurement. Of the HPLC methods available, electrochemical detection is preferred, with its high selectivity and sensitivity. However, this method does require a dedicated instrument and an experienced operator (Washko et al., 1989). Other simpler methods use HPLC coupled with an ultraviolet detector, but they have a low sensitivity (Washko et al., 1992).

Analysis of dehydroascorbic acid by HPLC is more difficult, because direct electrochemical detection of dehydroascorbic acid is not possible. Instead, samples must first be analyzed for ascorbic acid and then reduced for measurement of ascorbate plus dehydroascorbic acid. Dehydroascorbic acid is then determined by subtraction. To differentiate ascorbic acid and D-erythorbic (isoascorbic acid) acid (the epimer of L-ascorbic acid without antiscorbutic activity), a method employing a reversed-phase HPLC system in conjunction with amperometric detection is recommended (Kutnink et al., 1985).

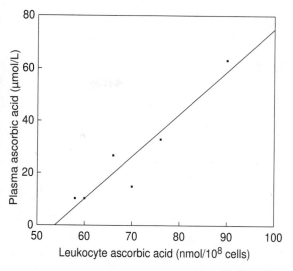

Figure 19.4: The relationship of mean plasma and leukocyte ascorbic acid concentrations measured at various stages during a depletion and repletion study of a group of six adult females. Data from Sauberlich et al., American Journal of Clinical Nutrition 50: 1039–1049, 1989 © Am J Clin Nutr. American Society for Clinical Nutrition.

19.2 Ascorbic acid in leukocytes and specific cell types

Leukocytes include lymphocytes, monocytes, and three classes of granulocytes: polymorphonuclear leukocytes or neutrophils, eosinophils, and basophils (Table 16.14). These cell types differ in their concentration of ascorbic acid and probably in their response to supplemental vitamin C, thus complicating the interpretation of ascorbic acid concentrations in leukocytes.

Leukocyte ascorbic acid

Levels of ascorbic acid in serum (or plasma) and leukocytes correlate (Figure 19.4), although ascorbic acid concentrations in leukocytes are at least 14 times greater than those in plasma (Levine et al., 1996). The concentrations range from 90 to 301 nmol/10^8 cells in adults (Omaye et al., 1979), and depend in

part on the heterogeneous nature of the leukocytes, and the methods used to analyze and isolate them.

Leukocyte ascorbic acid concentrations are commonly believed to be a more reliable index of tissue stores of ascorbic acid than are the corresponding levels in the serum, erythrocytes, or whole blood (Loh, 1972; Omaye et al., 1979; Turnbull et al., 1981). They do not exhibit the lower threshold effect that occurs for serum or plasma ascorbic acid levels, and hence they provide a more-sensitive measure of lower intakes. Further, leukocyte ascorbic acid concentrations are less responsive than serum to short-term fluctuations in recent vitamin C intakes. In the study shown in Figure 19.5, leukocyte ascorbic acid concentrations decreased about 33%, compared with the much larger and more rapid decline in plasma. Similar trends have been reported by others (Jacob et al., 1987).

Concentrations of ascorbic acid in leukocytes reflect changes in tissue ascorbic acid concentrations and the ascorbic acid body pool, but not dietary intakes. Indeed, animal studies (i.e., monkeys and guinea pigs) have

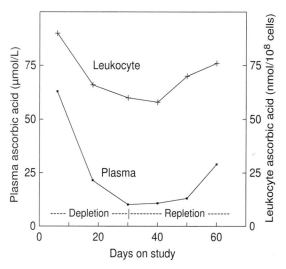

Figure 19.5: Mean plasma and leukocyte ascorbic acid concentrations during a depletion and repletion study of a group of six adult females. Ascorbic acid intakes were ad libitum for days 1–6; 0 mg/d for days 6–30; 30 mg/d for days 31–40; 60 mg/d for days 41–50; and 90 mg/d for days 51–60. Data from Sauberlich et al., American Journal of Clinical Nutrition 50: 1039–1049, 1989 © Am J Clin Nutr. American Society for Clinical Nutrition.

confirmed that leukocyte ascorbic acid concentrations provide an accurate reflection of ascorbic acid concentrations in the liver and body pool (Omaye et al., 1987).

Several factors can influence the levels of ascorbic acid in leukocytes, notably the platelet/leukocyte ratio (Vallance, 1986). Platelets should be completely separated from leukocytes prior to the leukocyte ascorbic acid assays, although this is not often achieved; the contribution of platelets to the leukocyte ascorbic acid content is often ignored (Vallance, 1986). Choice of the anticoagulant used may influence binding of platelets to leukocytes (Healy and Egan 1984).

Some additional non-dietary factors that influence concentrations of ascorbic acid in leukocytes are smoking, sex, infection, and certain drugs, as discussed for serum ascorbic acid concentrations. In some cases, these effects are due to alterations in cell populations (e.g., acute infection) or, alternatively, to differences in ascorbic acid uptake (Lee et al., 1988).

Ascorbic acid in specific cell types

The specific cell type that is most useful for assessing vitamin C status is presently uncertain. As noted earlier, both ascorbic acid concentrations in individual leukocytes and their response to vitamin C supplements vary. Mononuclear cells (lymphocytes and monocytes) have concentrations that are two- to threefold higher than granulocytes (i.e., polymorphonuclear leukocytes). Furthermore, the ascorbic acid pool in mononuclear cells is depleted more slowly than that from other blood compartments (Jacob, 1990). In addition, it is difficult to obtain homogeneous and reproducible fractions of specific cell types, so that their reported ascorbic acid concentrations vary widely and are sometimes inaccurate.

Lymphocyte ascorbic acid concentrations of 120–250 nmol/10^8 cells have been reported for healthy adults not consuming supplemental ascorbic acid (Evans et al., 1982; Yew, 1984). Jacob et al. (1991) measured lymphocyte ascorbic acid levels in a depletion–repletion study of some healthy men that was designed to induce moderate vitamin C deficiency. The mean baseline lymphocyte ascorbic acid concentration in the men was 209 nmol/10^8 cells. After 60 d of depletion, lymphocyte ascorbic acid concentrations fell significantly and consistently to a mean level of 87 nmol/10^8 cells. Moreover, the levels distinguished (with no overlap) the group of subjects receiving 5, 10, or 20 mg ascorbic acid (74–145 nmol/10^8 cells) from those subjects receiving either 60 or 250 mg/d (182–261 nmol/10^8 cells). Strong correlations of plasma and lymphocyte ascorbic acid levels were noted within the individual subjects when ascorbic acid intakes ranged from 5 to 250 mg/d (Table 19.2). There was no evidence of scorbutic symptoms in the depletion phase of this study, but there was evidence of greater oxidative damage, based on alterations in indices of oxidant status (Jacob et al., 1991).

In a later ascorbic acid depletion–repletion study, Levine et al. (1996) measured concentrations of ascorbic acid in neutrophils (polymorphonuclear leukocytes), as well as

Metabolic Period	Length (d)	Ascorbic acid intake (mg/d)	n	Plasma (μmol/L)	Mononuclear leukocyte (nmol/10^8 cells)
1	4	250†	8	59.6 ± 3.3^a	209 ± 9^a
2	32	5	8	6.6 ± 0.3^b	$117 \pm 7\ddagger^b$
3	28	10	4	5.3 ± 0.3^b	87 ± 9^c
		20	4	5.9 ± 0.5^b	95 ± 5^c
4	28	60	3	26.7 ± 8.8^c	201 ± 2^a
		250	5	64.2 ± 4.5^a	217 ± 11^a

Table 19.2: Ascorbic acid levels of healthy men after periods of various ascorbic acid intakes. Ascorbic acid levels are means $\pm$ SEM at the end of each period, n = number of subjects. Means within vertical columns not sharing the same subscript letter are significantly different (< 0.05) by t test. †Subjects consumed a supplement of 250 mg ascorbic acid in addition to their free-living diet for 1–2 wk before entering the study. ‡$n = 7$, one value deleted because of platelet contamination. From Jacob et al., American Journal of Clinical Nutrition 54: 1302S–1309S, 1991 © Am J Clin Nutr. American Society for Clinical Nutrition.

in purified monocytes and lymphocytes. Neutrophil ascorbic acid concentrations increased markedly in response to supplemental vitamin C intakes of between 30 and 100 mg/d but showed little further rise at higher doses. This trend is similar to that observed for plasma ascorbic acid levels (Figure 19.2), although the latter appear to reach a plateau at higher daily doses. The concentrations of ascorbic acid in purified monocytes and lymphocytes also followed a similar trend, again reaching a plateau at doses of 100 mg/d.

19.2.1 Interpretive criteria for leukocytes and other cell types

Confusion exists over the interpretive criteria used for leukocyte ascorbic acid concentrations, in part because they can be expressed in different ways: per 10^8 cells, per mL, per DNA level, or per unit of protein. This makes comparisons among laboratories difficult. The most common method is in terms of cell numbers (nmol/10^8 cells). The heterogeneous nature of the leukocytes and various technical difficulties with their analyses, are further complicating factors.

Table 19.1 presents the interpretive criteria used by Jacob (1994) and given in Sauberlich (1999), expressed in terms of cell numbers. When expressed in this way, clinical signs of scurvy — such as swollen or bleeding

gums, petechial hemorrhages, and so on — have been associated with leukocyte concentrations of about 11 nmol/10^8 cells. Even at levels as high as 50 nmol/10^8 cells, scorbutic changes including inflammation, tenderness, bleeding of the gums, and petechiae have sometimes been described (Sauberlich et al., 1989). For this reason, the cutoff shown in Table 19.1 that is indicative of deficiency is < 57 nmol/10^8 cells. This cutoff is for concentrations in mononuclear leukocytes (i.e. lymphocytes + monocytes). Cutoff values for ascorbic acid levels in specific cell types such as neutrophils, monocytes, and lymphocytes are less certain. Levine et al. (1996) showed that intracellular ascorbic acid levels in neutrophils were less than half of corresponding leukocyte concentrations.

The interpretation of leukocyte ascorbic acid concentrations may be particularly difficult in surgical patients or in cases of acute infection; these conditions are often associated with leukocytosis (MacLennan and Hamilton, 1977; Schorah et al., 1986; Vallance, 1988).

19.2.2 Measurement of ascorbic acid in leukocytes and other cell types

The isolation and assay of the leukocytes for ascorbic acid is technically difficult, and presently requires relatively large blood samples (2–5 mL), making the assay unsuitable for serial measurements on infants. Leukocytes can be isolated with density-gradient sedimentation. Monoclonal antibodies to various cell types can also be used (Field, 1996).

Analysis of the ascorbic acid in leukocytes or specific cell types is best performed by HPLC with electrochemical detection, after deproteinization (Washko et al., 1989).

19.3 Ascorbic acid in erythrocytes and whole blood

Erythrocyte ascorbic acid concentrations are not widely used as an index of ascorbic acid status. Levels are higher than in serum but only respond to changes in vitamin C intake over a narrow range. Hence, they are not as sensitive as serum ascorbic acid concentrations (Hodges et al., 1971). Moreover, both within- and between-variation and analytical variance are greater than for serum ascorbic acid, perhaps because of the method used to prepare the erythrocytes and the potential for oxidation of vitamin C by hemoglobin iron (Jacob et al., 1987).

Whole blood ascorbic acid concentrations have also been investigated in ascorbic acid depletion–repletion studies. Again, levels in whole blood are not as sensitive as plasma for assessing ascorbic acid depletion (Jacob et al., 1987). Levels < 17 μmol/L are defined as deficient because they have been associated with scorbutic signs (Sauberlich et al., 1989); those of 17–28 μmol/L are considered low. Levels > 28 μmol/L are interpreted as acceptable (Sauberlich, 1999).

19.4 Urinary excretion of ascorbic acid and metabolites

Urine is the major excretory route for absorbed ascorbic acid and its metabolites. If dietary intakes are normal, about half of the absorbed ascorbic acid is excreted as oxalic acid, with dehydroascorbate, 2,3-diketo-L-gluconate, and ascorbate-2-sulfate making up the remainder. When intakes >1 g/d, there is some increase in oxalate excretion, but

most of the ascorbic acid is excreted in the urine in its unmetabolized form (Olson and Hodges, 1987).

Urinary excretion of ascorbic acid reflects the recent dietary intake. Experimental depletion–repletion studies have demonstrated that concentrations in the urine decline progressively with increasing depletion of vitamin C until, in persons with scurvy, levels are undetectable. Nevertheless, urinary excretion is not a very sensitive index of ascorbic acid status; differences between persons with adequate or deficient intakes of ascorbic acid are small. For example, in the depletion–repletion study of 11 young men shown in Figure 19.6, although urinary ascorbic acid excretion was significantly lower during the depletion periods (weeks 3–6) than in the initial 2-wk 65 mg/d baseline period, the differences were small.

The specificity of urinary ascorbic acid is also low. The drugs aminopyrine, aspirin, barbiturates, hydantoins, and paraldehyde all increase urinary ascorbic acid excretion (Sauberlich, 1981). An additional disadvantage of this test as a measure of vitamin C status in humans is the requirement for 24-h urine specimens. The latter are impractical in field studies and best collected in clinical or research settings.

The ascorbic acid saturation test is some-

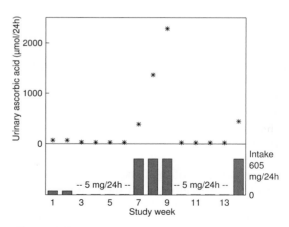

Figure 19.6: Mean urinary ascorbic acid during times of varied ascorbic acid intake. Data from a study of 11 adult men by Jacob et al., American Journal of Clinical Nutrition, 46, 818–826, 1987 © Am J Clin Nutr. American Society for Clinical Nutrition.

times used as an alternative index of vitamin C status in research studies. Ascorbic
acid is rapidly absorbed from the gastrointestinal tract, and any excess above the renal
threshold appears in the urine. In this test,
ascorbic acid is administered orally (usually
0.50–2.0 g of ascorbic acid per day) in divided doses for four consecutive days, and
the amount of the dose excreted in the urine
is determined. Recovery of the test dose in
the urine should be between 60% and 80%
for subjects with normal tissue saturation of
ascorbic acid (Lowry et al., 1946).

Measurement of urinary ascorbic acid

Ascorbic acid is very unstable in urine and
samples must be stabilized with metaphosphoric acid immediately after collection. In
the past, a colorimetric method was used for
the analysis, but HPLC with electrochemical
detection is now preferred.

19.5 Salivary and buccal cell ascorbic acid

The use of saliva as a biopsy material for
assessing vitamin C status has been investigated: the collection of saliva is noninvasive and simple to perform in population
surveys. Results have not been promising.
Ascorbic acid concentrations in whole mixed
saliva are relatively low, ranging from 1.1 to
22.7 µmol/L (Hess and Smith, 1949); they do
not correlate with levels of ascorbic acid in
plasma, leukocytes, or dietary intakes (Leggott et al., 1986; Jacob et al., 1987)

Buccal cell ascorbic acid concentrations
have also been investigated as a potential
biomarker of vitamin C status. In a vitamin C depletion–repletion study on healthy
men, buccal cell ascorbic acid levels were
significantly lower in subjects receiving low
ascorbic acid intakes (5, 10, 20 mg/d) compared with repletion intakes (60 or 250 mg/d)
(Jacob et al., 1991). Nevertheless, the investigators concluded that buccal cells are
probably not suitable as a marker of ascorbic
acid status over a broad range of population

intakes. More work is needed to standardize this method, to improve its sensitivity,
and to establish its validity as a noninvasive
screening test for ascorbic acid deficiency in
free-living populations (Jacob et al., 1991).

Measurement of buccal cell ascorbic acid

Buccal cells can be collected as discussed
in Section 15.1.11. After centrifuging the
cells, the cell pellet must be washed with
0.15 NaCl, and then the ascorbic acid can be
extracted from the pellet with metaphosphoric acid to stabilize the vitamin C. This mixture can be stored at −70°C prior to the assay
of ascorbic acid, preferably by HPLC, and the
analysis of protein (Jacob et al., 1991). Results are expressed as pmol/mg protein.

19.6 Body pool size

Isotope dilution techniques can be used to
determine the size of the body pool of vitamin
C. The method involves administering an oral
dose of ^{14}C-labeled or ^{13}C-labeled ascorbic
acid, followed by the measurement of the
specific activity of blood or urine ascorbate
within 24–48 h (Baker et al., 1971; Kallner et
al., 1977). Of the two radioactive isotopes,
^{14}C has a long half-life, so ^{13}C, a shorter-
lived isotope, is preferred.

In young healthy male adults, the pool size
of ascorbic acid is ~1500 mg (i.e., 20 mg/kg
body weight) (Baker et al., 1971; Kallner et
al., 1979). In adult men, the total body pool
of vitamin C ranges in size from < 20 mg
to approximately 3000 mg, depending on the
daily intake of L-ascorbate. When pool sizes
are < 600 mg of vitamin C, psychological
abnormalities have been reported (Kinsman
and Hood, 1971), whereas at levels < 300 mg
(1.7 mmol), scurvy symptoms have been observed (Baker et al., 1971).

19.7 Capillary fragility

Capillary fragility has been used as a functional test of vitamin C deficiency. For the

test, pressure is applied to veins of the upper arm, and the venous pressure at which petechial hemorrhages appear is measured with a blood pressure cuff (Hess, 1913; Göthlin, 1933). An alternative method involves applying a pressure of 100 mm Hg to the upper arm with a sphygmomanometer, and petechiae appearing after 5 min are counted. This test can produce inconsistent results in individuals with a deficiency of vitamin C and is not specific to vitamin C deficiency states: other diseases may also increase capillary fragility (Vilter, 1967). Consequently alternative functional tests of ascorbic acid status need to be developed.

19.8 Summary

Ascorbic acid is involved in a variety of biological processes, although for some of them, its precise mechanism is unclear. Clinical deficiency of vitamin C produces scurvy, a rare disease in industrialized countries today. Nevertheless, marginal vitamin C deficiency has been described in selected vulnerable groups such as institutionalized elderly and alcoholic patients; gingival inflammation and fatigue appear to be the most sensitive clinical markers for moderate vitamin C deficiency. Excess intakes of vitamin C may produce a range of adverse effects, including osmotic diarrhea, uricosuria, oxaluria, hypoglycemia, and allergic skin reactions.

There are no reliable functional indices of vitamin C nutriture. Static biochemical indices such as serum or leukocyte ascorbic acid concentrations are most frequently used. The former reflect recent dietary intake within a limited range (30–80 mg/d). Serum ascorbic acid levels increase linearly with dietary intake but only up to a plateau of about 80 μmol/L, and thus are unsuitable for detecting excessive intakes of vitamin C. Some non-nutritional factors, including sex, smoking, oral contraceptive use, and acute infection, affect serum ascorbic acid concentrations and, hence, reduce their specificity and sensitivity.

Cutoff points for low serum ascorbic acid

concentrations indicative of moderate risk for development of overt vitamin deficiency signs and symptoms are disputed, and values from 11.4 to 22.8 μmol/L have been used; levels <11.4 μmol/L are associated with scorbutic signs. Fasting blood samples are preferred for analysis of serum ascorbic acid concentrations.

Mixed leukocyte ascorbic acid concentrations (expressed as nmol/10^8 cells) are a more reliable index of tissue ascorbic acid stores; they are less responsive than serum to short-term fluctuations in vitamin C intakes, but their assay is difficult and requires a relatively large blood sample. A cutoff point of < 57 nmol/10^8 cells, indicative of deficiency, is recommended for leukocyte ascorbic acid concentrations, whereas concentrations of 57 to 114 nmol/10^8 cells are said to be indicative of low vitamin C status.

Urinary excretion of ascorbic acid is also influenced by recent dietary intake. Moreover, the sensitivity and specificity of this test is low, and 24-h urine samples are required. In a research environment, the ascorbic acid saturation test is sometimes used. The most reliable method for assessing body pool size of ascorbic acid involves isotope dilution techniques. Capillary fragility is the only functional physiological test for assessing vitamin C status, but it is rarely used because of its low specificity.

The method of choice for assaying ascorbic acid in all biological fluids and tissues is HPLC with electrochemical detection. This method is also capable of both measuring and distinguishing between ascorbic acid and D-erythorbic (isoascorbic) acid; the latter has no antiscorbutic activity. There is no direct method for measuring dehydroascorbic acid. More research is needed to identify a more useful functional test of ascorbic acid status.

References

Anderson R, Oosthuizen R, Maritz R, Theron A, Van Rensburg AJ. (1980). The effects of increasing weekly doses of ascorbate on certain cellular and humoral immune functions in normal volunteers. American Journal of Clinical Nutrition 33: 71–76.

Baker EM, Hodges RE, Hood J, Sauberlich HE, March SC, Canham JE. (1971). Metabolism of ^{14}C- and ^{3}H-labeled L-ascorbic acid in human scurvy. American Journal of Clinical Nutrition 24: 444–454.

Basu TK. (1981). The influence of drugs with particular reference to aspirin on the bioavailability of vitamin C. In: Counsell JN, Hornig DH (eds.) Vitamin C (Ascorbic Acid). Applied Science Publishers, London, pp. 273–281.

Bates CJ, Rutishauser IH, Black AE, Paul AA. (1979). Long-term vitamin status and dietary intake of healthy elderly subjects. 2: Vitamin C. British Journal of Nutrition 42: 43–56.

Bates CJ, Prentice AM, Paul AA. (1994). Seasonal variations in vitamins A, C, riboflavin and folate intakes and status of pregnant lactating women in a rural Gambian community: some possible implications. European Journal of Clinical Nutrition 48: 660–668.

Bates CJ, Thurnham DI, Bingham SA, Margetts BM, Nelson M. (1997). Biochemical markers of nutrient status. In: Margetts BM, Nelson M (eds.) Design Concepts in Nutritional Epidemiology. 2nd ed. Oxford University Press, Oxford. pp. 170–240.

Blanchard J. (1991). Effects of gender on vitamin C pharmocokinetics in man. Journal of the American College of Nutrition 10: 453–459.

Block G. (1991). Vitamin C and cancer prevention: the epidemiologic evidence. American Journal of Clinical Nutrition 53: 270S–282S.

Carr AC, Frei B. (1999). Toward a new recommended dietary allowance for vitamin C based on antioxidant and health effects in humans. American Journal of Clinical Nutrition 69: 1086–1107.

Cheng L, Cohen N, Bhagavan HN. (1985). Vitamin C and the elderly. In: Watson RR (ed.) Handbook of Nutrition in the Aged. CRC Press, Boca Raton, FL, pp. 157–185.

Davies HE, Davies JE, Hughes RE, Jones E. (1984). Studies on the absorption of L-xyloascorbic acid (vitamin C) in young and elderly subjects. Human Nutrition Clinical Nutrition 38: 463–471.

Dodds ML. (1969). Sex as a factor in blood levels of ascorbic acid. Journal of the American Dietetic Association 54: 32–33.

Dodds ML, MacLeod FL. (1947). Blood plasma ascorbic acid levels on controlled intakes of ascorbic acid. Science 106: 67.

Drewnowski A, Rock CL, Henderson SA, Shore AB, Fischler C, Galan P, Preziosi P, Hercberg S. (1997). Serum beta-carotene and vitamin C as biomarkers of vegetable and fruit intakes in a community-based sample of French adults. American Journal of Clinical Nutrition 65: 1796–1802.

Erdman JW Jr, Klein BP. (1982). Harvesting, processing and cooking influences on vitamin C in foods. In: Seib PA, Tolbert BM (eds.) Ascorbic Acid: Chemistry, Metabolism and Uses. Advances in Chemistry, Ser. 200. American Chemical Society, Washington, DC, pp. 499–532.

Evans RM, Currie L, Campbell A. (1982). The distribution of ascorbic acid between various cellular components of blood in normal individuals, and its relation to the plasma concentration. British Journal of Nutrition 47: 473–482.

Field CJ. (1996). Using immunological techniques to determine the effect of nutrition on T-cell function. Canadian Journal of Physiology and Pharmacology 74: 769–777.

Finch S, Doyle W, Lowe C, Bates CJ, Prentice A, Smithers G, Clarke PC. (1998). National Diet and Nutrition Survey: People Aged 65 Years or Over. Volume 1: Report of the Diet and Nutrition Survey. The Stationery Office, London.

Galan P, Hercberg S, Keller HE, Bellio JP, Bourgeois CF, Fourlon CH. (1988). Plasma ascorbic acid determination: is it necessary to centrifuge and to stabilize blood samples immediately in the field? International Journal for Vitamin and Nutrition Research 58: 473–474.

Garland D. (1991). Ascorbic acid and the eye. American Journal of Clinical Nutrition 54: 1198S–1202S.

Garry PJ, Goodwin JS, Hunt WC, Gilbert BA. (1982). Nutritional status in a healthy elderly population: vitamin C. American Journal of Clinical Nutrition 36: 332–339.

Gershoff SN. (1993). Vitamin C (ascorbic acid): new roles, new requirements? Nutrition Reviews 51: 313–326.

Göthlin GF. (1933). Outline of a method for the determination of the strength of the skin capillaries and the indirect estimation of the individual vitamin C standard. Journal of Laboratory and Clinical Medicine 18: 484–490.

Gregory J, Foster K, Tyler H, Wiseman M. (1990). The Dietary and Nutritional Survey of British Adults. Her Majesty's Stationery Office, London.

Gregory J, Collins DL, Davies PSW, Hughes JM, Clarke PC. (1995). National Diet and Nutrition Survey: Children Aged One-and-a-Half to Four-and-a-Half Years. Volume 1: Report of the Diet and Nutrition Survey. Her Majesty's Stationery Office, London.

Gregory J, Lowe S, Bates CJ, Prentice A, Jackson LV, Smithers G, Wenlock R, Farron M. (2000). National Diet and Nutrition Survey: Young People Aged 4 to 18 Years. Volume 1: Report of the Diet and Nutrition Survey. The Stationery Office, London.

Hallberg L, Brune M, Rossander-Hulten L. (1987). Is there a physiological role of vitamin C in iron absorption? Annals of the New York Academy of Sciences 498: 324–332.

Health and Welfare Canada. (1973). Nutrition Canada National Survey. Health and Welfare Canada, Ottawa.

Healy DT, Egan EL. (1984). Centrifugal and anticoagulant induced variations in platelet rich plasma and their influence on platelet aggregation. Scandinavian Journal of Haematology 32: 452–456.

Hemila H, Herman ZS. (1995). Vitamin C intake and the common cold: a retrospective analysis of Chalmer's review. Journal of the American College of Nutrition 14: 116–123.

Herbert V. (1995). Vitamin C supplements and disease: counterpoint. Journal of the American College of Nutrition 14: 112–113.

Hess AF. (1913). Involvement of the blood and blood vessels in infantile scurvy. Proceedings of the Society for Experimental Biology and Medicine 11: 130–132.

Hess WC, Smith BT. (1949). Ascorbic acid content of saliva of carious and noncarious individuals. Journal of Dental Research 28: 507–511.

Hodges RE, Baker EM, Hood J, Sauberlich HE, March SC. (1969). Experimental scurvy in man. American Journal of Clinical Nutrition 22: 535–548.

Hodges RE, Hood J, Canham JE, Sauberlich HE, Baker EM. (1971). Clinical manifestations of ascorbic acid deficiency in man. American Journal of Clinical Nutrition 24: 432–443.

Hornig D, Vuilleumier JP, Hartmann D. (1980). Absorption of large, single, oral intakes of ascorbic acid. International Journal for Vitamin and Nutrition Research 50: 309–314.

IOM (Institute of Medicine). (2000). Dietary Reference Intakes for Vitamin C, Vitamin E, Selenium and Carotenoids. National Academy Press, Washington, DC.

Jacob RA. (1990). Assessment of human vitamin C status. Journal of Nutrition 120: 1480–1485.

Jacob RA. (1994). Vitamin C. In: Shils ME, Olson JA, Shike M (eds.) Modern Nutrition in Health and Disease. 8th ed. Volume 1. Lea & Febiger, Philadelphia, pp. 432–448.

Jacob RA. (1999). Vitamin C. In: Shils ME, Olson JA, Shike M (eds.) Modern Nutrition in Health and Disease. 9th ed. Williams & Williams, Baltimore, MD. pp. 467–483.

Jacob RA, Skala JH, Omaye ST. (1987). Biochemical indices of human vitamin C status. American Journal of Clinical Nutrition 46: 818–826.

Jacob RA, Otradovec CL, Russell RM , Munro HN, Hartz SC, McGandy RB, Morrow FD, Sadowski JA. (1988). Vitamin C status and nutrient interactions in a healthy elderly population. American Journal of Clinical Nutrition 48: 1436–1442.

Jacob RA, Kelley DS, Pianalto FS, Swendseid ME, Henning SM, Zhang JZ, Ames BN, Fraga CG, Peters JH. (1991). Immunocompetence and oxidant defense during ascorbic acid depletion of healthy men. American Journal of Clinical Nutrition 54: 1302S–1309S.

Johnston CS. (1999). Biomarkers for establishing a tolerable upper intake level for vitamin C. Nutrition Reviews 57: 71–77.

Johnston CS, Martin LJ, Cai X. (1992). Antihistamine effect of supplemental ascorbic acid and neutrophil chemotaxis. Journal of the American College of Nutrition 11: 172–176.

Kallner A, Hartmann D, Hornig DH. (1977). Determi-nation of bodypool size and turnover rate of ascorbic acid in man. Nutrition and Metabolism 21(Suppl. 1): 31–35.

Kallner A, Hartmann D, Hornig D. (1979). Steady-state turnover and body pool of ascorbic acid in man. American Journal of Clinical Nutrition 32: 530–539.

Kallner AB, Hartmann D, Hornig DH. (1981). On the requirements of ascorbic acid in man: steady-state turnover and body pool in smokers. American Journal of Clinical Nutrition 34: 1347–1355.

King CG, Waugh WA. (1932). Chemical nature of vitamin C. Science 75: 357–358.

Kinsman RA, Hood J. (1971). Some behavioral effects of ascorbic acid deficiency. American Journal of Clinical Nutrition 24: 455–464.

Kutnink MA, Skala JH, Sauberlich HE, Omaye ST. (1985). Simultaneous determination of ascorbic acid, isoascorbic acid (erythorbic acid) and uric acid in human plasma by high performance liquid chromatography with amperometric detection. Journal of Liquid Chromatography 8: 31–46.

Lee W, Davis KA, Rettmer RL, Labbe RF. (1988). Ascorbic acid status: biochemical and clinical considerations. American Journal of Clinical Nutrition 48: 286–290.

Leggot PJ, Robertson PB, Rothman DL, Murray PA, Jacob RA. (1986). The effect of controlled ascorbic acid depletion and supplementation on periodontal health. Journal of Periodontology 57: 480–485.

Lehr HA, Weyrich AS, Saetzler R, Jurek A, Arfors KE, Zimmerman GA, Prescott SM, McIntyre TM. (1997) Vitamin C blocks inflammatory platelet-activating factor mimetics created by cigarette smoking. Journal of Clinical Investigations 99: 2358–2364.

Lemoine A, Le Devehat C, Codaccioni JL, Monges A, Bermond P, Salkeld RM. (1980). Vitamin B_1, B_2, B_6, and C status in hospital inpatients. American Journal of Clinical Nutrition 33: 2595–2600.

Levine M, Conry-Cantilena C, Wang Y, Welch RW, Washko PW, Dhariwal KR, Park JB, Lazarev A, Graumlich JF, King J, Cantilena LR. (1996). Vitamin C pharmacokinetics in healthy volunteers: evidence for a recommended dietary allowance. Proceedings of the National Academy of Sciences of the United States of America 93: 3704–3709.

Loh HS. (1972). The relationship between dietary ascorbic acid intake and buffy coat and plasma ascorbic acid concentrations at different ages. International Journal for Vitamin and Nutrition Research 42: 80–85.

Loria CM, Whelton P, Caulfield LE, Szklo M, Klag MJ. (1998). Agreement among indicators of vitamin C status. American Journal of Epidemiology 147: 587–596.

Lowry OH, Bessey OA, Brock MJ, Lopez JA. (1946). The interrelationship of dietary, serum, white blood cell and total ascorbic acid. Journal of Biological Chemistry 166: 111–119.

MacLennan WJ, Hamilton JC. (1977). The effect of acute illness on leukocyte and plasma ascorbic acid levels. British Journal of Nutrition 38: 217–223.

Maiani G, Azzini E, Ferro-Luzzi A. (1993). Vitamin C: FLAIR Concerted Action No. 10, Status Papers. International Journal for Vitamin and Nutrition Research 63: 289–295.

Mangels AR, Block G, Frey CM, Patterson BH, Taylor PR, Norkus EP, Levander OA. (1993). The bioavailability to humans of ascorbic acid from oranges, orange juice and cooked broccoli is similar to that of synthetic ascorbic acid. Journal of Nutrition 123: 1054–1061.

Margolis SA, Davis TP. (1988). Stabilization of ascorbic acid in human plasma, and its liquid-chromatographic measurement. Clinical Chemistry 34: 2217–2223.

Margolis SA, Duewer DL. (1996). Measurement of ascorbic acid in human plasma and serum stability, intralaboratory repeatability, and interlaboratory reproducibility. Clinical Chemistry 42: 1257–1262.

Moertel CG, Fleming TR, Creagan ET, Rubin J, O'Connell MJ, Ames MM. (1985). High-dose vitamin C versus placebo in the treatment of patients with advanced cancer who have had no prior chemotherapy: a randomized double-blind comparison. New England Journal of Medicine 312: 137–141.

Monget AL, Galan P, Preziosi P, Keller H, Bourgeois C, Arnaud J, Favier A, Hercberg S. (1996). Micronutrient status in elderly people. International Journal for Vitamin and Nutrition Research 66: 71–76

Ness AR, Khaw KT, Bingham S, Day NE. (1999). Plasma vitamin C: what does it measure? Public Health Nutrition 2: 51–54.

Newton HM, Schorah CJ, Habibzadeh N, Morgan DB, Hullin RP. (1985). The cause and correction of low blood vitamin C concentrations in the elderly. American Journal of Clinical Nutrition 42: 656–659.

Okamura M. (1980). Improved method for determination for L-ascorbic and L-dehydroascorbic acid in blood plasma. Clinica Chimica Acta 103: 259–268.

Olson JA, Hodges RE. (1987). Recommended dietary intakes (RDI) of vitamin C in humans. American Journal of Clinical Nutrition 45: 693–703.

Omaye ST, Turnbull JD, Sauberlich HE. (1979). Selected methods for the determination of ascorbic acid in animal cells, tissues, and fluids. Methods in Enzymology 62: 3–11.

Omaye ST, Schaus EE, Kutnink MA, Hawkes WC. (1987). Measurement of vitamin C in blood components by high-performance liquid chromatography: implications in assessing vitamin C status. Annals of the New York Academy of Sciences 498: 389–401.

Oreopoulos DG, Linderman RD, VanderJagt DJ, Tzamaloukas AH, Bhagavan HN, Garry PJ. (1993). Renal excretion of ascorbic acid: effect of age and sex. Journal of the American College of Nutrition 12: 537–542.

Pauling L. (1971). The significance of the evidence about ascorbic acid and the common cold. Proceedings of the National Academy of Sciences of the United States of America 68: 2678–2681.

Pfitzenmeyer P, Guilland JC, d'Athis P. (1997). Vitamin B6 and vitamin C status in elderly patients with infections during hospitalization. Annals on Nutrition and Metabolism 41: 344–352.

Rivers JM. (1975). Oral contraceptives and ascorbic acid. American Journal of Clinical Nutrition 28: 550–554.

Rivers JM. (1987). Safety of high-level vitamin C ingestion. Annals of the New York Academy of Sciences 498: 445–454.

Sauberlich HE. (1981). Ascorbic acid (vitamin C). Clinics in Laboratory Medicine 1: 673–684.

Sauberlich HE. (1999). Laboratory Tests for the Assessment of Nutritional Status. 2nd ed. CRC Press, Cleveland, OH.

Sauberlich HE, Kretch MJ, Taylor PC, Johnson HL, Skala JH. (1989). Ascorbic acid and erythorbic acid metabolism in nonpregnant women. American Journal of Clinical Nutrition 50: 1039–1049.

Schorah CJ, Habibzadeh N, Hancock M, King RF. (1986). Changes in plasma and buffy layer vitamin C concentrations following major surgery: what do they reflect? Annals of Clinical Biochemistry 23: 566–570.

Stein HB, Hasan A, Fox IH. (1976). Ascorbic acid-induced uricosuria: a consequence of megavitamin therapy. Annals of Internal Medicine 84: 385–388.

Svirbely JL, Szent-Györgyi A. (1932). Chemical nature of vitamin C. Biochemistry Journal 26: 865–870.

Tribble DL, Giuliano LJ, Fortmann SP. (1993). Reduced plasma ascorbic acid concentrations in nonsmokers regularly exposed to environmental tobacco smoke. American Journal of Clinical Nutrition 58: 886–890.

Tsao CS. (1997). An overview of ascorbic acid chemistry and biochemistry. In: Packer L, Fuchs J (eds.) Vitamin C in Health and Disease. Marcel Dekker, New York, pp. 25–58.

Turnbull JD, Sudduth JH, Sauberlich HE, Omaye ST. (1981). Depletion and repletion of ascorbic acid in the Rhesus monkey: relationship between ascorbic acid concentration in blood components with total body pool and liver concentration of ascorbic acid. International Journal for Vitamin and Nutrition Research 51: 47–53.

Vallance S. (1986). Platelets, leucocytes and buffy layer vitamin C after surgery. Human Nutrition: Clinical Nutrition 40: 35–41.

Vallance S. (1988). Changes in plasma and buffy layer vitamin C following surgery. British Journal of Surgery 75: 366–370.

VanderJagt DJ, Garry PJ, Bhagavan HN. (1987). Ascorbic acid intake and plasma levels in healthy elderly people. American Journal of Clinical Nutrition 46: 290–294.

Vilter RW. (1967). Effects of ascorbic acid deficiency in man. In: Sebrell WH Jr, Harris RS (eds.) The Vitamins: Chemistry, Physiology, Pathology, Methods. Volume I. Academic Press, New York, pp. 457–485.

Washko PW, Hartzell WO, Levine M. (1989). Ascorbic acid analysis using high-performance liquid chromatography with coulometric electrochemical detection. Analytical Biochemistry 181: 276–282.

Washko PW, Welch RW, Dhariwal KR, Wang Y, Levine M. (1992). Ascorbic acid and dehydroascorbic acid analyses in biological samples. Analytical Biochemistry 204: 1–14.

Weber C, Erl W, Weber K, Weber PC. (1996). Increased adhesiveness of isolated monocytes to endothelium is prevented by vitamin C intake in smokers. Circulation 93: 1488–1492.

Yew MS. (1984). Megadose vitamin C supplementation and ascorbic acid and dehydroascorbic acid levels in plasma and lymphocytes. Nutrition Reports International 30: 597–601.

20

Assessment of the status of thiamin, riboflavin, and niacin

The B vitamins — thiamin, riboflavin, and niacin — participate as coenzymes or prosthetic groups in a variety of reactions involved in the catabolism of carbohydrates, fats, and proteins. All three vitamins are stored in the body for a relatively short time, have no major tissue storage pool, are water soluble and rapidly excreted in the urine, and have a fast rate of catabolism. Consequently, deficiencies develop more quickly than for the fat-soluble vitamins or vitamin B_{12}.

Clinical deficiency signs for these B vitamins are not very specific. Hence, static and functional biochemical tests are frequently used to confirm the clinical diagnosis and to detect subclinical deficiency states. The latter may generate nonspecific subjective effects such as insomnia, irritability, loss of appetite, and weight loss. In addition, mild deficiencies of each of these vitamins may alter the metabolism of certain drugs.

Static biochemical tests for thiamin, riboflavin, and niacin measure the vitamin or its metabolites in blood and urine. Functional biochemical tests for thiamin and riboflavin measure the activity of an enzyme that requires the vitamin as a coenzyme. No comparable functional test exists for niacin.

The choice of the biochemical test depends on the objectives of the study. Some of the tests for these three B vitamins are only appropriate at specific levels of vitamin B nutriture. Further, in many cases, the within-subject variability of the test is large, even when subjects are on a constant diet. Hence for each of these B vitamins, a combination

of tests is often required to gain a more complete understanding of the nutritional status of an individual.

20.1 Thiamin

The isolation and synthesis of thiamin was carried out in 1932 by Williams and Cline (1936). The structure of thiamin was determined subsequently. It consists of a pyrimidine and thiazole ring linked by a methylene bridge (Figure 20.1). Phosphorylated forms of thiamin include thiamin monophosphate

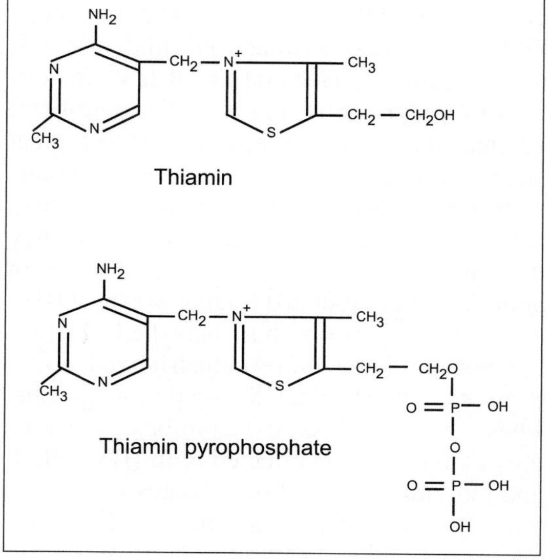

Figure 20.1: Structure of thiamin and the coenzyme thiamin pyrophosphate.

545

(TMP), thiamin pyrophosphate (TPP), and thiamin triphosphate (TTP), all of which can be interconverted in the tissues. Of these forms, TPP accounts for about 80% and TTP for about 5%–10% of total thiamin in the tissues; the remainder is present as thiamin and TMP.

Functions of thiamin

Thiamin, when converted to thiamin pyrophosphate (TPP) (Figure 20.1), has a major role in carbohydrate metabolism. Thiamin pyrophosphate is required for the oxidative decarboxylation of α-keto acids and for the action of transketolase in the pentose phosphate pathway. It also functions as a cofactor in the condensation of glyoxylate and α-ketoglutarate to form 2-hydroxy-3-ketoadipate. New research suggests that thiamin pyrophosphate is involved in the α-oxidation of 3-methyl-substituted fatty acids (Casteels et al., 2003). In addition, thiamin may be intimately involved in neurological function, although the precise mechanism is unclear.

Deficiency of thiamin in humans

The classical syndrome of thiamin deficiency is beriberi, which used to occur where polished rice was the staple food. The deficiency affects the cardiovascular, muscular, nervous, and gastrointestinal systems. It is characterized by polyneuritis, bradycardia, peripheral edema, muscle tenderness, and neurological signs. In areas where the local diet contains significant amounts of fermented raw fish, tea leaves, or betal nut, thiamin deficiency may also occur because these foods contain antithiamin compounds (Butterworth, 2001).

Food fortification has banished thiamin deficiency in the more-industrialized countries, except in selected population groups. These include chronic alcoholics, some of the elderly, persons infected with HIV-AIDS, and individuals with disease states associated with chronic emesis, diarrhea, and marked anorexia (Anderson et al., 1985; Wilkinson et al., 1997; Butterworth, 2001). Patients with chronic renal failure are also at risk as a result of dietary restrictions and loss of thiamin during dialysis (Talwar et al., 2000). Subclinical and clinical thiamin deficiency has also been described in Japan among university students (Kawai et al., 1980; Hatanaka and Ueda, 1981), and among some displaced persons, especially women during the postpartum period (McGready et al., 2001). This vitamin deficiency was also shown to be a contributing factor in an outbreak of neuropathy in Cuba in 1992–1993 (Macias-Matos et al., 1996).

Severe deficiency in alcoholics is often associated with Wernicke's encephalopathy. The latter is a genetic neurological disorder: subjects have a variant of transketolase, which requires a higher than normal concentration of thiamin diphosphate for activity (Bender, 1999).

Decreased activities of thiamin-dependent enzymes, notably α-ketoglutarate dehydrogenase, have been observed in the brain of patients with Alzheimer's disease and Parkinson's disease. However, the effect has been attributed to direct toxic effects of oxidative stress and β-amyloid deposition, and not to systemic thiamin deficiency in these patients (Butterworth, 2003). Lower levels of erythrocyte transketolase activity (Lemoine et al., 1986), and erythrocyte thiamin pyrophosphate and plasma thiamin monophosphate (Patrini et al., 2004) have also been observed in obese compared to nonobese women, but they have not been associated with any signs or symptoms of thiamin deficiency.

The effects of mild thiamin deficiency are nonspecific and thus easily overlooked, especially in the elderly. They include sleeplessness, depression, weight loss, malaise, anorexia, fatigue, and irritability (Hart and Reynolds, 1957; Smidt et al., 1991).

Food sources and dietary intakes

Whole grain cereals, pork, and legumes are the richest food sources of thiamin, followed by other meats, fish, green vegetables, fruits, and milk. Polished rice, sugar, alcohol, fat, and other refined foods are poor sources of thiamin. At present, data on bioavailability for thiamin from foods are limited (IOM, 2000).

Thiamin is rapidly destroyed at elevated temperatures unless the pH is below 5. Thus the addition of sodium bicarbonate to green vegetables to retain their green color destroys thiamin. Thiamin can also be destroyed by the presence of peroxides from fat oxidation (Gregory, 1996). Thiamin is lost when cooking water is discarded because it is a water-soluble vitamin. In alkaline solution, thiamin may be oxidized to the fluorescent compound thiochrome. This reaction is widely used for measuring thiamin in biological tissues and fluids.

In many industrialized countries, thiamin-fortified foods contribute as much as 25% of the total thiamin intake. In the U.S. 1995 Continuing Survey of Food Intakes by Individuals, the major food sources of thiamin for adults were bread and bread products, mixed foods with grains as the main ingredient, and ready-to-eat cereals. Other less-important sources were pork and ham products (IOM, 2000). In the U.K. and Australian national surveys, cereals and cereal products were also the most important source of thiamin in adults, followed in the United Kingdom by vegetables, especially potatoes (Gregory et al., 1990), and in Australia, by meat and meat products (McLennan and Podger, 1995).

Effects of high intakes of thiamin

No adverse effects of excessive intakes of thiamin have been described, except some occasional anaphylactoid responses (Stephen et al., 1992). The relatively few studies conducted on the adverse effects of taking large doses of thiamin did not allow a Tolerable Upper Intake Level (UL) for thiamin to be set by the U.S. Food and Nutrition Board (IOM, 2000).

Indices of thiamin status

Currently, there are no reliable physiological functional indices of thiamin status. The most widely used biochemical index of thiamin status is the activity of the transketolase

enzyme in erythrocytes; it reflects the adequacy of body stores and is very sensitive to marginal thiamin deficiency. Measurements of total thiamin in urine, whole blood, and erythrocytes, described below, are also used but do not adequately assess the status of body stores. In the future, measurement of thiamin pyrophosphate in erythrocytes or whole blood may become the biomarker of choice.

20.1.1 Erythrocyte transketolase

Transketolase (EC 2.2.1.1) is a TPP-dependent enzyme. Measurement of the activity of this enzyme in the erythrocytes is most frequently used as an index of thiamin nutritional status, as the erythrocytes are among the first tissues to be affected by thiamin depletion. In outline, this test and similar procedures used for riboflavin and pyridoxine, involves the following stages:

1. The basal activity of the enzyme (transketolase) in erythrocytes is measured. This represents the endogenous enzyme activity and depends on the amount of the coenzyme (TPP) in the erythrocytes.
2. The enzyme activity with excess coenzyme added in vitro is then determined. This equates to the maximum potential enzyme activity and is referred to as total or "stimulated" activity.
3. (1) and (2) are then compared to indicate the degree of unsaturation of the enzyme with the coenzyme.

The results are best expressed in terms of the activity coefficient (AC):

$$AC = \frac{\text{enzyme activity (with excess coenzyme)}}{\text{basal enzyme activity (without coenzyme)}}$$

When the vitamin status is adequate, the added coenzyme has little effect on the total enzyme activity, so the activity coefficient is very close to 1.0. However, in vitamin-deficiency states, the added coenzyme increases the enzyme activity. Larger increases are associated with greater degrees of deficiency and higher values for the activity coefficient. Sometimes the "percentage of stimulation" (PS) is calculated from the activity coefficient as follows:

$$PS = (\text{activity coefficient} \times 100) - 100$$

The basal and stimulated enzyme activities can be expressed per gram of hemoglobin, per number of erythrocytes, or in terms of the volume of erythrocytes (in mL).

The ratio of stimulated to basal enzyme activity is used as the primary measure because (*a*) the between-subject variation in basal erythrocyte enzyme activity is large, and (*b*) it is assumed that apoenzyme levels are not affected by vitamin deficiencies. This latter assumption may not be correct, however. Vitamin deficiency or excess, and other factors such as the presence of certain diseases and the administration of hormones and drugs, may affect apoenzyme levels and confound the interpretation. Hence, when interpreting the results, it is advisable to take into account the basal enzyme activity, as well as its activation with coenzyme (Bamji, 1981).

Transketolase, a TPP-requiring enzyme, catalyzes the following two reactions in the pentose phosphate pathway:

xylulose-5-phosphate + ribose-5-phosphate $\rightleftharpoons$

sedoheptulose-7-phosphate

+ glyceraldehyde-3-phosphate

xylulose-5-phosphate + erythrose-4-phosphate $\rightleftharpoons$

fructose-6-phosphate

+ glyceraldehyde-3-phosphate

In thiamin deficiency, the basal level of erythrocyte transketolase activity is low, and an enhancement in the enzyme activity after the addition of TPP in vitro is generally observed. This is known as the "TPP effect." Prolonged thiamin deficiency, however, induces a reduction in the apotransketolase enzyme level. Consequently, both the basal and stimulated erythrocyte transketolase activities tend to fall, with no change in TPP effect, giving rise to misleading "normal" erythrocyte transketolase AC values (Schrijver, 1991). In such cases, the basal enzyme activity should also be considered (Nixon et al., 1990).

Factors affecting erythrocyte transketolase activity

A variety of factors affect erythrocyte transketolase activity: some are independent of changes in thiamin status, while others may be linked to such changes.

Age of the erythrocytes influences enzyme activity; levels decline as the cells age. As a result, the basal enzyme activity depends on the mean age of the erythrocytes (Powers and Thurnham, 1981). Hence, in patients undergoing treatment for iron deficiency, for example, the basal level of erythrocyte transketolase activity will be increased as a result of the reticulocytosis. A similar effect is observed in patients who respond positively to treatment for pernicious anemia (Kjøsen and Seim, 1977).

Age affects transketolase activity. Older subjects tend to have lower activities, possibly as a result of a defect in the apoenzyme rather than inadequate activity of the coenzyme TPP (O'Rourke et al., 1990).

Certain disease states are associated with low erythrocyte transketolase activity. In some cases (e.g., diabetes and liver disease), the reduced activity results from a reduced apoenzyme level associated with the disease. In others (e.g., certain cancers), the TPP effect is enhanced despite adequate thiamin intakes because the conversion of thiamin to thiamin pyrophosphate is impaired (Basu and Dickerson, 1976; Nichols and Basu, 1994). Patients with polyneuritis, uremic neuropathy, and disorders of the gastrointestinal tract also have low transketolase activity (Kjøsen and Seim, 1977), although the cause is uncertain. Erythrocyte transketolase activity is also lower in obese compared to nonobese subjects (Lemoine et al., 1986).

Certain drugs such as 5-fluorouracil and cytotoxins used in the treatment of cancer, furosemide (a diuretic used in the treatment of congestive heart failure), and antacids may all influence the activity of erythrocyte trans-ketolase (Thurnham, 1981). Their precise mechanism is unclear.

Within-subject variation in erythrocyte transketolase activity can be large, even in subjects with fixed thiamin intakes (van Dok-kum et al., 1990) (Table 20.1). Such large variations occur because individuals differ in their sensitivity to thiamin deficiency. This leads to difficulties in interpreting transke-tolase activity coefficients between values indicative of adequacy (i.e., 1.0) and those indicative of thiamin deficiency (i.e., >1.25). Hence, correlation of transketolase activity coefficients and intakes within this range may be poor (Vir and Love, 1979).

When one considers these uncertainties, it is perhaps not surprising that erythrocyte trans-ketolase activity coefficients may not corre-late significantly with thiamin intakes. In general, such relationships have only been re-ported in surveys of population groups known to be vulnerable to thiamin deficiency, such as the elderly (Bailey et al., 1994; Finch et al., 1998). Significant correlations are much less

obvious in groups such as adolescents (Gans and Harper, 1991; Bailey et al., 1994), who are more likely to have an adequate thiamin status.

Likewise, abnormal erythrocyte transke-tolase activity may not be associated with clinical signs of thiamin neuropathy. For ex-ample, in a study of displaced Karen women in refugee camps on the northern Thai border, symptoms such as paresthesia were not assoc-iated with abnormal erythrocyte transketolase activity at 30 wk gestation or at delivery (Mc-Gready et al., 2001). Similar inconsisten-cies were reported among school children and adults during a neuropathy epidemic in Cuba, although in both the displaced women and the school children, initial thiamin status correlated with clinical outcome after treat-ment (Macias-Matos et al., 1996).

There is evidence that marginal thiamin deficiency may be associated with a vari-ety of clinical features including anorexia, weight loss, fatigue, sleep disorders, and de-pression. Smidt et al. (1991) studied the ef-fect of thiamin supplementation on both the health and general well-being of an elderly Irish population with marginal thiamin defi-ciency. They noted that after supplementation with thiamin for 6 wk, there were significant improvements in appetite, fatigue, and gen-eral well-being (how they felt) (Table 20.2), but not in sleep, tenseness, or concentration, (data not shown) in the supplemented com-pared with the placebo group. Further, the change in the TPP effect in the supplemented group was significantly correlated with chan-ges in general well-being ($r = -0.71$) and fatigue ($r = 0.78$), together with changes in energy intake ($r = -0.91$), appetite (via a subjective assessment) ($r = -0.93$), and body weight ($r = -0.89$). No differences in any of the clinical assessment parameters between or within the two groups at baseline and after treatment were observed. The criteria used in this study to denote marginal (TPP 14%–35%) and deficient (TPP > 35%) sta-tus differed from those recommended by the IOM (2000), suggesting that age-dependent cutoffs may be necessary, but this requires more investigation.

Indicator	Analytical variability: reference sample (CV %)	Within-subject variability range from 4 subjects (CV %)
Blood thiamin	4.8	8.1–11.4
Basal erythrocyte transketolase activity	7.8	4.3–5.8
Stimulated erythrocyte transketolase activity	5.3	3.1–4.9

Table 20.1: Variability of some indices of thiamin. The figures for the analytical variability are from analysis of a reference sample. The figures for the within-subject variability are from 20 samples from each subject over a 60-d period on a constant diet. Data from van Dokkum et al., European Journal of Clini-cal Nutrition 44: 665–674, 1990 © with permission of the Nature Publishing Group.

	Placebo group (n = 40)	Supplemented group (n = 40)
Appetite		
Baseline	5.9 ± 0.31	6.0 ± 0.36
Treatment	6.1 ± 0.52	9.5 ± 0.32*
Concentration		
Baseline	9.4 ± 0.72	9.1 ± 1.1
Treatment	9.4 ± 0.72	9.1 ± 1.1
Desired activities		
Baseline	8.4 ± 0.92	9.0 ± 1.0
Treatment	8.4 ± 0.92	9.0 ± 1.0
Fatigue		
Baseline	5.0 ± 0.91	5.4 ± 0.50
Treatment	4.9 ± 0.86	1.2 ± 0.54[a]
General well-being		
Baseline	4.8 ± 6.1	5.2 ± 0.74
Treatment	4.8 ± 6.1	8.8 ± 1.1[a]
Sleep		
Baseline	5.4 ± 1.1	4.9 ± 1.2
Treatment	5.4 ± 1.1	4.9 ± 1.2

Table 20.2: The effect of thiamin supplementation on some subjective assessments of health and well-being. The numbers listed are the mean score ± SD. Subjects rated each parameter on a scale from 0 (never have the condition or problem) to 10 (have the condition or problem all the time). [a] indicates significantly different from placebo ($p < 0.05$) at that time and for that specific parameter. Data from Smidt et al., Journal of Gerontology 46: M16–M22, 1991, Copyright © The Gerontological Society of America. Reproduced by permission of the publisher.

Interpretive criteria

Criteria for interpreting transketolase activity vary. Poor between-assay precision and the difficulty of standardizing the method may contribute, in part, to some of this lack of agreement in interpretive criteria; those recommended by the U.S. Food and Nutrition Board (IOM, 2000) are shown in Table 20.3. These same criteria for erythrocyte transketolase activity were used by Bates et al. (1999) in a U.K. study of people ≥ 65 y, and by McGready et al. (2001) to define marginal and severe thiamin deficiency in Karen mothers. Lower cutoffs were used by Hercberg et al. (1994) for a healthy French population.

The U.K. national surveys present data for

Indicator	Deficiency
Erythrocyte transketolase activity coefficient	> 1.25
Thiamin pyrophosphate effect (TPP) (%)	> 25
Erythrocyte thiamin (nmol/L)	< 70

Table 20.3: Interpretive criteria for some primary measures of thiamin status. Data from the U.S. Food and Nutrition Board (IOM, 2000), who also define marginal deficiency states.

erythrocyte transketolase activity coefficients for young people aged 4–18 y (Gregory et al., 2000) and for persons aged ≥ 65 y (Finch et al., 1998). Mean, median, and critical percentiles by age and sex are presented.

Measurement of erythrocyte transketolase activity

The measurement of erythrocyte transketolase activity is rather difficult. The packed erythrocytes must first be washed and care taken to remove the buffy coat, as leukocytes in the buffy coat are a rich source of thiamin pyrophosphate. Several different assay methods have been developed (e.g., Basu et al., 1974; Bayoumi and Rosalki, 1976), some including quality control and features that increase sensitivity and precision (Buttery et al., 1982). Spectrophotometric procedures measure either the synthesis of a product (sedoheptulose-7-phosphate) per unit time or the amount of the substrate (ribose-5-phosphate) used in the reaction, before and after the addition of TPP. Preferred methods are semi-automated, use glyceraldehyde-3-phosphate as an internal standard, and eliminate the interference by hemoglobin by incorporating dialyzers in the system (Waring et al., 1982).

Erythrocyte hemolysates rather than intact erythrocytes are used for the assay because they can be stored in the frozen state at −72°C for over a year without loss of transketolase activity. Storage at −20°C may lead to reduced activity (Puxty et al., 1985). To assess the reproducibility of the erythrocyte transketolase assay, pools of washed erythrocytes can be prepared and stored frozen in small aliquots at $-72°C$.

More work is required to standardize the assay of erythrocyte transketolase activity in order to facilitate the interpretation of the results among studies. In general, the test appears to be most useful as an indicator of thiamin status in population groups at risk of deficiency, but the large between-subject and analytical variability may limit its usefulness in populations with adequate thiamin status.

The activity of transketolase in leukocytes appears to be a sensitive and specific index of thiamin status in the rat, responding to dietary intakes of thiamin (Cheng et al., 1976). However, little subsequent work has been completed on transketolase activity in human leukocytes.

20.1.2 Urinary thiamin excretion

In thiamin-replete subjects, when the main tissue compartment is saturated and the urinary excretion threshold is exceeded, thiamin levels in the urine do not generally reflect body stores; instead, they parallel recent dietary intakes. In contrast, when the tissues are unsaturated, excretion is limited as the body conserves thiamin.

Oldham (1962) noted positive correlations between the intake of thiamin and the excretion in 24-h urine specimens in young adults receiving controlled diets. These ranged from 0.6 to 2.0 mg/d thiamin. At lower intakes, however, urinary excretion of thiamin is no longer linearly related to intake. Further, most of the thiamin excretion is in the form of metabolites.

The within-subject variability for urinary thiamin excretion based on a single 24-h urine sample is high, with coefficients of variation ranging from 11% to 13%, even for subjects on a constant diet for 60 d (van Dokkum et al., 1990). Furthermore, urinary thiamin excretion is increased by the use of certain drugs, particularly diuretics (Suter and Vetter, 2000). Hence, at the individual level, use of a single 24-h urine sample is limited. Instead, for evaluating the thiamin

status of an individual, more than one 24-h urine sample per subject should be collected (Van Dokkum et al., 1990).

Collection of 24-h urine samples in population studies is difficult. As a result, in several earlier studies — ICCND, Nutrition Canada, and the first U.S. Nutrition Examination Survey (NHANES I) — casual urine samples were collected. Thiamin excretion, expressed in terms of thiamin per gram of creatinine, was then related to intake (Figure 20.2). However, at the individual level, the interpretation of urinary thiamin excretion is difficult when based on a single casual urine sample. In particular, children have higher levels than adults of thiamin excretion, when it is expressed on a creatinine basis, so age-specific interpretive criteria are necessary. In addition, the within-subject variability for urinary excretion of thiamin, even when expressed on the basis of creatinine, remains high (van Dokkum et al., 1990).

Severe tissue depletion of thiamin can be detected by a thiamin load test. In this test, excretion of thiamin over a 4-h or 24-h period is measured after oral or intramuscular administration of a loading dose of 1–5 mg of thiamin. If subjects are deficient in thiamin, usually less than 20 µg of the 5-mg thiamin load during the 4-h period is excreted (Table 20.4). This test serves as a

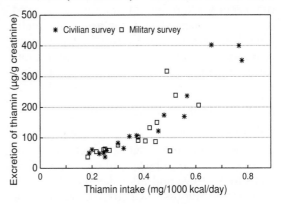

Figure 20.2: Relationship between thiamin intake and thiamin urinary excretion in adults as observed in nutrition surveys conducted in 18 countries by the Interdepartmental Committee on Nutrition for National Defense (ICNND). From FAO/WHO (1967), with permission.

Subjects	Less than acceptable (at risk)		Acceptable (low risk)
	Deficient (high risk)	Low (med. risk)	
Children	(μg/g creatinine)		
1–3 y	< 120	120–175	≥176
4–6 y	< 85	85–120	≥121
7–9 y	< 70	70–180	≥181
10–12 y	< 60	60–180	≥181
13–15 y	< 50	50–150	≥151
Adults	< 27	27–65	≥66
Preg. 2nd tri.	< 23	23–54	≥55
Preg. 3rd tri.	< 21	21–49	≥50
Adults	Other interpretive guidelines		
μg/24 h	< 40	40–99	≥100
μg/6 h	< 10	10–24	≥25
μg in 4 hr after thiamin load	< 20	20–79	≥80

Table 20.4: Interpretive guidelines for the urinary excretion of thiamin. From Sauberlich (1999).

useful index of low intakes and tissue deficits of the vitamin but does not indicate the severity of a thiamin deficiency.

Interpretive criteria

Table 20.4 presents guidelines for interpreting urinary excretion of thiamin expressed over a 24-h period and per gram of creatinine. Guidelines are also given on the amount of thiamin excreted over varying time frames following a loading dose of 5 mg of thiamin.

Measurement of urinary thiamin

The classical method for measuring thiamin in urine is the fluorometric thiochrome procedure. In the direct method, thiamin is measured before and after destruction of the thiochrome fluorescence, by the addition of benzylsulfonyl chloride (Leveille, 1972). The interfering compounds in the urine can be removed by using a cation-exchange resin, before the conversion of the eluted thiamin to the fluorescent thiochrome derivative. The

latter is then measured with a spectrofluorometer (ICNND, 1963).

Urinary thiamin can also be measured with a microbiological assay using *Lactobacillus viridescens*, *L. fermenti*, or *Ochromonas danica*; some of these assays have now been automated (Icke and Nicol, 1994). High-performance liquid chromatography (HPLC) techniques have had limited use (Roser et al., 1978). Urine samples for thiamin analyses are stable for at least 2 y when frozen at −20°C.

20.1.3 Total thiamin in whole blood and erythrocytes

Levels of total thiamin in whole blood and erythrocytes have been investigated as potential indices of thiamin status. Early studies suggested that whole blood thiamin concentrations were insensitive indices of thiamin status; only modest declines were observed, even in cases of clinical deficiency (Kawai et al., 1980). However, with improved HPLC assay methods that have increased sensitivity and reduced variability, reliable measurements of total thiamin concentrations in erythrocytes are now possible.

Some investigators have noted significant correlations of erythrocyte thiamin concentrations with erythrocyte transketolase activity coefficients (Warnock et al., 1978; Baines and Davis, 1988; Fidanza et al., 1989), but these findings have not been consistent (Bailey et al., 1994; Herve et al., 1995). Such discrepancies may arise from either analytical or biological variability. Certainly, large variability in erythrocyte thiamin values exists among individuals, even when they are consuming similar thiamin intakes, as noted earlier for erythrocyte transketolase activity (van Dokkum et al., 1990). Such differences may result from marked variations in the use of medications, physical activity, and — most important — alcohol consumption, smoking (Finglas, 1993; Bailey et al., 1997), and body weight (Patrini et al., 2004). In a study of U.K. free-living elderly women, for example, the correlation of thiamin intake with erythrocyte thiamin only became significant

	Persistently low thiamin			Isolated low thiamin		
	Supplemented ($n = 18$)	Placebo ($n = 17$)	Sig. p	Supplemented ($n = 20$)	Placebo ($n = 21$)	Sig. p
Nottingham Health Profile, total score	−17.0 (−40.6, 6.5)	7.6 (−17.3, 32.5)	0.13	−8.6 (−42.0, 24.8)	−14.8 (−33.8, 4.1)	0.74
Nottingham Health Profile, energy subscale	−5.7 (−17.2, 5.9)	7.4 (−2.1, 16.9)	0.07	7.9 (−3.0, 18.8)	6.9 (−1.7, 15.5)	0.9
Nottingham Health Profile, sleep subscale	−9.5 (−15.9, 3.2)	−0.7 (−9.1, 7.7)	0.07	−8.1 (−18.3, 2.0)	−4.4 (−15.0, 6.3)	0.6
Quality of life by visual analogue scale (mm)	−9 (−18, 0)	4 (−2, 10)	0.02	3 (−4, 10)	0 (−6, 6)	0.5
Systolic blood pressure (mm Hg)	−6.9 (−19.5, 5.7)	7.6 (−0.9, 16.2)	0.05	−3.4 (−14.6, 7.3)	7.0 (−4.5, 18.5)	0.16
Weight (kg)	−1.2 (2.4, 0.0)	0.6 (−0.1, 1.4)	< 0.01	−0.9 (−1.9, 0.0)	0.1 (−0.7, 1.0)	0.08

Table 20.5: Effect of thiamin supplementation on elderly people with isolated or persistently low erythrocyte thiamin pyrophosphate concentrations. Results are the mean change, with the 95% CI in parentheses. Negative changes in the Nottingham Health Profile scales indicate improvement. Data from Wilkinson et al., American Journal of Clinical Nutrition, 66, 925–928, 1997 © Am J Clin Nutr. American Society for Clinical Nutrition.

when smoking was taken into account (Bailey et al., 1997).

Thiamin pyrophosphate (TPP) concentrations can also be measured in erythrocytes or whole blood using HPLC with UV detection (Talwar et al., 2000). Thiamin pyrophosphate is the major form of thiamin coenzyme in erythrocytes. Concentrations fall at about the same rate as in other tissues when thiamin status declines (McCormick and Greene, 1994).

In a study of New Zealand elderly, erythrocyte TPP values were successfully used to screen individuals with subclinical thiamin deficiency for entry into a supplementation trial. In this study, only subjects who had persistently low erythrocyte TPP concentrations (i.e., < 140 nmol/L), benefited from supplemental thiamin, with improved quality of life and lower blood pressure and weight. Those with only one isolated low erythrocyte thiamin pyrophosphate value prior to randomization did not benefit from treatment (Table 20.5) (Wilkinson et al., 1997).

Interpretive criteria

At present, only limited data are available to clearly establish cutoff values for concentrations of total thiamin or thiamin pyrophosphate in erythrocytes. As a result, some discrepancies exist among published studies over the cutoff values used.

Bailey et al. (1994, 1997) used a value near the bottom of the normal range for adults (< 148 nmol/L) as a cutoff to denote "low" erythrocyte thiamin concentrations in a study of U.K. adolescents and free-living elderly. In marked contrast, Schrijver (1991) used 70–90 nmol/L as indicating marginal deficiency, and < 70 nmol/L as indicative of deficiency.

For TPP in erythrocytes, a cutoff value of < 140 nmol/L has been used to indicate risk of suboptimal thiamin status. This value is actually a reference limit as it is based on the 2.5 percentile of a healthy blood donor population (Wilkinson et al., 1997). Others have used a cutoff of < 120 nmol/L for erythrocyte

TPP as indicative of high risk for deficiency, and 120–150 nmol/L as marginally deficient (Bailey and Finglas, 1990). More research is required to establish cutoff values for both erythrocyte thiamin and erythrocyte thiamin pyrophosphate.

Erythrocyte thiamin and TPP measurement

To measure total thiamin, a microbiological assay using *L. fermenti* and employing microtiter plates can be used (Icke and Nicol, 1993, 1994). Use of a microtiter plate reduces the volume required and is fast, precise, sensitive, and relatively easy. As an alternative, total thiamin in erythrocytes can be determined via HPLC with UV detection (Bailey and Finglas, 1990). Values for total thiamin derived from microbiological methods, however, are higher than those determined using HPLC. The latter measures only the oxidized form of thiamin — thiochrome — whereas the microbiological methods measure all biologically active thiamin metabolites (Bui, 1999).

A reversed-phase HPLC method with post-column derivatization with alkaline ferricyanide and fluorescence detection can be used for the measurement of TPP in erythrocytes (Talwar et al., 2000). The method is simple, robust, and precise with a between-run coefficient of variation (CV) of < 8%. Quality-control samples can be prepared from pools of washed erythrocytes for the assay of both total thiamin and TPP, and stored frozen at −70°C in small aliquots.

Concentrations of erythrocyte TPP are said to be more stable in frozen erythrocytes and less susceptible to factors that influence enzyme activity, and the assay is more readily standardized than that of erythrocyte transketolase activity (Section 20.1.2) (Baines and Davies, 1988).

Some investigators have suggested measuring TPP in whole blood rather than washed erythrocytes because it is more convenient (Talwar et al., 2000). Thiamin pyrophosphate is stable in whole blood for 48 h at room temperature; when it is stored at −70°C, it is stable for at least 7 mo. It can also be measured by the same HPLC method as that used for TPP in erythrocytes. Moreover, a strong correlation between the measurement of thiamin pyrophosphate in erythrocytes and whole blood ($r = 0.97$) has been reported (Talwar et al., 2000).

20.2 Riboflavin

Riboflavin (7,8-dimethyl-10-ribityl-isoalloxazine) was first synthesized in 1935. Its structure consists of an isoalloxazine ring attached to a ribityl side chain (Figure 20.3). A detailed review of riboflavin and health is given in Powers (2003).

Functions of riboflavin

Riboflavin is a component of two important coenzymes, flavin mononucleotide (FMN) and flavin adenine dinucleotide (FAD), both of which are essential for a number of oxidative enzyme systems involved in electron transport (Figure 20.3). Of the two coenzymes, FMN is formed first, from free riboflavin, by ATP-dependent phosphorylation; a reaction catalyzed by cytosolic flavokinase (EC 2.7.1.26). Next, most of this FMN is combined with a molecule of ATP to form FAD; this step is catalyzed by the FAD-dependent FAD synthetase (EC 2.7.7.2). In turn, FAD can be converted into forms covalently bound to tissue proteins.

Both FMN and FAD are also cofactors for several enzymes, including glutathione reductase, L-gulonolactone oxidase, xanthine oxidase, L-amino oxidase, and nicotinamide adenine dinucleotide (NAD) dehydrogenase. Results from animal studies also suggest that flavins are cofactors in the cyclical β-oxidation of fatty acids (Olpin and Bates, 1982).

Riboflavin coenzymes are also involved in the metabolism of four other vitamins — vitamin B_{12}, folic acid, pyridoxine, and niacin. Flavin adenine dinucleotide is a cofactor for 5,10-methylenetetrahydrofolate reductase (EC 1.7.99.5), an enzyme involved in the conversion of methylene tetrahydrofolate to methyl tetrahydrofolate, which is required for

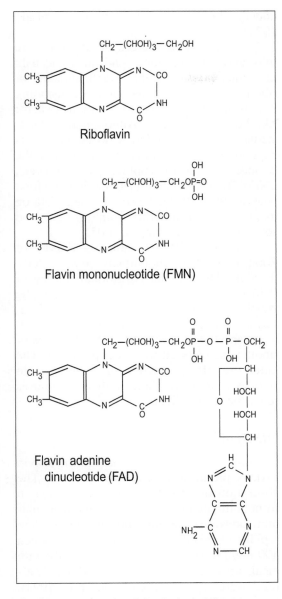

Figure 20.3: Structure of riboflavin and the two coenzymes derived from flavin, FMN and FAD.

the remethylation of homocysteine to methionine (Section 22.1.5). Vitamin B_6 requires FMN for conversion to the coenzyme pyridoxal-5'-phosphate, whereas the conversion of tryptophan to niacin involves FAD-dependent kynurenine hydroxylase. As a result, severe riboflavin deficiency can cause disturbances in the metabolic pathways of many enzyme systems in addition to those directly requiring flavin coenzymes.

Absorption of riboflavin occurs mainly in the proximal small intestine by an active or facilitated transport system, although a small amount may also be absorbed in the large intestine (Powers, 2003). The vitamin is transported in plasma as free riboflavin complexed with albumin and other proteins, mainly immunoglobulins, which also bind flavin coenzymes (Innis et al., 1985).

Deficiency of riboflavin in humans

The classical signs of riboflavin deficiency, termed ariboflavinosis, are angular stomatitis, cheilosis, and glossitis. Corneal vascularization, dermatological changes, and neurological alterations may also occur but are not specific for ariboflavinosis (Thurnham, 1981). Some environmental factors may also influence the clinical signs and symptoms of riboflavin deficiency.

Some evidence suggests that riboflavin deficiency is linked with impaired handling of iron, possibly by an effect on absorption or mobilization of iron stores (Powers, 2003).

Ariboflavinosis is rarely encountered in isolation, usually occurring in association with other vitamin deficiency states. In a study of Irish elderly, 49% had suboptimal riboflavin status, 39% had suboptimal vitamin B_6 status, and 21% had concurrent riboflavin and vitamin B_6 deficiencies. After supplementation with riboflavin alone, both the riboflavin deficiency and the low plasma pyridoxal-5'-phosphate levels were corrected (Madigan et al., 1998).

Riboflavin deficiency has been described in undernourished populations in several low-income countries, notably among women and children in The Gambia (Bates et al., 1981, 1994), some elderly persons in Guatemala (Boisvert et al., 1993), and in some adolescent refugees from Bhutan living in southeastern Nepal (Blanck et al., 2002). Infants of mothers with a low riboflavin status during gestation are also likely to be born riboflavin deficient (Bates et al., 1982). In industrialized countries, vulnerable population groups include the elderly (Leske et al., 1995; Bailey et al., 1997; Bates et al., 1999), and adolescents, especially girls of low socioeconomic status (Lopez et al., 1980; Nichoalds, 1981; Gregory et al., 2000).

Several conditions, including alcoholism, diabetes mellitus, liver disease, thyroid and adrenal insufficiency, and gastrointestinal and biliary obstruction, may precipitate or exacerbate riboflavin deficiency (Nichoalds, 1981). Alcohol causes deficiency by interfering with both the digestion and the intestinal absorption of riboflavin (Pinto et al., 1978). Psychotropic drugs such as chlorpromazine, imipramine, and amitriptyline, as well as some antimalarial drugs such as quinacrine, all inhibit the conversion of riboflavin to its active coenzyme derivatives. Drugs, such as tetracycline, theophylline, and caffeine, as well as metals, such as zinc, copper, and iron, may chelate or form complexes with riboflavin and, hence, affect its bioavailability (Sauberlich, 1985).

Riboflavin deficiency has been implicated as a risk factor for cancer in some animal studies (Power, 2003), but the epidemiological evidence is less consistent (Foy et al., 1984; Siassi et al., 2000). Because of the role of riboflavin in homocysteine homeostasis, a link between riboflavin deficiency and increased risk of cardiovascular disease has also been proposed (Jacques et al., 2001; Rozen, 2002). Persons with the genetic predisposition to thermolabile methylenetetrahydrofolate reductase (EC 1.7.99.5) may be especially sensitive to riboflavin deficiency. This genetic polymorphism affects approximately 12% of the Caucasian population and is associated with increased plasma homocysteine concentrations (Kang et al., 1991; McNulty et al., 2002).

Food sources and dietary intakes

Most of the riboflavin in foods is present as FAD, with a smaller amount as FMN. Small amounts of flavins bound covalently to protein are also found in some foods but are largely unavailable as nutritional sources of riboflavin; only limited amounts apparently undergo digestion and absorption (Chia et al., 1978).

The major food sources of riboflavin are milk and dairy products, and meat and fish; most plants contain only small amounts of riboflavin. As a result, individuals consuming mainly plant-based diets may be at risk for riboflavin deficiency. Although it is heat-stable, losses of riboflavin do occur if it is exposed to the light and, as it is water soluble, by leaching into the cooking water (Powers, 2003). Bioavailability of riboflavin from food is about 95% (IOM, 2000), although data on its relative bioavailability from different food sources is limited (Powers, 2003).

In the U.S. 1995 Continuing Survey of Food Intakes by Individuals (IOM, 2000), the U.K. Dietary and Nutritional Survey of British Adults (Gregory et al., 1990), and the Australian national nutrition survey (McLennan and Podger, 1995), milk and milk products were the most important food source of riboflavin, followed by cereal products. The latter are often enriched or fortified with riboflavin in many industrialized countries (e.g., the United States).

Effects of high intakes of riboflavin

In humans, there is no evidence for riboflavin toxicity produced by excessive intakes. The absorption of orally administered riboflavin from both vitamin supplements and from natural foodstuffs is poor, and high intakes are rapidly excreted in the urine. Even when 400 mg/d of riboflavin was given orally with meals for at least 3 mo, no short-term side effects were reported (Schoenen et al., 1994). In view of the limited data on adverse effects from high intakes of riboflavin, no Tolerable Upper Intake Level for riboflavin was set by the U.S. Food and Nutrition Board (IOM, 2000).

Indices of riboflavin status

As the signs and symptoms of riboflavin deficiency are not very specific, diagnosis of a deficiency state is difficult when based exclusively on clinical assessment. Consequently, biochemical tests are essential for confirming clinical cases of riboflavin deficiency and for establishing subclinical deficiencies. Several tests are available, and these are discussed in the following sections. A combination of indices is generally preferred: erythrocyte glutathione reductase activity and urinary riboflavin excretion are most commonly used.

20.2.1 Erythrocyte glutathione reductase activity

The measurement of the activity coefficient of erythrocyte glutathione reductase (EGR) (EC 1.6.4.1), an erythrocyte enzyme that depends on a cofactor derived from riboflavin, is the preferred method for assessing riboflavin status. It provides a measure of tissue saturation and long-term riboflavin status.

Glutathione reductase is a nicotinamide adenine dinucleotide phosphate (NADPH), a FAD-dependent enzyme, and the major flavoprotein in erythrocytes. It catalyzes the oxidative cleavage of the disulfide bond of oxidized glutathione (GSSG) to form reduced glutathione (GSH):

$$GSSG + NADPH + H^+ \rightarrow 2\,GSH + NADP^+$$

The activity of erythrocyte glutathione reductase is measured spectrophotometrically by monitoring the oxidation of NADPH to $NADP^+$ at 340 nm, with and without the presence of added FAD coenzyme. As an alternative, the production of GSH can be monitored colorimetrically. The activity coefficient, or the percentage of stimulation, is then derived, as described for erythrocyte transketolase activity (Section 20.1.1):

$$EGR\ AC = \frac{\text{activity (with added FAD)}}{\text{basal activity (without added FAD)}}$$

The degree of in vitro stimulation of EGR activity depends on the FAD saturation of the apoenzyme, which, in turn, depends on the availability of riboflavin. In persons with riboflavin deficiency, erythrocyte glutathione reductase activity falls and the in vitro stimulation by FAD rises.

Animal and human depletion–repletion studies have confirmed that the EGR AC is a useful, stable, and sensitive measure of impaired riboflavin status, reflecting for most subjects, the degree of tissue saturation ranging from marginal to severe deficiency. It is not very satisfactory as an index of optimum riboflavin status, however. In experimentally controlled human studies, concomitant increases in EGR AC in response to decreases in intakes of riboflavin have been reported (Figure 20.4; Tillotson and Baker, 1972). Nevertheless, the increase in the EGR AC does not continue indefinitely; riboflavin intakes below 0.5 mg/1000 kcal do not produce any further increases in EGR AC (Sterner and Price, 1973).

Consequently, the extent to which the EGR AC is elevated does not necessarily indicate the degree of riboflavin deficiency. Hence, it is not surprising that consistent correlations between EGR AC values and clinical signs of riboflavin deficiency have not always been observed (Bates et al., 1981).

Measurement of EGR AC has been used to monitor riboflavin status in studies in both industrialized and disadvantaged countries. In the United Kingdom, for example, EGR AC

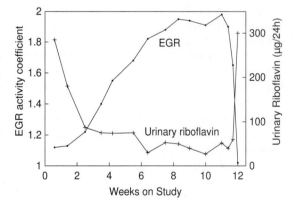

Figure 20.4: Relationship during depletion/repletion of riboflavin intake to urinary riboflavin excretion and erythrocyte glutathione reductase activity (EGR) coefficients. The depletion phase (wk 2–10) involved riboflavin intakes of 0.07 mg/d. From Tillotson and Baker, American Journal of Clinical Nutrition 25: 425–431, 1972 © Am J Clin Nutr. American Society for Clinical Nutrition.

has been assessed in community-based studies of adolescents (Bailey et al., 1994), and the elderly (Bailey et al., 1997). The assay was also used in the U.K. national surveys to assess the riboflavin status of children (Gregory et al., 1995), young people 4–18 y (Gregory et al., 2000), adults (Gregory et al., 1990), and people aged 65 y and over (Finch et al., 1998; Bates et al., 1999). The riboflavin status of the elderly in France and Ireland has also been investigated by measuring EGR AC (Hercburg et al., 1994; Madigan et al., 1998).

Comparison of the prevalence of suboptimal riboflavin status among these studies is often difficult because the cutoff values used to denote suboptimal status vary. In the studies of elderly in the United Kingdom by Bailey et al. (1997) and in Ireland by Madigan et al. (1998), however, the same cutoff value was used (i.e., EGR AC >1.2). Of the subjects, 78% in the United Kingdom and 49% in Ireland were reported to have suboptimal riboflavin status. Further, supplementation with physiological doses of riboflavin in a subsample of the Irish elderly reversed the biochemical abnormalities, confirming that riboflavin was indeed limiting (Madigan et al., 1998).

In some of these surveys, significant inverse relationships between the EGR AC and riboflavin intakes have been observed (Gregory et al., 1990; Hercburg et al., 1994; Bailey et al., 1997; Bates et al., 1999); results of the U.K. survey of British adults are given in Table 20.6. In the U.K. study of Norwich elderly (Bailey et al., 1997), initial EGR AC values for both males and females were significantly correlated with those measured 2 y later (Table 20.7), suggesting that EGR AC may be a reliable measure of long-term biochemical riboflavin status of individuals. This finding is consistent with earlier studies (Rutishauser et al., 1979).

The EGR AC has also been used in many low-income countries to confirm riboflavin deficiency, including some in Africa (Bates et al.,1981, 1994; Ajayi, 1984, 1985; Ajayi and James, 1984), Central America (Boisvert et al., 1993), and Asia (Thurnham et al.,1982;

Dietary intake	Erythrocyte glutathione reductase activity coefficient	
	Men	Women
Total riboflavin (incl. supplements)	–0.13 ($p < 0.01$)	–0.24 ($p < 0.01$)
Riboflavin from food sources	–0.23 ($p < 0.01$)	–0.31 ($p < 0.01$)

Table 20.6: Correlation coefficients between the erythrocyte glutathione reductase activity coefficient and dietary riboflavin intakes for U.K. adults. Data from Gregory et al. (1990).

Blanck et al., 2002). In a study of adolescent Bhutanese refugees living in Nepal, for example, in whom the prevalence of angular stomatitis was 27%, those with angular stomatitis had significantly higher EGR AC values than those without (i.e., 2.2 ± 0.4 vs. 2.0 ± 0.3; $p = 0.02$). The adjusted odds ratio for angular stomatitis and low riboflavin status was 5.1 (95% CI: 1.55, 16.5) (Blanck et al., 2002). Environmental factors may also influence the clinical manifestations of riboflavin deficiency.

There have been several attempts to establish a relationship in humans between a specific physiological function and EGR AC values, but the results have been inconclusive. Some reports of effects on work performance, neurovascular coordination, and iron handling with EGR AC values $\geqslant 1.7$ have been reported (Prasad et al., 1990; Fairweather-Tait et al., 1992; Bates et al., 1994) but need to be confirmed. In some supplementation

Elderly subjects	n	r	Significance
Males	37	0.411	< 0.02
Females	62	0.359	< 0.01

Table 20.7: The correlation of EGR activity coefficients measured on 99 subjects initially and after 2 y. Significant correlation does not imply agreement between initial and follow-up mean values. Data from Bailey et al., British Journal of Nutrition 77: 225–242, 1997.

studies of subjects with subclinical riboflavin deficiency, no improvement in physical performance or endurance has been reported (Prasad et al., 1990; Winters et al., 1992; van der Beek et al., 1994).

Factors affecting EGR AC values

FAD concentrations used in the assay to stimulate EGR can affect the EGR AC values obtained. Concentrations of FAD $> 5\,\mu mol$ result in lower normal ranges of EGR ACs, in comparison with FAD concentrations ranging from 1 to 3 μmol (Garry and Owen, 1976; Rutishauser et al., 1979).

Age of erythrocytes may also influence the EGR activity (Powers and Thurnham, 1981), concentrations declining as cells age, as noted for transketolase activity.

Age of the subjects may affect the EGR activity. In some (Garry et al., 1982; Wright et al., 1995), but not all (Hercberg et al., 1994) studies, a trend toward higher EGR ACs with increasing age, irrespective of sex, has been observed. If this trend is more firmly established, specific guidelines for EGR AC values for the elderly may be required.

Genetic disturbances, including glucose-6-phosphate dehydrogenase deficiency and heterozygous beta thalassemia, are associated with disturbances in erythrocyte flavin metabolism (Prentice et al., 1981; Anderson et al., 1987, 1993), which can result in misleading EGR AC test results. For example, in cases of glucose-6-phosphate dehydrogenase deficiency, there is increased avidity of the EGR for FAD, resulting in EGR AC values within the normal range, even in the presence of clinical signs of riboflavin deficiency (Thurnham, 1972). Glucose-6-phosphate dehydrogenase deficiency affects approximately 10% of Americans of African descent. In contrast, in heterozygous beta thalassemia, there is an inherited slow red-cell metabolism of riboflavin to FMN and FAD and a high stimulation of the erythrocyte glutathionine reductase by extraneous FAD (Anderson et al., 1993).

Pyridoxine deficiency also interferes with the EGR AC test, resulting in a decreased erythrocyte glutathione reductase activity but no change in the activity coefficient, probably arising from a decrease in apoenzyme. No comparable effects have been observed for other vitamin deficiencies such as thiamin and vitamin C.

Disease states, including iron-deficiency anemia (Ramachandran and Iyer, 1974), severe uremia, and cirrhosis of the liver, lead to increased erythrocyte glutathione reductase activity.

Conditions of negative nitrogen balance lead to a fall in EGR AC values. In pregnant women in The Gambia, for example, EGR AC values fell in association with a decline in body weight during the rainy season, despite evidence that malnutrition had actually increased (Bates et al., 1981). Similar findings have been reported in preschool children with upper respiratory tract infections and measles (Bamji et al., 1987).

Interpretive criteria

There is still uncertainty regarding the most appropriate threshold value indicative of normal riboflavin status. An EGR AC value of < 1.2 is generally considered to represent complete saturation of the tissues with riboflavin (Bates et al., 1997) (Table 20.8). Sadowski (1992), however, used an upper

	EGR activity coefficient			
	18–24 y	25–34 y	35–49 y	50–64 y
Men				
Median	1.09	1.09	1.09	1.07
95th percentile	1.20	1.20	1.19	1.19
Women				
Median	1.09	1.10	1.09	1.07
95th percentile	1.25	1.22	1.20	1.16

Table 20.8: Median and 95th percentile values for the activity coefficient (AC) of erythrocyte glutathione reductase (EGR) in U.K. adults by age and sex. Data from Gregory et al. (1990).

limit of 1.34 in a study of apparently healthy elderly. This value was based on the mean plus 2 SD of the EGR AC value derived from a large sample of Boston elderly aged 60 y and older. At such levels, the sensitivity of EGR AC is low.

Similarly, the cutoff points for abnormal EGR AC are poorly defined; they appear to be independent of sex. Cutoff values for marginal (medium risk, 1.2–1.4), or severe (high risk, >1.4) deficiency states are often used (McCormick and Greene, 1994). Generally, EGR AC values range from 1.5 to 2.5 in population groups consuming very low intakes of riboflavin, and who have evidence of clinical riboflavin deficiency (Bates et al., 1981; Thurnham et al., 1982; Low, 1985). In a study of adolescent Bhutanese refugees, Blanck et al. (2002) used an EGR AC cutoff of >1.7, and based on this value, 86% had low riboflavin status.

Information on the erythrocyte glutathione reductase activity coefficients from the U.K. surveys for young children (Gregory et al., 1995), young people aged 4–18 y (Gregory et al., 2000), and British adults and persons aged 65 y and over (Gregory et al., 1990; Finch et al., 1998) is available. Mean, median, and lower and upper 2.5 or 5.0 percentiles by age and sex are presented.

Measurement of erythrocyte glutathionine reductase activity

Only small samples of blood are required for the EGR assay, and fasting samples are not necessary (Komindr and Nicholalds, 1980). Either EDTA or heparin can be used as an anticoagulant. Erythrocytes must be washed and lysed, and the assay must be performed immediately after blood samples are drawn because FAD is a labile compound (McCormick and Greene, 1994). Alternatively, the hemolyzed samples can be kept frozen for over a year at −70°C without loss of EGR activity.

Generally, glutathione reductase activity is measured using an enzyme-coupled kinetic assay, although some colorimetric methods are also available (Sauberlich, 1984). An automated method involving the use of a centrifugal analyzer has been developed (Mak and Swaminathan, 1988; La Rue et al., 1997). An alternative procedure, using well plates and a plate reader, has also been described (Sauberlich, 1999). Very small volumes of whole blood instead of erythrocytes can be used for the measurement of glutathionine reductase activity, but the method, although simpler, is less sensitive. Care must be taken to ensure that the protocols for the assay are carefully specified and followed so that results can be compared among studies. As noted previously, the EGR assay is invalid for persons with glucose-6-phosphate dehydrogenase deficiency.

20.2.2 Urinary riboflavin excretion

Flavins are excreted in urine mainly in the form of riboflavin or other metabolites, such as 7-hydroxymethylriboflavin (7-α-hydroxyriboflavin) and lumiflavin (Chastain and McCormick, 1987). Very little riboflavin can be stored in the body, so urinary excretion reflects dietary intake until tissues become saturated.

Experimental balance studies indicate that urinary riboflavin excretionary rates increase slowly with increasing intakes, until intake levels approach 1.0 mg/d, when tissue saturation occurs. At higher intakes, the rate of excretion increases dramatically, as shown in Figure 20.5. Once intakes of 2.5 mg/d are reached, excretion becomes approximately equal to the rate of absorption (Horwitt et al., 1950). At such high intakes, a significant proportion of the riboflavin intake is not absorbed.

Urinary riboflavin was measured in several early population studies in North America: in the Nutrition Canada survey, the U.S. Ten State Nutrition Survey, and in NHANES I. In these surveys, casual urine samples — not 24-h urine samples — were collected, although the latter are preferred. As a result, riboflavin concentrations were expressed per gram of creatinine. For children, the rate of riboflavin excretion, when expressed per gram of creatinine is greater than for adults.

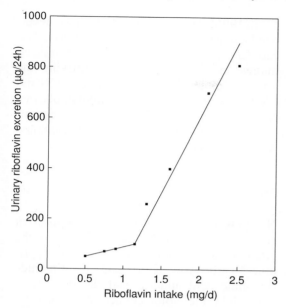

Figure 20.5: Relationship of riboflavin intake to urinary excretion. From Sauberlich (1999).

Occasionally, a riboflavin load test is used to assess the degree to which the body is saturated with riboflavin. An oral dose of 5 mg riboflavin is given, and again the timed excretion of riboflavin in the urine is measured, usually over a 4-h period (Lossy et al., 1951; ICNND, 1963); the results should be compared with the level in the urine before the test load.

Factors affecting riboflavin excretion

Physical activity and sleep can decrease riboflavin excretion (Soares et al., 1993).

Negative nitrogen balance and infection induce a breakdown of tissue protein and, hence, increase urinary excretion of riboflavin (Tucker et al., 1960). Consequently, measurement of urinary riboflavin is not very useful in circumstances where intakes of protein are low or where chronic infection is common.

Drugs including some antibiotics and psychotropic drugs such as phenothiazines can increase the excretion of riboflavin (Goldsmith, 1975).

Oral contraceptive agents and pregnancy influence riboflavin excretion. Concentrations decrease when oral contraceptive agents are used, and during the third trimester of pregnancy, as tissue retention of the vitamin is increased in response to increased need. However, during the second trimester, excretion increases.

Within-subject variability can be large for 24-h urinary riboflavin excretion. Coefficients of variation range from 13% to 25%, which are not reduced when results are expressed in terms of creatinine (van Dokkum et al., 1990).

Interpretive criteria

Interpretive criteria for urinary riboflavin excretion for adults and children are shown in Table 20.9. For adults, when dietary intakes are adequate, $\geqslant 120\,\mu g$ of riboflavin per day should be excreted. After a loading dose of 5 mg riboflavin, then $\geqslant 1400\,\mu g$ of riboflavin should be excreted in a 4-h period under conditions of adequate riboflavin intake. In a

Subjects	Less than acceptable (at risk)		Acceptable (low risk)
	Deficient (high risk)	Low (med. risk)	
Children	(μg/g creatinine)		
1–3 y	< 150	150–499	≥ 500
4–6 y	< 100	100–299	≥ 300
7–9 y	< 85	85–269	≥ 270
10–15 y	< 70	70–199	≥ 200
Adults	< 27	27–79	≥ 80
Preg. 1st tri.	< 27	27–65	66–129
Preg. 2nd tri.	< 23	23–54	55–109
Preg. 3rd tri.	< 21	21–49	50–99
Adults	Other interpretive guidelines		
μg/24 h	< 40	40–119	≥ 120
μg/6 h	< 10	10–29	≥ 30
μg in 4 h after ribofl. load	< 1000	1000–1399	≥ 1400

Table 20.9: Interpretive criteria for the urinary excretion of riboflavin. From Sauberlich HE (1999).

deficiency state, $< 1000\,\mu g$ of riboflavin will be excreted during the same time period. Interpretive criteria for riboflavin excretion in casual urine samples expressed as $\mu g/g$ creatinine for children, adults, and pregnant women are also given in Table 20.9.

Measurement of urinary riboflavin

In the past, fluorometric and microbiological assays have generally been used to determine riboflavin concentrations in urine. The fluorometric method measures the fluorescence of the flavins directly or converts the flavins to lumiflavin and then determines the fluorescence. The microbiological methods use *Ochromonas danica* or the protozoan *Tetrahymena pyriformis*.

Measurement of urinary riboflavin using HPLC with fluorometry (Gatautis and Naito, 1981) or competitive protein-binding assays (Tillotson and Bashor, 1980) is also possible. The protein-binding assays are rapid, sensitive, and require no treatment of the urine sample prior to analysis. Discrepancies among the analytical methods have been documented. Results for the HPLC method with fluorometry tend to be lower than those with the older fluorometric method alone because, in the HPLC method, riboflavin is separated from the other flavins (Smith, 1980).

20.2.3 Riboflavin and FAD in blood

No consensus exists on the value of riboflavin concentrations in blood or its components. Zempleni et al. (1996) suggest that riboflavin concentrations in serum and erythrocytes are changed only modestly by intake, and serum levels are probably too variable to serve as a useful index. Bates et al. (1999), however, reported a good relationship between EGR AC and erythrocyte riboflavin, provided the latter is expressed as a ratio to hemoglobin or to packed cell volume. Fluorometric and microbiological assays have been used to determine riboflavin in erythrocytes.

Concentrations of FAD in serum show low between-subject variation and only a modest response to changes in intake (Zempleni

et al., 1996). Hustad et al. (1999) have developed a sensitive and robust method, based on capillary electrophoresis and laser-induced fluorescence detection, for quantifying the low physiological concentrations of FMN and FAD, as well as riboflavin, in human plasma. Measurement of these in plasma, erythrocytes, and whole blood has potential and warrants further exploration.

20.3 Niacin

Niacin is the term used to describe a group of compounds with the biological activity of the vitamin. They include nicotinic acid (pyridine-3-carboxylic acid) and nicotinamide (nicotinic acid amide), and the derivatives that exhibit the biological activity of nicotinamide. The structure of nicotinic acid and nicotinamide is shown in Figure 20.6. Both

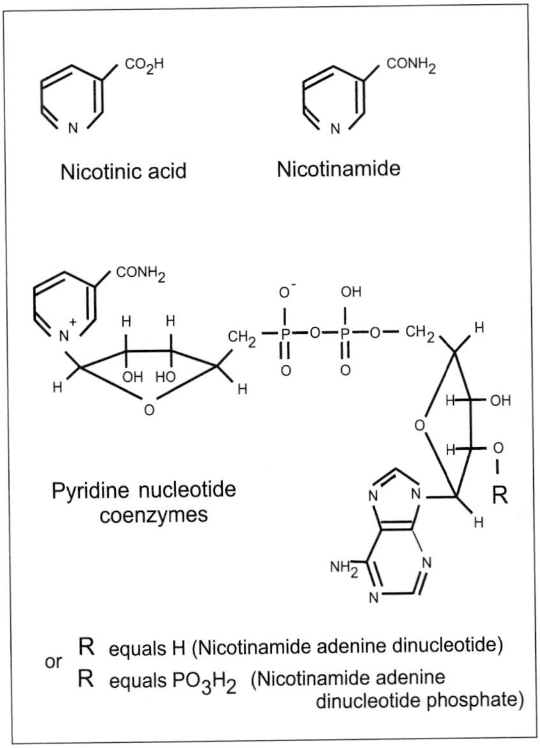

Figure 20.6: Structure of nicotinic acid and nicotinamide, as well as the two coenzyme forms containing the nicotinamide moiety.

compounds have similar but not identical properties. The body readily converts nicotinic acid to nicotinamide.

Functions of niacin

Both nicotinic acid and nicotinamide are substrates for the synthesis of the coenzymes, nicotinamide adenine dinucleotide (NAD), and its phosphorylated derivative, nicotinamide adenine dinucleotide phosphate (NADP) (Figure 20.6). These two coenzymes are synthesized in all tissues of the body, although concentrations are greatest in the liver, where some storage may occur. The nicotinamide moiety serves as an electron carrier or hydrogen donor in many biological redox reactions.

NAD functions as an electron carrier for intracellular respiration and as a codehydrogenase with enzymes involved in oxidation of glyceraldehyde 3-phosphate, lactate, alcohol, 3-hydroxybutyrate, pyruvate, and α-ketoglutarate. It is also required for important nonredox reactions. NAD is the substrate for three classes of enzymes that cleave the β-N-glycosylic bond of NAD to free nicotinamide and catalyze the transfer of ADP-ribose. More details are given in Jacob and Swendseid (1996).

NADP functions as a hydrogen donor in both fatty acid and steroid synthesis and, like NAD, also acts as a codehydrogenase in the oxidation of glucose 6-phosphate to ribose 5-phosphate in the pentose phosphate pathway (Swendseid and Jacob, 1994).

Absorption of nicotinamide or nicotinic acid takes place rapidly in the stomach and small intestine. At low intakes, absorption consists of a saturable transport component, which is dependent on sodium, energy, and pH, but at higher intakes, passive diffusion predominates (Jacob and Swendseid, 1996).

The amino acid tryptophan is converted in part to nicotinamide coenzymes, mainly in the liver. The conversion rate is controlled by the activities of tryptophan pyrrolase, the FAD-dependent kynurenine hydroxylase, and kynureninase (Section 20.3.1). Pyridoxal 5'-phosphate and iron are also involved in this conversion (McCormick, 1989).

Deficiency of niacin in humans

Pellagra is the characteristic syndrome of niacin deficiency. Early symptoms include lassitude, anorexia, weakness, depression, digestive disturbances, anxiety, and irritability. Later, photosensitive dermatitis and a depressive psychosis develop. No known metabolic lesion has been associated with the photosensitive dermatitis. The neurological symptoms have been associated with a relative deficit of tryptophan, which reduces synthesis of the monoamine neurotransmitter 5-hydroxytryptamine (Bender and Bender, 1986).

The absence of pellagra in most industrialized countries today results, in part, from fortifying certain foods (e.g., flour) with niacin. Some cases of pellagra still occur in association with chronic alcoholism, when the absorption of niacin is impaired. Pellagra can also develop as a result of prolonged use of isoniazid and 3-mercaptopurine, drugs used in the treatment of tuberculosis and leukemia, respectively. These drugs interfere with the conversion of tryptophan to niacin.

Pellagra continues to be a major problem in the parts of Southern Africa, Egypt, India, and China where maize and millet jowar (*Sorghum vulgare*) are dietary staples (Sauberlich, 1999). An outbreak of pellagra occurred among Mozambican refugees in 1990 in Malawi, a country where more than 50% of energy is provided by maize (Malfait et al., 1993).

Several etiological factors are linked with endemic pellagra. Poor bioavailability of bound forms of niacin in cereals, together with a relatively low tryptophan content are implicated (Bender and Bender, 1986). High concentrations of leucine in both maize and millet jowar may be an additional factor; excess leucine in the diet may inhibit the conversion of tryptophan to niacin, especially when niacin intake is low (Gopalan and Krishnaswamy, 1976; Bender, 1983). Some uncertainty exists about this interaction, however.

Additional factors possibly involved in the development of pellagra include lipid-soluble toxins, mycotoxins resulting from the fungal spoilage of maize and other grains, and other carcinogenic alkylating agents. Deficiencies of other micronutrients required in the tryptophan-to-niacin conversion pathway (e.g., pyridoxine, riboflavin, and iron) may also be implicated (Jacob and Swendseid, 1996).

Patients with the genetic disorder Hartnup disease develop pellagra because of a defect in the absorption of tryptophan and other monocarboxylic amino acids in the intestine and kidney (Halvorsen and Halvorsen, 1963). Secondary deficiency can also occur in patients with malignant carcinoid tumors, as a result of tryptophan being diverted to form 5-hydroxytryptamine.

Food sources and dietary intakes

Most of the niacin in food is present as a component of NAD or NADP; very little exists as free forms of niacin. Meat (especially liver), poultry, and fish are rich sources of niacin, followed by dairy products, oilseeds, cereals, and legumes. Niacin in mature cereal grains is largely bound to complex carbohydrates as niacytin; most of the niacytin is biologically unavailable, although a small fraction may be biologically available if it is hydrolyzed by gastric acid (Bender and Bender, 1986). Treatment of cereals with alkali (e.g., lime water), baking with alkaline baking powders, and roasting whole grain maize all result in the release of niacin from the bound form (Kodicek et al., 1974). Roasting green coffee also increases its nicotinic acid content, by removing the methyl group from trigonelline (1-methyl nicotinic acid). Tea, like coffee, also contains an appreciable amount of niacin. In some countries, such as the United States, wheat flour is enriched with niacin, so bread becomes an important dietary source of niacin (Swendseid and Jacob, 1994). Fortified ready-to-eat breakfast cereals are also an important dietary source (IOM, 2000).

In industrialized countries, meat and meat products often contribute as much as one-third of the total intake of niacin, closely followed by enriched and whole-grain breads and bread products, and fortified ready-to-eat cereals (Gregory et al., 1990; McLennan and Podger, 1995; IOM, 2000). Both vegetables and milk + milk products contribute about one-tenth of the total niacin intake in industrialized countries such as the United Kingdom (Gregory et al., 1990) and Australia (McLennan and Podger, 1995).

Because niacin can be derived from the amino acid L-tryptophan, normally obtained from dietary protein, intakes are usually expressed in terms of niacin equivalents (NE) (Section 4.4.5). About 60 mg of tryptophan yields 1 mg of niacin following digestion and absorption (Horwitt et al., 1981).

Effects of high intakes of niacin

Niacin toxicity may occur when large pharmacological doses of niacin, especially the nicotinic acid form, are taken. The central nervous and cardiovascular systems, blood lipids, and blood sugar levels may all be affected. The marked adverse effects of taking large doses of niacin led the U.S. Food and Nutrition Board (IOM, 2000) to set the Tolerable Upper Intake Level for persons $\geqslant 19$ y at 35 mg/d; details of the levels set for the other life-stage groups are given in IOM (2000).

Indices of niacin status

Functional biochemical tests that reflect body stores of niacin are not available at present. Likewise, no physiological functional tests responsive to changes in niacin intake have been identified. The measurement of cytogenetic damage and NAD-dependent ADP-ribosyltransferase in lymphocytes both have potential as indices (Hageman et al., 1998). Currently, the tests used reflect only recent dietary intakes of niacin and therefore may not identify all persons at risk to deficiency. The measurement of the urinary metabolite of niacin — N′-methylnicotinamide — in combination with one or more of the urinary pyridone turnover products is most useful. These tests and the measurement of niacin and its nucleotides in erythrocytes or whole blood are described below.

Metabolic period	Niacin intake (NE/d)	n	Day	Urinary metabolites		
				NMN (mg/d)	2-Pyr (mg/d)	2-Pyr/NMN*
Stabilization	19.6	7	11–13	2.90 ± 0.41	7.21 ± 1.86	2.07 ± 0.28
Depletion	6.1	3	47–49	0.8 ± 0.13	1.00 ± 0.05	1.21 ± 0.27
	10.1	4	47–49	0.81 ± 0.14	3.10 ± 0.71	4.02 ± 1.20
Repletion	19.2	6	62–64	1.82 ± 0.08	6.25 ± 0.04	3.12 ± 0.18
High intake	25	3	77–79	2.56 ± 0.04	11.40 ± 1.92	4.01 ± 0.68
	32	3	77–79	4.57 ± 0.38	19.36 ± 0.55	3.87 ± 0.36

Table 20.10: Variation in the concentration of urinary metabolites during a niacin depletion–repletion study on healthy young men. The concentrations are the mean $\pm$ SEM for the metabolites at the end of each metabolic period. NMN, N$'$-methylnicotinamide; 2-Pyr, 2-pyridone; *molar ratio. Data from Jacob et al., Journal of Nutrition 119: 591–598, 1989, with permission of the American Society for Nutritional Sciences.

20.3.1 Urinary excretion of niacin metabolites

The major end products of niacin metabolism in humans are N$'$-methylnicotinamide and N$'$-methyl-2-pyridone-5-carboxamide (2-pyridone); minor amounts of other urinary pyridone turnover products are also excreted. These products are derived from either preformed niacin or niacin obtained from dietary tryptophan (Figure 20.7).

Healthy adults generally excrete 20% to 30% of nicotinic acid as the N$'$-methylnicotinamide form and 40%–60% as 2-pyridone (de Lange and Joubert, 1964), although this pattern does vary with the amount and form of niacin ingested and the niacin status of the subject. Measurement of these two urinary metabolites is a reliable way of assessing very low niacin intakes. Of the two, however, N$'$-methylnicotinamide excretion is the easiest to measure, and is more sensitive to marginal intakes than urinary 2-pyridone (Jacob et al., 1989) (Table 20.10). These metabolites can be measured in a timed urine sample or expressed in terms of creatinine concentration in a casual sample.

Measurement of urinary N$'$-methylnicotinamide is not appropriate for pregnant subjects, in whom elevated excretion levels of N$'$-methylnicotinamide occur as a result of alterations in pyridoxine metabolism. In addition, it should not be used for diabetic

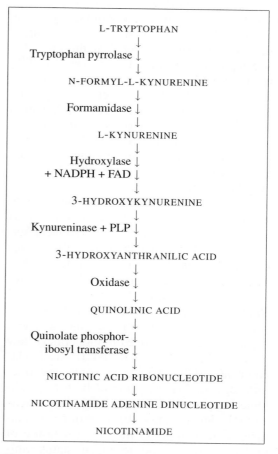

Figure 20.7: Metabolic pathway for conversion of trytophan to nicotinamide in the human. PLP, pyridoxal-5$'$-phosphate; FAD, flavine adenine diphosphate; NADPH, nicotinamide dinucleotide phosphate. Modified from Sauberlich (1999).

Metabolite	Control ($n = 9$)	No signs of pellagra ($n = 9$)	With pellagra ($n = 10$)
N′-methyl-6-pyridone-3-carboxamide (mmol/24h urine)	557 ± 199	152 ± 104	42 ± 9
N′-methylnicotinamide (mmol/24h urine)	273 ± 50	162 ± 17	213 ± 41
N′-methyl-6-pyridone-3-carboxamide / N′-methylnicotinamide (molecular ratio)	1.95	0.90	0.18

Table 20.11: Urinary excretion of niacin metabolites by Mozambican women. Data from Dillon et al., Annals of Nutrition and Metabolism 36: 181–185, 1992.

subjects, who excrete reduced amounts of urinary N′-methylnicotinamide.

Some studies have used a nicotinamide load test involving the intramuscular administration of a 50-mg test dose of nicotinamide, followed by measurement of N′-methylnicotinamide in urine collected at the end of a 4–5-h post-dose period. Gontzea et al. (1976) reported a 14% recovery of the test dose in well-nourished subjects over a 3-h period, compared with 8% for a rural population whose basal excretion of N′-methylnicotinamide was at the lower end of the normal range. Loading tests are impractical, however, for field surveys, where they have had very little use.

The ratio of 2-pyridone to N′-methylnicotinamide (Table 20.10) has been proposed as a convenient alternative index of niacin status, independent of age and creatinine excretion, and applicable to casual urine samples (De Lange and Joubert, 1964). More recently, however, use of this ratio has been challenged. In an experimental depletion–repletion study in adult males, the ratio was found to be insensitive to moderately low intakes of niacin (e.g., 6 and 10 NE/d) (Jacob et al., 1989). Moreover, some investigators suggest that excretion of both N′-methylnicotinamide and 2-pyridone in the urine is strongly dependent on the level of protein intake, so that the ratio may be a measure of protein adequacy and not niacin status (Shibata and Matuso, 1989a, 1989b). In view of these uncertainties, its use is not recommended in marginal niacin deficiency states.

Increasingly, with the development of new analytical methods, relationships between the other urinary pyridone turnover products including N′-methyl-4-pyridone-3-carboxamide (4-pyridone) and N′-methyl-6-pyridone-3-carboxamide (6-pyridone) and niacin intakes are being examined. During an outbreak of pellagra in Mozambican refugees, for example, French researchers measured 4-pyridone and 6-pyridone as well as N′-methylnicotinamide in 24-h urine collections (Dillon et al., 1992). They noted that the ratio of 6-pyridone to N′-methylnicotinamide in 24-h urine specimens correlated well with the development of clinical symptoms of pellagre, mainly dermatitis, as shown in Table 20.11 (Dillon et al., 1992).

Interpretive criteria

Interpretive criteria for adults for the urinary excretion of N′-methylnicotinamide, expressed as mg/g creatinine, are shown in Table 20.12. Jacob et al. (1989) report using a single cutoff value for the rate of excretion of either N′-methylnicotinamide or 2-pyridone, or both in a 24-h period; excretion levels of < 8.8 µmol/24-h (1.2 mg/24-h) are indicative

	Deficient	Low	Normal	High
mg/g creat.	< 0.5	0.5–1.59	1.6–4.29	≥ 4.3
mg/6 h g creat.	< 0.2	0.2–0.59	0.6–1.59	≥ 1.6

Table 20.12: Interpretive criteria for urinary N′-methylnicotinamide and N′-methyl-2-pyridone-3-carboxamide in adults. From Sauberlich HE (1999).

of niacin intakes below 6 NE/d. Such a low intake is likely to induce deficiency in adults.

Measurement of urinary excretion of N′-methylnicotinamide and 2-pyridone

Measurement of urinary N′-methylnicotin-amide is relatively simple, using fluorometric methods (Clark, 1980) or HPLC (Shaikh and Pontzer, 1979). Alternatively, microbiolog-ical methods can be used (Hankes, 1984). In contrast, until recently, measurement of 2-pyridone has been more difficult and time consuming. The most widely used method involves removing interfering compounds by column chromatography, followed by deter-mination of the absorption at 285–310 nm (Price, 1954).

With the development of improved HPLC techniques, several urinary pyridones, includ-ing 2-pyridone, 4-pyridone, and 6-pyridone together with N′-methylnicotinamide can be readily separated and measured, with im-proved accuracy and sensitivity (McKee et al., 1982; Terry and Simon, 1982).

20.3.2 Niacin and niacin coenzymes in plasma and erythrocytes

The concentrations of niacin compounds or derivatives in the plasma, erythrocytes, and leukocytes have also been studied as potential measures of niacin nutriture. Results have been inconsistent. Levels in plasma are low and reflect dietary intake rather than body stores: they do not appear to be very useful measures of niacin status. Methods for the analysis of niacin in both erythrocytes and leukocytes are presently unsatisfactory.

Erythrocyte or whole blood concentrations of NAD and NADP may be useful as mea-sures of niacin status. Experimental niacin depletion – repletion studies have shown that erythrocyte concentrations of NAD in young men are sensitive to short-term changes in niacin intake, even in the absence of clinical signs of deficiency.

Figure 20.8 shows a continuous decrease in erythrocyte NAD concentrations during a

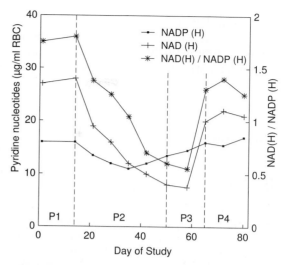

Figure 20.8: Mean concentration of erythrocyte nicoti-namide (NAD) and nicotinamde adenine dinucleotide phosphate (NADP), and the NAD/NADP ratio during four dietary periods: P1, stabilization; P2, depletion (6.1 or 10.1 NE/d); P3, repletion; and P4, high intake (25 or 32 NE/d). Data from Fu et al., Journal of Nu-trition 119: 1949–1955, 1989, with permission of the American Society for Nutritional Sciences.

5-wk depletion period, levels falling by 70% in men fed low-niacin diets containing either 6 or 10 NE/d (Fu et al., 1989). In contrast, NADP levels remained relatively unchanged when the subjects were fed the same low-niacin diets. These trends in NAD relative to NADP concentrations parallel those in fi-broblasts grown in niacin-restricted cultures (Jacobson et al., 1979). These results indi-cate that erythrocyte NAD levels may serve as a sensitive and reliable indicator of niacin sta-tus. Moreover, the ratio of NAD to NADP of <1.0 in erythrocytes or whole blood may also identify subjects at risk of developing niacin deficiency. The use of NAD and NADP con-centrations in erythrocytes in populations at risk to niacin deficiency should be explored further.

Measurement of niacin coenzymes in erythrocytes

The niacin coenzymes can be quantified both by enzyme-linked reactions or by making use of their natural fluorescence in alkaline solu-tion; micromethods can be used (Nisselbaum and Green, 1969). The methods are very sensitive and can be used on fingerprick blood samples. Alternatively, the niacin coenzymes can be separated and measured by HPLC.

20.4 Summary

Thiamin

Beriberi, the classical syndrome of thiamin deficiency, is rare in Western countries except for persons with conditions such as alcoholism, chronic emesis, diarrhea, and marked anorexia. Thiamin is a component of the coenzyme thiamin pyrophosphate (TPP), which has a role in carbohydrate metabolism.

Measurement of the erythrocyte activity of the transketolase enzyme, with and without added TPP, expressed as a ratio, is currently the most reliable test of thiamin status. The ratio, expressed as the activity coefficient or percentage of stimulation, provides a better measure of tissue stores of thiamin than do static biochemical tests such as thiamin concentrations in either urine or serum. Thiamin in urine can be measured in both 24-h and casual urine specimens, although the former is preferred. Concentrations in urine reflect dietary intakes, except at very low levels. The high within-subject variation in urinary thiamin excretion limits the use of a single 24-h urine sample for evaluating the thiamin status of individuals. Measurement of total thiamin or thiamin pyrophosphate in erythrocytes or whole blood by HPLC with UV detection appears promising and warrants further study.

Riboflavin

Riboflavin is a component of two coenzymes, flavin adenine dinucleotide (FAD) and flavin mononucleotide (FMN). Both are essential in some oxidative enzyme systems involving electron transport. Additionally, a number of flavocoenzymes are required for the synthesis of niacin, pyridoxine, folic acid, and vitamin B_{12}. Classical signs of riboflavin deficiency (ariboflavinosis) generally occur in association with other nutrient deficiencies, notably vitamin B_6.

Measurement of the activity of glutathione reductase, with and without the prosthetic group FAD, is the best method for assessing tissue riboflavin status in the absence of confounding factors, particularly in cases of impaired riboflavin status. The test measures tissue saturation and long-term riboflavin status. Urinary riboflavin excretion levels on casual or 24-h urine specimens reflect dietary intake but vary widely because concentrations are affected by many non-nutritional factors. Concentrations of riboflavin in erythrocytes — or FAD in plasma, whole blood, or erythrocytes — appear promising and warrant further exploration.

Niacin

The term "niacin" refers to two compounds: nicotinamide and nicotinic acid. The former is a component of two coenzymes, nicotinamide adenine dinucleotide (NAD) and nicotinamide adenine dinucleotide phosphate (NADPH), both of which function in a variety of oxidation and reduction reactions. Pellagra, the syndrome of niacin deficiency, is rare in industrialized countries but is prevalent where maize and an Indian variety of sorghum known as jowar are the dietary staples.

No functional biochemical test of niacin status exists. At present, the best marker is the measurement by HPLC of the urinary excretion of N′-methylnicotinamide, in conjunction with one or more of the pyridone turnover products: 2-pyridone, 4-pyridone, or 4-pyridone. If niacin intakes are < 6 NE/d, urinary excretion of either N′-methylnicotinamide or 2-pyridone, or both falls below $8.8\,\mu mol/d$ in adults. In cases of marginal niacin deficiency, measurement of these urinary metabolites is less useful. In the future, measurement of a reduction in the ratio of erythrocyte NAD : NADP to < 1.0 may prove useful as an index of niacin deficiency.

References

Ajayi OA. (1984). Biochemical ariboflavinosis among Nigerian rural school children. Human Nutrition: Clinical Nutrition 38: 383–389.

Ajayi OA. (1985). Incidence of biochemical riboflavin deficiency in Nigerian pregnant women. Human Nutrition: Clinical Nutrition 39: 149–153.

Ajayi OA, James OA. (1984). Effect of riboflavin supplementation on riboflavin nutriture of a secondary school population in Nigeria. American Journal of Clinical Nutrition 39: 787–791.

Anderson BB, Clements JE, Perry GM, Studds C, Vullo C, Salsini G. (1987). Glutathione reductase activity and its relationship to pyridine phosphate activity in G6PD deficiency. European Journal of Haematology 38: 12–20.

Anderson BB, Giuberti M, Perry GM, Salsini G, Casadio I, Vullo C. (1993). Low red blood cell glutathione reductase and pyridoxine phosphate activities not related to dietary riboflavin: selection by malaria? American Journal of Clinical Nutrition 57: 666–672.

Anderson SH, Charles TJ, Nicol AD. (1985). Thiamine deficiency at a district general hospital: report of five cases. Quarterly Journal of Medicine 55: 15–32.

Bailey AL, Finglas PM. (1990). A normal phase high performance liquid chromatographic method for determination of thiamin in blood and tissue samples. Journal of Micronutrient Analysis 7: 147–157.

Bailey AL, Finglas PM, Wright AJ, Southon S. (1994). Thiamin intake, erythrocyte transketolase activity and total erythrocytes thiamin in adolescents. British Journal of Nutrition 72: 111–115.

Bailey AL, Maisey S, Southon S, Wright A, Finglas P, Fulcher RA. (1997). Relationships between micronutrient intake and biochemical indicators of nutrient adequacy in a "free-living" elderly U.K. population. British Journal of Nutrition 77: 225–242.

Baines M, Davies G. (1988). The evaluation of erythrocyte thiamin diphosphate as an indicator of thiamin status in man and its comparison with erythrocyte transketolase activity measurements. Annals of Clinical Biochemistry 25: 698–705.

Bamji MS. (1981). Laboratory tests for the assessment of vitamin nutritional status. In: Briggs MH (ed.) Vitamins in Human Biology and Medicine. CRC Press, Boca Raton, FL, pp. 1–27.

Bamji MS, Bhaskaram P, Jacob CM. (1987). Urinary riboflavin excretion and erythrocyte glutathione reductase activity in preschool children suffering from upper respiratory tract infections and measles. Annals of Nutrition and Metabolism 31: 191–196.

Basu TK, Dickerson JW. (1976). The thiamin status of early cancer patients with particular reference to those with breast and bronchial carcinomas. Oncology 33: 250–252.

Basu TK, Patel DR, Williams DC. (1974). A simplified microassay of transketolase in human blood. International Journal for Vitamin and Nutrition Research 44: 319–326.

Bates CJ, Prentice AM, Paul AA, Sutcliffe BA, Watkinson M, Whitehead RG. (1981). Riboflavin status in Gambian pregnant and lactating women and its implications for Recommended Dietary Allowances. American Journal of Clinical Nutrition 34: 928–935.

Bates CJ, Prentice AM, Paul AA, Prentice A, Sutcliffe BA, Whitehead RG. (1982). Riboflavin status in infants born in rural Gambia, and the effects of a weaning food supplement. Transactions of the Royal Society of Tropical Medicine and Hygiene 76: 253–258.

Bates CJ, Evans PH, Allison G, Sonko BJ, Hoare S, Goodrich S, Aspray T. (1994). Biochemical indices and neuromuscular function tests in rural Gambian children given a riboflavin, or multivitamin plus iron, supplement. British Journal of Nutrition 72: 601–610.

Bates CJ, Thurnham DI, Bingham SA, Margetts BM, Nelson M. (1997). Biochemical markers of nutrient intake. In: Margetts BM, Nelson M (eds.) Design Concepts in Nutritional Epidemiology. Oxford University Press, Oxford, pp. 170–240.

Bates CJ, Prentice A, Cole TJ, van der Pols J, Doyle W, Finch S, Smithers G, Clarke PC. (1999). Micronutrients: highlights and research challenges from the 1994–5 National Diet and Nutrition Survey of people aged 65 years and over. British Journal of Nutrition 82: 7–15.

Bayoumi RA, Rosalki SB. (1976). Evaluation of methods of coenzyme activation of erythrocyte enzymes for detection of deficiency of vitamins B_1, B_2, and B_6. Clinical Chemistry 22: 327–335.

Bender DA. (1983). Effects of a dietary excess of leucine on the metabolism of tryptophan in the rat: a mechanism for the pellagragenic action of leucine. British Journal of Nutrition 50: 25–32.

Bender DA. (1999). Optimum nutrition: thiamin, biotin and pantothenate. Proceedings of the Nutrition Society 58: 427–433.

Bender DA, Bender AE. (1986). Niacin and tryptophan metabolism: the biochemical basis of niacin requirements and recommendations. Nutrition Abstracts and Reviews (Series A) 56: 695–719.

Blanck HM, Bowman BA, Serdula MK, Khan LK, Kohn W, Woodruff BA, Bhutanese Refugee Investigation Group (2002). Angular stomatitis and riboflavin status among adolescent Bhutanese refugees living in southeastern Nepal. American Journal of Clinical Nutrition 76: 430–435.

Boisvert WA, Castaneda C, Mendoza I, Langeloh G, Solomons NW, Gershoff SN, Russell RM. (1993). Prevalence of riboflavin deficiency among Guatemalan elderly people and its relationship to milk intake. American Journal of Clinical Nutrition 58: 85–90

Bui MA. (1999). A microbiological assay on microtitre plates of thiamine in biological fluids and foods. International Journal for Vitamin and Nutrition Research 69: 362–366.

Butterworth RF. (2001). Maternal thiamine deficiency:

still a problem in some world communities. American Journal of Clinical Nutrition 74: 712–713.

Butterworth RF. (2003). Thiamin deficiency and brain disorders. Nutrition Research Reviews 16: 277–283.

Buttery JE, Milner CR, Chamberlain BR. (1982). The NADH-dependent transketolase assay: a note of caution. Clinical Chemistry 28: 2184–2185.

Butterworth. (2003). Thiamin deficiency and brain disorders. Nutrition Research Reviews 16: 277–283.

Casteels M, Foulon V, Mannaerts GP, Van Veldhoven P. (2003). Alpha-oxidation of 3-methyl-substituted fatty acids and its thiamine dependence. European Journal of Biochemistry 270: 1619–1627.

Chastain JL, McCormick DB. (1987). Flavin catabolites: identification and quantification in human urine. American Journal of Clinical Nutrition 46: 830–834.

Cheng CH, Koch M, Shank RE. (1976). Leukocyte transketolase activity as an indicator of thiamin nutriture in rats. Journal of Nutrition 106: 1678–1685.

Chia CP, Addison R, McCormick DB. (1978). Absorption, metabolism and excretion of α-(amino acid) riboflavins in the rat. Journal of Nutrition 108: 373–381.

Clark BR. (1980). Fluorometric quantitation of picomole amounts of l-methylnicotinamide and nicotinamide in serum. Methods of Enzymology 66: 5–8.

de Lange DJ, Joubert CP. (1964). Assessment of nicotinic acid status of population groups. American Journal of Clinical Nutrition 15: 169–174.

Dillon JC, Malfait P, Demaux G, Foldi-Hope C. (1992). Urinary metabolites of nicotinamide during the course of pellagra. Annals of Nutrition and Metabolism 36: 181–185.

Fairweather-Tait SJ, Powers H, Minski M, Whitehead J, Downes R. (1992). Riboflavin deficiency and iron absorption in adult Gambian men. Annals of Nutrition and Metabolism 36: 34–40.

FAO/WHO (Food and Agriculture Organization/World Health Organization). (1967). Requirements of Vitamin A, Thiamine, Riboflavin, and Niacin. Report of a Joint Food and Agriculture Organization/World Health Organization Expert Committee. FAO Nutrition Meetings Report Series No. 41. WHO Technical Report Series No. 362. World Health Organization, Geneva.

Fidanza F, Simonetti MS, Floridi A, Codini M, Fidanza R. (1989). Comparison of methods for thiamin and riboflavin nutriture in man. International Journal for Vitamin and Nutrition Research 59: 40–47.

Finch S, Doyle W, Lowe C, Bates CJ, Prentice A, Smithers G, Clarke PC. (1998). National Diet and Nutrition Survey: People Aged 65 Years and Over. Volume 1: Report of the Diet and Nutrition Survey. The Stationery Office, London.

Finglas PM. (1993). Thiamin. International Journal for Vitamin and Nutrition Research 63: 270–274.

Foy H, Kondi A. (1984). The vulnerable oesophagus: riboflavin deficiency and squamous cell dysplasia of the skin and oesophagus. Journal of the National Cancer Institute 72: 941–948.

Fu CS, Swendseid ME, Jacob RA, McKee RW. (1989). Biochemical markers for assessment of niacin status in young men: levels of erythrocyte niacin coenzymes and plasma tryptophan. Journal of Nutrition 119: 1949–1955.

Gans DA, Harper AE. (1991). Thiamin status of incarcerated and nonincarcerated adolescent males: dietary intake and thiamin pyrophosphate response. American Journal of Clinical Nutrition 53: 1471–1475.

Garry PJ, Owen GM. (1976). An automated flavin adenine dinucleotide-dependent glutathione reductase assay for assessing riboflavin nutriture. American Journal of Clinical Nutrition 29: 663–674.

Garry PJ, Goodwin JS, Hunt WC. (1982). Nutritional status in a healthy elderly population: riboflavin. American Journal of Clinical Nutrition 36: 902–909.

Gatautis VJ, Naito HK. (1981). Liquid-chromatographic determination of urinary riboflavin. Clinical Chemistry 27: 1672–1675.

Goldsmith GA. (1975). Vitamin B complex: thiamine, riboflavin, niacin, folic acid (folacin), vitamin B12, biotin. Progress in Food and Nutrition Science 1: 559–609.

Gontzea I, Rujinski A, Sutzesco P. (1976). Rapide évaluation biochimique de l'état de nutrition niacinique. Bibliotheca Nutritio et Dieta 23: 95–104.

Gopalan C, Krishnaswamy K. (1976). Effect of excess leucine on tryptophan niacin pathway and pyridoxine (letter). Nutrition Reviews 34: 318–319.

Gregory JF. (1996). Vitamins. Food Chemistry. 3rd edition. Marcel Decker, New York, p.532.

Gregory J, Foster K, Tyler H, Wiseman M. (1990). The Dietary and Nutritional Survey of British Adults. Her Majesty's Stationery Office, London.

Gregory J, Collins DL, Davies PSW, Hughes JM, Clarke PC. (1995). National Diet and Nutrition Survey: Children Aged One-and-a-Half to Four-and-a-Half Years. Volume 1: Report of the Diet and Nutrition Survey. Her Majesty's Stationery Office, London.

Gregory J, Lowe S, Bates CJ, Prentice A, Jackson LV, Smithers G, Wenlock R, Farron M. (2000). National Diet and Nutrition Survey: Young People Aged 4 to 18 Years. Volume 1: Report of the Diet and Nutrition Survey. The Stationery Office, London.

Hageman GJ, Stierum RH, van Herwijnen MHM, van der Veer MSE, Kleinjans JCS. (1998). Nicotinic acid supplementation: effects on niacin status, cytogenetic damage, and poly(ADP-Ribosylation) in lymphocytes of smokers. Nutrition and Cancer 32: 113–120.

Halvorsen K, Halvorsen S. (1963). Hartnup disease. Pediatrics 31: 29–38.

Hankes LV. (1984). Nicotinic acid and nicotinamide. In: Machlin LJ (ed.) Handbook of Vitamins. Marcel Dekker, New York, pp. 329–377.

Hart M, Reynolds MS. (1957). Thiamine requirement of adolescent girls. Journal of Home Economics 49: 35–37.

Hatanaka Y, Ueda K. (1981). High incidence of sub-clinical hypovitaminosis of B_1 among university students found by a field study in Ehime, Japan. Medical Journal of Osaka University 31: 83–91.

Hercberg S, Preziosi P, Galan P, Devanlay M, Keller H, Bourgeois C, Potier de Courcy G, Cherouvrier F. (1994). Vitamin status of a healthy French population: dietary intakes and biochemical markers. International Journal for Vitamin and Nutrition Research 64: 220–232.

Herve C, Beyne P, Letteron P, Delacoux E. (1995). Comparison of erythrocyte transketolase activity with thiamine and thiamine phosphate ester levels in chronic alcoholic patients. Clinica Chimica Acta 234: 91–100.

Horwitt MK, Harvey CC, Hills OW, Liebert E. (1950). Correlation of urinary excretion with dietary intake and symptoms of ariboflavinosis. Journal of Nutrition 41: 247–264.

Horwitt MK, Harper AE, Henderson LM. (1981). Niacin – tryptophan relationships for evaluating niacin equivalents. American Journal of Clinical Nutrition 34: 423–427.

Hustad S, Ueland PM, Schneede J. (1999). Quantification of riboflavin, flavin mononucleotide, and flavin adenine dinucleotide in human plasma by capillary electrophoresis and laser-induced fluorescence detection. Clinical Chemistry 45: 862–868.

Icke GC, Nicol DJ. (1993). Thiamin status in pregnancy as determined by direct microbiological assay. International Journal for Vitamin and Nutrition Research 63: 33–35.

Icke GC, Nicol DJ. (1994). Automated microbiological assay of thiamin in serum and red cells. Journal of Clinical Pathology 47: 639–641.

ICNND (Interdepartmental Committee on Nutrition for National Defense). (1963). Manual for Nutrition Surveys. 2nd ed. U.S. Government Printing Office, Washington, DC.

Innis WS, McCormick DB, Merrill AH Jr. (1985). Variations in riboflavin binding by human plasma: identification of immunoglobulin as the major proteins responsible. Biochemical Medicine 34: 151–165.

IOM (Institute of Medicine). (2000). Dietary Reference Intakes for Thiamin, Riboflavin, Niacin, Vitamin B_6, Folate, Vitamin B_{12}, Pantothenic Acid, Biotin, and Choline. National Academy Press, Washington, DC.

Jacob RA, Swendseid ME. (1996). Niacin. In: Ziegler EE, Filer LJ, Jr. (eds.) Present Knowledge in Nutrition. International Life Sciences Institute Press, Washington, DC, pp.184–190.

Jacob RA, Swendseid ME, McKee RW, Fu CS, Clemens RA. (1989). Biochemical markers for assessment of niacin status in young men: urinary and blood levels of niacin metabolites. Journal of Nutrition 119: 591–598.

Jacobson EL, Lange RA, Jacobson MK. (1979). Pyridine nucleotide synthesis in 3T3 cells. Journal of Cell Physiology 99: 417–425.

Jacques PF, Bostom AG, Wilson PW, Rich S, Rosenberg IH, Selhub J. (2001). Determinants of plasma homocysteine concentration in the Framingham Offspring cohort. American Journal of Clinical Nutrition 73: 613–621.

Kang SS, Wong P, Susmano A, Sora J, Norusis M, Ruggie N. (1991). Thermolabile methylene tetrahydrofolate reductase: an inherited risk factor for coronary heart disease. American Journal of Human Genetics 48: 536–545.

Kawai C, Wakabayashi A, Matsumura T, Yui Y. (1980). Reappearance of beriberi heart disease in Japan: a study of 23 cases. American Journal of Medicine 69: 383–386.

Kjøsen B, Seim SH. (1977). The transketolase assay of thiamine in some diseases. American Journal of Clinical Nutrition 30: 1591–1596.

Kodicek E, Ashby DR, Muller M, Carpenter KJ. (1974). The conversion of bound nicotinic acid to free nicotinamide on roasting sweet corn. Proceedings of the Nutrition Society 33: 105A–106A.

Komindr S, Nichoalds GE. (1980). Clinical significance of riboflavin deficiency. In: Brewster MA, Naito HK (eds.) Nutritional Elements and Clinical Biochemistry. Plenum Press, New York, pp. 15–68.

La Rue A, Koehler KM, Wayne SJ, Chiulli SJ, Haaland KY, Garry PJ. (1997). Nutritional status and cognitive functioning in a normally aging sample: a 6-y reassessment. American Journal of Clinical Nutrition 65: 20–29.

Lemoine A, Le Devehat C, Herbeth B. (1986). Vitamin status in three groups of French adults: controls, obese subjects, alcohol drinkers. Annals of Nutrition and Metabolism 30(Suppl): 3–94.

Leske MC, Wu S, Hyman L, Sperduto R, Underwood B, Chylac LT, Milton RC, Srivastava S, Ansari N. (1995). Biochemical factors in the lens opacities: case-control study. Archives of Ophthalmology 113: 1113–1119.

Leveille GA. (1972). Modified thiochrome procedure for the determination of urinary thiamin. American Journal of Clinical Nutrition 25: 273–274.

Lopez R, Schwartz JV, Cooperman JM. (1980). Riboflavin deficiency in an adolescent population in New York City. American Journal of Clinical Nutrition 33: 1283–1286.

Lossy FT, Goldsmith GA, Sarett HP. (1951). Study of test dose excretion of 5 B complex vitamins in man. Journal of Nutrition 45: 213–224.

Low CS. (1985). Riboflavin status of adolescent southern Chinese: riboflavin saturation studies. Human Nutrition: Clinical Nutrition 39: 297–301.

Macias-Matos C, Rodriguez-Ojea A, Chi N, Jimenez S, Zulueta D, Bates CJ. (1996). Biochemical evidence of thiamine depletion during the Cuban neuropathy epidemic, 1992–1993. American Journal of Clinical Nutrition 64: 347–353.

Madigan SM, Tracey F, McNulty H, Eaton-Evans J, Coulter J, McCartney H, Strain JJ. (1998). Riboflavin and vitamin B_6 intakes and status and biochemical response to riboflavin supplementation in free-living elderly people. American Journal of Clinical Nutrition 68: 389–395.

Mak YT, Swaminathan R. (1988). Assessment of vitamin B_1, B_2, and B_6 status by coenzyme activation of red cell enzymes using a centrifugal analyser. Journal of Clinical Chemistry and Clinical Biochemistry 26: 213–217.

Malfait P, Moren A, Dillon JC, Brodel A, Begkoyian G, Etchegony MG, Malenga G, Hakewill P. (1993). An outbreak of pellagra related to changes in dietary niacin among Mozambican refugees in Malawi. International Journal of Epidemiology 22: 504–511.

McCormick DB. (1989). Two interconnected B vitamins: riboflavin and pyridoxine. Physiology Reviews 69: 1170–1198.

McCormick DB, Greene HL. (1994). Vitamins. In: Burtis CA, Ashwood ER (eds.) Tietz Textbook of Clinical Chemistry. W.B. Saunders, Philadelphia, pp. 366–375.

McGready R, Simpson JA, Cho T, Dubowitz L, Changbumrung S, Bøhm V, Munger RG, Sauberlich HE, White NJ, Nosten F. (2001). Postpartum thiamine deficiency in a Karen displaced population. American Journal of Clinical Nutrition 74: 808–813.

McKee RW, Kang-Lee YA, Panaqua M, Swendseid ME. (1982). Determination of nicotinamide and metabolic products in urine by high performance liquid chromatography. Journal of Chromatography 230: 309–318.

McLennan W, Podger A. (1995). Nutrient Intakes and Physical Measurements, Australia. Australian Bureau of Statistics, Canberra.

McNulty H, McKinley MC, Wilson B, McPartlin JM, Strain JJ, Weir DG, Scott JM. (2002). Impaired functioning of the thermolabile methylenetetrahydrofolate reductase is dependent on riboflavin status: implications for riboflavin requirements. American Journal of Clinical Nutrition 76: 436–441.

Nichoalds GE. (1981). Riboflavin. In: Labbac RF (ed.) Symposium on Laboratory Assessment of Nutritional Status: Clinics in Laboratory Medicine. W.B. Saunders, Philadelphia, pp. 685–698.

Nichols HK, Basu TK. (1994). Thiamin status of the elderly: dietary intake and thiamin pyrophosphate response. Journal of the American College of Nutrition 13: 57–61.

Nisselbaum JS, Green S. (1969). A simple ultramicromethod for determination of pyridine nucleotides in tissues. Analytical Biochemistry 27: 212–217

Nixon PF, Price J, Norman-Hicks M, Williams GM, Kerr RA. (1990). The relationship between erythrocyte transketolase activity and the "TPP effect" in Wernicke's encephalopathy and other thiamin deficiency states. Clinica Chimica Acta 192: 89–98.

Oldham HG. (1962). Thiamine requirements of women. Annals of the New York Academy of Sciences 98: 542–549.

Olpin SE, Bates CJ. (1982). Lipid metabolism in riboflavin-deficient rats. I. Effect of dietary lipids on riboflavin status and fatty acid profiles. British Journal of Nutrition 47: 577–588.

O'Rourke NP, Bunker VW, Thomas AJ, Finglas PM, Bailey AL, Clayton BE. (1990). Thiamine status of healthy and institutionalized elderly subjects: analysis of dietary intake and biochemical indices. Age and Aging 19: 325–329.

Patrini C, Griziotti A, Ricciardi L. (2004). Obese individuals as thiamin storers. International Journal of Obesity 28: 920–924.

Pinto J, Huang YP, McConnell R, Rivlin RS. (1978). Increased urinary riboflavin excretion resulting from boric acid ingestion. Journal of Laboratory and Clinical Medicine 92: 126–134.

Powers HJ, Thurnham DI. (1981). Riboflavin deficiency in man: effects on haemoglobin and reduced glutathione in erythrocytes of different ages. British Journal of Nutrition 46: 257–266.

Powers HJ. (2003). Riboflavin (Vitamin B_2) and health. American Journal of Clinical Nutrition 77: 1352–1360.

Prasad PA, Bamji MS, Lakshmi AV, Satyanarayama K. (1990). Functional impact of riboflavin supplementation in urban school children. Nutrition Research 10: 275–282.

Prentice AM, Bates CJ, Prentice A, Welch SG, Williams K, McGregor IA. (1981). The influence of G-6-PD activity on the response of erythrocyte glutathione reductase to riboflavin deficiency. International Journal for Vitamin and Nutrition Research 51: 211–215.

Price JM. (1954). The determination of N'-methyl-2-pyridone-5-carboxyamide in human urine. Journal of Biological Chemistry 211: 117–124.

Puxty JA, Haskew AE, Ratcliffe JG, McMurray J. (1985). Changes in erythrocyte transketolase activity and the thiamine pyrophosphate effect during storage of blood. Annals of Clinical Biochemistry 22: 423–427.

Ramachandran M, Iyer GY. (1974). Erythrocyte glutathione reductase in iron-deficiency anemia. Clinica Chimica Acta 52: 225–229.

Roser RL, Andrist AH, Harrington WH, Naito HK, Lonsdale D. (1978). Determination of urinary thiamine by high-pressure liquid chromatography utilizing the thiochrome fluorescent method. Journal of Chromatography 146: 43–53.

Rozen R. (2002). Methylenetetrahydrofolate reductase: a link between folate and riboflavin? American Journal of Clinical Nutrition 76: 301–302.

Rutishauser IHE, Bates CJ, Paul AA, Black AE, Mandel AR, Patnaik BK. (1979). Long term vitamin status and dietary intake of healthy elderly subjects. I. Riboflavin. British Journal of Nutrition 42: 33–42.

Sadowski JA. (1992). Riboflavin. In: Hartz SC, Russell RM, Rosenberg IH (eds.) Nutrition in the Elderly. The Boston Nutritional Status Survey. Smith-Gordon, London, pp. 119–125.

Sauberlich HE. (1984). Newer laboratory methods of assessing nutriture of selected B-complex vitamins. Annual Review of Nutrition 4: 377–407.

Sauberlich HE. (1985). Bioavailability of vitamins. Progress in Food and Nutrition Science 9: 1–33.

Sauberlich HE. (1999). Laboratory Tests for the Assessment of Nutritional Status. CRC Press, Boca Raton, FL.

Schoenen J, Lenaerts M, Bastings E. (1994). Rapid communication. High dose riboflavin as a prophylactic treatment of migraine: results of an open pilot study. Cephalalgia 14: 328–329.

Schrijver J. (1991). Biochemical markers for micronutrient status and their interpretation. In: Pietrzik K (ed.) Modern Lifestyles, Lower Energy Intake and Micronutrient Status. Springer-Verlag, London, pp. 55–85.

Shaikh B, Pontzer NJ. (1979). Direct urinary assay method of N′-methylnicotinamide by soap chromatography. Journal of Chromatography 162: 596–600.

Shibata K, Matsuo H. (1989a). Correlation between niacin equivalent intake and urinary excretion of its metabolites, N′-methylnicotinamide, N′-methyl-2-pyridone-5-carboxamide and N′-methyl-4-pyridone-3-carboxamide in humans consuming a self-selected food. American Journal of Clinical Nutrition 50: 114–119.

Shibata K, Matsuo H. (1989b). Effect of supplementing low protein diets with the limiting amino acids on the excretion of N′-methylnicotinamide and its pyridones in rats. Journal of Nutrition 19: 896–901.

Siassi F, Powansari Z, Ghadirian P. (2000). Nutrient intake and oesophageal cancer in the Caspian littoral of Iran: a case-control study. Cancer Detection and Prevention 24: 295–303.

Smidt LJ, Cremin FM, Grivetti LE, Clifford AJ. (1991). Influence of thiamin supplementation on the health and general well-being of an elderly Irish population with marginal thiamin deficiency. Journal of Gerontology 46: M16–M22.

Smith MD. (1980). Rapid method for determination of riboflavin in urine by high-performance liquid chromatography. Journal of Chromatography 182: 285–291.

Soares MJ, Satyanarayana K, Bamji MS, Jacob CM, Ramana YV, Rao SS. (1993). The effect of exercise on the riboflavin status of adult men. British Journal of Nutrition 69: 541–551.

Stephen JM, Grant R, Yeh CS. (1992). Anaphylaxis from administration of intravenous thiamine. American Journal of Emergency Medicine 10: 61–63.

Sterner RT, Price WR. (1973). Restricted riboflavin: within-subject behavioral effects in humans. American Journal of Clinical Nutrition 26: 150–160.

Suter PM, Vetter W. (2000). Diuretics and vitamin B_1: are diuretics a risk factor for thiamin malnutrition? Nutrition Reviews 58: 319–323.

Swendseid ME, Jacob RA. (1994). Niacin. In: Shils ME, Olson JA, Shike M (eds.) Modern Nutrition in Health and Disease. 8th ed. Lea & Febiger, Philadelphia, pp. 376–382.

Talwar D, Davidson H, Cooney J, O'Reilly D. (2000). Vitamin B_1 status assessed by direct measurement of thiamin pyrophosphate in erythrocytes or whole blood by HPLC: comparison with erythrocyte trans-

ketolase activation assay. Clinical Chemistry 46: 704–710.

Terry RC, Simon M. (1982). Determination of niacin metabolites 1-methyl-5-carboxlamide-2-pyridone and N-1-methylnicotinamide in urine by high performance liquid chromatography. Journal of Chromatography 232: 261–274.

Thurnham DI. (1972). Influence of glucose-6-phosphate dehydrogenase deficiency on the glutathione reductase test for ariboflavinosis. Annals of Tropical Medicine and Parasitology 66: 505–508.

Thurnham DI. (1981). Red cell enzyme tests of vitamin status: do marginal deficiencies have any physiological significance? Proceedings of the Nutrition Society 40: 155–163.

Thurnham DI, Rathakette P, Hambidge KM, Mumoz N, Crespi M. (1982). Ribolfavin, vitamin A, and zinc status in Chinese subjects in a high-risk area for oesophageal cancer in China. Human Nutrition: Clinical Nutrition 36: 337–349.

Tillotson JA, Baker EM. (1972). An enzymatic measurement of the riboflavin status in man. American Journal of Clinical Nutrition 25: 425–431.

Tillotson JA, Bashor M. (1980). Fluorometric apoprotein titration of urinary riboflavin. Analytical Biochemistry 107: 214–219.

Tucker RG, Mickelsen O, Keys A. (1960). The influence of sleep, work, diuresis, heat, acute starvation, thiamine intake and bed rest on human riboflavin excretion. Journal of Nutrition 72: 251–261.

van der Beek EJ, van Dokkum W, Wedel M, Schrijver J, van den Berg H. (1994). Thiamin, riboflavin and vitamin B_6: impact of restricted intake on physical performance in man. Journal of the American College of Nutrition 13: 629–640.

van Dokkum W, Schrijver J, Wesstra JA. (1990). Variability in man of levels of some indices of nutritional status over a 60-d period on a constant diet. European Journal of Clinical Nutrition 44: 665–674.

Vir SC, Love AH. (1979). Nutritional status of institutionalized and noninstitutionalized aged in Belfast, Northern Ireland. American Journal of Clinical Nutrition 32: 1934–1947.

Waring PP, Fisher D, McDonnell J, McGown EL, Sauberlich HE. (1982). A continuous-flow (Auto Analyzer II) procedure for measuring erythrocyte transketolase activity. Clinical Chemistry 28: 2206–2213.

Warnock LG, Prudhomme CR, Wagner C. (1978). The determination of thiamin pyrophosphate in blood and other tissues, and its correlation with erythrocyte transketolase activity. Journal of Nutrition 108: 421–427.

Wilkinson TJ, Hanger HC, Elmslie J, George PM, Sainsbury R. (1997). The response to treatment of subclinical thiamine deficiency in the elderly. American Journal of Clinical Nutrition 66: 925–928.

Williams RR, Cline JK. (1936). Synthesis of vitamin B-1. Journal of the American Chemical Society 58: 1504–1505.

Winters LR, Yoon JS, Kalkwarf HJ, Davies JC, Berk-
    owitz MG, Haas J, Roe DA. (1992). Riboflavin re-
    quirements and exercise adaptation in older women.
    American Journal of Clinical Nutrition 56: 526–532.
Wright AJA, Southon S, Bailey AL, Finglas PM,
    Maisey S, Fulcher RA. (1995).   Nutrient intake
    and biochemical status of non-institutionalized el-
derly subjects in Norwich: comparison with younger
    adults and adolescents from the same general com-
    munity. British Journal of Nutrition 74: 453–475.
Zempleni J, Galloway JR, McCormick DB. (1996).
    Pharmacokinetics of orally and intravenously ad-
    ministered riboflavin in healthy humans. American
    Journal of Clinical Nutrition 63: 54–66.

21

Assessment of vitamin B_6 status

The term "vitamin B_6" is used as the generic descriptor for 3-hydroxy-2-methylpyridine derivatives that exhibit the biological activity of pyridoxine in rats. The requirement for vitamin B_6 is linked to the intake of protein and the function of the vitamin in amino acid metabolism. The adult human has only a small body pool of this vitamin (20–30 mg), which is rapidly depleted when intakes of the vitamin are inadequate. Most of the vitamin B_6 in the body pool is in the form of pyridoxal-5'-phosphate (PLP) in muscle bound to phosphorylase.

Vitamin B_6 is found in foods mainly as pyridoxal (the aldehyde), pyridoxamine (the amine), and pyridoxine (the alcohol). These three dietary forms of vitamin B_6 are then converted, after absorption, into pyridoxal-5'-phosphate or pyridoxamine-5'-phosphate (PMP), the two active coenzyme forms of vitamin B_6 (Figure 21.1). These two coenzymes catalyze a variety of enzyme systems as discussed briefly below.

Functions of vitamin B_6

Pyridoxal-5'-phosphate is the most important coenzyme form in the body. It is a coenzyme for more than 100 enzymes that are involved mainly in protein and amino acid metabolism. These enzymes include decarboxylases, aminotransferases, racemases, and dehydratases.

Several PLP-dependent reactions involving the decarboxylation of precursor amino acids give rise to neurotransmitters, including serotonin (from tryptophan), taurine, dopamine, norepinephrine, histamine, and γ-aminobutyric acid. Pyridoxal-5'-phosphate is also a coenzyme for kynureninase, an enzyme involved in the conversion of tryptophan to niacin (Figure 20.7).

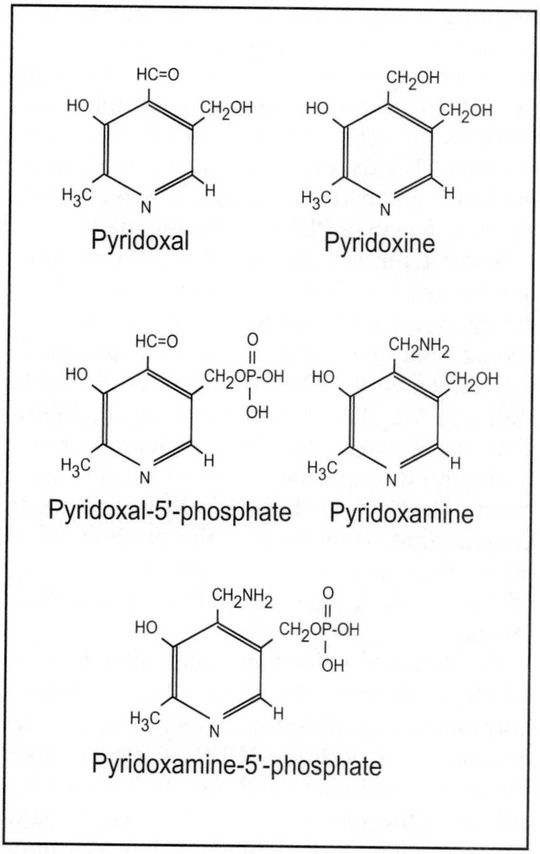

Figure 21.1: Structure of the forms of vitamin B_6.

Type of reaction	Examples
Aminotransferase	Alanine aminotransferase Aspartate aminotransferase
Decarboxylation	Tryptophan decarboxylase Tyrosine decarboxylase
Decarboxylation with carbon–carbon bond formation	δ-amino-levulinate synthetase Serine palmitoyltransferase
Side chain cleavage	Serine hydroxymethyltrans- ferase, Cystathionase
Dehydratase	L-serine dehydratase
Racemyization	Interconversion of D and L amino acids (bacteria only)

Table 21.1: Enzyme reactions catalyzed by pyridoxal 5′-phosphate. From Lecklem (1996).

In carbohydrate metabolism, the production of glucose involves PLP through its role in transamination reactions and its association with glycogen phosphorylase. The role of PLP in lipid metabolism is complex and involves the action of several PLP-dependent enzymes. For example, the synthesis of phospholipids and carnitine requires serine palmitoyltransferase, a PLP-dependent enzyme.

Several human studies suggest that vitamin B_6 influences the immune system; both the humoral and cell-mediated immune responses may be affected (Talbot et al., 1987; Ockhuizen et al., 1990; Meydani et al., 1991; Rall and Meydani, 1993; Kwak et al., 2002). The mechanisms involved remain unclear, but it may be through the action of serine trans-hydroxymethyltransferase, a PLP-dependent enzyme that is involved in the production of one-carbon units necessary for the synthesis of the nucleic acids (Axelrod and Trakatellis, 1964).

Pyridoxal-5′-phosphate may also have a role in modulating the action of some steroid hormones, thus affecting endocrine-mediated diseases. In addition, PLP is a coenzyme for aminolevulinate synthase, an enzyme involved in the synthesis of heme. As a result, in severe vitamin B_6 deficiency, hypochromic microcytic anemia occurs. In some circum-

stances, deficiency of vitamin B_6 may also lead to an accumulation of homocysteine in the blood, because the initial step in the transsulfuration cycle is mediated by the enzyme cystathione β-synthase and requires PLP (Section 22.1.5).

Table 21.1 summarizes the cellular processes and systems in which PLP has a role; more specific details are given in Lecklem (1994). A detailed review of the role of vitamin B_6 in metabolism is also given in Dolphin et al. (1986).

Deficiency of vitamin B_6 in humans

In the early stages, pyridoxine deficiency may cause fatigue and headaches. Later, seborrheic dermatitis, oral lesions (glossitis, cheilosis, angular stomatitis), epileptiform convulsions, and depression and confusion may develop (IOM, 2000). Whether the convulsions are due to the reduced level of one or more neurotransmitters is uncertain. Hypochromic, microcytic anemia may also occur, as noted earlier.

Vulnerable population groups at risk for suboptimal vitamin B_6 status include the elderly, adolescents, pregnant and lactating women, and probably weanlings (Schuster et al. 1981; Bates et al., 1999; IOM, 2000 FAO/WHO, 2002). Certain genetic defects of PLP-dependent enzymes may occur which mimic vitamin B_6 deficiency. These include homocystinuria and cystathionuria, xanthurenic aciduria (a defect of kynureninase), and a defect in ornithine aminotransferase that produces gyrate atrophy (Lecklem, 1994).

Alterations in vitamin B_6 status have also been associated with alcohol addiction, estrogen therapy, uremia, and liver disease. Patients with rheumatoid arthritis and those infected with HIV also appear to be at risk, despite apparently adequate dietary intakes (Rall and Meydani, 1993).

The drug isoniazid (used in the treatment of tuberculosis), and cycloserine, penicillamine, and hydrocortisone all interfere with vitamin B_6 metabolism. These drugs may form a complex with vitamin B_6 that is inhibitory for pyridoxal kinase, or they may positively displace PLP from binding sites; more specific information can be found in Bhagavan (1985). Vitamin B$_6$ antagonists also occur naturally in some foods. They include agaritine and gyromitrin (in some varieties of mushrooms), linatine (in flaxseed meal), canaline and canavanine (in jack beans), and mimosine (in mimosa) (Rechcigl, 1983).

Several (McCully, 1969; Selub et al., 1993) but not all (Vermaak et al., 1987) investigators, consider vitamin B$_6$ deficiency to be a risk factor for coronary heart disease, via its role in the metabolism of homocysteine (Section 22.1.5). In most cases, however, inadequate intake of folic acid appears to be the main determinant of the homocysteine-related increase in coronary heart disease (Selub et al., 1995). Suboptimal vitamin B$_6$ status may also occur with riboflavin deficiency, as noted earlier, because riboflavin is required for the formation of the coenzyme PLP (Section 20.2).

Food sources and dietary intakes

Vitamin B$_6$ is widely distributed in foods, so frank dietary deficiencies are rare. The form most common in plant foods is pyridoxine, whereas pyridoxal and pyridoxamine predominate in animals products.

Good food sources of vitamin B$_6$ are fish, meat, poultry, yeast, certain seeds, and bran. The application of dry heat, for example during baking and toasting, may lead to some losses of vitamin B$_6$.

In some industrialized countries, ready-to-eat cereals may be fortified with vitamin B$_6$. As a result, cereal products, as well as meat and meat products, are often the most important food sources of vitamin B$_6$ (Gregory et al.,1990; IOM, 2000).

The bioavailability of vitamin B$_6$ in a normal mixed diet is about 75%; limiting factors include dietary fiber causing incomplete digestion, food processing, and the existence of some less available forms of vitamin B$_6$ (e.g., 6-hydroxypyridoxine). Gregory (1997) has reviewed the bioavailability of vitamin B$_6$ in detail; data on the factors that influence vitamin B$_6$ bioavailability in foods and overall diets are lacking.

Effect of high intakes of vitamin B$_6$

The toxicity of vitamin B$_6$ is quite low. No adverse effects have been linked to high intakes of vitamin B$_6$ from food sources. Daily megadoses (2–6 g) of vitamin B$_6$ supplements have been associated with both sensory neuropathy and dermatological lesions (Schaumburg et al., 1983).

The U.S. Food and Nutrition Board has set the Tolerable Upper Intake Level (UL) for adults, including pregnant and lactating women, at 100 mg/d as pyridoxine; details for the other life-stage groups are given in IOM (2000).

Indices of vitamin B$_6$ status

The biochemical assessment of vitamin B$_6$ status is essential, as the clinical signs and symptoms of vitamin B$_6$ deficiency are very nonspecific. The three biochemical tests most widely used are the activation coefficient for the erythrocyte enzyme aspartate aminotransferase, plasma PLP concentrations, and the urinary excretion of vitamin B$_6$ degradation products, specifically urinary pyridoxic acid. Of these, plasma PLP is probably the best single measure because it reflects tissue stores (Liu et al., 1985; van den Berg et al., 1993), although concentrations of this biochemical marker are affected by many confounding factors. In view of the lack of concordance between tests, use of all three is often recommended, together with an assessment of the dietary intake of both vitamin B$_6$ and protein.

In future, functional tests for vitamin B$_6$ involving neurological and immunological measurements may be used (Reynolds, 1995). In the interim, three biochemical tests and some additional indices are described below.

21.1 Erythrocyte aminotransferases

The two enzymes alanine aminotransferase (AlAT) (EC 2.6.1.2, also known as glutamate pyruvate transaminase) and aspartate aminotransferase (AsAT) (EC 2.6.1.1, also known as glutamate oxaloacetate transaminase) both require pyridoxal phosphate as a coenzyme. AlAT catalyzes the following transamination reaction:

$$\text{L-alanine} + \alpha\text{-ketoglutarate} \rightleftharpoons$$
$$\text{pyruvate} + \text{L-glutamate}$$

whereas AsAT catalyzes the reaction:

$$\text{L-aspartate} + \alpha\text{-ketoglutarate} \rightleftharpoons$$
$$\text{oxaloacetate} + \text{L-glutamate}$$

Both aminotransferase enzymes transfer the amino group from their respective amino acid to α-ketoglutarate, forming L-glutamate and the keto acid corresponding to the original amino acid.

The activity of aminotransferase enzymes is greater in erythrocytes than in plasma. Consequently, the activity of the enzymes in erythrocytes is used as a measure of vitamin B_6 nutriture. In vitamin B_6 deficiency, the basal activity of these aminotransferase enzymes falls, but the in vitro stimulation of the enzymes with added pyridoxal phosphate increases. The activities are expressed in terms of activity coefficients (ACs) or percentage stimulation, as described for erythrocyte transketolase (Section 20.1.1). This test is most useful when intakes of vitamin B_6 are marginal or low; when intakes are higher, the sensitivity is low, as discussed earlier for the ACs for erythrocyte transketolase and erythrocyte glutathione reductase (Section 20.2.1).

To determine both the AC and the percentage stimulation of erythrocyte AlAT, the red blood cell hemolysate is incubated with α-ketoglutarate and DL-alanine to yield the transamination product pyruvate, in the presence and absence in vitro of PLP. The amount of pyruvate formed during the enzyme reaction is then measured spectrophotometrically:

erythrocyte AlAT AC =

$$\frac{\mu\text{g pyruvate/mL/hr (with added PLP)}}{\mu\text{g pyruvate/mL/hr (without added PLP)}}$$

percentage stimulation =

$$(\text{activity coefficient} \times 100) - 100$$

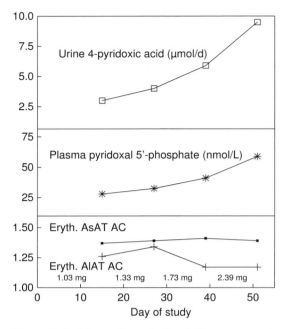

Figure 21.2: Mean values of vitamin B_6 measures at the end of four successive experimental periods with progressively increasing intakes of vitamin B_6. Data from Hansen et al., *American Journal of Clinical Nutrition* 66: 1379–1387, 1997 © Am J Clin Nutr. American Society for Clinical Nutrition.

The relationship of the activities of both erythrocyte AlAT and AsAT to other measures of vitamin B_6 status, including clinical manifestations of deficiency, has been evaluated in both experimental and epidemiological studies. These studies have shown that of the two enzymes, erythrocyte AlAT is much more responsive than erythrocyte AsAT to changes in dietary intakes of vitamin B_6 (Figure 21.2) and thus is a more sensitive marker of vitamin B_6 status (Cinnamon and Beaton, 1970; Brown et al., 1975; Kretsch et al., 1995; Hansen et al., 1997). Further, the activities of these two enzymes reflect the vitamin B_6 status over about the last 4 wk, which is the half-life of circulating erythrocytes (Leklem, 1990). Hence, in experimental studies, the response of erythrocyte AlAT is delayed, generally by about 1–2 wk relative to corresponding changes in both plasma PLP (Section 21.2), and urinary excretion of vitamin B_6 and 4-pyridoxic acid (Section 21.3 and 21.4) (Kretsch et al., 1995).

	Erythrocyte AlAT AC	
	Mean	SD
Age (y)		
⩽ 18 ($n = 37$)	1.37	1.24
> 18 ($n = 90$)	1.34	1.20
Trimester		
First ($n = 43$)	1.33	1.20
Second ($n = 64$)	1.35	1.23
Third ($n = 20$)	1.40	1.29
Race		
African American ($n = 99$)	1.36	1.21
Caucasian ($n = 28$)	1.28	1.18

Table 21.2: Mean erythrocyte alanine aminotransferase (AlAT) stimulation activity coefficients (ACs) of low-income pregnant women presented by age, stage of pregnancy, and race. The means within each category do not differ significantly ($p > 0.05$). However, the large standard deviations may result from large between-subject variation, which may mask true within-category differences. From Schuster et al., American Journal of Clinical Nutrition 34: 1731–1735, 1981 © Am J Clin Nutr. American Society for Clinical Nutrition.

In epidemiological studies, the activities of erythrocyte AlAT and AsAT may not reflect the degree of deficiency of vitamin B$_6$, especially in cases of marginal deficiency, because the activity may vary widely among individuals, as shown in Table 21.2 (Schuster et al., 1981).

Schuster et al. (1981) measured erythrocyte AlAT stimulation to assess the vitamin B$_6$ status of some low-income pregnant adolescent and adult women. The mean erythrocyte AlAT stimulation ACs were elevated at the first clinic visit and again at the 30th week of pregnancy (Table 21.2), consistent with the findings for pregnant Hispanic teenage girls by Martner-Hewes et al. (1986). Similar trends indicative of lower vitamin B$_6$ status during pregnancy have been observed for other biochemical indices (Section 21.2).

The clinical significance of these elevated AlAT stimulation ACs during pregnancy is uncertain. The decline in vitamin B$_6$ status may actually represent a normal physiological response and not a vitamin deficiency (Reynolds and Leklem, 1985). Nevertheless,

Schuster et al. (1981) reported significantly lower developmental Apgar scores for infants whose mothers had higher erythrocyte AlAT stimulation ACs (> 1.25) than for those infants whose mothers had normal values (< 1.25). Other variables, however, unrelated to vitamin B$_6$ may have also been involved.

Notwithstanding the greater sensitivity of erythrocyte AlAT, the activity of AsAT in erythrocytes is more frequently measured in population studies. It is about 20 times more active and, hence, easier to measure, and it is less affected by pregnancy and oral contraceptive use (Löwik et al., 1990; Bates et al., 1999). Nevertheless, care must be taken when interpreting such epidemiological data because several factors, unrelated to vitamin B$_6$ nutriture, may influence erythrocyte AsAT ACs, reducing the specificity.

21.1.1 Factors affecting activity of erythrocyte aminotransferases

Age affects AsAT AC. Activities in Finnish children were lowest at 4 mo, then increased gradually during childhood and adolescence. Figure 21.3 depicts the 10th and 90th percentile ranges and medians for erythrocyte AsAT activation coefficient, at selected ages, for Finnish children followed from 2 mo to

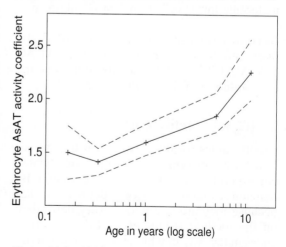

Figure 21.3: 10th, Median, and 90th percentiles for erythrocyte aspartate transaminase activation coefficients at selected ages. Data from Heiskanen et al., Journal of Nutrition 125: 2985–2992, 1995, by permission of the American Society for Nutritional Sciences.

11 y of age (Heiskanen et al., 1995). A similar age-related trend was also noted for boys 4–18 y in the U.K. Diet and Nutrition Survey, but not for girls (Bates et al., 1999; Gregory et al., 2000).

Alcohol intake lowers erythrocyte AsAT AC values, the change being independent of vitamin B_6 intake, and thus possibly masking suboptimal vitamin B_6 status. The exact mechanism is unclear. It may be due to higher PLP concentrations in plasma and erythrocytes arising from a high content of bioavailable vitamin B_6 in alcoholic beverages. Alternatively, it may be related to the metabolism of vitamin B_6. Inverse relationships between erythrocyte AsAT ACs and alcohol intake have been reported in several community-based studies (Löwik et al., 1990; Hercberg et al., 1994).

Acute-phase status has been reported to influence AsAT AC in some studies. Bates et al. (1999) noted a strong inverse association between plasma α_1-antichymotrypsin and erythrocyte AsAT AC in young people aged 4–18 y participating in the U.K. National Diet and Nutrition Survey ($r = -0.11$; $p = 0.0008$), but not in those aged $\geqslant 65$ y. Whether this relationship reflects a long-term metabolic factor or is transient is unknown.

Certain drugs and diseases that affect the liver and heart alter erythrocyte AsAT AC (and AlAT AC) and, hence, may confound the interpretation of the results (Bamji, 1981).

21.1.2 Interpretive criteria

Cutoff values for the activities of the aminotransferase enzymes in erythrocytes which correspond to marginal or severe vitamin B_6 deficiency states are poorly defined, in part because they are likely to be very dependent on the method (Bates et al., 1999). Differences in the way in which the enzyme activity is expressed across studies is another complicating factor. In some cases activities are given as μmol of product per mL of red blood cells, per g of hemoglobin, or per

Interpretive guideline	Erythrocyte AsAT activity coefficient
Acceptable	< 1.70
Marginal	1.70–1.85
Deficient	> 1.85

Table 21.3: Criteria for the interpretation of erythrocyte AsAT AC values. Data from Sauberlich (1999).

number of red blood cells. Standardization of the units for expressing activity is urgently required.

Table 21.3 presents the criteria reported by Sauberlich (1999) for evaluating erythrocyte AsAT AC values. Bates et al. (1999) used one cutoff ($\geqslant 1.80$) for erythrocyte AsAT AC, as indicative of poor vitamin B_6 status, for their study of U.K. young people and persons aged $\geqslant 65$ y. Leklem (1990) recommends the use of this same cutoff but provides a single cutoff value for erythrocyte AlAT AC indicative of inadequate status (i.e., $\geqslant 1.25$).

Sauberlich (1999) cautions that because the activity of erythrocyte AlAT is so low, it is more difficult to measure reliably. Moreover, its use as a marker of suboptimal vitamin B_6 status is limited by the genetic polymorphism of this enzyme (Ubbink et al., 1989a).

More work is needed to establish interpretive guidelines for pregnant and lactating women. Currently, cutoff values must be assessed by comparing erythrocyte transaminase activities with other tests of vitamin B_6 status, including plasma PLP and tests of lymphocyte function (Löwik et al., 1990; Heiskanen et al., 1995; Brussaard et al., 1997; Bates et al., 1999; Kwak et al., 2002).

Data on the median and percentile distribution for erythrocyte AsAT stimulation tests in lactating mothers ($n = 198$) and their infants from Finland are presented in Table 21.4 (Heiskanen et al., 1994). Infants in this study had an adequate vitamin B_6 status because they were breastfed by mothers who took a vitamin B_6 supplement during pregnancy.

The U.K. National Diet and Nutrition Surveys also include erythrocyte AsAT ACs data for young people aged 4–18 y (Gregory et al.,

Duration of lactation or age (mo)	Percentile		
	10th	50th	90th
Mothers			
0	1.59	1.80	2.22
2	1.72	1.92	2.24
4	1.67	1.88	2.09
6	1.67	1.85	2.07
9	1.67	1.85	2.08
Infants			
2	1.35	1.52	1.76
4	1.34	1.45	1.54
6	1.46	1.57	1.68
9	1.43	1.50	1.64
12	1.49	1.62	1.84

Table 21.4: Median, 10th, and 90th percentile erythrocyte aspartate transaminase activation coefficients in lactating females and their infants at selected ages. Data from Heiskanen et al., Journal of Nutrition 125: 2985–2992, 1995, with permission of the American Society for Nutritional Sciences.

2000) and persons aged $\geqslant 65$ y (Finch et al., 1998). Mean, median, and lower and upper 2.5 percentiles by age and sex are presented.

21.1.3 Measurement of erythrocyte transaminase activities

In the past, the activities of erythrocyte AlAT and AsAT (and the in vitro stimulation effect of PLP) have often been measured with colorimetry and coupled-enzyme spectrophotometry (Sauberlich, 1984). Both of these procedures lack specificity and sensitivity, suffer from severe matrix effects, and lack a suitable reference standard for quality control.

An automated method based on a continuous flow procedure has been developed for the analysis of AsAT activity before and after in vitro stimulation with PLP (Vuilleumier et al., 1990). The method measures the rate of oxidation of the pyridine nucleotide coenzyme, coupled to the aminotransferase reaction. A freeze-dried erythrocyte pool can be used for quality control. Bates et al. (1999) report between assay CVs of 3.7% and 1.8%, for the basal activity and AsAT AC, respectively, for this method. The activity of AsAT is best measured in fresh erythrocytes

(Hansen and Shultz, 2001), but this is not always practical. Bates et al. (1999) performed the erythrocyte AsAT assay within 6 mo in frozen samples that had not been previously thawed.

For the analysis of AlAT, the automated procedure of Skala et al. (1987) is recommended. This method can also be used for the simultaneous measurement of AsAT activity; only a small sample of packed erythrocytes is required (i.e., 0.25 mL). Quality-control samples for the assay can be prepared from a pool of erythrocytes that have been stored frozen in aliquots at −70°C or lower (Sauberlich, 1999). Erythrocyte samples for AlAT analysis may be frozen for 28 d at −20°C, and even longer (84 d) at −80°C before analysis. The activities of AlAT and AsAT have also been measured in leukocytes, but large blood samples are required and the method of isolating the leukocytes is too tedious for routine use.

21.2 Plasma pyridoxal-5′-phosphate

Pyridoxal-5′-phosphate (PLP) is the major transport form of vitamin B₆ in plasma, accounting for 70%–90% of the total vitamin B₆ in the plasma. Concentrations of plasma PLP are a direct measure of the active coenzyme form of vitamin B₆, and, in rats, reflect levels in the skeletal muscle (Lumeng et al., 1978).

Results of experimental depletion–repletion trials support the use of plasma PLP as a marker of vitamin B₆ intake and tissue status (Kretsch et al., 1995; Hansen et al., 1997, 2001; Huang et al., 1998; Kwak et al., 2002). A strong positive relationship between plasma PLP concentrations and vitamin B₆ intake has been observed, as shown in Figure 21.4 (IOM, 2000). In addition, significant correlations between plasma PLP and urinary total vitamin B₆ and plasma total vitamin B₆ have been reported (Hansen et al., 1997).

As a result, some investigators consider plasma PLP to be the method of choice for assessing vitamin B₆ status (Reynolds and Leklem, 1985). Indeed, in two depletion–

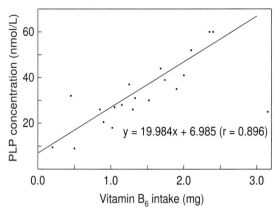

Figure 21.4: The regression relationship between plasma pyridoxal phosphate (PLP) concentrations and vitamin B$_6$ intake. Data derived from a compilation by Leklem (1990), Hansen et al. (1997), Huang et al. (1998), Kretch et al. (1995), and Ribaya-Mercado et al. (1991).

repletion studies, abnormal values for neurological and immunological measures were associated with low plasma PLP concentrations (Kretsch et al., 1995; Kwak et al., 2002). In the study of Kretsch et al. (1995), some subjects with plasma PLP < 9 nmol/L had abnormal electroencephalogram patterns. Positive correlations ($r = 0.456$; $p \leqslant 0.01$) between plasma PLP values and lymphocyte function, based on measurements of lymphocyte proliferation in response to mitogen stimulation, have also been noted in young women ($n = 7$) consuming diets with vitamin B$_6$ levels ranging from 1.5 to 2.7 mg/d (Kwak et al., 2002).

Several population surveys have included plasma PLP as a measure of vitamin B$_6$ status (Manore et al., 1989; Löwik et al., 1990; Vermaak et al., 1990; Brussaard et al., 1997; Bates et al., 1999). In general, correlations with dietary intakes have been rather disappointing; only modest correlations have been reported in most of these surveys (e.g., Brussaard et al., 1997), probably because of confounding factors weakening the correlation. For some of these factors (e.g., aging and pregnancy), it is unclear whether the changes in plasma PLP levels that arise, reflect a poorer vitamin B$_6$ status or represent a normal physiological change.

21.2.1 Factors affecting plasma PLP levels

Age-related changes have been noted. Values are high in the fetus, decreasing rapidly in the first year, after which they decline more gradually with age. Table 21.5 compares plasma PLP concentrations in young and older persons, based on results from the U.K. national surveys (Bates et al., 1999). Reasons for the low plasma PLP values in the elderly are unclear. They may be due to lower vitamin B$_6$ absorption and increased metabolism during aging, both leading to increased requirements (Russell, 1992). Alternatively, reductions in energy intake, increased use of multiple medications, and morbidity may be implicated.

Pregnancy influences plasma PLP concentrations, as noted for erythrocyte aminotransferase activities. The concentrations decrease progressively, especially during the third trimester, sometimes to below 10 nmol/L. Hemodilution does not appear to be responsible, because vitamin B$_6$ supplementation during pregnancy does not arrest the fall in plasma PLP levels (Reynolds and Leklem, 1985).

Alcohol intake reduces plasma PLP concentrations, sometimes to levels associated with clinical signs such as convulsions and peripheral neuropathy. The low vitamin B$_6$ status of alcoholics is not related to poor diets or liver disease. Instead, it is probably related to a systemic effect induced by acetaldehyde

Age (y)	n	PLP (nmol/L) G-mean (95% CI)	PA (nmol/L) G-mean (95% CI)
4–18	1006	56.5 (54.5–58.5)	10.6 (8.6–12.6)
$\geqslant$65	919	34.0 (32.0–36.0)	15.5 (13.5–17.5)
		$t = 13.0$; $p < 0.0001$	$t = 10.1$; $p < 0.0001$

Table 21.5: Comparison between young and older people for plasma pyridoxal-5′-phosphate (PLP) and 4-pyridoxic acid (PA). G-mean, geometric mean. Data from Bates et al., Public Health Nutrition 2: 529–535, 1999, with permission of the Nutrition Society.

that results in a reduction in the formation of cellular PLP by cells (Lumeng and Li, 1974).

Alkaline phosphatase activity is inversely related to plasma PLP concentrations, especially in older people (Bates et al., 1999). The effect is associated with the hydrolysis of PLP to pyridoxal by alkaline phosphatase (Black et al., 1978). Hence, when alkaline phosphatase activity is elevated (e.g., in bone or hepatic disorders), plasma PLP concentrations are generally, but not always reduced (Hansen et al., 2001).

Cigarette smoking reduces the concentrations of plasma PLP (Vermaak et al., 1990). This trend may be associated with increased alkaline phosphatase activity, although a low dietary intake among smokers may also have a role.

Aerobic exercise can increase plasma PLP concentrations, because in conditions of high muscle turnover, the muscle in the body becomes a source of plasma PLP in addition to that of the liver.

Infection has been linked to lower plasma PLP levels in some large epidemiological studies. For example, in the U.K. national surveys, infection, based on elevated plasma α-1-antichymotrypsin levels, was associated with lower PLP concentrations in both young people and those $\geqslant 65$ y (Bates et al., 1999). The results suggest that acute phase status may confound plasma PLP in all age groups.

Prolonged fasting results in the release of PLP from glycogen phosphorylase, causing increased levels in the plasma (Black et al., 1978).

Disease states in which decreased plasma PLP concentrations have been reported include coronary heart disease, breast cancer, Hodgkin's disease, and diabetes. In most cases, it is unclear whether vitamin B₆ status is really affected in these conditions as, often, plasma PLP was the only index of vitamin B₆ status measured (Leklem, 1990). For subjects with chronic renal failure and those on dialysis, low plasma PLP levels may be due to increased metabolic clearance of PLP.

Medications may alter plasma PLP levels (Ubbink et al., 1989b; Driskell, 1994). Such effects may be particularly important in the elderly who are much more dependent on medications than are younger people. A significant inverse relationship between the use of medications for respiratory diseases (bronchodilators, antihistamine, etc) and plasma PLP concentrations was observed in a U.K. survey of the elderly (Bates et al., 1999). However, for beta-blockers or antiplatelet drugs, a positive relationship was seen.

Other factors known to affect vitamin B₆ metabolism include oral contraceptive agents. However, the use of low-dose oral contraceptives does not appear to have long-term effects on serum PLP concentrations (Masse et al., 1996). Increased protein intake may decrease plasma PLP concentrations (Leklem, 1990).

21.2.2 Interpretive criteria

There are no universally accepted guidelines for interpreting plasma PLP concentrations, and age-specific criteria have not been developed. Reported concentrations range from 14.2 to 109.0 nmol/L in healthy unsupplemented women consuming self-selected diets (Hansen et al., 2001).

The U.S. Food and Nutrition Board (IOM, 2000) chose a cutoff of < 20 nmol/L for plasma PLP as indicative of inadequacy, based on the absence of any data suggesting clinical or functional consequences at or above this level. The Euronut investigators selected this same cutoff for use in a study of the elderly living in 11 European countries (Euronut SENECA Investigators, 1991). They noted an overall prevalence of deficiency of 23%, when a cutoff of < 20 nmol/L was used, although the prevalence varied markedly among the different geographical centers. Whether this same cutoff is appropriate during infancy is unclear. The higher plasma PLP values noted for neonates and infants could reflect ample body stores of vitamin B_6 or, alternatively, normal status for this age.

A slightly lower cutoff ($< 19 \, nmol/L$) was applied by some Dutch investigators, who reported a prevalence of only 3%–7% for low plasma PLP values among 444 adults aged 20–79 y (Brussaard et al., 1997). Other investigators have chosen higher cutoffs. Leklem (1990) and Hansen et al. (2001) both advocate the use of $< 30 \, nmol/L$ as indicative of biochemical deficiency, whereas an even higher cutoff (i.e., $< 34.4 \, nmol/L$) was chosen for use in two U.K. studies (Bailey et al., 1997; Bates et al., 1999). From this discussion, it is clear that data are urgently required to better define interpretive criteria for plasma PLP levels. Such data should be based on studies that include measures of other biochemical markers of vitamin B_6 status, as well as adverse functional health outcomes (Hansen et al., 2001).

Measurement of plasma pyridoxal-5′-phosphate

The normal procedure for the assay of plasma pyridoxal-5′-phosphate uses tyrosine apodecarboxylase (EC 4.11.25) (Leklem, 1990; Euronut SENECA Investigators, 1991). Details of this reaction are given by Sauberlich (1999). The assay should be carried out under yellow light to prevent photodecomposition. This method is now well standardized so that agreement among laboratories is good.

Various methods using HPLC have also been tried to separate and quantify plasma PLP. Both cation-exchange HPLC and cation-exchange open column chromatography followed by fluorometric assay have been used (Sharma and Dakshinamurti, 1992). Problems of sample extraction, sensitivity, and sample throughput still limit the application of HPLC methods at present.

Some loss of PLP occurs when plasma is frozen at –20°C (i.e., 2.2%), but when stored at –30°C, plasma PLP is stable for up to 2 y (Borschel et al., 1987).

21.3 Erythrocyte pyridoxal-5′-phosphate

The site of PLP coenzyme function is intracellular, so erythrocyte PLP concentrations may be a promising index of vitamin B_6 status (Vermaak et al., 1990), but at present, only a few studies have included this measurement. In the experimentally controlled metabolic study of Hansen et al. (2001), erythrocyte PLP concentrations correlated with plasma total vitamin B_6, urinary total vitamin B_6, 4-pyridoxic acid, and erythrocyte AlAT basal activity. They also correlated with dietary intakes of vitamin B_6 in term and preterm infants (Heiskanen et al., 1994). When large doses of vitamin B_6 are consumed, erythrocyte PLP concentrations increase to much higher values than those noted for plasma PLP (Bhagavan et al., 1975), reflecting the high binding capacity of hemoglobin for PLP.

Reference ranges for erythrocyte PLP concentrations have been published for Finnish lactating mothers and for young children aged from 2 mo to 11 y (Heiskanen et al., 1995). Kant et al. (1988) also reported erythrocyte PLP concentrations in adults for three age groups: 25–35 y, 45–55 y, 65–75 y. More work is required to validate erythrocyte PLP as a measure of vitamin B_6 status in humans and to establish interpretive criteria. A modification of the method of Reinken (1972) used for serum PLP has been used for this assay.

Concentrations of pyridoxal-5′-phosphate in whole blood, stored at $-20°C$, remain unchanged for at least several months.

21.4 Urinary vitamin B_6

Of the vitamin B_6 excreted in urine, about 50%–75% is present in a "free" form, an the remainder in a bound form. The excretion of both forms follows the same trend, so sometimes only the free form is measured. Concentrations in urine reflect recent dietary intake rather than tissues reserves of the vitamin. Of the daily intake of vitamin B_6, about 8% to 1% is excreted as the free and bound forms.

Several experimental depletion–repletion studies in adults have shown that urinary excretion of free vitamin B$_6$ reflects recent dietary intake, but only down to a critical point, as shown in Figure 21.5; below this level further reductions in intake result in only small and variable changes in urinary vitamin B$_6$ excretion (Sauberlich, 1981; Kretsch et al., 1995). A similar trend has been noted for the total amount of the vitamin ("free" plus "bound" vitamin B$_6$) excreted in the urine (Figure 21.5).

Unlike the activity of erythrocyte aminotransferases, between-subject variability for total and free urinary vitamin B$_6$ excretion is low when subjects follow metabolic diets in depletion–repletion studies (Kretsch et al., 1995). Moreover, both total and free urinary vitamin B$_6$, and plasma PLP concentrations respond similarly to depletion, and more quickly than erythrocyte aminotransferases, so that measurements of either total or free urinary vitamin B$_6$ can be used.

In studies of populations, morning fasting urine samples are preferred to minimize variations associated with both fluid intake

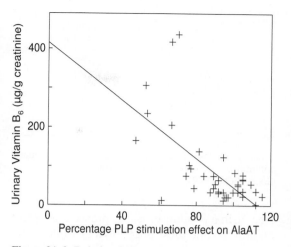

Figure 21.6: Relationship between urinary vitamin B$_6$ levels and percentage stimulation of erythrocyte AlaAT in 41 samples from U.S. female marine personnel. From Sauberlich (1981).

and physical activity. However, casual urine samples were collected in several early surveys (e.g., U.S. Ten-State Nutrition Survey) and total urinary vitamin B$_6$ concentrations were determined. Results were expressed as urinary B$_6$ per μg/g of creatinine. When expressed in this way, vitamin B$_6$ concentrations based on casual urine samples appear to be related to erythrocyte AlAT percentage stimulation (Sauberlich, 1981), as shown in Figure 21.6.

For studies of individuals, several 24-h urine collections over 1–3 wk are required to correctly reflect the long-term vitamin B$_6$ status, limiting the usefulness of urinary vitamin B$_6$ concentrations as a measure of status at the individual level (Leklem, 1990).

Drugs such as isoniazid, penicillamine, and cycloserine increase the excretion of vitamin B$_6$ in the urine, confounding the use of urinary concentrations as a measure of vitamin B$_6$ status. Data are limited on other factors affecting urinary vitamin B$_6$ excretion.

Generally, in 24-h urine samples, a urinary excretion of total vitamin B$_6$ of < 0.5 μmol/d is indicative of deficiency (Leklem, 1990). When casual urine samples are collected, interpretive critera are available for levels of

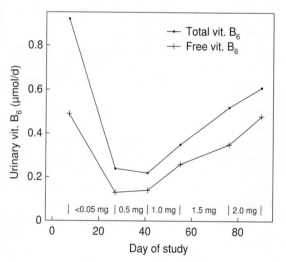

Figure 21.5: The response of total and free urinary vitamin B$_6$ concentrations to controlled intakes of vitamin B$_6$. The varying intakes (mg/d) and the duration of each regimen are also shown. Data from Kretsch et al., American Journal of Clinical Nutrition 61: 1091–1101, 1995 © Am J Clin Nutr. American Society for Clinical Nutrition.

Age group (years)	Acceptable levels (µg/g creatinine)
1–3+ y	⩾ 90
4–6+ y	⩾ 80
7–9+ y	⩾ 60
10–12+ y	⩾ 40
13–15+ y	⩾ 30
⩾16 y	⩾ 20

Table 21.6: Guidelines for evaluating "free" urinary vitamin B_6 excretion in casual urine samples. From Sauberlich (1999).

free urinary vitamin B_6 expressed as µg/g creatinine, and these are shown in Table 21.6.

Measurement of urinary vitamin B_6

To analyze total vitamin B_6, the bound form in the urine must first be converted to the "free" form by acid hydrolysis. The analysis of total and free vitamin B_6 in urine is commonly performed by microbiological assays using yeast *Saccharomyces uvarum* (*Sacch. Carlsbergensis*, ATCC No. 9080) as the test organism (Miller and Edwards, 1981). In the future, HPLC may be used, provided that problems of sample extraction, sensitivity, and throughput can be resolved.

21.5 Urinary 4-pyridoxic acid

When the adult intake of vitamin B_6 ranges from about 1 to 5 mg, about 40% to 60% is excreted as 4-pyridoxic acid (2-methyl-3-hydroxy-4-carboxy-methylpyridine), the proportion changing with age and the nature of the diet (Pannemans et al., 1994). Concentrations of 4-pyridoxic acid in urine reflect the recent dietary intake rather than tissue reserves. Levels respond very rapidly to changes in intakes within the normal range (Brown et al., 1975; Leklem, 1990; Huang et al., 1998; Hansen et al., 2001), but at low intakes, the sensitivity of urinary 4-pyridoxic acid is poor (Figure 21.7).

In some experimental depletion–repletion studies, strong correlations between urinary 4-pyridoxic acid and both vitamin B_6 intake

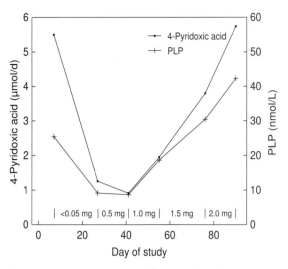

Figure 21.7: The response of urinary 4-pyridoxic acid and plasma PLP concentrations to controlled intakes of vitamin B_6. The varying intakes (mg/d) and the duration of each regimen are also shown. Data from Kretsch et al., American Journal of Clinical Nutrition 61: 1091–1101, 1995 © Am J Clin Nutr. American Society for Clinical Nutrition.

and the dietary vitamin B_6 to protein ratio have been reported at intakes ranging from 1 to 2.7 mg/d. Correlations between urinary 4-pyridoxic acid and total urinary vitamin B_6 or plasma PLP have also been strong (Figure 21.7) (Kretsch et al., 1995; Huang et al., 1998; Hansen et al., 2001).

Collection of casual urine samples appears to be a valid alternative to the measurement of 4-pyridoxic acid excretion in 24-h urine samples, provided results are expressed in terms of creatinine. Schuster et al. (1984) noted a positive correlation between 4-pyridoxic acid and 4-pyridoxic acid : creatinine ratios in the 24-h urine samples. Moreover, ratios of 4-pyridoxic acid : creatinine derived from 24-h urine samples and casual urine samples taken the next day were similar.

Interpretive criteria

Leklem (1990) suggest that a urinary 4-pyridoxic acid excretion level of ⩽ 3.0 µmol/d in males and females is associated with inadequate vitamin B_6 status. Whether such low excretion levels are associated with any adverse health consequence is uncertain.

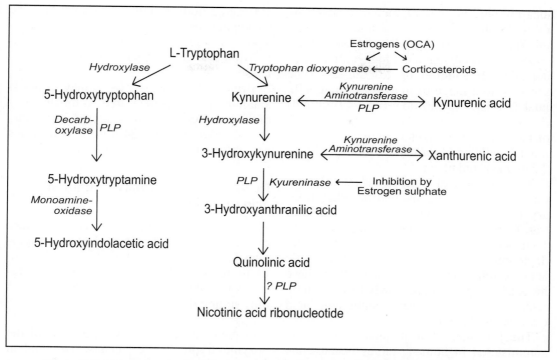

Figure 21.8: Tryptophan metabolic pathways. Reproduced with permission from Bamji (1981).

Measurement of 4-pyridoxic acid

The preferred method for the analysis of 4-pyridoxic acid in urine uses HPLC with fluorometric detection. Sample preparation is minimal: urine samples are first treated with trichloroacetic acid to precipitate any protein and are then injected directly into the HPLC system. Thereafter, the 4-pyridoxic acid is detected fluorometrically (Sharma and Dakshinamurti, 1992). In urine samples stored at −20°C, 4-pyridoxic acid is stable for at least 20 mo (Arend and Brown, 1981).

21.6 Tryptophan load test

Pyridoxal phosphate, one of the forms of vitamin B₆, is a coenzyme for kynureninase and kynurenine aminotransferase in the kynurenine pathway (Figure 21.8). Normally these enzymes act on both kynurenine and 3-hydroxykynurenine to form anthranilic and 3-hydroxyanthranilic acids, and the quinoline derivatives kynurenic and xanthurenic acids. In vitamin B₆ deficiency, the activities of the enzymes kynureninase and kynurenine aminotransferase are reduced. As a result, 3-hydroxykynurenine and kynurenine accumulate, leading to increased formation and excretion of xanthurenic and kynurenic acids, as well as kynurenine, hydroxykynurenine, and quinolinic acid, particularly if preceded by an oral loading dose of tryptophan.

Of the metabolites excreted, xanthurenic acid is usually determined after a tryptophan load as it is the most easily measured. Moreover, it is reported to be the most sensitive biochemical test for evaluating vitamin B₆ status under experimentally controlled conditions (Brown, 1981; Kretsch et al., 1995).

Several investigators have examined the response of multiple measures of vitamin B₆ status, including urinary excretion of xanthurenic acid after a tryptophan load, to the changes in vitamin B₆ status induced by depletion–repletion studies. Results have emphasized that net urinary xanthurenic acid measurement after a tryptophan load is the most sensitive biochemical index of vitamin B_6 status (Brown, 1981; Kretsch et al., 1995). Levels are markedly higher after 7 d of depletion. In addition, the test appears to be sensitive to a range of intakes of vitamin B_6 intakes when they are low (i.e., < 0.8 mg/d) (Figure 21.9). Nonetheless, the sensitivity of the tryptophan load test to intakes of vitamin B_6 within the normal adult range (1.0 to 2.5 mg/d) is unknown.

The response of other measures of vitamin B_6 status, such as plasma PLP, urinary total and free vitamin B_6, and aminotransferase activities, all lag approximately 1-wk behind the point of maximal vitamin B_6 depletion indicated by urinary xanthurenic acid excretion (Kretsch et al., 1995); these measures respond more slowly to vitamin B_6 repletion than to urinary xanthurenic acid (Hansen et al., 1997).

The L-isomer of tryptophan is normally administered in human studies because the D-isomeric form is not metabolized via the tryptophan-niacin pathway. For adults, a loading dose of 2 or 5 g of L-tryptophan is sufficient to cause increased urinary excretion of the metabolites of the kynurenine pathway. For infants and children, a loading dose of

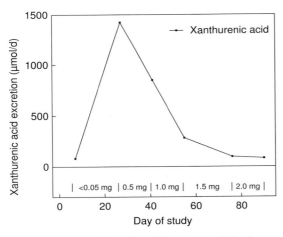

Figure 21.9: Xanthuranic acid excretion following a 4-g tryptophan load in relation to various controlled intakes. These include protein intake, exercise, lean body mass, and the size of the tryptophan loading dose. Data from Kretsch et al., American Journal of Clinical Nutrition 61: 1091–1101, 1995 © Am J Clin Nutr. American Society for Clinical Nutrition.

100 mg/kg body weight is appropriate. The tryptophan can be given as a tablet or as a powder suspended in milk, with breakfast, to avoid side effects such as somnolence and nausea.

Urine collections over 6–8 h may suffice if xanthurenic acid is measured, as the majority of the xanthurenic acid is excreted during this period. Nevertheless, 24-h urine collections are preferred (Luhby et al., 1971).

Factors affecting urinary xanthurenic acid excretion

A variety of other factors affect the urinary excretion of xanthurenic acid after a tryptophan load and interfere with this test, limiting its usefulness. These factors have been reviewed in detail by Bender (1987) and are only summarized briefly below.

Estrogens directly inhibit the activity of the enzyme tryptophan oxygenase (tryptophan pyrrolase) and, hence, the tryptophan load test is not appropriate for pregnant subjects and women taking oral contraceptive agents.

Certain drugs such as hydrocortisone also interfere with the tryptophan load test by increasing the tryptophan oxygenase activity in the liver and, hence, urinary kynurenine excretion. Some drugs also interfere with the analytical procedures (e.g., sulfonamides and para-aminosalicylic acid). Colorimetric methods in association with ion-exchange chromatography are severely affected (Price et al., 1965).

Cancer and other factors. Cancer tends to increase the urinary excretion of xanthurenic acid and the other metabolites of tryptophan after a tryptophan load (Rose and Randall, 1973). Other factors, such as protein intake, exercise, and the lean body mass may also interfere with the test (Bender, 1987).

Interpretive criteria

Leklem (1990) has suggested that a level of $\geqslant 65$ µmol/d after a 2-g tryptophan load is indicative of inadequate vitamin B$_6$ status in adults. Sauberlich (1999) notes that other investigators studying adults have used larger doses of up to 5 g L-tryptophan.

Measurement of xanthurenic acid

Several methods have been used to measure xanthurenic acid in the urine. The most frequently used techniques employ thin layer or ion-exchange chromatography for the separation of xanthurenic acid, followed by either colorimetry, spectrophotometry, or fluorometry. These methods are capable of analyzing many samples quickly and also are sensitive, specific, and reproducible (Brown, 1981; Liu et al., 1996).

Urine samples used for the measurement of the excretion of xanthurenic acid or kynurenic acid must be acidified to pH 3–4 to reduce bacterial growth and to stabilize the metabolites. Samples should be frozen at $-15°$C. Tryptophan metabolites are stable for 2–3 mo if frozen, after which significant losses of both 3-hydroxykynurenine and 3-hydroxyanthranilic acid may occur.

21.7 Kynurenine load test

The kynurenine load test was developed for use with pregnant women and subjects with disease or under stress, when interpretation of the tryptophan load test is difficult (Section 21.6). The test bypasses the enzyme tryptophan oxygenase (tryptophan pyrrolase) (Figure 21.8).

An oral dose of 200 mg of L-kynurenine sulfate produces modest and reproducible increases in the excretion of several urinary metabolites in normal subjects. Excretion levels of 3-hydroxykynurenine, kynurenine, and quinolinic acid are comparable to those seen after a 2.0 g tryptophan load, although no increase in xanthurenic acid excretion occurs. This test has also been used with oral contraceptive users and postmenopausal women receiving small doses of estradiol (Brown, 1981). However, because of the high cost of L-kynurenine sulfate, this load test has received little use.

Interestingly, Hansen et al. (1997) measured kynurenine excretion after a tryptophan load in women fed a constant protein diet with varying levels of vitamin B$_6$. The variation in kynurenine excretion among subjects was so great that although a downward trend was observed with increasing intakes of vitamin B$_6$ intakes, the changes were not significant.

21.8 Methionine load test

In vitamin B$_6$ deficiency, there is also an increase in the excretion of cystathionine that can be prevented with vitamin B$_6$ supplementation. Cystathionine is a metabolite of methionine and depends on vitamin B$_6$ for its synthesis and degradation. Figure 21.10 shows the PLP-dependent steps in an abbreviated pathway of methionine metabolism.

The urinary excretion of cystathionine, cysteine, cysteine-sulfinic acid, and homocysteine are all elevated in a vitamin B$_6$ deficient state after a loading dose of 3 g of L-methionine, whereas excretion of taurine is reduced (Park and Linkswiler, 1970). Urine samples must be collected over 24 h for the test.

The methionine load test has been used in pregnant women, in adult men suffering from neuropathy, and in patients being treated with isonicotinic acid hydrazide (Park and Linkswiler, 1970; Krishnaswamy, 1972; Shin and Linkswiler, 1974). It has been used in only a few experimental vitamin B$_6$ depletion–repletion studies. Based on these results, a cystathionine excretion concentration of > 350 µmol/d has been tentatively suggested as indicating vitamin B$_6$ deficiency (Leklem, 1990).

The potential of this test as a measure of vitamin B$_6$ status in the general population is unknown. The use of dose–response tests in population studies is difficult because timed urine samples are required. The analysis of methionine metabolites in the urine conventionally uses an amino acid analyzer.

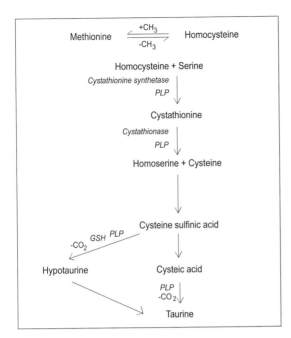

Figure 21.10: An abbreviated pathway of methionine metabolism showing the pyridoxal-5′-phosphate-dependent steps. From Bamji (1981).

A modification of the methionine load test has recently been developed by Graham et al. (1997). For this test, 100 mg of methionine per kg of body weight is given. Next, blood samples are taken fasting and 6 h after the loading dose, for analysis of plasma homocysteine and plasma PLP. Any increases in plasma homocysteine post load are assessed in relation to vitamin B_6 status, based on plasma PLP.

21.9 Multiple indices

A minimum of three biochemical tests is recommended to adequately evaluate vitamin B_6 status, over a range of intakes. The tests should include plasma PLP, together with the activation coefficient for erythrocyte AsAT, and a urinary metabolite. For epidemiological studies, urinary 4-pyridoxic acid, a short-term measure that reflects recent dietary intake, should be used; for experimental laboratory-based studies, the tryptophan load test is preferred. These biochemical tests

should be accompanied by a dietary assessment of the usual intakes of both vitamin B_6 and protein. Care must be taken to ensure that the factors known to confound these biochemical tests can be taken into account when interpreting the results.

Currently, no reliable physiological functional tests exist for assessing subclinical vitamin B_6 status. In the future, however, a test of lymphocyte function based on lymphocyte proliferation may be used in combination with the biochemical tests (Kwak et al., 2002).

Subclinical vitamin B_6 status is likely to be associated with riboflavin deficiency. Co-existence of these two vitamin deficiencies will lead to particularly adverse consequences because riboflavin is involved in vitamin B_6 metabolism. Hence, future epidemiological studies on vitamin B_6 status should include an assessment of both vitamin B_6 and riboflavin status. In a study of free-living Irish elderly, 21% had suboptimal status for both vitamin B_6 and riboflavin. Riboflavin supplementation corrected both the riboflavin deficiency and the low plasma PLP concentrations (Madigan et al., 1998).

21.10 Summary

Vitamin B_6 is present in foods mainly as pyridoxal, pyridoxine, and pyridoxamine. All of these are converted after absorption into pyridoxal-5′-phosphate (PLP) or pyridoxamine 5′-phosphate (PMP). These are the two active coenzyme forms of vitamin B_6 that catalyze a variety of enzyme systems involved in the metabolism of protein and amino acids and, to a lesser extent, carbohydrates and lipids.

Several biochemical tests for vitamin B_6 status exist. Their selection depends on both the study objectives and the characteristics of the study group. The tests most widely used are the activation coefficient for erythrocyte AsAT, plasma PLP concentrations, and urinary 4-pyridoxic acid excretion. Activity of erythrocyte AsAT reflects vitamin B_6 status over about the last month. Plasma PLP concentrations provide a more direct measure of the active coenzyme and reflect dietary intake and tissue status of vitamin B$_6$. In epidemiological studies, however, plasma PLP levels are affected by many factors, confounding the interpretation of the results. In contrast, urinary excretion levels of free vitamin B$_6$ and 4-pyridoxic acid reflect recent dietary intakes of vitamin B$_6$ rather than tissue levels.

The tryptophan load test is a sensitive functional biochemical test that is used in clinical settings to provide an indirect measure of low tissue vitamin B$_6$ levels. At present, the evaluation of vitamin B$_6$ status should include a combination of dietary intake and three biochemical tests (plasma PLP, erythrocyte AsAT AC, and a urinary metabolite). Future studies may include a test of lymphocyte function based on lymphocyte proliferation in addition to the three biochemical tests recommended.

References

Arend RA, Brown RR. (1981). Comparison of analytical methods for urinary 4-pyridoxic acid. American Journal of Clinical Nutrition 34: 1984–1985.

Axelrod AE, Trakatellis AC. (1964). Relationship of pyridoxine to immunological phenomena. Vitamins and Hormones 22: 591–607.

Bailey AL, Maisey S, Southon S, Wright A, Finglas P, Fulcher RA. (1997). Relationships between micronutrient intake and biochemical indicators of nutrient adequacy in a "free-living" elderly U.K. population. British Journal of Nutrition 77: 225–242.

Bamji MS. (1981). Laboratory tests for the assessment of vitamin nutritional status. In: Briggs MH (ed.) Vitamins in Human Biology and Medicine. CRC Press, Boca Raton, FL, pp. 2–27.

Bates CJ, Pentieva KD, Prentice A. (1999). An appraisal of vitamin B$_6$ status indices and associated confounders, in young people aged 4–18 years and in people aged 65 years and over, in two national British surveys. Public Health Nutrition 2: 529–535.

Bender DA. (1987). Oestrogens and vitamin B$_6$: actions and interactions. World Review of Nutrition and Dietetics 51: 140–188.

Bhagavan HN. (1985). Interaction between vitamin B$_6$ and drugs. In: Reynolds RD, Leklem JE (eds.) Vitamin B$_6$: Its Role in Health and Disease. Liss, New York, pp. 401–415.

Bhagavan HN, Coleman M, Coursin DB. (1975). The effect of pyridoxine hydrochloride on blood sero-

tonin and pyridoxal phosphate contents in hyperactive children. Pediatrics 55: 437–441.

Black AL, Guirard BM, Snell EE. (1978). The behavior of muscle phosphorylase as a reservoir for vitamin B$_6$ in the rat. Journal of Nutrition 108: 670–677.

Borschel MW, Kirksey A, Hamaker BR. (1987). A micromethod for determination of plasma pyridoxal phosphate and its use in assessment of storage stability of the vitamer. Journal of Pediatric Gastroenterology and Nutrition 6: 409–413.

Brown RR. (1981). The tryptophan load test as an index of vitamin B$_6$ nutrition. In: Leklem JE, Reynolds RD (eds.) Methods in Vitamin B$_6$ Nutrition. Plenum Press, New York, pp. 321–340.

Brown RR, Rose D, Leklem J, Linkswiler H, Anand R. (1975). Urinary 4-pyridoxic acid, plasma pyridoxal phosphate, and erythrocyte aminotransferase levels in oral contraceptive users receiving controlled intakes of vitamin B$_6$. American Journal of Clinical Nutrition 28: 10–19.

Brussaard JH, Lowik MR, van den Berg H, Brants HA, Kistemaker C. (1997). Micronutrient status, with special reference to Vitamin B$_6$. European Journal of Clinical Nutrition 51: S32–S38.

Cinnamon AD, Beaton JR. (1970). Biochemical assessment of vitamin B$_6$ status in man. American Journal of Clinical Nutrition 23: 696–702.

Dolphin D, Poulson R, Avarmovic O (eds.). (1986) Vitamin B$_6$ Pyridoxal Phosphate: Chemical, Biochemical and Medical Aspects. John Wiley and Sons, New York.

Driskell JA. (1994). Vitamin B$_6$ requirement of humans. Nutrition Research 14: 293–324.

Euronut SENECA Investigators. (1991). Nutritional status: blood vitamins A, E, B$_6$, B$_{12}$, folic acid and carotene. European Journal of Clinical Nutrition 45: 63–82.

FAO/WHO (Food and Agriculture Organization/World Health Organization (2002). Human Vitamin and Mineral Requirements. Report of a Joint FAO/WHO Expert Consultation, Bangkok, Thailand. World Health Organization, Food and Agricultural Organization of the United Nations, Rome.

Finch S, Doyle W, Lowe C, Bates CJ, Prentice A, Smithers G, Clarke PC. (1998). National Diet and Nutrition Survey: People Aged 65 Years and Over. Volume 1: Report of the Diet and Nutrition Survey. The Stationery Office, London.

Graham IM, Daly LE, Refsum HM, Robinson K, Brattstrom LE, Ueland PM, Palma-Reis RJ, Boers GH, Sheahan RG, Israelsson B, Uiterwaal C, Meleady R, et al. (1997). Plasma homocysteine as a risk factor for vascular disease. Journal of the American Medical Association 277: 1775–1781.

Gregory J, Foster K, Tyler H, Wiseman M. (1990). The Dietary and Nutritional Survey of British Adults. Her Majesty's Stationery Office, London.

Gregory J, Lowe S, Bates CJ, Prentice A, Jackson LV, Smithers G, Wenlock R, Farron M. (2000). National Diet and Nutrition Survey: Young People Aged 4 to 18 Years. Volume 1: Report of the Diet and Nutrition Survey. The Stationery Office, London.

Gregory JF 3rd. (1997). Bioavailability of vitamin B$_6$. European Journal of Clinical Nutrition 51: S43–S48.

Hansen CM, Shultz TD. (2001). Stability of vitamin B$_6$-dependent aminotransferase activity in frozen packed erythrocytes is dependent on storage temperature. Journal of Nutrition 131: 1581–1583.

Hansen CM, Leklem JE, Miller LT. (1997). Changes in vitamin B$_6$ status indicators of women fed a constant protein diet with varying levels of vitamin B$_6$. American Journal of Clinical Nutrition 66: 1379–1387.

Hansen CM, Shultz TD, Kwak H-K, Memon HS, Leklem JE. (2001). Assessment of vitamin B$_6$ status in young women consuming a controlled diet containing four levels of vitamin B$_6$ provides an estimated average requirement and recommended dietary allowance. Journal of Nutrition 131: 1777–1786.

Heiskanen K, Salmenperä L, Perheentupa J, Siimes M. (1994). Infant vitamin B$_6$ status changes with age and with formula feeding. American Journal of Clinical Nutrition 60: 907–910.

Heiskanen K, Kallio M, Salmenperä L, Siimes MA, Ruokonen I, Perheentupa J. (1995). Vitamin B$_6$ status during childhood: tracking from 21 months to 11 years of age. Journal of Nutrition 125: 2985–2992.

Hercberg S, Preziosi P, Galan P, Devanlay M, Keller H, Bourgeois C, Potier de Courcy G, Cherouvrier F. (1994). Vitamin status of a healthy French population: dietary intakes and biochemical markers. International Journal for Vitamin and Nutrition Research 64: 220–232.

Huang YC, Chen W, Evans M, Mitchell M, Shultz T. (1998). Vitamin B$_6$ requirement and status assessment of young women fed a high-protein diet with various levels of vitamin B$_6$. American Journal of Clinical Nutrition 67: 208–220

IOM (Institute of Medicine). (2000). Dietary Reference Intakes for Thiamin, Riboflavin, Niacin, Vitamin B$_6$, Folate, Vitamin B$_{12}$, Pantothenic Acid, Biotin, and Choline. National Academy Press, Washington, DC.

Kant AK, Moser-Veillon PB, Reynolds RD. (1988). Effect of age on changes in plasma, erythrocyte, and urinary B$_6$ vitamers after an oral vitamin B$_6$ load. American Journal of Clinical Nutrition 48: 1284–1290.

Kretsch M, Sauberlich H, Skala J, Johnson HL. (1995). Vitamin B$_6$ requirements and status assessment: young women fed a depletion diet followed by a plant- or animal-protein diet with graded amounts of vitamin B$_6$ American Journal of Clinical Nutrition 61: 1091–1101.

Krishnaswamy K. (1972). Methionine load test in pyridoxine deficiency. International Journal for Vitamin and Nutrition Research 42: 468–475.

Kwak HK, Hansem C, Leklem J, Hardin K, Shultz T. (2002). Improved vitamin B$_6$ status is positively related to lymphocyte proliferation in young women

consuming a controlled diet. Journal of Nutrition 132: 3308–3313.

Leklem JE. (1990). Vitamin B$_6$: a status report. Journal of Nutrition 120: 1503–1507.

Leklem JE. (1994). Vitamin B$_6$. In: Shils ME, Olson JA, Shike H (eds.) Modern Nutrition in Health and Disease. 8th ed. Lea & Febiger, Philadelphia, pp. 383–394.

Leklem JE. (1996). Vitamin B$_6$. In: Ziegler EE, Filer LJ (eds.) Present Knowledge in Nutrition. 7th ed. International Life Sciences Institute Press, Washington, DC. pp. 174–183.

Leklem JE, Hollenbeck CB. (1990). Acute ingestion of glucose decreases plasma pyridoxal-5′-phosphate and total vitamin B$_6$ concentrations. American Journal of Clinical Nutrition 51: 832–836.

Liu A, Lumeng L, Aronoff GR, Li T-K. (1985). Relationship between body store of vitamin B$_6$ and plasma pyridoxal-P clearance: metabolic balance studies in humans. Journal of Laboratory and Clinical Medicine 106: 491–497.

Liu M, Wang GR, Liu TZ, Tsai KJ. (1996) Improved fluorometric quantification of urinary xanthurenic acid. Clinical Chemistry 42: 397–401.

Löwik MRH, van Poppel G, Wedel M, van den Berg H, Schrijver J. (1990). Dependence of vitamin B$_6$ status assessment on alcohol intake among elderly men and women (Dutch Nutrition Surveillance System). Journal of Nutrition 120: 1344–1351.

Luhby AL, Brin M, Gorden M, Davis P, Murphy M, Spiegel H. (1971). Vitamin B$_6$ metabolism in users of oral contraceptive agents. I: Abnormal urinary xanthurenic acid excretion and its correction by pyridoxine. American Journal of Clinical Nutrition 24: 684–693.

Lumeng L, Li TK. (1974). Vitamin B$_6$ metabolism in chronic alcohol abuse. Pyridoxal phosphate levels in plasma and the effects of acetaldehyde on pyridoxal phosphate synthesis and degradation in human erythrocytes. Journal of Clinical Investigation 53: 693–704.

Lumeng L, Ryan MP, Li T-K. (1978). Validation of the diagnostic value of plasma pyridoxal-5′-phosphate measurements in vitamin B$_6$ nutrition of the rat. Journal of Nutrition 108: 545–553.

Madigan SM, Tracey F, McNulty H, Eaton-Evans J, Coulter J, McCartney H, Strain JJ. (1998). Riboflavin and vitamin B$_6$ intakes and status and biochemical response to riboflavin supplementation in free-living elderly people. American Journal of Clinical Nutrition 68: 389–395.

Manore MM, Vaughan LA, Carroll SS, Leklem JE. (1989). Plasma pyridoxal 5′-phosphate concentration and dietary vitamin B$_6$ intake in free-living, low-income elderly people. American Journal of Clinical Nutrition 50: 339–345.

Martner-Hewes PM, Hunt IF, Murphy NJ, Swendseid ME, Settlage RH. (1986). Vitamin B$_6$ nutriture and plasma diamine oxidase activity in pregnant Hispanic teenagers. American Journal of Clinical Nutrition 44: 907–913.

Masse PG, van den Berg H, Duguay C, Beaulieu G, Simard JM. (1996). Early effect of low dose (30 micrograms) ethinyl estradiol-containing Triphasil on vitamin B_6 status: a follow-up study on six menstrual cycles. International Journal for Vitamin and Nutrition Research 66: 46–54.

McCully KS. (1969). Vascular pathology of homocysteinemia: implications for the pathogenesis of arteriosclerosis. American Journal of Pathology 56: 111–128

Meydani SN, Ribaya-Mercado JD, Russell RM, Sahyoun N, Morrow FD, Gershoff SN. (1991). Vitamin B_6 deficiency impairs interleukin production and lymphocyte proliferation in elderly adults. American Journal of Clinical Nutrition 53: 1275–1280.

Miller LT, Edwards M. (1981). Microbiological assay of vitamin B_6 in blood and urine. In: Leklem JE, Reynolds RD (eds.) Methods in Vitamin B_6 Nutrition. pp. 45–55. Plenum Press, New York.

Ockhuizen T, Spanhaak S, Mares N, Veenstra J, Wedel M, Mulder J, van den Berg H. (1990). Short-term effects of marginal vitamin B deficiencies on immune parameters in healthy young volunteers. Nutrition Research 10: 483–492.

Pannemans DLE, van den Berg H, Westerterp KR. (1994). The influence of protein intake on vitamin B_6 metabolism differs in young and elderly humans. Journal of Nutrition 124: 1207–1214.

Park YK, Linkswiler H. (1970). Effect of vitamin B_6 depletion in adult man on the excretion of cystathionine and other methionine metabolites. Journal of Nutrition 100: 110–116.

Price JM, Brown RR, Yess N. (1965). Testing the functional capacity of the tryptophan-niacin pathway in man by analysis of urinary metabolites. Advances in Metabolic Disorders 2: 159–225.

Rall LC, Meydani SN. (1993). Vitamin B_6 and immune competence. Nutrition Reviews 51: 217–225.

Rechcigl M. Jr. (ed) (1983). CRC Handbook of Naturally Occurring Food Toxicants. CRC Press, Boca Raton, FL.

Reinken L. (1972). A microassay of pyridoxal phosphate in serum based on decarboxylation of L-tyrosine-I-14C. (German). International Journal of Vitamin and Nutrition Research 42: 476–481.

Reynolds RD. (1995). Biomedical methods for status assessment. In: Raiten DJ (ed.) Vitamin B_6 Metabolism in Pregnancy, Lactation, and Infancy. CRC Press, Boca Raton, FL. p.41–59.

Reynolds RD, Leklem JE. (1985). Vitamin B_6: Its Role in Health and Disease. Arthur R Liss, New York.

Ribaya-Mercado JD, Russell RM, Sahyoun N, Morrow FD, Gershoff SN. (1991). Vitamin B_6 requirements of elderly men and women. Journal of Nutrition 121: 1062–1074.

Rose DP, Randall ZC. (1973). Influence of the loading dose on the demonstration of abnormal tryptophan metabolism by cancer patients. Clinica Chimica Acta 47: 45–49.

Russell RM. (1992). Micronutrient requirements of the elderly. Nutrition Reviews 50: 463–466.

Sauberlich HE. (1981). Vitamin B_6 status assessment: past and present. In: Leklem JE, Reynolds RD (eds.) Methods in Vitamin B_6 Nutrition: Analysis and Status Assessment. Plenum Press, New York, pp. 203–239.

Sauberlich HE. (1984). Newer laboratory methods for assessing nutriture of selected B-complex vitamins. Annual Review of Nutrition 4: 377–407.

Sauberlich HE. (1999). Laboratory Tests for the Assessment of Nutritional Status. CRC Press, Boca Raton, FL.

Schaumburg H, Kaplan J, Windebank A, Vick N, Rasmus S, Pleasure D, Brown MJ. (1983). Sensory neuropathy from pyridoxine abuse: a new megavitamin syndrome. New England Journal of Medicine 309: 445–448.

Schuster K, Bailey LB, Mahan CS. (1981). Vitamin B_6 status of low-income adolescent and adult pregnant women and the condition of their infants at birth. American Journal of Clinical Nutrition 34: 1731–1735.

Schuster K, Bailey LB, Cerda JJ, Gregory JF. (1984). Urinary 4-pyridoxic acid excretion in 24-hour versus random urine samples as a measurement of vitamin B_6 status in humans. American Journal of Clinical Nutrition 39: 466–470.

Selhub J, Jacques PF, Bostom AG, D'Agostino RB, Wilson PW, Belanger AJ, O'Leary DH, Wolf PA, Schaefer EJ, Rosenberg IH. (1995). Association between homocysteine concentrations and extracranial carotid-artery stenosis. New England Journal of Medicine 332: 286–291

Sharma SK, Dakshinamurti K. (1992). Determination of vitamin B_6 vitamers and pyridoxic acid in biological samples. Journal of Chromatography 578:45–51

Shin HK, Linkswiler HM. (1974). Tryptophan and methionine metabolism of adult females as affected by vitamin B_6 deficiency. Journal of Nutrition 104: 1348–1355.

Skala JH, Gretz D, Waring PP. (1987). An automated continuous-flow procedure for simultaneous measurement of erythrocyte alanine and aspartate aminotranferase activities. Nutrition Research 7: 731–741.

Talbott MC, Miller LT, Kerkvleit NI. (1987). Pyridoxine supplementation: effect on lymphocyte responses in elderly persons. American Journal of Clinical Nutrition 46: 659–664.

Ubbink JB, Bissort S, van den Berg I, de Villiers L, Becker PJ. (1989a). Genetic polymorphism of glutamate-pyruvate transaminase (alanine aminotransaminase): influence on erythrocyte activity as a marker of vitamin B_6 nutritional status. American Journal of Clinical Nutrition 50: 1420–1428.

Ubbink JB, Delport R, Becker PJ, Bissport S. (1989b). Evidence of a theophylline-induced vitamin B_6 deficiency due to noncompetitive inhibition of pyridoxal kinase. Journal of Laboratory and Clinical Medicine 113: 15–22.

van den Berg H, Heseker H, Lamand M, Sandström B, Thurnham D. (1993). FLAIR Concerted Action

No. 10 status papers: introduction, conclusions and recommendations. International Journal for Vitamin and Nutrition Research 63: 247–251.

Vermaak WJ, Barnard HC, Potgieter G, du Theron H. (1987). Vitamin B_6 and coronary artery disease: epidemiological observations and case studies. Atherosclerosis 63: 235.

Vermaak WJ, Ubbink JB, Barnard HC, Potgieter GM, van Jaarsveld H, Groenewald AJ. (1990). Vitamin B_6 nutrition status and cigarette smoking. American Journal of Clinical Nutrition 51: 1058–1061.

Vuilleumier JP, Keller HE, Keck E. (1990). Clinical chemical methods for the routine assessment of the vitamin status in human populations. Part III: The apoenzyme stimulation tests for vitamins B_1, B_2, and B_6 adapted to the Cobas-Bio analyzer. International Journal for Vitamin and Nutrition Research 60: 126–135.

22

Assessment of folate and vitamin B_{12} status

Deficiencies of the two related vitamins, folic acid and vitamin B_{12}, cause megaloblastic anemia, an anemia characterized by abnormally large red-cell precursors (megaloblasts) in the bone marrow and larger than normal red cells (macrocytic cells) in the peripheral blood. These abnormalities in cell morphology arise because a deficiency of either vitamin B_{12} or folate impairs the production of 5,10-methylene tetrahydrofolate, which is essential for the biosynthesis of deoxyribonucleic acid (DNA). Interference with DNA synthesis induces abnormal cell replication, especially in rapidly dividing cells.

Vitamin B_{12} deficiency may also produce neurological disorders and spinal cord dysfunction, even in the absence of anemia. These abnormalities, attributed to the role of vitamin B_{12} in the synthesis of myelin in the nervous system, may not be reversible. Demyelination of nerves arises because of the interruption in the methylation cycle, specifically by the interference in the production of S-adenosylmethionine from methionine.

In folate deficiency, demyelinating neuropathy occurs surprisingly rarely, probably because nervous tissue has the ability to accumulate folate. As a result, the supply of S-adenosylmethionine (SAM) is preserved during folate deprivation. When folate deficiency is very severe and very prolonged, however, a folate-responsive neuropathy may develop (Manzoor and Runcie, 1976).

Other neuropsychiatric disturbances such as depression and dementia have been associated with both folate and vitamin B_{12} deficiencies, even when serum concentrations are within the low-to-normal range (Bottiglieri, 1996).

Even in the absence of overt clinical signs and symptoms, some biochemically detectable changes common to both folate and vitamin B_{12} deficiency occur. Of these, probably the most notable is the elevation in total plasma homocysteine concentration that occurs even with only modest dietary inadequacies (Selhub et al., 1993; Mason, 2003).

Accumulation of homocysteine in blood arises because of an interruption in the methylation cycle, shown by step D in Figure 22.1, whereby homocysteine is remethylated back to methionine (Carmel, 2000). Interruption of methylation may occur because of a reduced supply of 5-methyltetrahydrofolate as a methyl donor or because of reduced activity of the vitamin B_{12}-dependent enzyme methionine synthetase. In certain settings, deficiencies of vitamin B_6 and riboflavin may also interfere with methylation reactions, leading to a rise in plasma homocysteine levels. An elevated homocysteine concentration is important because it is known to be an independent risk factor for premature cardiovascular disease or stroke (Pancharuniti et al., 1994). Moreover, the risk appears to be associated with an apparently "normal" folate or vitamin B_{12} status (Scott, 1999).

It is possible that other complications that have been associated with vitamin B_{12} and folate deficiency — including both gastrointestinal and immunological disorders (Chanarin, 1980; Green and Miller, 1999), some

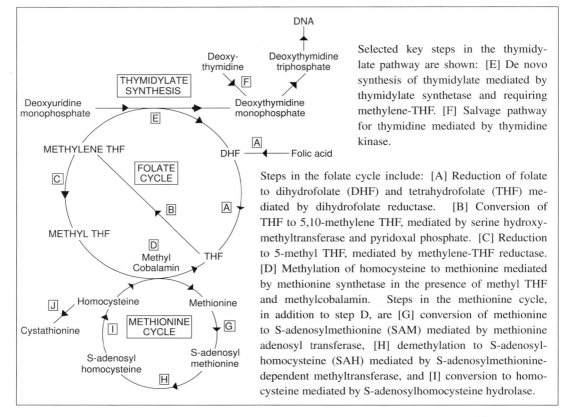

Selected key steps in the thymidylate pathway are shown: [E] De novo synthesis of thymidylate mediated by thymidylate synthetase and requiring methylene-THF. [F] Salvage pathway for thymidine mediated by thymidine kinase.

Steps in the folate cycle include: [A] Reduction of folate to dihydrofolate (DHF) and tetrahydrofolate (THF) mediated by dihydrofolate reductase. [B] Conversion of THF to 5,10-methylene THF, mediated by serine hydroxymethyltransferase and pyridoxal phosphate. [C] Reduction to 5-methyl THF, mediated by methylene-THF reductase. [D] Methylation of homocysteine to methionine mediated by methionine synthetase in the presence of methyl THF and methylcobalamin. Steps in the methionine cycle, in addition to step D, are [G] conversion of methionine to S-adenosylmethionine (SAM) mediated by methionine adenosyl transferase, [H] demethylation to S-adenosylhomocysteine (SAH) mediated by S-adenosylmethionine-dependent methyltransferase, and [I] conversion to homocysteine mediated by S-adenosylhomocysteine hydrolase.

Figure 22.1: The folate metabolic cycle and its interaction with cobalamin, the thymidylate pathway, and the methionine cycle. Also shown: [J] is the initial step in the unrelated transsulfuration pathway of homocysteine mediated by cystathionine β-synthase and requiring pyridoxal 5-phosphate. From Carmel, Annual Review of Medicine, Volume 51, 2000 © by Annual Reviews, with permission.

cancers (Choi, 1999), orofacial clefts (Tolarova and Harris, 1995), and neural tube defects (Daly et al., 1995) — also occur when levels for these two vitamins are within the normal range. Certainly, these complications often precede or occur in the absence of hematological disturbances (Green and Miller, 1999). With the exception of neural tube defects, these complications are less well characterized than the hematological defects associated with vitamin B_{12} and folate deficiencies. More research is required to confirm these interrelationships.

Folate deficiency usually develops more rapidly than vitamin B_{12} deficiency because of differences in turnover rates. Inadequate dietary intake is a major factor associated with folate deficiency. In contrast, the amount of vitamin B_{12} in omnivorous diets usually

greatly exceeds the estimated daily requirements. As a result, vitamin B_{12} deficiency generally arises in a variety of other ways. For example, defects in absorption per se or failure to secrete the gastric intrinsic factor necessary for the absorption of the vitamin may induce the deficiency (Stabler and Allen, 2004).

Diagnosis of megaloblastic anemia can be confirmed by the presence of macro-ovalocytic erythrocytes in peripheral blood and megaloblasts in the bone marrow. Conventional biochemical assessment techniques can be used to establish whether the megaloblastic anemia results from folic acid or vitamin B_{12} deficiency and to detect consequences from deficiencies of these two vitamins.

There is growing emphasis on the use of more sensitive biochemical tests for these two vitamins. These include homocysteine in plasma for folate and methylmalonic acid in plasma for vitamin B$_{12}$. Their use has increased with the knowledge that even modest dietary inadequacies of folate and vitamin B$_{12}$ contribute to important diseases such as neural tube defects, cardiovascular disease, and cancer. These biochemical tests are discussed in the following sections.

22.1 Folate

"Folate" is the term used as a generic descriptor for folic acid (pteroylmonoglutamic acid) and related compounds that exhibit the biological activity of folic acid. The pteroylmonoglutamic acid (PGA) molecule consists of a pterin nucleus (also called pteridine) linked via a methylene bridge to para-aminobenzoic acid (PABA) and glutamic acid (Figure 22.2). Reduced forms of this molecule are called dihydrofolate and tetrahydrofolate.

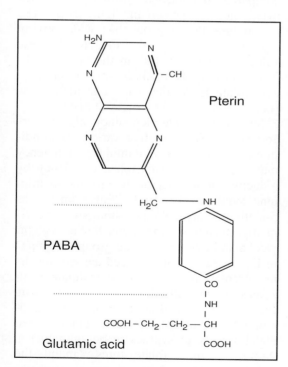

Figure 22.2: Structure of folic acid showing the pterin nucleus, and para-aminobenzoic acid (PABA) and glutamic acid components.

Functions of folate

Folates function as coenzymes only in the polyglutamate form. Hence, the folate monoglutamate forms in the blood are first reduced by folylpolyglutamate synthase and then resynthesized to the polyglutamate form. Folate coenzymes are involved in the transfer of single-carbon atom groups [e.g., methyl (CH$_3$), methylene (CH$_2$), methenyl (CH), forminino (CH=NH), and formyl (CHO)] in intermediary metabolism. These single-carbon atom groups are involved in five key metabolic functions of folate. For example, the methylene group participates in the metabolism of both serine and glycine and also in thymidylate synthesis. The forminino group is involved in histidine catabolism, the methyl group has a role in methionine synthesis, and both the methenyl and formyl groups are involved in purine synthesis. Metabolic intraconversion of these forms occurs via oxidation – reduction reactions (Klee, 2000). The reader is referred to Bailey (1995) for a detailed review of the functions of folate.

Absorption and metabolism of folate

Folate absorption takes place by an active process, primarily from the proximal third of the small intestine. Before absorption, the polyglutamate forms of folate are deconjugated to the monoglutamate form in the gut by the enzyme γ-glutamylhydrolase (more commonly termed folate conjugase). The monoglutamates are then taken up by the mucosal cells (Steinberg, 1984).

Most of the monoglutamates that are absorbed, including 5-methyltetrahydrofolate, are transported to the liver and then metabolized to polyglutamate derivatives by the enzyme folylpolyglutamate synthetase. These polyglutamate derivatives are stored in the liver or converted to 5-methyltetrahydrofolate for secretion into the bile. They are then reabsorbed by way of the enterohepatic circulation. This recirculation process may account for as much as 50% of the total folate that reaches the peripheral tissues. In the blood, folate is found as a monoglutamate, mainly as the reduced form — methyltetrahydrofolate.

Folate deficiency in humans

Rapidly proliferating cells are especially sensitive to abnormalities in DNA synthesis. Hence, clinical manifestations of folate deficiency appear first in the hematopoietic system and then in the epithelial cell surfaces and the gonads. Thus, one of the earliest signs of folate deficiency in humans is hypersegmentation of neutrophils, first in the bone marrow and then in the peripheral blood. This is eventually followed by macrocytosis of the erythrocytes. Some additional signs and symptoms that are associated with clinical folate deficiency include fatigue, angular cheilosis, anorexia, insomnia, glossitis, recurrent aphthous ulcers, and pallor of the skin and mucous membranes.

The prevalence of megaloblastic anemia, characteristic of severe folate deficiency, may be particularly high in pregnant and lactating women in developing countries. Here, dietary intakes of folate are often inadequate to meet the high requirements of pregnancy (O'Connor, 1994).

Marginal folate status, indicated mainly by low serum or erythrocyte folate concentrations, has also been reported in some low birth-weight and premature infants (Worthington-White et al., 1994). Women (Wartanowicz et al., 2001), especially if pregnant and lactating (Bailey et al., 1980), the elderly (Wagner et al., 1981; Rosenberg et al., 1982), and adolescents of low socioeconomic status (Bailey et al., 1982) are also at risk.

The role of folate in the prevention of neural tube defects is now established (MRC Vitamin Study Research Group, 1991; IOM, 2000), although the mechanism is still uncertain. Risk of neural tube defects is inversely associated with folate intake (Werler et al., 1993; Shaw et al., 1995), and erythrocyte folate concentration (Daly et al., 1995; Scott, 1999). However, it appears that the risk of neural tube defects may be associated with a folate status that would not conventionally be classed as deficient. In a prospective study of

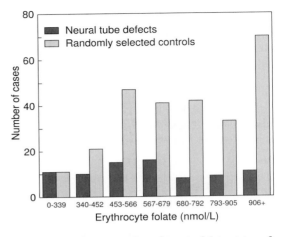

Figure 22.3: The maternal erythrocyte folate status of 84 cases of neural tube defects compared with that of 247 randomly selected controls. Data from Scott, Proceedings of the Nutrition Society 58: 441–448, 1999, with permission of the Nutrition Society.

women in Ireland, erythrocyte (and plasma) folate concentrations were measured in cases of neural tube defects during pregnancy and compared to controls; results for erythrocyte folate are shown in Figure 22.3. The neural tube defect group had wide-ranging erythrocyte folate levels; in general, these values were lower than in the control subjects, but only 12 of the cases had erythrocyte folate levels that were considered low (i.e., < 340 nmol/L) (Scott et al., 1994).

Secondary folate deficiency also occurs and is associated with a variety of conditions. For example, vitamin B_{12} deficiency may induce secondary folate deficiency by reducing the activity of the enzyme methionine synthase (EC 2.1.1.13 also known as 5-methyltetrahydrofolate—homocysteine *S*-methyltransferase) an enzyme that uses methylcobalamin as a prosthetic group for step D in Figure 22.1. This reduced activity results in a decrease in all the tetrahydrofolate coenzymes except methylfolate. Hence, the folate cofactors in the cell become "trapped" as 5-methyltetrahydrofolate, which cannot be used metabolically to synthesize polyglutamates. As a result, tissue folate stores — mainly the polyglutamates — decrease, and short-chain-length folates leak from the cells, resulting in tissue folate depletion.

Fragile X syndrome and 5,10-methylene-tetrahydrofolate reductase deficiency, two genetic disorders, are also associated with folate deficiency. High levels of folate supplements may provide some benefit to patients with severe mental retardation caused by fragile X syndrome. Therapy with 5-formyl-tetrahydrofolate may help in preventing the neurological deterioration associated with a 5,10-methylenetetrahydrofolate reductase deficiency.

Malabsorption of folate secondary to an infection with *Giardia lamblia* and bacterial overgrowth has been observed (Hjelt et al., 1992). Certain drugs affect the absorption of folate (e.g., sulfasalazine, aspirin, and perhaps cholestyramine), whereas others such as the antimalarial drug pyrimethamine, and possibly some anticonvulsants, interfere with the metabolism of folate. Folate deficiency is also seen in conditions of increased cellular turnover in cancer and hemolytic anemia.

Food sources and dietary intakes

Folates are widely distributed in food, especially in liver, yeast, leafy vegetables, fruits, pulses, and nuts, where they exist primarily as pteroylpolyglutamates. These contain up to nine glutamate residues linked in the form of a γ-polypeptide chain to PABA. The principal pteroylpolyglutamates in foods are 5-methyltetrahydrofolate and 10-formyltetra-hydrofolate, although numerous other forms have also been reported.

The nutritional activity of these polyglutamates remains intact as long as the essential subunit structure of PGA is not broken. Heat, air, and ultraviolet light cleave PGA, making it inactive. Folate may also be lost during food preparation because of leaching from the food into cooking water. Consequently, diets based on thoroughly cooked foods are generally low in folate. Estimated losses of folate from food preparation or processing range from 50% to 95% (Sauberlich, 1985).

Folic acid — pteroylmonoglutamic acid — is not present naturally in significant amounts in foods but is the form of folate commonly used in food fortification and supplementa-tion. The folic acid in fortified grain products is absorbed as well as supplemental folic acid (Pfeiffer et al., 1997).

The bioavailability of folate ranges from nearly 100% for folic acid supplements taken on an empty stomach to approximately 50% for pteroylpolyglutamates in food (Pfeiffer et al., 1997). These differences have led to the development of folate equivalents to estimate bioavailable folate in diets; more details are given in Section 4.8.8. So far there is no conclusive evidence that the bioavailability of dietary folate is influenced by other dietary components (Brouwer et al., 2001), although one study has reported a positive relationship between dietary fiber and folate status (Houghton et al., 1997).

In many industrialized countries, the most important food sources of folate are often ready-to-eat breakfast cereals, when these are fortified with folate, and vegetables (McLennan and Podger, 1998; Russell et al., 1999; IOM, 2000). The increasing trend to fortify cereal grains with folate in both industrialized and low-income countries will increase folate intakes in many countries. In 1998, the United States introduced fortification of enriched cereal grains at a level of 1.4 mg/kg grain (FDA, 1996), whereas Canada has chosen a level of 1.5 mg/kg for both wheat flour and cornmeal (Health Canada, 2003).

Effects of high intakes of folate

Generally, consumption of excess folate has not been accompanied by any adverse reactions. Indeed, folate is considered to be a nontoxic vitamin, except in epileptic patients, in whom very large doses may precipitate convulsions (Bailey, 1992). The U.S. Food and Nutrition Board has set the Tolerable Upper Intake Level (UL) for folate for adults, including pregnant and lactating women, at 1000 µg/d; details for children and adolescents are given in IOM (2000).

Indices of folate status

Static biochemical tests that measure folate levels in serum and erythrocytes are gener-

Disorder	Causes of macrocytosis	Comments
Alcoholism	Direct effect of alcohol on the bone marrow	Concurrent folate deficiency or liver disease may contribute to the macrocytosis
Liver disease	Defective DNA synthesis or accelerated erythropoiesis	Concurrent folate deficiency or alcoholism may contribute to the macrocytosis
Hemolysis	Accelerated erythropoiesis with reticulocytosis; hemolysis may also increase folate requirements	The presence of associated folate deficiency may be masked by an increase in the serum folate level caused by red blood cell lysis
Posthemorrhagic anemia	Accelerated erythropoiesis with reticulocytosis	
Hypothyroidism	Uncertain	Mean cell volume is usually normal or only slightly elevated; pernicious anemia is more prevalent in patients with autoimmune thyroid disease
Cold agglutin disease	Artifactual; clumping of red blood cells	
Severe hyperglycemia	Artifactual; swelling of red blood cells	

Table 22.1: Nonmegaloblastic causes of macrocytosis with or without anemia. From Snow, Archives of Internal Medicine 159: 1289–1298, 1999.

ally used to assess folate status, although homocysteine in serum or plasma is now increasingly used as a functional test of folate deficiency. As a coexisting deficiency of vitamin B_{12} may interfere with the diagnosis of folate deficiency, tests for folate deficiency should be performed together with an assessment of serum vitamin B_{12} concentrations.

22.1.1 Red cell indices

The abnormal morphological changes in the peripheral blood and bone marrow that occur in both folate and vitamin B_{12} deficiency are identical; they involve the development of megaloblastic anemia. The changes mark the final stages of chronic folate (or vitamin B_{12}) deficiency, and occur in adults after 3–4 mo of folate deprivation (O'Connor, 1994).

Macrocytosis can be tentatively diagnosed by identifying abnormally large red cells (macro-ovalocytic erythrocytes) in peripheral blood, and confirmed by the presence of an elevated mean cell volume. Several other conditions associated with bone marrow failure and other systemic diseases may also

result in abnormally large red cells (Green, 1999; Snow, 1999), as shown in Table 22.1. Usually, in the presence of macro-ovalocytic erythrocytes and an elevated MCV, a bone marrow biopsy is performed to confirm the presence of megaloblasts in the bone marrow.

Although there is no consensus on a cutoff indicative of macrocytosis, a mean cell volume of >100 fL has been most consistently used. Some investigators recommend >94 fL (Chanarin and Metz, 1997). Macro-ovalocytic erythrocytes occur when the anemia is severe, but their absence does not preclude less severe folate deficiency. If megaloblastic anemia is confirmed, additional tests must be used to differentiate folate from vitamin B_{12} deficiency. These tests are discussed in the following sections and in Section 22.2.

22.1.2 Serum folate concentrations

Approximately two-thirds of the folate in serum is bound to protein, of which about 50% is bound to albumin; low levels of high-affinity folate binders are also present. No polyglutamates are present in serum. Instead, the main folate derivative in serum is the reduced form — methyltetrahydrofolate.

Serum folate concentrations fluctuate with recent changes in folate intake, or temporary changes in folate metabolism, even when body stores remain stable. For example, serum folate values increase rapidly after the ingestion of folate-containing foods and supplements (Cooper and Lowenstein, 1964) and decrease rapidly on a folate-deficient diet, stabilizing at values of about 7 nmol/L after only 2–3 wk of negative folate balance (Herbert, 1962). Hence, serum folate levels reflect acute folate status but provide no information on the size of the folate tissue stores (Herbert, 1987b). Thus, serum folate levels cannot be used to distinguish between a transitory reduction in folate intake and chronic folate deficiency associated with depletion of tissue folate (Bailey, 1990).

Nevertheless, low serum folate values for an individual, over more than about a month, probably indicate low folate stores and folate depletion. At this stage, erythrocyte and liver folate concentrations are low (Herbert, 1987b, 1987c). Metabolic disturbances, indicated by an abnormal deoxyuridine suppression test (dUST) (Section 22.2.4) and elevated serum homocysteine concentrations, will also be evident at this stage. Abnormal hematological changes (e.g., macrocytosis) do not occur until after about 3–4 mo of folate deprivation, depending on the size of body stores. Most individuals with megaloblastic changes resulting from folate deficiency have low serum folate levels, but exceptions do occur. In vitamin B$_{12}$ deficiency uncomplicated by folate deficiency, serum folate levels are normal or raised.

Factors affecting serum folate

Age-related trends in serum folate concentrations were documented in the National Health and Examination Survey (NHANES) II (Table 22.2) and NHANES III. The percentages of persons with low serum folate levels in NHANES II were lowest in children aged 0.5–9 y (2%), followed by males aged 10–19 y (3%) (Senti and Pilch, 1985). Un-

Age	Males		Females	
	(*n*)	% with low values	(*n*)	% with low values
6 mo–9 y	294	2 ± 1.4	240	3 ± 2.1
10–19 y	204	3 ± 1.3	210	12 ± 3.1
20–44 y	362	18 ± 2.8	462	15 ± 3.1
45–74 y	606	10 ± 2.5	532	9 ± 2.6

Table 22.2: Percentage of persons aged 6 mo through 74 y with serum folate values < 6.8 nmol/L, by age and sex: NHANES II, 1976–1980. Value after the ± is the SEM of the percent. From Senti and Pilch (1985).

fortunately, this information cannot be compared with the NHANES III data, because of methodological problems with the serum and red blood cell folate assays (Raiten and Fisher, 1995). No age or gender differences in serum folate concentrations were reported in a Swedish survey of adults aged 35–80 y (Wahlin et al., 2002).

Neonates and infants have serum folate values that are significantly higher than maternal concentrations, but values fall during the first 6 mo of infancy.

Pregnancy usually results in a decline in serum folate values. The reason is not clear. Low values may be associated with physiological changes such as hemodilution and changes in renal tubular function, rather than negative folate balance (O'Connor, 1994).

Smoking appears to lower serum (and erythrocyte) folate concentrations (Senti and Pilch, 1985; Piyathilake et al., 1994; Benton et al., 1997), although not all studies have shown this (Wahlin et al., 2002). In NHANES II, significantly more of the women smokers than nonsmokers had low serum folate levels (Table 22.3) (Senti and Pilch, 1985). Low folate intakes rather than an increased requirement, may explain the poorer folate status of smokers (Subar et al., 1990).

Alcohol ingestion results in an acute drop in serum folate levels, because reabsorption of folate is impaired by alcohol (Hillman et al., 1977). However, these effects may

	No. of persons examined	Percent	Standard error of percent
	Serum folate < 6.8 nmol/L		
Smokers	381	18	3.1
Nonsmokers	587	13	3.0
	Erythrocyte folate < 317 nmol/L		
Smokers	312	11	2.9
Nonsmokers	490	6	2.4

Table 22.3: Percentage of persons classified as smokers and nonsmokers with low serum and red blood cell folate values: NHANES II, 1976–1980. From Senti and Pilch (1985).

be limited to excessive alcohol use; moderate consumption of alcohol does not result in lowered serum folate levels (Payette and Gray-Donald, 1991). In several European surveys of adults (Weggemans et al., 1997; Wahlin et al., 2002), no relationship between alcohol use and serum folate concentrations has been reported.

Oral contraceptive agents containing high levels of estrogens (Martinez and Roe, 1977), have been reported to reduce serum folate values, although this relationship has not been reported in more recent surveys, when oral contraceptive agents with a lower estrogen content have been used (Senti and Pilch, 1985; Green et al., 1998).

Hemolysis may produce misleadingly elevated serum folate values as the folate content of erythrocytes is much higher than serum.

Certain drugs have anti-folate activity and, hence, reduce serum folate concentrations. These include nonsteroidal anti-inflammatory drugs such as aspirin, ibuprofen, and acetaminophen when taken in large therapeutic doses. Methotrexate used in the treatment of nonneoplastic diseases such as psoriasis, rheumatoid arthritis, asthma, primary biliary cirrhosis, and inflammatory bowel disease also lowers serum folate levels, as do the anticonvulsants diphenylhydantoin and phenolbarbitol. Diphenylhydantoin inhibits

intestinal absorption of folate (Young and Ghadirian, 1989).

Other diseases that are often treated with drugs with antifolate activity include malaria with pyriethamine, bacterial infections with trimethoprim, hypertension with triamterene, *Pneumocystis carinii* infections with trimetrexate, and chronic ulcerative colitis with sulfasalazine (IOM, 2000).

Certain disease states such as stagnant-loop syndrome, acute renal failure, and liver damage result in elevated serum folate values.

Dietary folate intakes may only correlate weakly with plasma folate concentrations unless broad categories of folate intakes such as quintiles are used, as shown in the study of Jacques et al. (1993) (Table 22.4). This is because of the wide variety of factors noted above that affect serum folate concentrations, as well as additional factors that affect the bioavailability of dietary folate.

Interpretive criteria

Herbert (1967) defined a cutoff point for low serum folate concentrations of < 6.8 nmol/L, and this was used in NHANES II (Senti and Pilch, 1985). This cutoff level is known to be indicative of negative folate balance at the time of the sampling of the serum, but it does not necessarily indicate folate depletion unless the negative folate balance persists (Herbert, 1987b, 1987c). Hence, individuals may have normal biochemical function and no evidence of tissue folate depletion, despite serum folate concentrations below this cutoff point. This same cutoff is used for

	Folate intake quartiles			
	1	2	3	4
Plasma folate (nmol/L)	10	12	15	20
		$p = < 0.001$		

Table 22.4: Adjusted mean concentrations of plasma folate by quartile of folate intake for 139 adults. Data from Jacques et al., American Journal of Clinical Nutrition 57: 182–189, 1993 © Am J Clin Nutr. American Society for Clinical Nutrition.

low serum folate values during pregnancy, although data justifying its use are lacking (O'Connor, 1994).

Swedish reference data for serum folate levels are available for a population-based sample of healthy adults aged 35–80 y (Wahlin et al., 2002). The investigators excluded subjects who had hematological evidence of folate deficiency and those consuming folate supplements or medications likely to interfere with folate absorption or metabolism. Two reference intervals were defined as the concentration ranges between the 2.5–97.5th and 5–95th percentiles.

Age- and sex-specific means and selected percentiles for serum folate of U.S. persons aged 4 to > 70 y have been compiled from the NHANES III data and are shown in Appendix A22.1. These values have been corrected for a methodological problem which was associated with an inappropriate calibration used during the first 4 y of NHANES III (IOM, 2000).

The U.K. National Diet and Nutrition Surveys for young children, young people aged from 4 to 18 y, and people ⩾ 65 y also present data for the percentage distribution of serum folate, as well as the mean, median, and critical lower and upper percentiles for each sex and age group (Gregory et al., 1995; 2000; Finch et al., 1998).

In several countries, folate fortification of certain foods has been introduced in an effort to reduce the incidence of neural tube defects. For example, fortification of cereals was mandated by the U.S. government in 1998. In countries where folate fortification has been adopted, such policies may have a marked effect on "normal" reference ranges for folate (and homocysteine) (Klee, 2000). In addition, any reference range depends on the method used for the analysis of serum folate (see below).

Measurement of serum folate

Serum or plasma folate concentrations can be assayed using microbiological or competitive binding assays. Heparin or EDTA may be used as anticoagulants for plasma. As folate is susceptible to oxidation, suitable antioxidants must be added to stabilize folate in samples during collection and storage. Folate in serum or plasma can be stabilized by diluting the serum 1 in 20 with 0.5% sodium ascorbate solution. This solution is stable for 24 h when stored in a refrigerator. Samples should be protected from light until the sodium ascorbate is added to the sample. Note that the addition of sodium ascorbate makes it impossible to determine serum vitamin B$_{12}$ on the same sample. Serum or plasma should be stored frozen, preferably at −70°C.

The microbiological technique is the best method for assessing total folate activity in serum (and erythrocytes, tissues, and foods). In the past, *Lactobacillus rhamnosus* (ATCC 7469), formerly called *L. casei*, was used because it responds to the greatest number of different folate derivatives. However, this organism cannot be used with serum or plasma containing antibiotics or methotrexate because these compounds interfere with bacterial growth of the older strains. Hence, the preferred choice of organism is a new chloramphenicol resistant strain of *L. casei* (NCIB 10463).

Folate in serum is in the monoglutamate form, which can be analyzed directly without incubation. The microbiological assay involves adding aliquots of diluted serum to the assay medium that contains all the nutrients except the folate required for the growth of *L. casei*. The growth response of the organism, estimated by measuring the increase in turbidity of the medium or by automated sodium titration of lactic acid formed during a 48-h incubation, is then proportional to the folate concentration in the serum. If a non-drug-resistant strain of *L. casei* is used, the inhibition of growth induced by drugs can be determined by the addition of a known quantity of exogenous folate to some tubes along with the unknown sample.

Alternatively, 96-well microtiter plates and the same chloramphenicol resistant strain of *L. casei* (NCIB 10463) can be used in a semi-automated method. This is easier, quicker, and more reproducible than the conventional assay (O'Broin and Kelleher, 1992; Molloy and Scott, 1997).

A number of competitive binding assays can also be used for measuring folate in serum. The assays use a high-affinity binding protein derived from milk and labeled folic acid or methyltetrahydrofolate as the competing analyte (Brown et al., 1990), together with a variety of detection systems, including radioisotope dilution, enzyme-linked assays, and chemiluminescent tags. The assays are rapid and not affected by antibiotics, tranquilizers, or antimitotic agents, all of which inhibit the growth of some strains of *L. casei*.

A recent interlaboratory comparison of five methods among 20 research laboratories reported an overall coefficient of variation of 27.6% for serum folate concentrations, with the greatest variation occurring at critically low folate concentrations. Such comparisons emphasize the importance of rigorous quality-control procedures for all methods. Samples should be assayed in duplicate and quality-control pools included in each analytical run, as carried out in NHANES III (Raiten and Fisher, 1995).

Currently, comparing serum folate data among study populations measured by different methods is difficult. Method-specific reference ranges must be developed in which "deficient" status results have been confirmed clinically by other hematological indices, as noted earlier.

New methods for folate analysis include chemiluminescence, ion capture, and high performance liquid chromatography (HPLC) with fluorescence detection. For clinical research studies, mass spectrometry using gas chromatography (GC/MS) or liquid chromatography (LC/MS) is sometimes used.

22.1.3 Erythrocyte folate

Erythrocytes incorporate folate as they are formed in the bone marrow, and levels remain constant throughout the life span of the cell (about 120 d). Hence, erythrocyte folate concentrations are less sensitive than serum folate levels to short-term fluctuations in folate status and they decrease much more

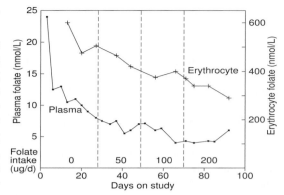

Figure 22.4: Plasma and erythrocyte folate concentrations in a single subject during a 92-day depletion–repletion trial. Data from Sauberlich et al., American Journal of Clinical Nutrition 46: 1016–1028, 1987 ⓒ Am J Clin Nutr. American Society for Clinical Nutrition.

slowly than serum or plasma folate during folate deprivation (Figure 22.4).

Erythrocyte folate concentrations correlate with liver folate levels (Wu et al., 1975) and thus reflect folate stores. Consequently, they are a more reliable measure of folate status than serum folate and should be used in population studies to estimate the prevalence of subjects with depleted folate stores (Senti and Pilch, 1985).

The initial stage of folate deficiency is a period of negative folate balance. If this is protracted, the stage of folate depletion is reached. This is characterized by declining liver stores and a fall in erythrocyte folate concentrations. No evidence of clinical impairment occurs at this stage.

With further folate deprivation, biochemical function is impaired, as indicated by an abnormal deoxyuridine (dU) suppression test and elevated concentrations of homocysteine (Section 22.1.5). Hypersegmented neutrophils may also be present, initially in the bone marrow cells and later in peripheral blood (Herbert, 1987c). These changes characterize the third stage of folate depletion, folate-deficient erythropoiesis, sometimes referred to as "subclinical deficiency." There is no evidence of anemia at this stage.

The final and fourth stage of folate depletion is folate-deficiency anemia. This stage is characterized by the appearance of macro-ovalocytic erythrocytes and low hemoglobin levels (Herbert, 1987c). Nearly all persons with folate-deficiency anemia will have low erythrocyte folate and serum folate concentrations.

It must be stressed that although the characteristics of the various stages of folate deficiency are clearly defined, the deficiency develops continuously and progressively. As a result, some overlap in the features of the different stages is to be expected.

Several investigators have compared the response of folate concentrations in serum and erythrocyte to changes in dietary folate intakes. Some of these studies have been experimentally controlled; others have been community-based. O'Keefe et al. (1995) conducted an experimental study using conventional foods in which they fed three groups of women constant diets, each containing different levels of folate for 70 d. Figure 22.5 shows the mean serum folate and erythrocyte folate concentrations at the end of the study period. In this experimental study, the mean serum and erythrocyte folate concentrations correlate positively with the folate intake.

In epidemiological studies, levels of erythrocyte folate generally more closely relate to dietary folate intakes than to plasma folate (Bates et al., 1980). Nevertheless, the correlations are often weak. In the U.K. National Diet and Nutrition surveys, for example, correlations between intakes of dietary folate and erythrocyte folate were 0.06 (ns) and 0.19 ($p < 0.01$) for preschool boys and girls (Gregory et al., 1995). Corresponding correlations for adults were 0.22 and 0.18 ($p < 0.01$) for males and females, respectively (Gregory et al., 1990). Such weak correlations are not unexpected. The dietary folate intakes in community-based surveys are based on relatively short-term measurements (e.g., over 7 d in the U.K. national surveys), which may fail to characterize the habitual intake. Moreover, folate is present in a variety of forms in the diet, and the bioavailability varies widely.

Factors affecting erythrocyte folate

Age-related trends in erythrocyte folate concentrations, comparable to those noted for serum folate have been observed (Senti and Pilch, 1985). In NHANES II, median erythrocyte folate concentrations were relatively high for infants and young children, but declined in later childhood and adolescence. A similar trend was noted for both sexes in the U.K. National Diet and Nutrition Survey for young people aged 4 to 18 y (Gregory et al., 2000).

Pregnancy and increasing parity tend to be associated with lower erythrocyte folate concentrations, as noted for serum folate.

Smoking may lower erythrocyte folate concentrations. In NHANES II, 11% of smokers compared to 6% of nonsmokers had erythrocyte folate concentrations < 317 nmol/L (Senti and Pilch, 1985) (Table 22.3), possibly arising from low intakes of folate (Subar et al., 1990).

Oral contraceptive use has been associated with lower erythrocyte folate values in earlier surveys, but not in more recent surveys (Green et al., 1998).

Vitamin B$_{12}$ deficiency blocks the uptake of folate by the tissues. Consequently, eryth-

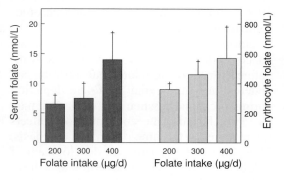

Figure 22.5: Serum and erythrocyte folate concentrations in three groups of young nonpregnant women fed controlled diets. These contained either 200 µg ($n = 5$), 300 µg ($n = 6$), or 400 µg ($n = 6$) of folate per day. Mean ($\pm$ SD) concentrations at the end of the 70-d study are shown. Data from O'Keefe et al., Journal of Nutrition 125: 2717–2725, 1995, with permission of the American Society for Nutritional Sciences.

rocyte folate concentrations fall, despite the presence of normal or sometimes even elevated serum folate levels (Hoffbrand et al., 1966; Chanarin, 1990). This disturbance in folate metabolism occurs because of the interaction of the folate metabolic cycle with vitamin B_{12}, as noted earlier (see also Figure 22.1). Hence, to identify folate deficiency, both erythrocyte folate and serum vitamin B_{12} concentrations should be measured.

Other disease states may also confound the interpretation of erythrocyte folate values. If patients have a raised reticulocyte count (e.g., when hemorrhage or hemolytic anemia is present), erythrocyte folate concentrations increase because reticulocytes tend to have higher folate concentrations than older cells (Hoffbrand et al., 1966).

Iron deficiency may result in increases in erythrocyte (and serum) folate values (Omer et al., 1970a), but the origin and magnitude of this effect are unknown. In such cases, the folate deficiency may be masked but can be indicated by an abnormal deoxyuridine suppression test (Section 22.2.4) and hypersegmentation in the peripheral blood (Section 22.1.6) (Herbert, 1985, 1987b, 1987c).

Interpretive criteria

The conventional cutoff points for classifying erythrocyte folate levels are based on data from subjects with biochemical and clinical signs associated with varying degrees of folate deficiency (Senti and Pilch, 1985). However, there is no consensus on the values that should be used to define each stage of folate deprivation. These discrepancies have arisen in part from differences in the analytical methods used for erythrocyte folate, often exacerbated by a failure to use a suitable certified reference material for comparing the accuracy of the methods.

Herbert (1987b, 1987c) has defined cutoffs that are indicative of sequential stages in the development of folate deficiency. The stages are negative folate balance, folate de-

pletion, folate-deficient erythropoiesis, and folate-deficiency anemia. Erythrocyte folate concentrations fall progressively during the first of these stages, and levels < 363 nmol/L indicate the onset of folate depletion, when liver folate stores are reduced. Concentrations < 272 nmol/L mark the beginning of the third stage of folate-deficient erythropoiesis. Folate-deficiency anemia, indicated by changes in red cell indices (Section 22.1.1), marks the fourth stage and this stage occurs when erythrocyte folate levels fall to < 227 nmol/L (Herbert, 1987c).

NHANES II used simpler criteria and only two cutoff points were defined. Erythrocyte levels of 317–363 nmol/L were designated as "low" and suggestive of an individual at risk, whereas an erythrocyte concentration below 317 nmol/L was taken to indicate deficiency. Using this criteria, the prevalence of erythrocyte folate levels indicative of deficiency among males and females was small in most age groups, as shown in Table 22.5.

The U.S. Food and Nutrition Board (IOM, 2000) recommends only one cutoff point for erythrocyte folate (i.e., < 305 nmol/L) as indicative of inadequate folate status. This cutoff point was based on reports of the appearance of hypersegmented neutrophils in peripheral blood (Herbert, 1962; Hoffbrand et al., 1966; Eichner et al., 1971), megaloblastic changes in the bone marrow (Varadi et al., 1966), and a measure of DNA and chromosome damage.

Cutoff values to interpret erythrocyte folate concentrations during pregnancy are still ill-defined. Erythrocyte folate concentration can underestimate the extent of folate depletion during pregnancy, when the depletion may be rapid, because the concentration reflects folate stores at the time of red cell synthesis. Thus, during the progressive development of a deficiency state, erythrocyte folate will always lag behind more acute markers such as serum folate.

Similarly, it is difficult to define the criteria for erythrocyte folate associated with increased risk of neural tube defects. It is possible that the risk of neural tube defects is associated with a folate status that would

Sex and age	Erythrocyte folate		Serum and erythrocyte folate	
	(n)	% with low values	(n)	% with low values
Males				
6 mo–9 y	243	2 ± 1.6	241	2 ± 1.6
10–19 y	178	5 ± 2.2	177	2 ± 1.1
20–44 y	299	8 ± 2.5	298	5 ± 2.3
45–74 y	503	8 ± 2.0	503	3 ± 1.2
Females				
6 mo–9 y	201	2 ± 1.5	200	2 ± 1.5
10–19 y	173	8 ± 2.8	173	2 ± 0.9
20–44 y	389	13 ± 2.4	388	6 ± 2.3
45–74 y	439	4 ± 0.8	439	2 ± 0.9

Table 22.5: Percentage of persons aged 6 mo through 74 y with erythrocyte folate < 317 nmol/L, and with both low erythrocyte and low serum folate values < 6.8 nmol/L, by age and sex: NHANES II, 1976–1980. Value after the ± is the SEM of the percent. From Senti and Pilch (1985).

not conventionally be classed as deficient, as noted earlier.

Tables of percentile values for erythrocyte folate values have been compiled for some recent national nutrition surveys. The mean and selected percentiles for persons ≥ 4 y for NHANES III are available and given in Appendix A22.2 (IOM, 2000). A correction was also applied to these erythrocyte folate values, as noted for serum folate. The U.K. National Diet and Nutrition Survey has also produced tables for erythrocyte folate values for young people aged 4 to 18 y, adults, and people ≥ 65 y (Gregory et al., 1990, 2000; Finch et al., 1998). The mean, median, and lower and upper 2.5th percentile values for erythrocyte folate values by age and sex are presented.

Measurement of erythrocyte folate

Although competitive binding and microbiological assays can both be used to measure erythrocyte folate concentrations, only the microbiological assay will be discussed here as it is now the method of choice. A chloramphenicol-resistant strain of *L. casei* (NCIB 10463) should be used, together with

96-well microtiter plates. This method is easier to perform, less time consuming, and also more reproducible than the conventional assay (O'Broin and Kelleher, 1992; Molloy and Scott, 1997). As erythrocytes contain the polyglutamate forms of folate, they must first be lysed and then treated with conjugase before analyzing for folate. These steps are outlined below.

1. Collect venous whole-blood samples in tubes containing either lithium-heparin or EDTA as an anticoagulant. Protect blood samples from light until the ascorbic acid is added to the sample.
2. Determine hematocrit on a subsample of the whole blood.
3. Hemolyze the remaining whole blood by 10-fold dilution in a hypotonic aqueous solution (usually a freshly prepared solution of 1% ascorbic acid). Incorporate a lysing agent (e.g., saponin) to guarantee complete hemolysis (Wright et al., 2000).
4. Incubate the hemolysate with plasma folate conjugase (γ-glu-x carboxypeptidase; EC 3.4.19.9) for a short period to ensure the complete hydrolysis of the erythrocyte polyglutamyl folates to the monoglutamate form. Generally, incubation periods are 2 h at 37°C, although Wright et al. (2000) suggest that the optimal pH, time, and temperature for this incubation should be determined before analysis.
5. If necessary, store red blood cell lysates frozen, preferably at –70°C.
6. Perform the assay by adding the hemolysate to the assay media.

Sources of variability during the preparation of the erythrocyte lysate include differences in the oxygenation state of the hemoglobin as a sample progresses through the assay procedure (Wright et al., 1998). The extent to which dilution of whole blood with hypotonic diluents produces complete hemolysis and release of folate is also important (Wright et al., 2000).

Interlaboratory comparisons have reported an overall coefficient of variation for erythrocyte folate of 35.7%, with the greatest variability occurring at critically low concentrations (Wright et al., 2000). In an effort to enhance the quality-control procedures for this assay, the U.K. National Institute of Biological Standards and Control has prepared lyophilized whole-blood reference materials. Investigators should use these or other appropriate reference materials to minimize the difficulties currently encountered when comparing erythrocyte folate data among study populations. Additional, method-specific reference ranges must be developed in which "deficient" status results have been confirmed clinically by other hematological indices, as noted for serum folate.

A method for whole blood folate based on dried blood spots on filter paper, followed by microbiological assay on microtiter plates using chloramphenicol-resistant *L. casei* has been developed and warrants further investigation for field-based studies. Details are given in O'Broin and Gunter (1999).

22.1.4 Formiminoglutamate excretion

Usually, histidine is converted to L-glutamic acid via the action of the enzyme formiminotransferase (EC 2.1.2.5) and tetrahydrofolic acid (Figure 22.6). In folate deficiency this conversion is inhibited and, as a result, the urinary excretion of formimino-glutamic acid (FIGLU) is increased, particularly when preceded by an oral loading dose of 2–15 g of L-histidine. The urine can be collected over 24-h or over an 8-h period (Wagner, 1984).

The sensitivity of the FIGLU test for folate deficiency is comparable to that of the erythrocyte folate assay. However, the test has had limited use because it offers no advantage over the serum or erythrocyte folate assays. Moreover, it is not specific to folate deficiency: a deficiency of vitamin B_{12} or of the enzyme formiminotransferase also produces abnormally high urinary excretion of FIGLU after a histidine load. High urinary excretion of FIGLU also occurs in patients with both liver and malignant diseases, or tuberculosis, regardless of the folate status (Herbert, 1967).

In contrast, FIGLU excretion is normal in kwashiorkor, even if severe folate deficiency

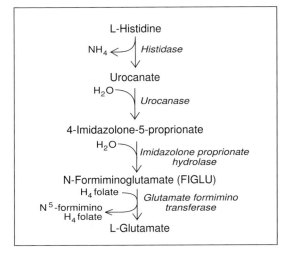

Figure 22.6: Pathway of histidine metabolism.

is also present. Excretion is also normal in persons with secondary folate deficiency arising from anticonvulsant drug therapy. Inconsistent results for the FIGLU excretion test have been reported during pregnancy. In lactation, however, FIGLU excretion does appear to be inversely associated with serum folate concentration and responds to folate supplementation (O'Connor, 1994).

Interpretive criteria and measurement

Normal levels of FIGLU in urine excreted by folate-replete adults are $< 35\,\mu mol/24\,h$ whereas following a 15 g histidine load, the level in urine rises to $< 144\,\mu mol/24\,h$. In folate-deficient adults, FIGLU excretion after a 15 g histidine load usually ranges from about 200–11,500 $\mu mol/24\,h$ (Biolab Medical Unit, London at www.biolab.co.uk).

The analysis of FIGLU in urine is normally carried out using an enzymatic method (Tabor and Wyngarden, 1958). A sensitive micromethod using thin layer chromatography can also be used (Bhatt et al., 1982).

22.1.5 Serum homocysteine

Homocysteine is a four-carbon amino acid $[HS(CH_2)_2CHNH_2COOH]$ derived from the remethylation of methionine. Multiple forms of homocysteine circulate in blood: the majority (65%) is disulfide linked to protein; about 30% is in an oxidized state, and about 15% is in the free reduced form. Total homocysteine is defined as the sum of all homocysteine species in serum or plasma, including free and protein-bound forms (Klee, 2000). Most analytical methods measure total homocysteine by including an initial pretreatment with a reductant.

Two biochemical pathways are involved in the metabolism of homocysteine: transsulfuration and the methionine cycle. The transsulfuration cycle is favored in the postprandial state. In this pathway, homocysteine is catabolized via cystathionine to cysteine, and eventually to the sulfate and then pyruvate, a source of energy. The initial step in this pathway, step J in Figure 22.1, is mediated by the enzyme cystathione β-synthase and requires the active form of vitamin B$_6$ (pyridoxal-5-phosphate).

Alternatively, under fasting conditions, the homocysteine can be metabolized by the remethylation pathway, which requires vitamin B$_{12}$ as a coenzyme and folate as cosubstrate (methyl donor). This pathway is step D in Figure 22.1. It involves the transfer of a methyl group to homocysteine to form methionine by methionine synthetase in the presence of methyltetrahydrofolate (from dietary folate) and methylcobalamin. Consequently, in folate or vitamin B$_{12}$ deficiency, homocysteine accumulates in the serum, and concentrations increase.

Riboflavin is also involved as a cofactor for 5,10-methylene tetrahydrofolate reductase (Hustad et al., 2000). This enzyme is involved in the conversion of methylene tetrahydrofolate to methyl tetrahydrofolate, which is required for the remethylation of homocysteine to methionine (Step D, Figure 22.1) (Jacques et al., 2001).

Of the vitamins involved in the metabolism of homocysteine, folate is reportedly the most important determinant of homocysteine concentrations in adults (Homocysteine Lowering Trialists' Collaboration, 1998; Pietrzik and Brønstrup, 1998), although in neonates, it may be vitamin B$_{12}$ (Minet et al., 2000).

Elevated circulating homocysteine concentrations have been associated with an increased risk of occlusive vascular disease and venous thrombosis (den Heijer et al., 1996; Refsum et al., 1998). For example, in the Physicians Heart Study, homocysteine concentrations 12% above reference values were associated with a threefold increase in the risk of myocardial infarction (Stampfer et al., 1992), whereas in NHANES III, participants in the highest quartile of homocysteine concentrations had a 2.9-fold increased odds ratio for stroke (Giles et al., 1998). In contrast, despite the role of occlusive vascular disease in the pathogenesis of age-related maculopathy, this condition was not related to increased homocysteine concentrations in the NHANES III population (Heuberger et al., 2002).

Pregnancy complications (Rajkovic et al., 1997) and Alzheimer's disease (Clarke et al., 1998) have also been linked to elevated serum homocysteine concentrations, but more studies are needed to confirm these findings.

Both experimental folate depletion – repletion studies and epidemiological studies have confirmed the relationship between folate deficiency and elevated homocysteine concentrations. In some reports, elevated serum homocysteine concentrations have been normalized by folate supplementation (Stabler et al., 1988). Jacob et al. (1994, 1998) have conducted experimental studies with adult men and postmenopausal women. The work showed that folate depletion leads to lower plasma folate levels and to a rise in plasma homocysteine. Results for postmenopausal women are shown in Figure 22.7.

Inverse correlations between plasma concentrations of folate and homocysteine have also been reported in several epidemiological studies among pre- and postmenopausal women, adult men, and the elderly, after controlling for confounding factors (Selhub et al., 1993; Tucker et al., 1996; Jacques et al., 2001).

The findings described above suggest that plasma homocysteine may serve to assess the adequacy of folate intakes. For example, data from the Framingham Heart Study

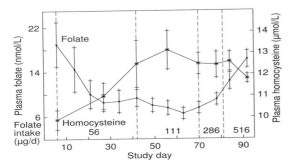

Figure 22.7: Plasma folate and homocysteine levels (mean ± SEM) for eight postmenopausal women in a 13-wk folate depletion–repletion trial. The total folate intake during the successive study periods is shown along the base of the figure. Data from Jacob et al., Journal of Nutrition 128: 1204–1212, 1998, with permission of the American Society for Nutritional Sciences.

showed an inverse correlation between folate intakes (based on a food frequency questionnaire) and plasma homocysteine levels. In this study, homocysteine concentrations appeared to fall and then remained constant as folate intakes reached about 400 µg/d (Tucker et al., 1996).

Factors influencing serum homocysteine

Other nutrient deficiencies, in addition to folate, can elevate serum homocysteine levels as noted in Table 22.6. Deficiencies of vitamin B_{12} (Stabler et al., 1996), vitamin B_6 (Ubbink et al., 1995), and riboflavin (Jacques et al., 2001) all act in this way. In elderly persons with a normal folate status, but who have shown a positive clinical response to vitamin B_{12} treatment, serum total homocysteine concentrations are generally elevated (Stabler et al., 1996). In addition, there is at least one report of elevated homocysteine concentrations associated with diminished riboflavin (Hustad et al., 2000), and low plasma pyridoxal-5'-phosphate levels (Bates et al., 1999), although in experimental vitamin B_6 depletion–repletion studies, results have been inconsistent (Miller et al., 1992; Ubbink et al., 1996).

These results emphasize that only in the absence of deficiencies of vitamin B_{12}, riboflavin, and probably vitamin B_6 can plasma

homocysteine concentrations serve as a useful functional test of folate status (Ueland et al., 1993).

Age-related trends are important. In young children, serum homocysteine levels tend to increase with age (Must et al., 2003). A similar trend occurs with adults (Jacques et al., 1999), but during adolescence hormonal determinants of plasma homocysteine may be more significant (Must et al., 2003).

Gender influences fasting serum homocysteine concentrations. In NHANES III, values for boys were higher than girls from 10 y and throughout adolescence (Must et al., 2003), which is consistent with findings noted for Belgian (De Laet et al., 1999), but not German, children (Rauh et al., 2001). In adults, fasting concentrations are higher in men than in women (Brattström et al., 1994; Bates et al., 1997a).

Race and ethnicity appear to impact on serum homocysteine levels (Ubbink et al., 1995). In NHANES III, Mexican American adolescent girls had lower homocysteine concentrations than boys (Must et al., 2003), which is consistent with the race and ethnic pattern observed in the same survey in adults (Jacques et al., 1999).

Intake of food affects serum homocysteine concentrations. Small increases associated with meals have been documented, which persist and reach a maximum after 6–8 h after the meal (Ueland et al., 1993).

Storage of blood samples can result in a progressive increase in serum homocysteine concentrations, through leakage of homocysteine from the erythrocytes, especially if samples are stored at room temperature (Kittner et al., 1995). For example, the 1 h of storage of whole blood at room temperature may increase serum or plasma homocysteine concentrations by about 10% (Ueland et al., 1993). Therefore, rigorous precautions must be taken when collecting blood samples for homocysteine analysis. Blood samples must be rapidly chilled to 4°C, and the plasma or serum must be separated as quickly as possible. Bates et al. (1997a) reported that such treatment is effective and prevents the higher plasma homocysteine concentrations observed when samples were separated after 6–10 h.

Position of the subject during the blood sampling may influence serum homocysteine concentrations because most homocysteine is bound to albumin. Serum albumin is about 9% greater in blood samples collected from subjects who are standing than in those in the supine position (Young and Bermes, 1998).

Pregnancy decreases fasting serum homocysteine levels by 30% to 50%, but concentrations normalize within a few days postpartum (Andersson et al., 1992).

Estrogen-containing preparations reduce fasting serum homocysteine concentrations, perhaps as a result of the role of these preparations in homocysteine metabolism (van der Mooren et al., 1994).

Alcohol intake raises fasting plasma homocysteine levels. The effect has been associated with the consumption of liquor or red wine, but not beer (van der Gaag et al., 2000; Jacques et al., 2001).

Caffeine-rich beverages, when consumed, may lead to higher plasma homocysteine concentrations (Nygård et al., 1997; Stolzenberg-Solomon et al., 1999; Jacques et al., 2001; Verhoef et al., 2002), although these findings are not consistent (Stampfer et al., 1992). In a randomized trial, 1 L unfiltered coffee per day for 2 wk increased fasting plasma homocysteine by 10% (i.e., 1.2 µmol/L (Grubben et al., 2000). Caffeine is only partly responsible, however, for the homocysteine-raising effect of coffee (Verhoef et al., 2002).

Cigarette smoking has been linked to serum or plasma homocysteine levels. In a U.K. study of adults ⩾ 65 y, the association was with the number of years smoked and not

the number of cigarettes smoked (Bates et al., 1997a).

Certain enzyme defects involved in homocysteine metabolism can cause abnormally elevated serum homocysteine concentrations. These enzymes are 5,10-methylene-tetrahydrofolate reductase (MTHFR), cystathionine β-synthase, and possibly methionine synthase (Table 22.6). The frequency of homozygosity for the MTHFR T^{677} allele among white populations ranges from 2% to 16% (van der Put et al., 1995). In a study of French adults, plasma homocysteine concentrations were higher in men but not in women homozygous for the 5,10-MTHFR T^{677} allele, but dietary folate intake was not measured (Chango et al., 2000).

Renal function may control the observed relationship between circulating concentrations of homocysteine and serum creatinine, although increased homocysteine production during creatine metabolism may also play a role (Brattström et al., 1994).

Vitamins	Cobalamin deficiency Folate deficiency Vitamin B$_6$ deficiency Riboflavin deficiency
Enzymes	Defects in cblC, D, E, F and G Cystathionine β-synthase deficiency MTHFR deficiency Methionine synthase deficiency Thermolabile MTHFR
Conditions	Renal insufficiency Hypothyroidism
Drugs	Colestipol Niacin L-dopa
Characteristics	Older age Male sex Increased muscle mass
Artifacts	Volume contraction Cellular release in vitro

Table 22.6: Causes of abnormally elevated serum homocysteine levels. MTHFR, 5,10-methylenetetrahydrofolate reductase. From Carmel, Annual Review of Medicine, Volume 51, 2000 © by Annual Reviews. with permission.

Medications, particularly antihypertensive medications, can affect serum or plasma homocysteine levels which are also related to blood pressure (Nygård et al., 1995).

Interpretive criteria

Serum homocysteine levels can become elevated during the early stages of tissue folate deficiency in the absence of macrocytosis and anemia, when the only other metabolic abnormality is an abnormal dUST test (Section 22.2.4). Caution must be used, however, in interpreting elevated homocysteine levels, particularly in the absence of biochemical evidence of folate, vitamin B_{12}, vitamin B_6, or riboflavin status, because of the large number of factors modifying homocysteine concentrations. Normalization of elevated serum homocysteine concentrations after treatment with folate is the best way to confirm a diagnosis of folate deficiency (Zittoun and Zittoun, 1999).

Numerous age- and gender-specific reference intervals for normal healthy adults have been proposed for plasma total homocysteine (Rasmussen et al., 1996; Bates et al., 1997a). A summary of earlier interpretive criteria is given in Ueland et al. (1993). The differences in the proposed reference intervals may be related to analytical methods used, method of sample processing, or existence of confounding factors, as discussed earlier. Confounding factors may be responsible for the occurrence of elevated homocysteine levels, even in apparently healthy normal subjects. This is illustrated by the skewed frequency distribution for total plasma homocysteine concentrations in a study of 3000 apparently healthy Norwegian men (Figure 22.8).

Usually values for serum or plasma homocysteine concentrations of 5–15 µmol/L are considered normal. Ubbink et al. (1995) proposed 4.9–11.7 µmol/L as the reference interval for homocysteine in males 20–65 y, based on a prediction model. The upper reference limit is slightly lower than that defined for elderly persons (mean age 75 y) by Joosten et al. (1996).

Several cutoff values are used to define

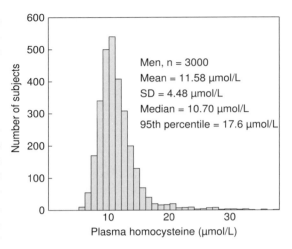

Figure 22.8: Frequency distribution for total plasma homocysteine for 3000 Norwegian men 40–42 y. Data from Ueland et al., Clinical Chemistry 39: 1764–1779, 1993, with permission of the AACC.

elevated serum homocysteine concentrations (Boushey et al., 1995). Some examples are summarized in Table 22.7. Of these, the most often cited cutoff for adults is >16 µmol/L, although levels >15 µmol/L (Refsum et al., 2001), >14 µmol/L (Selhub et al., 1993), and >12 µmol/L (Rasmussen et al., 1996) have also been used. Selhub et al. (1993) found that in elderly subjects, the risk of extracranial carotid-stenosis was elevated when plasma homocysteine levels were between 11.4 and 14.3 µmol/L.

Age and sex-specific means and selected percentiles for serum homocysteine (µmol/L) of U.S. persons aged 12 to 70+ y have been compiled from the NHANES III data; they are given in Appendix A22.3.

There is little information on homocysteine

	µmol/L
Framingham Heart Study (Selhub et al., 1995)	⩾ 14.4
United States Physicians Study (Stampfer et al., 1992)	⩾ 15.8
International Study of Elderly (Joosten et al., 1993)	⩾ 13.9

Table 22.7: Some interpretive criteria used for evaluating elevated plasma homocysteine levels.

Age (y)	n	Mean	SD	SEM	50th Pct
Boys					
4–5	139	4.6	1.1	0.15	4.6
6–11	161	5.2	1.1	0.14	5.0
12–15	347	7.2	3.1	0.27	6.6
16–19	295	8.7	2.8	0.27	8.3
Girls					
4–5	151	4.5	0.9	0.13	4.4
6–11	174	5.3	1.1	0.15	5.2
12–15	415	6.5	2.6	0.23	6.0
16–19	345	7.2	2.7	0.26	6.7

Table 22.8: Means and fiftieth percentiles (50th Pct) of serum total homocysteine concentrations (μmol/L) for children by age and sex for combined race and ethnicity groups from NHANES III. SD, complex sample standard deviation. SEM, smoothed standard error. Abstracted from more comprehensive data of Must et al., Journal of Nutrition 133: 2643–2649, 2003, with permission of the American Society for Nutritional Sciences.

Sample	Storage conditions	Stability
Whole blood	Room temp. 0–2°C	< 1 h 4–12 h
Plasma or serum	Room temp. 0–2°C –20°C	At least 4 days Several weeks Years

Table 22.9: Some guidelines used for storing whole blood, serum, or plasma samples for homocysteine analysis. From Ueland et al., Clinical Chemistry 39: 1764–1769, 1993, with permission of the AACC.

levels in children. Must et al. (2003) have presented means and selected percentiles of serum total homocysteine concentrations by age group and by sex, race, and ethnicity for children and adolescents 4–19 y using results from NHANES III (Table 22.8).

For neonates, a cutoff of >11.0 μmol/L for serum total homocysteine has been defined by Minet et al. (2000).

Measurement of serum homocysteine

Fasting blood samples are preferred for serum or plasma homocysteine analysis because intake of food may affect the levels. As noted above, rigorous precautions must be taken when collecting the blood samples. These must be rapidly chilled to 4°C, and the plasma or serum must be separated as quickly as possible. After separation, serum or plasma samples for homocysteine analyses can be stored at –20°C for several years (Table 22.9). Repeated freeze–thaw cycles, which may increase the homocysteine levels, should be avoided.

Several methods have been developed for the assay of total homocysteine levels in serum or plasma. Of these, a reverse-phase HPLC method with fluorescence detection is the most widely used. Prior to the HPLC analysis, the serum thiols are modified, often using SBD-F (ammonium 7-fluorobenzo-2-oxa-1,3-diazole-4-sulfonate). The latter is a commercially available thiol-specific fluorogenic probe, which yields thiols with high fluorescence and excellent stability. Retention of SBD-homocysteine is sensitive to pH; by using a mobile phase with pH 2.1, baseline separation of serum thiols within 6 min can be achieved. This method has a between-run CV of 6.6% and is suitable for routine determination of serum homocysteine concentrations (Ubbink et al., 1991).

A commercial kit has been developed for analysis of plasma homocysteine using electrochemical detection. Only 200 μL of sample is needed (Solomon and Duda, 1998). A method based on gas chromatography and mass spectrometry can also be used, but it is not fully automated and the equipment is costly (Stabler et al., 1993). In the future, electrospray tandem mass spectrometry may be used; this procedure does not require immunodiagnostic reagents or chromatographic columns. It has a high throughput (2.5 min per analysis), and the labor time is less than that required for most automated immuno-assays. The major limitation is the high cost of the equipment (Klee, 2000).

22.1.6 Neutrophil lobe count

Usually, neutrophils (also referred to as polymorphonuclear leukocytes) have three or four segments. However, in megaloblastic anemia, the number increases. Such hypersegmentation of neutrophils in the peripheral blood may be the earliest morphological change to appear in the blood in folate and vitamin B_{12} deficiency. Hypersegmentation generally but not always (Carmel et al., 1996a) precedes the development of macrocytosis (Herbert, 1962). Unfortunately, no relationship exists between the severity of the megaloblastic anemia and the presence of hypersegmentation.

Jägerstad and Pietrzik (1993) investigated the relationship between the neutrophil lobe count and serum and erythrocyte folate concentrations; results for the latter are shown in Figure 22.9. It appears that when erythrocyte folate concentrations are < 550 nmol/L (and serum folate < 10 nmol/L), the average neutrophil lobe count increases and is indicative of biochemical folate deficiency.

Neutrophil hypersegmentation also occurs in other conditions such as uremia, myeloproliferative disorders (e.g., myelogenous leukemia), and myelofibrosis and as a congenital lesion in approximately 1% of the population, even when vitamin B_{12} and folate stores are adequate. The occasional reported cases of hypersegmentation of neutrophils in iron deficiency (Beard and Weintraub, 1969; Westerman et al., 1999) probably result from the existence of a masked folate deficiency (Das et al., 1978).

Neutrophil hypersegmentation is not useful as a reliable index of folate deficiency in pregnancy when there is an underlying tendency to hyposegmentation. Gadowksy et al. (1995) noted only a weak negative correlation between serum or erythrocyte folate concentrations and neutrophil lobe counts in pregnant adolescents.

Neutrophil hypersegmentation can be evaluated in smears of peripheral blood or in white blood cells obtained from the interface between the serum or plasma and the sedimented red cells (i.e., the buffy coat). Several evaluation techniques can be used. Indeed, in the study by Gadowsky et al. (1995), the number of subjects classified as functionally folate deficient was critically dependent on the criteria used to evaluate neutrophil hypersegmentation. Criteria include calculating the average number of lobes per neutrophil, or the percentage of cells with five or more lobes. Abnormal hypersegmentation is when a lobe average of > 3.5 lobes per cell is found, or when 5% or more of the cells have five or more lobes (Colman, 1981). Such methods are very time consuming. A more practical approach involves examining smears for the existence of any six-lobed cells within a random sample of 100 cells. Six-lobed cells are a consistent feature of smears in nearly all persons with megaloblastic anemia (Lindenbaum and Nath, 1980).

For persons with concomitant iron and folate deficiency, evaluation of neutrophil hypersegmentation is especially useful because it occurs even when macrocytosis is masked by a coexisting iron deficiency (Das and Herbert, 1978).

22.1.7 Multiple indices

The stages in the development of folate deficiency were defined in a model of Herbert (1987c). This has now been revised to include tests to detect mild preclinical folate deficiency (Table 22.10). In this revised model, serum folate is the only test that reflects a negative folate balance, as indicated by a serum folate value < 6.8 nmol/L. If the negative balance persists, then a folate depletion stage is reached, when folate stores are reduced and erythrocyte folate concentrations fall to

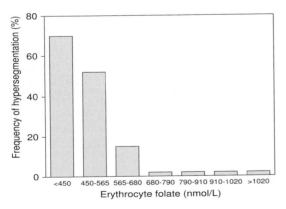

Figure 22.9: Frequency (%) of hypersegmentation of polymorphonuclear granulocytes (lobe average > 3.6) at different erythrocyte folate concentrations. Data from Jägerstad and Pietrzik, *International Journal for Vitamin and Nutrition Research* 63: 285–289, 1993.

	Normal	Negative folate balance	Folate depletion	Folate-deficient erythro-poiesis	Folate-deficiency anemia
Serum homocysteine (μmol/L)	< 10	< 10	10–15	>15	>15
Serum folate (nmol/L)	>11.3	< 6.8	< 6.8	< 6.8	< 6.8
Red blood cell folate (nmol/L)	> 453	> 453	< 363	< 272	< 227
Deoxyuridine suppression	Normal	Normal	Normal	Abnormal	Abnormal
Lobe average	< 3.5	< 3.5	< 3.5	> 3.5	> 3.5
Liver folate (nmol/g)	> 7	> 7	< 3.6	< 2.7	< 2.3
Erythrocytes	Normal	Normal	Normal	Normal	Macro-ovalocytic
Mean cell volume	Normal	Normal	Normal	Normal	Elevated
Hemoglobin	Normal	Normal	Normal	Normal	Low

Table 22.10: Sequential stages in the development of folate deficiency. The critical features of each stage are outlined. Adapted from Herbert, American Journal of Clinical Nutrition 46: 387–402, 1987 © Am J Clin Nutr. American Society for Clinical Nutrition.

< 363 nmol/L. It takes longer for erythrocyte folate concentrations than serum folate to decrease below the normal range because of the 120-d lifespan of erythrocytes.

Abnormal metabolic changes become evident at the stage of folate depletion when there is insufficient tissue folate to support folate-dependent biochemical pathways. Impaired biochemical function can be detected by an abnormal dU suppression test in bone marrow cells (Section 22.2.4), but the test is cumbersome and not suitable for routine clinical use. Instead, plasma homocysteine can be measured (Section 22.1.5) and any abnormally high levels can be detected, sometimes even before serum folate levels have fallen below the reference range.

The stage of folate-deficient erythropoiesis is characterized by low serum and erythrocyte folate concentrations, abnormal dU suppression test on peripheral blood lymphocytes, and elevated plasma homocysteine concentrations. When tissue folate stores are severely depleted in the third and final stage of folate deficiency anemia, macro-ovalocytic erythrocytes appear in the circulating blood and megaloblasts in the bone marrow. At this stage, hypersegmented neutrophils in the peripheral blood smear and abnormal red cell indices are apparent; mean red cell volume and mean cell hemoglobin are elevated, and hemoglobin is low (i.e., < 130 g/L in men; < 120 g/L in women).

Therefore, the recommended combination of indices required to detect one or more of the stages in the development of folate deficiency include serum and erythrocyte folate concentrations, plasma homocysteine, mean cell volume (Section 17.3.1) and hemoglobin (Section 17.1). Serum vitamin B$_{12}$ should be measured to distinguish between folate and vitamin B$_{12}$ deficiency.

New methods for assaying folate coenzymes in small tissue biopsy samples may allow routine coenzyme analysis of specific tissues in the future (Bagley and Selhub, 2000). Such analyses may provide important information because some tissues are particularly susceptible to folate depletion (Varela-Moreiras and Selhub, 1992).

22.2 Vitamin B$_{12}$

The term "vitamin B$_{12}$" is a generic descriptor for all the corrinoids that exhibit the biological activity of cyanocobalamin. The latter was first isolated in the crystalline form in

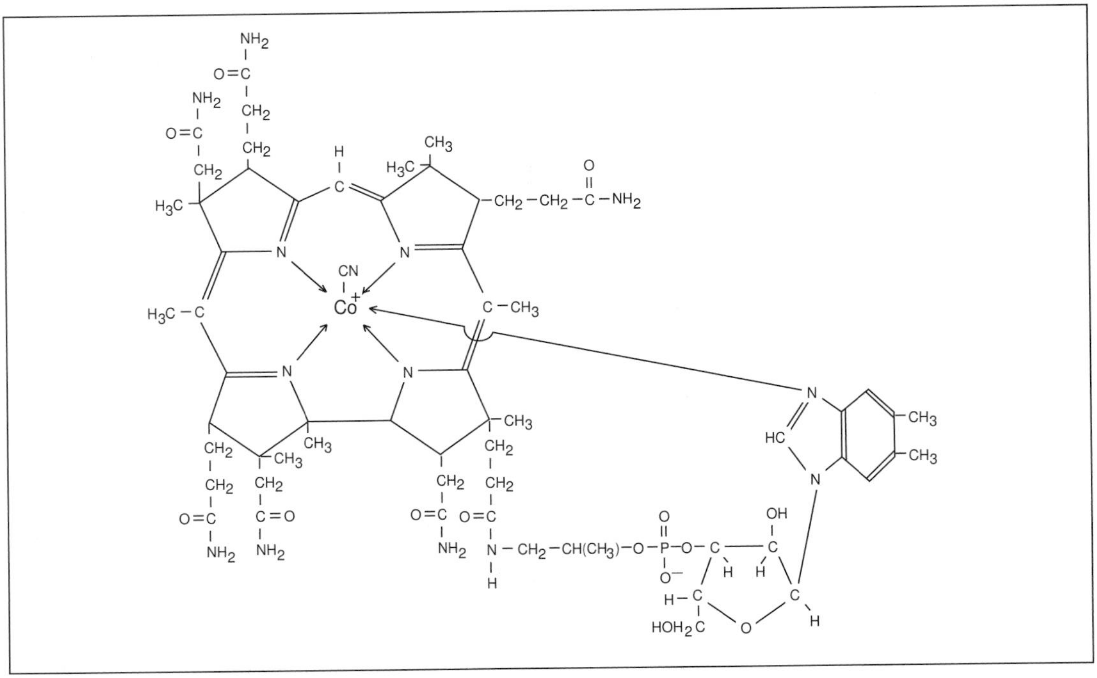

Figure 22.10: The structure of cyanocobalamin. The molecule is made up of a planar group, consisting of a corrin ring with a cobalt atom at the center and a nucleotide set at right angles to the corrin ring. The nucleotide is made up of the base, 5,6-dimethylbenzimidazole, and a phosphorylated sugar (ribose-3-phosphate).

1948 (Rickes et al., 1948; Smith, 1948), and the structure is shown in Figure 22.10.

Functions of vitamin B_{12}

There are two naturally occurring cobalamin-containing coenzymes: methylcobalamin, the main form in plasma, and 5′-deoxyadenosyl-cobalamin, found in the liver, most body tissues, and foods. In humans, methylcobalamin functions in the folate-dependent methylation of homocysteine to methionine (see Step D in Figure 22.1), whereas 5′-deoxy-adenosyl-cobalamin plays a major part in the conversion of L-methylmalonyl-coenzyme A to succinyl-coenzyme A in an isomerization reaction. The latter is a common pathway for the degradation of certain amino acids and odd-chain fatty acids.

Vitamin B_{12} also has a link with nucleic acid metabolism via its role in the conversion of 5-methyltetrahydrofolate to tetrahydrofolate (Step C in Figure 22.1). Consequently,

a deficiency of vitamin B_{12}, like folic acid, impairs the production of tetrahydrofolate, which is required for thymidine and thus DNA synthesis. Impaired DNA synthesis is responsible for the megaloblastic bone marrow, a characteristic of deficiencies of both vitamin B_{12} and folic acid.

The role of cobalamin-containing coenzymes in the conversion of methylmalonyl-coenzyme A to succinyl-coenzyme A is probably associated with the neurological defects that may arise in vitamin B_{12} deficiency, as well as in the accumulation of methylmalonic acid in the urine.

Absorption and metabolism

In nature, vitamin B_{12} is produced almost entirely by bacterial synthesis. In the human, this synthesis takes place in the colon and small intestine, although probably only the vitamin B_{12} synthesized in the small intestine is absorbed (Albert et al., 1980).

Absorption of vitamin B$_{12}$ mainly takes place through receptor sites in the ileum, at an alkaline pH, and in the presence of calcium. It is mediated by the gastric intrinsic factor, a highly specific binding glycoprotein of molecular weight 45,000–60,000, which is synthesized and secreted by the parietal cells of the gastric mucosa, after being stimulated by food. Absorption of small amounts of vitamin B$_{12}$ (generally 1% to 3% in normal diets) may also occur by simple diffusion (Herbert, 1987a).

The main storage site for vitamin B$_{12}$ is the liver; total body stores in healthy omnivorous subjects are about 2–3 mg. Loss of vitamin B$_{12}$ takes place via desquamation of epithelium and also through secretion in the bile. Most of the vitamin B$_{12}$ secreted in the bile, however, is reabsorbed and is thus available for metabolic functions. Losses in adults approximate 1–3 µg/d (about 0.1% of body stores) (Hughes-Jones and Wickramasinghe, 1996). Excretion of vitamin B$_{12}$ in the stool is proportional to stores, so that deficiency develops more slowly in vegetarians with low body stores than in persons with no intrinsic factor or with malabsorption.

Deficiency of vitamin B$_{12}$ in humans

The clinical signs of vitamin B$_{12}$ deficiency occur in the hematopoietic, gastrointestinal, and neurological systems. The hematological effects are indistinguishable from those of folate deficiency and include megaloblastic anemia, accompanied by the classical anemia symptoms of diminished energy and tolerance to exercise, fatigue, shortness of breath, and palpitations. The megaloblastic changes result from an interference with normal DNA synthesis, arising from lack of 5,10-methylene tetrahydrofolate, as described for folate deficiency.

The gastrointestinal effects of vitamin B$_{12}$ deficiency include atrophic glossitis, papillary atrophy of the tongue, loss of appetite, flatulence, and constipation.

The neurological complications progress gradually and are variable. They may precede or occur in the absence of anemia (Linden-baum et al., 1988). Indeed, it appears that the occurrence of neurological complications may be inversely correlated with the degree of anemia (Healton et al., 1991). Manifestations include tingling and numb extremities, motor disturbances such as abnormalities of gait, and cognitive changes that range from memory loss and depression to frank dementia, with or without mood changes (Goodman and Salt, 1990). The neurological complications are not always reversible after treatment with vitamin B$_{12}$.

Deficiency of vitamin B$_{12}$, like folate, has also been linked to an increased risk of occlusive vascular disease and stroke via its role in methylation of homocysteine to methionine (Step D: Figure 22.1), although folate concentrations are reportedly the most significant determinant of homocysteine concentrations in adults, as noted earlier (Pietrzik and Brønstrup, 1998). Dietary deficiency of vitamin B$_{12}$ in most industrialized countries is relatively rare, and the deficiency usually results from malabsorption (Stabler and Allen, 2004). Indeed, malabsorption is said to account for > 95% of the vitamin B$_{12}$ deficiency cases documented in the United States (Herbert, 1985). In developing countries, the deficiency may occur among children, as well as pregnant and lactating women, who either exclude or consume low amounts of animal products in their diets (Allen, 1994). There are also some reports of deficiency symptoms developing among infants born to mothers deficient in vitamin B$_{12}$ (Allen, 1994).

A variety of disease states may result in the malabsorption of vitamin B$_{12}$ and, thus, secondary vitamin B$_{12}$ deficiency. For example, in patients with pernicious anemia and those who have had a gastrectomy, malabsorption of vitamin B$_{12}$ occurs as a result of a lack of intrinsic factor. Megaloblastic anemia may not appear until a long period after total gastrectomy (5–10 y), because of the capacity of the body to reutilize the vitamin.

In subjects with intestinal lesions such as jejunal diverticulosis or some anatomical abnormalities (e.g., fistulas and blind-loops), vitamin B$_{12}$ deficiency may develop because bacteria in the colon competitively utilize all the available vitamin (Cooke et al., 1963). The fish tape worm (*Diphyllobothrium latum*) also sequesters vitamin B_{12} and was a well-recognized cause of vitamin B_{12} deficiency in Finland in the past.

Patients with either tropical or nontropical (gluten-sensitive) sprue and regional ileitis may also develop vitamin B_{12} deficiency, because of alterations in the brush border structure of the ileal mucosa, which contains the receptor for intrinsic factor. In addition, alcoholism may result in vitamin B_{12} deficiency, arising from inadequate ingestion and absorption of vitamin B_{12}, as well as enhanced utilization and excretion (Kanazawa and Herbert, 1985). The deficiency may also occur in pancreatic insufficiency due to an inability to digest protein-bound vitamin B_{12}.

Some drugs, including para-aminosalicylic acid and colchicine, also cause malabsorption of vitamin B_{12}, although the specific mechanisms are unclear (Hoffbrand, 1998). Some genetic diseases that involve defects of transcobalamin II, methylmalonyl CoA mutase, or enzymes in the pathway of cobalamin adenosylation, may also result in vitamin B_{12} deficiency (IOM, 2000).

Food sources and dietary intakes

Plant products do not contain vitamin B_{12} unless they are rich in bacteria. For example, bacteria forms vitamin B_{12} during the manufacture of fermented tempeh; fermented Thai fish sauce is also said to contain significant amounts of vitamin B_{12} (Stabler and Allen, 2004). The richest food sources of vitamin B_{12} are the organ meats of liver and kidney. The vitamin is also found in shellfish, muscle meats, fish, and chicken; lesser amounts are found in eggs and dairy products (Gimsing and Nexø, 1983). Ruminants and rabbits are richer sources of vitamin B_{12} than is poultry.

Vitamin B_{12} is fairly stable and not usually destroyed by cooking at normal temperatures, although in an alkaline pH some loss may occur. Prolonged boiling of milk can reduce its vitamin B_{12} content by 50%. Data on the bioavailability of naturally occur-

ring vitamin B_{12} are limited. The U.S. Food and Nutrition Board (IOM, 2000) assumed that absorption of dietary vitamin B_{12} was 50% for persons with normal gastric function, whereas for crystalline vitamin B_{12}, absorption may range from 60% for a low dose to 0.5% for a high dose consumed with food.

Data from the 1995 U.S. Continuing Survey of Food Intakes showed that mixed foods in which meat, poultry, or fish was the main ingredient provided the greatest amount of dietary vitamin B_{12}, followed by beef for men and milk and milk drinks for women. The latter foods were also the main contributor of dietary vitamin B_{12} in the U.K. survey of young people 4–18 y (Gregory et al., 2000).

Effects of high intakes of vitamin B_{12}

There appears to be no evidence that excessive intakes of vitamin B_{12} from food or supplements causes adverse effects in healthy persons (IOM, 2000). The U.S. Food and Nutrition Board (IOM, 2000) concluded that insufficient data are available to set a Tolerable Upper Intake Level for vitamin B_{12}.

Indices of vitamin B_{12} status

The biochemical methods for assessing vitamin B_{12} status are given below, together with tests for determining the cause of the vitamin B_{12} deficiency. If subclinical vitamin B_{12} deficiency is suspected, then total serum vitamin B_{12} should be measured first, followed by serum methylmalonic acid and, if feasible, serum transcobalamin II.

22.2.1 Serum vitamin B_{12}

Of the vitamin B_{12} in the serum, 20% is attached to the transport protein transcobalamin (TC II), and the remaining 80% is distributed among a mixture of glycoprotein B_{12} binders, designated as TC I and TC III. Of the three transcobalamins (TC I, II, and III), holoTC II is the only circulating transport protein that delivers vitamin B_{12} to receptors on cell membranes and, hence, is the only biologically active form of the vitamin.

The function of TC I and III, known jointly as haptocorrin, is uncertain. Human serum also contains a variable quantity of nonfunctional analogs of vitamin B$_{12}$ (Klee, 2000).

In early vitamin B$_{12}$ deficiency, when subjects are in negative balance, the amount of vitamin B$_{12}$ attached to the transport protein TC II falls, but there is no concomitant decline in the total serum vitamin B$_{12}$ concentrations. The latter often remain normal for weeks or months despite low serum holo-TC II levels. Serum vitamin B$_{12}$ concentrations only decline when the percentage saturation of total TC II with vitamin B$_{12}$ falls below 5% (Herbert, 1987b). At this point, serum vitamin B$_{12}$ concentrations start to fall below the normal levels of 130 pmol/L, to values between 111 and 74 pmol/L, which are indicative of vitamin B$_{12}$ depletion, but biochemical function is normal (Section 22.2.8).

Total serum vitamin B$_{12}$ is the biochemical test used for routine screening for vitamin B$_{12}$ deficiency; concentrations reflect both the vitamin B$_{12}$ intake and body stores. Nevertheless, it has low sensitivity. Some persons, notably the elderly, with serum vitamin B$_{12}$ concentrations apparently within the low to normal range (111–295 pmol/L) have abnormalities in biochemical function (Metz et al., 1996). Indeed, about 5% to 15% of the elderly with serum vitamin B$_{12}$ concentrations within this range are functionally vitamin B$_{12}$ deficient (Stabler et al., 1997). The measurement of serum methylmalonic acid (Section 22.2.5) and possibly holoTC II appear to be effective methods of detecting these subtle deficiencies (Savage et al., 1994).

Clinical cases of vitamin B$_{12}$ deficiency have been reported in persons with low-to-normal serum vitamin B$_{12}$ levels (Lindenbaum et al., 1988). Many, but not all, of these subjects have shown a positive response to treatment with vitamin B$_{12}$, based on improvements in abnormal metabolite levels and clinical indices (Stabler et al., 1990).

Factors affecting serum vitamin B$_{12}$

Age influences levels of serum vitamin B$_{12}$, which tend to decrease with age (Wahlin et al., 2002). This decline probably arises from the gradual decrease in both gastric acidity and the production of intrinsic factor with aging (van Asselt et al., 1996; Carmel, 1997). An age-related decrease in the intake of vitamin B$_{12}$ may be an additional factor (Johnson et al., 2003).

Gender may affect serum vitamin B$_{12}$ concentrations, although results are not consistent. In studies that controlled for factors that could affect serum vitamin B$_{12}$ concentrations, levels were higher in women than in men (Metz et al., 1971; Fernandes-Costa et al., 1985). In other smaller, less well controlled studies, levels for men and women have been similar, irrespective of age (de Carvalho et al., 1996; Wahlin et al., 2002).

Pregnancy can lead to a steady fall in vitamin B$_{12}$ concentration in the serum due to the rapid transfer of the vitamin to the fetal circulation. This decline commences in the first trimester (Allen, 1994).

Folate deficiency may result in moderately low serum vitamin B$_{12}$ concentrations because both folate as a cosubstrate (methyl donor) and vitamin B$_{12}$ (as a coenzyme) are required in the remethylation metabolic pathway of homocysteine (step D in Figure 22.1) (Klee, 2000).

Bacterial overgrowth of the small intestine may lead to vitamin B$_{12}$ deficiency because of bacterial uptake and conversion of vitamin B$_{12}$. However, serum vitamin B$_{12}$ concentrations may appear normal because of the production of biologically inactive noncobalamin corrinoids by the bacteria (Stabler and Allen, 2004).

Lack of intrinsic factor caused by pernicious anemia or gastrectomy leads to low serum vitamin B$_{12}$ levels. Intrinsic factor is a glycoprotein synthesized by the gastric parietal cells, and it is required for the absorption of vitamin B$_{12}$ in the small intestine. In pernicious anemia, parietal cell autoantibodies against H$^+$K$^+$-adenosine triphosphate results in loss of parietal cells, which, in turn, prevents production of intrinsic factor (IOM, 2000). The incidence of pernicious anemia increases with age, and is especially common among persons of European or African descent (Stabler and Allen, 2004).

Other disease states are associated with alterations in the levels of vitamin B_{12}-binding proteins, causing misleading results. For example, in patients with myeloproliferative disorders (e.g., chronic myelogenous leukemia, polycythemia vera) or severe liver diseases, apparently normal or elevated serum vitamin B_{12} concentrations occur despite low tissue vitamin B_{12} concentrations, because of increases in the amount of unsaturated TC I and TC III (Begley and Hall, 1975).

Low serum vitamin B_{12} values occur in some disease states, because of an inability to absorb (e.g., terminal ileal disease or resection, celiac and tropical sprue) or to digest (e.g., atrophic gastritis, pancreatic insufficiency) protein-bound vitamin B_{12}. Tropical sprue is endemic in South India, and is also prevalent in the Philippines and in the Caribbean (Stabler and Allen, 2004).

Genetic diseases that cause defects in TC II or deficiencies of serum haptocorrins can cause false low values for serum vitamin B_{12} (Amos et al., 1994). Individuals with defects of methylmalonyl CoA mutase or enzymes in the cobalamin adenosylation pathway may also have low serum vitamin B_{12} levels (Kano et al., 1985).

Body mass index may be inversely related to serum vitamin B_{12} levels, but the results are not consistent (Hanger et al., 1991; Weggemans et al., 1997; Wahlin et al., 2002).

Dietary intakes of omnivores are not generally strongly related to serum vitamin B_{12} levels. In the U.K. National Diet and Nutrition Survey of British adults, weak but positive correlations of 0.11 ($p < 0.01$) and 0.10 ($p < 0.01$) for males and females, respectively, were reported (Gregory et al., 1990). Such low correlations have been linked to

the large size of liver vitamin B_{12} stores in relation to daily intakes of the vitamin. As a result, the amount in the diet may only influence circulating levels of vitamin B_{12} very slowly (Bates et al., 1997b).

Vegetarians may have low serum or plasma vitamin B_{12} levels. Indeed, there have been several reports of low plasma vitamin B_{12} levels among Asian Indians in Great Britain (Antony 2003) and the United States (Carmel et al., 2002), as well as the Indian Subcontinent (Antony, 2001; 2003).

Analytical method may affect the reported serum vitamin B_{12} concentrations. Some of the nonfunctional analogs of vitamin B_{12}, as well as the cobalamins, were measured in earlier radioassays. This led to apparently normal serum vitamin B_{12} concentrations in individuals who were vitamin B_{12} deficient (Kumar et al., 1989). This problem has now been overcome by the use of purified intrinsic factor as the binder in the commercial radioassay kits. This does not react with these vitamin B_{12} analogs (Klee, 2000). Nevertheless, the recent introduction of non-isotopic serum vitamin B_{12} assays has led to an increase in the cutoff point for serum vitamin B_{12} deficiency, again limiting comparisons across studies (Rauma et al., 1995).

Interpretive criteria

It is recommended that each laboratory analyzing serum vitamin B_{12} establish its own lower reference limits or cutoff points based on its own assay method. Values said to be indicative of deficiency and those classified as "moderately low" and "normal" are inconsistently defined in the literature and vary with the analytical method used, the laboratory conducting the analysis, the sample size, and the study design.

Values indicating deficiency are not well defined. The WHO Scientific Group on Nutritional Anemias (FAO/WHO Expert Consultation, 1988) has suggested using a cutoff of < 59 pmol/L to indicate vitamin B_{12} deficiency. Carmel and Herbert (1969) note that concentrations <74 pmol/L almost always indicate a vitamin B$_{12}$ deficiency state, irrespective of the assay procedure used. At these low levels, biochemical function is generally affected, as indicated by an abnormal deoxyuridine suppression test (Section 22.2.4), elevated levels of homocysteine (Section 22.1.5) and methylmalonic acid (Section 22.2.6) in serum, and hypersegmented neutrophils (Section 22.1.6). In addition, a clinical deficiency state, characterized by the appearance of macro-ovalocytic erythrocytes and a low hemoglobin, usually occurs.

Moderately low values for vitamin B$_{12}$ concentrations in serum are often defined as 100–150 pmol/L. Such levels are much more difficult to interpret (Amos et al., 1994). They can occur in association with megaloblastic anemia produced by folate deficiency, in iron deficiency (Layrisse et al., 1959), and with other disease states and conditions, as noted earlier.

As a result of these difficulties, many investigators now recommend measuring concentrations of serum methylmalonic acid or serum homocysteine if serum vitamin B$_{12}$ concentrations are <225 pmol/L. These two additional tests are more sensitive and specific indicators of functional vitamin B$_{12}$ deficiency (Sections 22.1.5 and 22.2.6). Both serum methylmalonic acid and homocysteine concentrations may be elevated in subjects with serum vitamin B$_{12}$ levels in the low-to-normal range (100–300 pmol/L) (Nexø et al., 1994; Stabler et al., 1996).

Normal levels for serum vitamin B$_{12}$ concentrations in healthy persons also vary markedly according to the method used and the laboratory. Only a few studies have been large and well controlled, and excluded other factors that could influence serum vitamin B$_{12}$ values.

Reference data for serum vitamin B$_{12}$ concentrations have been published for a population-based sample of Swedish adults aged 35–80 y (Wahlin et al., 2002). In this study, exclusion criteria based on hemoglobin and mean cell volume, use of certain drugs known to interfere with folate or vitamin B$_{12}$, and use of folate or vitamin B$_{12}$ supplements, were applied. Nevertheless, the investigators did not exclude subjects with other biochemical anomalies that might result from vitamin B$_{12}$ deficiency that occur in the absence of abnormal hematology, as recommended by Patel and Briddon (2000). As a consequence, if biochemical functional tests such as measurement of plasma homocysteine and methylmalonic acid had been included, more individuals with values in the low-to-normal range of serum vitamin B$_{12}$ concentrations may have been excluded.

Table 22.11 presents the mean, median, and reference range for serum vitamin B$_{12}$ concentrations for these Swedish adults classified into five age groups, based on a radio-isotope dilution assay using a commercial kit (Bio-rad Diagnostics, CA, USA). Two reference intervals are defined as the ranges between the concentrations for the 2.5th–97.5th and 5th–95th percentiles. Note that the median declines markedly with age.

The distribution of serum vitamin B$_{12}$ concentrations for a sample of clinical patients is shown Figure 22.11. Analysis in this study was based on an immunoanalyzer used in the Mayo Clinic. Note that the distribution is skewed, with a number of anomalously high concentrations, emphasizing the importance of controlling for other factors that could influence serum vitamin B$_{12}$ values, when compiling reference limits for healthy persons.

Age- and sex-specific means and selected percentiles for serum vitamin B$_{12}$ of U.S.

Age	n	Median	P$_{2.5}$–P$_{97.5}$	P$_5$–P$_{95}$
35 and 40	197	316	167–573	178–517
45 and 50	194	308	146–582	168–500
55 and 60	194	300	129–552	156–473
65 and 70	193	279	118–579	151–533
75 and 80	183	268	113–515	134–457

Table 22.11: Serum vitamin B$_{12}$ concentrations (pmol/L) stratified by age group for 961 healthy Swedish adults of both sexes. Data from Wahlin et al., Public Health Nutrition 5: 505–511, 2002, with permission of the authors.

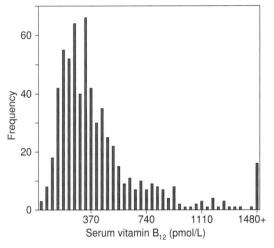

Figure 22.11: The distribution of serum vitamin B$_{12}$ concentrations in a survey of clinical patients using a method based on an immunoanalyzer (Bayer ACS:180); the reference range for this method is 148–480 pmol/L. Data from Klee, Clinical Chemistry 46: 1277–1283, 2000, with permission of the AACC.

persons aged 4–70+ y have been compiled from the NHANES III data; they are given in Appendix A22.4 (IOM, 2000). Serum vitamin B$_{12}$ values by sex and age, as well as the mean, median, and critical lower and upper percentiles for children, young people aged 4 to 18 y, and people $\geqslant$ 65 y in the U.K. National Diet and Nutrition Surveys are also available (Gregory et al., 1995; 2000; Finch et al., 1998). In these surveys, serum vitamin B$_{12}$ assays were carried out on a semiautomated analyzer using microparticle enzyme immunoassay (MEIA) technology. The lower limit of normal for adults was taken as 118 pmol/L in these surveys.

Measurement of serum vitamin B$_{12}$

Microbiological and competitive-binding assays are generally used for the measurement of serum vitamin B$_{12}$. For the microbiological assay, *Lactobacillus delbrueckii* subsp. *lactis* (ATCC 4797), also known as *L. leichmannii*, or *Euglena gracilis* are used; both having relatively specific requirements for vitamin B$_{12}$ for growth (Herbert et al., 1984). The microbiological assay is based on the same principle as that for the analysis of

serum or erythrocyte folate (Section 22.1.3) and has comparable limitations. For example, bacteriostatic substances in the blood, including antibiotics or cancer chemotherapeutic agents, inhibit the growth of the microorganism and interfere with the assay, producing misleadingly low serum vitamin B$_{12}$ concentrations. Furthermore, long incubation times may be necessary, making the procedure very time consuming.

A microbiological method using 96-well microtiter plates that are read with an automatic plate reader is now available (Kelleher and O'Broin, 1991). The presence of antibiotics in the serum samples can be overcome by enzyme inactivation (Kelleher et al., 1990), or by use of a collistin sulfate resistant organism (Kelleher et al., 1987).

Competitive-binding assays that use radioisotope dilution methods for detection are simpler and less time consuming than the microbiological assays. Many of the methods available can be automated (Chan, 1996), and unlike the microbiological assays, they are not affected by antibiotics or cancer chemotherapeutic agents. The coefficient of variation among the six laboratories for serum vitamin B$_{12}$ analyzed by automated competitive-binding assays has been reported to vary from 4.4% to 10.0% (Klee, 2000).

The competitive-binding methods depend on the addition of radioactive cyanocobalamin which competes with vitamin B$_{12}$ in the serum for the binding sites on an added cobalamin-binding protein. Purified hog intrinsic factor is now often used as the binding protein. Alkaline conditions are used to disrupt the vitamin B$_{12}$ from the binding proteins, after which the vitamin B$_{12}$ is generally converted to cyanocobalamin by potassium cyanide, prior to measurement (Klee, 2000).

Radioassays that measure serum folic acid and vitamin B$_{12}$ simultaneously are available (Gutcho and Mansbach, 1977), but should not be used if sodium ascorbate has been added to stabilize the folate in serum. Some of these radioassays can be semiautomated (Chen et al., 1982).

Both serum and plasma samples in which EDTA has been used as the anticoagulant can

	< 100 pmol/L (n = 50)	100–150 pmol/L (n = 46)	150–200 pmol/L (n = 43)	≥ 200 pmol/L (n = 65)	p
Cobalamin (pmol/L)	77 (47–95)	115 (101–145)	163 (151–197)	274 (205–964)	< 0.001
MMA (µmol/L)	0.68 (0.33–2.64)	0.63 (0.12–1.75)	0.47 (0.13–1.76)	0.26 (0.05–0.84)	< 0.001
MMA > 0.26 µmol/L (%)	98	78	74	49	< 0.001
HoloTC II (pmol/L)	11 (6–30)	18 (9–34)	22 (10–58)	55 (18–304)	< 0.001
Low holoTC II (%)	98	98	81	28	< 0.001
tHcy (µmol/L)	29.8 (13.6–80.1)	22.9 (10.4–42.1)	19.7 (11.7–37.3)	15.5 (8.5–27.1)	< 0.001
tHcy > 15 µmol/L (%)	96	83	84	55	< 0.001
Serum folate (nmol/L)	12.2 (6.3–26.0)	12.6 (5.3–27.2)	11.6 (2.2–29.3)	11.3 (3.5–37.9)	0.26
Hemoglobin (g/L)	149 (106–182)	144 (103–170)	144 (104–162)	144 (124–168)	0.78
Anemia (%)	19	11	19	22	0.55
MCV (fL)	80.7 (37.1–99.0)	81.8 (26.5–92.6)	82.2 (43.6–98.8)	82.2 (26.8–113.1)	0.71
Macroytosis (%)	0	3	0	3	0.45
Vegetarian diet (%)	42	57	23	32	0.007

Table 22.12: Differences in selected variables by serum cobalamin concentration in 204 men and women from India. Values are medians or percentages with the 5th–95th percentiles in parentheses. MMA, methylmalonic acid in serum; Holo TC II, holotranscobalamin II in serum; tHcy, serum total homocysteine; MCV, mean cell volume. Data from Refsum et al., American Journal of Clinical Nutrition 74: 233–241, 2001 © Am J Clin Nutr. American Society for Clinical Nutrition.

be used for all the analytical methods for vitamin B$_{12}$. Heparinized plasma samples cannot be used for the microbiological assay because heparin interferes with the assay. Generally, agreement between the vitamin B$_{12}$ microbiological assay and the more recent commercially available protein-binding kits involving radioisotope dilution is good, provided purified hog intrinsic factor is used as the binder for vitamin B$_{12}$ (Gilois et al., 1986).

22.2.2 Erythrocyte vitamin B$_{12}$

Erythrocyte assays for vitamin B$_{12}$ appear to have had limited use; variable results have been obtained, with a large overlap in values for normal and vitamin B$_{12}$-deficient subjects (Omer et al., 1970b). Moreover, erythrocyte vitamin B$_{12}$ concentrations also tend to be low in folate deficiency (Harrison, 1971), because vitamin B$_{12}$ is necessary for the uptake of folate by red blood cells.

22.2.3 Serum holotranscobalamin II

Serum holotranscobalamin II (holoTC II) is the physiologically active metabolite of vitamin B$_{12}$ that delivers the vitamin to all DNA-synthesizing cells, as discussed earlier. Holo-TC II is made in the ileal enterocytes from intracellularly synthesized TC II and absorbed vitamin B$_{12}$. Because holoTC II has a short half-life, concentrations quickly fall below normal after vitamin B$_{12}$ absorption ceases. Consequently, low holoTC II concentrations in serum are the earliest indicator of negative vitamin B$_{12}$ balance, and levels fall long before those of total serum vitamin B$_{12}$.

Unfortunately, the assay of holoTC II is difficult, so very few studies have included this measurement. Therefore, at the present time, the clinical utility of holoTC II is not well established (Wickramasinghe and Ratnayaka, 1996; Lindgren et al., 1999).

Table 22.12 shows data on the concentrations of vitamin B$_{12}$, holoTC II, methylmalonic acid, total homocysteine, and folate in serum, along with hemoglobin and mean cell volume concentrations in relation to the serum vitamin B$_{12}$ levels in a group of Asian Indians (Refsum et al., 2001). In this cross-sectional study, holoTC II was analyzed with a radioimmunoassay based on monoclonal antibodies against transcobalamin. The total serum vitamin B_{12} and holoTC II levels were strongly correlated ($r = 0.78$), with both variables demonstrating a significant inverse association with serum methylmalonic acid and total homocysteine concentrations. At higher serum vitamin B_{12} concentrations, holoTC II was also elevated. Hence, for subjects with serum vitamin B_{12} levels of > 300 pmol/L, the proportion with low holoTC II concentrations was $< 5\%$. Even subjects with normal to relatively normal serum vitamin B_{12} values had concentrations of serum methylmalonic acid and total homocysteine that were frequently high.

Low serum holoTC II concentrations have also been reported in patients with macrocytosis arising from causes not related to vitamin B_{12} deficiency, but perhaps resulting from factors such as erythroid hyperplasia (Zittoun and Zittoun, 1999).

Low serum holoTC II has been proposed as a surrogate for the Schilling test (a measure of vitamin B_{12} absorption) (Section 22.2.7) (Herbert et al., 1990). Technical concerns over the assay of holoTC II in serum must be resolved, however, before it can be used reliably in this way (Herbert et al., 1990).

Measurement of serum holoTC II

Radioimmunoassay methods are available for the analysis of holoTC II in serum (Vu et al., 1993). The assays are based on monoclonal antibodies against transcobalamin. To date, they have had limited use in routine clinical investigations (Wickramsinghe and Ratnayaka, 1996).

22.2.4 Deoxyuridine suppression test

This sensitive in vitro test has been used to diagnose early vitamin B_{12} (or folate) deficiency even in the absence of morphological changes in the blood. It was developed by Killman (1964) and Metz et al. (1968).

Abnormal deoxyuridine suppression is the biochemical expression of disordered DNA metabolism. Although either lymphocytes or whole blood can be used for this test to detect past vitamin B_{12} or folate status,

generally bone marrow cells are preferred because they measure the acute status (Colman, 1981). The test is used rarely today because it requires bone marrow cultures, uses a radioactive label, and is difficult to control (Carmel et al., 1996b; Chanarin and Metz, 1997).

Figure 22.1 depicts the folate metabolic cycle with its interactions with vitamin B_{12}, the thymidylate pathway, and the methionine cycle. The key pathways by which deoxyuridine is converted to thymidylate are shown. The preferred de novo pathway (E) uses thymidylate synthetase and 5,10-methylene-tetrahydrofolate (THFA). The salvage pathway (F) uses preformed thymidylate. If the supply of vitamin B_{12} (and folate) is adequate, the addition of nonradioactive deoxyuridine to bone marrow cells in vitro will promote de novo synthesis of thymidylate, suppressing the incorporation of the radioactive thymidylate into DNA via the salvage pathway. However, in vitamin B_{12} (or folate) deficiency, de novo biosynthesis of the thymidylate is blocked, and, instead, the salvage pathway is used. As a result, more radioactive thymidylate is incorporated into DNA, compared with the nutrient replete control.

Elevated dU-suppression values ($> 20\%$) characterize both vitamin B_{12}- and folate-deficient bone marrow cultures. To distinguish between these two vitamin deficiencies, either cobalamin or methyltetrahydrofolate is added to the bone marrow cultures. The uptake of ^{3}H-thymidine radioactivity is then compared in the absence or presence of the in vitro additional cobalamin or methyltetrahydrofolate (Wickramasinghe and Longland, 1974; Carmel, 1983). In this way, the vitamin that corrects the deficiency can be identified (Figure 22.12).

The modification described above is useful in diagnosing early folate and vitamin B_{12} deficiency before anemia has developed (Wickramasinghe and Saunders, 1975; Das and Herbert, 1978). It can also diagnose vitamin B_{12} and folate deficiency in the presence of concomitant iron deficiency, liver disease, myeloproliferative disorder, or hemoglobinopathy. Although these conditions do not

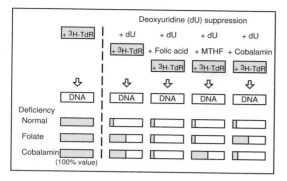

Figure 22.12: Deoxyuridine suppression test. Hatched bars represent ^{3}H-thymidine (^{3}H-TdR) radioactivity; results are expressed in percentage radioactivity incorporated into DNA, as compared with baseline 100% in the first column. The second column illustrates the normal value of < 10%, as compared with values of > 20% in deficiency. Folate-deficient marrow is not corrected by cobalamin (column 5), whereas cobalamin-deficient marrow is not corrected by methyltetra hydrofolate (MTHF in column 4). For unexplained reasons, cobalamin-deficient marrow is always corrected more completely by folic acid than by cobalamin. From Carmel R (1983). Clinical and laboratory features of the diagnosis of megaloblastic anemia. In: Lindenbaum J (ed). Nutrition in Hematology © Churchill Livingstone Inc., with permission.

confound the results of the dUST, they may result in normal erythrocyte and serum folate or serum vitamin B$_{12}$ concentrations, despite the presence of vitamin B$_{12}$ and folate deficiency. Unfortunately, the dUST is too cumbersome and not very reliable for routine laboratory diagnosis.

Measurement of dU suppression

For the test measurement of dU suppression, pairs of bone marrow cultures (or lymphocytes or whole blood), one with and one without nonradioactive dU, are preincubated. This preparatory step suppresses the ability of the bone marrow cells from a normal healthy individual to incorporate the subsequently added radioactive thymidine (^{3}H-thymidine) into DNA. Next, radioactive thymidine is added, and its uptake in each culture is counted on a scintillation counter. The results are expressed as a percentage of the uptake without preincubation with dU. This percentage is called the "dU-suppressed value." If > 20%

of total DNA in the culture is radioactive, vitamin B$_{12}$ or folate deficiency is present.

22.2.5 Methylmalonic acid excretion

Vitamin B$_{12}$ serves as a cofactor for methylmalonyl CoA mutase (EC 5.4.99.2). This enzyme acts in the conversion of methylmalonyl CoA to succinyl CoA (Figure 22.13). Therefore, in vitamin B$_{12}$ deficiency, methylmalonic acid accumulates in the blood and is excreted in increased amounts in the urine, resulting in methylmalonic aciduria (Norman and Morrison, 1993).

This test is sensitive and it detects early functional vitamin B$_{12}$ deficiency before the onset of macrocytic anemia. Nevertheless, the level of methylmalonic acid excretion is not necessarily related to the severity of the deficiency. Sensitivity can be enhanced by administering a loading dose of L-valine (5 g for children < 6 y; 10 g for adults) or isoleucine, precursors of methylmalonic acid. In normal adult subjects, < 254 μmol/24 h methylmalonic acid is excreted postload; in patients with vitamin B$_{12}$ deficiency, the postload excretion is > 423 μmol/24 h.

The test is also highly specific and is not affected by folate deficiency. Only rare congenital enzyme defects (e.g., methylmalonic aciduria) interfere with the test. In elderly patients with renal disease, however, urinary methylmalonic acid levels should be adjusted for creatinine excretion (Norman and Morrison, 1993).

Interpretive criteria for both endogenous

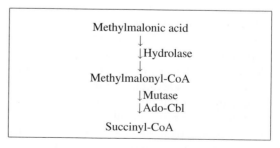

Figure 22.13: Conversion of methylmalonyl-coenzyme A (CoA) to succinyl-CoA via methylmalonyl CoA mutase (mutase). Ado-Cbl indicates adenosyl-cobalamin.

	Endogenous MMA excretion	Post 10 g valine
Normal	< 42.3 µmol/24 h (< 5.0 mg/24 h)	< 254 µmol/L (< 30.0 mg/L)
Borderline		254–423 µmol/24 h (30–50 mg/h)
Vit. B$_{12}$-deficient	> 33.9 µmol/24 h (> 4.0 mg/24 h)	> 423 µmol/24 h (> 50 mg/h)

Table 22.13: Expected values for urinary methylmalonic acid excretion. Data from Biolab Medical Unit, London. (http://www.biolab.co.uk/)

excretion of methylmalonic acid and after a loading dose of 10 g valine are given in Table 22.13.

Measurement of methylmalonic acid in urine

Combined gas-chromatography mass-spectrometry techniques are sensitive and reliable for measuring methylmalonic acid in urine (Norman and Morrison, 1993). Unfortunately, this procedure is technically difficult. The test is best performed on a 24-h urine sample, although spot urine samples can be used for screening. Methylmalonic acid is stable at room temperature, provided concentrated hydrochloric acid is added to the urine sample, and is stable for several years, when urine specimens are frozen at −70°C.

22.2.6 Serum methylmalonic acid

Methylmalonic acid also accumulates in the serum or plasma when the supply of vitamin B$_{12}$ is reduced; it does not rise in folate deficiency (Savage et al., 1994). Hence, the measurement of methylmalonic acid in serum or plasma, like urine, is a sensitive and specific marker of vitamin B$_{12}$ deficiency. Concentrations are elevated in vitamin B$_{12}$ deficiency, even in the absence of clinical signs or symptoms or of morphological changes in the blood. In a study of 70 elderly subjects, for example, Lindenbaum et al. (1994) reported that > 40% with serum vitamin B$_{12}$ < 150 pmol/L had serum methylmalonic acid levels > 376 nmol/L (> 0.38 µmol/L).

Elevated serum methylmalonic acid (and homocysteine) concentrations have been reported, even in patients with apparently "normal" serum vitamin B$_{12}$ concentrations. The results summarized in Figure 22.14 show that methylmalonic acid and homocysteine levels in serum were elevated in > 20% of patients with serum vitamin B$_{12}$ levels within the "normal" reference laboratory range (Holleland et al., 1999). A similar trend was noted in a study of 72 patients studied by Klee (2000). In this study, elevated concentrations of serum methylmalonic acid were reported even in patients with serum vitamin B$_{12}$ concentrations as high as 295 pmol/L.

In some cases, elevated serum methylmalonic acid (and homocysteine) concentrations have been reduced by vitamin B$_{12}$ therapy, thus confirming a vitamin B$_{12}$ deficiency (Lindenbaum et al., 1990; Joosten et al., 1993). Bolann et al. (2000), noted that patients in their study (n = 196) with elevated serum concentrations and urinary excretion levels for methylmalonic acid (> 376 nmo/L; > 0.38 µmol/24 h) all showed a reduction in serum methylmalonic acid of more than 50% after cobalamin supplementation.

The validity of serum or plasma methylmalonic acid concentrations as a sensitive and specific test for the diagnosis of nutritional vitamin B$_{12}$ deficiency during infancy has

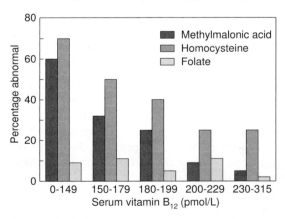

Figure 22.14: Abnormalities in serum methylmalonic acid, homocysteine, and folate concentrations found with various concentrations of serum vitamin B$_{12}$. Plotted from data in Holleland et al., Clinical Chemistry 45: 189–198, 1999, with permission of the AACC.

	Macrobiotics (n = 41)	Controls (n = 50)
MMA (μmol/L)	1.44 (0.17–12.15)	0.18 (0.06–0.51)
	$p < 0.0001$	
Hcy (μmol/L)	13.5 (6.8–26.8)	7.59 (5.3–11.0)
	$p < 0.0014$	
Cobalamin (pmol/L)	141 (59–340)	399 (194–821)
	$p < 0.0001$	
Cysteine (μmol/L)	164 (119–226)	184 (145–233)
	$p = 0.0001$	
Methionine (μmol/L)	6.0 (1.5–23.8)	6.9 (1.1–41.9)
	$p = 0.44$	

Table 22.14: Plasma levels of cobalamin and metabolites in macrobiotic and healthy control infants. MMA, methylmalonic acid; Hcy, homocysteine. Data from Schneede et al., Pediatric Research 36: 194–201, 1994.

also been confirmed. The results of a study of 41 Dutch infants on macrobiotic diets and 50 healthy omnivorous controls (Table 22.14) showed markedly higher plasma methylmalonic acid concentrations in the infants on macrobiotic diets compared to the controls (Schneede et al., 1994). Moreover, plasma methylmalonic acid concentrations were inversely related to plasma vitamin B$_{12}$ levels. Logistic regression showed that methylmalonic acid followed by total homocysteine and cobalamin in plasma, in that order, were the strongest predictors of vitamin B$_{12}$ deficiency in the macrobiotic group.

Several other investigators have compared the sensitivity of serum or plasma methylmalonic acid in diagnosing vitamin B$_{12}$ or folate deficiency with that of serum or plasma total homocysteine. Results of a study by Savage et al. (1994) (Table 22.15) emphasize the high sensitivity of both serum methylmalonic acid concentrations and total homocysteine levels for the diagnosis of functional vitamin B$_{12}$ deficiency.

Serum methylmalonic acid concentrations are also considered to be a very specific measure of functional vitamin B$_{12}$ deficiency. Only a few conditions confound their use. Levels may rise in cases of hypovolemia

(decrease in the volume of circulating blood), renal insufficiency, some inherited metabolic defects, and small bowel overgrowth and with concurrent use of antibiotics. Of these confounding conditions, renal failure results in more modest changes than those produced by vitamin B$_{12}$ deficiency (Savage et al., 1994). If small-bowel overgrowth with bacteria that produce high levels of propionic acid (the precursor of methylmalonic acid) is the condition suspected, treatment with antibiotics should result in a decline in serum methylmalonic acid concentrations (Snow, 1999).

In adults, decreases in serum methylmalonic acid concentrations with increasing age have been reported. This trend is said to reflect the increasingly inadequate absorption of vitamin B$_{12}$ that occurs with aging (Stabler and Allen, 2004). This arises from the gradual decrease in gastric acidity and production of intrinsic factor (van Asselt et al., 1996), as noted earlier, although inadequate intakes may be a contributing factor (Joosten et al., 1996; Johnson et al., 2003).

Interpretive criteria

Currently there is no consensus for the cutoff value for serum methylmalonic acid concentrations indicative of vitamin B$_{12}$ deficiency. Joosten et al. (1993) used > 376 nmol/L as abnormal in a study of elderly subjects. Klee

Serum level	Prevalence in cobalamin deficient patients (%)	Prevalence in folate deficient patients (%)
Elevated MMA	98	12
Elevated Hcy	96	91
Elevated MMA, Hcy normal	4	2
Elevated Hcy, MMA normal	1	80
Hcy and MMA both normal	0.2	7

Table 22.15: Performance of serum metabolite assays in patients with clinically defined cobalamin or folate deficiency. Data from Savage et al., American Journal of Medicine 96: 239–246, 1994.

	Geometric mean	Central 95% reference interval
M	107	50–227
F	132	59–296
M + F	123	55–278

Table 22.16: Geometric mean and reference intervals for serum methylmalonic acid (nmol/L) in 143 elderly subjects after a 3-wk vitamin supplementation period. Data from Joosten et al., European Journal of Haematology 57: 222–226, 1996.

(2000) cautions that a serum methylmalonic acid level > 400 nmol/L, in the presence of a serum vitamin B_{12} concentration ranging from 110 to 220 pmol/L, warrant further investigation.

Joosten et al. (1996) have compiled reference intervals for elderly males and females, based on a group who were supplemented with a combination of vitamin B_{12}, folate, and vitamin B_6, in an effort to ensure that their serum methylmalonic acid concentrations reflected "normal" values. These intervals are shown in Table 22.16.

Note that if both serum methylmalonic acid and homocysteine are analyzed, a distinction can be made between vitamin B_{12} and folate deficiencies. Elevated levels of both metabolites are expected in vitamin B_{12} deficiency, whereas in folate deficiency, only increases in serum homocysteine concentrations occur.

Measurement of methylmalonic acid

The analytical procedures most frequently used for serum methylmalonic acid involve capillary gas chromatography and mass spectrometry. A method based on capillary electrophoresis with laser-induced fluorescence detection has been developed for routine use (Schneede and Ueland, 1995), but it does not appear to have been widely adopted. Caution must be used when interpreting older data for serum methylmalonic acid because of recent improvements in the analytical method (Green and Kinsella, 1995). A new method, based on electrospray tandem mass spectrometry, as described for plasma homocysteine,

is being developed to measure serum methylmalonic acid (Klee, 2000). Levels in serum are stable for several years, when samples are stored at $-70°C$.

22.2.7 The Schilling and other tests

Once vitamin B_{12} deficiency has been diagnosed, it is essential to establish if malabsorption is the cause. This can be achieved by a two-stage process. First, a small oral dose (0.5–2 µg) of radioactive vitamin B_{12} is given, followed by a flushing dose of nonradioactive vitamin B_{12}. The percentage of radiolabel excreted in a 24-h urine sample is then measured. Second, intrinsic factor is given along with the radioactive vitamin B_{12}. Administration of the flushing dose and measurement of the radiolabel in the urine follows, as before. This two-stage procedure is called the Schilling test (Schilling, 1953).

One major disadvantage of the conventional Schilling test is that it measures the absorption of crystalline vitamin B_{12} rather than absorption of vitamin B_{12} bound to food. To overcome this limitation, the "food Schilling test" (or the protein-bound cobalamin absorption test) has been developed. The modification involves using radioactive B_{12} incorporated into foods such as eggs, chicken, egg albumin, and chicken serum instead of into crystalline vitamin B_{12}. Use of this modified approach is especially important for the elderly, when a conventional Schilling test may appear normal, despite the existence of low serum vitamin B_{12} concentrations. This arises because elderly subjects may have adequate intrinsic factor to absorb free crystalline vitamin B_{12}, but not vitamin B_{12} in foods (Doscherholmen et al., 1976; Carmel, 1997).

A further modification of the Schilling test involves performing both stages of the test simultaneously, to eliminate the 2–3 d delay. Further, a diagnosis of pernicious anemia can be made using this test, even when urine collections are incomplete. The reliability of this combined method, however, has been questioned (Domstad et al., 1981).

Joosten et al. (1993) used a protein-bound cobalamin absorption procedure with a group of 34 elderly patients with low serum vitamin B_{12} concentrations (i.e., <125 pmol/L) and 27 elderly control patients, then compared the results to those obtained with the conventional Schilling test. The 24-h urinary [57]Co-cobalamin excretion was significantly higher in the control group than in the elderly patients with low serum vitamin B_{12} (median 1.42% vs. 0.46%; $p = 0.0005$) (Figure 22.15). Of the 34 elderly patients, 9 (26%) had an abnormal protein-bound cobalamin absorption test with a [57]Co-cobalamin excretion $<0.18\%$. Comparison of the protein-bound cobalamin absorption test with the Schilling test, however, revealed concordant results in 80% of these elderly patients. This suggests that the protein-bound cobalamin absorption test offered little advantage over the conventional Schilling test in diagnosing vitamin B_{12} malabsorption in these elderly patients.

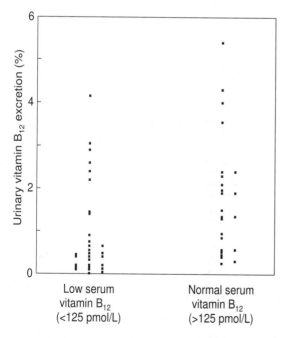

Figure 22.15: Urinary [57]Co-cobalamin excretion following protein-bound cobalamin absorption test in patients with low serum vitamin B_{12} and controls. Data from Joosten et al., European Journal of Haematology 51: 25–30, 1993.

Measurement of vitamin B_{12} absorption

To perform the conventional Schilling test, first a dose (0.5–2 µg) of radioactive vitamin B_{12} (labeled with [57]Co or [58]Co) is given orally to the fasting patient. One hour later, a large flushing dose (1000 µg) of nonradioactive vitamin B_{12} is given parenterally, followed by the collection of 24-h or 48-h urine samples.

The purpose of the flushing dose is to saturate both tissue-binding stores and circulating vitamin B_{12}-binding protein, enhancing the urinary excretion of the absorbed radioactive vitamin B_{12}. Although most of the radioactivity appears in the urine within the first 24-h when renal function is normal, it is delayed with renal insufficiency. Hence urine should be collected preferably for a 48-h period.

If the results are abnormal, stage two of the conventional test is carried out 2–3 d later, but with the addition of a commercial preparation of intrinsic factor with the oral radioactive dose. The urinary excretion should then be restored to near-normal values if the low vitamin B_{12} absorption arises from intrinsic factor deficiency. If, however, the vitamin B_{12} deficiency is associated with intestinal disease or infestation with fish tapeworm, the test results will not be normalized by the addition of intrinsic factor. In such circumstances, further investigations must be undertaken.

Unfortunately, the Schilling test is not well standardized among laboratories; the timing of the flushing dose of vitamin B_{12}, the level of the isotope dose, and the duration of the urine collection may all vary (Chanarin and Waters, 1974). Furthermore, the flushing dose of parenterally administered vitamin B_{12} is therapeutic and, as a result, may subsequently interfere with the diagnosis. Therefore, alternative techniques that do not necessitate a flushing dose have been developed. These include measurement of plasma radioactivity, stool excretion, hepatic radioactivity, or whole body counting (1 wk postdose). Such methods are not widely used because they require specialized equipment. It is also necessary in the whole body counting and the stool excretion tests

	Normal	Negative vitamin B_{12} balance	Vitamin B_{12} depletion	Vitamin B_{12}-deficient erythro-poiesis	Vitamin B_{12}-deficiency anemia
HoloTC II (pmol/L)	> 37	Low	Low	Low	Low
TC II % sat.	> 5%	< 4%	< 4%	< 4%	< 4%
dU suppression	Normal	Normal	Normal	Abnormal	Abnormal
Hypersegmentation	No	No	No	Yes	Yes
TBBC % sat.	> 15%	> 15%	> 15%	< 15%	< 10%
RBC folate (nmol/L)	> 363	> 363	> 363	< 317	< 227
Erythrocytes	Normal	Normal	Normal	Normal	Macro-ovalocytic
MCV	Normal	Normal	Normal	Normal	Elevated
Hemoglobin	Normal	Normal	Normal	Normal	Low
TC II	Normal	Normal	Normal	Elevated	Elevated
Methylmalonic acid	Normal	Normal	Normal	High	High
Homocysteine	Normal	Normal	Normal	High	High
Myelin damage	No	No	No	?	Frequent

Table 22.17: Sequential stages in the development of vitamin B_{12} deficiency. HoloTC II, holotranscobalamin II; TC II % sat, percentage of total TC II with attached cobalamin; dU suppression, deoxyuridine suppression test; TBBC % sat; percentage of total B_{12} binding capacity of plasma with attached B_{12}; RBC, red blood cells; MCV, mean cell volume. From Herbert, American Journal of Clinical Nutrition 46: 387–402, 1987c © Am J Clin Nutr. American Society for Clinical Nutrition.

to ensure complete excretion of unabsorbed vitamin B_{12}.

In view of the limitations discussed above, and the necessity for using radioactive isotopes, the Schilling test is rarely used today. Instead, measurements of methylmalonic acid and homocysteine are being used as more sensitive tests of early pernicious anemia. Some alternative procedures that can help diagnose pernicious anemia include a combination of anti-intrinsic factor antibodies, and gastrin and pepsinogen A and C in serum (Toh et al., 1997). These three tests can all be performed using serologic assays, and used in combination they can identify most cases of pernicious anemia (Lindgren et al., 1998).

22.2.8 Multiple indices

Table 22.17 depicts the sequential stages in the development of vitamin B_{12} deficiency developed initially by Herbert (1987c), and modified in 1996. Modifications to the model include the newer, more sensitive, and

specific functional tests of mild preclinical vitamin B_{12} deficiency (i.e., serum methylmalonic acid and homocysteine).

Unlike folate deficiency, the first stage of vitamin B_{12} deficiency (negative balance), cannot be detected by analysis of total serum vitamin B_{12}. Instead, this early stage can be detected only by a reduction in holoTC II in serum (Section 22.2.3), although technical difficulties still exist with this assay. If the negative balance persists, the second stage occurs, vitamin B_{12} depletion. At this stage, total serum vitamin B_{12} concentrations are reduced to 75–110 pmol/L, but biochemical function is still normal.

Abnormalities in biochemical function do not occur until the third stage, vitamin B_{12} deficient erythropoiesis. Until recently, this stage was characterized by an abnormal dU suppression test or hypersegmented neutrophils (or both), as described for folate deficiency. Today, measurement of two metabolites — homocysteine and methylmalonic acid — in serum can now be performed to

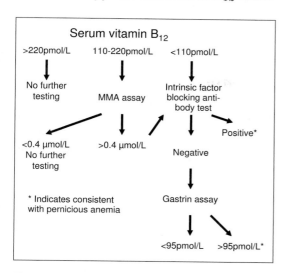

Serum vitamin B$_{12}$

>220pmol/L   110-220pmol/L   <110pmol/L

No further
testing   MMA assay   Intrinsic factor
                                      blocking anti-
                                      body test

<0.4 µmol/L   >0.4 µmol/L   Positive*
No further
testing   Negative

* Indicates consistent   Gastrin assay
with pernicious anemia

                        <95pmol/L   >95pmol/L*

Figure 22.16: Algorithm for the laboratory evaluation of patients with suspected pernicious anemia, beginning with serum vitamin B$_{12}$ measurements and cascading to tests for methylmalonic acid (MMA), intrinsic factor blocking antibodies, and serum gastrin. From Klee, Clinical Chemistry 46: 1277–1283, 2000, with permission of the AACC.

detect this early stage of functional vitamin B$_{12}$ deficiency. Serum concentrations of these two metabolites rise when cellular vitamin B$_{12}$ stores fall below the levels required to maintain normal metabolism. Of the two, serum methylmalonic acid is more sensitive and specific for vitamin B$_{12}$-deficient erythropoiesis than is homocysteine. Concentrations of total serum vitamin B$_{12}$ at this stage are even lower.

Hematopoietic defects associated with the deficiency do not occur until the fourth stage, vitamin B$_{12}$-deficiency anemia. At this stage, symptoms similar to those of folic acid deficiency can be observed. These include macro-ovalocytic erythrocytes, abnormal red cell indices, and a low hemoglobin.

The recommended combination of tests, therefore, to detect the stages in the development of vitamin B$_{12}$ deficiency includes serum vitamin B$_{12}$ and methylmalonic acid, mean cell volume, and hemoglobin. Serum folate should also be measured to establish whether folate deficiency coexists.

To diagnose pernicious anemia, a sequence of tests shown in Figure 22.16 can be used. In

this sequence, serum vitamin B$_{12}$ levels are first assayed. Specimens with test concentrations < 110 pmol/L are subjected to intrinsic factor antibody testing, and, if positive, they are considered consistent with pernicious anemia. Specimens testing negative for antibodies should be followed up with gastrin testing, as shown in Figure 22.16, when, again, increased levels (> 200 ng/L) are considered consistent with pernicious anemia. Specimens with serum vitamin B$_{12}$ values of 110–220 pmol/L can be analyzed for serum methylmalonic acid. If the latter are elevated (i.e., > 400 nmol/L), then intrinsic factor antibody testing should be performed, followed by gastrin testing for those negative for antibodies (Klee, 2000).

22.3 Summary

Folate

Megaloblastic anemia associated with nutritional folate deficiency may occur in pregnant and lactating women in low-income countries. In industrialized countries, subclinical folate deficiency is more widespread, again especially in pregnant and lactating women and in the presence of certain diseases and drugs.

Folate coenzymes are involved in the transfer of single-carbon atom groups, including methylene (CH$_2$), forminino (CH=NH), methyl (CH$_3$), methenyl (CH), and formyl (CHO), in intermediary metabolism. These single-carbon atom groups are involved in five key metabolic functions: (*a*) serine and glycine metabolism; (*b*) histidine catabolism; (*c*) thymidylate synthesis; (*d*) methionine synthesis; and (*e*) purine synthesis. Both folate and vitamin B$_{12}$ deficiency can lead to megaloblastic anemia arising from impairment in the production of 5,10-methylene tetrahydrofolate, which is essential for the biosynthesis of DNA. Hence, abnormal cell replication in the hematopoietic system, manifested by hypersegmented neutrophils, is one of the early morphological changes associated with folate deficiency. Later, macrocytes appear in the peripheral blood and megaloblasts appear in the bone marrow.

In the past, serum and erythrocyte folate concentrations were the most frequently used biochemical tests of folate status, but now serum homocysteine concentrations are often measured as well. Serum folate levels reflect folate balance, fluctuate rapidly with recent changes in folate intakes, and provide no information on the size of tissue folate stores. The latter can be estimated by measuring erythrocyte folate concentrations, which only fall in subjects in persistent negative folate balance. Concentrations of folate in erythrocytes, but not serum, also fall in vitamin B_{12} deficiency. Consequently, both serum and erythrocyte folate concentrations must be measured to distinguish between folate and vitamin B_{12} deficiency.

The initial stage of folate deficiency — termed negative folate balance — is consistent with serum folate values of < 6.8 nmol/L. If the negative balance persists, serum folate values fall below the reference range, and then tissue folate becomes depleted (as indicated by erythrocyte folate levels falling below the normal range to < 363 nmol/L). At this second stage — termed folate depletion — there is little evidence that biochemical function is impaired, although plasma homocysteine levels may be slightly elevated (Table 22.10). Functional impairment is usually evident at the third stage — termed folate-deficient erythropoiesis — when erythrocyte folate values are < 272 nmol/L. At this stage, the dU suppression test is abnormal, and concentration of plasma homocysteine is markedly elevated.

Identification of folate deficiency at this third stage has gained increasing importance because during pregnancy it can cause neural tube defects in the developing fetus. In addition, the compensatory increase in homocysteine levels that occurs in folate-deficient erythropoiesis is known to be a significant risk factor for cardiovascular disease.

Tissue folate stores are severely depleted in the fourth and final stage of folate deficiency — folate-deficiency anemia. At this stage, the classical hematological changes occur. These include macro-ovalocytic erythrocytes in the circulating blood and megaloblasts in the bone marrow. At this stage, hypersegmented neutrophils in the peripheral blood smear and abnormal red cell indices are also apparent; mean red cell volume and mean cell hemoglobin are elevated and hemoglobin is low. These sequential stages in the development of folate deficiency are summarized in Table 22.10.

Vitamin B_{12}

In contrast to folate, dietary deficiencies of vitamin B_{12} in industrialized countries are relatively rare and usually arise from atrophic gastritis and malabsorption, particularly in the elderly. In developing countries, dietary vitamin B_{12} deficiency may occur among children and pregnant and lactating women who exclude or consume low amounts of animal foods. A variety of disease states may cause malabsorption and thus secondary vitamin B_{12} deficiency.

There are two major metabolic roles for vitamin B_{12}: (*a*) the synthesis of methionine from homocysteine and (*b*) the conversion of methylmalonyl coenzyme A to succinyl coenzyme A.

Deficiency of vitamin B_{12} occurs in four stages. The first stage — termed negative vitamin B_{12} balance — can only be detected by a reduction in holoTC II (Table 22.17). If the negative balance persists, then the second stage — termed vitamin B_{12} depletion — is reached, indicated by a fall in serum vitamin B_{12} concentrations to low-to-normal levels. Even at this stage, there may be some evidence of biochemical impairment, as indicated by an elevated serum methylmalonic acid (> 400 nmol/L) and homocysteine concentration.

At the third stage — termed vitamin B_{12}-deficient erythropoiesis — serum concentrations of vitamin B_{12} are even lower, whereas serum methylmalonic acid and homocysteine are even further elevated. As well, the dU suppression test is now abnormal, and hypersegmented neutrophils exist, as described for folate deficiency. Urinary excretion of methylmalonic acid is also often elevated at this stage.

In the fourth and final stage — termed vitamin B_{12}-deficiency anemia — defects in the hematopoietic system, similar to those of folic acid deficiency arise. Macro-ovalocytic erythrocytes, abnormal red cell indices, and a low hemoglobin occur, together with elevated serum and urine concentrations of methylmalonic acid and serum homocysteine.

Vitamin B_{12} has an important role in the metabolism of methylmalonate and thus may be responsible for the neurological disorders that can arise in vitamin B_{12} deficiency. In the past, the Schilling test was used to ascertain the cause of vitamin B_{12} deficiency. This test is rarely used today. It has been replaced by the measurement of serum methylmalonic acid in conjunction with serological assays of anti-intrinsic factor antibodies, gastrin, and pepsinogen A and C. These three tests can together identify most causes of pernicious anemia.

References

Albert MJ, Mathan VI, Baker SJ. (1980). Vitamin B_{12} synthesis by human small intestinal bacteria. Nature 283: 781–782.

Allen LH. (1994). Vitamin B_{12} metabolism and status during pregnancy, lactation and infancy. In: Allen L, King J, Lønnerdal B (eds.) Nutrient Regulation during Pregnancy, Lactation and Infant Growth. Plenum Press, New York. pp. 173–186.

Amos RJ, Dawson DWI, Fish DI, Leeming RJ, Linnell JC. (1994). Guidelines on the investigation and diagnosis of cobalamin and folate deficiencies. Clinical and Laboratory Haematology 46: 101–115.

Andersson A, Hultberg B, Brattström L, Isaksson A. (1992). Decreased serum homocysteine in pregnancy. European Journal of Clinical Chemistry and Clinical Biochemistry 30: 377–379.

Antony AC. (2001). Prevalence of cobalamin (vitamin B_{12}) and folate deficiency in India: audi alteram partem. American Journal of Clinical Nutrition 74: 157–159.

Antony AC. (2003). Vegetarianism and vitamin B_{12} (cobalamin) deficiency. American Journal of Clinical Nutrition 78: 3–6.

Bagley PJ, Selhub J. (2000). Analysis of folate form distribution by affinity followed by reversed-phase chromatography with electrical detection. Clinical Chemistry 46: 404–411.

Bailey LB. (1990). Folate status assessment. Journal of Nutrition 120: 1508–1511.

Bailey LB. (1992). Evaluation of a new recommended dietary allowance for folate. Journal of the American Dietetic Association 92: 463–468.

Bailey LB (ed). (1995). Folate in Health and Disease. Vol. 1, Marcel Dekker, New York.

Bailey LB, Mahan CS, Dimperio D. (1980). Folacin and iron status in low-income pregnant adolescents and mature women. American Journal of Clinical Nutrition 33: 1997–2001.

Bailey LB, Wagner PA, Christakis GJ, Davis CG, Appledorf H, Araujo PE, Dorsey E, Dinning JS. (1982). Folacin and iron status and hematological findings in black and Spanish-American adolescents from urban low-income households. American Journal of Clinical Nutrition 35: 1023–1032.

Bates CJ, Fleming M, Paul AA, Black AE, Mandal AR. (1980). Folate status and its relation to vitamin C in healthy elderly men and women. Age and Ageing 9: 241–248.

Bates CJ, Mansoor MA, van der Pols J, Prentice A, Cole TJ, Finch S. (1997a). Plasma total homocysteine in a representative sample of 972 British men and women aged 65 and over. European Journal of Clinical Nutrition 51: 691–697.

Bates CJ, Thurnham DI, Bingham SA, Margetts BM, Nelson M. (1997b). Biochemical markers of nutrient intake. In: Margetts BM, Nelson M (eds.) Design Concepts in Nutritional Epidemiology, 2nd ed. Oxford University Press, Oxford, pp. 170–241.

Bates CJ, Pentieva KD, Prentice A, Mansoor MA, Finch S. (1999). Plasma pyridoxal phosphate and pyridoxic acid and their relationship to plasma homocysteine in a representative sample of British men and women aged 65 years and over. British Journal of Nutrition 81: 191–201.

Beard ME, Weintraub LR. (1969). Hypersegmented neutrophilic granulocytes in iron-deficiency anemia. British Journal of Haematology 16: 161–163.

Begley JA, Hall CA. (1975). Measurement of vitamin B_{12}-binding proteins of plasma. II: Interpretation of patterns of disease. Blood 45: 287–293.

Benton D, Haller J, Fordy J. (1997). The vitamin status of young British adults. International Journal for Vitamin and Nutrition Research 67: 34–40.

Bhatt HR, Green A, Linnell JC. (1982). A sensitive micromethod for the routine estimation of methylmalonic acid in body fluids and tissues using thin layer chromatography. Clinica Chimica Acta 118: 311–321.

Bolann BJ, Solli JD, Schneede J, Grottum K, Lorass A, Stokkeland M, Stallemo A, Schjøth A, Bie RB, Refsum H, Ueland PM. (2000). Evaluation of indicators of cobalamin deficiency defined as cobalamin-induced reduction in increased serum methylmalonic acid. Clinical Chemistry 46: 1744–1750.

Bottiglieri T. (1996). Folate, vitamin B_{12} and neuropsychiatric disorders. Nutrition Reviews 54: 382–390.

Boushey CJ, Beresford SA, Omenn GS, Motulsky AG.

(1995). A quantitative assessment of plasma homocysteine as a risk factor for vascular disease: probable benefits of increasing folic acid intakes. Journal of the American Medical Association 274: 1049–1057.

Brattström L, Lindgen A, Israelsson B, Andersson A, Hulthberg B. (1994). Homocysteine and cysteine: determinants of plasma levels in middle-aged and elderly subjects. Journal of Internal Medicine 236: 633–641.

Brouwer IA, van Dusseldorp M, West CE, Steegers-Theunissen RPM. (2001). Bioavailability and bioefficacy of folate and folic acid in man. Nutrition Research Reviews 14: 267–293.

Brown RD, Jun R, Hughes W, Watman R, Arnold B, Kronenberg H. (1990). Red cell folate assays: some answers to current problems with radioassay variability. Pathology 22: 82–87.

Carmel R. (1983). Clinical and laboratory features of the diagnosis of megaloblastic anemia. In: Lindenbaum J (ed.) Nutrition in Hematology. Churchill Livingstone, New York, pp. 1–31.

Carmel R. (1997). Cobalamin, the stomach, and aging. American Journal of Clinical Nutrition 66: 750–759.

Carmel R. (2000). Current concepts in cobalamin deficiency. Annual Review of Medicine 51: 357–375.

Carmel R, Herbert V. (1969). Deficiency of vitamin B_{12}-binding alpha globulin in two brothers. Blood 33: 1–12.

Carmel R, Green R, Jacobsen DW, Qian GD. (1996a). Neutrophil nuclear segmentation in mild cobalamin deficiency: relation to metabolic tests of cobalamin status and observations on ethnic differences in neutrophil segmentation. American Journal of Clinical Pathology 106: 57–63.

Carmel RC, Mallidi PV, Vinarskiy S, Brar S, Frouhar Z. (2002). Hyperhomocysteinemia and cobalamin deficiency in young Asian Indians in the United States. American Journal of Hematology 70: 107–114.

Carmel R, Rasmussen K, Jacobsen DW, Green R. (1996b). Comparison of the deoxyuridine suppression test with serum levels of methylmalonic acid and homocysteine in mild cobalamin deficiency. British Journal of Haematology 93: 311–318.

Chan DA (ed.). (1996). Immunoassay Automation: An Updated Guide to Systems. Academic Press, New York.

Chanarin I. (1980). The folates. In: Barker BM Bender D (eds.) Vitamins in Medicine. Heinemann Medical Books, London, pp. 247–314.

Chanarin I. (1990). The Megaloblastic Anaemias. 3rd ed. Blackwell Scientific, Oxford.

Chanarin I, Metz J. (1997). Diagnosis of cobalamin deficiency: the old and the new. British Journal of Haematology 97: 695–700.

Chanarin I, Waters DA. (1974). Failed Schilling tests. Scandinavian Journal of Haematology, 12: 245–248.

Chango A, Potier de Courcy G, Boisson F, Guilland JC, Barbé F, Perrin MO, Christidès, Rabhi K, Pfister M, Galan P, Hercberg S, Nicolas JP. (2000).

5,10-methylenetetrafolate reductase common mutations, folate status and plasma homocysteine in healthy French adults of the Supplementation en Vitamines et Mineraux Antioxydants (SU.VI.MAX) cohort. British Journal of Nutrition 84: 891–896.

Chen IW, Silberstein EB, Maxon HR, Volle CP, Sohnlein BH. (1982). Semiautomated system for simultaneous assays of serum vitamin B_{12} and folic acid in serum evaluated. Clinical Chemistry 28: 2161–2165.

Choi SW. (1999). Vitamin B_{12} deficiency: a new risk factor for breast cancer? Nutrition Reviews 57: 250–253.

Clarke R, Smith AD, Jobst KA, Refsum H, Sutton L, Ueland P. (1998). Folate, vitamin B_{12}, and serum total homocysteine levels in confirmed Alzheimer disease. Archives of Neurology 55: 1449–1455.

Colman N. (1981). Laboratory assessment of folate status. Clinics in Laboratory Medicine 1: 755–796.

Cooke WT, Cox EV, Fone OJ, Meynell MJ, Gaddie R. (1963). The clinical and metabolic significance of jejunal diverticuli. Gut 4: 115–131.

Cooper BA, Lowenstein L. (1964). Relative folate deficiency of erythrocytes in pernicious anemia and its correction with cyanocobalamin. Blood 24: 502–521.

Daly LE, Kirke PN, Molloy A, Weir DG, Scott JM. (1995). Folate levels and neural tube defects: implications for prevention. Journal of the American Medical Association 274: 1698–1702.

Das KC, Herbert V. (1978). The lymphocyte as a marker of past nutritional status: persistence of abnormal lymphocyte deoxyuridine (dU) suppression test and chromosomes in patients with past deficiency of folate and vitamin B_{12}. British Journal of Haematology 38: 219–233.

Das KC, Herbert V, Colman N, Longo DL. (1978). Unmasking covert folate deficiency in iron-deficient subjects with neutrophil hypersegmentation: dU suppression tests on lymphocytes and bone marrow. British Journal of Haematology 39: 357–375.

de Carvalho MJ, Guilland JC, Moreau D, Boggio V, Fuchs F. (1996). Vitamin status of healthy subjects in Burgundy (France). Annals of Nutrition and Metabolism 40: 24–51.

De Laet C, Wautrecht JC, Brasseur D, Dramaix M, Boeynaems J, Decuyper J, Kahn A. (1999). Plasma homocysteine concentration in a Belgian school-age population. American Journal of Clinical Nutrition 69: 968–972.

den Heijer M, Koster T, Blom HJ, Bos GM, Briet E, Reitsma PH, Vandenbroucke JP, Rosendaal FR, (1996). Hyperhomocysteinema as a risk factor for deep-vein thrombosis. New England Journal of Medicine 334: 759–762.

Domstad PA, Choy YC, Kim EE, DeLand FH. (1981). Reliability of the dual-isotope Schilling test for the diagnosis of pernicious anemia or malabsorption syndrome. American Journal of Clinical Pathology 75: 723–726.

Doscherholmen A, McMahon J, Ripley D. (1976). Inhibitory effect of eggs on vitamin B$_{12}$ absorption: description of a simple ovalbumin ^{57}Co-vitamin B$_{12}$ absorption test. British Journal of Haematology 33: 261–272.

Eichner ER, Pierce HI, Hillman RS. (1971). Folate balance in dietary-induced megaloblastic anemia. New England Journal of Medicine 284: 933–938.

FDA (U.S. Food and Drug Administration) (1996). Food standards: amendment of the standards of identity for enriched grain products to require addition of folic acid. Federal Register 61: 8781–8797.

Fernandes-Costa F, van Tonder S, Metz J. (1985). A sex difference in serum cobalamin and transcobalamin levels. American Journal of Clinical Nutrition 41: 784–786.

FAO/WHO (Food and Agricultural Organization/World Health Organization) Expert Consultation (1988). Requirements of Vitamin A, Iron, Folate and Vitamin B$_{12}$. Food and Nutrition Series No. 23. FAO, Rome.

Finch S, Doyle W, Lowe C, Bates CJ, Prentice A, Smithers G, Clarke PC. (1998). National Diet and Nutrition Survey: People Aged 65 Years and Over. Volume 1: Report of the Diet and Nutrition Survey. The Stationery Office, London.

Gadowsky SL, Gale C, Wolfe SA, Jory J, Gibson R, O'Connor DL. (1995). Biochemical folate, B$_{12}$, and iron status of a group of pregnant adolescents accessed through the public health system in Southern Ontario. Journal of Adolescent Health 16: 465–474.

Giles WH, Croft JB, Greenlund KJ, Ford ES, Kittner SJ. (1998). Total homocyst(e)ine concentration and the likelihood of nonfatal stroke: results from the Third National Health and Examination Survey, 1988–1994. Stroke 29: 2473–2477.

Gilois CR, Beattie G, Mills SP. (1986). Measurement of vitamin B$_{12}$ and serum folic acid: a comparison of methods. Medical Laboratory Sciences 43: 140–144.

Gimsing P, Nexø E. (1983). The forms of cobalamin in biological materials. In: Hall CA (ed.) The Cobalamins. Churchill-Livingstone, New York, pp. 7–30.

Goodman KI, Salt WB. (1990). Vitamin B$_{12}$ deficiency: important new concepts in recognition. Postgraduate Medicine 88: 147–158.

Green R. (1999). Macrocytic and marrow failure anemias. Laboratory Medicine 30: 595–599.

Green R, Kinsella IJ. (1995). Current concepts in the diagnosis of cobalamin deficiency. Neurology 45: 1435–1440.

Green R, Miller JW. (1999). Folate deficiency beyond megaloblastic anemia: hyperhomocysteinemia and other manifestations of dysfunctional folate metabolism. Seminars in Hematology 36: 47–64.

Green TJ., Houghton LA, Donovan U, Gibson RS, O'Connor DL. (1998). Oral contraceptives did not affect biochemical folate indexes and homocysteine concentrations in adolescent females. Journal of the American Dietetic Association 98: 49–55.

Gregory J, Foster K, Tyler H, Wiseman M. (1990). The Dietary and Nutritional Survey of British Adults. Her Majesty's Stationery Office, London.

Gregory J, Collins DL, Davies PSW, Hughes JM, Clarke PC. (1995). National Diet and Nutrition Survey: Children Aged One-and-a-Half to Four-and-a-Half years. Volume 1: Report of the Diet and Nutrition Survey. Her Majesty's Stationery Office, London

Gregory J, Lowe S, Bates CJ, Prentice A, LV Jackson L, Smithers G, Wenlock R, Farron M. (2000). National Diet and Nutrition Survey: Young People Aged 4 to 18 Years. Volume 1: Report of the Diet and Nutrition survey. The Stationery Office, London

Grubben MJ, Boers GH, Blom HJ, Broekhuizen R, de Jong R, van Rijt L, de Ruijter E, Swinkels DW, Nagengast FM, Katan MB. (2000). Unfiltered coffee increases plasma homocysteine concentrations in healthy volunteers: a randomized trial. American Journal of Clinical Nutrition 71: 480–484.

Gutcho S, Mansbach L. (1977). Simultaneous radioassay of serum in vitamin B$_{12}$ and folic acid. Clinical Chemistry 23: 1609–1614.

Hanger HC, Sainsbury R, Gilchrist NL, Beard MEJ, Duncan JM. (1991). A community study of vitamin B$_{12}$ and folate levels in the elderly. Journal of the American Geriatrics Society 39: 1155–1159.

Harrison RJ. (1971). Vitamin B$_{12}$ levels in erythrocytes in anaemia due to folate deficiency. British Journal of Haematology 20: 623–628.

Health Canada. (2003). Departmental Consolidation of the Food and Drugs Act and the Food and Drug Regulations with Amendments to Jan 1, 2003. Health Canada, Ottawa.

Healton EB, Savage DG, Brust JC, Garrett TJ, Lindenbaum J. (1991). Neurologic aspects of cobalamin deficiency. Medicine 70: 229–245.

Herbert V. (1962). Experimental nutritional folate deficiency in man. Transactions of the Association of American Physicians 75: 307–320.

Herbert V. (1967). Biochemical and hematological lesions in folic acid deficiency. American Journal of Clinical Nutrition 20: 562–569.

Herbert V. (1985). Megaloblastic anemias. Laboratory Investigation 52: 3–19.

Herbert V. (1987a). Recommended dietary intakes (RDI) of folate in humans. American Journal of Clinical Nutrition 45: 661–670.

Herbert V. (1987b). Making sense of laboratory tests of folate status: folate requirements to sustain normality. American Journal of Hematology 26: 199–207.

Herbert V. (1987c). The 1986 Herman Award Lecture. Nutrition Science as a continually unfolding story: the folate and vitamin B$_{12}$ paradigm. American Journal of Clinical Nutrition 46: 387–402.

Herbert V. (1996). Vitamin B$_{12}$. In: Ziegler EE, Filer LJ. Jr (eds.) Present Knowledge in Nutrition. 7th ed. International Life Sciences Institute Press, Washington, DC, pp. 191–205.

Herbert V, Colman N, Palat D, Manusselis C, Drivas G, Block E, Akerkar A, Weaver D, Frenkel E. (1984). Is there a "gold" standard for human serum vitamin B_{12} assay? Journal of Laboratory and Clinical Medicine 104: 829–841.

Herbert V, Fong W, Gulle V, Stopler T. (1990). Low holotranscobalamin II is the earliest serum marker for subnormal vitamin B_{12} (cobalamin) absorption in patients with AIDS. American Journal of Hematology 34: 132–139.

Heuberger RA, Fisher AI, Jacques PF, Klein R, Klein BEK, Palta M, Mare-Perlman JA. (2002). Relation of blood homocysteine and its nutritional determinants to age-related maculopathy in the third National Health and Nutrition Examination Survey. American Journal of Clinical Nutrition 76: 897–902.

Hillman RS, McGuffin R, Campbell C. (1977). Alcohol interference with the folate enterohepatic cycle. Transactions of the Association of American Physicians 90: 145–156.

Hjelt K, Paerregaard A, Krasilnikoff PA. (1992). Giardiasis: haematological status and the absorption of vitamin B_{12} and folic acid. Acta Paediatrica 81: 29–34.

Hoffbrand AV. (1998). Megaloblastic anemia. In: Hoffbrand AV, Lewis SM, Tuddenham EDG (eds.) Postgraduate Haematology. Hodder Arnold, London.

Hoffbrand AV, Newcombe BFA, Mollin DL. (1966). Method of assay of red cell folate activity and the value of the assay as a test for folate deficiency. Journal of Clinical Pathology 19: 17–28.

Holleland G, Schneede J, Ueland PM, Lund PK, Refsum H, Sandberg S. (1999). Cobalamin deficiency in general practice: assessment of diagnostic utility and cost-benefit analysis of methylmalonic acid determination in relation to current diagnostic strategies. Clinical Chemistry 45: 189–198.

Homocysteine Lowering Trialists' Collaboration. (1998). Lowering blood homocysteine with folic acid based supplements: meta-analysis of randomized trials. British Medical Journal 316: 894–898.

Houghton LA, Green TJ, Donovan UM, Gibson RS, Stephen AM, O'Connor DL. (1997). Association between dietary fiber intake and the folate status of a group of female adolescents. American Journal of Clinical Nutrition 66: 1414–1421.

Hughes-Jones NC, Wickramasinghe SN. (1996). Lecture Notes on Haematology. 6th ed. Blackwell Publishing, Oxford.

Hustad S, Ueland PM, Vollset SE, Zhang Y, Bjorke-Monsen AL, Schneede J. (2000). Riboflavin as a determinant of plasma total homocysteine: effect modification by the methylenetetrahydrofolate reductase C677T polymorphism. Clinical Chemistry 46: 1065–1071.

IOM (Institute of Medicine). (2000). Dietary reference intakes for Thiamin, Riboflavin, Niacin, Vitamin B_6, Folate, Vitamin B_{12}, Pantothenic Acid, Biotin, and Choline. National Academy Press, Washington, DC.

Jacob RA, Wu M-M, Henning SM, Swendseid ME. (1994). Homocysteine increases as folate decreases in plasma of healthy men during short-term dietary folate and methyl group restriction. Journal of Nutrition 124: 1072–1080.

Jacob RA, Gretz DM, Taylor PC, James SJ, Pogribny IP, Miller BJ, Henning S, Swendseid M. (1998). Moderate folate depletion increases plasma homocysteine and decreases lymphocyte DNA methylation in postmenopausal women. Journal of Nutrition 128: 1204–1212.

Jacques PF, Sulsky SI, Sadowski JA, Phillips JC, Rush D, Willet WC. (1993). Comparison of micronutrient intake measured in a dietary questionnaire and biochemical indicators of micronutrient status. American Journal of Clinical Nutrition 57: 182–189.

Jacques PF, Rosenberg IH, Rogers G, Selhub J, Bowman BA, Gunter EW, Wright JD, Johnson CL. (1999). Serum total homocysteine concentrations in adolescent and adult Americans: results from the third National Health and Nutrition Examination Survey. American Journal of Clinical Nutrition 69: 482–489.

Jacques PF, Bostom AG, Wilson PWF, Rich S, Rosenberg IH, Selhub J. (2001). Determinants of plasma total homocysteine concentration in the Framingham Offspring cohort. American Journal of Clinical Nutrition 73: 613–621.

Jägerstad M, Pietrzik K. (1993). Folate: Flair Concerted Action No.10 Status Papers. International Journal for Vitamin and Nutrition Research 63: 285–289.

Johnson MA, Hawthorne NA, Brackett WR, Fischer JG, Gunter EW, Allen RH, Stabler SP. (2003). Hyperhomocysteinemia and vitamin B_{12} deficiency in elderly using Title IIIc nutrition services. American Journal of Clinical Nutrition 77: 211–220.

Joosten E, Pelemans W, Devos P, Lesaffre E, Goossens W, Criel A, Verhaeghe R. (1993). Cobalamin absorption and serum homocysteine and methylmalonic acid in elderly subjects with low serum cobalamin. European Journal of Haematology 51: 25–30.

Joosten E, Lesaffre E, Riezler R. (1996). Are different reference intervals for methylmalonic acid and total homocysteine necessary in elderly people? European Journal of Haematology 57: 222–226.

Kanazawa S, Herbert V. (1985). Total corrinoid, cobalamin (vitamin B_{12}), and cobalamin analogue levels may be normal in serum despite cobalamin in liver depletion in patients with alcoholism. Laboratory Investigation 53: 108–110.

Kano Y, Sakamoto S, Miura Y, Takaku F. (1985). Disorders of cobalamin metabolism. Critical Reviews in Oncology/Hematology 3: 1–34.

Kelleher BP, O'Broin SD. (1991). Microbiological assay for vitamin B_{12} performed in 96-well microtiter plates. Journal of Clinical Pathology 44: 592–595.

Kelleher BP, Walshe KG, Scott JM, O'Broin SD. (1987). Microbiological assay for vitamin B_{12} with use of a colistin-sulfate-resistant organism. Clinical Chemistry 33: 52–54.

Kelleher BP, Scott JM, O'Broin SD. (1990). Use of beta-lactamase to hydrolyse interfering antibiotics in vitamin B$_{12}$ microbiological assay using *Lactobacillus leichmannii*. Clinical and Laboratory Haematology 12: 87–95.

Killmann SA. (1964). Effect of deoxyuridine on incorporation of tritiated thymidine: difference between normoblasts and megaloblasts. Acta Medica Scandinavica 175: 483–488.

Kittner SJ, Malinow MR, Seipp MJ, Upson B, Hebel JR. (1995). Stability of blood homocyst(e)ine under epidemiological field conditions. Journal of Clinical Laboratory Analysis 9: 75–76.

Klee GG. (2000). Cobalamin and folate evaluation: measurement of methylmalonic acid and homocysteine vs vitamin B$_{12}$ and folate. Clinical Chemistry 46: 1277–1283.

Kumar S, Ghosh K, Das KC. (1989), Serum vitamin B$_{12}$ levels in an Indian population: an evaluation of three assay methods. Medical Laboratory Sciences 46: 120–126.

Layrisse M, Blumenfeld N, Dugarte I, Roche M.(1959). Vitamin B$_{12}$ and folic acid metabolism in hookworm-infected patients. Blood 14: 1269–1279.

Lindenbaum J, Nath BJ.(1980). Megaloblastic anaemia and neutrophil hypersegmentation. British Journal of Haematology 44: 511–513.

Lindenbaum J, Healton EB, Savage DG, Brust JC, Garrett TJ, Podell ER, Marcell PD, Stabler SP, Allen RH.(1988). Neuropsychiatric disorders caused by cobalamin deficiency in the absence of anemia or macrocytosis. New England Journal of Medicine 318: 1720–1728.

Lindenbaum J, Savage DG, Stabler SP, Allen RH. (1990). Diagnosis of cobalamin deficiency. 2: Relative sensitivities of serum cobalamin, methylmalonic acid, and total homocysteine concentrations. American Journal of Hematology 34: 99–107.

Lindenbaum J, Rosenberg IH, Wilson PW, Stabler SP, Allen RH. (1994). Prevalence of cobalamin deficiency in the Framingham elderly population. American Journal of Clinical Nutrition 60: 2–11.

Lindgren A, Lindstedt G, Kilander AF. (1998). Advantages of serum pepsinogen A combined with gastrin or pepsinogen C as first-line analytes in the evaluation of suspected cobalamin deficiency: a study in patients previously not subjected to gastrointestinal surgery. Journal of Internal Medicine 244: 341–349.

Lindgren A, Kilander A, Bagge E, Nexø E. (1999). Holotranscobalamin: a sensitive marker of cobalamin malabsorption. European Journal of Clinical Investigation 29: 321–329.

Manzoor M, Runcie J. (1976). Folate-responsive neuropathy: report of 10 cases. British Medical Journal 1(6019): 1176–1178.

Martinez O, Roe DA. (1977). Effect of oral contraceptives on blood folate levels in pregnancy. American Journal of Obstetrics and Gynecology 128: 255–261.

Mason JB. (2003). Biomarkers of nutrient exposure and status in one-carbon (methyl) metabolism. Journal of Nutrition 133: 941S–947S.

McLennan W, Podger A. (1998). National Nutrition Survey: Nutrient Intakes and Physical Measurements, Australia 1995. Australian Bureau of Statistics, Canberra.

Metz J, Kelly A, Swett VC, Waxman S, Herbert V. (1968). Deranged DNA synthesis by bone marrow from vitamin B$_{12}$-deficient humans. British Journal of Haematology 14: 575–592.

Metz J, Hart D, Harpending HC. (1971). Iron, folate, and vitamin B$_{12}$ nutrition in a hunter-gatherer people: a study of the King Bushmen. American Journal of Clinical Nutrition 24: 229–242.

Metz J, Bell AH, Flicker L, Bottiglieri T, Ibrahim J, Seal E, Schultz D, Savoia H, McGrath KM. (1996). The significance of subnormal serum vitamin B$_{12}$ concentration in older people: a case control study. Journal of American Geriatrics Society 44: 1355–1361.

Miller JW, Ribaya-Mercado JD, Russell RM, Shepard DC, Morrow FD, Cochary EF, Sadowski JA, Gershoff SN, Selhub J. (1992). Effect of vitamin B$_6$ deficiency on fasting plasma homocysteine concentrations. American Journal of Clinical Nutrition 55: 1154–1160.

Minet J-C, Bissé E, Aebischer C-P, Beil A, Wieland H, Lütschg J. (2000). Assessment of vitamin B$_{12}$, folate, and vitamin B$_6$ status and relation to sulfur amino acid metabolism in neonates. American Journal of Clinical Nutrition 72: 751–757.

Molloy AM, Scott JM. (1997). Microbiological assay for serum, plasma, and red-cell folate using cryopreserved, microtiter plate method. Methods in Enzymology 281: 43–53.

MRC Vitamin Study Research Group. (1991). Prevention of neural tube defects: results of the Medical Research Council Vitamin Study. Lancet 338: 131–137.

Must A, Jacques PF, Rogers G, Rosenburg IH, Selhub J. (2003). Serum total homocysteine concentrations in children and adolescents: results from the Third National Health and Nutrition Examination Survey (NHANES III). Journal of Nutrition 133: 2643–2649.

Nexø E, Hansen M, Rasmussen K, Lindgren A, Grasbeck R. (1994). How to diagnose cobalamin deficiency. Scandinavian Journal of Clinical Laboratory Investigation Supplement 219: 61–76.

Norman EJ, Morrison JA. (1993). Screening elderly populations for cobalamin (vitamin B$_{12}$) deficiency using the urinary methylmalonic acid assay by gas chromatography mass spectrometry. American Journal of Medicine 94: 589–594.

Nygärd O, Vollset SE, Refsum H, Stensvold I, Tverdal A, Nordrehaug JE, Ueland M, Kvale G. (1995). Total plasma homocysteine and cardiovascular risk profile: the Hordaland Homocysteine Study. Journal of the American Medical Association 274: 1526–1533.

Nygärd O, Refsum H, Ueland PM, Stensvold I, Nordrehaug JE, Kvale G, Vollset FE. (1997). Coffee consumption and plasma total homocysteine: the Hordaland Homocysteine Study. American Journal of Clinical Nutrition 65: 136–143.

O'Broin SD, Gunter EW. (1999). Screening of folate status with use of dried blood spots on filter paper. American Journal of Clinical Nutrition 70: 359–367.

O'Broin S, Kelleher B. (1992). Microbiological assay on microtiter plates of folate in serum and red cells. Journal of Clinical Pathology 45: 344–347.

O'Connor DL. (1994). Folate status during pregnancy and lactation. In: Allen L, King J, Lønnerdal B (eds.) Nutrient Regulation during Pregnancy, Lactation, and Infant Growth. Plenum Press, New York, pp.157–173.

O'Keefe CA, Bailey LB, Thomas EA, Hofler SA, Davis BA, Cerda JJ, Gregory JF 3rd. (1995). Controlled dietary folate affects folate status in nonpregnant women. Journal of Nutrition 125: 2717–2725.

Omer A, Finlayson NDC, Shearman DJC, Samson RR, Girdwood RH. (1970a). Plasma and erythrocyte folate in iron deficiency and folate deficiency. Blood 35: 821–828.

Omer A, Finlayson NDC, Shearman DJC, Samson RR, Girdwood RH. (1970b). Erythrocyte vitamin B_{12} activity in health, polycythemia, and in deficiency of vitamin B_{12} and folate. Blood 35: 73–82.

Pancharuniti N, Lewis CA, Sauberlich HE, Perkins LL, Go RC, Alvarez JO, Macaluso M, Acton RT, Copeland RB, Cousins AL, et al. (1994). Plasma homocyst(e)ine, folate, and vitamin B_{12} concentrations and risk for early-onset coronary artery disease. American Journal of Clinical Nutrition 59: 940–980. Erratum in American Journal of Clinical Nutrition 63: 609.

Patel N, Briddon A. (2000). Moderately low vitamin B_{12} does not compromise transmethylation in adults on a free diet: implications for assessment of vitamin B_{12} status. Annals of Clinical Biochemistry 37: 686–689.

Payette J, Gray-Donald K. (1991). Dietary intake and biochemical indices of nutritional status in an elderly population, with estimates of the precision of the 7-d food record. American Journal of Clinical Nutrition 54: 478–488.

Pfeiffer CM, Rogers LM, Bailey LB, Gregory JF. (1997). Absorption of folate from fortified cereal-grain products and of supplemental folate consumed with or without food determined using a dual-label stable isotope protocol. American Journal of Clinical Nutrition 66: 1388–1397.

Pietrzik K, Brønstrup A. (1998). Vitamins B_{12}, B_6 and folate as determinants of homocysteine concentration in the healthy population. European Journal of Pediatrics 157: S135–S138.

Piyathilake CJ, Macaluso M, Hine RJ, Richards EW, Krumdieck CL. (1994). Local and systemic effects of cigarette smoking on folate and vitamin B_{12}. American Journal of Clinical Nutrition 60: 559–566.

Raiten DJ, Fisher KD. (1995). Assessment of folate methodology used in the Third National Health and Nutrition Examination Survey (NHANES III, 1988–1994). Journal of Nutrition 125: 1371S–1379S.

Rajkovic A, Catalano PM, Malinow MR. (1997). Elevated homocysteine levels with preeclampsia. Obstetrics and Gynecology 90: 168–171.

Rasmussen K, Moller J, Lyngbak M, Pedesen A-M, Dybkjaer L. (1996). Age- and gender-specific reference intervals for total homocysteine and methylmalonic acid in plasma before and after vitamin supplementation. Clinical Chemistry 42: 630–636.

Rauh M, Verwied S, Knerr I, Dorr HG, Sonnichsen A, Koletzko B. (2001). Homocysteine concentrations in a German cohort of 500 individuals: reference ranges and determinants of plasma levels in healthy children and their parents. Amino Acids 20: 409–418.

Rauma AL, Torronen R, Hanninen O, Mykkanen H. (1995). Vitamin B_{12} status of long-term adherents of a strict uncooked vegan diet ("living food diet") is compromised. Journal of Nutrition 125: 2511–2515.

Refsum H, Ueland PM, Nygärd O, Vollset SE. (1998). Homocysteine and cardiovascular disease. Annual Review of Medicine 49: 31–62.

Refsum H, Yajnik CS, Gadkari M, Schneede J, Vollset SE, Orning L, Guttormsen AB, Joglekar A, Sayyard MG, Ulvik A, Ueland PM. (2001). Hyperhomocysteinemia and elevated methylmalonic acid indicate a high prevalence of cobalamin deficiency in Asian Indians. American Journal of Clinical Nutrition 74: 233–241.

Rickes EL, Brink NG, Koniuszy FR., Ward TR, Folkers K. (1948). Crystalline vitamin B_{12}. Science 107: 396-397.

Rosenberg IH, Bowman BB, Cooper BA, Halsted CH, Lindenbaum J. (1982). Folate nutrition in the elderly. American Journal of Clinical Nutrition 36: 1060–1066.

Russell D, Parnell W, Wilson N. (1999). NZ Food: NZ People. Key results of the 1997 National Nutrition Survey. Ministry of Health, Wellington.

Sauberlich HE. (1985). Bioavailability of vitamins. Progress in Food Nutrition Science 9: 1–33.

Sauberlich HE, Kretch MJ, Skala JH, Johnson HL, Taylor PC. (1987). Folate requirement and metabolism in nonpregnant women. American Journal of Clinical Nutrition 46: 1016–1028.

Savage DG, Lindenbaum J, Stabler SP, Allen RH. (1994). Sensitivity of serum methylmalonic acid and total homocysteine determinations for diagnosing cobalamin and folate deficiencies. American Journal of Medicine 96: 239–246.

Schilling RF. (1953). Intrinsic factor studies II: the effect of gastric juice on the urinary excretion of radioactivity after oral administration of radioactive vitamin B_{12}. Journal of Laboratory and Clinical Medicine 42: 860–866.

Schneede J, Ueland PM. (1995). Application of capillary electrophoresis with laser-induced fluorescence detection for routine determination of methylmalonic acid in human serum. Analytical Chemistry 67: 812–819.

Schneede J, Dagnelie PC, van Staveren WA, Vollset SE, Refsum H, Ueland PM. (1994). Methylmalonic acid and homocysteine in plasma as indicators of functional cobalamin deficiency in infants on macrobiotic diets. Pediatric Research 36: 194–201.

Scott JM. (1999). Folate and vitamin B$_{12}$. Proceedings of the Nutrition Society 58: 441–448.

Scott JM, Dinn JJ, Wilson P, Weir DG. (1981). Pathogenesis of subacute combined degeneration: a result of methyl group deficiency. Lancet 2(8242): 334–337.

Scott J, Kirke P, Molloy A, Daly L, Weir D. (1994). The role of folate in the prevention of neural tube defects. Proceedings of the Nutrition Society 53: 631–636.

Selhub J, Jacques PF, Wilson PWF, Rush D, Rosenberg IH. (1993). Vitamin status and intake as primary determinants of homocysteinemia in an elderly population. Journal of the American Medical Association 270: 2693–2698.

Selhub J, Jacques PF, Boston AG, D'Agostino RB, Wilson PWF, Belanger AJ, O'Leary DH, Wolf PA, Schaefer EJ, Rosenberg IH. (1995). Association between plasma homocysteine concentrations and extracranial carotid-artery stenosis. New England Journal of Medicine 332: 286–291.

Senti FR, Pilch SM. (1985). Assessment of the Folate Nutritional Status of the U.S. Population Based on Data Collected in the Second National Health and Nutrition Examination Survey 1976–1980. Life Sciences Research Office, Federation of American Societies for Experimental Biology, Bethesda, MD.

Shaw GM, Schaffer D, Velie EM, Morland K, Harris JA. (1995). Periconceptional vitamin use, dietary folate, and the occurrence of neural tube defects. Epidemiology 6: 219–226.

Smith EL. (1948). Purification of antipernicious anaemia factors from liver. Nature 161: 638–639.

Snow CF. (1999). Laboratory diagnosis of vitamin B$_{12}$ and folate deficiency: a guide for the primary care physician. Archives of Internal Medicine 159: 1289–1298.

Solomon BP, Duda CT. (1998). Homocysteine determination in plasma. Current Separations 17: 3–7.

Stabler SP, Allen RH. (2004). Vitamin B$_{12}$ deficiency as a worldwide problem. Annual Review of Nutrition 24: 299–326.

Stabler SP, Marcell PD, Podell ER, Allen RH, Savage DG, Lindenbaum J. (1988). Elevation of total homocysteine in the serum of patients with cobalamin or folate deficiency detected by capillary gas chromatography–mass spectrometry. Journal of Clinical Investigation 81: 466–474.

Stabler SP, Allen RH, Savage DG, Lindenbaum J. (1990). Clinical spectrum and diagnosis of cobalamin deficiency. Blood 76: 871–881.

Stabler SP, Lindenbaum J, Savage DG, Allen RH. (1993). Elevation of serum cystathionine levels in patients with cobalamin and folate deficiency. Blood 81: 3403–3413.

Stabler SP, Lindenbaum J, Allen RH. (1996). The use of homocysteine and other metabolites in the specific diagnosis of vitamin B$_{12}$ deficiency. Journal of Nutrition 126: 1266S–1272S.

Stabler SP, Lindenbaum J, Allen RH. (1997). Vitamin B$_{12}$ deficiency in the elderly: current dilemmas. American Journal of Clinical Nutrition 66: 741–749.

Stampfer MJ, Malinow MR, Willett WC, Newcomer L, Upson B, Ullman D, Tishler PV, Hennekens CH. (1992). A prospective study of plasma homocyst(e)ine and risk of myocardial infarction in U.S. physicians. Journal of the American Medical Association 268: 877–881.

Steinberg SE. (1984). Mechanisms of folate homeostasis. American Journal of Physiology 246: G319–G324.

Stolzenberg-Solomon RZ, Miller ER 3rd, Maguire MG, Selhub J, Appel LJ. (1999). Association of dietary protein intake and coffee consumption with serum homocysteine concentrations in an older population. American Journal of Clinical Nutrition 69: 467–475.

Subar AF, Harlan LC, Mattson ME. (1990). Food and nutrient intake differences between smokers and non-smokers in the U.S. American Journal of Public Health 80: 1323–1329.

Tabor H, Wyngarden L. (1958). A method for the determination of formiminoglutamic acid in urine. Journal of Clinical Investigation 37: 824–828.

Toh BH, van Driel IR, Gleeson PA. (1997). Mechanisms of disease: pernicious anemia [Review]. New England Journal of Medicine 337: 1441–1448.

Tolarova M, Harris J. (1995). Reduced recurrence of orofacial clefts after periconceptional supplementation with high dose folic acid and multivitamins. Teratology 51: 71–78.

Tucker KL, Selhub J, Wilson PWF, Rosenberg IH. (1996). Dietary intake pattern relates to plasma folate and homocysteine concentrations in the Framingham Heart Study. Journal of Nutrition 126: 3025–3031.

Ubbink JB, Vermaak WJH, Bissbort S. (1991). Rapid high-performance liquid chromatographic assay for total homocysteine levels in human serum. Journal of Chromatography 565: 441–446.

Ubbink JB, Becker PJ, Vermaak WJ, Delport R. (1995). Results of B-vitamin supplementation study used in a prediction model to find a reference range for plasma homocysteine. Clinical Chemistry 41: 1033–1037.

Ubbink JB, van der Merwe A, Delport R, Allen RH, Stabler SP, Riezler R, Vermaak WJ. (1996). The effect of a sub-normal vitamin B$_6$ status on homocysteine metabolism. Journal of Clinical Investigation 98: 177–184.

Ueland PM, Refsum H, Stabler SP, Malinow MR, Andersson A, Allen RH. (1993). Total homocysteine in plasma or serum: methods and clinical applications. Clinical Chemistry 39: 1764–1769.

van Asselt DZ, van den Broek WJ, Lamers CB, Corstens FH, Hoefnagels WH. (1996). Free and protein-bound cobalamin absorption in healthy middle-aged and older subjects. Journal of American Geriatric Society 44: 949–953.

van der Gaag M, Ubbink JB, Sillanaukee P, Nikkari S, Hendriks HF. (2000). Effect of consumption of red wine, spirits, and beer on serum homocysteine [Letter]. Lancet 355: 1522.

van der Mooren MJ, Wouters MG, Blom HJ, Schellekens LA, Eskes TK, Rolland R. (1994). Hormone replacement therapy may reduce high serum homocysteine in postmenopausal women. European Journal of Clinical Investigation 24: 733–736.

van der Put NM, Steegers-Theunissen RP, Frosst P, Trijbels FJ, Eskes TK, van den Heuvel LP, Mariman EC, den Heyer M, Rozen R, Blom HJ. (1995). Mutated methylenetetrahydrofolate reductase as a risk factor for spina bifida. Lancet 346: 1070–1071.

Varadi S, Abbott D, Elwis A. (1966). Correlation of peripheral white cell and bone marrow changes with folate levels in pregnancy and their clinical significance. Journal of Clinical Pathology 19: 33–36.

Varela-Moreiras G, Selhub J. (1992). Long-term folate deficiency alters folate content and distribution differentially in rat tissues. Journal of Nutrition 122: 986–991.

Verhoef P, Pasman WJ, Van Vliet T, Urgert R, Katan M. (2002). Contribution of caffeine to the homocysteine-raising effect of coffee: a randomized controlled trial in humans. American Journal of Clinical Nutrition 76: 1244–1248.

Vu T, Amin J, Ramos M, Flener V, Vanyo L, Tisman G. (1993). New assay for the rapid determination of plasma holotranscobalamin II levels: preliminary evaluation in cancer patients. American Journal of Hematology 42: 202–211.

Wagner C. (1984). Folic acid. In: Olsen RE (ed.) Present Knowledge in Nutrition. 5th ed. The Nutrition Foundation Inc., Washington, DC, pp. 332–346.

Wagner PA, Bailey LB, Krista ML, Jernigan JA, Robinson JD, Cerda JJ. (1981). Comparison of zinc and folacin status in elderly women from differing socioeconomic backgrounds. Nutrition Research 1: 565–570.

Wahlin A, Backmän L, Hultdin J, Adolfsson R, Nilsson L-G. (2002). Reference values for serum levels of vitamin B_{12} and folic acid in a population-based sample of adults between 35 and 80 years of age. Public Health Nutrition 5: 505–511.

Wartanowicz M, Ziemlański Ś, Bulhak-Jachymczyk B, Konopka L. (2001). Assessment of nutritional folate status and selected vitamin status of women of child-bearing age. European Journal of Clinical Nutrition 55: 743–747.

Weggemans RM, de Groot LC, Haller J. (1997). Factors related to plasma folate and vitamin B_{12}: the SENECA study. International Journal of Food Science and Nutrition 48: 141–150.

Werler MM, Shapiro S, Mitchell AA. (1993). Periconceptual folic acid exposure and risk of occurrent neural tube defects. Journal of the American Medical Association 269: 1257–1261.

Westerman DA, Evans D, Metz J. (1999). Neutrophil hypersegmentation in iron deficiency anaemia: a case-control study. British Journal of Haematology 107: 512–515.

Wickramasinghe SN, Longland JE. (1974). Assessment of deoxyuridine suppression test in diagnosis of vitamin B_{12} or folate deficiency. British Medical Journal 3(924): 148–150.

Wickramasinghe SN, Saunders JE. (1975). Letter: deoxyuridine suppression test. British Medical Journal 2(5962): 87.

Wickramsinghe SN, Ratnayaka ID. (1996). Limited value of serum holotranscobalamin II measurements in the differential diagnosis of macrocytosis. Journal of Clinical Pathology 49: 755–758.

Worthington-White DA, Behnke M, Gross S. (1994). Premature infants require additional folate and vitamin B_{12} to reduce the severity of anemia of prematurity. American Journal of Clinical Nutrition 60: 930–935,

Wright AJA, Finglas PM, Southon S. (1998). Erythrocyte folate analysis: a cause for concern? Clinical Chemistry 44: 1886–1891.

Wright AJA, Finglas PM, Southon S. (2000). Erythrocyte folate analysis: saponin added during lysis of whole blood can increase apparent folate concentrations depending on hemolysate pH. Clinical Chemistry 46: 1978–1986.

Wu A, Chanarin I, Slavin G, Levi AJ. (1975). Folate deficiency in the alcoholic: its relationship to clinical and hematological abnormalities, liver disease and folate stores. British Journal of Haematology 29: 469–478.

Young DS, Bermes EW. (1998). Specimen collection and processing: sources of biological variation. In: Burtis CA, Asherwood ER (eds.) Tietz Textbook of Clinical Chemistry. W.B. Saunders, Philadelphia, pp. 42–72.

Young SN, Ghadirian AM. (1989). Folic acid and psychopathology. Progress in Neuropsychopharmacology and Biological Psychiatry 13: 841–863.

Zittoun J, Zittoun R. (1999). Modern clinical testing strategies in cobalamin and folate deficiency. Seminars in Hematology 36: 35–46.

23

Assessment of calcium, phosphorus, and magnesium status

Calcium, magnesium, and phosphorus are the major mineral components of the body. The distribution of these elements in the body compartments of a 70-kg reference man is shown in Table 23.1. All three minerals occur in combination with organic and inorganic compounds. Calcium and magnesium also exist as free ions and phosphorus as phosphate in circulation. They have two major roles: structural components in bone and soft tissues, and regulatory agents in body fluids.

Bone serves as the major reservoir for these minerals, containing 99% of the total body calcium, 88% of total body phosphorus, and about 55% of total body magnesium. Calcium and phosphorus exist in the bones mostly as calcium hydroxyapatite and octacalcium phosphate: more than half of the magnesium in bone is present within the apatite crystal structure.

The fractional absorption of calcium and magnesium is generally inversely related to dietary intake, whereas that of phosphorus is relatively constant and varies little with the diet. In adults consuming a typical mixed diet, absorption of calcium and magnesium approximates 25% and 55%, respectively, compared to 55%–70% for phosphorus. The vitamin D status of the individual affects the efficiency of absorption of both calcium and phosphorus but has a smaller effect on magnesium. The absorption of calcium is also influenced by dietary components such as phytate, dietary fiber, oxalate, and lactose. Calcium, and to a lesser degree aluminium and strontium, can affect phosphorus absorption, but such effects are probably relatively minor in human nutrition.

The dietary factors influencing magnesium absorption are not well characterized, but they probably include phytate, dietary fiber, phosphorus, and protein. The gastrointestinal tract is the main site for the regulation of calcium absorption, mainly via 1,25-dihydroxy-vitamin D, although the kidney may have a role. In contrast, most of magnesium regulation is at the site of the kidney and not the gastrointestinal tract. There is very little regulation of phosphorus absorption, and only a very small fraction is facilitated by 1,25-dihydroxyvitamin D.

Calcium deficiency, characterized by demineralization of the skeleton (osteopenia), can occur slowly and insidiously as a result of a combination of coexisting dietary, genetic, endocrine, and age-related factors. Dietary factors have no role in the development of phosphorus deficiency and probably only a minor role for magnesium. Instead, these deficiencies most frequently occur in association with disease states or drugs, or in

Element	Mass (g)	Percentage in the skeleton	Percentage in soft tissues
Ca	1200	99	1
Mg	24	55	40
P	900	88	12

Table 23.1: Calcium, phosphorus, and magnesium distribution in an adult weighing 70 kg.

patients receiving prolonged total parenteral nutrition deficient in phosphorus or magnesium.

23.1 Calcium

The most abundant mineral in the body is calcium, accounting for 10–20 g per kg body weight in adults. Bone is the main reservoir for calcium. The remainder is located in body tissues (10 g), blood, and the extracellular fluids (900 mg) (Table 23.1).

Functions of calcium

Calcium has a structural role in bones and teeth, where it exists primarily as calcium hydroxyapatite $[Ca_{10}(PO_4)_6(OH)_2]$. Bone is a dynamic tissue that undergoes remodeling throughout life except for the teeth. Bone formation is under the control of osteoblasts (bone-forming cells), whereas bone resorption is initiated by osteoclasts (bone-resorbing cells). During growth, bone formation exceeds resorption, but in later life bone resorption often occurs at a faster rate than bone formation, and this results in age-related bone loss (Frost, 1997).

The remaining 1% of total body calcium in the soft tissues has a regulatory role in several metabolic processes, including enzyme activation, vascular contraction and vasodilation, muscle contractibility, nerve transmission, hormone function, and membrane transport. When the levels of absorbed calcium from the diet are insufficient to balance the obligatory fecal and urinary losses, calcium is drawn from the bone and blood calcium levels are maintained within narrow limits. This homeostatic regulation of the calcium level in the blood is achieved by the interaction of the parathyroid hormone, 1,25-dihydroxycholcalciferol, and calcitonin, the three major calcium-regulating hormones. Phosphorus, protein, estrogen, and other hormones, including glucocorticoids, thyroid hormones, growth hormone, and insulin also have a role; details are given in Allen and Wood (1994).

Absorption and metabolism of calcium

Calcium is absorbed across the intestinal mucosa in two ways: active transport and passive diffusion. Active absorption of calcium is influenced by calcium and vitamin D status of the individual, age, pregnancy, and lactation. Active absorption occurs when intakes of calcium are low or moderate and is regulated primarily via 1,25-dihydroxyvitamin D and its intestinal receptors. Passive absorption is more important at high intakes of calcium.

The absorption of calcium is highest when dietary calcium intakes are low and the requirements for calcium are high, as occurs during periods of rapid growth in infancy, early childhood, and adolescence, and during pregnancy and lactation. Indeed, absorption is very high during infancy (about 60%) (Abrams et al., 1997) and about 34% during puberty (Abrams and Stuff, 1994), stabilizing at about 25% in young adults. Subsequently, the intestinal absorption of calcium decreases progressively with age (Heaney et al., 1989). Urinary excretion of calcium is also regulated in response to need. As a result of both these adaptive mechanisms, severe nutritional deficiency of calcium is rare.

Several other dietary variables affect both calcium absorption and retention and, hence, calcium status. Diets high in protein increase the urinary excretion of calcium (hypercalciurea), which is not compensated by increased calcium absorption (Heaney, 2000). The importance of this effect on the calcium status of persons consuming a typical mixed high-protein diet depends mainly on the amount of calcium in the habitual diet (Heaney, 2000). Dietary sodium also influences urinary calcium losses. Indeed, negative consequences of high sodium intakes on bone density have been been reported in a longitudinal study of postmenopausal women (Devine et al., 1995). Caffeine, like protein and sodium, also increases urinary calcium loss and hence has a small negative effect on calcium retention, which can be offset by increasing dietary calcium intakes (Barger-Lux et al.,1990; Barrett-Connor et al., 1994).

In contrast to protein, sodium, and caffeine, high phosphorus intakes reduce urinary calcium losses (i.e., have a hypocalciuric effect), but because they increase losses of endogenous fecal calcium at the same time (Heaney and Recker, 1994), their net effect on calcium balance is probably zero.

Several components of the diet, including phytates and oxalates, can inhibit the absorption of calcium by forming insoluble calcium complexes in the gastrointestinal tract (Barger-Lux et al.,1995). Hence they may have a negative effect on calcium status, although their overall effect seems small. Some other dietary components, including lactose, enhance passive calcium absorption by increasing calcium solubility in the ileum (Schuette and Linkswiler, 1984).

Several clinical conditions are associated with disturbances in calcium absorption. Calcium malabsorption is associated with gastrointestinal diseases such as Crohn's and celiac disease, and intestinal resection or bypass. Intestinal absorption of calcium is also impaired in patients with renal failure, caused by the reduced synthesis of 1,25-dihydroxyvitamin D. Excessive intestinal absorption of calcium and hypercalcemia occur in sarcoidosis, in vitamin D intoxication, and in patients with calcium kidney stones.

Calcium deficiency in humans

Chronic calcium deficiency, arising from an habitually inadequate intake or poor absorption of calcium is one of the many important factors associated with reduced bone mass. Bone mass in later life depends on the peak bone mass achieved during growth and the rate of the subsequent age-related bone loss. The age span over which peak bone mass is achieved is from 19 through 30 years of age, and varies with the skeletal site and sex (IOM, 1997). Optimization of bone mass is important because it reduces the risk of osteoporosis in later life. Osteoporosis is a condition characterized by a reduced bone mass, as well as increased bone fragility and risk of fracture (WHO, 1994). It can be quantified by the T-score, the measurement of the bone mineral content or density of the spine,

hip, or forearm expressed in standard deviation units. The T-score is calculated as the difference between a subject's measured bone mineral density and the mean bone mineral density of healthy young adults, matched for gender and ethnic group. The difference is expressed relative to the young adult (YA) population standard deviation. Thus the T-score equals:

$$(\text{measured BMD} - \text{YA mean BMD}) / \text{YA SD}.$$

WHO (1994) has defined both osteoporosis and osteopenia based on T-score values measured using dual X-ray absorptiometry (DXA) (Section 23.1.8) or other related techniques. An individual with a T-score less than -2.5 at the spine, hip, or forearm is classified as having osteoporosis; a T-score between -2.5 and -1 is classified as osteopenia; and a T-score greater than -1 is healthy. These WHO definitions should not be applied to other bone mineral density measurement sites or to other technologies. Approximately 30% of all Caucasian postmenopausal women may have T-scores below -1.0 (Kanis et al., 1997).

The International Society for Clinical Densitometry (ISCD) (Lewiecki et al., 2004) has established guidelines for bone density testing using DXA. The guidelines specify the skeletal sites to measure and the region(s) of interest within a skeletal site that should be used for diagnosis, because these details were not specified by WHO. In addition, they provide specific guidelines for diagnosing osteoporosis based on T-score values for postmenopausal women, men (20 y and older), premenopausal women (20 y to menopause), and children (males or females < 20 y).

The association between calcium intake and bone health has been the subject of intense debate (Prentice, 2004; Ginty and Prentice, 2004). Epidemiological studies have not always found a consistent relationship between calcium intake and bone density (Heaney et al., 1978; Matković et al., 1979). A meta-analysis of epidemiological studies conducted up to 1988, however, confirmed a positive relationship between calcium intake and bone status (Cummings, 1990). Moreover, a higher calcium intake does appear to be beneficial during peak bone mass development, and may even slow bone loss in older postmenopausal women, especially if their usual dietary intake of calcium has been low. There is also accumulating evidence that hip fractures may be prevented by increasing calcium intakes (Reid and New, 1997).

Several other factors affect bone loss. Possible nutritional risk factors, in addition to calcium, include high protein and phosphorus intakes, and suboptimal vitamin D and possibly potassium, magnesium, zinc, copper, and manganese status (Reid and New, 1997). Genetic and environmental factors also influence bone mass. Indeed, up to 75% of the variation in bone mass in the elderly is said to be influenced by genetic factors (Flicker et al., 1995). For a more detailed discussion of these factors see Ralston (1996).

There is some evidence that very low calcium intakes in children may induce rickets and osteomalacia, although the mechanism is still uncertain (Abrams, 2002). It may involve increased catabolism of 25-hydroxy-vitamin D in the liver (Clements et al., 1987). Case reports from the United States, South Africa, and Nigeria have described infants and children with radiological rickets, growth retardation, and biochemical signs of hyperparathyroidism but with normal vitamin D status. In all these cases of rickets, habitual calcium intakes were low but phosphorus intakes were adequate or high. Moreover, the children in the United States and South Africa responded to calcium-rich hospital diets (Pettifor, 1991), whereas the Nigerian children responded more to calcium or a combination of calcium and vitamin D than to vitamin D alone (Oginni et al., 1996; Thatcher et al., 1999). Low calcium intakes have also been linked with hypertension, but the effect is probably modest and rather variable (Allender et al., 1996).

Food sources and dietary intakes

Calcium is not widely distributed in foods. Milk and milk products (e.g., cheeses, yoghurt) are excellent sources of readily available calcium. Soymilk substitutes and canned fish with bones (e.g., salmon, sardines) are good sources of calcium. Leafy-green vegetables are also good sources, but absorption of calcium from some of these foods may be low. Meats, grains, and nuts are poor sources of calcium. Hence, if milk and milk products are not consumed regularly, intakes of available calcium may be inadequate.

Weaver (2004) has compared the bioavailability of calcium from a variety of food sources and the corresponding number of servings equivalent to that provided from a glass of milk (Weaver, 2001).

In most industrialized countries, dairy products are the major food source of calcium (NIN, 1995; Cleveland et al., 1996; McLennan and Podger, 1998; Russell et al., 1999). In surveys in the United Kingdom (Gregory et al., 1990), New Zealand (Russell et al., 1999), and Australia (McLennan and Podger, 1998), for example, milk and milk products provided approximately 50% of the total intake of calcium for adults, followed by cereals and cereal products. Increasingly, foods are being fortified with calcium (e.g., milk, orange juice) in these countries.

Effects of high intakes of calcium

Excessive intakes of calcium from food alone are unlikely to cause hypercalcemia (elevated serum calcium concentrations). Instead, this condition often results from hyperparathyroidism, excessive doses of vitamin D (Koutkia et al., 2001), or high intakes of calcium from both supplements and food (IOM, 1997). Nevertheless, persons who are predisposed to the formation of kidney stones and milk alkali syndrome should avoid excessive intakes of calcium. The U.S. Food and Nutrition Board has set the Tolerable Upper Intake Level (UL) for calcium at 2500 mg/d for all persons older than 1 y, including pregnant and lactating women (IOM, 1997).

Indices of calcium status

There is no satisfactory test to assess calcium status on a routine basis. Serum ionized calcium is increasingly used to assess disturbances in calcium metabolism. Several biochemical markers of bone remodeling can also be used to measure subtle changes in the rate of formation or degradation of the bone matrix brought about by dietary influences. Some monitor bone formation, by measuring enzymatic activity of the bone forming or resorbing cells in serum (e.g., bone alkaline phosphatase). Others measure bone-matrix components released into the circulation during bone formation (e.g., serum osteocalcin) or bone resorption (e.g., urinary pyridinoline, N-telopeptides) (Table 23.2). The sensitivity and specificity of these bone biomarkers varies (Demers and Kleerekoper, 1994; Seibel and Pols, 1996); those most frequently used are discussed in the following sections, with the exception of hydroxyproline. The latter is discussed in Section 16.3.2. When remodeling rates are changing, a combination of biomarkers, such as one formation marker and one resorption marker can give more information than a single marker (Watts, 1999).

Several noninvasive techniques can also be used to provide an indirect assessment of the bone mineral content of the appendicular skeleton, the axial skeleton, or the total skeleton. The mineral content of the skeleton relates directly to its calcium content. As almost all of the calcium in the body is stored in the skeleton, it follows that skeletal mineral content can be used as an indirect measure of body calcium stores. These techniques are described in Sections 23.1.6 to 23.1.12. They can also be used to monitor the response to changes in calcium intakes over relatively long time periods — months or even years.

Biomarkers in serum of bone formation (osteoblastic activity)	Biomarkers in urine of bone resorption (osteoclastic activity)
Total alk. phosphatase Bone alk. phosphatase Osteocalcin	Hydroxyproline Pyridinoline Deoxypyridoline N-telopeptide C-telopeptide

Table 23.2: Biochemical markers of bone turnover; alk, alkaline.

23.1.1 Serum calcium

Serum calcium concentrations cannot be used as a measure of calcium status because they are strongly homeostatically controlled and remain constant under most conditions: low levels of serum calcium only occur after prolonged periods of calcium deprivation or following interference with calcium absorption.

Fifty percent of the calcium in serum is ionized and physiologically active; it is this fraction that is under hormonal control. The remaining 50% is not ionized and is physiologically inert. Of the inert calcium fraction, 40%–50% is bound to protein, primarily albumin, and 5%–10% is complexed with citrate, bicarbonate, and phosphate. As such a large amount of calcium in serum is bound to albumin, it follows that concentrations can be influenced by changes in serum albumin levels. As a result, when serum albumin levels are outside the normal limits (Iqbal et al., 1988), as may occur in liver disease or malnutrition, serum calcium values should be corrected. The correction is approximate, and if there is uncertainty in the interpretation of the results, serum ionized calcium should be determined (see below).

Homeostatic regulation of serum calcium is achieved by the interaction of parathyroid hormone, 1,25-hydroxycholecalciferol, and calcitonin, the three calcium-regulating hormones that affect calcium transport in the kidney, bone, and intestine. If serum calcium concentrations are outside the normal range, pathological rather than nutritional problems should be suspected. For example, in cases of hypoparathyroidism, hypomagnesemia, and acute pancreatitis, serum calcium concentrations are low (hypocalcemia).

Hypercalcemia or elevated serum calcium values occur in association with hyperparathyroidism, hyperthyroidism, and sarcoidosis and when large parts of the body are immobilized (e.g., when a patient is hospitalized after spinal cord injury or major limb-bone fractures). In the latter cases, calcium from the rapidly atrophying bone is released into the circulating body fluids. In addition, hypercalcemia is one of the characteristic features of vitamin D intoxication. It arises from hyperabsorption of intestinal calcium and to a lesser degree from the release of calcium from bone (Chesney, 1989).

Interpretive criteria

Concentrations of calcium in serum of normal adults range from 2.20 to 2.64 mmol/L. Values decrease with age in men. Females usually have slightly lower concentrations (2.20–2.54 mmol/L), associated with small differences in serum albumin content and the calcium-reducing effect of estrogens. Serum calcium decreases by 5%–10% up to the end of the third trimester of pregnancy, after which concentrations rise.

Serum calcium levels were determined in both the National Health and Nutrition Examination Survey (NHANES) I (Harlan et al., 1984) and the Nutrition Canada National Survey (Health and Welfare Canada, 1973). Plasma calcium concentrations, determined on blood collected using lithium heparin as an anticoagulant, were measured in the U.K. Diet and Nutrition Surveys on British adults (Gregory et al., 1990) and people aged $\geqslant 65$ y (Finch et al., 1998). Mean and median values, as well as the lower and upper 5th percentile values by age and sex are given.

Measurement of serum calcium

Serum calcium levels are usually determined by flame atomic absorption spectrophotometry (AAS) (Zettner and Seligson, 1964) or by automated procedures that use the *o*-cresolphthalein complexone method (Bourke and Delaney, 1993). Earlier methods included flame photometry and a calcium oxalate titration procedure.

Considerable differences in the quality of serum calcium measurements among laboratories may occur, emphasizing the necessity for rigorous quality-control practices. In general, the coefficient of variation for the AAS method is less than that for flame photometry (Linko et al., 1998). Gallagher et al. (1989) reported that analytical variation for serum calcium via AAS ranges from 0.9%–3.04%.

Standard reference materials for serum calcium measurements are available from National Institute of Standards and Technology (NIST), Gaithersburg, MD. Serum rather than plasma should be used for calcium analysis. Most anticoagulants, with the notable exception of lithium heparin, interfere with the determination of calcium: they complex with or precipitate the calcium in the sample.

23.1.2 Serum ionized calcium

Ionized calcium makes up about 50% of the calcium in serum. It is the physiologically active form of calcium in blood, as noted above, and governs secretion of the three calcitropic hormones: parathyroid hormone, 1,25-hydroxycholecalciferol (vitamin D), and calcitonin. Parathyroid hormone and 1,25-hydroxycholecalciferol are secreted when the ionized calcium in the serum is low, whereas calcitonin is secreted when serum ionized calcium is high.

Changes in serum ionized calcium levels relate to disturbances in calcium metabolism. Reductions in ionized calcium occur in both hypoparathyroidism and vitamin D-deficient rickets, and result in increased neuromuscular irritability. Elevated ionized calcium values suggest functional hypercalcemia and occur in patients who have hyperparathyroidism or who are receiving chronic renal hemodialysis. In such conditions, total serum calcium levels may be normal (Ladenson and Bowers, 1973).

The levels of serum ionized calcium cannot be predicted from serum calcium because of the low correlation of ionized calcium with total calcium in the serum in healthy persons.

Factors affecting serum ionized calcium

Age-related trends exist and levels decline with age in men (Minisola et al., 1993). A similar trend is not apparent in women, perhaps because the trend is obscured by hormonal disturbances during menopause.

High levels of sodium and magnesium confound the measurement, although their effects can be eliminated by using calcium standards containing sodium and magnesium chloride in the same concentrations as those expected in the samples (Ladenson and Bowers, 1973).

Trypsin, triethanolamine, and heparin all bind calcium (Ladenson and Bowers, 1973) and should not be used.

Changes in the pH of the blood during collection and storage of the sample may alter the measurement. The affect can be minimized by collecting and handling the serum samples anerobically and by adjusting to pH 7.4 with CO_2 gas before the measurement (Ladenson and Bowers, 1973; Schwartz, 1976). Measurements should be made as soon as possible after the blood collection.

Interpretive criteria

Reported levels of serum ionized calcium in adults vary. Some of the discrepancies may be attributed to difficulties in collecting and handling serum samples anerobically and to differences in the electrode systems used. Ladenson and Bowers (1973) reported a mean serum ionized calcium concentration of 1.28 mmol/L (range: 1.18–1.38 mmol/L) for 86 apparently healthy adults 19–50 y. This mean value corresponds closely to that obtained in some earlier studies (Oreskes et al., 1968; Li and Piechocki, 1971).

In NHANES III, mean age-adjusted serum ionized calcium values are presented for male and female non-Hispanic Caucasians, African Americans, and Mexican Americans for two age groups: 25–59 y and 60–89 y; the reported mean age-adjusted value for serum ionized calcium was 1.237 mmol/L for males and 1.232 mmol/L for females (Vargas et al., 1998). Mean age-adjusted values for African Americans were slightly higher.

Measurement of serum ionized calcium

Fasting blood samples are recommended for the measurement of ionized calcium in serum, to eliminate the effect of a recent meal. The samples should be stored anerobically at 0°C–4°C prior to the assay. Serum ionized calcium can be measured using commercially available ion-specific electrodes (Wandrup and Kvetny, 1985). Care must be taken to ensure that the calcium standards used for the assay contain sodium and chloride at the same levels as in the test samples.

23.1.3 Bone alkaline phosphatase activity in serum

In adults approximately 50% of serum total alkaline phosphatase is present as bone alkaline phosphatase, an isoenzyme also known as bone-specific alkaline phosphatase or skeletal alkaline phosphatase. During childhood, however, the bone isoenzyme predominates. Bone alkaline phosphatase has a half-life in the serum of 24–48 h. The activity of bone alkaline phosphatase exhibits marked diurnal variation, with levels peaking in the afternoon and evening (Nielson et al., 1990a).

Bone alkaline phosphatase is essential for normal bone mineralization, and several techniques have been developed to measure the activity of this enzyme. The activity of bone alkaline phosphatase gradually rises in normal healthy women from the fourth to the tenth decade of life, along with increases in osteocalcin and urinary hydroxyproline. These changes reflect increases in bone turnover. In patients with disturbances in bone metabolism, bone alkaline phosphatase activity in serum is markedly elevated. For example, Farley et al. (1981) reported a mean level of 10.4 U/L in 43 osteoporotic patients, compared with 7.1 U/L for healthy controls. Elevated bone alkaline phosphatase activity has also been observed in British Asians with osteomalacia (Nisbet et al., 1990). However, bone alkaline phosphatase is cleared by the liver so that the skeletal fraction may also be increased in patients with liver disease (Watts, 1999).

Studies have monitored the response of serum bone alkaline phosphatase to calcium supplementation. Responses have varied and depend on the usual calcium intake of the study subjects, the length of the supplementation period, the age of the subjects, and the number of years post-menopause (IOM, 1997; Ginty et al., 1998). Some investigators have observed no significant changes in serum bone alkaline phosphatase activity in calcium supplementation studies of young adults or elderly women. In these studies, intervention periods have ranged from 2 wk to as long as 4 y (Table 23.3) (Ginty et al., 1998; Riggs et al., 1998; Heaney et al., 1999).

Measurement of bone alkaline phosphatase activity

The activity of bone alkaline phosphatase is not usually measured in clinical chemistry laboratories. Most of the assays are difficult. In the simplest method, alkaline phosphatase is measured in serum with a spectrophotometric assay with *p*-nitrophenyl phosphate, before and after precipitation of bone alkaline phosphatase by wheat-germ agglutinin (Behr and Barnert, 1986). Alternatively, a two-site enzyme-linked immunosorbent assay (ELISA) technique can be used (Bailyes et al., 1987; Heaney et al., 1999).

An alternative method uses an immunoradiometric assay based on two monoclonal antibodies specific for bone alkaline phosphatase (Garnero and Delmas, 1993). A commercial kit is now available with intra- and interassay variations of between 3.7%–6.6% and 7.0%–8.1%, respectively (Woitge et al., 1996). Normal values using this assay are 11.6 ± 4.1 µg/L for premenopausal females and 12.4 ± 4.4 µg/L for males. Further studies with this new more specific assay are needed to establish the specificity and responsiveness of bone alkaline phosphatase to the activity of bone cells.

23.1.4 Serum osteocalcin

Osteocalcin is also called a bone γ-carboxyglutamic acid–containing protein because it contains up to three γ-carboxy-glutamic acid residues. This small noncollagenous protein is specific for bone tissue and dentin and comprises about 1%–2% of total bone protein. Osteocalcin is synthesized primarily by the osteoblasts mediated by a vitamin K–depend-

ent enzyme and 1,25-dihydroxycholecalciferol. Most of the osteocalcin is incorporated into the bone mineral immediately after synthesis, but a small fraction is released directly into the blood.

The precise physiological role of osteocalcin is unclear. Levels in serum appear to reflect the activity and number of osteoblasts. Studies in mice suggest that osteocalcin may have an inhibitory role in bone formation (Ducy et al., 1996). Osteocalcin is cleared by the kidneys so that serum levels depend on renal function. The half-life of serum osteocalcin is short (15–70 min).

Serum levels of osteocalcin are affected by a variety of factors, including both age and sex (Figure 23.1), alcohol intake (Laitinen and Valimaki, 1991), season (Thomsen et al., 1989), vitamin D status (Nielsen et al., 1991), diurnal and circadian variation (Gundberg et al., 1985; Watts, 1999). Changes in serum osteocalcin concentrations occur around menopause in women, as shown in Figure 23.1 (Eriksen, 1995). The circadian rhythm probably results from an increase in bone turnover during the night, as noted for other markers of bone turnover. A significant effect of the menstrual cycle has also been re-

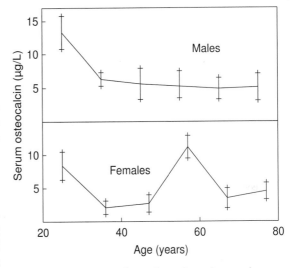

Figure 23.1: Age- and sex-dependent changes in osteocalcin concentrations. Data from Eriksen et al., European Journal of Endocrinology 132: 251–263, 1995 © Society for the European Journal of Endocrinology. Reproduced with permission.

ported, associated with an increase in serum osteocalcin during the luteal phase (Nielsen et al., 1990b).

Elevated levels of osteocalcin have been noted in postmenopausal osteoporosis (Delmas et al., 1985; Eastell et al., 1993). Indeed, serum osteocalcin may be the most useful single biomarker of bone turnover and, hence, rate of bone loss in postmenopausal women. Serum values correlate with the rate of bone loss assessed by sequential measurements of bone mineral content of the radius and the lumbar spine (Slemenda et al., 1987; Johansen et al., 1988).

Several investigators have shown serum osteocalcin as responding to changes in bone metabolism brought about by an increased calcium intake. For example, calcium supplementation (1600 mg/d) for 4 y significantly reduced serum levels of osteocalcin (and urinary pyridinoline, see below) in postmenopausal women with an average usual intake of calcium of 714 mg/d, while at the same time significantly reducing bone loss (Table 23.3) (Riggs et al., 1998).

Decreases in serum osteocalcin in response to supplemental calcium have also been seen in other age groups (e.g., prepubertal children and premenopausal women), especially when habitual calcium intakes have been low (Johnston et al., 1992; Elders et al., 1994; McKane et al., 1996). Table 23.4 shows the effect of calcium supplementation for 1 y on plasma

	Calcium group ($n = 80$)	Placebo group ($n = 80$)
Baseline	24.8 ± 12.1	24.3 ± 7.9
Outcome	17.9 ± 7.3	23.2 ± 9.5

Table 23.4: Mean ± SD plasma osteocalcin concentrations (μg/L) in Gambian children aged 8.3–11.9 y supplemented with 1000 mg Ca/d for 1 y. Data from Dibba et al., American Journal of Clinical Nutrition 71: 544–549, 2000 © Am J Clin Nutr. American Society for Clinical Nutrition.

osteocalcin concentrations in children from the Gambia who were accustomed to a low-calcium diet (i.e., 300 mg/d) (Dibba et al., 2000). Note the marked decrease in plasma osteocalcin concentrations in the calcium-supplemented group. This was accompanied by significant increases in both bone mineral content and bone mineral density, measured by single-photon absorptiometry (Section 23.1.7). These findings are consistent with those of Johnston et al. (1992), who studied 41 pairs of monozygotic twins residing in the same household. At the end of the 3-y trial, they reported mean serum osteocalcin concentrations in the calcium-supplemented versus placebo group of 48.5 vs. 54.0 μg/L ($p = 0.008$), respectively.

Nevertheless, there is still some question about whether the effects are maintained after the calcium supplementation stops. In the study of identical twins described above, the effect of the supplemental calcium on serum osteocalcin had all but disappeared 2 y later (Slemenda et al.,1997). Moreover, such changes in serum osteocalcin, indicative of bone formation, are not always seen in calcium supplementation studies. Results may depend on the duration and level of the calcium supplement, site of the skeletal measurements, the usual calcium intakes, age, and, where appropriate, number of years post-menopause of the subjects (IOM, 1997; Ginty et al., 1998).

	Calcium ($n = 88$)		Placebo ($n = 89$)		
	Bsl.	Diff.	Bsl.	Diff	p
Bone alkaline phosphatase U/L)	21.3	2.70	22.80	3.75	0.590
Osteocalcin (nmol/L)	1.04	−0.12	1.09	0.02	0.035
Free pyridoline (nmol/mmol Creat)	39.5	3.05	41.1	13.40	0.001

Table 23.3: Baseline (Bsl) and median changes (Diff) in serum and urine (free pyridinoline) biomarkers following 4 y of calcium supplementation in elderly women. Creat, creatinine. Data from Riggs et al., Journal of Bone and Mineral Research 13: 168–174, 1998.

Measurement of serum osteocalcin

Serum osteocalcin can be assessed by radio-immunoassay (Price and Nishimoto, 1980) and by commercially available ELISA methods (Shiraki et al., 1991; Garnero et al., 1992). Measurements should be made in the morning to avoid the later afternoon nadir. Caution must be used when comparing results across assay methods because assays for osteocalcin are not standardized. Measurements should be evaluated against a reference population determined using the same assay in the same laboratory (Delmas et al., 1990).

23.1.5 Urinary pyridinium cross-links

Most of the organic matrix of bone is type I collagen associated with noncollagenous proteins. Type I collagen is rich in the amino acid hydroxyproline. It has a triple helix structure, with strands connected by cross-links between lysine or hydroxylysine residues that join nonhelical amino- and carboxy-terminal ends of one collagen molecule to the helical portion of an adjacent molecule. The cross-links are hydroxylysylpyridinoline (known as pyridinoline) and lysylpyridinoline (known as deoxypyridinoline) and are important for the structural integrity of the collagen.

Pyridinoline is widely distributed in both type I collagen of bone and type II collagen of cartilage, as well as in smaller amounts in the other connective tissues. In contrast, deoxypyridinoline is found almost exclusively in type I collagen of bone. Neither of these two cross-links occurs in skin.

Both the cross-links are released into the circulation after mature tissue collagen is degraded. They are not re-utilized or metabolized in the liver but, instead, are excreted in the urine unchanged, in peptide-bound and free forms. Hence, their potential as markers of bone resorption has been extensively investigated (Table 23.2) (Delmas, 1992; Eyre, 1992). Of the two cross-links, total deoxypyridinoline correlates better than pyridinoline with estimates of bone resorption by calcium kinetics (Eastell et al., 1997).

Urinary excretion levels of the pyridinolines are elevated in diseases in which the catabolism of collagen is increased, such as osteoporosis, rheumatoid arthritis, osteoarthritis, Paget's disease, and primary hyperpara-

thyroidism (Uebelhart et al., 1990). Moreover, studies have shown significant correlations with bone turnover as assessed by both histomorphometry (Delmas et al., 1991) and radiotracer kinetics. For example, in a study of osteoporotic subjects, Eastell et al. (1993) reported a significant correlation between the levels of pyridinoline cross-links in urine and bone resorption rate ($r = 0.92$; $p < 0.001$), as measured by tracer kinetics.

Increases in urinary excretion of pyridinolines have also been reported in women during menopause because of an estrogen deficiency, followed by restoration to normal concentrations after hormone replacement therapy (Melton et al., 1997).

Urinary excretion of pyridinoline and deoxypyridinoline has also been used to monitor the response to certain treatments over varying time periods. Ginty et al. (1998) examined the response of increasing calcium intake over 2 wk in healthy young adults (mean age 23 y), by measuring the urinary excretion of pyridinoline cross-links and serum bone alkaline phosphatase and osteocalcin. Urinary excretion of both pyridinoline and deoxypyridinoline were lower in the calcium-supplemented group than in the unsupplemented group, indicating a reduction in bone resorption, although changes in bone alkaline phosphatase and osteocalcin in serum were not significant (Table 23.5). It appears that such changes in bone resorption are sustained during longer periods of calcium supplementation (Johnston et al., 1992; Riggs et al., 1998). A reduction in urinary pyridinoline excretion has been reported in response to antiresorptive treatment with bisphosphonates for 2 y by postmenopausal osteoporotic women (Garnero et al., 1994). Nevertheless there is still some question about whether the effect is maintained after the calcium supplementation stops.

In addition to pyridinoline and deoxypyridinoline, cross-linked N- and C-telopeptides are also used as markers of bone resorption. These are amino- and carboxy-terminal fragments of collagen which are excreted in the urine with cross-links attached. Comparative studies have shown that they are

	Unsupplemented (22 mmol Ca/d)	Ca-supplemented (40 mmol Ca/d)	*p* value
Urine			
Creatinine (Cr) (mmol/L)	13.4 ± 5.5	13.0 ± 5.6	0.736
Ca (mmol/mmol Cr)	0.25 ± 0.09	0.42 ± 0.17	< 0.001
Mg (mmol/mmol Cr)	0.30 ± 0.05	0.29 ± 0.07	0.637
Pyr (nmol/mmol Cr)	42.9 ± 12.9	36.9 ± 10.1	0.044
Dpyr (nmol/mmol Cr)	12.4 ± 3.4	10.4 ± 3.0	0.032
Serum			
Ca (mmol/L)	2.54 ± 0.30	2.58 ± 0.26	0.130
Mg (mmol/L)	0.83 ± 0.16	0.83 ± 0.14	0.965
B-Alkphos (U/L)	23.6 ± 9.4	23.9 ± 7.5	0.845
Osteocalcin (μg/L)	9.7 ± 5.7	10.5 ± 4.9	0.531

Table 23.5: Mean ($\pm$ SD) for urinary and serum biochemical variables in healthy young adults ($n = 18$) during a calcium supplementation study. Pyr, pyridoline; Dpyr, deoxypyridoline; B-Alkphos, bone-specific alkaline phosphatase. The significance (p) of each biochemical test was calculated using a two-sample t-test. Data from Ginty et al., British Journal of Nutrition 80: 437–443, 1998, with permission of the Nutrition Society.

both more responsive and specific markers of bone resorption than are the free cross-links themselves (Garnero et al., 1995; Gertz et al., 1998).

The urinary pyridinium cross-links appear to be more specific biomarkers of bone resorption than is urinary hydroxyproline excretion (Section 16.3.2). Dietary sources of pyridinium cross-links from collagen or gelatin, unlike urinary hydroxyproline, are not well absorbed, so there is no dietary contribution in the urine. In addition, in certain diseases, notably Paget's disease and primary hyperparathyroidism, urinary pyridinium cross-links are much more sensitive markers of bone resorption than is urinary hydroxyproline (Uebelhart et al., 1990; Seibel et al., 1992).

Together, the results of these studies undertaken over the past decade have confirmed the validity of pyridinium cross-links, either free or with fragments of the collagen molecule attached, as markers of bone resorption. Nevertheless, their response to relevant diseases and treatments differs according to the marker used. Continued research is needed to identify the best marker or combinations of markers for prediction of treatment response and for prediction of bone loss or fracture in un-

treated patients. In addition, several factors are known to influence the urinary excretion level of pyridinium cross-links, and these should be taken into account during interpretation of the results, especially when only subtle changes in bone metabolism are expected.

Factors affecting urinary pyridinium cross-links

Age-related changes in the urinary excretion of pyridinoline, deoxypyridinoline, and cross-linked telopeptides are significant. Concentrations increase during puberty and again after menopause (Eriksen et al., 1995; Watts, 1999).

Circadian variation in the urinary excretion of pyridinium cross-links can be 20% compared to about 10% for bone formation markers (Watts, 1999).

Diurnal variation in urinary excretion can be significant, ranging from 35% to 70% between individuals (Pagani and Panteghini, 1994), with peak excretion in the early morning and the nadir in the afternoon. Within individuals, urinary free deoxypyridinoline exhibits the least biological variability across a 24-h period compared with that observed for N- and C-cross-linked telopeptides (Ju et al., 1997).

Circannual rhythms related to variations in the hormonal regulation of skeletal homeostasis occur, and are especially significant in premenopausal women. Urinary excretion levels of total pyridinoline, deoxypyridinoline, and N-telopeptides (NTx) are increased in winter. These changes are accompanied by significant variations in serum 25-hydroxyvitamin D_3, 1,25-dihydroxyvitamin D_3, and parathyroid hormone (Woitge et al., 2000). At present, the biological significance of these seasonal changes in bone turnover is unknown.

Stage of the menstrual cycle influences urinary excretion, with levels being slightly higher in the luteal phase (Gorai et al., 1998).

Fracture elevates urinary excretion levels by 20% to 60% for 6 mo or more (Watts, 1999).

Prolonged bed rest increases urinary excretion by 40%–50%, but the patterns of recovery vary depending on the marker (Lueken et al., 1993).

Creatinine excretion influences urinary bone markers so results are often normalized to creatinine (Bettica et al., 1996).

Measurement of urinary pyridinium cross-links

Proper interpretation of the assay results for the urinary pyridinium cross-links requires an understanding of their biological variability and analytical performance. To minimize the effect of within-subject variation on urinary excretion of pyridinium cross-links, multiple measurements in 24-h urine collections should be performed (Eyre, 1992; Eastell et al., 1997; Ju et al., 1997).

Total urinary pyridinolines can be detected and measured using their natural fluorescence after reversed-phase HPLC of a cellulose-bound extract of hydrolyzed urine (Black et al., 1988). No synthetic standards are available to calibrate the assay, however, making it difficult to compare results among laboratories. This is a severe limitation because the method is complex, and the analytical variation can be large. In addition, the amplitude of the diurnal variation exhibited by urinary excretion of pyridinium cross-links measured by HPLC is greater than has been reported when determined by immunoassay (Schlemmer et al., 1992; Colwell et al., 1993; Blumsohn et al., 1994; Ju et al., 1997).

Radioimmunoassays, based on a high-affinity monoclonal antibody specific for free pyridinoline cross-links, have also been developed (Robins et al., 1994; Gomez et al., 1996). As an alternative, enzyme-linked immunosorbent assays that measure the urinary excretion of the free pyridinolines or the cross-linked N- and C-telopeptides are now available. Free pyridinoline and deoxypyridinoline can be assayed with the Pyrilinks (Gomez et al., 1996) and Pyrilinks-D assays, respectively (Robins et al., 1994) (Metra Biosystems). For the N-telopetides of type I collagen, the Osteomark assay (Ostex International) can be used (Hanson et al., 1992), whereas the C-telopeptides can be measured with CrossLaps (Osteometer BioTech A/S) (Bonde et al., 1994).

Ju et al. (1997) have compared the analytical performance and biological variability of commercially available bone resorption enzyme-linked immunosorbent assays for the measurement of urinary free deoxypyridinoline and cross-linked N- and C-telopeptides (CTx). The within and between-assay coefficients of variation for precision of the deoxypyridinoline and cross-linked NTx were < 10% for analyte concentrations greater than the second calibrator (i.e., 3 nmol/L deoxypyridinoline or 30 nmol bone collagen equivalents/L NTx). The CTx showed poor precision for analyte concentrations lower than the third calibrator (i.e., 200 μg/L). The analytes were stable up to five freeze-thaw cycles (Ju et al., 1997).

In the future, pyridinolines may be measured in sweat instead of urine. Sarno et al.

(1999) describe a sweat collection method and immunoassay, in which the within- and between-assay variation for pyridinolines is markedly smaller than that for urine specimens. Moreover, the sweat pyridinolines, normalized to potassium output, significantly increased by 36% in the population group experiencing bone resorption, compared with a healthy reference group. A sensitive immunoassay has also been developed to measure cross-linked N-telopeptides (NTx) in serum (Clemens et al., 1997; Gertz et al., 1998).

23.1.6 Radiogrammetry

Radiogrammetry, also known as radiographic absorptiometry, was developed to examine the peripheral skeleton (the limbs). It measures the thickness and the diameter of the cortex of the metacarpals or radius using standard anterior and posterior roentgenograms (X-rays). Quantitative measurements can be made with a dial caliper or a digitizer. Cortical bone volume can then be calculated (Health and Public Policy Committee, 1984). The radiographic image can also be captured digitally and processed to yield an estimate of the bone mineral density in the phalanges. Serial measurements can be used to monitor changes in cortical bone volume.

Radiogrammetry provides no information on trabecular bone (Cummings et al., 1985). Therefore, although the measurements are precise, they do not accurately reflect the total amount of bone present, so correlations with the total mass of the skeleton, as determined by neutron activation, are poor. In addition, changes in the bone mineral density of the phalanges and radius in response to treatment can be relatively small. In such cases, measurements on the axial skeleton are preferable (Faulkner, 1998).

23.1.7 Single-photon absorptiometry

Single-photon absorptiometry is a practical noninvasive method that was developed to examine the peripheral skeleton (Wahner et al., 1983); it is gradually being replaced by dual X-ray absorptiometry. The original method is based on the assumption that the bone mineral content is inversely proportional to the amount of photon energy transmitted through the bone under study. A monoenergetic photon source is used, usually ^{125}I or ^{241}Am. The technique is fast, taking approximately 5 min. With this method, bone mineral density is measured with a precision (%CV) of less than 2% and with an effective dose to the subject of only 0.1 μSv.

The site most frequently selected for measurements by single-photon absorptiometry is the lower radius, at approximately one-third of the distance from the styloid process to the olecranon. Single-photon absorptiometry is not suitable for measurements on the axial skeleton because the technique requires that a uniform thickness of soft tissue surrounds the bone. Only weak correlations between the bone mineral content of the lower radius and the amount of trabecular bone in the spine have been reported (Mazess, 1983). Hence, this method should not be used to predict bone mineral content or density of the vertebrae, especially in patients with metabolic bone disease (Mazess et al., 1984).

Bone mineral content is usually expressed as the bone mineral density, which corrects for projected bone area but is not a true density measurement. Instead, it is a measure of areal density (g/cm^2) and is derived by dividing bone mineral content (g) by the scanned bone area. Bone mineral density is calculated in this way to reduce the biological variation observed in values for bone mineral content at all ages and thus to increase the statistical power of detecting abnormal values. However, bone mineral density does not adequately correct for bone area and body size, and its use in epidemiological research has been questioned (Prentice et al., 1994). Nevertheless, measurements of bone mineral density using single-photon absorptiometry can still be used to assess fracture risk and to examine and monitor patients with osteoporosis.

Single-photon absorptiometry was used by Dibba et al. (2000) to monitor the effects of calcium supplementation over 12 mo on the bone mineral content (g/cm) and bone mineral density (g/cm^2) of the bones of the forearm in Gambian children consuming habitual diets with a low-calcium content. Significant increases in bone mineral density were apparent, ranging from 4.5% at the midshaft radius to 7.0% at the distal radius. This change represents a shift of about 0.3–0.4 of the population standard deviation for this age group, which in adults would represent a significant reduction in fracture risk. Unfortunately, because only single-photon absorptiometry was available for these measurements, the investigators were not able to monitor the effects of calcium supplementation at other skeletal sites. Furthermore, there is mounting evidence that such gains in bone mineral density are not retained postintervention (Lee et al., 1997).

23.1.8 Dual X-ray absorptiometry (DXA)

Originally this method, which is also termed dual-photon absorptiometry, used an isotopic source, typically ^{153}Gd emitting two low-energy gamma rays at 44 and 100 KeV. The method was used to determine total bone mineral content of the axial skeleton, generally using the lumbar vertebrae (L2 to L4) sites and parts of the femur. For example, Johnston et al. (1992) used this procedure to measure bone mineral density at two sites in the radius, three sites in the hip (femoral neck, Ward's triangle, and greater-trochanter region), and in the spine (from second to fourth lumbar vertebrae) in a 3-y calcium supplementation study of pairs of identical twins. They reported an overall mean increase in bone mineral density for all six sites that was 1.4% greater in the calcium-supplemented group, with the greatest increase occurring at the midshaft radius and distal radius. The age of the subjects relative to puberty was an important confounding factor (Table 23.6), with only prepubertal children responding to supplementation.

The short half-life of the isotopic source ^{153}Gd, however, limits the precision with which long-term changes in bone mineral content in the same subject can be made using this technique. Indeed, in the study

by Johnston et al. (1992), the ^{153}Gd source was replaced every 6 mo during the 3-y study (Table 23.6).

This limitation has led to the radioactive ^{153}Gd source being replaced with an X-ray tube behind a K-edge filter. The filter converts the polychromatic X-ray beam into one with two main energy peaks at 40 and 70 KeV. These two congruent X-ray beams are passed through the body, and the ratio of beam attenuation at the lower energy relative to that at the higher energy differentiates between bone mineral, bone-free mass, and the fat mass (Mazess et al., 1990). As a result, this modified instrument, known as a dual energy X-ray absorptiometer (DXA), is also used extensively to assess body composition, as described in Section 14.11. Only the measurements of bone mineral mass (g), bone mineral content (g/cm), and "areal" bone mineral density (g/cm^2) are discussed here.

The first commercial DXA scanner was marketed in 1987 and measured spine bone mineral content with greater precision and less radiation exposure than when the radio-isotope ^{153}Gd was used. There are now several commercial versions, each using similar measurement procedures. The most recent generation uses a slit collimator to generate a fanbeam coupled to a linear array of detectors, as shown in Figure 14.9. Fogelman and Blake (2000) provide further details. The

Site	Prepubertal twins (22 pairs)	Pubertal or post-pubertal twins (23 pairs)
Midshaft radius	5.1 (1.5 to 8.7)	−0.1 (−3.0 to 2.9)
Distal radius	3.8 (1.4 to 6.2)	2.9 (−0.7 to 6.5)
Lumbar spine	2.8 (1.1 to 4.5)	−1.0 (−3.2 to 1.2)
Femoral neck	1.2 (−1.6 to 4.0)	−0.4 (−3.4 to 2.5)
Ward's triangle	2.9 (−0.1 to 5.9)	−0.4 (−3.7 to 2.9)

Table 23.6: Percentage differences (95% confidence interval) in bone mineral density following calcium supplementation between the calcium-supplement and placebo groups according to pubertal status. The subjects were 45 sets of identical twins. Data from Johnston et al., New England Journal of Medicine 327: 82–87, 1992, with permission.

measurements are generally made in the antero-posterior position. Site-specific measurements of areal bone mass density can be made at the lumbar spine, femur, and forearm (Lunt et al., 1997). Measurements of body mineral density at the lumbar vertebrae (L2 to L4) are often favored because they are sensitive to the changes associated with aging, disease, and therapy. Nonetheless, such measurements are often affected by the presence of degenerative changes that may occur after the age of 70 y that lead to artificially elevated bone mineral density values. Among researchers, measurements of the total femur is becoming the preferred "gold standard" method for bone density measurements (Kanis and Gider, 2000).

Care must be taken when positioning the subject for the scan to ensure that precise and accurate data are obtained. Under some circumstances, it may be appropriate to make a whole-body scan. This is quick, taking from 3 min to 35 min, depending on the instrument used and the age of the subject, and requires very little cooperation from the subject. As a result, scans can be readily performed on young children, the elderly, and even persons who are sick, although pregnant women should be excluded.

Numerous DXA validation studies have been performed, although few have used analyses of human cadavers (Heymsfield et al., 1989; Svendsen et al., 1993; Ellis et al., 1994; Lunt et al., 1997). In general, the accuracy of DXA scanning is limited by the variable composition of soft tissue, as noted in Section 14.11 (Roubenoff et al., 1993). The attenuation coefficient of fat differs from that of lean tissue because of the higher hydrogen content of the fat. In a cadaver study, Svendsen et al. (1995) examined the impact of soft tissue on in vivo accuracy of bone mineral measurements in the spine, hip, and forearm. Reported results for the root mean square accuracy errors were 3% for forearm, 5% for spine, and 6% for femoral neck and total hip bone mineral density. Good agreement between DXA-derived values for bone mineral content (and lean tissue mass and fat mass) and those from a multicompartment model based on neutron activation analysis have also been reported (Heymsfield et al., 1991).

Strong correlations ($r = 0.94$; $p < 0.001$) have been reported between bone mineral content estimated by DXA and total body calcium determined by neutron activation analysis in healthy nonobese adults (Heymsfield et al., 1989). Nevertheless, in this study, as well as others (Pierson et al., 1995; Ellis et al., 1996), substantial differences in the slope of the regression equations have been noted. Such differences reflect discrepancies in the methods used for calibrating DXA.

Dual-energy x-ray absorptiometry is now the dominant method for measuring bone loss for clinical diagnosis of osteopenia and osteoporosis (Section 23.1) (Lasky, 1996). It is also used to measure changes in bone mineral density in intervention studies (Dawson-Huges et al., 1990; Riggs et al., 1998). Care must be taken to ensure that both the length of the intervention and the size of the study population are sufficient to allow the detection of small changes in bone mineral density. In the 4-y randomized, double-blind calcium supplementation trial in 236 normal postmenopausal women, reported earlier (Table 23.3), bone mineral density of the lumbar spine, proximal femur, and total body bone mineral (TBBM) content were measured by DXA every six months (Riggs et al. 1998). A significant small decrease in bone loss in the calcium-supplemented women was reported, with differences for the median total body bone mass of 0.9% ($p = 0.017$) at year 4 for the treatment compared to the placebo group. Larger decreases in bone loss have been observed after treatment with estrogen, calcitonin, or biphosphates.

Care must be taken when comparing measurements using DXA based on different instruments and technologies. Systematic differences arising from methodological factors must be distinguished from those associated with biological variation. The former may include differences in methods used to calibrate the instrument. Major sources of biological variation are body thickness, variation in fat distribution, and variation in the fat content of the bone marrow. Of these, DXA is especially sensitive to discrepancies in body thickness, which can lead to systematic differences in the bone mineral estimates on thin and obese subjects. The other sources of biological variation result in small errors, which can generally be corrected in the calculations (Mazess et al., 1990; Going et al., 1993).

The International Committee for Standards in Bone Measurements (ICSBM) have defined criteria for bone mineral density measurements in an effort to ensure consistency in the diagnosis of osteoporosis across centers (Hanson, 1997). The ICSBM recommends the use of the total femur as the region of interest instead of the femoral neck site, together with the reference range for hip bone mineral density derived from the NHANES III survey (Looker et al., 1998).

Unfortunately, DXA scanners from the different manufacturers have yet to be cross-validated with a standard phantom, so it is still difficult to compare the data generated across different machines (Roubenoff et al., 1993).

23.1.9 Computerized tomography

Computerized tomography (CT) can be used to measure bone mass of both the appendicular and axial skeleton (Section 14.9), but the method is not feasible for population studies. The equipment is not portable, and the radiation dose required per slice for imaging is relatively high (50–500 µSv), although it can be reduced if scans are limited to regions of specific interest. The cost of the equipment is high.

The advantage of computerized tomography is that a true three-dimensional (i.e., volumetric) bone density can be obtained, so results can be expressed in g/cm^3 rather than the two-dimensional areal density measured by DXA. Bone can also be identified as cortical or trabecular in nature on the basis of bone density measurements. This is an advantage because some forms of osteoporosis are predominantly trabecular in character.

Both single-energy and dual-energy scanning are possible with more modern equipment. Dual-energy scanning is preferred be-

cause it allows the variable composition of bone marrow to be taken into account. However, although it improves the accuracy, the radiation dose is higher, and the precision is poorer.

23.1.10 Quantitative ultrasound

Quantitative ultrasound is used increasingly for measurements of the bone density of the peripheral skeleton. A wide variety of equipment is now available to measure the attenuation of a sonographic pulse as it passes through bone and is scattered and absorbed by the trabeculae. The heel is the most frequently used measurement site because it encompasses a large volume of trabecular bone between relatively flat faces and is readily accessible for transmission measurements.

A major advantage of quantitative ultrasound devices is that they do not use ionizing radiation. In addition, the equipment is relatively inexpensive, and portable systems are available. Experience suggests that the equipment is useful in predicting hip-fracture risk in elderly patients (i.e., $> 70\,\mathrm{y}$) (Hans et al., 1996; Pluijm et al., 1999). In patients with osteoporosis, for example, the broadband ultrasonic attenuation (BUA), expressed in dB/MHz, is reduced because there are fewer trabeculae to attenuate the signal. Whether ultrasound measurements can also be used to predict fracture risk in younger patients is uncertain. Because the precision is poor relative to DXA, however, the equipment is unsuitable for monitoring the response to treatment.

23.1.11 Neutron activation

In contrast to the scanning methods described above, neutron activation in vivo measures the calcium content directly and is generally regarded as the "gold standard" method for total body calcium. Of total body calcium, 99% is in the skeleton, as noted earlier, and calcium is a relatively constant fraction (38%–39%) of bone mineral weight. Therefore, measurement of total body calcium can provide an estimate of total body bone mineral content, except in cases where extra-osseous deposits of calcium occur.

Neutron activation is based on the conversion of a proportion of ^{48}Ca in the body to ^{49}Ca by exposing the body of the patient to a low neutron flux for a few minutes in a neutron irradiation unit. A radioactive isotope is normally used as the neutron source — often ^{238}PuBe. The patient is then transferred to a whole-body counter where the gamma rays emitted by the ^{49}Ca are counted using an array of sodium iodide detectors. The gamma ray count is proportional to the mass of total body calcium; further details are given in Section 14.5.2.

The radiation exposure using this method varies from 2.5 to 25 mSv, depending on the neutron source. This range is considerably higher than photon absorptiometry and limits the general applicability of the method. Consequently, it is mainly used as a calibration tool for other techniques. The reported accuracy and precision is from 1% to 2%, suggesting that the method could be used to study longitudinal changes (Cohn et al., 1974).

Harrison et al. (1979) have developed a calcium bone index (CaBI) in which total body calcium content is normalized for body size. This index may be used to distinguish between normal (with CaBI 1.0 ± 0.12) and osteoporotic (0.69 ± 0.10) subjects. Mild osteoporosis in patients who have not yet experienced any vertebral fractures can be detected. Ma et al. (2000) have emphasized the problems of measuring total body calcium by neutron activation in obese subjects. The neutron attenuation through fat necessitates additional corrections or a special calibration when determining total body calcium using neutron activation in subjects with a BMI > 30.

23.2 Phosphorus

Phosphorus is the second most abundant mineral in the body and accounts for 6.5–11 g/kg body weight in adults. About 85% of phosphorus is present in the bones as calcium phosphate [$Ca_3(PO_4)_2$] and hydroxyapatite [$Ca_{10}(PO_4)_6(OH)_2$]. The rest is present in the cells and extracellular fluids as inorganic phosphate and in combination with nucleic acids and nucleotides, phosphorylated sugars, and phospholipids.

Functions of phosphorus

Phosphorus is an essential factor in all the energy-producing reactions of the cells. Other functional roles include the action of phosphorus in many physiological buffer systems and the activation of many catalytic proteins by phosphorylation.

Absorption and metabolism

About 55%–70% of all dietary phosphorus is absorbed by healthy adults consuming a typical mixed diet. Unlike calcium, there is no evidence that absorption of phosphorus varies with dietary intake. Most phosphorus in the diet is absorbed by a passive, concentration-dependent process, although a small portion is absorbed by active transport facilitated by 1,25-dihydroxyvitamin D (Chen et al., 1974). The mechanisms are not well understood.

The kidney has the major role in regulating phosphorus balance. More than 80% of absorbed phosphorus is excreted by the kidney, so that in healthy adults urinary phosphorus reflects the amount of absorbed dietary phosphorus. When dietary intakes of phosphorus are low, renal excretion of phosphorus is reduced by a mechanism that is not well established. The resultant hypophosphatemia (i.e., low serum phosphorus concentrations) is accompanied by increased production of the active metabolite of vitamin D (1,25-dihydroxyvitamin D) in the kidney, increased absorption of calcium, mild hypercalcemia (i.e., high serum calcium levels), and a decrease in parathyroid secretion and hypophosphaturia. The effect of diets high in phosphorus and low in calcium on hypocalcemia and secondary hyperthyroidism, and thus bone health is hotly debated (Whybro et al.,1998; Heaney, 2000; Anderson and Garner, 2001; Sax, 2001).

Deficiency of phosphorus in humans

Dietary deficiency of phosphorus is rare, as phosphorus intakes generally exceed requirements. Moreover, in the absence of disease, parathyroid and renal mechanisms function to conserve body phosphorus.

Growing low birth-weight preterm infants fed human milk are susceptible to suboptimal phosphorus status: the phosphate content of human milk is inadequate for their growth requirements. These infants may develop skeletal abnormalities, even in the presence of adequate vitamin D intakes (Pettifor, 1991). This rickets-like metabolic bone disease is characterized by hypophosphataemia, raised serum alkaline phosphatase levels, low urinary phosphorus excretion, and a reduction in calcium retention, as indicated by hypercalciuria. Supplementation with phosphate is said to reverse this disorder (Pettifor, 1991).

There is also some evidence that marginal phosphorus intakes in children in Northeast Thailand are associated with the incidence of bladder stones. Certainly, in infants and children living in areas where bladder stones are endemic, urinary excretion of phosphorus is low, but calcium is high and crystalluria is common (Valyesevi and Dhanamitta, 1967). Moreover, these features were reversed by phosphate supplementation (Valyesevi et al., 1967).

The absorption of dietary phosphorus is reduced by excessive intakes of aluminium, calcium, and strontium, all cations that form insoluble phosphates in the intestine. As a result, suboptimal phosphorus status may arise in persons taking prolonged and excessive intakes of the antacids aluminium hydroxide or aluminum carbonate (Lotz et al., 1968).

Phosphorus depletion may also occur in patients receiving long-term total parenteral nutrition unsupplemented with phosphorus, and in patients with diabetic keto-acidosis treated with insulin with no supplemental phosphate.

Depletion of phosphorus generates low serum phosphorus concentrations (i.e., hypophosphatemia). It is accompanied by a reduction in urinary phosphorus excretion and an increase in urinary excretion of calcium, magnesium, and potassium. As a result, phosphorus deficiency can result in a wide variety of clinical complications. These include impairment of oxygen delivery, failure of muscle contractility, severe muscle weakness, anorexia, bone pain, and cardiac and respiratory failure. All of the increased urinary calcium and most of the urinary magnesium are derived from the bone. Hence, in phosphorus deficiency, the skeleton tends to exhibit either rickets in children or osteomalacia in adults.

Food sources and dietary intakes

Protein-rich foods, such as meat, poultry, fish, eggs, milk, and milk products, are major sources of phosphorus in typical mixed diets of industrialized countries. In the 1995 survey in Australia, for example, milk and milk products provided nearly 25% of total dietary phosphorus for women aged 19 y and older, followed by meat and meat products (18%) (McLennan and Podger, 1998).

Whole grain cereals, legumes, and nuts are also good sources of phosphorus, although its bioavailability in these foods may be poor. Much of the phosphorus in cereals is in the form of phytic acid (inositol hexaphosphate), which is not absorbed because the intestinal mucosa does not secrete a phytase enzyme, essential for the hydrolysis of phytic acid. During fermentation, as may occur when making leavened bread with yeast, some phosphorus is liberated from the phytate moiety by phytase-induced hydrolysis of phytate (Gibson and Hotz, 2001).

Additional sources of phosphorus in the diet in recent years include polyphosphates added during the manufacture of foods such as frozen poultry, bacon, processed cheese, instant soups, deserts, and sauces. Carbonated cola beverages are also an important source of phosphorus (as phosphoric acid) for some age groups (e.g., adolescents) (Wyshak, 2000).

Patients with chronic renal failure are prescribed diets with low levels of phosphorus (800–1000 mg/d), although compliance to such diets is difficult. Consumption of high-protein foods and processed foods such as snacks and fast foods should be avoided.

Effect of high intakes of phosphorus

High phosphorus intakes may be associated with the consumption of commercially available foods containing phosphate additives (Calvo and Park, 1996). Animal studies have indicated that excessive dietary phosphorus in relation to calcium causes secondary hyperparathyroidism and bone loss (Calvo, 1994).

Some evidence suggests that high-phosphorus/low-calcium diets in humans also produce a significant sustained increase in serum parathyroid concentrations (Calvo et al.,1990; Whybro et al., 1998). Whether these higher parathyroid hormone levels cause increased bone resorption and accelerated bone loss is not clear. Long-term studies in growing children or the elderly are needed to establish whether such adverse skeletal effects occur (Sax, 2001).

The U.S. Food and Nutrition Board has set the Tolerable Upper Intake Level for phosphorus as 3.0 g/d for children 1–8 y, and 3.5, and 4.0 g/d for adults 19–70 y and pregnant and lactating women (IOM, 1997).

Indices of phosphorus status

Currently there is no ideal measure of phosphorus status. Serum phosphorus is used most frequently but is not very satisfactory. It is discussed below. New approaches need to be developed.

23.2.1 Serum phosphorus

Unlike calcium, only 10% of the circulating inorganic phosphorus is bound to protein in the serum. The rest is largely present as inorganic phosphates, of which 80% occurs as the divalent anion HPO_4^{2-}, and 20% is the monovalent anion, $H_2PO_4^-$; only very small amounts of trivalent phosphate are present in the serum (Harrison, 1984). Concentrations of phosphorus in serum are commonly termed "inorganic phosphate" (P_i) because the analytical methods measure only the inorganic fraction.

Serum phosphorus concentrations tend to fall within a narrow range (0.8–1.6 mmol/L). They are regulated largely by the tubular reabsorptive capacity of the kidney under the influence of the parathyroid hormone, growth hormone, and other factors that stimulate change in renal phosphorus clearance.

Factors affecting serum phosphorus

Dietary phosphorus levels usually correlate with serum phosphorus levels when intakes are low (< 20 mmol/d or < 619 mg/d). At higher intakes, serum concentrations only weakly reflect variations in habitual intake, as shown in Figure 23.2.

Age affects serum phosphorus levels. The high serum phosphorus levels of early infancy can be attributed to lower glomerular filtration rates. These high values decline quickly during infancy and then more gradually during childhood, but concentrations are still about 50% higher than values for adults. Such higher serum phosphorus values are probably necessary for the adequate

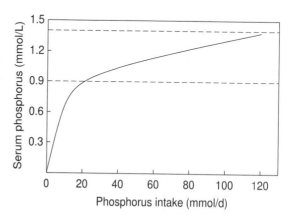

Figure 23.2: Schematic diagram showing the equilibrium relationship between phosphorus intake and serum phosphorus concentrations. From Heany (1997), with permission.

mineralization of the growing skeleton. Normal adult values are reached by about the third decade. However, the further decline in serum phosphorus that occurs in early adulthood (Figure 23.3) is not well understood but is probably a hormone-mediated effect.

Gender-related changes in the concentrations of serum phosphorus are marked. In women, serum phosphorus values decline progressively between 20 and 35 y, increasing after 40 y. In males, values decline progressively with age after the third decade.

Lactation is often associated with above-normal serum phosphorus concentrations, as shown in Figure 23.4. Such increases in serum phosphorus are independent of the dietary intake. They are attributed to a decrease in serum parathyroid hormone, which, in turn, leads to high serum ionized phosphorus. They occur at a time when there is an increase in bone resorption and, hence, mobilization of phosphorus from bone and decreased urinary excretion of phosphorus (Lopez et al., 1996). In contrast, during pregnancy, serum phosphorus concentrations are within the normal range (Cross et al., 1995).

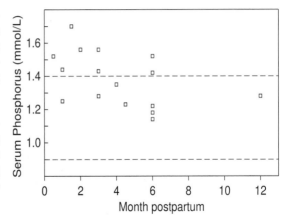

Figure 23.4: Serum phosphorus concentrations (mmol/L) in lactating women in relation to the normal range for nonlactating women (shown by dashed lines). Data from Chan et al. (1982); Bryne et al. (1987); Kent et al. (1990); Specker et al. (1991); Cross et al., (1995); Dobnig et al. (1995); Kalkwarf et al. (1996); Lopez et al. (1996).

Diurnal variation in serum phosphorus concentrations occur. There is a minor peak in the afternoon and a major peak just after midnight (Portale et al., 1987). This diurnal rhythm probably results in part from diurnal changes in plasma cortisol. The peak to trough concentrations may change the 24-h mean level by 30%.

Seasonal variations in serum phosphorus concentrations may occur. In children, levels tend to rise during the summer and decline in the winter, reflecting the seasonal changes in serum 25-0H-D concentrations, which, in turn, parallel seasonal changes in solar radiation (see Section 18.2.1).

Malabsorption syndromes such as short bowel syndrome, Crohn's disease, and celiac disease may reduce serum phosphorus concentrations. Hyperparathyroidism also results in low serum phosphorus values.

Renal tubular function abnormalities may result in hypophosphatemia; some of these conditions are listed in Table 23.7. The hypophosphatemia arises from excessive urinary losses of phosphorus.

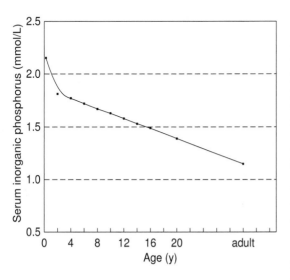

Figure 23.3: Diagram showing the decline in serum phosphorus with age during childhood.

Fanconi syndrome
  Cystinosis, tyrosinosis, heavy metal poisoning, nephrotoxic organic compounds, multiple myeloma
Renal tubular acidosis
Genetic primary hypophosphatemia
Acquired primary hypophosphatemia
  Connective tissue tumors

Table 23.7: Hypophosphatemia secondary to disorders of renal tubule reabsorption of phosphate. From Harrison, (1984). Phosphorus. In: Present Knowledge in Nutrition. 5th ed. © The Nutrition Foundation Inc., with permission.

Insulin administration to diabetic patients with ketosis can result in a large shift of phosphorus from extracellular to intracellular sites and result in frank hypophosphatemia, as noted earlier.

Rickets is associated with low serum phosphorus levels, possibly because the active vitamin D metabolite, 1,25-dihydroxyvitamin D, has an essential role in the efficacy of phosphorus absorption.

Genetic diseases, such as primary hypophosphatemia and hereditary hypophosphatemic rickets with hypercalciuria, involve impaired renal tubular reabsorption of filtered phosphorus (Rasmussen and Anast, 1983), that is attributed to defects in the proximal tubular Na-P_i transporters (Tenenhouse, 1997).

Other factors may significantly affect serum phosphorus levels. Hypophosphatemia may arise from rapid shifts of extracellular phosphorus into the intracellular compartment, markedly reduced intestinal absorption, increased intestinal losses, or increased losses of phosphorus in the urine. For example, nutritional repletion of phosphorus-depleted patients may increase intracellular phosphorus demand and can cause rapid shifts of extracellular phosphorus to intracellular sites.

Interpretive criteria

The U.S. Food and Nutrition Board defined the low end of the normal adult range for serum phosphorus as 0.8–0.9 mmol/L (IOM, 1997). Chronic moderate hypophosphatemia often results in rickets in children or osteomalacia in adults. Severe hypophosphatemia (serum phosphorus levels < 0.3–0.5 mmol/L) can cause muscle weakness, skeletal deformities, and growth retardation in children. Anorexia, increased susceptibility to infection, ataxia, and confusion have also been reported (Lotz et al., 1968). Concentrations < 0.3 mmol/L are often associated with red blood cell fragility and hemolysis (Klock et al., 1974). Serum alkaline phosphatase activity is generally elevated in cases of hypophosphataemia.

Serum phosphorus concentrations indicative of hyperphosphatemia are >1.5 mmol/L in adults and >2.0 mmol/L in children.

Measurement of serum phosphorus

Serum phosphorus is generally determined by a modification of the colorimetric molybdenum blue method of Fiske and Subbarow (1925). Automated procedures are available. The analytical CV for this method ranges between 2.0% and 6.1%. The within-subject CV for serum phosphorus ranges from 6.0% to 10.0% (Gallagher et al., 1989).

Only serum or heparinized plasma is suitable for this colorimetric procedure because EDTA and other anticoagulants interfere with the color reaction. Nonhemolyzed samples must be used for serum or plasma phosphorus analysis: erythrocytes contain about 17 times more phosphorus than plasma (Gallagher et al., 1989). Serum or plasma can be stored frozen for several months before analysis for phosphorus

23.3 Magnesium

The adult human body contains about 24 g of magnesium, of which approximately 55% is in the skeleton. The remainder is equally distributed between muscle and nonmuscular soft tissues (Table 23.1). One-third of skeletal magnesium resides on the surface of bone and is exchangeable. It is this fraction that may serve as a reservoir for maintaining normal extra-cellular magnesium concentrations (Elin, 1987a). The latter accounts for about 1% of the total body magnesium.

Functions of magnesium

Magnesium is the second most abundant cation in the intracellular fluid. It acts as a metal activator or cofactor in more than 300 enzyme systems, especially those involving energy metabolism, specifically phosphate-transfer reactions involving adenosine triphosphate (ATP) and nucleotide triphosphates (Rude, 1998).

Magnesium may also be required for the transport of other ions such as potassium and calcium and is involved in protein synthesis, specifically in the formation of cyclic adenosine monophosphate. Magnesium acts in the neuromuscular system by stabilizing nerve axons, as well as by influencing the release of neurotransmitters at myoneural junctions (Rude, 1998). Hence, in magnesium deficiency, abnormal neuromuscular function is probably the result of neuromuscular hyperexcitability. For further details see Shils (1994).

Absorption and metabolism

Magnesium homeostasis depends on the balance between intestinal absorption and renal excretion. Intestinal absorption of magnesium occurs along the entire intestinal tract, with maximal absorption in the distal jejunum and ileum (Kayne and Lee, 1993). Little is known about the factors controlling intestinal absorption of magnesium; vitamin D metabolites and parathyroid hormone have been implicated (Fine et al., 1991).

At low dietary intakes, fractional absorption of magnesium is increased by an active magnesium-transport system in the intestine (Kayne and Lee, 1993; Konrad et al., 2004). At high dietary intakes, absorption of magnesium continues at a lower fractional absorption rate by a passive cellular transport process (Fine et al., 1991).

Intestinal absorption may also be affected by other dietary components. For example, high intakes of dietary fiber, phytate, and phosphate bind magnesium and reduce magnesium absorption. Intakes of protein < 30 g/d may also reduce magnesium absorption (Hunt and Schofield, 1969). In contrast, some dietary components can enhance magnesium absorption. They include lactose and probably other carbohydrates that stimulate bacterial fermentation in the intestine (Schaafsma, 1997). Whether non-nutritional factors such as age, sex, pregnancy, and lactation affect magnesium absorption is unknown.

The kidney plays a role in magnesium homeostasis that is even more important than that of intestinal absorption. At low intakes tubular reabsorption increases markedly so that plasma magnesium concentration is maintained. Tubular reabsorption is regulated mainly by the plasma magnesium concentration; there is no tubular secretion of magnesium. Certain dietary factors also affect renal magnesium excretion. Diets high in sodium, calcium, and protein, and both caffeine and alcohol, all enhance magnesium excretion (Schaafsma, 1997).

Magnesium deficiency in humans

Dietary magnesium deficiency in humans is not very common. Nevertheless, studies have shown that the elderly may be at risk for inadequate intakes of magnesium, perhaps because of poor appetite or poor food choices (Mountokalakis, 1987). Decreases in magnesium absorption with age combined with increases in urinary magnesium may be exacerbating factors (Lowik et al., 1993).

Magnesium deficiency, especially when it is moderate to severe, generally develops in association with predisposing and complicating disease states. These disease states may result in low intakes of magnesium, or impaired intestinal or renal absorption, or both, leading to increased losses; some examples are shown in Box 23.1.

The signs and symptoms characterizing magnesium deficiency in humans may in-

Conditions associated with inadequate intakes of magnesium

> Protein-energy malnutrition (usually with infection)
> Nursing multiple infants
> Prolonged infusion or ingestion of nutrient solutions or diets low in magnesium
> Alcoholism

Disorders associated with reductions in magnesium absorption

> Prolonged nasogastric suction or periods of vomiting
> Acute and chronic diarrhea
> Malabsorption syndromes
> > Inflammatory bowel disease
> > Gluten enteropathy; sprue
> > Crohn's disease; ulcerative colitis
> > Whipple's disease; celiac disease
> > Gastrointestinal infections
> Extensive bowel resection
> Intestinal and biliary fistulae
> Acute hemorrhagic pancreatitis
> Intestinal hypomagnesemia

Conditions in which reabsorption of magnesium in the kidney is reduced

> Chronic parenteral fluid therapy
> Osmotic diuresis involving glucose, mannitol, or urea
> Hypercalcemia
> Drugs, including amphotericin B, viomycin, capreomycin, pentamidine, and cisplatin
> Metabolic acidosis (starvation, alcoholism, ketoacidosis)
> Various renal diseases, including interstitial nephritis, glomerulonephritis, renal tubular acidosis

Genetic diseases resulting in hypomagnesemia

> Bartter syndrome
> Gitelman syndrome
> Hypomagnesemia with secondary hypocalcemia
> Primary hypomagnesemia with hypercaliuria
> Renal hypomagnesemia 2

Box 23.1: Conditions associated with magnesium depletion. Compiled from Rude (1998), Shils (1994), Fleet and Cashman (2001).

clude neuromuscular, gastrointestinal, and personality changes. The former include positive Trousseau's and Chvostek's signs, spontaneous generalized muscle spasm, muscle fasciculations, tremor, and anorexia, nausea, and vomiting (Shils, 1964). Personality changes include apathy, depression, nervousness, delirium, hallucinations, and even psychosis (Rude, 1998). Convulsions occur more frequently in acute magnesium deficiency in infants than in adults. Some of these signs and symptoms have been induced in experimental studies of magnesium deficiency in human volunteers (Shils, 1964), and all have been reversed with magnesium supplementation.

The results of some experimental depletion studies have emphasized the important interrelationships between magnesium and other cations, including potassium, calcium, and sodium, as well as with vitamin D metabolism. For example, magnesium depletion affects potassium homeostasis and results in hypokalemia. Indeed, hypokalemia may be the cause of the electrocardiographic changes that have been reported in magnesium depletion. Hypocalcemia is also prominent in magnesium deficiency and may contribute to the neurological signs. Magnesium may also have a role in the metabolism or action of vitamin D (Medalle and Waterhouse, 1973).

Evidence is emerging that a habitually low intake of magnesium may be an etiological factor in hypertension and in some cardiovascular diseases. These include coronary artery disease, cardiac arrhythmias, heart disease, and myocardial infarction (Quamme, 1993; Antman, 1996). Certainly, intracellular Mg^{2+} is known to modulate the vasoconstrictive effects of intracellular Ca^{2+} in vascular smooth muscle cells. Intracellular Mg^{2+} also has a role in the myocardial vasoconstriction/vasorelaxation cycle, but the precise mechanism is not fully understood.

There have been several investigations of the effects of magnesium supplementation on markers of bone formation, rate of bone loss, and bone mass. Results are conflicting; further studies are needed into the role of magnesium in bone metabolism and osteoporosis (Stendig-Lindberg et al., 1993; Sojka and Weaver, 1995).

Food sources and dietary intakes

Magnesium is widely distributed in both plant and animal foodstuffs, especially in nuts, green vegetables, soybeans, chocolate, and whole grain cereals. Hard drinking water may also be an important source of dietary magnesium (Gibson et al., 1987). In contrast to calcium, dairy products tend to be low in magnesium. In the U.S. 1989 Total Diet Study, 45% of dietary magnesium was contributed by vegetables, fruits, grains, and nuts and about 29% from milk, meat, and eggs (Pennington and Young, 1991). Intakes of magnesium in the United States have tended to decrease with the increased consumption of refined and processed foods. Net absorption of dietary magnesium in a typical mixed diet is about 50%.

Effects of high intakes of magnesium

Magnesium toxicity, arising from excessive intake of oral $MgSO_4$, generally occurs only when kidney function is impaired (Venugopal and Luckey, 1978). Osmotic diarrhea and dehydration may result. In cases of acute magnesium toxicity via the parenteral route, nausea, depression, and paralysis may occur.

Magnesium toxicity arising from excessive dietary magnesium intakes is unlikely. The Tolerable Upper Intake Level for magnesium set by the U.S. Food and Nutrition Board (IOM, 1997) is 350 mg/d of supplemental magnesium for individuals >8 y and for pregnant and lactating women. Lower levels have been set for infants and children ⩽ 8 y.

Indices of magnesium status

Assessment of the magnesium status of an individual is difficult because of uncertainty about which tissue pool is in equilibrium with the total body magnesium (Elin, 1987a). Table 23.8 shows the distribution of magnesium among the body compartments. The equilibrium among tissue pools of magnesium is only reestablished slowly.

The biological half-life for magnesium in the body ranges from 41 to 181 d, and thus the different individual tissue pools become depleted in magnesium over varying time periods. For example, in magnesium deficiency, concentrations in serum decrease rapidly, followed by a slower decline in erythrocytes. Within a few days, urinary and fecal magnesium levels fall to very low levels (Shils, 1994). The magnesium content of individual tissue pools are also affected by many nonnutritional factors. As a result, to define magnesium status, a combination of laboratory tests, in conjunction with a clinical assessment, is recommended. At present, no physiological functional tests of magnesium status exist, so it is difficult to relate magnesium status to health outcomes.

Tissue	Body mass (kg wet wt.)	Mg conc. (mmol/kg wet wt.)	Mg content (mmol)
Serum	3.0	0.8	2.6
Erythrocytes	2.0	2.5	5.0
Soft tissues	22.7	8.5	193.0
Muscle	30.0	9.0	270.0
Bone	12.3	43.2	530.1

Table 23.8: Distribution of magnesium in adult humans. From Quamme, Clinics in Laboratory Medicine 13: 209–223, 1993.

23.3.1 Serum magnesium

Serum magnesium concentration is the most frequently used measure of magnesium status, even though only about 1% of total body magnesium exists in the serum. Of this, 55% is in the free ionized Mg^{2+} form, 13% is complexed, and 32% is bound nonspecifically to albumins and 8% to globulins (Kroll and Elin, 1985).

Experimental magnesium depletion in humans is consistently associated with an early and progressive fall in serum magnesium. Fatemi et al. (1991) demonstrated a significant decline in serum magnesium levels from 0.80 mmol/L at the baseline to 0.61 mmol/L ($p < 0.001$) after 3 wk on a low-magnesium diet. This decline was accompanied by a significant increase in magnesium retention (Figure 23.5) and a fall in erythrocyte-ionized Mg^{2+} levels.

Nevertheless, in clinical studies involving patients with diabetes mellitus, alcoholism, and malabsorption syndromes, the serum magnesium concentrations are often normal, despite low magnesium concentrations in erythrocytes, mononuclear cells, and muscle (Ryzen et al., 1986; Nadler et al., 1992; Abbott et al., 1994; Rude and Olerich, 1996). Further, in five cases of cardiac arrhythmias subsequently dispelled by parenteral administration of magnesium, serum magnesium concentrations were also normal (Cohen and Kitzes, 1983). Hence, a normal serum magnesium concentration does not preclude tissue magnesium deficiency. Conversely, low serum magnesium concentrations have been reported in patients with normal cellular magnesium and no clinical signs of deficiency (Ryzen et al., 1986). Consequently, use of serum magnesium as an indicator of body magnesium status is questionable.

Factors affecting serum magnesium

Age, gender, and race influence serum magnesium concentrations. In NHANES I, values for males declined from 1 to 18 y, after which levels remained fairly stable. In females, values decreased, and then increased after 24 y (Lowenstein and Stanton, 1986). Small sex differences were observed in adults aged 18–45 y; males had higher concentrations than females (Figure 23.6). Caucasians had consistently higher serum magnesium concentrations than comparably aged persons of African descent.

In the U.K. National Diet and Nutrition Survey of young people aged 4–18 y, boys had higher plasma magnesium concentrations than girls, which varied little with age. In the girls, plasma magnesium concentration was highest in the youngest age group (4–6 y) (Gregory et al., 2000).

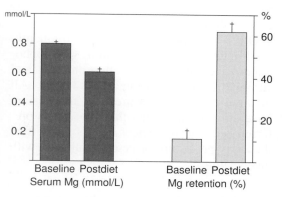

Figure 23.5: Mean ± SEM serum Mg (n = 26) and Mg retention (n = 16) before and after a 3-week low-Mg dietary trial on adults. Data from Fatemi et al., Journal of Clinical Endocrinology and Metabolism 73: 1067–1072, 1991.

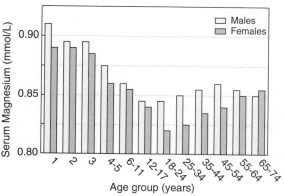

Figure 23.6: Variations in serum magnesium concentrations with age and sex, United States, 1971–1974. Data from Lowenstein and Stanton, Journal of the American College of Nutrition 5: 399–414, 1986.

Pregnancy results in lower serum magnesium concentrations following hemodilution (Chesley, 1972).

Diurnal variation in serum magnesium concentrations occurs: values are slightly lower in the morning than in the evening. The observed trends are probably associated with food intake and physical activity level, although some changes in the function of the parathyroid gland may also play a part.

Strenuous exercise reduces serum magnesium concentrations. This arises from a shift of magnesium from the plasma into the red blood cells and an increase in the urinary excretion of magnesium, together with loss of magnesium in sweat and cellular exfoliation (Lukaski, 2000).

Hemolysis affects serum magnesium values because the magnesium concentration of the erythrocytes is much higher than for serum.

Serum albumin concentrations are related to serum magnesium in a linear fashion when they are high or low, but not when they are within the normal range (Kroll and Elin, 1985). Hence, the presence of hypo- or hyperalbuminemia will confound the interpretation of serum magnesium concentrations.

Drugs such as diuretics and antibiotics may decrease serum magnesium levels, but the magnesium-rich drugs such as antacids or cathartics result in elevated serum magnesium concentrations.

Disease states such as renal failure have been associated with elevated serum magnesium concentrations (Elin, 1991). In contrast, in postmenopausal women with osteoporosis, a significant reduction in serum magnesium concentrations has been reported (Stendig-Lindberg et al., 1993).

Interpretive criteria

The mean serum magnesium concentration in adults is approximately 0.85 mmol/L, with a reference interval of 0.7–1.0 mmol/L (Yang et al., 1990). Hypomagnesemia is usually defined as a serum magnesium concentration < 0.75 mmol/L (Elin, 1987a).

Serum magnesium levels were measured in NHANES I, but not in NHANES II or NHANES III. Concentrations in nonfasting blood samples of U.S. adults 18–74 y ranged from 0.75 to 0.95 mmol/L. Tables of mean and selected percentiles by race, age, and sex for NHANES I are given in Lowenstein and Stanton (1986).

Plasma magnesium was also measured in the U.K. National Diet and Nutrition Survey of young people aged 4–18 y (Gregory et al., 2000). Data on the mean, median, and lower and upper 2.5th percentiles by age and sex are presented. No data on plasma magnesium are available for the surveys of young children (Gregory et al., 1995) or U.K. adults (Gregory et al., 1990; Finch et al., 1998).

Measurement of serum magnesium

Serum magnesium can be readily measured using atomic absorption spectrophotometry (AAS) or a colorimetric method that uses either calmagite or methylthymol blue as the chromophore. Results of the colorimetric assay are comparable to those obtained using AAS. Analytical CVs for serum magnesium using AAS range from 2.0% to 7.6%, whereas the within-subject coefficient of variation ranges from 3.8% to 6.9% (Gallagher et al., 1989).

Other analytical methods less frequently used include atomic emission spectrophotometry, compleximetry, fluorometry, and chromatography (Deuster et al., 1987). All of these methods measure total magnesium in serum. Serum, rather than plasma, is preferred because the anticoagulants may affect the assay procedure or be contaminated with magnesium.

23.3.2 Ionized magnesium in serum and erythrocytes

Only the free or ionized form of magnesium is physiologically active, participates in metabolic interactions, activates biochemical processes, and is transported across the cell membranes. Consequently, efforts have been made to utilize recently developed methods for ionized magnesium in both the serum and erythrocytes.

Handwerker et al.(1996) documented small but significant decreases in ionized serum magnesium (and total) concentrations during pregnancy (Figure 23.7), which were not correlated with changes in albumin or total protein in the serum. Hence, the decline does not result from hemodilution. Such measurements may be of clinical significance because magnesium deficiency during pregnancy may have a role in pregnancy-induced hypertension, intrauterine growth retardation, and preterm delivery (Conradt et al., 1985). Nevertheless, additional studies are needed to confirm these findings and to establish the validity of plasma-ionized magnesium as a measure of magnesium status.

Ryzen et al. (1989) measured ionized magnesium in erythrocytes and serum magnesium in 20 normal subjects and 22 hypomagnesemic patients. The mean erythrocyte ionized magnesium concentration was significantly lower in the hypomagnesemic patients compared with the value for the normal subjects (Table 23.9). In addition, there was a signifi-

	Normal Subjects ($n = 20$)	Hypomagnesemic Subjects ($n = 22$)
Serum Mg (mmol/L)	0.90 ± 0.016	0.62 ± 0.016
RBC Mg^{2+} (μM)	178 ± 6.3	146 ± 7.1

Table 23.9: Serum Mg and erythrocyte ionized Mg concentrations in 20 normal subjects and 22 hypomagnesemic subjects (serum Mg < 0.74 mmol/L). Data from Ryzen et al., Journal of the American College of Nutrition 8: 580–587, 1989.

cant positive correlation between erythrocyte ionized magnesium and serum magnesium in these subjects (Figure 23.8). Nevertheless, the existence of some overlap of erythrocyte ionized magnesium values within the normal range for some of the hypomagnesemic patients suggests that erythrocyte ionized magnesium may not always reflect the status of magnesium.

Measurement of ionized magnesium

Serum ionized magnesium can be measured using commercial ion-specific electrodes, as described for serum ionized calcium (Section 23.1.2). Erythrocyte ionized magnesium

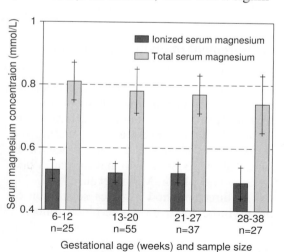

Figure 23.7: Variations in pregnancy in ionized and total serum magnesium concentrations with gestational age. Data from Handwerker et al., Journal of the American College of Nutrition 15: 36–43, 1996.

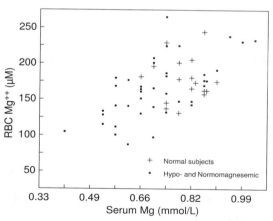

Figure 23.8: Correlation of serum magnesium (Mg) and erythrocyte (RBC) ionized Mg concentrations in normal, hypo-, and normomagnesemic subjects. For all subjects $r = 0.54$, $p < 0.001$. Data from Ryzen et al., Journal of the American College of Nutrition 8: 580–587, 1989.

is usually measured with metallochromic and fluorescent indicators (London, 1991). Of these, a fluorescent dye, Furaptra (mag-fura-2), can be used to determine millimolar concentrations of ionized magnesium, provided the calcium concentration does not rise above 5 μM. The acetoxymethyl form of the fluorescent dye passes across the cell membrane and is used to load the indicator into the cells (Quamme, 1993).

Alternatively, nuclear magnetic resonance (NMR) spectroscopy can be used to measure ionized magnesium without damage to the erythrocyte (Ryzen et al. 1989; Fatemi et al., 1991; London, 1991).

More research is needed to establish if serum or erythrocyte ionized magnesium concentrations are useful for diagnosing magnesium depletion in clinical disorders.

23.3.3 Erythrocyte magnesium

Magnesium exists in erythrocytes in three forms: free, complexed, and protein-bound. Concentrations are about three times greater than in serum. Erythrocyte magnesium concentrations reflect chronic rather than acute magnesium status because of the long erythrocyte lifespan (120 d). Hence, decreases in erythrocyte magnesium concentrations are not observed until some weeks after the onset of a dietary deficiency.

In a study of nonobese elderly subjects ($n = 12$, 78 ± 2 y), erythrocyte magnesium levels were markedly lower than for young healthy control subjects aged 36 ± 0.4 y (1.86 vs. 2.18 mmol/L). Moreover, after 4 wk of supplementation with magnesium, there was an increase in both erythrocyte magnesium concentrations and insulin secretion and action in the elderly subjects, suggesting that the low erythrocyte magnesium concentrations were of physiological significance.

Nevertheless, erythrocyte magnesium concentrations do not correlate with concentrations in other tissue pools of magnesium such as mononuclear blood cells or muscle, limiting their usefulness for assessing magnesium status (Ryzen et al., 1986; Elin, 1987b). For example, in a boy with selective magnesium

malabsorption who was treated with oral supplements, erythrocyte magnesium did not accurately reflect magnesium status (Guillard et al., 1992).

Concentrations of magnesium in erythrocytes are dependent on the age of the cells; the magnesium content slowly declines as the erythrocytes age (Elin et al., 1980). Nevertheless, in most cases, the erythrocyte magnesium content is not seriously affected by the age distribution of cells in the erythrocyte pellet prepared for analysis (Deuster et al., 1987). Exceptions are conditions in which the survival time of erythrocytes is reduced, such as during chronic renal failure, thalassemia, and sickle cell anemia. In these diseases, erythrocyte magnesium concentrations may be higher because magnesium-rich immature erythrocytes predominate.

The erythrocyte magnesium content is also altered in a variety of different clinical conditions including hyperthyroidism (Rizek et al., 1965), and chronic lymphatic leukemia (Rosner and Gorfien, 1968) and in women with premenstrual tension (Abraham and Lubran, 1981; Sherwood et al., 1986). All of these conditions may confound the interpretation of erythrocyte magnesium concentrations. Normal values for erythrocyte magnesium based on AAS are said to be 2.3 ± 0.24 mmol/L packed cells (Millart et al., 1995).

Measurement of erythrocyte magnesium

Both indirect and direct methods are used for erythrocyte magnesium analysis (Deuster et al., 1987). The indirect methods involve measuring the magnesium concentration in whole blood and serum and calculating the content in erythrocytes by difference (Refsum et al., 1973; Abraham and Lubran, 1981; Lukaski et al., 1983; Millart et al., 1995).

The direct method involves separation of the erythrocytes from whole blood followed by acid digestion of the erythrocyte pellet, and then analysis. In both methods, magnesium concentrations are usually measured by flame AAS.

Deuster et al. (1987) concluded that the indirect procedure, using nitric acid to lyse the erythrocytes, is reproducible, accurate, and much less time-consuming than the direct method.

23.3.4 Magnesium in leukocytes and other cell types

Concentrations of magnesium in leukocytes and in specific cell types (e.g., mononuclear blood cells) have been investigated as measures of intracellular magnesium status. The magnesium content of human blood leukocytes is higher than that of the mononuclear cells (lymphocytes + monocytes), probably because leukocytes include neutrophils which have a higher magnesium content than mononuclear blood cells (Rosner and Lee, 1972; Ross et al., 1980).

In initial experimental studies of magnesium depletion in rats, changes in peripheral mononuclear blood cell magnesium concentrations reflected those in cardiac and skeletal muscle (Ryan and Ryan, 1979). Comparable results were subsequently reported in some human clinical studies. For example, significant correlations between magnesium concentrations in lymphocytes and muscle were reported in patients with type I diabetes (Sjøgren et al., 1986), and mild hypertension (Dyckner and Wester, 1985), although not in those with congestive heart failure (Dyckner and Wester, 1984). Instead, in the patients with congestive heart failure, mononuclear blood cell magnesium concentrations were positively correlated with magnesium balance. Congestive heart failure patients receive diuretics that increase urinary losses of magnesium (Ryan et al., 1981). Lymphocyte magnesium concentrations were also shown to reflect a marked deficit in magnesium in a patient with congenital hypomagnesemia (Guillard et al., 1992). As a result of these findings, some investigators have used magnesium concentrations in lymphocytes alone or in mononuclear blood cells to evaluate magnesium status in certain clinical conditions (Ryzen et al., 1986; Abraham et al., 1988).

Martin et al. (1993) have cautioned against the use of magnesium concentrations in either lymphocytes or mononuclear blood cells to evaluate magnesium status, especially for patients with illnesses that may change the size and protein content of the cells. Table 23.10 compares the serum and mononuclear blood cell magnesium concentrations in a group of elderly hospitalized subjects with a control group from the community (Martin et al., 1993). Note that the mononuclear blood cell magnesium concentrations for the ill patients, when expressed as $\mu mol/mg$ protein (see below), were significantly lower than those for the control subjects ($p < 0.001$). There was no correlation, however, between the magnesium concentrations in the mononuclear blood cells, when they are expressed as $\mu mol/mg$ protein and as fmol/cell. Martin et al. (1993) attributed these conflicting results to the effects of illness on the size and protein content of cells in the lysate, which may have overshadowed the effects of illness on magnesium status per se.

Interpretive criteria

At present, three methods are used for quantifying the magnesium in leukocytes or mononuclear blood cell types (Elin, 1983, 1987b). The methods are:

- Mg per cell (fmol/cell)
- Mg per mg protein ($\mu mol/mg$ protein)
- Mg per kg dry weight (mmol/kg DW)

Unfortunately, there is no consensus on the preferred method or the interpretive criteria

	Serum Mg ($\mu mol/L$)	MBC Mg ($\mu mol/mg$ protein)
Community controls (n = 24)	0.75 (0.07)	0.049 (0.01)
Hospitalized patients (n = 21)	0.80 (0.11)	0.035 (0.01)

Table 23.10: Serum and mononuclear blood cell (MBC) magnesium (mean (SD)) in elderly community and hospitalized patients. Data from Martin et al., Annals of Clinical Biochemistry 30: 23–27, 1993.

to use. Elin and Hosseini (1985) reported a mean ($\pm$ SD) value of 2.91 ± 0.6 fmol/cell for the magnesium content of mononuclear blood cells from 20 apparently healthy adult volunteers. This value falls within the range noted by others (Elin and Johnson, 1982). When results are reported per unit mass of protein, the mean magnesium values range from 0.052–0.073 µmol/mg protein (Elin and Johnson 1982; Hosseini et al., 1983; Sjögren et al., 1986). For dry weight of cells, mean magnesium concentrations range from 31.0 to 43.4 mmol/kg dry weight (Elin, 1987a).

Care must be taken to ensure that the assay and units for reporting magnesium concentrations in leukocytes or mononuclear blood cells are standardized, so results among studies can be compared (Elin, 1987b).

Measurement of magnesium in leukocytes and other cell types

Large blood samples are required for harvesting the leukocytes or other cells for measurement of magnesium concentrations, limiting the use of this assay in pediatric populations.

Both the isolation of the cell types and the subsequent analysis for magnesium are complex. First, the process involves removing the platelets from whole blood and then separating the leukocytes, mononuclear blood cells, or lymphocytes generally with a discontinuous Ficoll-Hypaque gradient. Next, the separated cells are washed, centrifuged to form a pellet, and lysed by sonication with distilled water. The lysate can then be frozen until analysis.

The analysis is generally performed by AAS, after the addition of lanthanum oxide to the cell lysate to liberate the magnesium bound to cellular elements (Elin and Hosseini, 1985).

In view of the difficulty of isolating the different cell types, and the presence of residual platelet contamination, it is not surprising that measurement of the magnesium concentrations in both leukocytes and mononuclear blood cells is often associated with large CVs (often > 25%). Standardizing the centrifugal force used to harvest the leukocytes or cell

types after washing can reduce the analytical CV (Elin and Hosseini, 1985). However, the magnesium content of the leukocytes also varies with the age and size of the cells. As a result, the between-subject variation in leukocyte magnesium concentrations may also be large.

More work is necessary before the validity of magnesium concentrations in leukocytes or specific cell types as biomarkers of total body magnesium status is established.

23.3.5 Urinary magnesium and the magnesium load test

The major excretory route for absorbed magnesium is via the urine. Normal urinary magnesium excretion is from 120 to 140 mg/24 h for persons on a mixed diet (Aikawa, 1981). Excretion is reduced in persons with low or depleted magnesium stores as a result of a compensatory conservation of magnesium by the kidneys. Hence, urinary magnesium excretion has been used as a biomarker of magnesium status, primarily in association with a magnesium load test.

The magnesium load test is seen by some investigators as the most reliable screening method for diagnosing magnesium deficiency in adults. Its use, however, assumes that disease states in which a magnesium deficiency is generated by abnormal urinary losses, are absent. It also cannot be used in infants and children (Gullestad et al., 1992). Others, however, question the validity of this test for assessing magnesium status in patients at risk of magnesium deficiency but with no evidence of hypomagnesemia (Costello et al., 1997).

The intravenous magnesium load test is both invasive and cumbersome, and it requires a minimal 24-h time frame because of the diurnal variation in magnesium excretion by the kidney (Martin, 1990). It has been used to assess magnesium deficiency in postpartum U.S. women, patients with gastrointestinal disease, alcoholics, and patients who have had intestinal bypass operations for severe obesity (Thorén, 1963; Caddell, 1969; Caddell et al., 1975; Bøhmer and Mathiesen, 1982; Holm et al., 1987). An intravenous magnesium load test has also been used on some patients with ischemic heart disease, acute myocardial infarction (Rasmussen et al.,1988), and congestive heart failure (Costello et al., 1997). In most but not all of these investigations, no other corroborating index of magnesium status, with the exception of serum magnesium, was measured.

Use of the magnesium load test requires normal renal handling of magnesium as urinary magnesium losses associated with some conditions itemized in Section 23.3 may yield a false-negative test. Alternatively, impaired renal function may result in a positive test (Martin, 1990).

Age may be an important confounding variable in the magnesium load test, because older subjects may retain more magnesium than younger subjects, despite comparable dietary magnesium intake (Figure 23.9; Gullestad et al., 1994). After supplementing the elderly subjects with magnesium (225 mg/d) for 30 d, test results were normal.

In another study of elderly females (mean age 82 y), those with low serum magnesium levels (< 0.59 mmol/L) retained a higher proportion of the magnesium load than those with serum levels of 0.72 mmol/L (i.e., 61% vs. 43%). Nevertheless, retention levels for both groups were higher than those reported in younger women (Martin, 1990). Hence, care must be taken when interpreting the results of the magnesium load test in the elderly. Moreover, the sensitivity of this test in normal subjects is not yet known.

Interpretive criteria

The cutoff values used for net retention of magnesium that is associated with magnesium deficiency vary. Thorén (1963) claimed that magnesium retention >20%–50% after an intravenous magnesium load indicates a magnesium deficiency. Caddell et al. (1975) used 40% as their upper limit of normal for magnesium retention for postpartum U.S. women. Subjects with lower magnesium retention values (i.e., < 40%) had significantly higher plasma magnesium concentrations and correspondingly higher dietary magnesium intakes than their counterparts with retention values >40%.

Holm et al. (1987) showed that patients with magnesium retentions >20% had significantly lower retentions after treatment with magnesium chloride. Consequently, these investigators recommend a cutoff value of > 20% magnesium retention as indicative of suboptimal magnesium status. In a more recent review, however, a cutoff value of > 30% of intravenously administered magnesium was recommended in the absence of renal disease (Ryan, 1991). More data are urgently required on the normal retention of a magnesium load for different age groups.

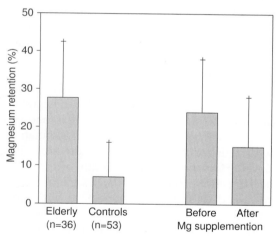

Figure 23.9: Twenty-four-hour magnesium (Mg) retention after a Mg load of 30 mmol given over 8 h to elderly and control subjects. Retention before and after oral Mg supplementation of a subsample (*n* = 14) of the elderly is also shown. Data from Gullestad et al., Journal of the American College of Nutrition 13: 45–60, 1994.

Measurement urinary magnesium

For the magnesium load test, basal urinary magnesium excretion is first determined on a timed preload urine collection. Three consecutive 24-h urine samples should be collected to counteract the effects of both diurnal and random day-to-day variation (Graham et al., 1960). A reduction in urinary excretion of magnesium at night has been reported. Magnesium is then administered, generally over an 8-h period, either intramuscularly for infants or intravenously for adults, at levels from 0.25 mmol/kg body weight (for infants) to an adult load of 1.0 mmol/kg. Parenteral administration is used to eliminate variability in intestinal absorption of magnesium. Following the load, the excretion of magnesium is measured over the subsequent 24–48-h period. Urine specimens should be collected with an acidifying agent to prevent precipitation of magnesium compounds at high pH.

The net retention of magnesium is calculated by comparing basal excretion data with net excretion after the load. Thorén (1963) recommended calculating retention over 48 h, and not 24 h, to better distinguish normal and pathological magnesium retention. Normal subjects excrete at least 80% of an intravenous magnesium load within 24 h, but patients with magnesium deficiency excrete much less (Gullestad et al., 1992).

There is an urgent need to standardize the protocol for this test, particularly the amount of the magnesium load, the length of time over which the load is infused, and the urine collection time.

23.3.6 Muscle magnesium

Magnesium concentrations of muscle have been used to assess magnesium status. The muscle is a major tissue storage site for magnesium with approximately 27% of total body magnesium stored there. Muscle magnesium concentrations were restored to normal levels after magnesium replacement therapy in patients with magnesium deficiency arising from long-term diuretic therapy for heart failure (Lim and Jacob, 1972).

Muscle specimens can be obtained by needle biopsy, but the procedure requires skill and is too invasive for community surveys or for routine clinical use. Moreover, very few studies have reported a correlation between concentrations of magnesium in muscle and serum or erythrocytes (Elin, 1991), although some significant correlations with mononuclear blood cells have been noted in certain

disease states. In patients with type 1 diabetes mellitus (Sjögren et al., 1986) or with mild arterial hypertension, magnesium concentrations in lymphocytes reflected those in skeletal muscle, as noted earlier (Section 23.3.4), but such a relationship was not observed in patients with congestive heart failure (Dyckner and Wester, 1984). Some of the inconsistencies observed could be attributed to biological variability in the assay.

More research is warranted to establish the validity of this test before it can be recommended for assessing magnesium status. In the meantime, it is preferable to use this test in association with other indices of magnesium status, such as serum magnesium and possibly ionized magnesium in serum.

23.4 Summary

Calcium

Calcium is the most abundant mineral in the body and is stored primarily in the bones and teeth where it has a structural role. The remaining calcium is involved in blood coagulation, enzyme activation, nerve transmission, muscle contractibility, membrane transport, and hormone function. Severe nutritional deficiency of calcium is rare because calcium absorption and urinary excretion are regulated in response to need. There is some evidence that very low calcium intakes in children may induce rickets and osteomalacia. Chronic calcium deficiency arising from inadequate calcium intakes or poor intestinal absorption does occur. Indeed, it is one of many important etiological factors associated with reduced bone mass and osteoporosis. Several factors influence calcium absorption and retention. Nutritional factors include calcium and vitamin D status, lactose, caffeine, and diets high in protein, phytates, or oxalates. Age and physiological status such as pregnancy and lactation are also important.

Serum ionized calcium concentration is the most promising index of calcium status and is superior to total serum calcium levels, which are under strict homeostatic control. Several new markers of bone turnover that measure enzymes or matrix proteins in serum or urine are now used. Biomarkers of bone formation include serum bone-specific alkaline phosphatase (EC 3.1.3.1) and osteocalcin in serum: serum osteocalcin is preferred. Biomarkers to assess bone resorption include hydroxylysyl pyridinoline (pyridinoline) and lysylpyridinoline (deoxypyridinoline), which are two naturally occurring cross-links of collagen that are excreted unchanged in the urine. Alternatively, two cross-linked telopeptides (N- and C-telopeptides) can be used. These are amino- and carboxy-terminal fragments of collagen which are excreted in the urine with cross-links attached. These biomarkers can be used together with serum osteocalcin to detect subtle changes in bone metabolism brought about by dietary influences.

Measurements of the bone mass of the appendicular or axial skeleton are also performed as an indirect assessment of bone calcium content and, hence, body calcium stores. Methods based on single-photon absorptiometry (SPA) are only used to measure the bone mineral content of the appendicular skeleton, whereas those using dual-energy X-ray absorptiometry (DXA) can be used to measure bone mineral content of the lumbar spine, forearm, and femur. Of these sites, researchers favor the total femur as the gold standard for bone densitometry measurements. Absorptiometric data are expressed as areal densities (bone mineral density), derived by dividing bone mineral content by bone width (for SPA) or area (for DXA). The bone mineral content is inversely related to the amount of transmitted radiation. Methods used less frequently include computerized tomography, quantitative ultrasound, radiogrammetry, and neutron activation measurements of total body calcium. Neutron activation is primarily used to validate bone mineral content estimated by DXA and other methods.

Phosphorus

Phosphorus is present in the bones, as well as in cells and extracellular fluids where it func-

tions in all the energy-producing reactions of the cells. Dietary deficiency of phosphorus is rare, although cases associated with excessive intakes of antacids and prolonged total parenteral nutrition have occurred. Growing low birth-weight preterm infants fed human milk are also susceptible to suboptimal phosphorus status. Serum phosphorus is the most frequently used measure of phosphorus status, but it has a low specificity and sensitivity. Concentrations are affected by many confounding factors unrelated to phosphorus status, such as insulin injections or abnormalities of renal tubular function. New approaches for assessing phosphorus status are required.

Magnesium

Approximately two-thirds of the total body magnesium content is in the bone, with the remainder in the muscle and nonmuscular soft tissues and intracellular fluid. Magnesium is involved in energy metabolism, protein synthesis, and neuromuscular transmission and activity. Secondary deficiency of magnesium may develop in clinical conditions associated with either gastrointestinal or renal loss of magnesium. A nutritional deficiency is rare, but suboptimal magnesium status may occur in the elderly.

No single test is available to accurately assess magnesium status. Serum magnesium concentrations are used most frequently, despite their low sensitivity and specificity. Measurement of ionized magnesium in serum using ion-selective electrodes is promising, but more studies are needed to confirm its use in clinical disease states. Measurements of intracellular magnesium, limited to erythrocytes, leukocytes, and specific cell types (e.g., mononuclear cells) reflect chronic magnesium status, but their analysis is complex and cumbersome, and as a result both biological and analytical variability are high.

Net retention of magnesium after an intravenous magnesium load test can be used to assess magnesium status in research studies, but only in those disease states where the magnesium deficiency is not due to urinary losses. In persons with depleted body stores of magnesium with normal renal handling of magnesium, urinary excretion will be low. Basal urinary magnesium excretion is first determined, followed by the measurement of magnesium concentrations in 2-h urine samples, post dose. The magnesium concentrations of muscle biopsy specimens may be useful in the future, provided the assay is validated and simplified. Muscle comprises a major tissue storage site for magnesium, and concentrations correlate with those of mononuclear blood cells in some studies.

References

Abbott L, Nadler J, Rude RK. (1994). Magnesium deficiency in alcoholism: possible contribution to osteoporosis and cardiovascular disease in alcoholics. Alcoholism, Clinical and Experimental Research 18: 1076–1082

Abraham GE, Lubran MM. (1981). Serum and red cell magnesium levels in patients with premenstrual tension. American Journal of Clinical Nutrition 34: 2364–2366.

Abraham AS, Rosenmann D, Zion MM, Eylath U. (1988). Lymphocyte potassium and magnesium concentrations as prognostic factors after acute myocardial infarction. Cardiology 75: 194–199.

Abrams SA. (2002). Nutritional rickets: an old disease returns. Nutrition Reviews 60: 111–115.

Abrams SA, Stuff JE. (1994). Calcium metabolism in girls: current dietary intakes lead to low rates of calcium absorption and retention during puberty. American Journal of Clinical Nutrition 60: 739–743.

Abrams SA, Silber TJ, Esteban NV, Vieira NE, Stuff JE, Meyers R, Majd M, Yergey AL. (1993). Mineral balance and bone turnover in adolescents with anorexia nervosa. Journal of Pediatrics 123: 326–331.

Abrams SA, Grusak MA, Stuff J, O'Brien KO. (1997). Calcium and magnesium balance in 9–14-y-old children. American Journal of Clinical Nutrition 66: 1172–1177.

Aikawa JK. (1981). Magnesium: its biological significance. CRC Press, Boca Raton, FL.

Allen LH, Wood RJ. (1994). Calcium and phosphorus. In: Shils ME, Olson JA, Shike M (eds.) Modern Nutrition in Health and Disease. 8th ed. Lea & Febiger, Philadelphia, pp. 144–161.

Allender PS, Cutler JA, Follmann D, Cappuccio FP, Pryer J, Elliott P. (1996). Dietary calcium and blood pressure: a meta-analysis of randomized clinical trials. Annals of Internal Medicine 124: 825–831.

Anderson JJ, Garner SC. (2001). Controversy over dietary phosphorus. Journal of the American College of Nutrition 20: 269–270.

Antman EM. (1996). Magnesium in acute myocardial infarction: overview of available evidence. American Heart Journal 132: 487–495.

Bailyes EM, Seabrook RN, Calvin J, Maguire GA, Price CP, Siddle K, Luzio JP. (1987). The preparation of monoclonal antibodies to human bone and liver alkaline phosphatase and their use in immunoaffinity purification and in studying these enzymes when present in serum. Biochemical Journal 244: 725–733.

Barger-Lux MJ, Heaney RP, Stegman MR. (1990). Effects of moderate caffeine intake on the calcium economy of premenopausal women. American Journal of Clinical Nutrition 52: 722–725.

Barger-Lux MJ, Heaney RP, Lanspa SJ, Healy JC, DeLuca HF. (1995). An investigation of sources of variation in calcium absorption efficiency. Journal of Clinical Endocrinology and Metabolism 80: 406–411.

Barrett-Connor E, Chang JC, Edelstein SL. (1994). Coffee-associated osteoporosis offset by daily milk consumption: the Rancho Bernardo Study. Journal of the American Medical Association 271: 280–283.

Behr W, Barnert J. (1986). Quantification of bone alkaline phosphatase in serum by precipitation with wheat-germ lectin: a simplified method and its clinical plausibility. Clinical Chemistry 32: 1960–1966.

Bettica P, Taylor AK, Talbot J, Moro L, Talamini R, Baylink DJ. (1996). Clinical performance of galactosyl hydroxylysine, pyridinoline, and deoxypyridinoline in postmenopausal osteoporosis. Journal of Clinical Endocrinology and Metabolism. 81: 542–546.

Black D, Duncan A, Robins SP. (1988). Quantitative analysis of the pyridinium crosslinks of collagen in urine using ion-paired reversed-phase high-performance liquid chromatography. Analytical Biochemistry 169: 197–203.

Blumsohn A, Herrington RA, Shao P, Eyre DR, Eastell R. (1994). The effect of calcium supplementation on the circadian rhythm of bone resorption. Journal of Clinical Endocrinology and Metabolism 79: 730–735.

Bøhmer T, Mathiesen B. (1982). Magnesium deficiency in chronic alcoholic patients uncovered by an intravenous loading test. Scandinavian Journal of Clinical and Laboratory Investigation 42: 633–636.

Bonde M, Qvist P, Fledelius C, Riis BJ, Christiansen C. (1994). Immunoassay for quantifying type I collagen degradation products in urine evaluated. Clinical Chemistry 40: 2022–2025.

Bourke E, Delaney V. (1993). Assessment of hypocalcemia and hypercalcemia. Clinics in Laboratory Medicine 13: 157–181.

Bryne J, Thomas MR, Chan GM. (1987). Calcium intake and bone density of lactating women in their late childbearing years. Journal of the American Dietetic Association 87: 883–887.

Caddell JL. (1969). The effect of magnesium therapy on cardiovascular and electrocardiograph changes in severe protein-calorie malnutrition. Tropical and Geographic Medicine 21: 33–38.

Caddell JL, Saier FL, Thomason CA. (1975). Parenteral magnesium load tests in postpartum American women. American Journal of Clinical Nutrition 28: 1099–1104.

Calvo MS. (1994). The effects of high phosphorus intake on calcium homeostasis. Advances in Nutritional Research 9: 183–207.

Calvo MS, Park YK. (1996). Changing phosphorus content of the U.S. diet: potential for adverse effects on bone. Journal of Nutrition 126: 1168S–1180S.

Calvo MS, Humar R, Heath H. (1990). Persistently elevated parathyroid hormone secretion and action in young women after four weeks of ingesting high phosphorus, low calcium diets. Journal of Clinical Endocrinology and Metabolism 70: 1334–1340.

Chan GM, Slater RN, Hollis J, Thomas MR. (1982). Decreased bone mineral status in lactating adolescent mothers. Journal of Pediatrics 101: 767–770.

Chen TC, Castillo L, Korycka-Dahl M, DeLuca HF. (1974). Role of vitamin D metabolites in phosphate transport of rat intestine. Journal of Nutrition 104: 1056–1060.

Chesley LC. (1972). Plasma and red blood cell volumes during pregnancy. American Journal of Obstetrics and Gynecology 112: 440–450.

Chesney RW. (1989). Vitamin D: can an upper limit be defined? Journal of Nutrition 119: 1825–1828.

Clements MR, Johnson L, Fraser DR. (1987). A new mechanism for induced vitamin D deficiency in calcium deprivation. Nature 325: 62–65.

Cleveland LE, Goldman JD, Borrud LG. (1996). Data Tables: Results from USDA's 1994 Continuing Survey of Food Intakes by Individuals and 1994 Diet and Health Knowledge Survey. (CD-ROM). Agricultural Research Service, U.S. Department of Agriculture, Riverdale, MD.

Cohen L, Kitzes R. (1983). Magnesium sulfate and digitalis-toxic arrhythmias. Journal of the American Medical Association 249: 2808–2810.

Cohn SH, Ellis KJ, Wallach S. (1974). In vivo neutron activation analysis: clinical potential in body composition analysis. American Journal of Medicine 57: 683–686.

Colwell A, Russell RGG, Eastell R. (1993). Factors affecting the assay of urinary 3-hydroxy pyridinium crosslinks of collagen as markers of bone resorption. European Journal of Clinical Investigation 23: 341–349.

Conradt A, Weindinger H, Algayer H. (1985). Magnesium therapy decreased the rate of intrauterine fetal retardation, premature rupture of membranes, and premature delivery in high risk pregnancies treated with betamimetics. Magnesium 4: 20–28.

Costello RB, Moser-Veillon PB, DiBianco R. (1997). Magnesium supplementation in patients with congestive heart failure. Journal of the American College of Nutrition 16: 22–31.

Cross NA, Hillman LS, Allen SH, Krasue GF, Vieira N. (1995). Calcium homeostasis and bone metabolism during pregnancy, lactation, and postweaning: a longitudinal study. American Journal of Clinical Nutrition 61: 514–523.

Cummings RB. (1990). Calcium intake and bone mass: a quantitative review of the evidence. Calcified Tissue International 47: 194–201.

Cummings SR, Kelsey JL, Nevitt MC, O'Dowd KJ. (1985). Epidemiology of osteoporosis and osteoporotic fractures. Epidemiologic Reviews 7: 178–208.

Dawson-Huges B, Dallal GE, Krall EA, Sadowski L, Sahyoun N, Tannenbaum S. (1990). A controlled trial of the effect of calcium supplementation on bone density in postmenopausal women. New England Journal of Medicine 323: 878–883.

Delmas PD. (1992). Clinical use of biomarkers of bone remodeling in osteoporosis. Bone 13: S17–S21.

Delmas PD, Malaval L, Arlot ME, Meunier PJ. (1985). Serum bone Gla-protein compared to bone histomorphometry in endocrine disease. Bone 6:339–341

Delmas PD, Christiansen C, Mann K, Price P. (1990). Bone Gla protein (osteocalcin): assay standardization report. Journal of Bone and Mineral Research 5: 5–11.

Demers LM, Kleerekoper M. (1994). Recent advances in biochemical markers of bone turnover [Editorial]. Clinical Chemistry 40: 1994–1995.

Delmas PD, Schlemmer A, Gineyts E, Riis B, Christiansen C. (1991). Urinary excretion of pyridinoline crosslinks correlates with bone turnover measured on iliac crest biopsy in patients with vertebral osteoporosis. Journal of Bone and Mineral Research 6: 639–644.

Deuster PA, Trostmann UH, Bernier LL, Dolev E. (1987). Indirect vs direct measurement of magnesium and zinc in erythrocytes. Clinical Chemistry 33: 529–532.

Devine A, Criddle RA, Dick IM, Kerr DA, Prince RL. (1995). A longitudinal study of the effect of sodium and calcium intakes on regional bone density in postmenopausal women. American Journal of Clinical Nutrition 62: 740–745.

Dibba B, Prentice A, Ceesay M, Stirling DM, Cole TJ, Poskitt EME. (2000). Effect of calcium supplementation on bone mineral accretion in Gambian children accustomed to a low-calcium diet. American Journal of Clinical Nutrition 71: 544–549.

Dobnig H, Kainer F, Stepan V, Winter R, Lipp R, Schaffer M, Kahr A, Nocnik S, Patterer G, Leb G. (1995). Elevated parathyroid hormone-related peptide levels after human gestation: Relationship to changes in bone and mineral metabolism. Journal of Clinical Endocrinology and Metabolism 80: 3699–3707.

Drinkwater BL, Bruemner B, Chesnut C. (1990). Menstrual history as a determinant of current bone density in young athletes. Journal of the American Medical Association 263: 545–548.

Ducy P, Desbois C, Boyce B, Pinero G, Story B, Dunstan C, Smith E, Bonadio J, Goldstein S, Gundberg C, Bradley A, Karsenty G. (1996). Increased bone formation in osteocalcin-deficient mice. Nature 382: 448–452.

Dyckner T, Wester PO. (1984). Intracellular magnesium loss after diuretic administration. Drugs 28(Suppl. 1): 161–166.

Dyckner T, Wester PO. (1985). Skeletal muscle magnesium and potassium determinations: correlation with lymphocyte contents of magnesium and potassium. Journal of the American College of Nutrition 4: 619–625.

Eastell R, Hampton L, Colwell A. (1993). Urinary collagen crosslinks are highly correlated with radioisotopic measurements of bone resorption. In: Christiansen C, Overgaard K (eds.) Osteoporosis. Osteopress, Copenhagan, pp. 469–470.

Eastell R, Colewell A, Hampton L, Reeve J. (1997). Biochemical markers of bone resorption compared with estimates of bone resorption from radiotracer kinetic studies in osteoporosis. Journal of Bone and Mineral Research 12: 59–65.

Elders PJM, Lips P, Netelenbos JC, van Ginkel FC, Khoe E, van der Vijgh WJF, van der Stelt PF. (1994). Long-term effect of calcium supplementation on bone loss in perimenopausal women. Journal of Bone and Mineral Research 9: 963–970.

Elin RJ. (1983). The status of cellular analysis. Journal of the American College of Nutrition 4: 329–330.

Elin RJ. (1987a). Assessment of magnesium status. Clinical Chemistry 33: 1965–1970.

Elin RJ. (1987b). Status of the mononuclear blood cell magnesium assay. Journal of the American College of Nutrition 6: 105–107.

Elin RJ. (1991). Laboratory tests for the assessment of magnesium status in humans. Magnesium and Trace Elements 10: 172–181.

Elin RJ, Hosseini JM. (1985). Magnesium content of mononuclear blood cells. Clinical Chemistry 31: 377–380.

Elin RJ, Johnson E. (1982). A method for the determination of the magnesium content of blood mononuclear cells. Magnesium 1: 115–121.

Elin RJ, Utter A, Tan HK, Corash L. (1980). Effect of magnesium deficiency on erythrocyte aging in rats. American Journal of Pathology 100: 765–778.

Ellis KJ, Shypailo RJ, Pratt JA, Pond WG. (1994). Accuracy of dual-energy x-ray absorptiometry for body composition measurements in children. American Journal of Clinical Nutrition 60: 660–665.

Ellis KJ, Shypailo RJ, Hergenroeder A, Perez M, Abrams S. (1996). Total body calcium and bone mineral content: comparison of dual-energy x-ray absorptiometry with neutron activation analysis. Journal of Bone and Mineral Research 11: 843–848.

Eriksen EF, Brixen K, Charles P (1995). New markers of bone metabolism: clinical use in metabolic bone disease. European Journal of Endocrinology 132: 251–263.

Eyre DR. (1992). New biomarkers of bone resorption. Journal of Clinical Endocrinology and Metabolism 74: 470–471.

Farley JR, Chestnut CH, Baylink DJ. (1981). Improved method for quantitative determination in serum of alkaline phosphatase of skeletal origin. Clinical Chemistry 27: 2002–2007.

Fatemi S, Ryzen E, Flores J, Endres DB, Rude RK. (1991). Effect of experimental human magnesium depletion on parathyroid hormone excretion and 1,25-dihydroxyvitamin D metabolism. Journal of Clinical Endocrinology and Metabolism 73: 1067–1072.

Faulkner KG. (1998). Bone densitometry: choosing the proper skeletal site to measure. Journal of Clinical Densitometry 1: 279–285.

Finch S, Doyle W, Lowe C, Bates CJ, Prentice A, Smithers G, Clarke PC. (1998). National Diet and Nutrition Survey: People Aged 65 Years and Over. The Stationery Office, London.

Fine KD, Santa Ana CA, Porter JL, Fordtran JS. (1991). Intestinal absorption of magnesium from food and supplements. Journal of Clinical Investigation 88: 396–402.

Fiske CH, Subbarow Y. (1925). The colorimetric determination of phosphorus. Journal of Biological Chemistry 66: 375–400.

Fleet JC, Cashman KD. (2001). Magnesium. In: Bowman BA, Russell RM. (eds.) Present knowledge in Nutrition (Eighth Edition). International Life Sciences Institute Press, Washington, DC, pp. 292–301.

Flicker L, Hopper JL, Rodgers L, Kaymakci B, Green RW, Wark JD. (1995). Bone density in elderly women: a twin study. Journal of Bone and Mineral Research 10: 1607–1613.

Fogelman I, Blake GM. (2000). Different approaches to bone densitometry. Journal of Nuclear Medicine 41: 2015–2025.

Frost HM. (1997). On our age-related bone loss: insights from a new paradigm. Journal of Bone Mineral Research 12: 1539–1546.

Gallagher SK, Johnson LK, Milne DB. (1989). Short-term and long-term variability of indices related to nutritional status. I: Ca, Cu, Fe, Mg, and Zn. Clinical Chemistry 35: 369–373.

Garnero P, Delmas PD. (1993). Assessment of the serum levels of bone alkaline phosphatase with a new immunoradiometric assay in patients with metabolic bone disease. Journal of Clinical Endocrinology 77: 1046–1053.

Garnero P, Grimaux M, Demiaux B, Preaudat C, Seguin P, Delmas PD. (1992). Measurement of serum osteocalcin with a human-specific two-site immunoradiometric assay. Journal of Bone and Mineral Research 7: 1389–1398.

Garnero P, Shih WJ, Gineyts E, Karpf DB, Delmas PD. (1994). Comparison of new biochemical markers of bone turnover in late postmenopausal osteoporotic women in response to alendronate treatment. Journal of Clinical Endocrinology and Metabolism 79: 1693–1700.

Garnero P, Gineyts E, Arbault P, Christiansen C, Delmas PD. (1995). Different effects of bisphosphonates and estrogen therapy on free and peptide-bound cross-links excretion. Journal of Bone Mineral Research 10: 641–649.

Gertz BJ, Clemens JD, Holland SD, Greenspan S. (1998). Application of a new serum assay for type 1 collagen cross-linked N-telopeptides: assessment of diurnal changes in bone turnover with and without alendronate treatment. Calcified Tissue International 63: 102–106.

Gibson RS, Hotz C. (2001). Dietary diversification/modification strategies to enhance micronutrient content and bioavailability of diets in developing countries. British Journal of Nutrition 85(Suppl. 2): S159–S166.

Gibson RS, Smit Vanderkooy PD, McLennan CE, Mercer NM. (1987). Contribution of tap water to mineral intakes of Canadian preschool children. Archives of Environmental Health 42: 165–169.

Ginty F, Prentice A. (2004). Can osteoporosis be prevented with dietary strategies during adolescence? British Journal of Nutrition 92; 5–6.

Ginty F, Flynn A, Cashman KD. (1998). The effect of short-term calcium supplementation on biochemical markers of bone metabolism in healthy adults. British Journal of Nutrition 80: 437–443.

Going SB, Massett MP, Hall MC, Bare LA, Root PA, Williams DP, Lohman TG. (1993). Detection of small changes in body composition by dual-energy X-ray absorptiometry. American Journal of Clinical Nutrition 57: 845–850.

Gomez B Jr, Ardakani S, Evans BJ, Merrell LD, Jenkins DK, Kung VT. (1996). Monoclonal antibody assay for free urinary pyridinium cross-links. Clinical Chemistry 42: 1168–1175.

Gorai I, Taguchi Y, Chaki O, Kikuchi R, Nakayama M, Yang BC, Yokata S, Minaguchi H. (1998). Serum soluble interleukin-6-receptor and biochemical markers of bone metabolism show significant variations during the menstrual cycle. Journal of Clinical Endocrinology and Metabolism 83: 326–332.

Graham LA, Caesar JJ, Burgen AS. (1960). Gastrointestinal absorption and excretion of Mg28 in man. Metabolism 9: 646–659.

Gregory J, Foster K, Tyler H, Wiseman M. (1990). The Dietary and Nutritional Survey of British Adults. Office of Population Censuses and Surveys, Social Survey Division. Her Majesty's Stationery Office, London.

Gregory J, Collins DL, Davies PSW, Hughes JM, Clarke PC. (1995). National Diet and Nutrition Survey: Children aged One-and-a-Half to Four-and-a-Half Years. Volume 1: Report of the Diet and Nutrition Survey. Her Majesty's Stationery Office, London.

Gregory J, Lowe S, Bates CJ, Prentice A, Jackson LV, Smithers G, Wenlock R, Farron M. (2000). National Diet and Nutrition Survey: Young People Aged 4 to 18 Years. Volume 1: Report of the Diet and Nutrition Survey. The Stationery Office, London.

Guillard O, Mettey R, Lecron JC, Pineau A. (1992). Congenital hypomagnesemia: alternatives to tissue biopsies for monitoring magnesium status. Clinical Biochemistry 25: 463–465.

Gullestad L, Dolva L, Waage A, Falch D, Fagerthun H, Kjekshus J. (1992). Magnesium deficiency diagnosed by an intravenous loading test. Scandinavian Journal of Clinical and Laboratory Investigation 52: 245–253.

Gullestad L, Nes M, Ronneberg R, Midtvedt K, Falch D, Kjekshsu J. (1994). Magnesium status in healthy free-living elderly Norwegians. Journal of the American College of Nutrition 13: 45–50.

Gundberg CM, Markowitz ME, Mizruchi M, Rosen JF. (1985). Osteocalcin in human serum: a circadian rhythm. Journal of Clinical Endocrinology and Metabolism 60: 736–739.

Handwerker SA, Altura BT, Altura BM. (1996). Serum ionized magnesium and other electrolytes in the antenatal period of human pregnancy. Journal of American College of Nutrition 15: 36–43.

Hans D, Dargent-Molina P, Schott AM, Sebert JL, Cormier C, Kotzki PO, Delmas PD, Pouilles JM, Breart G, Meunier PJ. (1996). Ultrasonographic heel measurements to predict hip fracture in elderly women: the EPIDOS prospective study. Lancet 348: 511–514.

Hanson J. (1997). Standardization of femur BMD [letter to the editor]. Journal of Bone and Mineral Research 12: 1316–1317.

Hanson D, Weis M, Bollen A, Maslan S, Singer F, Eyre D. (1992). A specific immunoassay for monitoring human bone resorption: quantitation of type I collagen cross-linked N-telopeptides in urine. Journal of Bone and Mineral Research 7: 1251–1258.

Harlan WR, Hull AL, Schmouder RL, Landis JR, Thompson FE, Larkin FA. (1984). Blood pressure and nutrition in adults: the National Health and Nutrition Examination Survey. American Journal of Epidemiology 120: 17–28.

Harrison HE. (1984). Phosphorus. In: Present Knowledge in Nutrition. 5th ed. Nutrition Foundation, Washington, DC, pp. 413–421.

Harrison JE, NcNeil KG, Hitchman AJ, Britt BA. (1979). Bone mineral measurements of the central skeleton by in vivo neutron activation analysis for routine investigation of osteopenia. Investigative Radiology 14: 27–34.

Health and Public Policy Committee, American College of Physicians. (1984). Radiologic methods to evaluate bone mineral content. Annals of Internal Medicine 100: 908–911.

Health and Welfare Canada. (1973). Nutrition Canada National Survey. Health and Welfare, Ottawa.

Heany RP. (1997). Phosphorous. In: IOM (Institute of Medicine). Dietary Reference Intakes for Calcium, Phosphorus, Magnesium, Vitamin D, and Fluoride. National Academy Press, Washington, DC.

Heaney RP. (2000). Dietary protein and phosphorus do not affect calcium absorption. American Journal of Clinical Nutrition 72: 758–761.

Heaney RP, Recker RR. (1994). Determinants of endogenous fecal calcium in healthy women. Journal of Bone and Mineral Research 9: 1621–1627.

Heaney RP, Recker RR, Saville PD. (1978). Menopausal changes in calcium balance performance. Journal of Laboratory and Clinical Medicine 92: 953–963.

Heaney RP, Recker RR, Stegman MR, Moy AJ. (1989). Calcium absorption in women: relationships to calcium intake, estrogen status, and age. Journal of Bone and Mineral Research 4: 469–475.

Heaney RP, McCarron D, Dawson-Hughes B, Oparil S, Berga SL, Stern JS, Barr SI, Rosen CJ. (1999). Dietary changes favorably affect bone remodeling in older adults. Journal of the American Dietetic Association 99: 1228–1233.

Hegsted M, Schuette SA, Zemel MB, Linkswiler HM. (1981). Urinary calcium and calcium balance in young men as affected by level of protein and phosphorus intake. Journal of Nutrition 111: 553–562.

Heymsfield SB, Wang J, Heshka S, Kehayias JJ, Pierson RN. (1989). Dual photon absorptiometry: comparison of bone mineral and soft tissue mass measurements in vivo with established methods. American Journal of Clinical Nutrition 49: 1283–1289.

Heymsfield SB, Waki M, Kehayias J, Lichtman S, Dilmanian FA, Kamen Y, Wang J, Pierson RN Jr. (1991). Chemical and elemental analysis of humans in vivo using improved body composition models. American Journal of Physiology 261: E190–E198.

Holm CN, Jepsen JM, Sjogaard G, Hessov I. (1987). A magnesium load test in the diagnosis of magnesium deficiency. Human Nutrition: Clinical Nutrition 41: 301–306.

Hosseini JM, Johnson E, Elin RJ. (1983). Comparison of two separation techniques for the determination of blood mononuclear cell magnesium content. Journal of the American College of Nutrition 4: 361–368.

Hunt SM, Schofield FA. (1969). Magnesium balance and protein intake in adult human female. American Journal of Clinical Nutrition 22: 367–373.

IOM (Institute of Medicine). (1997). Dietary Reference Intakes for Calcium, Phosphorus, Magnesium, Vitamin D, and Fluoride. National Academy Press, Washington, DC.

Iqbal SJ, Giles M, Ledger S, Nanji N, Howl T. (1988). Need for albumin adjustments of urgent total serum calcium. Lancet 2(8626–8627): 1477–1478.

Johansen JS, Riis BJ, Delmas PD, Christiansen C. (1988). Plasma BGP: an indicator of spontaneous bone loss and of the effect of oestrogen treatment in postmenopausal women. European Journal of Clinical Investigation 18: 191–195.

Johnston CC Jr, Miller JZ, Slemenda CW, Reister TK, Hui S, Christian JC, Peacock M. (1992). Calcium supplementation and increases in bone mineral density in children. New England Journal of Medicine 327: 82–87.

Ju H-S, Leung S, Brown B, Stringer MA, Leigh S, Scherrer C, Shepard K, Jenkins D, Knudsen J, Cannon R. (1997). Comparison of analytical perfor-

mance and biological variability of three bone resorption assays. Clinical Chemistry 43: 1570–1576.

Kalkwarf HJ, Specker BL, Heubi JE, Viera NE, Yergey AL. (1996). Intestinal calcium absorption of women during lactation and after weaning. American Journal of Clinical Nutrition 63: 526–531.

Kanis JA, Gider C-C. (2000). An update on the diagnosis and assessment of osteoporosis with densitometry. Osteoporosis International 11: 192–202.

Kanis JA, Delmas P, Burckhardt P, Cooper C, Torgerson D. (1997). Guidelines for diagnosis and treatment of osteoporosis: European Foundation for Osteoporosis and Bone Disease. Osteoporosis International 7: 390–406.

Kayne LH, Lee DBN (1993). Intestinal magnesium absorption. Mineral and Electrolyte Metabolism 19: 210–217.

Kent GN, Price RI, Gutteridge DH, Smith M, Allen JR, Bhagat CI, Barnes MP, Hickling CJ, Retallack RW, Wilson SG, Devlin RD, Davies C, St. John A. (1990). Human lactation: Forearm trabecular bone loss, increased bone turnover, and renal conservation of calcium and inorganic phosphate with recovery of bone mass following weaning. Journal of Bone and Mineral Research 5: 361–369.

Klock JC, Williams HE, Mentzer WC. (1974). Hemolytic anemia and somatic cell dysfunction in severe hypophosphatemia. Archives of Internal Medicine 134: 360–364.

Konrad M, Schlingmann KP, Gudermann T. (2004). Insights into the molecular nature of magnesium homeostasis. American Journal of Renal Physiology 286: F599–F605.

Koutkia P, Chen TC, Holick MF. (2001). Vitamin D intoxication associated with an over-the-counter supplement. New England Journal of Medicine 345: 66–67.

Kroll MH, Elin RJ. (1985). Relationships between magnesium and protein concentrations in serum. Clinical Chemistry 31: 244–246.

Ladenson JH, Bowers GN. (1973). Free calcium in serum. II: Rigor of homeostatic control, correlations with total serum calcium, and review of data on patients with disturbed calcium metabolism. Clinical Chemistry 19: 575–582.

Laitinen K, Valimaki M. (1991). Alcohol and bone. Calcified Tissue International 49: S70–S73

Laskey MA. (1996). Dual-energy x-ray absorptiometry and body composition. Nutrition 12: 45–51.

Ledger GA, Burritt MF, Kao PC, O'Fallon WM, Riggs BL, Khosla S. (1995). Role of parathyroid hormone in mediating nocturnal and age-related increases in bone resorption. Journal of Clinical Endocrinology and Metabolism 80: 3304–3310.

Lee WT, Leung SS, Leung DM, Wang SH, Xu YC, Zeng WP, Cheng JC. (1997). Bone mineral acquisition in low calcium intake children following the withdrawal of calcium supplement. Acta Paediatrica 86: 570–576.

Lewiecki EM, Watts NB, McClung MR, Petak SM, Bachrach LK, Shepherd JA, Downs RW Jr., for the International Society for Clinical Densitometry. (2004). Official Positions of the International Society for Clinical Densitometry. Journal of Clinical Endocrinology and Metabolism 89: 3651–3655.

Li T-K, Piechocki JT. (1971). Determination of serum ionic calcium with an ion-selective electrode: evaluation of methodology and normal values. Clinical Chemistry 17: 411–416.

Lim P, Jacob E. (1972). Magnesium deficiency in patients on long-term diuretic therapy for heart failure. British Medical Journal 3(827): 620–622.

Linko S, Himberg JJ, Thienpont L, Støøckl D, De Leenheer A. (1998). Assessment of the state-of-the-art trueness and precision of serum total-calcium and glucose measurements in Finnish laboratories: the QSL-Finland study. Scandinavian Journal of Clinical and Laboratory Investigation 58: 229–239.

London RE. (1991). Methods for measurement of intracellular magnesium: NMR and fluorescence. Annual Review of Physiology 53: 241–258.

Looker AC, Wahner HW, Dunn WL et al. (1998). Updated data on proximal femur bone mineral levels of U.S. adults. Osteoporosis International 8: 468–489.

Lopez JM, Gonzalez G, Reyes V, Campino C, Diaz S. (1996). Bone turnover and density in healthy women during breastfeeding and after weaning. Osteoporosis International 6: 153–159.

Lotz M, Zisman E, Bartter FC. (1968). Evidence for a phosphorus-depletion syndrome in man. New England Journal of Medicine 278: 409–415.

Lowenstein FW, Stanton MF. (1986). Serum magnesium levels in the United States, 1971–1974. Journal of the American College of Nutrition 5: 399–414.

Lowik M, van Dokkum W, Kistemaker C, Schaafsma G, Ockhuizen T. (1993). Body composition, health status and urinary magnesium excretion among elderly people (Dutch Nutrition Surveillance System). Magnesium Research 6: 223–232.

Lueken SA, Arnaud SB, Taylor AK, Baylink DJ. (1993). Changes in markers of bone formation and resorption in a bed rest model of weightlessness. Journal of Bone Mineral Research 8: 1433–1438.

Lukaski HC. (2000). Magnesium, zinc, and chromium nutriture and physical activity. American Journal of Clinical Nutrition 72: 585S–5893S.

Lukaski HC, Bolonchuk WW, Klevay LM, Milne DB, Sandstead HH. (1983). Maximal oxygen consumption as related to magnesium, copper, and zinc nutriture. American Journal of Clinical Nutrition 37: 407–415.

Lunt MD, Felsenberg D, Adams J, Benevolenskaya L, Cannata J, Dequeker J, Dodenhof C, Falch JA, Johnell O, Khaw KT, Masaryk P, Pols H, Poor G, Reid D, Scheidt-Nave C, Weber K, Silman AJ, Reeve J. (1997). Population-based geographic variations in DXA bone density in Europe: the EVOS study. European vertebral osteoporosis. Osteoporosis International 7: 175–189.

Ma R, Stamatelatos IE, Yasumura S. (2000). Calibration of the Brookhaven National Laboratory delayed gamma neutron activation facility to measure total body calcium. Annals of the New York Academy of Sciences 904: 148–151.

Martin BJ. (1990). The magnesium load test: experience in elderly subjects. Aging 2: 291–296.

Martin BJ, Lyon TDB, Walker W, Fell GS. (1993). Mononuclear blood cell magnesium in older subjects: evaluation of its use in clinical practice. Annals of Clinical Biochemistry 30: 23–27.

Matković V, Kostial K, Simonović I, Buzina R, Brodarec A, Nordin BE. (1979). Bone status and fracture rates in two regions of Yugoslavia. American Journal of Clinical Nutrition 32: 540–549.

Mazess RB. (1983). Errors in measuring trabecular bone by computed tomography due to marrow and bone composition. Calcified Tissue International 35: 148–152.

Mazess RB, Peppler WW, Chesney RW, Lange TA, Lingren U, Smith E Jr. (1984). Does bone measurement on the radius indicate skeletal status: concise communication. Journal of Nuclear Medicine 25: 281–288.

Mazess RB, Burden HS, Bisek JP, Hanson J. (1990). Dual-energy X-ray absorptiometry for total-body and regional bone-mineral and soft-tissue composition. American Journal of Clinical Nutrition 51: 1106–1112.

McKane WR, Khosla S, Egan KS, Robins SP, Burritt MF, Riggs BL. (1996). Role of calcium intake in modulating age-related increases in parathyroid function and bone resorption. Journal of Clinical Endocrinology and Metabolism 81: 1699–1703.

McLennan W, Podger A. (1998). National Nutrition Survey: Nutrient Intakes and Physical Measurements, Australia 1995. Australian Bureau of Statistics, Canberra.

Medalle R, Waterhouse C. (1973). A magnesium-deficient patient presenting with hypocalcemia and hyperphosphatemia. Annals of Internal Medicine 79: 76–79.

Melton LJ 3rd, Khosla S, Atkinson EJ, O'Fallon WM, Riggs BL. (1997). Relationship of bone turnover to bone density and fractures. Journal of Bone and Mineral Research 12: 1092–1099.

Millart H, Durlach V, Durlach J. (1995). Red blood cell magnesium concentrations: analytical problems and significance. Magnesium Research 8: 65–76.

Minisola S, Pacitti MT, Scarda A, Rosso R, Romagnoli E, Carnevale V, Scarnecchia L, Mazzuoli GF. (1993). Serum ionized calcium, parathyroid hormone and related variables: effect of age and sex. Bone and Mineral 23: 183–193.

Mountokalakis TD. (1987). Effects of aging, chronic disease, and multiple supplements on magnesium requirements. Magnesium 6: 5–11.

Nadler JL, Malayan S, Luong H, Shaw S, Natarjan R, Rude RK. (1992). Intracellular free magnesium deficiency plays a key role in increased platelet reactivity in type 2 diabetes mellitus. Diabetes Care 15: 835–841.

Nielsen HK, Brixen K, Mosekilde L. (1990a). Diurnal rhythm in serum activity of wheat-germ lectin-precipitable alkaline phosphatase: temporal relationships with the diurnal rhythm of serum osteocalcin. Scandinavian Journal of Clinical Laboratory Investigation 50: 851–856.

Nielsen HK, Brixen K, Bouillon R, Mosekilde L. (1990b). Changes in biochemical markers of osteoblastic activity during the menstrual cycle. Journal of Clinical Endocrinology and Metabolism 70: 1431–1437

Nielsen HK, Brixen K, Kassem M, Mosekilde L. (1991). Acute effects of 1,25-dihydroxyvitamin D 3, prednisone, and 1,25-dihydroxyvitamin D 3 plus prednisone on serum osteolcalcin in normal individuals. Journal of Bone and Mineral Research 6: 435–441.

NIN (National Institute of Nutrition). (1995). Dairy Products in the Canadian Diet. NIN Review No. 24. NIN, Ontario, Canada.

Nisbet JA, Eastwood JB, Colston KW, Ang L, Flanagan AM, Chambers TJ, Maxwell JD. (1990). Detection of osteomalacia in British Asians: a comparison of clinical score with biochemical measurements Clinical Science 78: 383–389.

Oginni LM, Worsfold M, Oyelami OA, Sharp CA, Powell DE, Davie MW. (1996). Etiology of rickets in Nigerian children. Journal of Pediatrics 128: 692–694.

Oreskes I, Hirsch C, Douglas KS, Kupfer S. (1968). Measurement of ionized calcium in human plasma with a calcium selective electrode. Clinica Chimica Acta 21: 303–313.

Pagani F, Panteghini M. (1994). Diurnal rhythm in urinary excretion of pyridinium crosslinks. Clinical Chemistry 40: 952–953.

Pennington JA, Young BE. (1991). Total diet study nutritional elements, 1982-1989. Journal of the American Dietetic Association 91: 179–183.

Pettifor JM. (1991). Dietary calcium deficiency. In: Glorieux FH (ed.) Rickets. Vevey: Nestec/New York, Raven Press, pp. 123–143.

Pierson RN Jr, Wang J, Thorton JC, Kotler DP, Heymsfield SB, Weber DA, Ma RM. (1995). Bone mineral and body fat measurements by two absorptiometry systems: comparisons with neutron activation analysis. Calcified Tissue International 56: 93–98.

Pluijm SMF, Graafmans WC, Bouter LM, Lips P. (1999). Ultrasound measurements for the prediction of osteoporotic fractures in elderly people. Osteoporosis International 9: 550–556.

Portale AA, Halloran BP, Morris RC. (1987). Dietary intake of phosphorus modulates the circadian rhythm in serum concentration of phosphorus: implications for the renal production of 1,25-dihydroxyvitamin D. Journal of Clinical Investigation 80: 1147–1154.

Prentice A. (2004). Diet, nutrition, and the prevention of osteoporosis. Public Health Nutrition 7: 227–243.

Prentice A, Parsons TJ, Cole TJ. (1994). Uncritical use of bone mineral density in absorptiometry may lead to size-related artifacts in the identification of bone

mineral determinants. American Journal of Clinical Nutrition 60: 837–842.

Price PA, Nishimoto SK, (1980). Radioimmunoassay for the vitamin K-dependent protein of bone and its discovery in plasma. Proceedings of the National Academy of Sciences of the United States of America 77: 2234–2238.

Quamme GA. (1993). Laboratory evaluation of magnesium status: renal function and free intracellular magnesium concentration. Clinics in Laboratory Medicine 13: 209–223.

Ralston SH. (1996). Pathophysiology of osteoporosis. In: Compston JE. (ed.) Osteoporosis: New Perspectives on Prevention and Treatment. Royal College of Physicians, London. pp. 31–40.

Rasmussen H, Anast C. (1983). Familial hypophosphatemic rickets and vitamin D-dependent rickets. In: Stanbury JB, Wyngarden JB, Frederickson DS, Goldstein JL, Brown MS (eds.) The Metabolic Basis of Inherited Bone Disease. 5th ed. McGraw Hill, New York, pp. 17431773.

Rasmussen HS, McNair P, Gøransson L, Balslov S, Larsen OG, Aurup P. (1988). Magnesium deficiency in patients with ischemic heart disease with and without acute myocardial infarction uncovered by an intravenous loading test. Archives of Internal Medicine 148: 329–332.

Refsum HE, Meen HD, Strømme SB. (1973). Whole blood, serum and erythrocyte magnesium concentrations after repeated heavy exercise of long duration. Scandinavian Journal of Clinical and Laboratory Investigation 32: 123–127.

Reid DM, New SA. (1997). Nutritional influences on bone mass. Proceedings of the Nutrition Society 56: 977–987.

Riggs BL, O'Fallon WM, Muhs J, O'Connor MK, Kumar R, Melton LJ III. (1998). Long-term effects of calcium supplementation on serum parathyroid hormone level, bone turnover, and bone loss in elderly women. Journal of Bone and Mineral Research 13: 168–174.

Rizek JE, Dimich A, Wallach S. (1965). Plasma and erythrocyte magnesium in thyroid disease. Journal of Clinical Endocrinology and Metabolism 25: 350–358.

Robins SP, Woitge H, Hesley R, Ju J, Seyedin S, Seibel MJ. (1994). Direct, enzyme-linked immunoassay for urinary doxypyridinoline as a specific marker for measuring bone resorption. Journal of Bone and Mineral Research 9: 1643–1649.

Rosner F, Gorfien PC. (1968). Erythrocyte and plasma zinc and magnesium levels in health and disease. Journal of Laboratory and Clinical Medicine 72: 213–219.

Rosner F, Lee SL. (1972). Zinc and magnesium content of leukocyte alkaline phosphatase isoenzymes. Journal of Laboratory and Clinical Medicine 79: 228–239.

Ross PS, Seelig MS, Berger AR. (1980). Isolation of leukocytes for magnesium determination. In: Cantin M, Seelig MS (eds.) Magnesium in Health and Disease. Spectrum Publications, New York, pp. 7–15.

Roubenoff R, Kehayias JJ, Dawson-Hughes B, Heymsfield SB. (1993). Use of dual-energy x-ray absorptiometry in body-composition studies: not yet a "gold standard." American Journal of Clinical Nutrition 58: 589–591.

Rude RK. (1998). Magnesium deficiency: a cause of heterogenous disease in humans. Journal of Bone and Mineral Research 13: 749–758.

Rude RK, Olerich M. (1996). Magnesium deficiency: possible role in osteoporosis associated with gluten-sensitive enteropathy. Osteoporosis International 6: 453–461.

Russell D, Parnell W, Wilson N, Faed J, Ferguson E, Herbison P, Horwath C, Nye T, Walker R, Wilson B. (1999). New Zealand Food: New Zealand People. Key results of the 1997 National Nutrition Survey. Ministry of Health, Wellington, New Zealand.

Ryan MF. (1991). The role of magnesium in clinical biochemistry: an overview. Annals of Clinical Biochemistry 28: 19–26.

Ryan MP, Ryan MF. (1979). Lymphocyte electrolyte alterations during magnesium deficiency in the rat. Irish Journal of Medical Science 148: 108–109.

Ryan MP, Ryan MF, Counihan TB. (1981). The effect of diuretics on lymphocyte magnesium and potassium. Acta Medica Scandinavica Supplement 647: 153–161.

Ryzen E, Elkayam U, Rude RK. (1986). Low blood mononuclear cell magnesium in intensive cardiac care unit patients. American Heart Journal 3: 475–480.

Ryzen E, Servis KL, DeRusso P, Kershaw A, Stephen T, Rude RK. (1989). Determination of intracellular free magnesium by nuclear magnetic resonance in human magnesium deficiency. Journal of the American College of Nutrition 8: 580–587.

Sarno M, Powell H, Tjersland G, Schoendorfer D, Harris H, Adams K, Ogata P, Warnick GR. (1999). A collection method and high-sensitivity enzyme immunoassay for sweat pyridinoline and deoxypyridinoline cross-links. Clinical Chemistry 45: 1501–1509.

Sax L. (2001). The institute of medicine's "dietary reference intake" for phosphorus: a critical perspective. Journal of the American College of Nutrition 20: 271–278.

Schaafsma G. (1997). Bioavailability of calcium and magnesium. European Journal of Clinical Nutrition 51: (Suppl. 1): S13–S16.

Schlemmer A, Hassager C, Jensen SB, Christiansen C. (1992). Marked diurnal variation in urinary excretion of pyridinium cross-links in premenopausal women. Journal of Clinical Endocrinology and Metabolism 74: 476–480.

Schuette SA, Linkswiler HM. (1984). Calcium. In: Present Knowledge in Nutrition. 5th ed. Nutrition Foundation, Washington, DC, pp. 410–412.

Schwartz HD. (1976). New techniques for ion-selective measurements of ionized calcium in serum after pH

adjustment of aerobically handled sera. Clinical Chemistry 22: 461–467.

Seibel MJ, Gartenberg F, Silverberg SJ, Ratcliffe A, Robins SP, Bilezikian JP. (1992). Urinary hydroxypyridinium cross-links of collagen in primary hyperparathyroidism. Journal of Clinical Endocrinology and Metabolism 74: 481–486.

Seibel MJ, Pols HAP. (1996). Clinical application of biochemical markers of bone metabolism. In: Bilezikian JP, Raisz LG, Rodan GA (eds.) Principles of Bone Biology. Academic Press, San Diego, pp. 1293–1311.

Sherwood RA, Rocks BF, Stewart A, Saxton R. (1986). Magnesium and the premenstrual syndrome. Annals of Clinical Biochemistry 23: 667–670.

Shils ME. (1964). Experimental human magnesium depletion. I: Clinical observations and blood chemistry alterations. American Journal of Clinical Nutrition 15: 133–143.

Shils ME. (1994). Magnesium. In: Shils ME, Olson JA, Shike M (ed.) Modern Nutrition in Health and Disease. 8th ed. Volume 1. Lea & Febiger, Philadelphia, pp.164–184.

Shiraki M, Rosado K, Seino Y. (1991). The region specific sandwich enzyme immunoassays for intact and N-fragment osteocalcin. Journal of Bone and Mineral Research 6(Suppl. 1): S245.

Sjögren A, Floren CH, Nilsson A. (1986). Magnesium deficiency in IDDM related to level of glycosylated hemoglobin. Diabetes 35: 459–463.

Slemenda C, Hui SL, Longcope C, Johnston C. (1987). Sex steroids and bone mass: a study of changes about the time of menopause. Journal of Clinical Investigation 80: 1261–1269.

Slemenda CW, Peacock M, Hui S, Zhou L, Johnston C. (1997). Reduced rates of skeletal remodeling are associated with increased bone mineral density during the development of peak skeletal mass. Journal of Bone and Mineral Research 12: 676–682.

Sojka JE, Weaver CM. (1995). Magnesium supplementation and osteoporosis. Nutrition Reviews 53: 71–74.

Specker BL, Tsang RC, Ho ML. (1991). Changes in calcium homeostasis over the first year post-partum: Effect of lactation and weaning. Obstetrics and Gynecology 78: 56–62.

Stendig-Lindberg G, Tepper R, Leichter I. (1993). Trabecular bone density in a two year controlled trial of peroral magnesium in osteoporosis. Magnesium Research 6: 155–163.

Svendsen OL, Haarbo J, Hassager C, Christiansen C. (1993). Accuracy of measurements of body composition by dual-energy-ray absorptiometry in vivo. American Journal of Clinical Nutrition 57: 605–608.

Svendsen OL, Hassager C, Skody V, Christiansen C. (1995). Impact of soft tissue on in-vivo accuracy of bone mineral measurements in the spine, hip, and forearm: a human cadaver study. Journal of Bone and Mineral Research 10: 868–873.

Tenenhouse HS. (1997). Cellular and molecular mechanisms of renal phosphate transport. Journal of Bone Mineral Research 12: 159–164.

Thacher TD, Fischer PR, Pettifor JM, Lawson JO, Isichei CO, Reading JC, Chan GM. (1999). A comparison of calcium, vitamin D, or both for nutritional rickets in Nigerian children. New England Journal of Medicine 341: 563–568.

Thomsen K, Eriksen EF, Jørgensen JCR, Charles P, Mosekilde L. (1989). Seasonal variation of serum bone GLA protein. Scandinavian Journal of Clinical Laboratory Investigation 49: 605–611.

Thorén L. (1963). Magnesium deficiency in gastrointestinal fluid loss. Acta Chirurgica Scandinavica Supplement 306: 1–65.

Uebelhart D, Gineyts E, Chapuy M-C, Delmas PD. (1990). Urinary excretion of pyridinium crosslinks: a new marker of bone resorption in metabolic bone disease. Bone and Mineral 8: 87–96.

Valyesevi A, Dhanamitta S. (1967). Studies of bladder stone disease in Thailand. VII: Urinary studies in newborn and infants of hypo- and hyper-endemic areas. American Journal of Clinical Nutrition 20: 1369–1379.

Valyesevi A, Halstead SB, Pantuwatana S, Tankayui C. (1967). Studies of bladder stone disease in Thailand. IV: Dietary habits, nutritional intake, and infant feeding practices among residents of hypo- and hyper-endemic areas. American Journal of Clinical Nutrition 20: 1340–1351.

Vargas CM, Obisesan T, Gillum RF. (1998). Association of serum albumin concentration, serum ionized calcium concentration, and blood pressure in the Third National Health and Nutrition Examination Survey. Journal of Clinical Epidemiology 51: 739–746.

Watts NB. (1999). Clinical utility of biochemical markers of bone remodeling. Clinical Chemistry 45: 1359–1368.

Venugopal B, Luckey TD. (1978). Metal Toxicity in Mammals. Volume 2. Plenum Press, New York, pp. 41–100.

Wahner HW, Dunn WL, Riggs BL. (1983). Noninvasive bone mineral measurements. Seminars in Nuclear Medicine 13: 282–289.

Wandrup J, Kvetny J. (1985). Potentiometric measurement of ionized calcium in anaerobic whole blood, plasma, and serum evaluated. Clinical Chemistry 31: 856–860.

Weaver CB. (2001). Caclium. In: Bowman BA, Russell RM. (eds.) Present Knowledge in Nutrition. 8th ed. International Life Sciences Institute Press, Washington, DC, pp. 273–2 80.

WHO (World Health Organization). (1994). Assessment of fracture risk and its application to screening for postmenopausal osteoporosis. Technical Report Series no. 843. Geneva: WHO.

Whybro A, Jagger H, Barker M, Eastell R. (1998). Phosphate supplementation in young men: lack of effect on calcium homeostasis and bone turnover. European Journal of Clinical Nutrition 52: 29–33.

Woitge HW, Seibel MJ, Ziegler R. (1996). Comparison of total and bone-specific alkaline phosphatase in patients with non-skeletal disorder or metabolic bone diseases. Clinical Chemistry 42: 1796–1804.

Woitge HW, Knothe A, Witte K, Schmidt-Gayk H, Ziegler R, Lemmer B, Seibel MJ. (2000). Circannual rhythms and interactions of vitamin D metabolites, parathyroid hormone, and biochemical markers of skeletal homeostasis: a prospective study. Journal of Bone and Mineral Research 15: 2443–2450.

Wyshak G. (2000). Teenaged girls, carbonated beverage consumption, and bone fractures. Archives of Pediatrics and Adolescent Medicine 154: 610–613.

Yang XY, Hosseini JM, Ruddel ME, Elin RJ. (1990). Blood magnesium parameters do not differ with age. American College of Nutrition 9: 308–313.

Zettner A, Seligson D. (1964). Application of atomic absorption spectrophotometry in the determination of calcium in serum. Clinical Chemistry 10: 869–890.

24

Assessment of chromium, copper and zinc status

Trace elements occur in the body in small or "trace" amounts, typically milligrams or micrograms per kilogram body weight; they generally constitute $< 0.01\%$ of the body mass. Certain trace elements have been identified as essential for life, and these are listed in Table 24.1. Of these, chromium, copper, and zinc are reviewed in this chapter; iron was discussed in Chapter 17. Iodine and selenium are considered together in Chapter 25 in view of the interactions that occur between these two trace elements.

In the past, trace elements were considered to be essential when a deficient intake produced an impairment of function, and when supplementation with physiological levels of that element reversed the impaired function or prevented an impairment (Mertz, 1981a). This conventional definition has now been abandoned in favor of a less rigid concept of essentiality. This change has arisen because of the increasing recognition that even modest dietary inadequacies, of a degree insufficient to cause classical deficiency syndromes, can contribute to the risk of certain disease states such as cardiovascular disease and cancer. Further, some trace elements may confer specific health benefits when taken in nonphysiological or pharmacological doses.

Trace elements vary in their properties and biological functions; many act primarily by forming metallo-enzymes. Deficiencies of trace elements produce multiple and diverse clinical signs and symptoms. Many of these classical symptoms were first identified in

Essential in humans and animals	Essential in some animals	Possibly essential in some animals
Chromium Cobalt Copper Fluorine Iodine Iron Manganese Molybdenum Selenium Zinc	Arsenic Lithium Nickel Silicon Vanadium	Bromine Cadmium Lead Tin

Table 24.1: The essential trace elements. Reproduced from Casey and Robinson (1983) © Marcel Dekker, Inc., with permission.

patients receiving total parenteral nutrition (TPN) unsupplemented with trace elements. Even today, only some of the clinical manifestations of trace-element deficiencies have been explained in biochemical terms.

Trace-element deficiencies may arise from low intakes or poor bioavailability in the diet, or they may be associated with disease states in which decreased absorption, excessive excretion, and excessive utilization occur. Numerous interactions, both between trace elements (e.g., zinc and copper; zinc and iron) and with other micronutrients (e.g., zinc and vitamin A), have been identified, some of which induce suboptimal trace element status in humans (Prasad et al., 1978a; Yadrick et al., 1989; Christian et al., 2001; Lind et al., 2003).

Genetic defects in trace-element metabolism resulting in deficiency syndromes have also been described. Some of the more common defects relate to copper (Menkes' kinky hair syndrome), iron (congenital atransferrinemia), and zinc (acrodermatitis enteropathica).

Some trace elements have a high toxicity; for example, the daily intake of selenium associated with the appearance of toxicity is only 10 times the nutritional requirement. For others (e.g., trivalent chromium), adverse effects associated with excess intakes from food or supplements have rarely been reported.

Major advances in the collection, preparation, and analysis of trace elements in biological samples have greatly improved the quality of analytical data on biological tissues and fluids. Precautions introduced to avoid adventitious contamination include the use of trace-element-free syringes and evacuated tubes fitted with siliconized needles, laminar flow hoods, 18-Mohm deionized water, ultrapure reagents which are often distilled at sub-boiling temperatures, acid-washed glassware, and plastic storage containers made of polyethylene or polypropylene for sample preparation and analysis (Veillon and Patterson, 1999). If possible, all sample preparation for the analysis of trace elements in biological samples should be carried out in a clean room or in a class-100 laminar-flow hood.

Presently, the most widely used method for trace-element analysis in biological samples is atomic absorption spectrophotometry (AAS). For the ultra-trace elements such as chromium, graphite furnace AAS with Zeeman-effect background correction has the sensitivity required for making measurements at levels of 1.0 nmol/L.

Several multi-element methods, including X-ray fluorescence, instrumental neutron activation analysis (INAA), inductively coupled plasma (ICP) spectroscopy, and ICP mass spectrometry, have been developed for trace-element analysis. Multi-element analytical methods are especially useful for investigating potential trace-element interactions. For some (e.g., INAA), matrix effects are nonexistent, and treatment of the sample by ashing or digestion is usually unnecessary, reducing the risk of contamination. Others (e.g., graphite furnace AAS) are susceptible to interference from the sample matrix, so that for ultra trace elements, such as chromium in urine, the method of additions should be used to minimize matrix effects (Veillon and Patterson, 1999).

Efforts continue to reduce interferences (if present) and to increase both the precision and sensitivity of all of these methods. Checks on the accuracy of trace-element analytical work can be made by analyzing reference materials, with certified values for each element, in parallel with routine samples.

The static biochemical tests currently used to assess chromium, copper, and zinc status still depend on measuring the total quantity of the trace element in various accessible tissues (e.g., hair, fingernails) and body fluids (whole blood or some fraction, urine, etc.); details are given in Section 15.1. These tests, however, are generally not very sensitive or specific; hence, new functional tests have been developed for some of the trace elements. The best functional tests measure the changes associated with the first limiting biochemical system that affects health and well-being; they are discussed in Section 15.2.

Other functional tests measure more general trace-element-dependent behavioral or physiological functions. Such tests are often easier to perform and are more directly related to health status than are the functional biochemical tests noted above. However, tests based on general physiological or behavioral functions are not very specific; they may be affected by more than one nutrient. For example, immune function is impaired by deficiencies of copper, zinc, iron, iodine, and selenium, whereas glucose tolerance may be affected by copper and manganese status, as well as chromium depletion (Turnlund, 1994; Strain, 1999).

In general, a combination of tests is recommended for each trace element. Ideally, the combination should include a test that reflects total body trace-element content or tissue stores, together with the best discrete functional test.

For some trace elements (e.g., chromium and zinc), the most reliable method currently available for detecting a marginal deficiency state is still supplementation, followed by an evaluation of improvement or reversal of a previously impaired trace-element-dependent function. This approach is time consuming and tedious and therefore unsuitable for use in surveys.

Frank or marginal nutritional deficiencies of iron, chromium, copper, zinc, and iodine and selenium have been reported in certain population groups that consume self-selected diets. Chromium, copper, and zinc are discussed below; selenium and iodine are considered in Chapter 25, iron in Chapter 17. Trace elements with known toxic effects but which have yet to be demonstrated as essential for humans (e.g., arsenic, lead, and cadmium) are not discussed (Table 24.1).

24.1 Chromium

Estimates of the total adult body pool of chromium are from 4 to 6 mg, which is probably all in the trivalent form. To function physiologically, absorbed chromium is first converted to a biologically active form. The precise structure and the function of this molecule remains uncertain (Mertz, 1993). In early studies this molecule was called glucose tolerance factor (Frieden, 1985), but more recently, the existence of a chromium-containing protein, termed chromodulin, has been proposed (Vincent, 2000). Details of the physiology and functions of chromium are reviewed in Anderson (2003) and Vincent (2004); only a brief outline is given below.

Functions of chromium

The biologically active form of chromium has a role in normal glucose metabolism and insulin activity. It potentiates the action of insulin in cellular glucose uptake, thus reducing the susceptibility to diabetes. Some individuals, especially the elderly, appear to lose the ability to convert inactive chromium complexes to the active form. Hence, they become dependent solely on intake of pre-formed biologically active complexes from the diet.

The specific nature of the relationship between chromium and insulin function is still not resolved. Chromium may act directly on insulin or its receptor. Alternatively, it may regulate the synthesis of a molecule such as chromodulin that potentiates insulin action; details are given in Vincent (2000, 2004).

Chromium may also be implicated in fat metabolism as a result of its role in insulin resistance, which is known to promote hyper-triglyceridemia and to increase secretion of very-low-density lipoprotein (VLDL) cholesterol from the liver (Kraegen et al., 2001).

Absorption and metabolism of chromium

The absorption of trivalent chromium, the form of chromium in foods, is very poor, ranging from 0.5% to 2.5% (Offenbacher et al., 1986). There is some evidence that chromium absorption is regulated by the level in the diet. Absorption is approximately 2% at dietary intakes of 10 µg/d, but only 0.5% at intakes ranging from 40 to 240 µg/d (Anderson and Kolzlovsky, 1985). At present, the mechanism whereby chromium is absorbed from the intestine is not clear.

Some components of the diet can affect chromium absorption. Ascorbic acid and amino acids promote absorption (Dowling et al., 1990; Offenbacher, 1994). Some medications are also significant in this respect: aspirin increases absorption, whereas antacids appear to have the reverse effect (Davis et al., 1995).

Absorbed chromium is excreted rapidly in the urine, primarily through the kidney (Anderson et al., 1983a). Consumption of diets high in simple sugars increases urinary chromium excretion (Kozlovsky et al., 1986). Increases in urinary excretion also occur during aerobic exercise, physical trauma, and lactation (Anderson et al., 1988; Rubin et al., 1998).

The unabsorbed chromium is excreted in

the feces; very little is excreted via the bile (Offenbacher et al., 1986; Davis-Whitenack et al., 1996). Hair and skin may account for relatively large losses.

Once absorbed, the trivalent chromium is bound mainly to transferrin, the main transport protein for iron, although albumin and some degradation products also act as chromium carriers. As a result, interactions between chromium and iron have been investigated. In hemochromatosis, when all the metal transport sites on transferrin are saturated with iron, chromium transport is decreased. This effect may explain, in part, the glucose intolerance that may occur in hemochromatosis and other diseases characterized by elevated levels of iron (Anderson, 2003).

Chromium deficiency in humans

A chromium-responsive deficiency syndrome has been reported in three cases of adults receiving long-term total parenteral nutrition (Jeejeebhoy et al., 1977; Freund et al., 1979; Brown et al., 1986). Clinical manifestations of chromium deficiency seen in all three cases included impaired glucose tolerance with pronounced insulin resistance, hyperglycemia, and unexplained weight loss; neuropathy was not a consistent finding (Brown et al., 1986).

Marginal chromium deficiency, confirmed by an improvement in glucose tolerance after chromium supplementation, has been noted in some population groups and is reviewed in detail in Mertz (1993) and Anderson (1998). The studies have included malnourished children (Carter et al., 1968; Hopkins et al., 1968; Gürson and Saner, 1971), diabetics (Glinsmann and Mertz, 1966; Nath et al., 1979), the elderly (Levine et al., 1968; Offenbacher and Pi-Sunyer, 1980; Martinez et al., 1985), and apparently normal healthy individuals (Riales and Albrink, 1981; Anderson et al., 1983a).

Results of these studies have also confirmed that normal glucose tolerance is not further improved with chromium supplementation (Mertz, 1993; Anderson, 2003). However, some discrepancies have been noted when comparing these studies that may be associated not only with the differing chrom-

ium status of the subjects, but also with differences in the amount and form of the chromium supplement used (Evans and Bowman, 1992; Anderson, 1998). Differences in the degree of glucose intolerance and stage and duration of diabetes may be additional factors.

The effect of chromium supplementation on subjects with type 2 diabetes has been inconsistent and warrants further study (Anderson, 2000). Several uncontrolled clinical studies have been performed (Hellerstein, 1998), but only a few randomized controlled chromium supplementation trials have been conducted in China on subjects with type 2 diabetes (Anderson et al., 1997; Cheng et al., 1999) and India (Ghosh et al., 2002). Results suggest that chromium may be efficacious in treating type 2 diabetes, provided the amount given is adequate (Anderson, 2000). Indeed, the metabolic improvements described in the first large scale randomized controlled trial in China (Figure 24.1) when subjects received 1000 μg (19.2 μmol/L) supplemental chromium daily (as chromium picolinate) (Anderson et al., 1997) were comparable to those for

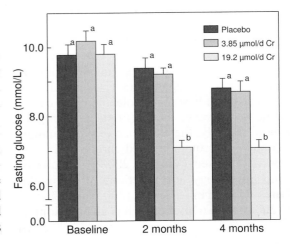

Figure 24.1: Supplemental chromium effects on mean (± SD) fasting serum glucose. Placebo group, $n = 50$; 3.85 μmol/d (200 μg/d) group, $n = 53$; 19.2 μmol/d (1000 μg/d) group, $n = 52$. Bars with different letters are significantly different from other groups for the same time period at $p < 0.05$. Data from Anderson et al.© American Diabetes Association. From Diabetes, Vol. 46, 1997; 1786–1791. Reprinted with permission from the American Diabetes Association.

oral hypoglycemic agents or insulin. Nevertheless, some uncertainties still exist about the interpretation of these results that may limit their applicability to type 2 diabetes in Western countries. Large clinical trials in Western diabetic populations are urgently required.

Marginal chromium deficiency in humans has sometimes been associated with disturbances in lipid metabolism, although these findings are still equivocal (Mertz, 1993; Greenburg, 2000). Changes in serum lipids in response to chromium supplementation have been investigated in both nondiabetic and diabetic subjects (Abraham et al., 1992; Greenburg, 2000). Long-term chromium supplementation trials are needed, however, to confirm a role for chromium in the prevention of cardiovascular disease and to establish its mode of action.

Food sources and dietary intakes

Reliable data on the chromium content of foodstuffs are limited, but some of the best food sources of chromium are brewers' yeast, liver, processed meats, spices, whole-grain cereals including some ready-to-eat bran cereals, legumes such as dried beans, and some vegetables such as broccoli and mushrooms. The chromium content of cereals tends to decrease with refining and processing. Dairy products and most fruits and vegetables contain only very small amounts of chromium (Anderson et al., 1988, 1992). Some brands of beer and wine may contain significant quantities of chromium (Cabrera-Vique et al., 1997).

Food composition values for chromium determined before 1980 are often unreliable and only those based on recent analyses should be used (Hunt and Stoecker, 1996). Release 16 of the USDA Nutrient Database for Standard Reference does not include data for chromium (USDA, 2003). Some values for selected foods are listed in Thomas (2003). No recent national nutrition surveys have generated results on chromium intakes. Anderson et al. (1992) reported that U.S. self-selected and institutionalized diets had an average chromium density of 13.4 µg/1000 kcal and ranged from 8.4 to 23.7 µg/1000 kcal.

Effects of high intakes of chromium

There is no evidence that excessive intakes of trivalent chromium from food or supplements are associated with adverse effects. High doses fed to rodents, fish, and cats (Schroeder et al., 1962) had no apparent toxic responses. Likewise, intravenous chromium supplementation of 250 µg/d to chromium-deficient, malnourished children produced no toxicity (Hopkins et al., 1968). Hence, the U.S. Food and Nutrition Board concluded that data are insufficient to establish an Tolerable Upper Intake Level for soluble chromium III salts. More studies are required to more completely assess the safety of high-doses of trivalent chromium from supplements (IOM, 2001).

In contrast, the toxicological effects of hexavalent chromium, which can penetrate biological membranes relatively easily and cause oxidative damage to cell contents, are well known. Exposure to industrial hexavalent chromium in chrome plate workers and welders is a particular problem (Vaglenov et al., 1999). Toxic effects include contact dermatitis, skin ulcers, perforation of the nasal septum, bronchial asthma, and increased incidence of bronchogenic carcinoma (Langard, 1980).

Indices of chromium status

One of the biggest difficulties faced by all chromium researchers today is the absence of an accepted, simple, reliable test to assess chromium status. As a result, it is difficult to quantify the incidence and severity of chromium deficiency in the population. At present, no chromium-dependent enzyme has been identified, in part because the specific biological function of chromium is still unclear. Instead, chromium concentrations in serum, urine, and hair have been investigated as potential measures of chromium status. Only those analytical values reported after 1980 and which have been generated using appropriate quality-control procedures, should be considered.

Further studies are needed to establish the usefulness of chromium concentrations in these biological fluids and tissues as biomarkers of chromium status. At present, the best method of identifying marginal chromium deficiency is still a retrospective diagnosis based on an improvement in glucose tolerance after chromium supplementation at physiological levels. Implementation of such a procedure, however, is limited by the difficulty of identifying potentially chromium-responsive individuals. The tests currently used are discussed in the following sections.

24.1.1 Serum chromium

Chromium in serum exists largely as Cr^{3+}. It is bound competitively to transferrin, which transports chromium in the blood to body tissues. Serum chromium concentrations reflect recent intake and are not necessarily indicative of tissue chromium stores. The latter are markedly higher than those in serum and not in equilibrium with serum concentrations. Reported values for serum chromium have declined dramatically since the 1970s (Table 24.2). Early values are probably unreliable and associated with contamination during sample preparation and analysis (Brune et al., 1993).

Serum chromium concentrations respond to chromium supplementation (Lukaski et al., 1996) but do not necessarily correlate with serum glucose or insulin in the fasting state or after a glucose load (Offenbacher et al., 1985).

Factors affecting serum chromium

Gender may influence the concentration of chromium in serum, but only at certain ages. In a study of 11,715 U.K. ambulatory, non-hospitalized patients aged $\leqslant 75$ y, Davies et al. (1997) reported significantly higher values in males than in females aged 35 to 54 y. Further, serum chromium levels were significantly correlated with hair chromium in both males and females in this study.

Year	Serum chromium (µg/L)
1948–1970	28–1000
1971	13
1972	10
1974	1.6
1974	150
1976	1.3
1978	6.1
1980	1.7
1983	0.43
1984	0.13
1984	0.12
1985	0.13

Table 24.2: Changes in the reported mean concentrations of chromium in serum or plasma. Data from Kobla and Volpe, Critical Reviews in Food Science and Nutrition 40: 291–308, 2000. Conversion factor to SI units (nmol/L) = × 19.31.

Age-related decreases in serum or plasma chromium levels for males and females have been described. In U.K. ambulatory, nonhospitalized outpatients, concentrations declined from about 9.6 nmol/L in early childhood to about 5.8 nmol/L at 70 y (Davies et al., 1997). Whether this age-related decline is a normal physiological development or due to poor nutrition is uncertain.

Diurnal variation in both serum and plasma chromium concentrations occur. The changes appear to be dominated by the effects of an insulin response to meals. Note the inverse relationship ($r=-0.39$; $p<0.001$) between plasma chromium and plasma insulin concentrations over a 24-h period shown in Figure 24.2. This inverse relationship was also evident after a 75-g glucose load (Morris et al., 1992). Plasma chromium levels exhibit a sharp decline between breakfast and early afternoon, after which they increase, falling again after the evening meal. However, during sleep plasma chromium is approximately constant.

Pregnancy appears to be associated with a decline in serum chromium concentrations, possibly due to increased requirements for chromium at this time (Wallach and Verch, 1984), although these results require confirmation. Serum chromium does not predict

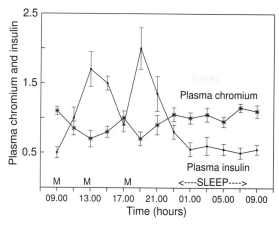

Figure 24.2: Plasma chromium (nmol/L) and plasma insulin (nmol/L) over a 24-h period. Normalized data, normalized to mean of individual. M, meal times; mean ± SE; All data points, $n = 117$. Data from Morris et al., American Journal of Clinical Nutrition 55: 989–991, 1992 © Am J Clin Nutr. American Society for Clinical Nutrition.

	Tannery workers	Control subjects
Serum Cr (ng/ml)	0.49 (0.37–0.81)	0.15 (0.12–0.20)
Urinary Cr (ng/ml)	0.96 (0.62–2.75)	0.24 (0.16–0.31)
Urinary Cr/Cre (ng/mg)	0.83 (0.48–1.82)	0.18 (0.13–0.26)

Table 24.3: Serum and urinary chromium and urinary chromium creatinine (Cre) ratios in tannery workers and controls. Median and 1st–3rd Quartiles). Levels for tannery workers are significantly higher than those for the controls for each measure ($p < 0.0001$, Kruskal-Wallis test). Data from Randall and Gibson, Proceedings of the Society for Experimental Biology and Medicine 185: 16–23, 1987.

glucose tolerance during pregnancy however. In a study of 79 women with abnormal results for a 50-g glucose challenge test during the third trimester, serum chromium levels did not correlate with glucose intolerance, insulin resistance, or serum lipids (Gunton et al., 2001).

Type I and type 2 diabetes mellitus have not been consistently associated with lower serum chromium concentrations (Vanderlinde et al., 1979; Rabinowitz et al., 1983; Morris et al., 1988). Such discrepancies may be related in part to analytical inadequacies.

Dietary chromium supplements increase serum chromium levels (Lukaski et al., 1996), although the size of the increase depends on the type of supplement, dose, and chromium nutriture of the subjects (Thomas, 2003). In two studies in which a daily supplement of 200 μg/d of chromium as chromium chloride was given for 10 or 12 wk, significant increases were observed (Anderson et al., 1985; Offenbacher et al., 1985).

Industrial exposure to trivalent and hexavalent chromium increases serum chromium concentrations (Alsbirk et al., 1981; Randall and Gibson, 1987). Table 24.3 shows a significant increase in serum chromium concentrations in tannery workers exposed to industrial trivalent chromium. Further, concentrations of serum chromium were positively correlated with hair ($r = 0.52$; $p < 0.01$), and urine ($r = 0.72$, $p < 0.0001$) chromium levels (Randall and Gibson, 1987, 1989). These findings suggest that serum chromium may provide an index of industrial exposure to trivalent chromium.

Interpretive criteria

Data are insufficient to establish interpretive criteria for serum chromium concentrations. Even subjects with a marginal chromium status who have showed improved glucose tolerance following chromium supplementation, have not had consistently lower serum chromium concentrations than those showing no such response (Anderson et al., 1985, 1987; Morris et al., 1992).

A tentative range for serum chromium concentrations of 1–3 nmol/L for adults with no known exposure to either tri- or hexavalent chromium has been suggested by Brune et al. (1993). Davies et al. (1997) present data for serum chromium (μg/L) (mean ± SD) for U.K. ambulatory non-hospitalized male and female patients ($n = 11,715$) aged ≤ 75 y in 16 age groups.

Measurement of serum chromium

Analysis of chromium in serum is difficult, and the reader is advised to consult the review by Veillon and Patterson (1999) for specific details. Blood samples must be collected in plastic syringes (Safety Monovette, Sarstedt Inc.) with silicon-treated needles. Sample preparation and analysis must be conducted in ultra-clean rooms to avoid adventitious contamination, and precision and accuracy of the analytical methods must be controlled by using certified reference materials. A standard reference material (Bovine serum, SRM 1598) certified for chromium is available from the U.S. National Institute of Standards and Technology (NIST), Gaithersburg, MD. Versieck et al. (1988) have also produced a certified freeze-dried chromium reference material for serum. Some other agencies producing biological reference materials with established chromium levels are listed in Appendix A4.1. Graphite furnace AAS with Zeeman-effect background correction is now generally used for serum chromium analyses. Care must be used because this method is very susceptible to matrix interferences, Other methods, less frequently used, include neutron activation analysis and mass spectrometry. Inductively-coupled plasma-mass spectrometry can also be used; details are given in Veillon and Patterson (1999).

24.1.2 Changes in serum chromium after a glucose load

Changes in serum chromium concentrations 1 h after a glucose load have been advocated as an index of chromium status (Mertz, 1981b). The change is expressed as the ratio of the 1-h serum chromium to the fasting serum chromium and is termed the "relative chromium response." This approach is based on the apparent increase in serum chromium values after a glucose load in normal subjects, but not in diabetic patients, who are assumed to have a suboptimal chromium status. Increases in diabetic subjects were only observed after chromium supplementation (Glinsmann et al., 1966). These results

suggest that subjects with adequate chromium stores release chromium from tissues after a glucose load, resulting in increased serum chromium concentrations. Unfortunately, such a response in healthy subjects has not been a consistent finding (Doisy et al., 1971; Davidson and Burt, 1973; Liu and Morris, 1978; Liu and Abernathy, 1982; Anderson et al., 1985). Hence, the physiological interpretation of acute changes in serum chromium after a glucose load is still uncertain, and the relative chromium response cannot be considered a reliable index.

24.1.3 Erythrocyte and whole blood chromium

Data on erythrocyte and whole blood chromium concentrations are limited. The physiological levels of chromium in erythrocytes appear to be 20 times higher than in plasma, thus facilitating chromium analysis (Manthey and Kübler, 1980; Rabinowitz et al., 1980). Nevertheless, reported erythrocyte chromium concentrations have a wide range, and there is a considerable overlap of values for diabetics and normal persons. Some investigators have suggested that erythrocyte chromium concentrations may serve as a biomarker of industrial exposure to hexavalent chromium (Lewalter et al., 1985; Wiegand et al., 1985; Vaglenov et al., 1999).

Whole blood chromium concentrations approximate 56 nmol/L in normal healthy adults (Nomiyama et al., 1980; Zober et al., 1984). A few studies have used whole blood chromium concentrations as an index of industrial chromium exposure (Kiilunen et al., 1983; Rahkonen et al., 1983; Edme et al., 1997). Data on whole blood chromium concentrations in studies of suboptimal chromium status are sparse.

24.1.4 Urinary chromium

Urine is the major excretory route for absorbed chromium, accounting for about 95% of chromium excretion (Mertz, 1969). Small amounts of absorbed chromium are lost in the hair, perspiration, and bile (Doisy et al.,

Authors and year	Urinary Cr : Creatinine (ng/mg)
Davidson et al., 1974	1.65
Gürson and Saner, 1978	7.43
Anderson et al., 1982a	0.10

Table 24.4: Post-1966 data for urinary chromium : creatinine ratios in adults.

Subjects	Males	Females
Control		
Self-selected diets	4.05 ± 1.42	4.81 ± 1.35
4 wk low-Cr diet	1.75 ± 0.56	2.56 ± 0.46
Placebo	2.92 ± 0.88	3.35 ± 0.88
Cr supplementation	8.04 ± 2.08	13.7 ± 2.12
Hyperglycemic		
Self-selected diets	3.12 ± 0.62	2.69 ± 0.44
4 wk low-Cr diet	2.52 ± 0.81	2.14 ± 0.52
Placebo	2.71 ± 0.77	2.14 ± 0.44
Cr supplementation	19.35 ± 6.56	11.83 ± 2.48

Table 24.5: Effect of the diet and chromium supplementation on mean ($\pm$ SE) 24-h chromium excretion (mmol/d). Data from Anderson et al., American Journal of Clinical Nutrition 54: 909–916, 1991 © Am J Clin Nutr. American Society for Clinical Nutrition.

1971). Hence, theoretically, urine could be a useful index of recent chromium intake, with data expressed in terms of ng/mg creatinine (Table 24.4). Certainly both urinary chromium concentration and 24-h excretion are responsive to chromium supplementation. However, they are questionable biomarkers of chromium status because urinary chromium concentrations do not correlate with glucose or insulin concentrations (Offenbacher et al., 1985).

The average urinary chromium excretion for normal healthy adults is about 0.2 μg/d (Anderson et al., 1982b). Like serum, reported urinary chromium excretion values have decreased with improved sampling and analytical procedures (Table 24.4) and control of adventitious contamination (Veillon and Patterson., 1999). Values that are accepted as likely to be accurate are < 1.0 μg/d for normal healthy subjects.

Factors affecting urinary chromium

Level of recent chromium intake influences urinary chromium excretion. Studies by Anderson et al. (1982a, 1983a) have reported urinary chromium excretion levels that were approximately 0.5%, and 2% of the amount of dietary chromium, when daily intakes were 40 μg and 10 μg of chromium, respectively. Moreover, in this range of dietary intakes, a negative linear relationship has been reported between the intake and urinary excretion of chromium (Anderson and Kozlovsky, 1985).

One experimentally controlled chromium depletion–repletion study has been carried out to date. In this study, urinary chromium losses tended to be lower after 4 wk of a low-chromium diet compared with levels on the self-selected diets, as shown in Table 24.5,

but differences were not significant (Anderson et al., 1991b). After supplementation with chromium for 4 wk in this study, urinary chromium excretion levels increased significantly ($p < 0.05$) in males and females in both groups.

Industrial exposure to both tri- (Randall and Gibson, 1987) and hexavalent (Vaglenov et al.,1999) chromium increases the urinary chromium concentrations, as noted in the tannery worker study shown in Table 24.3. The urinary chromium : creatinine ratios were also elevated in these tannery workers compared to controls, and positively correlated with hair chromium levels (Randall and Gibson, 1989).

Consumption of diets high in simple sugars increases the urinary chromium excretion, with the rise occurring within 90 min of the high sugar intake (Kozlovsky et al. 1986). The effect is related to the insulinogenic properties of carbohydrates: simple sugars lead to a greater increase in circulating insulin, which in turn results in greater urinary chromium losses (Anderson et al., 1990).

Diurnal variation strongly influences urinary chromium concentrations. In a study of 9 healthy adults, urinary chromium excretion, expressed in terms of creatinine, declined

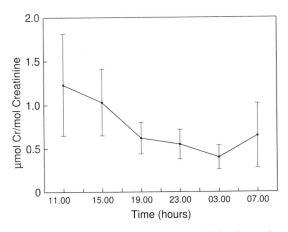

Figure 24.3: Urine chromium (µmol Cr/mol creatinine) excretion over 24 h. Sampling frequency, 4 h; results (mean ± SE) plotted mid-point between sampling. From Morris et al., American Journal of Clinical Nutrition 55: 989–991, 1992 © Am J Clin Nutr. American Society for Clinical Nutrition.

steadily throughout a 24-h period but then returned to near their initial values over the last collection period, as shown in Figure 24.3 (Morris et al., 1992).

Acute strenuous exercise increases urinary chromium excretion. The magnitude of the increase is related to the duration and intensity of the exercise. Anderson et al. (1984) reported a nearly 5-fold increase in urinary chromium concentrations in nine male runners 2 h after a 6-mile run. Increases in serum glucose and glucagon also occurred (Anderson et al., 1982a).

Such increases in urinary chromium levels after acute strenuous exercise result from the mobilization of chromium induced by the increased uptake of glucose by muscle during exercise. The increases have been related to the level of stress as measured by post-exercise serum cortisol (Anderson et al., 1991a). Some suggest that increased urinary losses following exercise may be offset by increased chromium absorption (Rubin et al., 1998).

Stress, infection, and physical trauma (including disease), like physical exercise, all lead to increased urinary chromium losses

(Anderson et al., 1991a). Again, the magnitude of the increase depends on the degree of stress (Anderson et al., 1991a).

Type 1 and type 2 diabetes elevate urinary chromium excretion compared with levels in healthy subjects (Morris et al., 1988; Morris et al., 1999). The increase in excretion probably results from chromium mobilization in response to increased glucose metabolism or an elevated insulin response. The magnitude of this effect depends on the degree of glucose intolerance (Anderson et al., 1987, 1990; Morris et al., 1988, 1999).

Use of medications including aspirin, antacids, and corticosteroids may alter urinary chromium excretion (Thomas, 2003). However, some of these reported urinary chromium values are suspiciously high, and hence the importance of these factors remains uncertain.

Interpretive criteria

Urinary chromium levels in normal healthy persons are very low and approach the limits of detection for many analytical methods. In general, urinary chromium excretion is more useful as an index of overexposure than as an index of suboptimal chromium status (Table 24.3). Correlations of urinary chromium excretion with selected clinical parameters of chromium depletion have produced inconclusive results (Anderson et al., 1983b). As a result, interpretive criteria for urinary chromium indicative of chromium depletion have not been defined. Tentative reference ranges for normal healthy subjects with no known exposure to chromium range from 2 to 10 nmol/L or 0.2 to 1.0 µmol/mol creatinine (Brune et al., 1993).

Measurement of urinary chromium

Graphite furnace AAS with Zeeman-effect background correction is often used for urinary chromium analysis. The method of additions must be used (Veillon and Patterson, 1999), in view of the susceptibility of this method to interference from the sample matrix.

Twenty-four-hour urine samples are preferred, although urinary chromium concentrations can also be determined on casual urine samples, when they are expressed as a chromium : creatinine ratio, as shown in Table 24.4 (Anderson et al., 1983b; Randall and Gibson, 1987).

24.1.5 Changes in urinary chromium after a glucose load

Changes in urinary chromium excretion after a glucose load have also been examined as a potential index of chromium status. Subjects with depleted chromium stores are postulated not to show an increase in urinary chromium losses after a glucose load, whereas those with sufficient chromium stores lose additional chromium in response to a glucose load.

However, changes in urinary chromium excretion in normal healthy and diabetic subjects following a glucose load have not been consistent (Anderson et al., 1982a, 1991b, Morris et al., 1988). In the study shown in Table 24.6, urinary chromium losses after a glucose challenge were significantly greater after chromium supplementation, and the response of both control and hyperglycemic subjects was similar (Anderson et al., 1991a).

The magnitude of the increase probably depends on the glucose tolerance of the subjects. Hence, a suboptimal chromium status may not be detected by changes in urinary chromium excretion after an oral glucose tolerance test.

24.1.6 Hair chromium concentrations

Studies of the use of hair as a biopsy material for assessing chromium status are limited. Because scalp hair is exposed to adventitious contamination, standardized collection and washing procedures are essential prior to analysis. Concentrations of chromium in hair are markedly higher than those in serum and urine, thus facilitating analyses. Davies et al. (1997) analyzed hair chromium concentrations in a large group ($n = 40,872$) of ambulatory, nonhospitalized patients. Concentrations declined significantly with age (Figure 24.4), in parallel with serum chromium concentrations.

Additional confounding factors that affect trace-element concentrations in hair include hair color, hair beauty treatments, pregnancy, season, geographical location, parity, smoking, and the presence of certain disease states (Section 15.1.9). To date, the effects of only

Subjects	Placebo	Chromium
Control		
0–90 min Cr	0.30 ± 0.05	1.10 ± 0.29
90–180 min Cr	0.30 ± 0.05	0.87 ± 0.19
Hyperglycemic		
0–90 min Cr	0.24 ± 0.06	0.93 ± 0.20
90–180 min Cr	0.26 ± 0.04	0.82 ± 0.20

Table 24.6: Effect of supplemental chromium and glucose on mean ($\pm$ SE) urinary chromium excretion (nmol/90 min) after a glucose load in both control and hyperglycemic subjects. The urine samples were collected at the designated times after the glucose load. Data from Anderson et al., American Journal of Clinical Nutrition 54: 909–916, 1991 © Am J Clin Nutr. American Society for Clinical Nutrition.

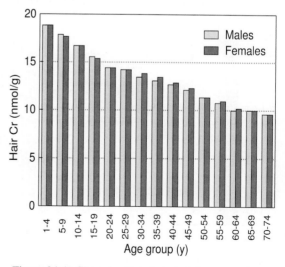

Figure 24.4: Chromium levels in hair by age and sex. Data from Davies et al., Metabolism 46: 469–473, 1997.

some of these factors on hair chromium concentrations are known.

Evidence that hair chromium concentrations may provide a chronic index of chromium status comes from a variety of sources:

- Hair chromium concentrations are low in persons with non-insulin-dependent diabetes, a disease associated with marginal chromium deficiency.
- Decreases in hair chromium concentrations with age apparently parallel those in serum (Davies et al., 1997) and tissue chromium (Schroeder et al., 1962).
- Low hair chromium concentrations were noted in a long-term TPN patient with a chromium-responsive deficiency syndrome (Jeejeebhoy et al., 1977).
- A dose/effect relationship in tannery workers between the area of work in the tannery and hair chromium concentrations was documented by Randall and Gibson (1989) (Figure 24.5).
- Hair chromium concentrations correlated positively with serum and urinary chromium levels in tannery workers exposed to industrial trivalent chromium (Randall and Gibson, 1989).

These findings suggest that hair chromium concentrations may be a useful biomarker

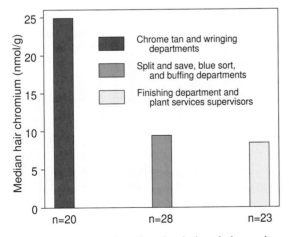

Figure 24.5: Hair chromium levels in relation to industrial exposure in a tannery. From Randall and Gibson, British Journal of Industrial Medicine 46: 171–175, 1989, with permission.

of chronic chromium status. Nevertheless, interpretive criteria for hair chromium concentrations are not yet available. Instead, values derived from the at-risk subjects must be compared with an age- and sex-matched healthy control group.

Davies et al. (1997) have compiled data for hair chromium for males and females aged $\leqslant 75\,y$ in 16 age groups. Data are based on hair samples from 22,013 ambulatory, non-hospitalized U.K. patients and hence do not represent a true "healthy reference sample."

Measurement of hair chromium

Standardized procedures are necessary for the sampling, washing, and analysis of hair samples for chromium (Section 15.1.9). Several washing procedures have been investigated. These include using nonionic or anionic detergents such as sodium lauryl sulfate (SLS), hexane-methanol, acetone, triton-X10, water, and a mixture of hexane and ethanol (Hambidge et al., 1972b). Kumpulainen et al. (1982) suggest using two 20-min washes in SLS after a hexane rinse for hair chromium analysis.

Hair samples must be ashed or digested prior to analysis by graphite furnace AAS with Zeeman-effect background correction. A certified reference material for human hair (Community Bureau of Reference Certified Reference Material #397) can be obtained from the Institute for Reference Materials and Measurements, Retieseweg, B-2440, Geel, Belgium, and this or a similar standard should always be used to confirm the accuracy of the analytical method.

24.1.7 Oral glucose tolerance test

At present, an abnormal result of a glucose tolerance test is taken as suggestive of a low chromium status, because of the absence of a more specific test to diagnose chromium deficiency. However, impaired glucose tolerance has many causes and, hence, is inadequate as the sole diagnostic criterion for suboptimal chromium status. Therefore, normally, the existence of chromium deficiency is only confirmed if at physiological levels, an improvement in glucose tolerance follows supplementation with chromium.

Such an approach has been used in most of the placebo-controlled chromium supplementation studies reported in the literature (Mertz, 1993). Results have been variable, as noted earlier. Only some of these studies have shown improvements in impaired glucose tolerance after chromium supplementation; in some cases they have shown beneficial effects on serum insulin or blood lipid profiles. In part, these discrepancies have arisen from including normal, hypoglycemic, hyperglycemic, and diabetic subjects in a single group. Such inconsistent results have emphasized the limitations of using an abnormal result of a glucose tolerance test to diagnose chromium-responsive individuals.

To better assess the validity of the glucose tolerance test in truly chromium-responsive individuals, Anderson et al. (1991b) carried out glucose tolerance tests on 17 subjects participating in an experimentally controlled chromium depletion – repletion study. All subjects received a low chromium diet for 14 wk, and after a 4-wk adaptation period, they were assigned to either a placebo or chromium supplementation group for 5 wk, followed by a crossover for another 5 wk. Four-hour glucose tolerance tests were performed after weeks 1, 4, 9, and 14 using a glucose dose of 1 g/kg body weight. Blood was taken at 0, 30, 60, 90, 120, 180, and 240 minutes.

Results for the glucose tolerance test and serum insulin concentrations for eight subjects (22–65 y) in the control group fed the low-chromium diet (5 µg/1000 kcal Cr) for 9 wk, followed by a supplement of 200 µg/d chromium as chromium chloride ($CrCl_3$) for 5 wk, are given in Table 24.7. All these control subjects had baseline 90-min glucose values < 5.56 mmol/L.

After 4 wk on the depletion diet, there were no significant changes; after 9 wk, there was a significant increase in the sums of glucose (i.e., area index total) and in glucose 90 min after the glucose load. In addition, following supplementation with chromium for 5 wk (wk

9–14), there was a tendency ($p < 0.10$) for the sums of glucose and insulin concentrations to be reduced. These results strongly support the role of chromium in regulating blood glucose concentrations in subjects who are chromium depleted.

Several studies have examined the effect of chromium supplementation on glucose tolerance in individuals with type 2 diabetes (Anderson, 1998, 2000). For example, a 2-h glucose tolerance test with a 75-g glucose load was performed in the large-scale chromium supplementation study of 180 Chinese with type 2 diabetes (Anderson et al., 1997). The subjects took either a placebo, 200 µg/d (3.85 µmol/d), or 1000 µg/d (19.2 µmol/d) of chromium as chromium picolinate for 4 mo. Compared to the placebo group, fasting and 2-h glucose concentrations (and oral glucose tolerance test insulin values) decreased in both treatment groups, with greater changes in the high-dose chromium supplement group. Some changes were evident after 2 mo (Figure 24.6), although, in general, 4 mo were

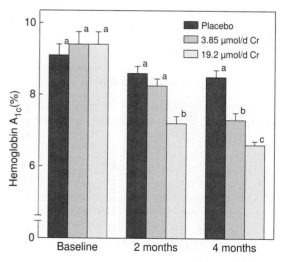

Figure 24.6: Supplemental chromium effects on mean ($\pm$ SD) glycosylated hemoglobin in subjects with type 2 diabetes. Placebo group, $n = 50$; 3.85 µmol (200 µg) group, $n = 53$; 19.2 µmol (1000 µg) group, $n = 52$. Bars with different letters are significantly different from other groups for the same time period at $p < 0.05$. Data from Anderson et al. Diabetes, 46, 1997, 1786–1791 © American Diabetes Association. Reprinted with permission from the American Diabetes Association.

	Week 0	Week 4	Week 9	Week 14
Glucose (nmol/L)				
Fasting	4.9 ± 0.2	4.8 ± 0.1	4.9 ± 0.1	5.1 ± 0.1
90 minute	4.2 ± 0.4	4.5 ± 0.4	5.0 ± 0.6	4.4 ± 0.4
Sums (0–240 min)	33.6 ± 1.6	35.1 ± 1.4	37.0 ± 2.2	34.6 ± 1.6
Insulin (pmol/L)				
Fasting	38 ± 5	33 ± 5	48 ± 6	49 ± 7
Sums (0-240 min)	1146 ± 130	1214 ± 167	1577 ± 354	1319 ± 281

Table 24.7: Glucose and insulin concentrations of eight subjects fed low-chromium (5 µg/1000 kcal) diets for 9 wk, followed by 200 µg/d $CrCl_3$ for 5 wk. The tendency was for reduced sums of glucose and insulin concentration in the subjects at the end of the study. Data from IOM (2001) based on a reanalysis of Anderson et al. (1991b).

needed to produce consistent glucose and insulin-lowering effects. Moreover, at this time glycosylated hemoglobin was also reduced to values of 7.5% and 6.6% in the low-dose and high-dose supplement groups, respectively, whereas it remained quite high at 8.5% in the placebo group at the end of the 4-mo trial. The glycosylated hemoglobin percentage is used to measure long-term glycemic control in individuals with diabetes (Bunn, 1981). It is noteworthy that the final values observed for glycosylated hemoglobin in the chromium-supplemented groups are similar in magnitude to those seen after treatment with diabetes medications (Thomas, 2003).

Measuring glucose tolerance

The glucose tolerance test involves taking a venipuncture blood sample after an overnight fast, to give baseline data on fasting plasma glucose levels. A glucose load is then given orally, after which venipuncture blood samples for plasma glucose analysis are taken at varying time intervals. Sometimes, blood is taken 30, 60, 90, and 120 min after the glucose drink (Levine et al., 1968; National Diabetes Data Group, 1979; Offenbacher and Pi-Sunyer, 1980), or at 45 and 90 min (Offenbacher et al., 1985). When the former intervals are used, the total areas under the curve for glucose are calculated using the following formula:

$$(A/2) + B + C + D + (E/2) = \text{area index total (AIT)}$$

where A is the fasting value, and B, C, D, and

E are the 30, 60, 90, and 120 min values, respectively (Vecchio et al., 1965).

Alternatively, to ease screening in community studies, a single blood glucose level, at 90 min (Anderson et al., 1985) or 120 min (Martinez et al., 1985; Anderson et al., 1997) after the glucose load can be used.

The level of the oral glucose load used has also varied. Oral loading doses of 75 g (Martinez et al., 1985; Offenbacher et al., 1985; Anderson et al., 1997), as recommended by the National Diabetes Data Group (1979), 100 g (Offenbacher and Pi-Sunyer, 1980), or a load of 1 g of glucose per kilogram body weight (Anderson et al., 1985) have all been used. These large differences in glucose load apparently have little effect on blood glucose levels (National Diabetes Data Group, 1979), but higher glucose loads do have a greater effect on stimulating insulin secretion.

Plasma glucose can be analyzed by the glucose oxidase method (Loft and Turner, 1975). Automated procedures are now available. Insulin is now normally analyzed with a commercial radioimmunoassay kit and glycosylated hemoglobin using BioRad HbA$_{lc}$ columns (BioRad Laboratories, Richmond, CA).

24.1.8 Multiple indices

No single reliable biomarker of chromium status exists. Abnormal results of a glucose tolerance test, although tentatively used to identify chromium-responsive individuals, are inadequate as the sole diagnostic criterion for chromium status. Instead, at present, improvement in glucose tolerance after supplementation with chromium at physiological levels is still the best criteria to confirm the existence of chromium deficiency.

In the future, with improvements in analytical techniques, chromium concentrations in serum or hair may be used as a screening tool to identify subjects at risk for chromium deficiency, preferably in combination with evidence of impaired glucose tolerance. Chromium concentrations in different blood fractions may prove to be useful biomarkers of chromium status (Rükgauer and Zeyfang, 2002). Hopefully, once the specific biological function of chromium has been identified, surrogate functional markers of chromium status may be developed, which will have greater diagnostic significance than the determination of total chromium levels in serum and other tissues (Mertz, 1993).

Enzyme and Function

Ceruloplasmin (Ferroxidase I)
    Copper transport, iron mobilization,
    antioxidant

Cytochrome c oxidase   Electron transport, terminal oxidase
Superoxide dismutase   Free radical detoxication
Tyrosinase   Synthesis of melanin
Lysyl oxidase   Collagen and elastin cross-linking
Amine oxidases   Deamination of primary amines
Dopamine-β-monooxygenase   Dopamine → norepinephrine
Peptidylglycine monooxygenase   α-Amidation of neuropeptides

Table 24.8: Function of some copper enzymes with oxidation and reduction activity in humans. From Uauy et al., American Journal of Clinical Nutrition 67S: 952S–959S, 1998 © Am J Clin Nutr. American Society for Clinical Nutrition.

24.2 Copper

The adult human body contains 70–80 mg of copper. Of this, approximately 25% is in the skeletal muscle, 15% in the skin, 15% in the bone marrow, 19% in the skeleton, 8.0 to 15% in the liver, and 8.0% in the brain. The liver and brain contain the highest concentrations of copper. Copper is an essential component of numerous enzyme systems shown in Table 24.8, including many that catalyze oxidation-reduction reactions (Harris, 1997).

Functions of copper

Many clinical features of copper deficiency can be explained by changes in the activities of cuproenzymes. For instance, a reduction in ceruloplasmin (ferroxidase I) (EC 1.16.3.1) impairs the transport of iron to the erythropoietic sites, leading to hypochromic anemia. Deficiency of the cuproenzyme lysyl oxidase (EC 1.4.3.13) may be responsible for the skeletal and vascular defects reported in copper deficiency. Lysyl oxidase is essential for the normal maturation of collagen, spec-

ifically in the steps involving the formation of lysine-derived cross-links (O'Dell, 1976). The latter are required for the formation of strong, flexible connective tissues (Rucker and Murray, 1978).

Depigmentation is often associated with a deficiency of tyrosinase (EC 1.14.18.1), an enzyme involved in the production of melanin. The latter is necessary for protection against excess ultraviolet exposure. The central nervous system disturbances in copper deficiency are the result of myelinization derangements or of abnormal catecholamine levels and associated decreased activity of dopamine-β-monooxygenase (EC 1.14.17.1) or reduced activity of cytochrome c oxidase (EC 1.9.3.1) (Mason, 1979).

Absorption and metabolism of copper

The major site of copper absorption is the small intestine, although some copper is also absorbed from the stomach. Absorption is inversely related to the amount of copper

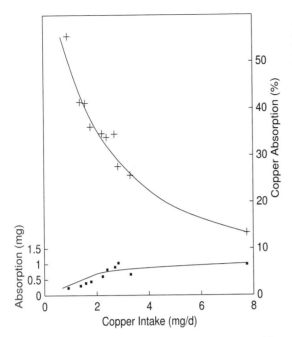

Figure 24.7: Copper absorption as a percentage and in mg/d in relation to a dietary copper intake varying from 0.8–7.5 mg/d. Redrawn from Turnlund et al., American Journal of Clinical Nutrition 67: 960S–964S, 1998 © Am J Clin Nutr. American Society for Clinical Nutrition.

in the diet, decreasing the likelihood of deficiency and toxicity (Turnlund et al., 1989). For dietary intakes above 5 mg/d, absorption is < 20%, whereas for intakes < 1 mg/d, absorption is as high as 50% (Figure 24.7).

Once absorbed, copper is transported via the portal blood bound to albumin and transcuprein, mainly to the liver. In the liver, copper is incorporated into ceruloplasmin, and then distributed to other tissues. For further details, see the review by Linder et al. (1998).

At present, the mechanisms of copper regulation are poorly understood. Tissue copper concentrations are maintained within a narrow range, through homeostatic mechanisms that operate at the level of intestinal absorption and biliary excretion. Of the two levels, biliary excretion is the more important. As more copper is absorbed, turnover is faster, and, hence, more copper is excreted into the

gastrointestinal tract. Very little copper is excreted in the urine, and urinary losses do not help regulate copper stores. Relatively little copper is stored in the body, compared with other trace elements such as iron (Turnlund, 1998).

Copper deficiency in humans

Copper deficiency in humans is rare. It has been described in infants recovering from malnutrition (Graham and Cordano, 1969) and in premature and low-birth-weight infants fed cow's milk (al-Rashid and Spangler, 1971; Griscom et al., 1971; Ashkenazi et al., 1973). Copper deficiency has also been reported in patients receiving prolonged total parenteral nutrition (TPN) unsupplemented with copper (Karpel and Peden, 1972; Dunlap et al., 1974; Vilter et al., 1974) and in a woman receiving a normal diet supplemented with antacids (Anonymous, 1984a). Severely handicapped patients ($n = 60$) receiving an enteral diet with only 15 µg/1000 kcal Cu for 12 to 66 mo also developed copper deficiency (Higuchi et al., 1988).

The earliest clinical manifestation of copper deficiency in humans is persistent neutropenia, usually followed by hypochromic microcytic anemia, scurvy-like bone changes, and osteoporosis (in infants) (Cordano et al., 1964; al-Rashid and Spangler, 1971; Karpel and Peden, 1972; Higuchi et al., 1988). The anemia probably results from defective iron mobilization and hemoglobin formation related to lower ceruloplasmin activity (Danks, 1988), or to increased susceptibility to oxidative damage (Johnson and Kramer, 1987).

Less frequent features of copper deficiency include hypopigmentation of the hair and hypotonia (low muscle tone), as well as impaired growth, the increased incidence of infections, and changes in the phagocytic capacity of the neutrophils (Uauy et al., 1998). In some experimental depletion–repletion studies, changes in blood clotting factors (Milne and Nielsen, 1996) and in markers of bone metabolism (Baker et al., 1999a) have also been reported. Low copper intakes have been implicated as a risk factor in the development of cardiovascular disease (Lukaski et al., 1988, Klevay, 2000).

A few cases of adults with sickle cell disease who were receiving prolonged zinc therapy have developed hematological signs of copper deficiency (Prasad et al., 1978a). Clinical features of copper deficiency, with the exception of anemia, occur in infants with Menkes' kinky hair syndrome (KHS), an X-linked, recessive, hereditary disorder of copper metabolism with an intracellular defect of copper utilization (Danks et al., 1972).

Most of the reports of copper deficiency in humans have resulted from inadequate dietary intakes of copper, often associated with prolonged diarrhea, which prevents reabsorption of copper from the bile. Hence, it is not surprising that subjects with malabsorption syndromes — including tropical sprue, celiac disease, cystic fibrosis, and short-bowel syndrome resulting from intestinal resection — are at risk of copper deficiency (Rodriguez et al., 1985).

Diseases associated with chronic loss of proteins, such as nephritic syndrome and protein-losing enteropathy, may also cause copper deficiency as a result of loss of ceruloplasmin and of copper bound to albumin. High intakes of fructose and sucrose exacerbate the effects of copper deficiency, but the importance of this effect in humans is unclear (O'Dell, 1990).

Food sources and dietary intakes

Copper is widely distributed in foods; the richest food sources are oysters, other shellfish, organ meats (e.g., liver, kidney), nuts, and dried legumes. Milk and dairy products are low in copper. The copper level in plants is not influenced by the copper content of the soil in which they grow (Pennington et al., 1995). Drinking water may contribute a relatively large amount of copper to the daily intake, especially if the water is slightly acidic or very soft and is supplied from copper pipes (Lönnerdal, 1996).

Copper deficiency among the general population has not been described. Dietary intakes of copper for adult European populations range from 0.9 to 2.3 mg/d (van Dokkum, 1995). Data are available on the copper intakes of the U.S. population based on the Continuing Survey of Food Intakes by Individuals (CSFII) 1994–1996 and NHANES III (IOM, 2001) and for the U.K. population, based on the National Diet and Nutrition Surveys (Gregory et al., 1990, 1995, 2000; Finch et al., 1998; Henderson et al., 2003). Copper intakes of infants fed breast milk or cow's milk are often low.

The composition of mixed western diets has little effect on the bioavailability of copper in humans. Copper deficiency has been observed in some cases of excessively high intakes of iron or zinc supplements (Fischer et al., 1984; Barclay et al., 1991; Botash et al., 1992), induced by their adverse effect on copper absorption. There is some evidence that the adverse effect of high dietary iron intake on copper absorption may occur only when copper status is low or marginal (Cohen et al., 1985).

Effect of high intakes of copper

Several cases of accidental copper toxicity in humans have been described, arising from ingestion of copper sulfate (Chuttani et al., 1965), acidic drinks in prolonged contact with copper (Paine, 1968), or drinking water with an unusually high copper concentration (800 µg/L) (Salmon and Wright, 1971). Adverse effects include nausea, gastrointestinal effects (nausea, diarrhea, cramps, abdominal pain), and, in some cases, liver damage (O'Donohue et al., 1993; Pizarro et al., 1999).

Patients suffering from Wilson's disease, a copper-related genetic defect, also exhibit symptoms of copper toxicity such as nausea, vomiting, diarrhea, acute hemolytic anemia, hepatic necrosis, hepatic central vein dilation, and jaundice (Zelkowitz et al., 1980). In Wilson's disease, copper accumulates in the liver because the copper in the liver cells can neither enter the bile nor participate in ceruloplasmin synthesis (Linder and Hazegh-Azam, 1996).

There is no evidence that high dietary copper intakes are a public health problem. The U.S Tolerable Upper Intake Level (UL) for copper for adults ≥19 y is 10 mg/d. For pregnant and lactating women and adolescents 14–18 y, the UL is set at 8 mg/d (IOM, 2001).

Indices of copper status

The methods used to assess copper status in humans include static tests, as well as the measurement of the activities of certain copper enzymes. These methods are discussed below. There is still no consensus on the best biomarker to use, in part, because of the efficiency of the homeostatic control that maintains tissue copper concentrations within a narrow range. As a result, measures of copper status tend to be resistant to change, except when dietary intakes are very low or very high.

Serum copper or serum ceruloplasmin are most often used to assess copper status, but the sensitivity and specificity of both these measures are poor. Hence, they should be combined with a more sensitive and specific functional measure such as cytochrome c oxidase in platelets or superoxide dismutase in erythrocytes. It is likely that in the future functional indicators, perhaps including antioxidant status, changes in immune function, and the lysyl oxidase activity in skin, will be used in conjunction with other biochemical markers.

24.2.1 Serum copper

There are two main forms of copper in serum; one is firmly bound to ceruloplasmin, the other is reversibly bound to serum albumin. Serum also contains the two copper enzymes cytochrome c oxidase and monoamine oxidase, a small amount of free copper, and copper bound to amino acids. The function of the amino acid–bound copper fraction is unknown.

Serum copper concentrations are a reliable biomarker in cases of severe copper deficiency, when they are almost always low. However, they are not sensitive enough to

be used as a measure of marginal copper status, as noted earlier, and do not reflect dietary intake, except when it is low. Normally, supplementation with copper does not increase serum copper because concentrations are under strict homeostatic control. Levels are only reduced after copper stores are significantly depleted. In healthy adults consuming diets adequate in copper, the lower end of the normal range for serum copper is 10 µmol/L.

Experimental studies have confirmed that serum copper is not a sensitive index of marginal copper status in adults (Reiser et al., 1985; Turnlund et al., 1989; Milne and Nielsen, 1996). In a depletion–repletion study of postmenopausal women fed a diet with only 0.57 mg/d Cu for 105 d, serum copper levels did not change significantly during the copper-depletion period (Figure 24.8), despite the presence of other biochemical changes (Milne and Nielsen, 1996).

Eventually serum copper concentrations do fall. In patients receiving prolonged TPN unsupplemented with copper, falls of about 1.7 µmol/L per week may occur (Solomons et al., 1976). Values < 9.5–11 µmol/L have been reported in infants with copper defi-

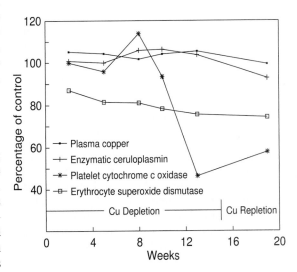

Figure 24.8: Changes in copper biomarkers during copper deprivation. Each data point is the mean of 3 wk surrounding date. Data from Milne and Nielsen, American Journal of Clinical Nutrition 63: 358–364, 1996 © Am J Clin Nutr. American Society for Clinical Nutrition.

ciency (Cordano et al., 1964; Castillo-Duran and Uauy, 1988). Low serum copper concentrations also occur with the two genetic disorders of copper metabolism: Menkes' kinky hair syndrome and Wilson's disease. In Menkes' kinky hair syndrome, low serum copper concentrations arise from an intracellular defect of copper utilization, as discussed earlier (Danks et al., 1972). In Wilson's disease, the low serum copper levels are induced by defects in the hepatic storage of copper and in ceruloplasmin metabolism.

Plasma copper concentrations appear to be consistently lower than corresponding values in serum (Table 24.9) (Smith et al., 1985). In contrast, concentrations of copper in serum and erythrocytes are comparable, so slight hemolysis does not affect serum copper concentrations.

Age group (years)	Men	Women
Serum copper (µmol/L)		
25–34	14.7 ± 0.6	14.8 ± 0.5
35–44	15.0 ± 0.3	16.7 ± 0.4
45–54	16.2 ± 0.4	17.8 ± 0.6
55–64	16.3 ± 0.4	18.8 ± 0.7
65+	15.3 ± 1.0	16.8 ± 0.5
Ceruloplasmin (U/dL)		
25–34	9.9 ± 0.7	11.0 ± 0.6
35–44	10.8 ± 0.3	12.8 ± 0.4
45–54	11.9 ± 0.4	15.2 ± 1.1
55–64	11.8 ± 0.5	14.1 ± 0.8
65+	11.3 ± 1.2	12.3 ± 1.1

Table 24.10: Effect of age in men and women who were not taking estrogen-containing preparations on serum copper concentration and ceruloplasmin activity. Data from Fischer et al., Nutrition Research 10: 1081–1090, 1990.

Factors affecting serum copper

Age-related changes in serum copper concentrations are well documented. Newborn infants have low values, which rise to adult levels by 6 to 12 mo of age (Salmenperä et al., 1986). In men, and in women not taking estrogen-containing preparations, serum copper levels increase with age until 55–64 y,

after which they decline (Table 24.10) (Fischer et al., 1990; Milne and Johnson, 1993).

Gender influences serum copper. Levels in adult females tend to be higher than in males (Table 24.10).

Pregnancy influences serum copper concentrations. Higher serum copper concentrations are evident after the third month of pregnancy (Halsted et al., 1968; Hambidge and Droegemueller, 1974).

Estrogen-containing preparations, such as oral contraceptive agents and estrogen replacement therapy, elevate serum copper concentrations (hypercupremia) (Table 24.11) (Fischer et al., 1990; Nielsen et al., 1992). This effect is due to an estrogen-mediated rise in serum ceruloplasmin concentration. No differences in copper absorption or copper balance have been reported between users and non-users of oral contraceptive agents (King et al., 1978; Crews et al., 1980).

Subject no.	Serum (µmol/L)	Plasma (µmol/L)	Percentage difference
1	20.0	19.4	3
2	18.7	17.8	5
3	19.0	17.3	9
4	19.2	16.7	13
5	19.5	16.7	15
6	19.4	16.5	15
7	18.1	16.5	9
8	16.5	15.4	7
Mean $\pm$ SD	18.9 ± 1.1	17.0 ± 1.1	9 ± 4

Table 24.9: Copper concentrations of serum or citrated plasma prepared from single venipuncture samples of eight subjects. Plasma was prepared by adding 0.15 mL of 30% sodium citrate per 15 mL of whole blood. Percentage difference = [(serum – plasma)/serum] × 100. From Smith et al., Journal of the American College of Nutrition 4: 627–638, 1985 © John Wiley & Sons, Inc., with permission.

Diurnal variation in serum copper concentrations has been noted (Cartwright, 1950; Guillard et al., 1979); the highest levels occur in the morning (Lifschitz and Henkin, 1971).

| | Premenopausal women | |
	Non-users of OCA	Users of OCA
Serum copper (μmol/L)	16.2 ± 0.3	26.8 ± 1.3
Ceruloplasmin (U/dL)	12.2 ± 0.4	20.4 ± 0.9
	Postmenopausal women	
	Non-users of estrogens	Users of estrogens
Serum copper (μmol/L)	18.1 ± 0.4	25.9 ± 1.2
Ceruloplasmin (U/dL)	14.5 ± 0.7	19.7 ± 1.0

Table 24.11: Effect of oral contraceptive agents (OCA) and estrogen replacement therapy on serum copper concentration and ceruloplasmin activity. Data from Fischer et al., Nutrition Research 10: 1081–1090, 1990.

Regular strenuous exercise may also affect serum copper concentrations. Lukaski et al. (1983) showed values to be higher in male university athletes relative to controls.

Smoking raises serum copper concentrations (Kocyigit et al., 2001).

Infection, inflammation, and stress all elevate serum copper concentrations (Honkanen et al., 1991; Brown et al., 1993). This is a result of an increase in ceruloplasmin (an acute phase protein), effected by leukocytic endogenous mediators (Pekarek et al., 1972).

Malabsorption syndromes such as celiac disease, cystic fibrosis, and ulcerative colitis (Sternlieb and Janowitz, 1964) are often associated with low serum copper concentrations, arising from prolonged diarrhea which prevents reabsorption of copper from the bile (Rodriguez et al., 1985).

Certain disease states lead to alterations in serum copper concentrations. Levels increase in leukemia, Hodgkin's disease, various anemias, collagen disorders, hemochromatosis, and myocardial infarction and in patients with dilated cardiomyopathy (Mason, 1979; Oster, 1993). In other diseases (e.g., the nephrotic

syndrome), serum copper concentrations are low (Cartwright et al., 1954).

Interpretive criteria

Interpretive criteria used for serum copper concentrations for adults are 8.8–17.5 μmol/L for men and 10.7–26.6 μmol/L for women who are not taking oral contraceptive agents. A slightly higher range (15.7–31.5 μmol/L) has been proposed for women taking estrogen-containing preparations (Milne and Johnson, 1993).

Rükgauer et al. (1997) have published reference values for plasma copper for children ranging from 1 mo to 18 y, although the number of children studied in some of the age groups was small. These reference values are based on self-selected samples of apparently healthy subjects who were not taking any vitamin or mineral supplements (Table 24.12).

Salmenperä et al. (1986) have compiled reference values for serum copper in exclusively breastfed infants followed longitudinally for the first year of life. These reference values are shown in Figure 24.9.

Serum copper levels were measured in subjects from 3 to 74 y in the Canada Health Survey (Health and Welfare Canada, 1981). The National Health and Nutrition Examination Survey (NHANES II) survey also collected data on serum copper concentrations (Klasing and Pilch, 1985). Concentrations were not measured in the more recent U.K. national surveys.

Age group (years)	n	Serum Cu (μmol/L)
1 to < 2	15	21.1 ± 4.6
2 to < 4	23	21.5 ± 3.9
4 to < 6	19	19.4 ± 5.3
6 to < 10	25	23.4 ± 2.5
10 to < 14	21	21.1 ± 3.7
14 to < 18	17	20.5 ± 4.4

Table 24.12: Plasma copper concentrations in children, grouped according to age (mean ± SD). Data from Rükgauer et al., Journal of Trace Elements in Medicine and Biology 11: 92–98, 1997.

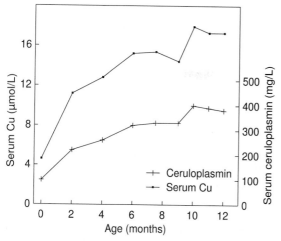

Figure 24.9: Median serum copper and ceruloplasmin concentrations in exclusively breastfed infants during the first year of life. Data from Salmenperä et al., American Journal of Clinical Nutrition 43: 251–257, 1986 © Am J Clin Nutr. American Society for Clinical Nutrition.

Measurement of serum copper

The most widely used method for measuring serum copper is AAS. Generally, a direct technique is used, involving sample dilution with deionized water (1 part plasma or serum to 1 part deionized water) (Osheim, 1983; Smith et al., 1985): a signal-enhancing mixture such as butanol and water is also sometimes used (Meret and Henkin, 1971). In some instances, use of a "high solids" burner head may be necessary (Boling, 1966). Sometimes, the protein in the blood sample is removed using an acid such as trichloroacetic acid (Kelson and Shamberger, 1978), but this procedure may introduce volume errors during the deproteinization step and adventitious contamination from the acid and is not recommended.

Analytical variation for serum copper by AAS is usually small; Gallagher et al. (1989) reported it to be < 2.6%. For very small pediatric samples, graphite furnace AAS, with Zeeman-effect background correction, may be used (Wang and Demshar, 1993). Increasingly inductively coupled plasma spectrometry (ICP) is being used because it is a multi-element technique with a detection limit and sensitivity better than flame AAS (Nixon et al., 1986). Standard reference materials for the analysis of copper in serum are available from NIST (Gaithersburg, MD).

24.2.2 Serum ceruloplasmin

Ceruloplasmin is the major copper-containing protein in the α_2-globulin fraction of human serum. More than 60% to 95% of serum copper is associated with ceruloplasmin (Wirth and Linder, 1985), so changes in serum copper generally parallel the level of ceruloplasmin in the blood.

Ceruloplasmin (EC 1.16.3.1) is a copper transport protein synthesized primarily in the liver. It is a single-chain glycoprotein with six copper atoms per molecule. A ferroxidase, it assists in iron transport by oxidizing intracellular Fe^{2+} to Fe^{3+}, which can then combine with transferrin. Ceruloplasmin is also among those enzymes involved in the acute-phase reaction of inflammation and in the scavenging of oxygen radicals to protect cells against oxidative damage (Linder and Hazegh-Azam, 1996).

Ceruloplasmin levels in serum, like copper, are significantly reduced in cases of severe copper deficiency that can occur with the hereditary diseases associated with disturbances in copper metabolism: Menkes' kinky hair syndrome and Wilson's disease. However, the response of ceruloplasmin to marginal copper deficiency or short-term copper depletion is variable (Milne and Nielsen, 1993,1996). In most short-term studies of copper depletion (e.g., Milne and Nielsen, 1996) or supplementation (e.g., Kehoe et al., 2000a), there has been little or no response by ceruloplasmin (Figure 24.8).

Many of the factors that influence serum copper also affect serum ceruloplasmin and limit its usefulness as a marker of copper status, except in cases of severe copper deficiency.

Factors affecting ceruloplasmin

Age and gender influence serum ceruloplasmin activity in the same manner as serum copper as shown in Table 24.10 (Fischer et al., 1990).

Estrogen-containing preparations tend to increase the serum ceruloplasmin activity, as shown in Table 24.11 (Fischer et al., 1990). Ceruloplasmin synthesis and secretion by the liver is regulated in the long term by estrogen, probably through stabilization of mRNA (Middleton and Linder, 1993).

Pregnancy can increase serum ceruloplasmin activity (Fischer et al., 1990), again via the effect of estrogen on ceruloplasmin synthesis. This effect may be related to the copper needs of the growing fetus during pregnancy (Lee et al., 1993).

Infection and inflammatory stress can lead to markedly elevated ceruloplasmin activity levels in serum (Brown, 1998). Ceruloplasmin is an acute-phase protein and the inflammatory hormones (interleukin-1 [IL-1], IL-6, and tissue necrosis factor) regulate its acute synthesis and secretion by the liver (Linder and Hazegh-Azam, 1996). Hence, it is not surprising that serum ceruloplasmin activity is also elevated in rheumatoid arthritis (DiSilvestro et al.,1992).

Interpretive criteria

Reference data for serum ceruloplasmin are limited. Salmenperä et al. (1986) have published reference values for exclusively breast-fed infants followed during the first year of life, and they are shown in Figure 24.9. Levels increase steadily during the first year of life, paralleling the trend for serum copper.

Milne (1994) suggests that a ratio of enzyme activity (ceruloplasmin oxidase activity) to ceruloplasmin protein concentration may be a useful index of copper status. The ratio has several advantages. Effects of age, sex, or hormone use are small (Table 24.13) (Milne and Johnson, 1993), and it appears to be more sensitive to changes in copper status than either the enzymatic activity or immunoreactive protein alone (Milne et al., 1988). Indeed, in some individuals, ceruloplasmin

Age (years)	Group	Enzyme activity (mg/L)	RID (mg/L)	ENZ/RID
20–29	M ($n = 10$)	408	266	1.56
	F ($n = 10$)	503	330	1.53
	FOC ($n = 10$)	612	371	1.71
30–39	M ($n = 10$)	416	296	1.49
	F ($n = 10$)	516	314	1.66
	FOC ($n = 11$)	744	525	1.42
40–49	M ($n = 11$)	442	337	1.31
	F ($n = 11$)	519	359	1.48
50–59	M ($n = 9$)	441	310	1.43
	F ($n = 13$)	516	370	1.44
	FE ($n = 4$)	593	384	1.57
60–69	M ($n = 8$)	470	284	1.70
	F ($n = 10$)	559	354	1.60
70+	M ($n = 7$)	485	332	1.51
	F ($n = 7$)	470	368	1.29
ANOVA				
	Gender	0.0001	0.0002	NS
	Decade	NS	0.03	NS

Table 24.13: Effect of age, gender, and hormone use on mean ceruloplasmin concentrations, measured both enzymatically (ENZ) and by radial immunodiffusion (RID). The ratio of ENZ/RID is also shown. FOC, females taking oral contraceptives; FE, females using estrogen therapy. Significance levels from analysis of variance (ANOVA) are also shown (interactions between gender and decade were nonsignificant in all three cases). Data from Milne and Johnson Clinical Chemistry: 39, 883–887, 1993, with permission of the AACC.

oxidase activity (but not ceruloplasmin protein concentration) was depressed during experimental copper depletion (Milne et al., 1988). Further, in young women, ceruloplasmin oxidase activity has been reported as inversely related to physiological changes due to copper depletion (e.g., autonomic cardiovascular function)(Lukaski et al., 1988).

Table 24.13 presents mean ceruloplasmin values measured both enzymatically (ENZ) and by radial immunodiffusion, and the ratio of the enzyme activity to the immunoreactive protein for males and females by age and hormone use (Milne and Johnson, 1993). Values for ceruloplasmin for the two assays were standardardized to mg/L by using purified human ceruloplasmin as a standard.

Measurement of serum ceruloplasmin

Serum ceruloplasmin can be assayed enzymatically by measuring *p*-phenylenediamine oxidase activity (Sunderman and Nomoto, 1970). Ceruloplasmin protein levels can be measured immunochemically by radial immunodiffusion techniques (Mancini et al., 1965; Buffone et al., 1979). Alternatively, nephelometry (Buffone et al., 1979), or immunoelectophoresis techniques (Gibbs and Walshe, 1979) can be used. Some discrepancies have been reported between radial immunodiffusion and nephelometry, which may be attributed to different sources of antibodies used for the assays (Buffone et al., 1979). Analytical variation for serum ceruloplasmin performed by radial immunodiffusion ranges up to 6% (Gallagher et al., 1989).

24.2.3 Erythrocyte superoxide dismutase

Approximately 60% of the copper found in erythrocytes is present in the cytosol as superoxide dismutase (Cu,Zn-SOD) (EC 1.15.1.1). This enzyme, which contains both divalent copper and divalent zinc, has a molecular weight of approximately 32,500. It is important as a scavenger of O_2^-, a free radical that causes damage to membranes and biological structures. It catalyzes the dismutation reaction, converting the highly reactive superoxide anion O_2^- to less reactive hydrogen peroxide and oxygen:

$$O_2^- + O_2^- + 2H^+ \xrightarrow{\text{SOD}} H_2O_2 + O_2$$

Studies with both animal models and humans have shown that the activity of erythrocyte Cu,Zn-SOD is depressed in copper deficiency and that the activity is often, but not always, restored during copper repletion (Bettger et al., 1979; Okahata et al., 1980; Uauy et al., 1985; Milne et al., 1990; Milne and Nielsen, 1996). Table 24.14 presents data on erythrocyte Cu,Zn-SOD activity in infants recovering from malnutrition and receiving marginal copper intakes: levels returned to normal after copper supplementation (Uauy

Measure	Study ($n=8$)	Control ($n=9$)
Plasma copper (μmol/L)		
Before	15.4 ± 10.5	22.4 ± 4.1
After	26.0 ± 5.4	
Ceruloplasmin (mg/L)		
Before	330 ± 260	540 ± 120
After	500 ± 140	
SOD (U/g Hb)		
Before	1073 ± 312	1461 ± 451
After	1371 ± 207	

Table 24.14: Effect of copper supplementation on mean ($\pm$ SD) serum copper, ceruloplasmin, and erythrocyte superoxide dismutase in infants recovering from malnutrition. Data from Uauy et al., Journal of Nutrition 115: 1650–1655, 1985, with permission of the American Society for Nutritional Sciences.

et al., 1985), and there was a significant positive correlation between erythrocyte Cu,Zn-SOD and plasma copper concentrations in these malnourished infants (Figure 24.10). Such a correlation was not reported by Fischer et al. (1990) in their study of healthy adults, probably because the individuals studied had a copper status within the normal range.

Positive correlations between erythrocyte Cu,Zn-SOD activity and other measures of

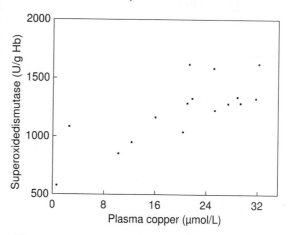

Figure 24.10: Correlation between erythrocyte cell superoxide dismutase activity and plasma copper ($r=0.78$, $p<0.001$) in eight malnourished infants studied before and after copper supplementation. Redrawn from Uauy et al., Journal of Nutrition 115: 1650–1655, 1985, with permission of the American Society for Nutritional Sciences.

copper status (e.g., liver cytochrome c oxidase) have also been observed in some animal studies (Bettger et al., 1979; Andrewartha and Caple, 1980).

Erythrocyte Cu,Zn-SOD activity appears to be a more sensitive index of copper depletion than serum copper or ceruloplasmin. In several experimental copper depletion–repletion studies in humans (Reiser et al., 1985; Milne and Nielsen, 1996), erythrocyte Cu,Zn-SOD activity declined significantly during the depletion phase, despite no detectable decrease in serum copper or ceruloplasmin. This trend is shown in Figure 24.8.

Nevertheless, the response of erythrocyte Cu,Zn-SOD activity to copper repletion in these experimental studies has not been consistent. Several investigators have failed to show a response by erythrocyte Cu,Zn-SOD to copper supplementation (Turnlund et al., 1990; Medeiros et al., 1991). Even in a later study by Kehoe et al. (2000a) involving two different copper compounds and two levels of copper supplementation, the activity of Cu,Zn-SOD in erythrocytes (and leukocytes) did not respond to the copper supplements.

It appears that the study duration, amount of copper fed, and probably rates of cell turnover all influence the response of erythrocyte Cu,Zn-SOD activity to copper repletion (Klevay et al., 1984; Milne et al., 1988; Turnlund et al., 1990; Medeiros et al., 1991; Milne and Nielsen, 1996; Kehoe et al.,2000a). In Figure 24.8, the erythrocyte Cu,Zn-SOD activity remained at a plateau during copper repletion, perhaps associated with the rate at which new erythrocytes were being synthesized. In contrast, in the study of malnourished copper-deficient infants (Table 24.14), erythrocyte Cu,Zn-SOD activity increased to normal levels after supplementation with copper (80 µg/kg/d) for 120 d.

Very few investigators have used erythrocyte Cu,Zn-SOD activity as an index of copper status in community-based studies. Fischer et al. (1990) measured erythrocyte Cu,Zn-SOD activity (and serum copper and ceruloplasmin) in 384 free-living adults and examined the relationships with age, sex, estrogen use, smoking, alcohol use, and ex-

Age group (years)	Men (Mean ± SEM)	Women (Mean ± SEM)
25–34	82.1 ± 6.3	74.7 ± 2.9
35–44	76.7 ± 1.4	75.3 ± 2.7
45–54	76.2 ± 2.1	79.0 ± 5.7
55–64	77.8 ± 1.8	75.5 ± 3.9
65+	77.4 ± 2.9	68.9 ± 3.9
Women Premenopausal	Non-users of oral contr. 75.1 ± 2.1	Users of oral contr. 77.2 ± 6.1
Postmenopausal	Non-users of estrogens 76.7 ± 3.5	Users of estrogens 73.8 ± 7.9

Table 24.15: Effect of age in men and women (not taking estrogen-containing preparations) on erythrocyte Cu,Zn-superoxide dismutase activity (U/mg Hb). The nonsignificant differences shown in the lower part of the table demonstrate the minimal impact of oral contraceptive use and estrogen replacement therapy on Cu,Zn-superoxide dismutase activity. Data from Fischer et al., Nutrition Research 10: 1081–1090, 1990.

ercise, as noted earlier. Table 24.15 presents the mean ± SEM for erythrocyte Cu,Zn-SOD activity for males and females by age. Unlike serum copper levels and ceruloplasmin activity, erythrocyte Cu,Zn-SOD activity appears to be unaffected by age, gender (Table 24.15), hormone use, or the acute phase status (Solomons, 1985; Fischer et al., 1990; Milne and Johnson, 1993).

In some conditions that produce oxidative stress (Lukaski et al., 1990), including alcoholism and Down's syndrome (Del Villano et al., 1980; Porstmann et al., 1990), erythrocyte Cu,Zn-SOD activity may be elevated. In rheumatoid arthritis patients, lower levels than those in controls have been observed (DiSilvestro et al., 1992).

Interpretive criteria

Interpretive criteria for erythrocyte Cu,Zn-SOD activity are limited. Laboratories should establish their own reference range for erythrocyte Cu,Zn-SOD activity. Milne and Johnson (1993) have compiled ranges for healthy adults based on the assay of Winterbourne et al. (1975). However, there were relatively small numbers of subjects in each age group. Activity levels are unaffected by age, gender, and hormone use.

The U.K. National Diet and Nutrition Survey of young people aged 4–18 y measured erythrocyte Cu,Zn-SOD activity; levels decreased for both boys and girls with increasing age. Mean, median, and the lower and upper 2.5 percentile values by age and sex are presented (Gregory et al., 2000). However, work is still required to confirm the utility of erythrocyte Cu,Zn-SOD activity in studies of the copper status of the general population.

Measuring erythrocyte Cu,Zn-SOD

There is no standard assay for the measurement of erythrocyte Cu,Zn-SOD activity. Several methods are available; some are very time consuming, require large samples, necessitate the removal of hemoglobin immediately after sample collection, and are subject to interferences.

The assay generally involves the inhibition of oxidation-reduction reactions which are catalyzed by the superoxide anion. The latter may be generated enzymatically by, for example, xanthine plus xanthine oxidase, which, in turn, reduces cytochrome c. The reduction of cytochrome c is followed spectrophotometrically (Marklund and Marklund, 1974).

Several of these procedures are now automated. L'Abbé and Fischer (1986) developed a method for determining Cu,Zn-SOD activity that can be used with small samples. Commercial kits based on either an enzyme-linked immunosorbent assay or on a spectrophotometric assay are now available for measuring Cu,Zn-SOD activity in human serum and urine.

The analytical coefficient of variation for the erythrocyte superoxide dismutase assay when determined using an automated method ranges from 1.9% to 11.9%. The within-subject variation for erythrocyte Cu,Zn-SOD activity is generally high (Gallagher et al., 1989).

24.2.4 Cytochrome C oxidase

Cytochrome c oxidase (EC 1.9.3.1) is present in most tissues of living organisms and is the terminal enzyme of the electron transport chain. It reacts directly with molecular oxygen in cellular respiration; it catalyzes the electron transfer from cytochrome c to O_2.

Cytochrome c oxidase activity in erythrocytes, platelets, or mononuclear leukocytes (lymphocytes and monocytes) has potential as a sensitive measure of copper status. Animal studies have generally reported reduced tissue cytochrome c oxidase activity as an early sign of copper deficiency (Underwood, 1971), in association with a reduction in the respiratory capacity of mitochondria, especially in the liver, heart, and brain. Coupling of respiration to phosphorylation is generally not affected (Linder and Hazegh-Azam, 1996). In some of these animal studies, cytochrome c oxidase activity in platelets correlated very strongly with liver copper levels ($r = 0.99$; $p < 0.0001$) (Johnson et al., 1993).

Genetic defects in the activity of cytochrome c oxidase, whereby activity is only about 50% of normal, may lead to neurological, cardiac, and muscle disease in children (DiMauro et al., 1985; Tulinius et al., 1991; Van Coster et al., 1991). Reduced activity of cytochrome c oxidase has also been reported in leukocytes in infants and children with Menkes' kinky hair syndrome, a genetic defect in copper metabolism (Garnica et al., 1977).

More recently, results of copper depletion–repletion studies have reported that platelet cytochrome c oxidase activity may be more sensitive than either serum copper or ceruloplasmin to changes in copper intake. In Figure 24.8, for example, the activity of cytochrome c oxidase in platelets was significantly lower ($p < 0.0001$) at the end of the copper-depletion period than at baseline (Milne and Nielsen, 1996); levels for many women were below the reference range for comparable healthy women (Table 24.16) (Milne and Johnson, 1993). Moreover, unlike erythrocyte Zn,Cu-SOD activity or levels of serum copper and ceruloplasmin, the activity

Age (years)	Group	Platelets U/10^9 cells	Mononuclear blood cells U/10^6 cells
20–29	M	2.75 (10)	0.33 (9)
	F	2.36 (9)	0.27 (7)
	FOC	2.87 (9)	0.32 (7)
30–39	M	2.94 (9)	0.31 (8)
	F	2.75 (9)	0.36 (10)
	FOC	3.87 (10)	0.39 (11)
40–49	M	3.52 (9)	0.40 (10)
	F	3.08 (10)	0.35 (9)
50–59	M	3.89 (9)	0.35 (9)
	F	3.88 (12)	0.38 (10)
	FE	3.54 (3)	0.42 (3)
60–69	M	4.92 (7)	0.43 (6)
	F	4.56 (9)	0.37 (9)
70+	M	4.51 (6)	0.45 (4)
	F	3.65 (5)	0.39 (7)
ANOVA			
	Gender	NS	NS
	Decade	0.0001	0.004

Table 24.16: Effect of age, gender, and hormone use on mean cytochrome-c oxidase concentrations, measured in both platelets and mononuclear blood cells. FOC, females taking oral contraceptives; FE, females using estrogen therapy. Significance levels from analysis of variance (ANOVA) are also shown (interactions between gender and decade were nonsignificant in both cases). Data from Milne and Johnson, Clinical Chemistry 39: 883–887, 1993, with permission of the AACC.

of platelet cytochrome c showed a positive response to copper repletion, with activity levels returning to about 60% of control values (Milne and Nielsen, 1996).

Cytochrome c activity responded similarly in both platelets and mononuclear leukocytes to copper repletion in young women fed a copper-depleted diet. However, baseline values were not measured, so that the response of these indices to depletion cannot be evaluated (Milne et al., 1988).

The activity of cytochrome c oxidase in both platelets and mononucleated leukocytes tends to be higher in older than in younger adults, and varies markedly between subjects (Table 24.16) (Milne and Johnson, 1993). The activity in mononuclear cells, but not

platelets, was affected by oral contraceptive use, and only in the 30–39 y age group. Adolescents with cystic fibrosis also have lower cytochrome c activity in mononucleated leukocytes, compared with age- and sex-matched controls (Percival et al., 1995). The postulated mechanism relates to the alterations in chloride transport in cystic fibrosis, which, in turn, impairs copper transport (Alda and Garay, 1990).

Interpretive criteria

Table 24.16 presents mean cytochrome-c oxidase activity in platelets and mononuclear blood cells (lymphocytes and monocytes) by age and sex for adults 20 to >70 y. Subjects were healthy, nonpregnant, and nonsmokers and were not taking any vitamin or mineral supplements, or prescribed medications, with the exception of estrogen.

Measurement of cytochrome-c oxidase

Platelets and mononuclear cells have a shorter lifespan ($\sim$10 d) than erythrocytes ($\sim$120 d) and therefore activities in these shorter-lived cell types better reflect the metabolically-active pool of endogenous copper. However, the isolation of such specific cell types is time consuming and complex, as noted in Section 15.1.3. Moreover, the enzyme cytochrome c oxidase is labile, and between-subject variation is large. Hence, before the test can be used in community studies, the assay method must be rigorously standardized. Currently, an assay developed by Prohaska and Wells (1974) is often used. Further work is needed to establish the validity and feasibility of this enzyme as a biomarker of copper deficiency in community studies.

24.2.5 Skin lysyl oxidase

Lysyl oxidase (EC 1.4.3.13) is another extracellular copper-containing enzyme that is essential for the normal maturation and function of collagen, specifically in the steps involving the formation of lysine-derived cross-links. The latter are required for the formation of

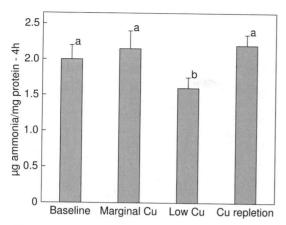

Figure 24.11: Lysyl oxidase activity in the skin of healthy male subjects fed different amounts of copper. Marginal Cu, 0.66 mg/d; Low Cu, 0.38 mg/d; Cu repletion, 2.49 mg/d. Bars with different letters differ significantly ($p < 0.05$). Values are mean ± SEM of 11 subjects at each time period. Redrawn from Werman et al., Nutritional Biochemistry 8: 201–204, 1997.

strong, flexible connective tissue (Rucker and Murray, 1978).

Copper deficiency in animals results in low lysyl oxidase activity in heart, aorta, connective tissue, lung, and skin, which increases with copper supplementation (O'Dell, 1976). Decreased lysyl oxidase activity may be responsible for the skeletal and cardiac abnormalities reported in copper deficiency (Kagan and Trackman, 1991).

To date, very few experimental copper depletion–repletion studies have examined the effect of low dietary copper on the activity of skin lysyl oxidase. Results shown in Figure 24.11 present the changes in mean lysyl oxidase activity in the skin of healthy males receiving diets containing four levels of dietary copper. There was a significant fall in activity when the subjects were fed a low copper diet (0.38 mg/d), which returned to baseline values after copper repletion. No such decline was observed when the marginal copper diet (0.66 mg/d) was fed. Plasma copper, ceruloplasmin, and urinary copper were also measured in this study; levels fell significantly on feeding the low-copper diet (Werman et al., 1997).

The results of this initial study suggest that

lysyl oxidase activity declines when dietary copper intake is inadequate, indicating that the cross-linking of collagen may be modulated by copper deficiency. Skin lysyl oxidase could be used as a biomarker of copper status in young men. Further studies are needed to assess whether the test can also be used in women and older subjects. Skin biopsies are invasive procedures, so that the test probably will have limited use in community-based studies. Lysyl oxidase activity was assayed using the method of Werman and Bhathena (1992).

24.2.6 Diamine oxidase

Diamine oxidase (EC 1.4.3.6) is a copper-metalloenzyme that is responsible for the deamination of putrescine, cadaverine, and histamine (Wolvekamp and de Bruin, 1994). The activity of this enzyme has been reported to be low in some studies in rats (Kehoe et al., 2000b) and renal dialysis patients with copper deficiency (DiSilvestro et al., 1997).

In an experimental copper supplementation study of healthy adults, the activity of diamine oxidase in serum increased significantly during all three Cu-supplementation

Group (n)	Mean	SE	Mean	SE
	3 mg CuSO$_4$/d		Placebo	
Men (7)	0.87	0.27	0.27	0.17
Women (9)	1.64	0.47	0.33	0.17
	3 mg CuGC/d		Placebo	
Men (9)	1.21	0.36	0.47	0.01
Women (11)	1.92	0.41	0.42	0.23
	6 mg CuGC/d		Placebo	
Men (7)	1.55	0.49	0.44	0.28
Women (10)	2.37	0.79	1.16	0.32

Table 24.17: Response of serum diamine oxidase (U/L) in men and women to three different regimens of copper supplementation. In all three cases and for both sexes, activity in the treatment group differed significantly from placebo ($p < 0.01$). CuGC: copper gluconate. Abstracted from Kehoe et al., British Journal of Nutrition 84: 151–156, 2000, with permission of the authors.

regimens in both males and females, as shown in Table 24.17 (Kehoe et al. 2000a). These results suggest that the activity of diamine oxidase in serum has the potential to be a sensitive indicator of copper status in adults and warrants further investigation. Whether there are any adverse health consequences associated with low serum diamine oxidase activity is unknown.

The activity of this enzyme is, however, modified by conditions other than copper status, including pregnancy (Kusche et al., 1974), uremia (Tam et al., 1979), malabsorption syndromes or gastrointestinal damage (Bayless et al., 1981), and kidney dialysis (DiSilvestro et al.,1997). Further studies are needed with other population groups to establish the specificity of this enzyme to changes in copper status. A sensitive automated colorimetric assay developed by Takagi et al. (1994) can be used for the assay of serum diamine oxidase.

24.2.7 Hair copper concentrations

Concentrations of copper in hair appear to correlate with levels in the liver (Jacob et al., 1978), heart, and kidney (Klevay, 1981) of rats. However, the validity of hair copper concentrations as a biomarker of copper status in humans is much less certain. In a detailed human study, hair copper concentrations did not correlate with the copper content of heart, muscle, liver, kidney, aorta, or rib (Aalbers and Houtman, 1985).

Many studies have confirmed that gender (in adults), pregnancy, lactation, prematurity, hair color, race, and age all affect hair copper concentrations (Petering et al., 1971; Creason et al., 1975; Gibson and DeWolfe, 1980; Taylor, 1986). The marked rise in hair (and serum) copper concentrations during early infancy is presumably associated with the redistribution of tissue copper which occurs at this time, and not with changes in dietary copper intake (Gibson and DeWolfe, 1980) (Figure 24.12).

Normal hair copper levels are found in two conditions in which copper accumulates in the liver — primary biliary cirrhosis (Epstein

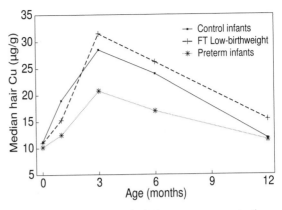

Figure 24.12: Changes in hair copper concentrations during infancy. From Gibson RS, (1982). The trace metal status of some Canadian full term and low birth-weight infants at one year of age. Journal of Radioanalytical Chemistry 70: 175–189, with permission.

et al., 1980) and Wilson's disease (Rice and Goldstein, 1961; Gibbs and Walshe, 1965). Additionally, infants with copper deficiency, characterized clinically by neutropenia and biochemically by concentrations of serum copper and ceruloplasmin below the detection limit, did not have lower hair copper levels than age- and sex-matched controls (Bradfield et al., 1980). Similarly, the copper content of the hair of children with Menkes' kinky hair syndrome is normal (Danks, 1980). It appears, therefore, that hair copper cannot be used as a biomarker of copper status in humans.

24.2.8 Other indices of copper status

Urinary copper is seldom used as an index of copper status; levels are very low in healthy subjects (10–60 µg/d) because copper is efficiently reabsorbed by the renal tubules. The main excretory route for copper is the biliary system. Urinary copper concentrations do decrease in persons receiving TPN copper-deficient solutions (Solomons, 1979), conserving body copper. However, in a 13-wk experimental depletion–repletion study in which men were fed three levels of dietary copper, urinary copper levels were unaffected by dietary copper levels (Turnlund et al., 1990).

Very limited data are available on copper concentrations in erythrocytes (Vitoux et al., 1999) and fingernails (Martin, 1964). Elevated values for erythrocyte copper have been reported in patients with the two inherited metabolic disorders associated with defects in copper metabolism (Wilson's disease and Menkes' syndrome), as well as in children with Down's syndrome and cystic fibrosis. Further studies are needed to ascertain the validity of these measures of copper status.

Studies on weanling rats have shown that the expression level of the copper chaperone for Cu,Zn-SOD (CCS) may be a promising biomarker of marginal copper status (Bertinato et al., 2003). More research is needed to establish whether CCS could also be used for diagnosing marginal copper deficiency in humans.

Changes in some biochemical markers of bone metabolism have been noted during experimental copper depletion–repletion (Baker et al. 1999a) and also in some supplementation trials (Baker et al., 1999b; Cashman et al., 2001). Results suggest that changes in both urinary pyridinoline and deoxypyridinoline (biomarkers of bone resorption) may serve as additional functional markers of copper status in populations that consume diets low in copper; details of these biomarkers of bone resorption are given in Section 23.1.5.

24.2.9 Multiple indices

Serum copper is frequently used to assess copper status in both clinical and community studies, but it is not very sensitive or specific. Increasingly, because of its higher sensitivity and specificity, the activity of Cu,Zn-SOD in erythrocytes is used in combination with serum copper. In the future, the activity of cytochrome c oxidase in platelets or diamine oxidase in serum may be used in combination with serum copper, instead of erythrocyte Cu,Zn-SOD, if their validity as biomarkers of copper status in a community setting is confirmed.

24.3 Zinc

In an adult 70-kg male there is approximately 1.5–2.5 g of zinc, of which over 80% is found in muscle and bone. Much smaller amounts are present in the liver, gastrointestinal tract, skin, kidney, lung, prostate, and other organs, as shown in Table 24.18.

Unlike other trace elements such as iron and copper, or minerals such as calcium, there are no large, readily mobilizable stores of zinc that can be rapidly released or sequestered in response to variations in dietary intakes of zinc. Instead, there may be a small pool of rapidly exchangeable zinc, located, at least in part, in bone, liver, and plasma (King et al., 2000). It is the loss of a critical but small amount of zinc from this pool that leads to the biochemical and clinical signs of zinc deficiency. Bone may also provide a passive reserve of zinc, especially during growth, so that when dietary zinc intakes are

Tissue	Zn conc. (mg/kg wet wt.)	Total content (mg)	Proportion of total body zinc (%)
Skeletal muscle	50	1400	63
Skeleton			
Bone	90	450	20
Marrow	20	60	3
Periarticular tissue	11	11	< 1
Cartilage	34	30	1
Liver	40	72	3
Lung	40	40	2
Skin	15	39	2
Whole blood	6	33	1
Kidney	50	15	1
Brain	10	14	1
Teeth	250	11.5	1
Hair	200	4	< 1
Spleen	20	3.6	< 1
Lymph nodes	14	3.5	< 1
Gastrointestinal tract	15	1.8	< 1
Prostate	100	1.6	< 1
Other organs/tissues	Variable	50	2
Total		2240	100

Table 24.18: Zinc content of major organs and tissues in adult (70 kg) man. Adapted from Iyengar, Radiation Physics and Chemistry 51: 545–560, 1998.

low, less of the zinc released during normal bone turnover, is re-deposited in the skeleton (Giugliano and Millward, 1984; Zhou et al., 1993; Hotz and Brown, 2004).

Functions of zinc

Zinc has multiple functions in cellular metabolism. More than 100 enzymes require zinc for function or regulation. In many cases the enzymes serve as an electron acceptor (Cousins, 1996), and they play an important role in the metabolism of proteins, nucleic acids, lipids, and carbohydrates; some examples are shown in Table 24.19. So far no consistent changes in the activity of any zinc metalloenzymes have been reported in experimental zinc depletion–repletion studies.

Zinc is essential for the maintenance of protein structure and for the synthesis and degradation of ribonucleic acid (RNA) and deoxyribonucleic acid (DNA) and ribosomes. As a result, disturbances in cell replication and differentiation occur in zinc deficiency (Cunnane, 1988).

Zinc is required to stabilize the structure of certain DNA-binding proteins (zinc-fingers) which regulate gene expression (Prasad, 1995). Zinc-dependent enzymes are also involved in the synthesis of certain proteins, such as collagen, that are important in wound healing. Zinc is required for thymulin (thymic hormone) activation and for metallothionein;

Zinc metalloenzymes
Alcohol dehydrogenase
Alkaline phosphatase
Carbonic anhydrase
Carboxypeptidase
Deoxynucleotidyl transferase
DNA polymerase
Glutamic acid dehydrogenase
Malic acid dehydrogenase
Nucleoside phosphorylase
RNA polymerase
Tyrosine kinase
Zinc-copper superoxide dismutase

Table 24.19: Selected zinc metalloenzymes. Adapted from Cunnane (1988) and Prasad (1995).

the latter has a role in regulating body zinc homeostasis (Cunnane, 1988).

In addition to their role in protein and nucleic acid metabolism, zinc-dependent enzymes are involved in lipid metabolism, particularly with the synthesis of long-chain fatty acids and various prostaglandins. Zinc also has a role in cholesterol metabolism and in maintaining the stability of lipids within cell membranes (Hotz and Brown, 2004).

Zinc also has a clear role in carbohydrate metabolism, with impaired glucose tolerance occurring in zinc deficiency. Zinc may interact with insulin by controlling glucose uptake by adipocytes. Zinc influences the activity of several other hormones, in addition to insulin. These include human growth hormone, the gonadotropins, sex hormones, prolactin, thyroid hormones, and corticosteroids (Cunnane, 1988).

Zinc is also essential for the optimum functioning of the immune system. This topic has been reviewed in detail by Shankar and Prasad (1998) and Fraker et al. (2000), who note that zinc plays a major role in cell-mediated immune function, especially in the thymic-dependent lymphocytes (T-cells).

Other biological actions of zinc include its role in reproduction, appetite, taste acuity, night vision, and vitamin A metabolism (Christian and West, 1998; Hotz and Brown, 2004). Nevertheless, explanations for many of the wide range of disturbances that occur in zinc deficiency have still not been firmly established. This is surprising in view of the new and extensive knowledge of the biochemical functions of zinc.

Absorption and metabolism of zinc

Zinc is absorbed in the small intestine, mainly by a transcellular process. Once inside the intestinal cells, much of the absorbed zinc becomes bound to metallothionein.

The transfer of absorbed zinc from the intestine to the liver is via the portal system. The liver is the main organ involved in zinc metabolism. About 30%–40% of zinc in portal blood is exchanged with the liver. From the liver, zinc is released into the systemic circulation for delivery to other tissues, bound mainly to albumin (Cousins, 1996).

Zinc homeostasis in the body is tightly regulated, in part by changes in zinc absorption and excretion in response to variation in the dietary intake. Zinc excretion is mainly via the feces, with fecal zinc losses being a combination of unabsorbed dietary and endogenous zinc. Sources of endogenous zinc include secretions from pancreatic and intestinal mucosal cells. During periods of low zinc intake, absorption is enhanced and secretion of endogenous zinc into the gastrointestinal lumen is suppressed. In contrast, when zinc intakes are high, absorption is decreased and secretion of endogenous zinc is enhanced. Adjustments in renal excretion of zinc also occur with extremely low or high intakes of zinc (King and Keen, 1999).

Zinc deficiency in humans

The first cases of dietary zinc deficiency in humans were described in the 1960s in male dwarfs from the Middle East (Prasad et al., 1963). Typical clinical features, which were corrected by zinc supplementation, included growth retardation, delayed secondary sexual maturation (hypogonadism), poor appetite, mental lethargy, and skin changes. In North America and New Zealand, overt and severe nutritional zinc deficiency was first recognized in hospital patients who received either parenteral nutrition or enteral feedings without zinc supplements (Kay and Tasman-Jones, 1975; Arakawa et al., 1976).

Two genetic disorders are known to induce zinc deficiency: acrodermatitis enteropathica (Barnes and Moynahan, 1973) and sickle cell disease (Prasad and Cossack, 1982).

Secondary zinc deficiency has been documented in the presence of malabsorption syndromes such as Crohn's disease, short bowel syndrome, and cystic fibrosis (Pironi et al., 1987). A variety of other diseases — including renal and liver diseases, diabetes, acquired immuno-deficiency syndrome, and alcoholism — also induce secondary zinc deficiency. In such cases, zinc deficiency may arise from either increased urinary excretion

of zinc (hyperzincuria) or excess loss of zinc via intestinal secretions and exudates (Aggett and Comerford, 1995).

Treatment with certain drugs has also been associated with secondary zinc deficiency. For example, long-term treatment with penicillamine for Wilson's disease (Smolarek and Stremmel, 1999), and administration of chlorthiazide and glucagon (Prasad and Oberleas, 1976) have all been implicated as iatrogenic causes of zinc deficiency.

In some industrialized countries, such as the United States and Canada, marginal zinc deficiency, characterized by slow physical growth, poor appetite, and by diminished taste acuity (hypogeusia), has been identified in apparently healthy infants and children (Hambidge et al., 1972a; Walravens and Hambidge, 1976; Walravens et al., 1983; Smit-Vanderkooy and Gibson, 1987; Gibson et al., 1989a).

More recently, several double-blind zinc supplementation studies been carried out with infants and children in low-income countries (Bhutta et al., 1999; Brown et al., 2002). Based on these results, an increasing range of functional impairments, in addition to impaired growth, have been associated with zinc deficiency. These include abnormalities of the immune system and increased risk of common childhood infections. For example, reductions in the incidence of acute and persistent diarrhea and acute lower respiratory infections (e.g., pneumonia) have been reported in children supplemented with zinc (Bhutta et al., 1999, 2000).

Accumulating evidence also suggests that zinc deficiency may be related to compromised neurobehavioral function in children (Sazawal et al., 1996; Bentley et al., 1997; Sandstead et al., 1998; Grantham-McGregor et al., 1999), and mortality in low birth-weight infants (Sazawal et al., 2001).

Zinc supplementation trials have also been conducted during pregnancy; these have been reviewed in detail by others (Tamura and Goldenberg, 1996; Caulfield et al.,1999; and King, 2000; Osendarp et al., 2003). Results have been inconsistent; only some have reported a positive effect of supplemental zinc on pregnancy outcome measures. Of these, improvements in fetal growth, based on birth weight (Garg et al., 1993; Goldenberg et al., 1995), and significant reductions in preterm deliveries (Cherry et al., 1989; Garg et al., 1993; Goldenberg et al., 1995), and the incidence of maternal complications (Hunt et al., 1984; Jameson, 1993) have been reported in some studies.

Zinc status is sometimes compromised in the elderly, probably because of low zinc intakes and age-related changes in physiological function. As well, the presence of certain disease states and the use of certain medications may have exacerbating roles (Aggett and Comerford, 1995). There are several reports of improvements in immune function in older adults following zinc supplementation (Duchateau et al., 1981; Bogden et al., 1994).

Food sources and dietary intakes

Nutritional deficiencies of zinc may arise from low intakes or poor bioavailability of dietary zinc. Food sources of readily absorbable zinc include meat, liver, fish, and shellfish; oysters are one of the richest food sources of available zinc. In general, the amount of zinc is higher in dark red meat than in white meat. Zinc is less readily available in whole grain cereals, nuts and legumes; further, their zinc content varies, depending on the zinc content of the soil or fertilizer treatment, growing location, and processing methods (e.g., milling of cereals). Starchy roots, tubers, fruits, and vegetables have a low zinc content. Loss of zinc from most foods during cooking is minimal.

Several dietary components affect zinc bioavailability by influencing either the absorption of exogenous zinc or the reabsorption of endogenous zinc. Phytate (myoinositol hexaphosphate) forms insoluble complexes with zinc, thus inhibiting its absorption. Fermentation of bread doughs hydrolyzes phytic acid and improves zinc absorption. Soaking unrefined cereal flours can reduce their phytate content, mainly by the diffusion of water-soluble phytate (Gibson and Hotz, 2001).

The degree to which phytate inhibits zinc absorption depends on both the molar ratio of phytate to zinc in the diet and the calcium content. In affluent countries, the phytate content of most omnivorous diets is generally low. Further, the inhibitory effect of phytate in such diets is probably readily counteracted by the enhancing effect of animal proteins on zinc absorption. In low-income countries, however, where diets are predominantly plant-based, and intakes of animal protein are low, diets are often high in phytate, so bioavailability of zinc is low (Gibson, 1994; Hotz and Brown, 2004).

Studies investigating the effects of calcium on zinc absorption have yielded equivocal results (McKenna et al., 1997; Wood and Zheng, 1997). In general, calcium does not have an inhibitory effect on zinc absorption, except, perhaps, in high-phytate meals (Lönnerdal, 2000).

The amount and type of protein in the diet and its zinc content may also influence zinc absorption. Fractional zinc absorption increases with increasing protein content, with animal protein from beef and eggs probably having a further enhancing effect. The total zinc content of a meal also influences zinc absorption; fractional zinc absorption, expressed as a percentage, decreases with increasing intake of zinc, although the absolute amount of zinc absorbed increases (Lönnerdal, 2000).

A competitive interaction between iron and zinc may occur, depending on the form of the iron, as well as the conditions and levels under which the iron and zinc are given (Lönnerdal, 2000). The interaction is especially evident when the ratio of iron to zinc is very high and when the iron is administered in water and fed under fasting conditions. It is less apparent when the iron is consumed with food or as part of a meal (Sandström et al., 1985; Rossander-Hultén et al., 1991; Whittaker, 1998).

In general, in omnivorous adult diets in affluent countries, the meat group supplies the greatest amount of zinc, followed by cereals and dairy products (Mares-Perlman et al., 1995), However, increasingly among young women in many of these countries, the major food sources of zinc are cereals, nuts, and legumes (Gibson et al., 2001).

Effects of high intakes of zinc

There are no reported cases of toxicity from excess intakes of dietary zinc, although toxicity arising from short-term exposure to very high levels of contaminant zinc (> 300 ppm) from the improper storage of food or beverages in galvanized vessels has been reported (Brown et al., 1964). Signs and symptoms include dehydration, vomiting, electrolyte imbalance, abdominal pain, nausea, lethargy, dizziness, and muscular incoordination (Fosmire, 1990).

Adverse effects of excess zinc on copper metabolism have been described (Prasad et al., 1978a; Fischer et al.,1984; Samman and Roberts, 1988; Yadrick et al., 1989), although the clinical significance of the depressed erythrocyte Cu,Zn-SOD activity observed is unknown.

High intakes of zinc have been associated with reductions in serum HDL cholesterol levels (Hooper et al., 1980), and perhaps with detrimental effects on the immune system (Chandra, 1984). As a result, excessive self-supplementation with zinc may have an adverse effect on health, although doses of 25–35 mg/d Zn in adults do not appear to pose a health hazard (Smith, 1994).

The Tolerable Upper Intake Level (UL) for zinc set by the U.S. Food and Nutrition Board for adults and pregnant and lactating women > 19 y, is 40 mg/d; details for children and adolescents are given in IOM (2001).

Indices of zinc status

Diagnosis of zinc deficiency at the individual level is still hampered by the lack of a single, specific, and sensitive biochemical index of zinc status that reflects the entire spectrum of "zinc status" from deficiency through adequacy to excess and toxicity. At the population level, serum or plasma zinc is useful for identifying subgroups at risk of zinc deficiency (Hotz and Brown, 2004).

Where possible, the use of a combination of dietary, biochemical, and functional physiological indices is recommended to evaluate zinc status, and these latter indices are discussed below.

24.3.1 Serum zinc

From 12% to 22% of the zinc in blood is in the serum; the remainder is within the erythrocytes. Zinc is transported in the serum bound principally to albumin (70%), so conditions that alter serum albumin levels will, in turn, affect serum zinc concentrations. Of the remaining zinc in serum, 18% is tightly bound to α2-macroglobulin, whereas the rest is bound to other proteins such as transferrin and ceruloplasmin and to amino acids, especially histidine and cystine (Cousins, 1985). Significant amounts of zinc bound to these plasma amino acids may be excreted via the urine.

Serum zinc is the most commonly used biochemical marker of zinc status. Several studies have confirmed its usefulness for assessing zinc status at the population level (Donovan and Gibson, 1995; Gregory et al., 2000; Gibson et al., 2001; Brown et al., 2002). In the U.K. national survey of young people aged 4–18 y (Gregory et al., 2000), significant but weak positive correlations between serum zinc and dietary zinc intakes (assessed by 7-d weighed diet records) were reported for girls, but not for boys; serum zinc values were not analyzed in the U.K. adult survey. In noninstitionalized Canadian elderly, a comparable relationship was reported in men but not in women (Payette and Gray-Donald, 1991).

In population groups where cereals rather than animal source foods are the major source of dietary zinc, significant inverse relationships between serum zinc and dietary phytate : zinc molar ratios have sometimes been observed (Donovan and Gibson, 1995; Gibson et al., 2001).

In individuals with severe zinc deficiency, serum zinc concentrations are usually low. Marked decreases have been reported in patients receiving TPN unsupplemented with

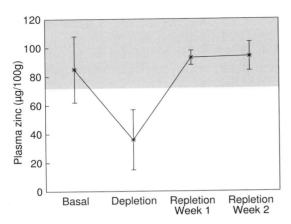

Age (years)	Male serum zinc (μmol/L)	Female serum zinc (μmol/L)
3–8	13.0	12.9
9–19	14.5	13.8
20–44	14.7	13.2
45–64	13.5	12.7
65–74	12.9	12.4

Table 24.20: Median serum zinc levels of males and females in a reference population, by age: United States, 1976–1980. Data are for an "a.m. nonfasting sample." From Pilch and Senti (1984).

Figure 24.13: Changes in plasma zinc (mean ± SD) at the end of basal, depletion, and repletion periods. The shaded area represents the normal range. From Baer and King, American Journal of Clinical Nutrition 39: 556–570, 1984 © Am J Clin Nutr. American Society for Clinical Nutrition.

zinc (Arakawa et al., 1976) and in subjects receiving very low zinc intakes (0.3 mg Zn/d) for 3–4 wk during experimentally induced zinc deficiency (Baer and King, 1984). Concentrations return to normal after zinc supplementation (Figure 24.13).

Serum zinc concentrations are homeostatically controlled, so that even in the presence of dietary zinc restriction, values may remain within the normal range (10–15 μmol/L) for many weeks, despite the existence of clinically important features of zinc deficiency (Fickel et al., 1986; Milne et al., 1987; Ruz et al., 1991). Consequently, serum zinc concentrations are an insensitive measure of zinc status (King, 1990), and values within the normal range do not exclude zinc deficiency. Maintenance of such normal circulating zinc levels is achieved by a reduction in growth rate or by a decrease in excretion (King, 1990)

Factors affecting serum zinc

Age-related changes in serum zinc concentrations occur. In NHANES II, serum zinc values were low in childhood, reaching a peak in adolescence and young adulthood (Pilch and Senti, 1984), after which they declined (Table 24.20). Similar trends in serum

zinc levels during infancy, childhood, and adulthood have been noted by others (Hambidge et al., 1972a; Kasperek et al., 1977; Butrimovitz and Purdy, 1978; Kirsten et al., 1985; Parnell et al., 2003).

Gender may influence serum zinc concentrations. During infancy and early childhood, boys tend to have lower serum zinc levels than girls (Smit-Vanderkooy and Gibson, 1987; Cavan et al., 1993a; Parnell et al., 2003), although in NHANES II, these differences were not apparent for children 3 to 8 y. In contrast, after adolescence, NHANES II males had higher mean serum zinc levels than females, the greatest differences being seen in adults 20–44 y (Table 24.20).

Pregnancy is associated with decreases in serum zinc concentrations, perhaps as early as the first trimester (Hambidge and Droegemueller, 1974). Figure 24.14 shows the median serum zinc concentrations by month of pregnancy, drawn from the NHANES II data. The decline in later pregnancy is attributed to hemodilution, but this effect does not explain the earlier decline (Breskin et al., 1983).

Acute infection and inflammation leads to spurious low serum zinc values because zinc is redistributed from the serum to the liver (Singh et al., 1991). This redistribution is mediated by the release of cytokines, probably interleukin-1 (IL-1), during the acute-phase response. Cytokines activate metallothionein synthesis in the liver (Schroeder and Cousins,

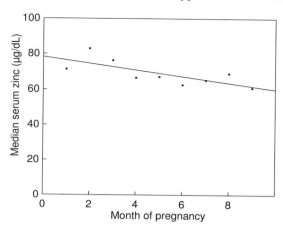

Figure 24.14: Median serum zinc concentrations during pregnancy at 1-mo intervals with the line of linear regression. From Hotz and Brown, Food and Nutrition Bulletin 25 (supp. 2): S94–S204, 2004.

Participants (n)	Mean serum zinc (μmol/L)	Mean serum alkaline phosphatase (U/L)
Non-users (202)	12.11	22.8
OC users (128)	11.81	19.5
Probability of significant dif.	0.05	0.01[a]

Table 24.21: The effect of oral contraceptive (OC) use on serum zinc and alkaline phosphatase concentrations. [a]After correction for age. Data from Gibson et al., British Journal of Nutrition 86: 71–80, 2001, with permission of the authors.

1990), which, in turn, alters the hepatic uptake of zinc (Rofe et al., 1996).

Diurnal variation in serum zinc concentrations has been reported. Levels are higher in serum in the morning, regardless of fasting status, compared to the afternoon (Guillard et al., 1979; Pilch and Senti, 1984; Markowitz et al., 1985; Goodall et al., 1988). As a result of these trends, interpretive criteria for serum zinc vary, depending on the time of day of the blood collection (Table 24.22).

Fasting status markedly affects serum zinc concentrations. Large changes in serum zinc, associated with meals and induced by hormone regulation, have been documented (Markowitz et al., 1985; Goodall et al., 1988; King et al., 1994). Zinc levels in serum increase immediately after a meal, but then decline progressively during the next 4 h, after which they rise again until food is eaten. During an overnight fast, serum zinc levels are slightly elevated, compared with levels of nonfasted individuals, possibly reflecting catabolic changes in muscle protein (Pilch and Senti, 1984).

Estrogen-containing preparations, such as oral contraceptive agents and other hormones, when used, can lead to markedly lower serum zinc concentrations (Table 24.21) (Swanson and King, 1982; Hobisch-Hagen et al., 1997; Gibson et al., 2001).

Hemolysis increases serum zinc concentrations because the concentration of zinc in erythrocytes is higher than that of serum. The effect of hemolysis may be particularly important in cases of zinc deficiency, when red cell fragility is increased (Bettger et al., 1978). Note that in NHANES II, serum zinc levels of "slightly" hemolyzed samples (by visual inspection) were not significantly different from those of nonhemolyzed samples (Pilch and Senti, 1984).

Storage of blood samples prior to separation of the serum affects zinc concentrations if separation is delayed. Changes cannot be detected during the first hour, but longer intervals prior to separation are associated with progressively increasing serum zinc concentrations, as zinc is released from platelets (English and Hambidge, 1988). Tamura et al. (1994) emphasize that the effect of these changes can be reduced by refrigerating the blood samples immediately after collection, and separating the serum as soon as possible, preferably within 30–40 min.

Prolonged use of a tourniquet may result in an increase in serum or plasma zinc levels. This occurs as a result of intravascular pressure caused by venous occlusion, which may cause movement of fluid into the interstitial space, thus increasing the concentration of

Collection time	Males			Females	
	3–9 y	10–64 y	65+ y	3–9 y	10–70 y
AM fasting	NA	15.0±14	14.1±13	NA	13.8±13
AM other	13.0±14	14.4±15	12.5±15	13.2±15	13.2±14
PM	11.8±17	12.5±15	11.6±16	11.5±15	11.9±14

Table 24.22: Geometric mean ± CV (%) for serum zinc (μmol/L) from NHANES II. For conversion to μg/dL, divide by 0.1530. Adult cutoffs based on data from subjects 20 y and older only. NA, not available. From Hotz and Brown, Food and Nutrition Bulletin 25 (supp. 2): S94–S204, 2004.

both serum zinc and proteins (Walker et al., 1979; Juswigg et al., 1982). Hence, a tourniquet should only be used for about 1 min.

Malabsorption syndromes such as celiac disease result in low serum or plasma zinc concentrations arising from a failure of intestinal uptake and transfer of zinc and increased loss of endogenous zinc (Crofton et al., 1983, 1990).

Chronic disease states resulting from hypoalbuminemia, such as alcoholic cirrhosis and protein-energy malnutrition, lead to lower serum zinc concentrations, because zinc is transported in the serum bound to albumin (Solomons, 1979).

Rapid synthesis of tissues during growth may lead to a fall in serum or plasma zinc. This effect has been reported in children during the anabolic phases of recovery from malnutrition (Golden and Golden, 1981) and during the rapid growth that occurs in preterm infants (Altigani et al., 1989). It probably arises because zinc is taken up from the exchangeable zinc pool in the plasma more rapidly than it can be replaced by intestinal absorption or from other body compartments (Aggett and Comerford, 1995).

Interpretive criteria

The International Zinc Consultative Group (IZiNCG) has recently reanalyzed serum zinc data from NHANES II. In this reanalysis, data for subjects with conditions significantly affecting serum zinc concentrations were excluded. These were subjects with low serum albumin (< 35 L); an elevated white blood cell count ($> 11.5 \times 10^9$/L); using oral contraceptive agents, hormones or steroids; or experiencing diarrhea. The IZiNCG also took age, gender, fasting status (i.e., > 8 h since the last meal), and time of day of the sample collection into account in the reanalysis; details are given in Hotz et al. (2003) and Hotz and Brown (2004).

Table 24.22 presents the geometric means for serum zinc for males and females for four age groups 3–9 y, 10–64 y and $\geqslant 65$ y (males) and 10–70 y (females) by fasting status and time of sampling. New reference limits were also determined by IZiNCG, based on the 2.5th percentile of serum zinc concentration for males and females aged < 10 y and $\geqslant 10$ y (by fasting status) and time of sampling. These are given in Table 24.23. Although data were not available from NHANES II for children < 3 y, IZiNCG suggests that the cutoffs for children < 10 y also be applied to children < 3 y, until appropriate reference data are available (Hotz and Brown, 2004).

Data for pregnant women examined during NHANES II are limited ($n = 61$). The

Collection time	Children < 10 y	Males $\geqslant 10$ y	Females $\geqslant 10$ y
AM fasting[a]	NA	11.3	10.7
AM other	9.9	10.7	10.1
PM	8.7	9.3	9.0

Table 24.23: Suggested lower reference limits (2.5[th] percentiles) (μmol/L) for serum zinc concentration based on age group, sex, fasting status, and time of day collection, derived from the NHANES II data. For conversion to μg/dL, divide by 0.1530. [a] Adult reference limits based on data from subjects 20 y and older only. NA, not available. From Hotz and Brown, Food and Nutrition Bulletin 25 (supp. 2): S94–S204, 2004.

2.5th percentile values for the first and second plus third trimesters of pregnancy were calculated by IZiNCG and are 8.6 and 7.6 μmol/L, respectively. No estimate for the 2.5th percentile serum zinc value for lactating women can be derived from the NHANES II survey results because of the limited sample size. Instead, the cutoff derived for nonpregnant women should be used for lactating women at this time (Hotz and Brown, 2004).

The time of blood collection and fasting status should always be recorded during large-scale surveys, to allow the appropriate cutoff values to be used.

Two prevalence levels for low serum zinc concentrations have also been proposed by IZiNCG. These are based on age, sex, time of day of sample collection, and fasting status, and can be used to indicate if zinc deficiency is a serious public health problem (Hotz and Brown, 2004). When the prevalence of low serum zinc values exceeds 20%, the risk of zinc deficiency is probably high, whereas a prevalence of 10%–20% indicates that some segments of the population may be at high risk. When the prevalence of low serum zinc concentrations is < 10%, zinc deficiency is probably not a public health concern.

Karr et al. (1997) have derived cutoffs for Australian children 0–5 y, based on the 2.5th percentile of serum zinc concentrations for children 9–23 mo ($n = 132$) and 24–35 mo ($n = 109$). These two cutoffs are 9.0 and 8.0 μmol/L, respectively, but neither time of day nor fasting status or the existence of possible confounders (e.g., infection) were taken into account in this analysis.

Measurement of serum zinc

Blood samples for serum or plasma zinc should be taken under carefully controlled, standardized conditions. Contamination from various sources such as preservatives, evacuated tubes, lubricants, anticoagulants, water, and rubber stoppers must be avoided. For venipuncture blood samples, trace-element-free evacuated tubes with siliconized rather than rubber stoppers must always be used. Stainless steel or siliconized needles and Tef-

lon or polypropylene catheters can all be used. For capillary blood samples, use of polyethylene serum separators with polyethylene stoppers and olefin-oligomer is recommended (Iyengar et al., 1998).

The following practices have been recommended by IZiNCG (Hotz and Brown, 2004) to minimize contamination during the collection and analysis of serum zinc:

- Disposable polyethylene gloves, free of talc or other coatings, should be worn by those handling blood samples.
- Samples should be processed in laminar flow class 100 clean rooms, laminar flow hoods, or otherwise in a clean, dust- and smoke-free laboratory.
- Stainless steel needles should be used.
- Anticoagulants, if required, should always be prescreened for adventitious zinc contamination prior to use; zinc-free heparin is preferred.
- Prescreen trace-element-free polyethylene evacuated tubes, stoppers, and serum separators for zinc contamination prior to use.
- Prescreen polyethylene storage vials and transfer pipets for zinc contamination before use.
- All equipment used, with the exception of the prescreened disposable items, should be decontaminated by washing procedures (soaked for 24 h in ultrapure 10%–20% HCl or HNO_3 solution and rinsed 3 or 4 times in distilled, deionized water).
- All materials and equipment should be covered or sealed during storage to avoid dust.

Some investigators prefer to use plasma because it is readily separated, less susceptible to platelet contamination, and not subject to contamination from a reaming instrument (Smith et al., 1985). Lower zinc values for plasma than for serum have been reported for samples collected simultaneously from the same persons (English and Hambidge, 1988). Such differences in zinc values in serum compared to plasma are probably due, in part, to discrepancies in the time between collection and separation. For serum, a longer time period between blood collection and separation is generally needed to allow samples to clot prior to separation. During this clotting time, zinc may be released from platelets, causing an increase in serum zinc concentrations. To avoid this effect, blood samples should be refrigerated while stored or kept on ice prior to separation within 30–40 minutes, if possible.

The most frequently used method for the analysis of serum zinc is AAS, using a direct method in which the sample is diluted with four or nine parts of deionized water, aqueous acid solution (e.g., 0.1 M HCl), organic acids (e.g., n-butanol or n-propanol), or with a signal enhancing mixture (Smith et al., 1979; Iyengar et al., 1998). Dilution of the serum reduces the viscosity of the sample, which minimizes both the matrix effect on the rate of aspiration and the tendency for the burner head to become blocked. The latter may be especially a problem with plasma because of precipitates that form in these samples.

To ensure that the viscosity of the samples and standards are similar, a 5% aqueous glycerol solution is sometimes used as the solvent for the standards (Smith et al., 1979) or, alternatively, a 6% aqueous solution of butanol as a sample diluent in a 5–10-fold dilution (Iyengar et al., 1998). A coefficient of variation of < 5% is attainable for zinc using flame AAS. Use of a trichloroacetic acid deproteinization technique is not recommended.

Sometimes the serum or plasma samples are ashed at low temperatures prior to analysis by flame AAS. For very small samples, flameless AAS can be used (Shaw et al., 1982). The U.K. National Diet and Nutrition Survey (Gregory et al., 2000) utilized a sensitive colorimetric determination for serum zinc using a water-soluble pyridylazo dye (Makino et al., 1982). Other techniques include ICP mass spectrometry, ICP atomic emission spectrometry, X-ray spectrometry, proton-induced X-ray emission, INAA, and anodic stripping voltammetry. These alternative methods and their corresponding sample preparation procedures are reviewed by Herber and Stoeppler (1994) and Iyengar et al. (1998).

Certified reference materials, suitable for use when analyzing serum zinc, are available — bovine serum (SRM 1598) from NIST (Gaithersburg, MD) or animal blood (IAEA-A-13) from the IAEA (Seibersdorf, Austria). Because these are expensive, in-house or bench reference materials such as a pooled serum sample, analyzed against a SRM to establish its zinc content, should be prepared and used with every run to monitor precision. In summary, the following procedures for the collection, preparation, and analysis of serum or plasma samples for zinc analysis by AAS, are recommended by IZiNCG (Hotz and Brown, 2004).

- Employ appropriate practices throughout the procedure to avoid adventitious trace element contamination.
- Arrange for the subject to be seated.
- Clean subject's skin with alcohol at the site of the antecubital vein.
- Restrict occlusion of subject's arm with tourniquet to about 1 min.
- Draw blood using a stainless steel needle, and collect into trace-element-free evacuated blood collection tubes *without* anticoagulant for processing serum.
- Place blood sample in refrigerator or on ice and allow to clot for 30–40 min.
- Centrifuge blood sample at 2000–3000 g for 10–15 min.
- Discard any obviously hemolyzed samples.
- Store samples frozen unless they are to be analyzed immediately.
- Dilute sample 5–10-fold in solvents such as 6% aqueous butanol or 10% aqueous propanol.
- Read sample zinc concentration using AAS with appropriate standard dilutions, along with in-house quality controls and standard reference materials.

Serum or plasma samples for zinc analyses can be refrigerated (4°C) for 2–3 wk prior to analysis. For longer storage periods, samples should be frozen at –25°C or lower. To prevent dehydration during long-term storage, especially if frost-free freezers are used, serum or plasma samples should be stored together with ice cubes in heat-sealed plastic bags.

24.3.2 Erythrocyte zinc

The concentration of zinc in erythrocytes is approximately ten times higher than in plasma. It is present mainly as carbonic anhydrase (EC 4.2.1.1) (80–88%), with a small amount bound to Cu,Zn-SOD (EC 1.15.1.1) (~5%). Approximately 2%–3% is bound to low molecular weight binding ligands. The lifespan of erythrocytes is about 120 d. As a result, erythrocyte zinc concentrations do not reflect short-term changes in dietary zinc intake or recent changes in body zinc stores (Neggers et al., 1997).

Few investigators have used erythrocytes to assess zinc status, although their preparation and analysis is not difficult (Milne et al., 1985). In diseases with evidence of tissue zinc depletion such as cirrhosis, severe burns, and histidinemia, as well as diabetes and Crohn's disease, the results for erythrocyte zinc have been conflicting (Vitoux et al., 1999). In experimental zinc depletion – repletion studies (Prasad et al., 1978b; Baer and King, 1984; Ruz et al., 1992; Thomas et al., 1992; Abdallah and Samman, 1993; Cao and Cousins, 2000; Davis et al., 2000), only a few have demonstrated a positive response by erythrocyte zinc or erythrocyte membrane zinc to changes in dietary zinc. For example, in a 49-d zinc depletion study, no changes in erythrocyte zinc were seen, despite evidence of impaired taste acuity and immune function (Ruz et al., 1992). In addition, no response was reported in zinc supplementation studies of 30 and 90 d duration, even when a dose of 50 mg/d Zn was used (Thomas et al., 1992; Davis et al., 2000). The results emphasize the low sensitivity of erythrocyte zinc.

Age-related changes in erythrocyte zinc have been reported. In Japanese subjects, concentrations were very low during infancy (18.7 ± 6.1 µg/g Hb) and increased gradually with age, reaching adult concentrations between 11 and 15 y (42.2 ± 5.6 µg/g Hb), after

which levels remained constant. Vitoux et al. (1999) observed a similar trend. In general, during pregnancy, the zinc content of erythrocytes increases to maintain overall activity of carbonic anhydrase, a zinc-dependent enzyme (Neggers et al., 1997).

Interpretive criteria

At present, no interpretive criteria for erythrocyte zinc have been established. Further, there are no standardized units for the expression of zinc concentrations in erythrocytes, making any comparisons among studies difficult. The units can be based on hemoglobin, volume of packed cells, and per cell. There are presently no accepted standards for conversion among these units.

Measurement of erythrocyte zinc

Erythrocytes for zinc analysis are first washed with isotonic phosphate-buffered saline and then lysed with deionized water. A diluted aliquot of the erythrocyte lysate is used for the analysis by flame or graphite furnace AAS (Whitehouse et al., 1982; Milne et al., 1985). Hemoglobin is also determined concurrently on the erythrocyte lysate, so the zinc content can be expressed in terms of µg per gram of hemoglobin. When graphite furnace AAS is used, standard solutions containing the same inorganic constituents as erythrocytes are required to compensate for matrix effects.

24.3.3 Leukocyte and neutrophil zinc

Leukocytes contain up to 25 times more zinc than erythrocytes, and have a very much shorter lifespan than the 120-d lifespan of erythrocytes. Hence, they are assumed to be more sensitive to changes in zinc supply. Indeed, results of earlier studies based on experimental zinc depletion – repletion, and patients with a number of diseases suggested that leukocyte zinc was a more reliable biomarker of zinc status than erythrocyte or plasma zinc (Meadows et al., 1981; Prasad 1982). It appears to reflect levels of soft tissue zinc (Jones et al., 1981). Later results, however, have been more equivocal (Ruz et al., 1992).

Some of the inconsistencies reported for leukocyte zinc may result from analyzing mixtures of cell types (e.g., neutrophils and lymphocytes), with different half-lives and zinc contents (Table 16.14). Leukocyte subpopulations, such as neutrophils, have been separated and analyzed, but, again, results of human depletion studies have been mixed (Prasad and Cossack, 1982; Ruz et al., 1992) and no interpretive criteria have been established.

Measurement of zinc in leukocytes or specific cell types

The separation of leukocytes and other specific cellular types is difficult. Further, they are prone to contamination from exogenous sources of zinc and from platelets. Milne et al. (1985) showed that the zinc content of leukocytes is a function of the type of separation used; cell suspensions must be free of residual erythrocytes and platelets, as they both have a relatively high zinc content.

Data are also difficult to interpret because no consensus exists for the method used to express zinc concentrations in leukocytes or specific cell types. Results can be expressed on a mg/kg dry weight basis to eliminate the effects of variable cell water content, but results expressed as $ng/10^6$ cells are generally preferred (Nishi, 1980; Prasad and Cossack, 1982; Milne et al., 1985). When the latter method is used, clump-free suspensions are essential; cell clumping results in an underestimate of the actual cell count.

The choice of the anticoagulant affects cell separation; EDTA is preferred (Milne et al., 1985). Cell types can be isolated from whole blood on discontinuous gradients of colloidal polyvinylpyrrolidone-coated silica (Percoll), as recommended by Milne et al. (1985), or Ficoll-Hypaque (English and Anderson, 1974). Alternatively, the separation can involve the use of monoclonal antibodies to various cell types.

Once the cells have been isolated, they must be treated to produce a homogeneous solution or suspension. This is then digested with nitric acid and diluted with deionized water, prior to analysis via AAS. A graphite furnace adapted for microsamples can also be used. When graphite furnace flameless AAS is used, standard solutions simulating the sample matrix are required to compensate for the matrix effects of the digested samples (Milne et al., 1985).

These methodological problems and the contradictory results obtained limit the use of zinc concentrations in these cell types as a valid measure of zinc status at the present time. Relatively large volumes of blood (i.e., about 5 ml) are also required, inhibiting the use of zinc concentrations in mixed leukocytes or specific cell types in infants and children.

24.3.4 Urine zinc concentrations

When intakes of zinc are adequate, the 24-h urinary excretion of zinc is relatively constant and does not reflect the day-to-day variation in zinc intake. Urinary excretion of zinc decreases only in cases of extremely severe zinc deficiency (Hess et al., 1977; Baer and King, 1984); it is unaffected by mild zinc deficiency states (Wada et al., 1985). A similar trend has been noted with zinc supplementation: again 24-h urinary zinc excretion shows a positive response when very high doses of elemental zinc are consumed for 1 wk (i.e., 100 gm/d), but not when lower doses (i.e., 50 mg/d) are given (Verus and Samman, 1994). These results emphasize that urinary zinc is only sensitive to extremes of zinc intake.

The urinary excretion of zinc is also confounded by a variety of clinical conditions that induce hyperzincuria. These include sickle cell disease, alcoholism and liver disease, certain renal diseases and infections, injury, and burns. Hypertensive patients on long-term therapy with chlorothiazide may also exhibit hyperzincuria and, hence, are vulnerable to zinc deficiency (Prasad, 1983). Muscle catabolism also increases urinary zinc excretion, whereas anabolism may depress excretion.

Measurement of urinary zinc excretion

The amounts of zinc excreted in the urine usually range from 300 to 600 µg/d. A 24-h urine collection is preferred because diurnal variation in urinary zinc excretion may be significant. Measurements of urinary zinc are usually performed by flame AAS.

24.3.5 Hair zinc concentrations

The available evidence suggests that low zinc concentrations in hair samples collected during childhood probably reflect a chronic suboptimal zinc status when the confounding effect of severe protein-energy malnutrition is absent (Hambidge et al., 1972a; Gibson, 1980; Smit-Vanderkooy and Gibson, 1987; Gibson et al., 1989a).

Low hair zinc concentrations were reported in the first documented cases of human zinc deficiency in young adult male dwarfs from the Middle East (Strain et al., 1966). Low hair zinc concentrations have also been observed among children with impaired taste acuity and those with low growth percentiles, both features of marginal zinc deficiency in childhood (Hambidge et al., 1972a; Buzina et al., 1980; Chen et al., 1985; Smit-Vanderkooy and Gibson, 1987; Gibson et al., 1989a; Cavan et al., 1993a; Ferguson et al., 1993). In addition, some studies have shown significant relationships between hair zinc concentrations and dietary zinc indices, especially dietary phytate : zinc molar ratios, in subjects consuming predominantly plant-based diets (Ferguson et al., 1989; Gibson and Huddle, 1998; Gibson et al., 2001).

In some but not all cases of suboptimal zinc status, hair zinc concentrations have increased in response to zinc supplementation. The discrepancies may arise from variations in the zinc nutriture of the subjects, duration and dose of the zinc supplementation period, and confounding effects of season on hair zinc concentrations in children. Periods < 6 wk are probably too short for a response in hair zinc, as the latter reflects chronic changes in zinc status (Greger and Geissler, 1978; Lane et al., 1982). Unfortunately, for longer-term studies, seasonal changes in hair zinc concentrations among children must also be taken into account (Hambidge et al., 1979; Gibson et al., 1989b). Hair zinc values in children tend to be lower in the spring and summer, possibly arising from seasonal changes in linear growth velocity that result in a gradual depletion of tissue zinc pools (Gibson et al., 1989b).

Some investigators have failed to find any positive correlations between the zinc content of hair and serum or plasma zinc concentrations (McBean et al., 1971) and relatively short-term (Lane et al., 1982) experimental zinc depletion or supplementation studies. These findings are not unexpected. The zinc content of the hair shaft reflects the quantity of zinc available to the hair follicles at the time of growth, not at the time of sampling. For example, assuming a normal rate of hair growth, the zinc concentrations in the proximal 1–2 cm of hair reflect the zinc uptake by the follicles 4–8 wk prior to sample collection. Hence, positive correlations between hair zinc concentrations and other biochemical indices are only observed in chronic zinc deficiency. Unfortunately, very few long-term zinc depletion – repletion human studies have simultaneously examined hair, serum, and tissue zinc concentrations.

Hair zinc cannot be used in cases when hair growth is arrested, as may occur in severe cases of protein-energy malnutrition or very severe zinc deficiency (e.g., acrodermatitis enteropathica). In such cases, hair zinc levels may be normal or even high (Erten et al., 1978; Bradfield and Hambidge, 1980).

Among malnourished children, impaired linear growth may not be induced by zinc deficiency per se but, instead, by environmental factors such as parasitic infections, morbidity, or deficiencies of other growth-limiting nutrients. Any reduction in growth rate in these children in turn, will reduce their requirements for zinc, and thus may explain apparently normal or even high hair zinc concentrations (Ferguson et al., 1993).

Variations in hair zinc concentrations with hair color, hair beauty treatments, age, site of sampling (scalp versus pubic), and rate of hair growth have also been described (Hambidge, 1982; Taylor, 1986; Klevay et al., 1987). Sex also influences hair zinc concentrations: boys often have lower levels than girls of the same age (Taylor, 1986; Smit-Vanderkooy and Gibson, 1987), perhaps resulting from the higher zinc requirements of boys or relations with growth hormone or testosterone concentrations (Nishi, 1996). The effects of all these possible confounding factors must be considered when interpreting hair zinc concentrations.

Interpretive criteria

Clinical signs of marginal zinc deficiency in childhood, such as impaired growth and poor appetite (anorexia), are usually associated with hair zinc concentrations < 1.07 μmol/g (Hambidge et al., 1972a; Smit-Vanderkooy and Gibson, 1987). Therefore, this value is frequently used as the cutoff point for hair zinc concentrations indicative of suboptimal zinc status in the spring or summer. In the winter, a cutoff point of < 1.68 μmol/g has been used for hair zinc values for young children (Gibson et al., 1989a).

Nevertheless, more work is required to establish age- and season-specific cutoffs for hair zinc concentrations in children. The validity of hair zinc as a chronic index of suboptimal zinc status in adults is uncertain. Conflicting results have been obtained, and no definite conclusions can be drawn.

Measurement of hair zinc

Standardized procedures for sampling, washing, and analyzing hair samples are essential (Section 15.1.9). Samples should be collected from close to the occipital portion of the scalp with stainless steel scissors, and only the proximal 1.0–1.5 cm of the hair strands retained for analysis. Next, any nits and lice must be removed before washing the hair samples using a standardized method; a nonionic detergent (e.g., Actinox) with (McKenzie, 1979) or without (Harrison et al. 1969) acetone is often used.

Hair zinc analysis is most frequently per-

formed by flame AAS, after the ashing of the hair samples. Instrumental neutron activation analysis can also be used (Gibson and De-Wolfe, 1979). A reference material for human hair (e.g., Community Bureau of Reference, Certified Reference Material #397; Institute for Reference Materials and Measurements, Retieseweg, B-2440 Geel, Belgium) must be used to assess the accuracy of the analytical method.

24.3.6 Salivary zinc

Concentrations of zinc in saliva have been investigated as a measure of zinc status because zinc appears to be a component of gustin, an essential protein involved in taste acuity. The latter is impaired by marginal zinc deficiency (Henkin et al., 1971). Zinc concentrations in mixed saliva, parotid saliva, salivary sediment, and salivary supernatant have all been investigated, but their use as biomarkers of zinc status is equivocal (Greger and Sickles, 1979; Freeland-Graves et al., 1981; Lane et al., 1982; Baer and King, 1984). As well, although the collection of saliva samples is quick and relatively noninvasive, the rate of flow and stimulation of saliva is difficult to control, and diurnal variation in zinc levels may occur (Warren et al., 1981). These problems, and the contradictory results observed, limit the use of salivary zinc as a marker of zinc status (Greger and Sickles, 1979).

24.3.7 Zinc-dependent enzymes

Although over one hundred zinc metallo-enzymes have been identified, no single zinc-dependent enzyme has gained widespread acceptance as a biomarker of zinc status in humans. Their response to zinc deficiency, even in experimental studies of zinc depletion – repletion, has been very variable, and none has consistently reflected zinc status. Indeed, their response depends on the biopsy material sampled, the affinity of the enzyme to zinc, the severity of the zinc deficient state, and their specificity.

Of the zinc metallo-enzymes, the activity of alkaline phosphatase (EC 3.1.3.1) in serum has been most frequently studied. Each sub-unit of this dimeric protein contains two Zn atoms. In general, the activity of serum alk-aline phosphatase is reduced in subjects with severe zinc deficiency resulting from acroder-matitis enteropathica (Weismann and Høyer, 1978, 1985), or from severely restricted zinc intakes, either experimentally-induced (Baer et al., 1985) or from total parenteral nutrition unsupplemented with zinc (Ishizaka et al., 1981). In contrast, when only moderately zinc-restricted diets have been fed, no sig-nificant changes in the activity of serum alk-aline phosphatase have been observed (Milne et al., 1987; Davis et al., 2000; Pinna et al., 2001).

The activity of alkaline phosphatase in neutrophils (Prasad, 1983, 1985), leukocytes (Baer et al., 1985; Schilirò et al., 1987), eryth-rocytes (Samman et al., 1996) and erythro-cyte membranes (Ruz et al.,1992; Davis et al., 2000) has also been investigated. In general the response has been positive in experi-mentally controlled zinc depletion – repletion studies, but not when used in community-based supplementation trials (Cavan et al., 1993b), in part because of the large between-subject variation. More studies are needed be-fore a definitive conclusions can be reached.

Several other zinc metallo-enzymes have been investigated as possible biomarkers of zinc status. They include δ-amino-levulinic acid dehydratase (EC 4.2.1.24) in erythrocy-tes (Faraji and Swendseid, 1983; Baer et al., 1985), angiotensin-1-converting enzyme (EC 3.4.15.1) (White et al., 1984; Reeves and O'Dell, 1985; Ruz et al., 1992), and α-D-mannosidase (EC 3.2.1.24) (Apgar and Fitzgerald, 1987) in serum or in neutrophils (Ruz et al., 1992).

The activity of Cu,Zn-SOD in both serum (Davis et al., 2000) and erythrocytes (Abdal-lah and Samman, 1993), nucleoside phos-phorylase (EC 2.4.2.1) in whole, lysed cells (Prasad and Rabbani, 1981; Ballester and Prasad, 1983; Anonymous, 1984b), and ecto purine 5'nucleotidase (EC 3.1,3,5) in red cell membranes (Everett and Apgar, 1986), plas-ma, or in specific cell types has also been studied (Meftah et al., 1991; Bales et al.,1994;

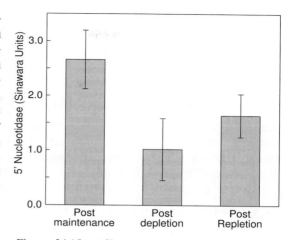

Figure 24.15: Changes in plasma ecto purine 5'nucleotidase after 15 d of zinc depletion followed by 9 d of repletion. Changes in plasma zinc in the same subjects over the same time interval were non-significant. Data from Bales et al., Journal of the American College of Nutrition 13: 455–462, 1994.

Blostein-Fujii et al., 1997; Davis et al., 2000; Pinna et al., 2001).

Of the enzymes investigated, measurement of the activity of ecto purine 5'nucleotidase in plasma or lymphocytes appears to be the most promising. This enzyme is derived from the CD73 cell-surface markers of B and T cells; details are given in Goldberg (1973) and Sunderman (1990). Three sepa-rate studies of postmenopausal women have reported significant changes in the activity of this enzyme in plasma in response to changes in zinc intake; in two cases over a rela-tively short-time period of 15 and 21 d re-spectively (Bales et al., 1994; Blostein-Fujii et al., 1997) (Figure 24.15) and the third after 90 d (Davis et al., 2000).

In an experimental zinc-depletion study by Meftah et al. (1991), the activity of ecto purine 5'nucleotidase in lymphocytes was also reported to be sensitive to changes in zinc intake after 4–8 wk of mild zinc restric-tion, whereas plasma zinc remained unaf-fected. Whether the activity of this enzyme in plasma or lymphocytes is useful in other age groups and in community settings remains to be confirmed. Certainly, in a study of young men consuming a zinc-restricted diet (4.6 mg/d) for 10 wk, no change in the activity of plasma ecto purine 5'nucleotidase was observed (Pinna et al., 2001). Hence, use of ecto purine 5'nucleotidase in plasma or lymphocytes warrants further study.

Measurement of zinc-dependent enzymes

Both alkaline phosphatase activity and 5'nucleotidase activity can be measured spectrophotometrically using commercial assay kits (e.g., Sigma Chemical, St. Louis, MO).

24.3.8 Serum thymulin

Thymulin is a zinc-containing polypeptide which activates T cells. It is secreted by thymic epithelial cells. Circulating thymulin levels in serum decrease in mild zinc deficiency, even when there is no change in serum zinc concentrations. This decrease in activity can be reversed by the in vitro addition of zinc. A decrease in serum thymulin has also been noted in patients with sickle-cell anemia (Prasad et al., 1988). The ability of zinc to enhance in vitro activity when serum thymulin is not saturated with zinc may provide a potentially useful marker for examining optimal zinc status in subjects of varying ages and warrants further investigation (Prasad, 1991).

24.3.9 Metallothionein

Concentrations of metallothionein in serum, erythrocytes, or monocytes have been investigated as potential markers of human zinc status. Metallothionein is a small, cysteine-rich, metal-binding protein that can bind zinc and other heavy metals with high affinity. It is found in most tissues, especially the liver, pancreas, kidney, and intestinal mucosa. Its functional significance is not well understood. Circulating levels respond to changes in zinc intake in both animals (Sato et al., 1984; Cousins and Lee-Ambrose, 1992) and in humans (Grider et al., 1990; Thomas et al., 1992; Sullivan et al., 1998).

The concentrations of metallothionein in serum reflect changes in hepatic metallothionein levels. Hence, any increase in hep-

atic levels in response to stress, inflammation, exercise, or hormonal changes will result in concomitantly elevated levels in serum. As a result, King (1990) recommends the use of a combination of serum zinc and serum metallothionein to assess zinc nutriture. Using this combination, a low level of both plasma zinc and metallothionein would indicate a reduction in the size of the exchangeable zinc pool, as a result of a decrease in zinc intake. In contrast, low plasma zinc concentrations in association with an elevated level of metallothionein could be indicative of redistribution of tissue zinc in response to infection and stress and not to suboptimal zinc status.

Measurement of erythrocyte metallothionein has also been investigated because it appears to be sensitive to changes in dietary zinc intake and, unlike levels in serum, is not responsive to stress. In an experimental zinc depletion – repletion study, levels fell after only 8 d of severe dietary zinc restriction (0.7 mg Zn/kg diet), rising again sevenfold in a 7-d repletion phase during which 50 mg/d Zn was given (Grider et al., 1990). In experimental studies of moderate rather than severe zinc deficiency, levels also declined (Figure 24.16), although the magnitude of the

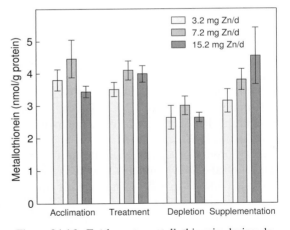

Figure 24.16: Erythrocyte metallothionein during depletion and supplementation. Bars represent mean concentrations ($\pm$ SEM) at the end of each phase. Data from Thomas et al., Journal of Nutrition 122: 2408–2414, 1992, with permission of the American Society for Nutritional Sciences.

response was greater when a longer depletion period was used (Thomas et al., 1992).

Nevertheless, more research is required to establish the sensitivity and specificity of erythrocyte metallothionein as a valid measure of zinc status. Activity increases during pregnancy, with oral contraceptive use, and with smoking. In addition, because young erythrocytes contain most of the erythrocyte metallothionein, circumstances that alter erythropoietin concentrations (e.g., iron deficiency; weight loss) may alter erythrocyte metallothionein levels. Metallothioneine can be assayed in serum and erythrocytes using a radioimmunoassay (Shaikh, 1991).

24.3.10 Monocyte metallothionein messenger RNA

Polymerase chain reaction assays are being increasingly used to measure mRNA for some of the proteins involved in zinc regulation. For example, metallothionein mRNA has been measured in a variety of tissues after zinc supplementation. Both mononuclear blood cells (lymphocytes plus monocytes), or monocytes alone have been used (Cao and Cousins, 2000). Results for the monocytes appear promising. Metallothionein mRNA in monocytes decreased markedly in response to mild zinc depletion (Allan et al., 2000). They have also been reported to respond to zinc supplementation. In a study by Sullivan and Cousins (1997), levels increased rapidly in subjects given a 50-mg zinc supplement, such that they were about five times those of controls, declining again within 4 d to control values after the supplement was discontinued (Sullivan et al., 1998). Even when a supplement of only 15 mg/d Zn was given, a four-fold increase in metallothionein mRNA levels in monocytes occurred (Figure 24.17). Note that after zinc supplementation, expression of metallothionein mRNA levels was markedly less in peripheral blood mononuclear cells compared to that in monocytes (Figure 24.18). Further, when zinc supplementation ceased, metallothionein mRNA levels decreased in both purified monocytes and mononuclear cells, confirming the sen-

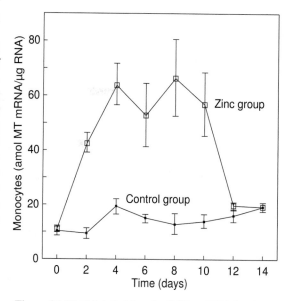

Figure 24.17: Metallothionein (MT) mRNA levels in purified monocytes from control and zinc supplemented men. The subjects were given 15 mg/d Zn or placebo for 10 d and no zinc supplementation for an additional 4 d. Monocytes were purified from venous blood by NycoPrep 1.068 gradient centrifugation and were the source of the total RNA used for reverse transcription. MT mRNA was measured by competitive reverse transcription-polymerase chain reaction (C-RT-PCR) and expressed as amol MT mRNA/μg total RNA. Values are means $\pm$ SE, $n = 8$. Zinc mean is significantly different from mean for control subjects for days 2–10 inclusive. From Cao and Cousins, Journal of Nutrition 130: 2180–2187, 2000, by permission of The American Society for Nutritional Sciences.

sitivity of these measures to changes in zinc intake (Figure 24.17 and 24.18) (Cao and Cousins, 2000). A similar trend was noted for metallothionein mRNA levels in dried blood spots (Cao and Cousins, 2000). More investigation is required of the response of metallothionein mRNA in monocytes to changes in dietary zinc intakes and to various stresses to assess the specificity of this biomarker, and to establish the reliability of the dried blood spot sampling method when investigating metallothionein mRNA levels in community-based and clinical studies.

Measurement of metallothionein mRNA

The assay of metallothionein mRNA levels in dried blood spots has potential for population

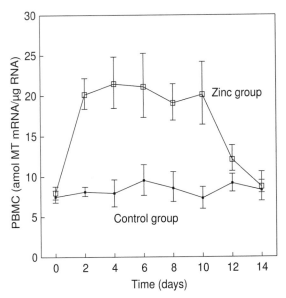

Figure 24.18: Metallothionein (MT) mRNA levels in purified peripheral blood mononuclear cells (PBMC) from control and zinc supplemented men. The subjects were given 15 mg/d Zn or placebo for 10 d and no zinc supplementation for an additional 4 d. PBMC were purified from venous blood by Histopaque 1.077 gradient centrifugation and were the source of the total RNA used for reverse transcription. MT mRNA was measured by competitive reverse transcription-polymerase chain reaction (C-RT-PCR) and expressed as amol MT mRNA/μg total RNA. Values are means ± SE, $n = 8$. Zinc mean is significantly different from mean for control subjects for days 2–10 inclusive. From Cao and Cousins, Journal of Nutrition 130: 2180–2187, 2000, with permission of the American Society for Nutritional Sciences.

studies. The blood samples could be easily collected in the field from a small finger prick or heel prick, dried on filter paper, and sent to a laboratory for subsequent analysis. Samples, once dried and stored in airtight bags, can be kept at –20°C for 1 mo or at 4°C for at least 10 d without any significant loss of metallothionein mRNA activity (Cao and Cousins, 2000). The assay is based on the competitive reverse transcriptase-polymerase chain reaction. Nevertheless, more research is required to confirm the specificity of this assay and to confirm whether these modern molecular techniques can be used routinely for the assessment of zinc status of individuals, as well as populations.

24.3.11 Kinetic markers: pool sizes and turnover rates

In the future, estimates of exchangeable zinc pools (EZP) may be used to confirm the zinc status of individuals with chronically low intakes. Currently, however, the conditions for assessing the EZP have not been standardized, and the test is not easily performed in clinical studies.

Isotope studies evaluating turnover rate in plasma or urine have identified a relatively small exchangeable pool of zinc, mainly in the plasma and liver (Wastney et al., 1986; Miller et al., 1994). This rapidly exchangeable pool of zinc appears to be responsive to acute zinc depletion (King et al., 2001) or chronically low zinc intakes (Sian et al., 1996), but not to modest short-term changes in zinc intake (Pinna et al., 2001).

The size of the EZP appears to correlate with the fat-free mass in adults (Pinna et al., 2001). This suggests that the body size of individuals should be taken into account when EZP values are compared. The size of the pool can be estimated from tracer–tracee disappearance curves using kinetic modeling software. However, such studies are invasive and costly, so that they cannot be used for population assessments. Instead, they may be useful for assessing the risk of zinc deficiency in small clinic-based studies.

Serum zinc turnover rates may also serve as an indicator of zinc status. When the total body zinc content is reduced, fractional plasma zinc turnover rates are increased to meet tissue needs. For example, a 50% increase in fractional plasma zinc turnover rates was noted in the zinc-deficient Egyptian dwarfs compared with normal controls (Prasad, 1966). Increases in the fractional plasma turnover from ~150 to ~200 times per day have also been reported in healthy men as a result of acute, severe zinc depletion (i.e., 0.23 mg/d) (King et al., 2001), but not when it was more modest (Pinna et al., 2001). In the study of acute depletion, there was also a decline in total zinc flux from ~475 to ~230 mg because of a marked decline in plasma zinc concentrations concomitant with the onset of clinical symptoms of zinc deficiency (King et al., 2001). More research is required to establish the validity of either fractional plasma turnover rate or total plasma zinc flux as a marker of zinc status and to standardize the conditions for making the measurements.

24.3.12 Oral zinc tolerance test

A zinc tolerance test, also referred to as a plasma appearance test, measures the increase in plasma zinc from the fasting level after the oral ingestion of a pharmacological dose of zinc. Samples of plasma are collected after a 12-h fast and at hourly intervals post-dose for a 5-h period. Subjects must refrain from eating or drinking during the post-dose period. Generally, a fixed oral dose (e.g., 25 or 50 mg Zn as zinc acetate) is used, irrespective of body weight, although it may be preferable to give the dose on a per kilogram body weight basis (Watson, 1988).

The zinc tolerance test is based on the assumption that it measures zinc status by assessing the overall zinc absorption, which increases in zinc deficiency (Capel et al., 1982; Bales et al., 1986; Fickel et al., 1986). Variable results among subjects in any given group have been noted, making the test most useful when each subject serves as his or her own control (Abu-Hamdan et al., 1986).

Valberg et al. (1985) confirmed that the test does reflect zinc absorption. They compared results of the oral zinc tolerance test with those obtained by direct measurements of ^{65}Zn absorption and retention over a 1-wk period and obtained good agreement. The oral zinc tolerance test has been used to assess the effects of different foods, meals, and vitamin mineral supplements (Solomons, 1982), disease processes (Crofton et al., 1983, 1990; Abu-Hamdan et al., 1986), and medications (Abu-Hamdan et al. 1986) on zinc absorption. It has also been used to determine whether intestinal zinc absorption is increased during pregnancy (Uckan et al., 2001).

Figure 24.19 shows the plasma response of seven subjects to an oral load of 50 mg zinc,

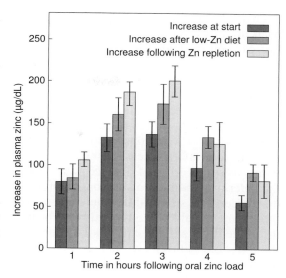

Figure 24.19: Plasma response to an oral load of 50 mg Zn. Values represent the mean ($\pm$ SEM) increase of plasma zinc over the fasting level for 7 subjects. From Fickel et al., American Journal of Clinical Nutrition 43: 47–58, 1986 © Am J Clin Nutr. American Society for Clinical Nutrition.

initially, after 8 wk on a zinc depleted diet, and after 12 d of zinc repletion. In all cases, the peak of the increase occurred at 3 hr post load. After the zinc-depleted diet, the peak percentage increase of plasma zinc was significantly greater than that of the initial test, but generally not higher than that after zinc repletion (Fickel et al., 1986). This persistent elevation of the zinc tolerance curve after repletion markedly decreases the reliability of the zinc tolerance test as an index of zinc status. In addition, use of pharmacological doses of zinc limit the usefulness of the test. Such doses may be handled differently than physiological levels of zinc by the gastrointestinal tract. Parotid saliva does not respond to a zinc tolerance test and cannot be used as an alternative to plasma (Fickel et al., 1986).

24.3.13 Taste acuity tests

Diminished taste acuity (hypogeusia) is one of the features of marginal zinc deficiency in children (Hambidge et al., 1972a; Buzina et al., 1980; Gibson et al., 1989a) and adults

(Henkin, 1984; Wright et al., 1981), and has been used as a functional index of zinc status. Several methods for testing taste acuity have been used (Bartoshuk, 1978), but for all methods, tests should preferably be performed midmorning, at least 2 h after a meal, and by the same person on each occasion.

The three-drop stimulus technique used by Henkin et al. (1963) consists of presenting a single drop of each test solution, together with two single drops of distilled water, onto the anterior two-thirds of the tongue, in random order. The size of the stimulated area of the tongue should be controlled when using the three-drop stimulus technique, because the threshold is inversely related to the size; this variable is very difficult to control (Bartoshuk, 1978). Test solutions of varying concentrations for each of the four taste qualities are used: for salt (sodium chloride), for sweet (sucrose), for bitter (urea), and for sour (hydrochloric acid).

Evaluation of taste acuity is usually based on the detection and recognition thresholds for each taste quality. The detection threshold is defined as the lowest concentration at which a taste can just be detected; the recognition threshold is the lowest concentration at which the quality of the taste stimulus can be recognized (Bartoshuk, 1978). The two thresholds are each determined for one taste quality before proceeding to the next. Several investigators have used this technique on young children (Hambidge et al., 1972a; Buzina et al., 1980; Siegler et al., 1981; Watson et al., 1983), with varying degrees of success.

An alternative technique, which assesses only recognition thresholds and which is better suited to young children, was developed by Desor and Maller (1975). This method was adapted by Gibson and co-workers in studies of Canadian boys with low height percentiles and with Guatemalan school children. In these two investigations, children with low hair zinc concentrations had higher recognition thresholds for salt than children with hair zinc concentrations indicative of "normal" zinc status (Gibson et al., 1989a; Cavan et al. 1993a). It was also used in a study of Canadian vegetarian adolescents, but comparable relationships were not observed (Donovan and Gibson, 1995).

A few studies have used an electrogustometer to measure taste acuity. The method measures the taste threshold by applying a weak electric current (Grant et al., 1987).

Recognition thresholds for salt

For the test of recognition taste thresholds, only one taste quality (salt) is determined, minimizing the potential problems with short attention span and distractions in children. Salt is selected because taste perception to moderately salty solutions changed significantly during a zinc-depletion study of young adult men (Wright et al., 1981).

Sodium chloride concentrations used for testing the Canadian children for recognition thresholds were 10, 15, 20, and 25 mmol/L. Subjects rinse a small amount (10 mL) of each solution around in their mouths, expectorate it, and are then asked to identify the presented sample as salty or plain water. Salt solutions of increasing or decreasing concentrations are used, where appropriate, until the subjects correctly identify salt at one concentration and fail to do so at the next lower concentration. Only 2 out of 10 judgments are allowed to be incorrect before moving to the next higher or lower salt concentration. The midpoint between these two concentrations is used as the recognition threshold for salt for each subject.

Many other factors affect taste function, and taste acuity alone should not be used to assess zinc status.

24.3.14 Multiple indices

The best approach to confirm the existence and magnitude of zinc deficiency involves the measurement of a static biochemical marker (i.e., serum zinc) in conjunction with a physiological test that depends on zinc for optimal function such as taste acuity. In practice, such a combination is often not available, especially at the population level. Hence, alternative combinations have been proposed for an initial assessment at the population level. These include estimates of the adequacy of zinc in the national food supply (Section 2.1.1), in conjunction with stunting, as a functional marker.

Stunting has been selected on the basis of a meta-analysis of 33 community-based zinc intervention trials completed throughout the world (Brown et al., 2002). As well, national data on stunting can be derived from the WHO Global Data Base on Child Growth and Malnutrition (WHO, 1997). Updated information on stunting is available on the internet from WHO. Estimates of the adequacy of zinc in the national food supply can be derived from national food balance sheet data as described earlier (Section 2.1.1) (Brown et al., 2001). Based on this combination, three levels of risk of zinc deficiency have been proposed by Hotz and Brown (2004) and are shown in Table 24.24.

After classifying a country in the intermediate or high risk category, then a more direct assessment via measurement of dietary zinc intake or serum zinc concentrations should be performed. Such an approach will permit the identification of the most vulnerable population groups and selection of an appropriate intervention strategy.

24.4 Summary

Chromium

Chromium, as an organic chromium complex, has a role in glucose metabolism and insulin activity, although its exact biological function is unknown. Clinical manifestations of deficiency can include impaired glucose tolerance, hyperglycemia, relative insulin resistance, peripheral neuropathy, and metabolic encephalopathy. These disturbances have been reported in adults on long-term TPN, and they respond to chromium supplementation. Marginal chromium deficiency states have also been reported in selected population groups, confirmed by an improvement in glucose tolerance after chromium supplementation at physiological levels. This is still the best method of diagnosing a marginal chromium deficiency state. Chromium has yet to be identified as a constituent of any enzyme and, hence, there are presently no enzyme-based tests for chromium status.

Alternative and less certain biomarkers of chromium status include the measurement of hair, serum, and urine chromium concentrations. These methods have been used successfully to assess overexposure to chromium; their use for identifying suboptimal chromium status is less certain. One study has shown strong correlations between hair and serum chromium. These results suggest that low concentrations of chromium in hair or serum, combined with an abnormal glucose tolerance test, may identify subjects at risk for chromium deficiency, at least until a functional marker based on a chromium-dependent enzyme is identified. Graphite furnace AAS with Zeeman-effect background correction is the analytical method most frequently used. Care must be taken to avoid all sources of adventitious contamination during the preparation and analysis of the samples and to use certified reference materials to control the accuracy of the analyses.

Risk of deficiency	Prevalence of stunting	Absorbable zinc in the food supply
High	$\geq 20\%$	$< 63\%$
Moderate	$\geq 10\%, < 20\%$	$< 63\%, < 75\%$
Low	$< 10\%$	$> 75\%$

Table 24.24: Index of the risk of zinc deficiency based on percent adequacy of the national food supply of zinc and the prevalence of stunting (height-for-age Z-score < -2.0. From Hotz and Brown, Food and Nutrition Bulletin 25 (supp. 2): S94–S204, 2004.

Copper

Copper deficiency is rare in humans, although the early hematological deficiency signs, including both neutropenia and hypochromic anemia, have been described in low-birth-weight infants fed cow's-milk-based diets and in some adults with sickle cell disease receiving prolonged zinc therapy. The majority of the clinical features of copper deficiency are associated with changes in the activities of cuproenzymes. A few cases of copper toxicity have also been described, arising either accidentally or in patients with a copper-related genetic defect (Wilson's disease). Toxicity arising from high dietary intakes of copper has not been described.

Serum copper is most frequently used to assess copper status, despite the limited sensitivity and specificity of the measure. Copper depletion – repletion studies suggest that the activity of Cu,Zn-SOD in erythrocytes is both more sensitive and specific than serum copper or serum ceruloplasmin. Nevertheless, its usefulness as a biomarker of copper status in the general population requires confirmation. Concentrations of copper in hair and urine are not valid indices of copper status. In cases of clinical copper deficiency, for example, hair copper levels are normal and urine copper concentrations are too low to measure accurately. In the future two copper-dependent enzymes, cytochrome c oxidase in platelets and diamine oxidase in serum, may prove to be valid and feasible biomarkers of copper status in humans. Assay of lysyl oxidase activity in skin is too invasive for community-based studies.

Zinc

As a constituent of over one hundred metalloenzymes, zinc is essential for many diverse functions, including optimal growth and development, normal reproduction, antioxidant protection, immune and sensory function, and the stabilization of membranes. Primary and secondary deficiencies of zinc are more prevalent in industrialized and low-income countries than are those of chromium and copper. Marginal zinc deficiency, characterized by slow physical growth, poor appetite, and diminished taste acuity, has been described in otherwise healthy infants and children, arising from inadequate intakes or poor availability of dietary zinc. Toxicity from excessive intakes of zinc from the diet has never been reported. Nevertheless, pharmacological doses of zinc supplements have produced hematological signs of copper deficiency, decreases in serum HDL cholesterol levels, and detrimental effects on the immune system.

A combination of biochemical and functional physiological functional indices is best for assessing zinc nutriture and should be used where possible. Serum zinc concentrations are the most frequently used biochemical marker, and can be used to identify population sub-groups at risk of zinc deficiency. Many non-nutritional factors reduce the specificity and sensitivity of serum zinc: infections, fever, estrogen-containing preparations and pregnancy lower serum zinc, but starvation and catabolism increase it. The IZiNCG have compiled lower reference limits for serum zinc based on age, sex, fasting status, and time of collection, derived from NHANES II data.

The validity of leukocyte, erythrocyte, and neutrophil zinc as indices of zinc status remains uncertain. Results have been inconsistent, perhaps because of difficulties with cell separation and analysis. Urine zinc concentrations in 24-h urine samples are only useful in disease-free subjects, when levels decrease as zinc deficiency develops. In the presence of certain diseases, however, hyperzincuria occurs, despite the presence of zinc deficiency. Hair zinc concentrations, measured during childhood, probably reflect chronic zinc status, provided that the effects of confounding factors such as age and season and hair growth rate are taken into account, and the hair is sampled, washed, and analyzed by standardized procedures. Their validity as a chronic index of suboptimal zinc status in adults is less certain.

Of the numerous zinc-dependent enzymes investigated, the activity of ecto purine 5′nucleotidase in plasma appears most promising as a sensitive index of zinc status. Measurement of metallothionein expression through the C-RT-PRC assay in cells from dried blood spot sampling also holds promise, especially for population studies where the collection of venipuncture blood samples is difficult. Isotopic measurements of the exchangeable zinc pool from tracer – tracee disappearance curves is the most definitive index of zinc status but this method is not yet standardized and is only suitable for clinical research studies. Many of the physiological functional tests (e.g., impaired taste acuity) are not conducted routinely and are nonspecific, so that they must be used in conjunction with biochemical zinc indices. An oral zinc tolerance test has also been used on the assumption that it reflects zinc absorption, but results have been inconsistent.

The IZiNCG has compiled an indicator based on the proportion of the population at risk of inadequate zinc intake and the prevalence of stunting to assess three levels at which risk of zinc deficiency is considered to be a public health risk: low, intermediate, and high. If a country falls within the intermediate or high risk levels, then a more direct population assessment, based on dietary zinc intake or serum zinc concentrations in a representative sample of the population, is required.

References

Aalbers TG, Houtman JP. (1985). Relationships between trace elements and atherosclerosis. Science of the Total Environment 43: 255–283.

Abdallah SM, Samman S. (1993). The effect of increasing dietary zinc on the activity of superoxide dismutase and zinc concentration in erythrocytes of healthy female subjects. European Journal of Clinical Nutrition 47: 327–332.

Abraham AS, Brooks BA, Eylath U. (1992). The effects of chromium supplementation on serum glucose and lipids in patients with and without non-insulin-dependent diabetes. Metabolism 41: 768–771.

Abu-Hamdan DK, Mahajan SK, Migdal S, Prasad AS, McDonald FD. (1986). Zinc tolerance test in uremia: effect of ferrous sulphate and aluminium hydroxide. Annals of Internal Medicine 104: 50–52.

Aggett PJ, Comerford JG. (1995). Zinc and human health. Nutrition Reviews 53: S16–S22.

Alda JO, Garay R. (1990). Chloride (or bicarbonate)-dependent copper uptake through the anion exchanger in human red blood cells. American Journal of Physiology 259: C570–C576.

Allan AK, Hawksworth GM, Woodhouse LR, Sutherland B, King JC, Beattie JH. (2000). Lymphocyte metallothionein mRNA responds to marginal zinc intake in human volunteers. British Journal of Nutrition 84: 747–756. Erratum 85: 247

al-Rashid RA, Spangler J. (1971). Neonatal copper

deficiency. New England Journal of Medicine 285: 841–843.

Alsbirk KE, Mogensen CE, Husted SE, Geday E. (1981). Liver and kidney function in stainless steel welders. Ugeskrift Laeger 143: 112–116.

Altigani M, Murphy JF, Gray OP. (1989). Plasma zinc concentration and catchup growth in preterm infants. Acta Paediatrica Scandinavica Suppl 357: 20–33.

Anderson RA. (1998). Chromium, glucose intolerance and diabetes. Journal of the American College of Nutrition 17: 548–555.

Anderson RA. (2000). Chromium in the prevention and control of diabetes. Diabetes and Metabolism 26: 22–27.

Anderson RA. (2003). Chromium and insulin resistance. Nutrition Research Reviews 16: 267–275.

Anderson RA, Kozlovsky AS. (1985). Chromium intake, absorption and excretion of subjects consuming self-selected diets. American Journal of Clinical Nutrition 41: 1177–1183.

Anderson RA, Polansky MM, Bryden NA, Roginski EE, Patterson KY, Reamer C. (1982a). Effect of exercise (running) on serum glucose, insulin, glucagon and chromium excretion. Diabetes 31: 212–216.

Anderson RA, Polansky MM, Bryden NA, Roginski EE, Patterson KY, Veillon C, Glinsmann W. (1982b). Urinary chromium excretion of human subjects: effects of chromium supplementation and glucose loading. American Journal of Clinical Nutrition 36: 1184–1193.

Anderson RA, Polansky MM, Bryden N, Patterson K, Veillon C, Glinsmann WH. (1983a). Effects of chromium supplementation on urinary Cr excretion of human subjects and correlation of Cr excretion with selected clinical parameters. Journal of Nutrition 113: 276–281.

Anderson RA, Polansky MM, Bryden NA, Roginski EE, Mertz W, Glinsmann W. (1983b). Chromium supplementation of human subjects: effect on glucose, insulin, and lipid variables. Metabolism 32: 894–899.

Anderson RA, Polansky MM, Bryden NA. (1984). Acute effects on chromium, copper, zinc and selected clinical variables in urine and serum of male runners. Biological Trace Element Research 6: 327–336.

Anderson RA, Bryden NA, Polansky MM. (1985). Serum chromium of human subjects: effects of chromium supplementation and glucose. American Journal of Clinical Nutrition 41: 571–577.

Anderson RA, Polansky MM, Bryden NA, Bhathena SJ, Canary JJ. (1987). Effects of supplemental chromium on patients with symptoms of reactive hypoglycemia. Metabolism 36: 351–355.

Anderson RA, Bryden NA, Polansky MM, Deuster PA. (1988). Exercise effects on chromium excretion of trained and untrained men consuming a constant diet. Journal of Applied Physiology 64: 249–252.

Anderson RA, Bryden NA, Polansky MM, Reiser S.

(1990). Urinary chromium excretion and insulinogenic properties of carbohydrates. American Journal of Clinical Nutrition 51: 864–868.

Anderson RA, Bryden NA, Polansky MM, Thorp JW. (1991a). Effects of carbohydrate loading and underwater exercise on circulating cortisol, insulin and urinary losses of chromium and zinc. European Journal of Applied Physiology and Occupational Physiology 63: 146–150.

Anderson RA, Polansky MM, Bryden NA, Canary JJ. (1991b). Supplemental-chromium effects on glucose, insulin, glucagon, and urinary chromium losses in subjects consuming controlled low-chromium diets. American Journal of Clinical Nutrition 54: 909–916.

Anderson RA, Bryden NA, Polansky MM. (1992). Dietary chromium intake: freely chosen diets, institutional diets, and individual foods. Biological Trace Element Research 32: 117–121.

Anderson RA, Cheng N, Bryden NA, Polansky MM, Cheng N, Chi J, Feng J. (1997). Elevated intakes of supplemental chromium improve glucose and insulin variables in individuals with type 2 diabetes. Diabetes 46: 1786–1791.

Andrewartha KA, Caple IW. (1980). Effects of changes in nutritional copper on erythrocyte superoxide dismutase activity in sheep. Research in Veterinary Science 28: 101–104.

Anonymous (1984a). Conditioned copper deficiency due to antacids. Nutrition Reviews 42: 319–321.

Anonymous (1984b). Nucleoside phosphorylase: a zinc metalloenzyme and a marker of zinc deficiency. Nutrition Reviews 42: 279–281.

Apgar J, Fitzgerald JA. (1987). Measures of zinc status in ewes given a low zinc diet throughout pregnancy. Nutrition Research 7: 1281–1290.

Arakawa T, Tamura T, Igarashi Y, Suzuki H, Sandstead HH. (1976). Zinc deficiency in two infants during total parenteral alimentation for diarrhea. American Journal of Clinical Nutrition 29: 197–204.

Ashkenazi A, Levin S, Djaldetti M, Fishel E, Benvenisti D. (1973). The syndrome of neonatal copper deficiency. Pediatrics 52: 525–533.

Baer MT, King JC. (1984). Tissue zinc levels and zinc excretion during experimental zinc depletion in young men. American Journal of Clinical Nutrition 39: 556–570.

Baer MT, King JC, Tamura T, Margen S, Bradfield RB, Weston WL, Daugherty NA. (1985). Nitrogen utilization, enzyme activity, glucose intolerance and leukocyte chemotaxis in human experimental zinc depletion. American Journal of Clinical Nutrition 41: 1220–1235.

Baker A, Harvey L, Majask-Newmann G, Fairweather-Tait S, Flynn A, Cashman K. (1999a). Effect of dietary copper intakes on biochemical markers of bone metabolism in healthy adult males. European Journal of Clinical Nutrition 53: 408–412.

Baker A, Turley E, Bonham MP, O'Connor JM, Strain J, Flynn A, Cashman K. (1999b). No effect of copper supplementation on biochemical markers of bone

metabolism in healthy adults. British Journal of Nutrition 82: 283–290.

Bales CW, Steinman LC, Freeland-Graves JH, Stone J, Young RK. (1986). The effect of age on plasma zinc uptake and taste acuity. American Journal of Clinical Nutrition 44: 664–669.

Bales CW, DiSilvestro RA, Currie KL, Plaisted CS, Joung H, Galanos AN, Lin PH. (1994). Marginal zinc deficiency in older adults: responsiveness of zinc status indicators. Journal of the American College of Nutrition 13: 455–462.

Ballester OF, Prasad AS. (1983). Anergy, zinc deficiency, and decreased nucleoside phosphorylase activity in patients with sickle cell anemia. Annals of Internal Medicine 98: 180–182.

Barclay SM, Aggett PJ, Lloyd DJ, Duffty P. (1991). Reduced erythrocyte superoxide dismutase activity in low birth weight infants given iron supplements. Pediatric Research 29: 297–301.

Barnes PM, Moynahan EJ. (1973). Zinc deficiency in acrodermatitis enteropathica: multiple dietary intolerance treated with synthetic diet. Proceedings of the Royal Society of Medicine 66: 327–329.

Bartoshuk LM. (1978). The psycho-physics of taste. American Journal of Clinical Nutrition 31: 1068–1077.

Bayless TM, Luk GD, Baylin SB, Thomas ME. (1981). Decreased plasma diamine oxidase levels in Crohn's disease and celiac disease. Gastroenterology 80: 1106.

Bentley ME, Caulfield LE, Ram M, Santizo MC, Hurtado E, Rivera JA, Ruel MT, Brown KH. (1997). Zinc supplementation affects the activity patterns of rural Guatemalan infants. Journal of Nutrition 127: 1333–1338.

Bertinato J, Iskandar M, L'Abbé MR. (2003). Copper deficiency induces the upregulation of the copper chaperone for Cu/Zn superoxide dismutase in weanling male rats.

Bettger WJ, Fish TJ, O'Dell BL. (1978). Effects of copper and zinc status of rats on erythrocyte stability and superoxide dismutase activity. Proceedings of the Society of Experimental Biology and Medicine 158: 279–282.

Bettger WJ, Savage JE, O'Dell BL. (1979). Effects of dietary copper and zinc on erythrocyte superoxide dismutase activity in the chick. Nutrition Reports International 19: 893–900.

Bhutta ZA, Black RE, Brown KH, Gardner JM, Gore S, Hidayat A, Khatun F, Martorell R, Ninh NX, Penny ME, Rosado JL, Roy SK, Ruel M, Sazawal S, Shankar A. (1999). Prevention of diarrhea and pneumonia by zinc supplementation in children in developing countries: pooled analysis of randomized controlled trials. Journal of Pediatrics 135: 689–697.

Bhutta ZA, Bird SM, Black RE, Brown KH, Gardner JM, Hidayat A, Khatun F, Martorell R, Ninh NX, Penny ME, Rosado JL, Roy SK, Ruel M, Sazawal S, Shankar A. (2000). Therapeutic effects of oral zinc in acute and persistent diarrhea in children in developing countries: pooled analysis of randomized controlled trials. American Journal of Clinical Nutrition 72: 1516–1522.

Blostein-Fujii A, DiSilvestro RA, Frid D, Katz C, Malarkey W. (1997). Short-term zinc supplementation in women with non-insulin-dependent diabetes mellitus: effects on plasma 5′nucleotidase activities, insulin-like growth factor I concentrations and lipoprotein oxidation rates in vitro. American Journal of Clinical Nutrition 66: 639–642.

Bogden JD, Bendich A, Kemp FW, Bruening KS, Shurnick JH, Denny T, Baker H, Louria DB. (1994). Daily micronutrient supplements enhance delayed-hypersensitivity skin test responses in older people. American Journal of Clinical Nutrition 60: 437–447.

Boling EA. (1966). A multiple slit burner for atomic absorption spectroscopy. Spectrochimica Acta 22: 425–431.

Botash AS, Nasca J, Dubowy R, Weinberger HL, Oliphant M. (1992). Zinc-induced copper deficiency in an infant. American Journal of Diseases of Children 146: 709–711.

Bradfield RB, Hambidge KM. (1980). Problems with hair zinc as an indicator of body zinc status. Lancet 1(8164): 363.

Bradfield RB, Cordano A, Baertl J, Graham G. (1980). Hair copper in copper deficiency. Lancet 2(8190): 343–344.

Breskin MW, Worthington-Roberts BS, Knopp RH, Brown Z, Plovie B, Mottet NK, Mills JL. (1983). First trimester serum zinc concentrations in human pregnancy. American Journal of Clinical Nutrition 38: 943–953.

Brown KH. (1998). Effect of infections on plasma zinc concentration and implications for zinc status assessment in low-income countries. American Journal of Clinical Nutrition 68: 425S–429S.

Brown KH, Lanata CF, Yuen ML, Peerson JM, Butron B, Lönnerdal B. (1993). Potential magnitude of the misclassification of a population's trace element status due to infection: example from a survey of young Peruvian children. American Journal of Clinical Nutrition 58: 549–554.

Brown KH, Wuehler SE, Peerson JM. (2001). The importance of zinc in human nutrition and estimation of the global prevalence of zinc deficiency. Food and Nutrition Bulletin 22: 113–125.

Brown KH, Peerson JM, Allen LH, Rivera J. (2002). Effect of supplemental zinc on the growth and serum zinc concentrations of prepubertal children: a meta-analysis of randomized, controlled trials. American Journal of Clinical Nutrition 75: 1062–1071.

Brown MA, Thom JV, Orth GL, Cova P, Juarez J. (1964). Food poisoning involving zinc contamination. Archives of Environmental Health 8: 657–660.

Brown RO, Forloines-Lynn S, Cross RE, Heizer WD. (1986). Chromium deficiency after long-term total parenteral nutrition. Digestive Diseases and Sciences 31: 661–664.

Brune D, Aitio A, Nordberg G, Vesterberg O, Gerhardsson L. (1993). Normal concentrations of chromium in serum and urine. Scandinavian Journal of Work and Environmental Health 19(Supp.1): 39–44.

Buffone GL, Brett EM, Lewis SA, Iosefsohn M, Hicks JM. (1979). Limitations of immunochemical measurements of ceruloplasmin. Clinical Chemistry 25: 749–751.

Bunn HF. (1981). Evaluation of glycosylated hemoglobin in diabetic patients. Diabetes 30: 613–617.

Butrimovitz GP, Purdy WC. (1978). Zinc nutrition and growth in a childhood population. American Journal of Clinical Nutrition 31: 1409–1412.

Buzina R, Jusic M, Sapunar J, Milanovic N. (1980). Zinc nutrition and taste acuity in school children with impaired growth. American Journal of Clinical Nutrition 33: 2262–2267.

Cabrera-Vique C, Teissedre PL, Cabanis MT, Cabanis JC. (1997). Determination and levels of chromium in French wine and grapes by graphite furnace atomic absorption spectrometry. Journal of Agricultural and Food Chemistry 45: 1808–1811.

Cao J, Cousins RJ. (2000). Metallothionein mRNA in monocytes and peripheral blood mononuclear cells and in cells from dried blood spots increases after zinc supplementation of men. Journal of Nutrition 130: 2180–2187.

Capel ID, Spencer EP, Davies AE, Levitt HN. (1982). The assessment of zinc status by the zinc tolerance test in various groups of patients. Clinical Biochemistry 15: 257–260.

Carter JP, Kattab A, Abd-el-Hadi K, Davis JT, el Gholmy A, Patwardhan VN. (1968). Chromium (3) in hypoglycemia and in impaired glucose utilization in kwashiorkor. American Journal of Clinical Nutrition 21: 195–202.

Cartwright GE. (1950). Copper metabolism in human subjects. In: McElroy WD, Glass B (eds.) Symposium in Copper Metabolism. Johns Hopkins University Press, Baltimore, pp. 274–314.

Cartwright GE, Gubler CJ, Wintrobe MM. (1954). Studies on copper metabolism; copper and iron metabolism in the nephrotic syndrome. Journal of Clinical Investigation 33: 685–698.

Casey CE, Robinson MF. (1983). Some aspects of nutritional trace element research. In: Sigel H (ed.) Metal Ions in Biological Systems. Volume 16: Methods Involving Metal Ions and Complexes in Clinical Chemistry. Marcel Dekker, New York, pp. 1–26.

Cashman KD, Baker A, Ginty F, Flynn A, Strain JJ, Bonham MP, O'Connor JM, Bügel S, Sandström B. (2001). No effect of copper supplementation on biochemical markers of bone metabolism in healthy young adult females despite apparently improved copper status. European Journal of Clinical Nutrition 55: 525–531.

Castillo-Duran C, Uauy R. (1988). Copper deficiency impairs growth of infants recovering from malnutrition. American Journal of Clinical Nutrition 47: 710–714.

Caulfield LE, Zavaleta N, Figueroa A, Leon Z. (1999). Maternal zinc supplementation does not affect size at birth or pregnancy duration in Peru. Journal of Nutrition 129: 1563–1568.

Cavan KR, Gibson RS, Grazioso CF, Isalgue AM, Ruz M, Solomons NW. (1993a). Growth and body composition of periurban Guatemalan children in relation to zinc status: a cross-sectional study. American Journal of Clinical Nutrition 57: 334–343.

Cavan KR, Gibson RS, Grazioso CF, Isalgue AM, Ruz M, Solomons NW. (1993b). Growth and body composition of periurban Guatemalan children in relation to zinc status: a longitudinal zinc intervention trial. American Journal of Clinical Nutrition 57: 344–352.

Chandra RK. (1984). Excessive intakes of zinc impairs immune responses. Journal of the American Medical Association 252: 1443–1446.

Chen XC, Yin TA, He JS, Ma QY, Han ZM, Li LX (1985). Low levels of zinc in hair and blood, pica, anorexia, and poor growth in Chinese preschool children. American Journal of Clinical Nutrition 42: 694–700.

Cheng N Zhu X, Shi H, Wu W, Chi J, Cheng J, Anderson RA (1999). Follow-up survey of people in China with type 2 diabetes mellitus consuming supplemental chromium. Journal of Trace Elements in Experimental Research 12: 55–60.

Cherry FF, Sandstead HH, Rojas P, Johnson LK, Batson HK, Wang XB. (1989). Adolescent pregnancy: associations among body weight, zinc nutriture, and pregnancy outcome. American Journal of Clinical Nutrition 50: 945–954.

Christian P, West KP Jr. (1998). Interactions between zinc and vitamin A: an update. American Journal of Clinical Nutrition 68(suppl): 435S–441S.

Christian P, Khatry S, Yamini S, Stallings R, LeClerq S, Shrestha SR, Pradhan EK, West KP Jr. (2001). Zinc supplementation might potentiate the effect of vitamin A in restoring night vision in pregnant Nepalese women. American Journal of Clinical Nutrition 73: 1045–1051.

Chuttani HK, Gupta PS, Gulati S, Gupta DN. (1965). Acute copper sulfate poisoning. American Journal of Medicine 39: 849–854.

Cohen N, Keen CL, Hurley LS, Lönnerdal B. (1985). Determinants of copper-deficiency anemia in rats. Journal of Nutrition 115: 710–725.

Cordano A, Baertl JM, Graham GG. (1964). Copper deficiency in infancy. Pediatrics 34: 324–336.

Cousins RJ. (1985). Absorption, transport, and hepatic metabolism of copper and zinc: special reference to metallothionein and ceruloplasmin. Physiology Reviews 65: 238–309.

Cousins RJ. (1996). Zinc. In: Ziegler EE, Filer Jr LJ (eds.) Present Knowledge in Nutrition, 7th ed. International Life Sciences Institute Press, Washington, DC, pp. 293–306.

Cousins RJ, Lee-Ambrose LM (1992). Nuclear zinc uptake and interactions and metallothionein gene expression are influenced by dietary zinc in rats. Journal of Nutrition 122: 56–64.

Creason JP, Hinners TA, Bumgarner JE, Pinkerton C. (1975). Trace elements in hair, as related to exposure in metropolitan New York. Clinical Chemistry 21: 603–612.

Crews MG, Taper LJ, Ritchey SJ. (1980). Effects of oral contraceptive agents on copper and zinc balance in young women. American Journal of Clinical Nutrition 33: 1940–1945.

Crofton RW, Glover SC, Ewen SW, Aggett PJ, Mowat NA, Mills CF. (1983). Zinc absorption in celiac disease and dermatitis herpetiformis: a test of small intestinal function. American Journal of Clinical Nutrition 38: 706–712.

Crofton RW, Aggett PJ, Gvozdanovic S, Gvozdanovic D, Mowat NA, Brunt PW. (1990). Zinc metabolism in celiac disease. American Journal of Clinical Nutrition 52: 379–382.

Cunnane SC. (1988). Zinc: Clinical and Biochemical Significance. CRC Press, Boca Raton, FL.

Danks DM. (1980). Copper deficiency in humans. Ciba Foundation Symposium 79: 209–225.

Danks DM. (1988). Copper deficiency in humans. Annual Review of Nutrition 8: 235–257.

Danks DM, Cambell PE, Stevens BJ, Mayne V, Cartwright E. (1972). Menkes' kinky hair syndrome: an inherited defect in copper absorption with widespread effects. Pediatrics 50: 188–201.

Davidson IW, Burt RL. (1973). Physiologic changes in plasma chromium of normal and pregnant women: effect of a glucose load. American Journal of Obstetrics and Gynecology 116: 601–608.

Davidson IW, Burt RL, Parker JC. (1974). Renal excretion of trace elements: chromium and copper. Proceedings of the Society of Experimental Biology and Medicine 147: 720–725.

Davies S, McLaren Howard J, Hunnisett A, Howard M. (1997). Age-related decreases in chromium levels in 51,665 hair, sweat, and serum samples from 40,872 patients: implications for the prevention of cardiovascular disease and type II diabetes mellitus. Metabolism 46: 469–473.

Davis ML, Seaborn CD, Stoecker BJ. (1995). Effects of over-the-counter drugs on 51chromium retention and urinary excretion in rats. Nutrition Research 15: 202–210.

Davis CD, Milne DB, Nielsen FH. (2000). Changes in dietary zinc and copper affect zinc-status indicators of postmenopausal women, notably extracellular superoxide dismutase and amyloid precursor proteins. American Journal of Clinical Nutrition 71: 781–788.

Davis-Whitenack ML, Adeleye BO, Rolf LL, Stoecker BJ. (1996). Biliary excretion of 51-chromium in bile-duct cannulated rats. Nutrition Research 16: 1009–1015.

Del Villano DC, Miller SI, Schacter LP, Tischfield JA. (1980). Elevated superoxide dismutase in black alcoholics. Science 207: 991–993.

Desor JA, Maller O. (1975). Taste correlates of disease

states: cystic fibrosis. Journal of Pediatrics 87: 93–96.

DiMauro S, Bonilla E, Zeviani M, Nakagawa M, De-Vivo DC. (1985). Mitochondrial myopathies. Annals of Neurology 17: 521–538.

DiSilvestro RA, Marten J, Skehan M. (1992). Effects of copper supplementation on ceruloplasmin and copper-zinc superoxide dismutase in free-living rheumatoid arthritis patients. Journal of the American College of Nutrition 11: 177–180.

DiSilvestro RA, Jones AA, Smith D, Wildman R. (1997). Plasma diamine oxidase activities in renal dialysis patients, a human with spontaneous copper deficiency and marginally copper deficient rats. Clinical Biochemistry 30: 559–563.

Doisy RJ, Streeten DHP, Sourma ML, Kalafer ME, Rekant SL, Dalakos TG. (1971). Metabolism of chromium in human subjects: normal, elderly and diabetic subjects. In: Mertz W, Cornazen WE (eds.) Newer Trace Elements in Nutrition. Marcel Dekker, New York, pp. 155–168.

Donovan UM, Gibson RS. (1995). Iron and zinc status of young women aged 14 to 19 years consuming vegetarian and omnivorous diets. Journal of the American College of Nutrition 14: 463–472.

Dowling HJ, Offenbacher EG, Pi-Sunyer FX. (1990). Effects of amino acids on the absorption of trivalent chromium and its retention by regions of the rat small intestine. Nutrition Research 10: 1261–1271.

Duchateau J, Delepesse G, Vrijens R, Collet H. (1981). Beneficial effects of oral zinc supplementation on the immune response of old people. American Journal of Medicine 70: 1001–1004.

Dunlap WM, James GW, Hume DM. (1974). Anemia and neutropenia caused by copper deficiency. Annals of Internal Medicine 80: 470–476.

Edme JL, Shirali P, Mereau M, Sobaszek A, Boulenguez C, Diebold F, Haguenoer JM. (1997). Assessment of biological chromium among stainless steel and mild steel welders in relation to welding processes. International Archives of Occupational and Environmental Health 70: 237–242.

English JL, Anderson BR. (1974). Single step separation of red blood cells, granulocytes and mononuclear leucocytes on discontinuous gradients of Ficoll-Hypaque. Journal of Immunological Methods 5: 249–252.

English JL, Hambidge KM. (1988). Plasma and serum zinc concentrations: effect of time between collection and separation. Clinica Chimica Acta 175: 211–215.

Epstein O, Boss AM, Lyon TDB, Sherlock S. (1980). Hair copper in primary biliary cirrhosis. American Journal of Clinical Nutrition 33: 965–967.

Erten J, Arcasoy A, Cavdar AO, Cin S. (1978). Hair zinc levels in healthy and malnourished children. American Journal of Clinical Nutrition 31: 1172–1174.

Evans GW, Bowman TD. (1992). Chromium picolinate increases membrane fluidity and rate of insulin internalization. Journal of Inorganic Biochemistry 46: 243–250.

Everett G, Apgar J. (1986). Comparison of four enzymes in zinc-deficient rats as possible indicators of marginal zinc status. Acta Pharmacologica et Toxicologica 59(suppl 7): 163–165.

Faraji B, Swendseid ME. (1983). Growth rate, tissue zinc levels and activities of selected enzymes in rats fed a zinc-deficient diet by gastric tube. Journal of Nutrition 113: 447–455.

Ferguson EL, Gibson RS, Thompson LU, Ounpuu S. (1989). Dietary calcium, phytate, and zinc intakes and the calcium, phytate, and zinc molar ratios of the diets of a selected group of East African children. American Journal of Clinical Nutrition 50: 1450–1456.

Ferguson EL, Gibson RS, Opare-Obisaw C, Ounpuu S, Thompson LU, Lehrfeld J. (1993). The zinc nutriture of preschool children living in two African countries. Journal of Nutrition 123: 1487–1496.

Fickel JJ, Freeland-Graves JH, Roby MJ. (1986). Zinc tolerance tests in zinc deficient and zinc supplemented diets. American Journal of Clinical Nutrition 43: 47–58.

Finch S, Doyle W, Lowe C, Bates CJ, Prentice A, Smithers G, Clarke PC. (1998). National Diet and Nutrition Survey: People Aged 65 Years or Older. Volume 1: Report of the Diet and Nutrition Survey. The Stationery Office, London.

Fischer PWF, Giroux A, L'Abbé MR. (1984). Effect of zinc supplementation on copper status in adult man. American Journal of Clinical Nutrition 40: 743–746.

Fischer PWF, L'Abbe MR, Giroux A. (1990). Effects of age, smoking, drinking, exercise and estrogen use on indices of copper status in healthy adults. Nutrition Research 10: 1081–1090.

Fosmire GJ. (1990). Zinc toxicity. American Journal of Clinical Nutrition 51: 225–227.

Fraker PJ, King LE, Laakko T, Vollmer TL. (2000). The dynamic link between the integrity of the immune system and zinc status. Journal of Nutrition 130: 1399–1406.

Freeland-Graves JH, Hendrickson PJ, Ebangit ML, Snowden JY. (1981). Salivary zinc as an index of zinc status in women fed a low-zinc diet. American Journal of Clinical Nutrition 34: 312–321.

Freund H, Atamian S, Fischer JE. (1979). Chromium deficiency during total parenteral nutrition. Journal of the American Medical Association 241: 496–498.

Frieden E. (1985). New perspectives on the essential trace elements. Journal of Chemical Education 62: 917–923.

Gallagher SK, Johnson LK, Milne DB. (1989). Short- and long-term variability of selected indices related to nutritional status. I: Ca, Cu, Fe, Mg, and Zn. Clinical Chemistry 35: 369–373.

Garg HK, Singhal KC, Arshad Z. (1993). A study of the effect of oral zinc supplementation during pregnancy on pregnancy outcome. Indian Journal of Physiology and Pharmacology 37: 276–284.

Garnica AD, Frias JL, Rennert OM. (1977). Menkes' kinky hair syndrome: is it a treatable disorder? Clinical Genetics 11: 154–161.

Ghosh D, Bhattacharya B, Mukherjee B, Manna B, Sinha M, Chowdhury J, Chowdhury S. (2002). Role of chromium supplementation in Indians with type 2 diabetes mellitus. Journal of Nutritional Biochemistry 13: 690–697.

Gibbs K, Walshe JM. (1965). Copper content of hair in normal families and those with Wilson's disease. Journal of Medical Genetics 2: 181–184.

Gibbs K, Walshe JM. (1979). A study of caeruloplasmin concentrations found in 75 patients with Wilson's disease, their kinships and various control groups. Quarterly Journal of Medicine 191: 447–463.

Gibson RS. (1980). Hair as a biopsy material for the assessment of trace element status in infancy: a review. Journal of Human Nutrition 34: 405–416.

Gibson RS. (1982). The trace metal status of some Canadian full term and low birth-weight infants at one year of age. Journal of Radioanalytical Chemistry 70: 175–189.

Gibson RS. (1994). Content and bioavailability of trace elements in vegetarian diets. American Journal of Clinical Nutrition 59: 1223S–1232S.

Gibson RS, DeWolfe MS. (1979). The zinc, copper, manganese, vanadium and iodine content of hair from 38 Canadian neonates. Pediatric Research 13: 959–962.

Gibson RS, DeWolfe MS. (1980). Changes in hair trace metal concentrations in some Canadian low birth-weight infants. Nutrition Reports International 21: 341–349.

Gibson RS, Hotz C. (2001). Dietary diversification/modification strategies to enhance micronutrient content and bioavailability of diets in developing countries. British Journal of Nutrition 85: S159–S166.

Gibson RS, Huddle JM. (1998). Suboptimal zinc status in pregnant Malawian women: its association with low intakes of poorly available zinc, frequent reproductive cycling, and malaria. American Journal of Clinical Nutrition 67: 702–709.

Gibson RS, Vanderkooy PD, MacDonald AC, Goldman A, Ryan BA, Berry M. (1989a). A growth limiting, mild zinc-deficiency syndrome in some southern Ontario boys with low height percentiles. American Journal of Clinical Nutrition 49: 1266–1273.

Gibson RS, Ferguson EL, Vanderkooy PD, MacDonald AC. (1989b). Seasonal variations in hair zinc concentrations in Canadian and African children. Science of Total Environment 84: 291–298.

Gibson RS, Heath AL, Limbaba ML, Prosser N, Skeaff CM. (2001). Are changes in food consumption patterns associated with lower biochemical zinc status among women from Dunedin, New Zealand? British Journal of Nutrition 86: 71–80.

Giugliano R, Millward DJ. (1984). Growth and zinc homeostasis in the severely Zn-deficient rat. British Journal of Nutrition 52: 545–560.

Glinsmann WH, Mertz W. (1966). Effect of trivalent chromium on glucose tolerance. Metabolism 15: 510–520.

Glinsmann WH, Feldman FJ, Mertz W. (1966). Plasma chromium after glucose administration. Science 152: 1243–1245.

Goldberg DM. (1973). 5′nucleotidase: recent advances in cell biology, methodology, and clinical significance. Digestion 8: 101–109.

Golden BE, Golden MH. (1981). Plasma zinc, rate of weight gain, and the energy cost of tissue deposition in children recovering from severe malnutrition on a cow's milk or soya protein based diet. American Journal of Clinical Nutrition 34: 892–899.

Goldenberg RL, Tamura T, Neggers Y, Copper RL, Johnston KE, DuBard MB, Hauth JC. (1995). The effect of zinc supplementation on pregnancy outcome. Journal of the American Medical Association 274: 463–468.

Goodall MJ, Hambidge KM, Stall C, Pritts J, Nelson D. (1988). Daily variations in plasma zinc in normal adult women. In: Hurley LS, Keen CL, Lönnerdal B, Rucker RB (eds.) Trace Elements in Man and Animals 6. Plenum Press, New York, pp. 491–492.

Graham GG, Cordano A. (1969). Copper depletion and deficiency in the malnourished infant. Johns Hopkins Medical Journal 124: 139–150.

Grant R, Ferguson MM, Strang R, Turner JW, Bone I. (1987). Evoked taste thresholds in a normal population and the application of electrogustometry to trigeminal nerve disease. Journal of Neurology, Neurosurgery and Psychiatry 50: 12–21.

Grantham-McGregor SM, Fernald LC, Sethuraman K. (1999). Effects of health and nutrition on cognitive and behavioral development in children in the first three years of life. Part 2: Infections and micronutrient deficiencies: iodine, iron, and zinc. Food and Nutrition Bulletin 20: 76–99.

Greenburg D. (2000). Chromium picolinate and cholesterol. Journal of the American College of Nutrition 19: 687.

Greger JL, Geissler AH. (1978). Effect of zinc supplementation on taste acuity of the aged. American Journal of Clinical Nutrition 31: 633–637.

Greger JL, Sickles VS. (1979). Saliva zinc levels: potential indicators of zinc status. American Journal of Clinical Nutrition 32: 1859–1866.

Gregory J, Foster K, Tyler H, Wiseman M. (1990). The Dietary and Nutritional Survey of British Adults. Her Majesty's Stationery Office, London.

Gregory J, Collins DL, Davies PSW, Hughes JM, Clarke PC. (1995). National Diet and Nutrition Survey: Children Aged One-and-a-Half to Four-and-a-Half Years. Volume 1: Report of the Diet and Nutrition Survey. Her Majesty's Stationery Office, London

Gregory J, Lowe S, Bates CJ, Prentice A, Jackson LV, Smithers G, Wenlock R, Farron M. (2000). National Diet and Nutrition Survey: Young People Aged 4 to 18 Years. Volume 1: Report of the Diet and Nutrition Survey. The Stationery Office, London.

Grider A, Bailey LB, Cousins RJ. (1990). Erythrocyte metallothionein as an index of zinc status in humans. Proceedings of the National Academy of Sciences of the United States of America 87: 1259–1262.

Griscom NT, Craig JN, Neuhauser EB. (1971). Systemic bone disease developing in small premature infants. Pediatrics 48: 883–895.

Guillard O, Piriou A, Gombert J, Reiss D. (1979). Diurnal variations of zinc, copper and magnesium in the serum of normal fasting adults. Biomedicine 31: 193–194.

Gunton JE, Hams G, Hitchman R, McElduff A. (2001). Serum chromium does not predict glucose tolerance in late pregnancy. American Journal of Clinical Nutrition 73: 99–104.

Gürson CT, Saner G. (1971). Effect of chromium on glucose utilization in marasmic protein-calorie malnutrition. American Journal of Clinical Nutrition 24: 1313–1319.

Gürson CT, Saner G. (1978). The effect of glucose loading on urinary excretion of chromium in normal adults, in individuals from diabetic families and in diabetics. American Journal of Clinical Nutrition 31: 1158–1161.

Halsted JA, Hackley BM, Smith JC Jr. (1968). Plasma-zinc and copper in pregnancy and after oral contraceptives. Lancet 2(7562): 278–279.

Hambidge KM. (1982). Hair analyses: worthless for vitamins, limited for minerals. American Journal of Clinical Nutrition 36: 943–949.

Hambidge KM, Droegemueller W. (1974). Changes in plasma and hair concentrations of zinc, copper, chromium and manganese during pregnancy. Journal of Obstetrics and Gynecology 44: 666–672.

Hambidge KM, Hambidge C, Jacobs M, Baum JD. (1972a). Low levels of zinc in hair, anorexia, poor growth, and hypogeusia in children. Pediatric Research 6: 868–874.

Hambidge KM, Franklin ML, Jacobs MA. (1972b). Hair chromium concentration: effect of sample washing and external environment. American Journal of Clinical Nutrition 25: 384–389.

Hambidge KM, Chavez MN, Brown RM, Walravens PA. (1979). Zinc nutritional status of young middle-income children and effects of consuming zinc-fortified breakfast cereals. American Journal of Clinical Nutrition 32: 2532–2539.

Harris ED. (1997). Copper. In: O'Dell BL, Sunde RA (eds.) Handbook of Nutritionally Essential Mineral Elements. Marcel Dekker, New York, pp. 231–273.

Harrison WW, Yurachek JP, Benson CA. (1969). The determination of trace elements in human hair by atomic absorption spectroscopy. Clinica Chimica Acta 23: 83–91.

Health and Welfare Canada. (1981). The Health of Canadians: Report of the Canada Health Survey. Ministry of Supply and Services, Ottawa.

Hellerstein MK. (1998). Is chromium supplementation effective in managing type 2 diabetes? Nutrition Reviews 56: 302–306.

Henderson L, Irving K, Gregory J, Bates CJ, Prentice A, Perks J, Swan G, Farron M. (2003). National Diet and Nutrition Survey: Adults Aged 19 to 64. Volume 3: Vitamin and Mineral Intake and Urinary Analytes. The Stationery Office, London.

Henkin RI. (1984). Zinc in taste function: a critical review. Biological Trace Element Research 6: 263–280.

Henkin RI, Gill JR, Bartter FC. (1963). Studies on taste thresholds in normal man and in patients with adrenal cortical insufficiency: the role of adrenal cortical steroids and of serum sodium concentration. Journal of Clinical Investigation 42: 727–735.

Henkin RI, Schechter PJ, Hoye R, Mattern CFT. (1971). Idiopathic hypogeusia with dysgeusia, hyposmia, and dysosmia: a new syndrome. Journal of the American Medical Association 217: 434–440.

Herber RFM, Stoeppler M. (1994). Trace Element Analysis in Biological Specimens: Techniques and Instrumentation in Analytical Chemistry. Volume 15. Elsevier, Amsterdam.

Hess FM, King JC, Margen S. (1977). Zinc excretion in young women on low zinc intakes and oral contraceptive agents. Journal of Nutrition 107: 1610–1620.

Higuchi S, Higashi A, Nakamura T, Matsuda I. (1988). Nutritional copper deficiency in severely handicapped patients on a low copper enteral diet for a prolonged period: estimation of the required dose of dietary copper. Journal of Pediatric Gastroenterology and Nutrition 7: 583–587.

Hobisch-Hagen P, Mortl M, Schobersberger W. (1997). Hemostatic disorders in pregnancy and the peripartum period. Acta Anaesthesiologica Scandinavica Suppl 111: 216–217.

Honkanen V, Konttinen YT, Sorsa T, Hukkanen M, Kemppinen P, Santavirta S, Saari H, Westermarck T. (1991). Serum zinc, copper and selenium in rheumatoid arthritis. Journal of Trace Elements and Electrolytes in Health and Disease 5: 261–263.

Hooper PL, Visconti L, Garry PJ, Johnson GE. (1980). Zinc lowers high-density lipoprotein-cholesterol levels. Journal of the American Medical Association 244: 1960–1961.

Hopkins LL, Ransome-Kuti O, Majaj AS. (1968). Improvement of impaired carbohydrate metabolism by chromium (III) in malnourished infants. American Journal of Clinical Nutrition 21: 203–211.

Hotz C, Brown KH. (eds.) (2004) International Zinc Nutrition Consultative Group (IZiNCG). Technical Document #1: Assessment of the risk of zinc deficiency in populations and options for its control. Food and Nutrition Bulletin 25(supp 2): S94–S204

Hotz C, Peerson JM, Brown KH. (2003). Suggested cut-offs of serum zinc concentrations for assessing zinc status: reanalysis of the second National Health and Nutrition Examination Survey data (1976–1980). American Journal of Clinical Nutrition 78: 756–764.

Hunt CD, Stoecker BJ. (1996). Deliberations and evaluations of the approaches, endpoints and paradigms for boron, chromium and fluoride dietary recommendations. Journal of Nutrition 126:2441S–2451S.

Hunt IF, Murphy NJ, Cleaver AE, Faraji B, Swendseid ME, Coulson AH, Clark VA, Browdy BL, Cabalum T, Smith JC Jr. (1984). Zinc supplementation during pregnancy: effects on selected blood constituents and on progress and outcome of pregnancy in low-income women of Mexican descent. American Journal of Clinical Nutrition 40: 508–521.

IOM (Institute of Medicine). (2001). Dietary Reference Intakes for Vitamin A, Vitamin K, Arsenic, Boron, Chromium, Copper, Iodine, Iron, Manganese, Molybdenum, Nickel, Silicon, Vanadium, and Zinc. National Academy Press, Washington, DC.

Ishizaka A, Tsuchida F, Ishii T. (1981). Clinical zinc deficiency during zinc supplemented parenteral nutrition. Journal of Pediatrics 99: 339–340.

Iyengar GV. (1998). Reevaluation of the trace element content in reference man. Radiation Physics and Chemistry 51: 545–560.

Iyengar GV, Subramanian KS, Woittiez JRW. (1998). Element Analysis of Biological Samples: Principles and Practice. CRC Press, Boca Raton, FL.

Jacob RA, Klevay LM, Logan GM Jr. (1978). Hair as a biopsy material. V: Hair metal as an index of hepatic metal in rats — copper and zinc. American Journal of Clinical Nutrition 31: 477–480.

Jameson S. (1993). Zinc status in pregnancy: the effect of zinc therapy on perinatal mortality, prematurity, and placental ablation. Annals of the New York Academy of Sciences 678: 178–192.

Jeejeebhoy KN, Chu RC, Marliss EB, Greenberg GR, Bruce-Robertson A. (1977). Chromium deficiency, glucose intolerance, and neuropathy reversed by chromium supplementation in a patient receiving long-term total parenteral nutrition. American Journal of Clinical Nutrition 30: 531–538.

Johnson WT, Kramer TR. (1987). Effect of copper deficiency on erythrocyte membrane proteins of rats. Journal of Nutrition 117: 1085–1090.

Johnson WT, Dufault SN, Thomas AC. (1993). Platelet cytochrome C oxidase activity is an indicator of copper status in rats. Nutrition Research 13: 1153–1162.

Jones RB, Keeling PW, Hilton PJ, Thompson RP. (1981). The relationship between leucocyte and muscle zinc in health and disease. Clinical Science 60: 237–239.

Juswigg T, Bates R, Solomons NW, Pineda O, Milne D. (1982). The effect of temporary venous occlusion on trace mineral concentrations in plasma. American Journal of Clinical Nutrition 36: 354–358.

Kagan HM, Trackman PC. (1991). Properties and function of lysyl oxidase. American Journal of Respiratory Cell and Molecular Biology 5: 206–210.

Karpel JT, Peden VH. (1972). Copper deficiency in long-term parenteral nutrition. Journal of Pediatrics 80: 32–36.

Karr M, Mira M, Causer J, Earl J, Alperstein G, Wood F, Fett MJ, Coakley J. (1997). Age-specific

reference intervals for plasma vitamins A, E and beta-carotene and for serum zinc, retinol-binding protein and prealbumin for Sydney children aged 9–62 months. International Journal for Vitamin and Nutrition Research 67: 432–436.

Kasperek K, Feinendegen LE, Lombeck I, Bremer HJ. (1977). Serum zinc concentrations during childhood. European Journal of Pediatrics 126: 199–202.

Kay RG, Tasman-Jones C. (1975). Acute zinc deficiency in man during intravenous alimentation. Australian and New Zealand Journal of Surgery 45: 325–330.

Kehoe CA, Turley E, Bonham MP, O'Connor JM, McKeown A, Faughnan MS, Coulter JS, Gilmore W, Howard AN, Strain JJ. (2000a). Response of putative indices of copper status to copper supplementation in human subjects. British Journal of Nutrition 84: 151–156.

Kehoe CA, Faughnan MS, Gilmore WS, Coulter JS, Howard AN, Strain JJ. (2000b). Plasma diamine oxidase activity is greater in copper adequate than copper marginal or copper deficient rats. Journal of Nutrition 130: 30–33.

Kelson JR, Shamberger RJ. (1978). Methods compared for determining zinc in serum by flame atomic absorption spectroscopy. Clinical Chemistry 24: 240–244.

Kiilunen M, Kivistö H, Ala-Laurila P, Tossavainen A, Aitio A. (1983). Exceptional pharmacokinetics of trivalent chromium during occupational exposure to chromium lignosulfonate dust. Scandinavian Journal of Work Environment and Health 9: 265–271.

King JC. (1990). Assessment of zinc status. Journal of Nutrition 120: 1474–1479.

King JC. (2000). Determinants of maternal zinc status during pregnancy. American Journal of Clinical Nutrition 71: 1334S–1343S.

King JC, Keen CL. (1999). Zinc. In: Shils ME, Olson JA, Shike M, Ross AC (eds.) Modern Nutrition in Health and Disease, 9th ed. Lea & Febiger, Philadelphia. pp. 223–239

King JC, Raynolds WL, Margen S. (1978). Absorption of stable isotopes of iron, copper, and zinc during oral contraceptive use. American Journal of Clinical Nutrition 31: 1198–1203.

King JC, Hambidge KM, Westcott JL, Kern DL, Marshall G. (1994). Daily variation in plasma zinc concentrations in women fed meals at six-hour intervals. Journal of Nutrition 124: 508–516.

King JC, Shames DM, Woodhouse LR. (2000). Zinc homeostasis in humans. Journal of Nutrition 130: 1360S–1366S.

King JC, Shames DM, Lowe NM, Woodhouse LR, Sutherland B, Abrams SA, Turnlund JR, Jackson MJ. (2001). Effect of acute zinc depletion on zinc homeostasis and plasma zinc kinetics in men. American Journal of Clinical Nutrition 74: 116–124.

Kirsten GF, de V Heese H, de Villiers S, Dempster WS, Pocock F, Varkevisser H. (1985). Serum zinc and copper levels in the 1st year of life. South African Medical Journal 67: 414–418.

Klasing SA, Pilch SM (eds.). (1985). Suggested Measures of Nutritional Status and Health Conditions for the Third National Health and Nutrition Examination Survey. Life Sciences Research Office, Federation of American Societies for Experimental Biology, Bethesda, MD.

Klevay LM. (1981). Hair as a biopsy material. VI: Hair copper as an index of copper in heart and kidney of rats. Nutrition Reports International 23: 371–376.

Klevay LM. (2000). Cardiovascular disease from copper deficiency — a history. Journal of Nutrition 130: 489S–492S.

Klevay LM, Inman L, Johnson LK, Lawler M, Mahalko JR, Milne DB, Lukaski HC, Bolonchuk W, Sandstead HH. (1984). Increased cholesterol in plasma in a young man during experimental copper depletion. Metabolism 33: 1112–1118.

Klevay LM, Bistrian BR, Fleming CR, Neumann CG. (1987). Hair analysis in clinical and experimental medicine. American Journal of Clinical Nutrition 46: 233–236.

Kobla HV. Volpe SL. (2000). Chromium, exercise, and body composition. Critical Reviews in Food Science and Nutrition 40: 291–308.

Kocyigit A, Erel O, Gur S. (2001). Effects of tobacco smoking on plasma selenium, zinc, copper and iron concentrations and related antioxidative enzyme activities. Clinical Biochemistry 34: 629–633.

Kozlovsky AS, Moser PB, Reiser S, Anderson RA. (1986). Effects of diets high in simple sugars on urinary chromium losses. Metabolism 35: 515–518.

Kraegen EW, Cooney GJ, Ye J, Thompson AL. (2001). Triglycerides, fatty acids and insulin resistance — hyperinsulinemia. Experimental and Clinical Endocrinology and Diabetes 109: S516–S526.

Kumpulainen J, Salmela S, Vuori E, Lehto J. (1982). Effects of various washing procedures on the chromium content of human scalp hair. Analytica Chimica Acta 138: 361–364.

Kusche J, Trotha UV, Muhlberger G, Lorenz W. (1974). The clinical-chemical application of the NADH test for the determination of diamine oxidase activity in human pregnancy. Agents and Actions 4: 188–189.

L'Abbé MR, Fischer PW. (1986). An automated method for the determination of Cu, Zn-superoxide dismutase in plasma and erythrocytes using an ABA-200 discrete analyzer. Clinical Biochemistry 19: 175–178.

Lane HW, Warren DC, Squyres NS, Cotham AC. (1982). Zinc concentrations in hair, plasma, and saliva and changes in taste acuity of adults supplemented with zinc. Biological Trace Element Research 4: 83–93.

Langard S. (1980). Chromium. In: Waldron HH (ed.) Metals in the Environment. Academic Press, London, pp. 111–132.

Lee SH, Lancey R, Montaser A, Madani N, Linder MC. (1993). Ceruloplasmin and copper transport during the latter part of gestation in the rat. Proceedings of the Society for Experimental Biology and Medicine 203: 428–439.

Levine RA, Streeten DHP, Doisy RJ. (1968). Effects of oral chromium supplementation on the glucose tolerance of elderly human subjects. Metabolism 17: 114–125.

Lewalter J, Korallus U, Harzdorf C, Weidemann H. (1985). Chromium bond detection in isolated erythrocytes: a new principle of biological monitoring of exposure to hexavalent chromium. International Archives of Occupational Environmental Health 55: 305–318.

Lifschitz MD, Henkin RI. (1971). Circadian variation in copper and zinc in man. Journal of Applied Physiology 31: 88–92.

Lind T, Lonnerdal B, Stenlund H, Ismail D, Seswandhana R, Ekstrom E-C, Persson L-A. (2003). A community-based randomized controlled trial of iron and zinc supplementation in Indonesian infants: interactions between iron and zinc. American Journal of Clinical Nutrition 77: 883–890.

Linder MC, Hazegh-Azam M. (1996). Copper biochemistry and molecular biology. American Journal of Clinical Nutrition 63: 797S–811S.

Linder MC, Wooten L, Cerveza P, Cotton S, Shulze R, Lomeli N. (1998). Copper transport. American Journal of Clinical Nutrition 67(Suppl): 965S–971S.

Liu VJ, Abernathy RP. (1982). Chromium and insulin in young subjects with normal glucose tolerance. American Journal of Clinical Nutrition 35: 661–667.

Liu VJK, Morris JS. (1978). Relative chromium response as an indicator of chromium status. American Journal of Clinical Nutrition 31: 972–976.

Loft JA, Turner K. (1975). Evaluation of Trinder's glucose oxidase method for measuring glucose in serum and urine. Clinical Chemistry 21: 1754–1760.

Lönnerdal B. (1996). Bioavailability of copper. American Journal of Clinical Nutrition 63: 821S–829S.

Lönnerdal B. (2000). Dietary factors influencing zinc absorption. Journal of Nutrition 130: 1378S–1383S.

Lukaski HC, Bolonchuk WW, Klevay LM, Milne DB, Sandstead HH. (1983). Maximal oxygen consumption as related to magnesium, copper, and zinc nutriture. American Journal of Clinical Nutrition 37: 407–415.

Lukaski HC, Klevay LM, Milne DB. (1988). Effects of dietary copper on human autonomic cardiovascular function. European Journal of Applied Physiology and Occupational Physiology 58: 74–80.

Lukaski HC, Hoverson BS, Gallagher SK, Bolonchuk WW. (1990). Physical training and copper, iron, and zinc status of swimmers. American Journal of Clinical Nutrition 51: 1093–1099.

Lukaski HC, Bolonchuk WW, Siders WA, Milne DB. (1996). Chromium supplementation and resistance training: effects on body composition, strength, and trace element status of men. American Journal of Clinical Nutrition 63: 954–965.

Makino T, Saito M, Horiguchi D, Kina K. (1982). A highly sensitive colorimetric determination of serum zinc using water-soluble pyridylazo dye. Clinica Chimica Acta 120: 127–135.

Mancini G, Carbonara AO, Hermans JF. (1965). Immunochemical quantitation of antigens by single radial immunodiffusion. Immunochemistry 2: 235–254.

Manthey J, Kübler W. (1980). High serum chromium levels after cardiac valve replacement: clinical significance and metabolic effects. American Journal of Cardiology 45: 940–944.

Mares-Perlman JA, Subar AF, Block G, Greger JL, Luby MH. (1995). Zinc intake and sources in the U.S. adult population: 1976–1980. Journal of the American College of Nutrition 14: 349–357.

Marklund S, Marklund G. (1974). Involvement of the superoxide anion radical in the autoxidation of pyrogallol and a convenient assay for superoxide dismutase. European Journal of Biochemistry 47: 469–474.

Markowitz ME, Rosen JF, Mizruchi M. (1985). Circadian variations in serum zinc (Zn) concentrations: correlation with blood ionized calcium, serum total calcium and phosphate in humans. American Journal of Clinical Nutrition 41: 689–696.

Martin GM. (1964). Copper content of hair and nails of normal individuals and of patients with hepatolenticular degeneration. Nature (London) 202: 903–904.

Martinez OB, MacDonald AC, Gibson RS, Bourn DM. (1985). Dietary chromium and effect of chromium supplementation on glucose tolerance of elderly Canadian women. Nutrition Research 5: 609–620.

Mason KE. (1979). A conspectus of research on copper metabolism and requirements of man. Journal of Nutrition 109: 1979–2066.

McBean LD, Mahloudji M, Reinhold JG, Halsted JA. (1971). Correlation of zinc concentrations in human plasma and hair. American Journal of Clinical Nutrition 24: 506–509.

McKenna AA, Ilich JZ, Andon MB, Wang C, Matkovic V. (1997). Zinc balance in adolescent females consuming a low- or high-calcium diet. American Journal of Clinical Nutrition 65: 1460–1464.

McKenzie JM. (1979). Content of zinc in serum, urine, hair, and toenails of New Zealand adults. American Journal of Clinical Nutrition 32: 570–579.

Meadows NJ, Ruse W, Smith MF, Day J, Keeling PW, Scopes JW, Thompson RP, Bloxam DL. (1981). Zinc and small babies. Lancet 2(8256): 1135–1137.

Medeiros DM, Milton A, Brunett E, Stacy L. (1991). Copper supplementation effects on indicators of copper status and serum cholesterol in adult males. Biological Trace Element Research 30: 19–35.

Meftah S, Prasad AS, Lee DY, Brewer GJ. (1991). Ecto 5'nucleotidase (5'NT) as a sensitive indicator of human zinc deficiency. Journal of Laboratory and Clinical Medicine 118: 309–316.

Meret S, Henkin RI. (1971). Simultaneous direct estimation by atomic absorption spectrophotometry of copper and zinc in serum, urine and cerebrospinal fluid. Clinical Chemistry 17: 369–373.

Mertz W. (1969). Chromium occurrence and function in biological systems. Physiological Reviews 49: 163–239.

Mertz W. (1981a). The essential trace elements. Science 213: 1332–1338.

Mertz W. (1981b). The scientific and practical importance of trace elements. Philosophical Transactions of the Royal Society of London Series B — Biological Sciences 294: 9–18.

Mertz W. (1993). Chromium in human nutrition: a review. Journal of Nutrition 123: 626–633.

Middleton RB, Linder MC. (1993). Synthesis and turnover of ceruloplasmin in rats treated with 17-β-estradiol. Archives of Biochemistry and Biophysics 302: 362–368.

Miller LV, Hambidge KM, Naake VL, Hong Z, Westcott JL, Fennessey PV. (1994). Size of the zinc pools that exchange rapidly with plasma zinc in humans: alternative techniques for measuring and relation to dietary zinc intakes. Journal of Nutrition 124: 268–276.

Milne DB. (1994). Assessment of copper nutritional status. Clinical Chemistry 40: 1479–1484.

Milne DB, Johnson PK. (1993). Assessment of copper status: effect of age and gender on reference ranges in healthy adults. Clinical Chemistry 39: 883–887.

Milne DB, Nielsen FH. (1993). Effect of high dietary fructose on Cu homeostasis and Cu status indicators in men during Cu deprivation. In: Anke M, Meisner D, Mills CF (eds.) Proceedings of the Conference on "Trace Element Metabolism in Man and Animals" (TEMA-8). Verlag Media Touristik, Gersdorf, Germany, pp. 370–373.

Milne DB, Nielsen FH. (1996). Effects of a diet low in copper on copper-status indicators in postmenopausal women. American Journal of Clinical Nutrition 63: 358–364.

Milne DB, Ralston NVC, Wallwork JC. (1985). Zinc content of cellular components of blood: methods for cell separation and analysis evaluated. Clinical Chemistry 31: 65–69.

Milne DB, Canfield WK, Gallagher SK, Hunt JR, Klevay LM. (1987). Ethanol metabolism in post-menopausal women fed a diet marginal in zinc. American Journal of Clinical Nutrition 46: 688–693.

Milne DB, Klevay LM, Hunt JR. (1988). Effects of ascorbic acid supplements and a diet marginal in copper on indices of copper nutriture in women. Nutrition Research 8: 865–873.

Milne DB, Johnson PE, Klevay LM, Sandstead HH. (1990). Effect of copper intake on balance, absorption, and status indices of copper in men. Nutrition Research 10: 975–986.

Morris BW, Griffiths H, Kemp GJ. (1988). Effect of glucose loading on concentrations of chromium in plasma and urine of healthy adults. Clinical Chemistry 34: 1114–1116.

Morris BW, Blumsohn A, Mac Neil S, Gray TA. (1992). The trace element chromium: a role in glucose homeostasis. American Journal of Clinical Nutrition 55: 989–991.

Morris BW, MacNeil S, Hardisty CA, Heller S, Burgin C, Gray TA. (1999). Chromium homeostasis in patients with type II (NIDDM) diabetes. Journal of Trace Elements in Medicine and Biology 13: 57–61.

Nath R, Minocha J, Lyall V, Sunder S, Kuman V, Kapoor S, Dhar KL. (1979). Assessment of chromium metabolism in maturity onset and juvenile diabetes using chromium-51 and therapeutic response of chromium administration on plasma lipids, glucose tolerance and insulin levels. In: Shapcott D, Hubert J (eds.) Chromium in Nutrition and Metabolism. Elsevier, Amsterdam, pp. 213–221.

National Diabetes Data Group. (1979). Classification and diagnosis of diabetes mellitus and other categories of glucose intolerance. Diabetes 28: 1039–1057.

Neggers YH, Goldenberg RL, Tamura T, Johnston KE, Copper RL, DuBard M. (1997). Plasma and erythrocyte zinc concentrations and their relationship to dietary zinc intake and zinc supplementation during pregnancy in low-income African-American women. Journal of the American Dietetic Association 97: 1269–1274.

Nielsen FH, Gallagher SK, Johnson LK, Nielsen EJ. (1992), Boron enhances and mimics some effects of estrogen therapy in post-menopausal women. Journal of Trace Elements in Experimental Medicine 5: 237–246.

Nishi Y. (1980). Zinc levels in plasma, erythrocyte and leucocyte in healthy children and adults. Hiroshima Journal of Medical Sciences 29: 7–13.

Nishi Y. (1996). Zinc and growth. Journal of the American College of Nutrition 15: 340–344.

Nixon DE, Moyer TP, Johnson P, McCall JT, Ness AB, Fjerstad WH, Wehde MB. (1986). Routine measurement of calcium, magnesium, copper, zinc, and iron in urine and serum by inductively coupled plasma emission spectroscopy. Clinical Chemistry 32: 1660–1665.

Nomiyama H, Yotoriyama M, Nomiyama K. (1980). Normal chromium levels in urine and blood of Japanese subjects determined by direct flameless atomic absorption spectrophotometry, and valency of chromium in urine after exposure to hexavalent chromium. American Industrial Hygiene Association Journal 41: 98–102.

O'Dell BL. (1976). Biochemistry of copper. Medical Clinics of North America 60: 687–703.

O'Dell BL. (1990). Dietary carbohydrate source and copper bioavailability. Nutrition Reviews 48: 425–434.

O'Donohue J, Reid MA, Varghese A, Portmann B, Williams R. (1993). Micronodular cirrhosis and acute liver failure due to chronic copper self-intoxication. European Journal of Gastroenterology and Hepatology 5: 561–562.

Offenbacher E. (1994). Promotion of chromium absorption by ascorbic acid. Trace Elements and Electectrolytes 11: 178–181.

Offenbacher EG, Pi-Sunyer FX. (1980). Beneficial effect of chromium-rich yeast on glucose tolerance and blood lipids in elderly subjects. Diabetes 29: 919–925.

Offenbacher EG, Rinko CJ, Pi-Sunyer FX. (1985). The effects of inorganic chromium and brewer's yeast on glucose tolerance, plasma lipids, and plasma chromium in elderly subjects. American Journal of Clinical Nutrition 42: 454–461.

Offenbacher EG, Spencer H, Dowling HJ, Pi-Sunyer FX. (1986). Metabolic chromium balances in man. American Journal of Clinical Nutrition 44: 77–82.

Okahata S, Nishi Y, Hatano S, Kobayashi Y, Usui T. (1980). Changes in erythrocyte superoxide dismutase in a patient with copper deficiency. European Journal of Pediatrics 134: 121–124.

Osendarp SJ, West CE, Black RE, The Maternal Zinc Supplementation Study Group. (2003). The need for maternal zinc supplementation in developing countries: an unresolved issue. Journal of Nutrition 133: 817S–827S.

Osheim DL. (1983). Atomic absorption determination of serum copper: collaborative study. Journal of the Association of Official Analytical Chemists 66: 1140–1142.

Oster O. (1993). Trace element concentrations (Cu, Zn, Fe) in sera from patients with dilated cardiomyopathy. Clinica Chimica Acta 214: 209–218.

Paine CH. (1968). Food-poisoning due to copper. Lancet 2(7566): 520.

Parnell W, Scragg R, Wilson N, Schaaf D, Fitzgerald E. (2003). NZ Food, NZ Children: Key Results of the 2002 National Children's Nutrition Survey. Ministry of Health, Wellington.

Payette H, Gray-Donald K. (1991). Dietary intake and biochemical indices of nutritional status in an elderly population with estimates of the precision of the 7-d food record. American Journal of Clinical Nutrition 54: 478–488.

Pekarek RS, Powanda MC, Wannemacher RW Jr. (1972). The effect of leukocytic endogenous mediator (LEM) on serum copper and ceruloplasmin concentrations in the rat. Proceedings of the Society of Experimental Biology and Medicine 141: 1029–1031.

Pennington JA, Schoen SA, Salmon GD, Young B, Johnson RD, Marts RW. (1995). Composition of core foods of the U.S. Food Supply, 1982–1991. III: Copper, manganese, selenium, and iodine. Journal of Food Composition and Analysis 8: 171–217.

Percival SS, Bowser E, Wagner M. (1995). Reduced copper enzyme activities in blood cells of children with cystic fibrosis. American Journal of Clinical Nutrition 62: 633–638.

Petering HG, Yeager DW, Witherup SO. (1971). Trace metal content of hair. I: Zinc and copper content of human hair in relation to age and sex. Archives of Environmental Health 23: 202–207.

Pilch SM, Senti FR (eds.) (1984). Assessment of the Zinc Nutritional Status of the U.S. Population Based on Data Collected in the Second National Health and Nutrition Examination Survey, 1976–1980. Life

Sciences Research Office, Federation of American Societies for Experimental Biology, Bethesda, MD.

Pinna K, Woodhouse LR, Sutherland B, Shames DM, King JC. (2001). Exchangeable zinc pool masses and turnover are maintained in healthy men with low zinc intakes. Journal of Nutrition 131: 2288–2294.

Pironi L, Miglioli M, Cornia GL, Ursitti MA, Tolomelli M, Piazzi S, Barbara L. (1987). Urinary zinc excretion in Crohn's disease. Digestive Diseases and Sciences 32: 358–362.

Pizarro F, Olivares M, Uauy R, Contreras P, Rebelo A, Gidi V. (1999). Acute gastrointestinal effects of graded levels of copper in drinking water. Environmental Health Perspectives 107: 117–121.

Porstmann T, Wietschke R, Cobet G, Larenz K, Grunow R, John S, Ballman R, Stamminger G, von Bachr R. (1990). Immunochemical quantification of Cu/Zn superoxide dismutase in prenatal diagnosis of Down's syndrome. Human Genetics 85: 362–366.

Prasad AS. (1966). Metabolism of zinc and its deficiency in human subjects. In: Prasad AS (ed.) Zinc Metabolism. Charles C. Thomas, Springfield, IL.

Prasad AS. (1982). Clinical and biochemical spectrum of zinc deficiency in human subjects. In: Prasad AS (ed.) Clinical, Biochemical and Nutritional Aspects of Trace Elements. Alan R Liss, New York, pp. 3–62.

Prasad AS. (1983). Clinical, biochemical and nutritional spectrum of zinc deficiency in human subjects: an update. Nutrition Reviews 41: 197–208.

Prasad AS. (1985). Diagnostic approaches to trace element deficiencies. In: Chandra RK (ed.) Trace Elements in Nutrition of Children. Nestlé Nutrition Workshop Series, Vol. 8. Raven Press, New York, pp. 17–34.

Prasad AS. (1991). Discovery of human zinc deficiency and studies in an experimental human model. American Journal of Clinical Nutrition 53: 403–412.

Prasad AS. (1995). Zinc: an overview. Nutrition 11(suppl.1): 93–99.

Prasad AS, Cossack ZT. (1982). Neutrophil zinc: an indicator of zinc status in man. Transactions of the Association of American Physicians 95: 165–176.

Prasad AS, Oberleas D. (1976). Trace elements in human health and disease. New York, Academic Press.

Prasad AS, Rabbani P. (1981). Nucleoside phosphorylase in zinc deficiency. Transactions of the Association of American Physicians 94: 314–321.

Prasad AS, Schulert AR, Miale A Jr., Farid Z, Sandstead HH. (1963). Zinc and iron deficiencies in male subjects with dwarfism and hypogonadism but without ancylostomiasis and schistosomiasis or severe anemia. American Journal of Clinical Nutrition 12: 437–444.

Prasad AS, Brewer GJ, Schoomaker EB, Rabbani P. (1978a). Hypocupremia induced by zinc therapy in adults. Journal of the American Medical Association 240: 2166–2168.

Prasad AS, Rabbani P, Abbasii A, Bowersox E, Fox M.

(1978b). Experimental zinc deficiency in humans. Annals of Internal Medicine 89: 483–490.

Prasad AS, Meftah S, Abdallah J, Kaplan J, Brewer GJ, Bach JF, Dardenne M. (1988). Serum thymulin in human zinc deficiency. Journal of Clinical Investigation 82: 1202–1210.

Prohaska JR, Wells WW. (1974). Copper deficiency in developing rat brain: a possible model for Menkes' steely-hair disease. Journal of Neurochemistry 23: 91–98.

Rabinowitz MB, Levin SR, Gonick HC. (1980). Comparisons of chromium status in diabetic and normal men. Metabolism 29: 355–364.

Rabinowitz MB, Gonick HC, Levin SR, Davidson MB. (1983). Effects of chromium and yeast supplements on carbohydrate and lipid metabolism in diabetic men. Diabetes Care 6: 319–327.

Rahkonen E, Junttila M, Kalliomaki P, Olkinouora M, Koponen M, Kalliomaki K. (1983). Evaluation of biological monitoring among stainless steel welders. International Archives of Occupational Environmental Health 52: 243–255.

Randall JA, Gibson RS. (1987). Serum and urine chromium as indices of chromium status in tannery workers. Proceedings of the Society for Experimental Biology and Medicine 185: 16–23.

Randall JA, Gibson RS. (1989). Hair chromium as an index of chromium exposure of tannery workers. British Journal of Industrial Medicine 46: 171–175.

Reeves PG, O'Dell BL. (1985). An experimental study of the effect of zinc on the activity of angiotensin converting enzyme in serum. Clinical Chemistry 31: 581–584.

Reiser S, Smith JC Jr, Mertz W, Holbrook JT, Scholfield DJ, Powell AS, Canfield W, Canary JJ. (1985). Indices of copper status in humans consuming a typical American diet containing either fructose or starch. American Journal of Clinical Nutrition 42: 242–251.

Riales R, Albrink MJ. (1981). Effect of chromium chloride supplementation on glucose tolerance and serum lipids including high-density lipoprotein of adult man. American Journal of Clinical Nutrition 34: 2670–2678.

Rice EW, Goldstein NP. (1961). Copper content of hair and nails in Wilson's disease (hepatolenticular degeneration). Metabolism 10: 1085–1087.

Rodriguez A, Soto G, Torres S, Venegas G, Castillo-Duran C. (1985). Zinc and copper in hair and plasma of children with chronic diarrhea. Acta Paediatrica Scandinavica 74: 770–774.

Rofe AM, Philcox JC, Coyle P. (1996). Trace metal, acute phase and metabolic response to endotoxin in metallothionein-null mice. Biochemical Journal 314: 793–797.

Rossander-Hultén L, Brune M, Sandstrom B, Lönnerdal B, Hallberg L. (1991). Competitive inhibition of iron absorption by manganese and zinc in humans. American Journal of Clinical Nutrition 54: 152–156.

Rubin MA, Miller JP, Ryan AS, Treuth MS, Patterson KY, Pratley RE, Hurley BF, Veillon C, Moser-Veillon PB, Anderson RA. (1998). Acute and chronic resistive exercise increase urinary chromium excretion in men as measured with an enriched chromium stable isotope. Journal of Nutrition 128: 73–78.

Rucker RB, Murray J. (1978). Cross-linking amino acids in collagen and elastin. American Journal of Clinical Nutrition 31: 1221–1236.

Rükgauer M, Zeyfang A. (2002). Chromium determinations in blood cells: clinical relevance demonstrated in patients with diabetes mellitus type 2. Biological Trace Element Research 86: 193–202.

Rükgauer M, Klein J, Kruse-Jarres JD. (1997). Reference values for the trace elements copper, manganese, selenium, and zinc in the serum/plasma of children, adolescents, and adults. Journal of Trace Elements in Medicine and Biology 11: 92–98.

Ruz M, Cavan KR, Bettger WJ, Thompson L, Berry M, Gibson RS. (1991). Development of a dietary model for the study of mild zinc deficiency in humans and evaluation of some biochemical and functional indices of zinc status. American Journal of Clinical Nutrition 53: 1295–1303.

Ruz M, Cavan KR, Bettger WJ, Gibson RS. (1992). Erythrocytes, erythrocyte membranes, neutrophils and platelets as biopsy materials for the assessment of zinc status in humans. British Journal of Nutrition 68: 515–527.

Salmenperä L, Perheentupa J, Pakarinen P, Siimes MA. (1986). Cu nutrition in infants during prolonged exclusive breast-feeding: low intake but rising serum concentrations of Cu and ceruloplasmin. American Journal of Clinical Nutrition 43: 251–257.

Salmon MA, Wright T. (1971). Chronic copper poisoning presenting as pink disease. Archives of Disease in Childhood 46: 108–110.

Samman S, Roberts DCK. (1988). The effect of zinc supplements on lipoproteins and copper status. Atherosclerosis 70: 247–252.

Samman S, Soto S, Cooke L, Ahmad Z, Farmakalidis E. (1996). Is erythrocyte alkaline phosphatase activity a marker of zinc status in humans? Biological Trace Element Research 51: 285–291.

Sandstead HH, Penland JG, Alcock NW, Dayal HH, Chen XC, Li JS, Zhao F, Yang JJ. (1998). Effects of repletion with zinc and other micronutrients on neuropsychologic performance and growth of Chinese children. American Journal of Clinical Nutrition 68: 470S–475S.

Sandstrom B, Davidsson L, Cederblad A, Lönnerdal B. (1985) Oral iron, dietary ligands and zinc absorption. Journal of Nutrition 115: 411–414.

Sato M, Mehra RK, Bremner I. (1984). Measurement of plasma metallothionein-I in the assessment of the zinc status of zinc-deficient and stressed rats. Journal of Nutrition 114: 1683–1689.

Sazawal S, Bentley M, Black RE, Dhingra P, George S, Bhan MK. (1996). Effect of zinc supplementation on observed activity in low socioeconomic Indian preschool children. Pediatrics 98: 1132–1137.

Sazawal S, Black RE, Menon VP, Dinghra P, Caulfield LE, Dhingra U, Bagati A. (2001). Zinc supplementation in infants born small for gestational age reduces mortality: a prospective, randomized, controlled trial. Pediatrics 108: 1280–1286.

Schilirò G, Russo A, Azzia N, Mancuso GR, Di Gregorio FD, Romeo MA, Fallico R, Sciacca S. (1987). Leucocyte alkaline phosphatase (LAP): a useful marker of zinc status in β-thalassemic patients. American Journal of Pediatric Hematology and Oncology 9: 149–152.

Schroeder HA, Balassa JJ, Tipton IH. (1962). Abnormal trace metals in man: chromium. Journal of Chronic Diseases 15: 941–964.

Schroeder JJ, Cousins RJ. (1990). Interleukin 6 regulates metallothionein gene expression and zinc metabolism in hepatocyte monolayer cultures. Proceedings of the National Academy of Sciences of the United States of America 87: 3137–3141.

Shaikh ZA. (1991). Radioimmunoassay for metallothioneine in body fluids and tissues. Methods in Enzymology 205: 120–130.

Shankar AH, Prasad AS. (1998). Zinc and immune function: the biological basis of altered resistance to infection. American Journal of Clinical Nutrition 68: 447S–463S.

Shaw JC, Bury AJ, Barber A, Mann L, Taylor A. (1982). A micromethod for the analysis of zinc in plasma or serum by atomic absorption spectrophotometry using graphite furnace. Clinica Chimica Acta 118: 229–239.

Sian L, Mingyan X, Miller LV, Tong L, Krebs NF, Hambidge KM. (1996). Zinc absorption and intestinal losses of endogenous zinc in young Chinese women with marginal zinc intakes. American Journal of Clinical Nutrition 63: 348–353.

Siegler RL, Eggert JV, Udomkesmalee E. (1981). Diagnostic indices of zinc deficiency in children with renal diseases. Annals of Clinical and Laboratory Science 11: 428–433.

Singh A, Smoak BL, Patterson KY, LeMay LG, Veillon C, Deuster PA. (1991). Biochemical indices of selected trace minerals in men: effect of stress. American Journal of Clinical Nutrition 53: 126–131.

Smit-Vanderkooy PD, Gibson RS. (1987). Food consumption patterns of Canadian preschool children in relation to zinc and growth status. American Journal of Clinical Nutrition 45: 609–616.

Smith JC Jr. (1994). Comparison of reference dose with recommended dietary allowances for zinc: methodologies and levels. In: Mertz W, Abernathy CO, Olin SS (eds.) Risk Assessment of Essential Elements. International Life Sciences Institute Press, Washington, DC, pp. 127–143.

Smith JC Jr, Butrimovitz GP, Purdy WC. (1979). Direct measurement of zinc in plasma by atomic absorption spectroscopy. Clinical Chemistry 25: 1487–1491.

Smith JC Jr, Holbrook JT, Danford DE. (1985). Analysis and evaluation of zinc and copper in human plasma and serum. Journal of the American College of Nutrition 4: 627–638.

Smolarek C, Stremmel W. (1999). [Therapy of Wilson disease.] Zeitschrift für Gastroenterologie 37: 293–300. German.

Solomons NW. (1979). On the assessment of zinc and copper nutriture in man. American Journal of Clinical Nutrition 32: 856–871.

Solomons NW. (1982). Biological availability of zinc in humans. American Journal of Clinical Nutrition 35: 1048–1075.

Solomons NW. (1985). Biochemical, metabolic, and clinical role of copper in human nutrition. Journal of the American College of Nutrition 4: 83–105.

Solomons NW, Layden TJ, Rosenberg IH, VoKhactu K, Sandstead HH. (1976). Plasma trace metals during total parenteral alimentation. Gastroenterology 70: 1022–1025.

Sternlieb I, Janowitz HD. (1964). Absorption of copper in malabsorption syndromes. Journal of Clinical Investigation 43: 1049–1055.

Stoecker BJ. (1994). Derivation of the estimated safe and adequate daily dietary intake for chromium. In Mertz W, Abernathy, Co O, Onin SS (eds.) Risk Assessment of Essential Elements. International Life Sciences Institute Press, Washington, DC, pp.197–205.

Strain JJ. (1999). Optimal nutrition: an overview. Proceedings of the Nutrition Society 58: 395–396.

Strain WH, Steadman LT, Lankau CA Jr, Berliner WP, Pories WJ. (1966). Analysis of zinc levels in hair for the diagnosis of zinc deficiency in man. Journal of Laboratory and Clinical Medicine 68: 244–249.

Sullivan VK, Cousins RJ (1997). Competitive reverse transcriptase-polymerase chain reaction shows that dietary zinc supplementation in humans increases monocyte metallothionein mRNA levels. Journal of Nutrition 127: 694–698.

Sullivan VK, Burnett FR, Cousins RJ (1998). Metallothionein expression is increased in monocytes and erythrocytes of young men during zinc supplementation. Journal of Nutrition 128: 707–713.

Sunderman FW. (1990). The clinical chemistry of 5'nuceotidase. Annals of Clinical Laboratory Science 20: 123–139.

Sunderman FW Jr, Nomoto S. (1970). Measurement of human serum ceruloplasmin by its p-phenylenediamine oxidase activity. Clinical Chemistry 16: 903–910.

Swanson CA, King JC. (1982). Zinc utilization in pregnant and nonpregnant women fed controlled diets providing the zinc RDA. Journal of Nutrition 112: 697–707.

Takagi K, Nakao M, Ogura Y, Nabeshima T, Kunii A. (1994). Sensitive colorimetric assay of serum diamine oxidase. Clinica Chimica Acta 226: 67–75.

Tam CF, Kopple JD, Wang M, Swendseid ME. (1979). Diamine oxidase activity in plasma and urine in uremia. Nephron 23: 23–27.

Tamura T, Goldenberg R L. (1996). Zinc nutriture and pregnancy outcome. Nutrition Research 16: 139–181.

Tamura T, Johnston KE, Freeberg LE, Perkins LL, Goldenberg RL. (1994). Refrigeration of blood samples prior to separation is essential for the accurate determination of plasma or serum zinc concentrations. Biological Trace Element Research 41: 165–173.

Taylor A. (1986). Usefulness of measurements of trace elements in hair. Annals of Clinical Biochemistry 23: 364–378.

Thomas EA, Bailey LB, Kauwell GA, Lee D-Y, Cousins RJ. (1992). Erythrocyte metallothionein response to dietary zinc in humans. Journal of Nutrition 122: 2408–2414.

Thomas PR. (2003). The enigmatic mineral. Nutrition Today 38: 120–133.

Tulinius MH, Holme E, Kristiansson B, Larsson NG, Oldfars A. (1991). Mitochondrial enceophalomyopathies in childhood. I : Biochemical and morphologic investigations. Journal of Pediatrics 119: 242–250.

Turnlund JR. (1994). Future directions for establishing mineral/trace element requirements. Journal of Nutrition 124: 1765S–1770S.

Turnlund JR. (1998). Human whole-body copper metabolism. American Journal of Clinical Nutrition 67(5 suppl.): 960S–964S.

Turnlund JR, Keyes WR, Anderson HL, Acord LL. (1989). Copper absorption and retention in young men at three levels of dietary copper by use of the stable isotope ^{65}Cu. American Journal of Clinical Nutrition 49: 870–878.

Turnlund JR, Keen CL, Smith RG. (1990). Copper status and urinary and salivary copper in young men at three levels of dietary copper. American Journal of Clinical Nutrition 51: 658–664.

Turnlund JR, Thompson KH, Scott KC. (1998). Key features of copper versus molybdenum metabolism models in humans. Advances in Experimental Medicine and Biology 445: 271–281.

Uauy R, Castillo-Duran C, Fisberg M, Fernandez N, Valenzuela A. (1985). Red cell superoxide dismutase activity as an index of human copper nutrition. Journal of Nutrition 115: 1650–1655.

Uauy R, Olivares M, Gonzalez M. (1998). Essentiality of copper in humans. American Journal of Clinical Nutrition 67S: 952S–959S.

Uckan D, Cetin M, Dincer N, Yetgin S, Cavdar A. (2001). Oral zinc tolerance test in pregnant women. Journal of Trace Elements in Experimental Medicine 14: 17–23.

Underwood EJ. (1971). Trace elements in human and animal nutrition. 3rd ed. Academic Press, New York.

USDA (U.S. Department of Agriculture). (2003). USDA National Nutrient Database for Standard Reference, Release 16. Nutrient Data Laboratory, U.S. Government Printing Office, Washington DC. http://www.nal.usda.gov/fnic/foodcomp/

Vaglenov A, Nosko M, Georgieva R, Carbonell E,

Creus A, Marcos R. (1999). Genotoxicity and radioresistance in electroplating workers exposed to chromium. Mutation Research 446: 23–34.

Valberg LS, Flanagan PR, Brennan J, Chamberlain MJ. (1985). Does the oral zinc tolerance test measure zinc absorption? American Journal of Clinical Nutrition 41: 37–42.

Van Coster R, Lombres A, De Vivo DC, Chi TL, Dodson WE, Rothman S, Orrechio EJ, Grover W, Berry GT, Schwartz JF, et al. (1991). Cytochrome c oxidase-associated Leigh syndrome: phenotypic features and pathogenetic speculations. Journal of Neurological Sciences 104: 97–111.

Vanderlinde RE, Kayne FJ, Komar G, Simmons MJ, Tsou JY, Lavine RL. (1979). Serum and urine levels of chromium. In: Shapcott D, Hubert J (eds.) Chromium in Nutrition and Metabolism. Elsevier, Amsterdam, pp. 49–58.

van Dokkum W. (1995). The intake of selected minerals and trace elements in european countries. Nutrition Research Reviews 8: 271–302.

Vecchio TJ, Oster HL, Smith DL. (1965). Oral sodium, tolbutamide and glucose tolerance tests. Archives of Internal Medicine 115: 161–166.

Veillon C, Patterson KY. (1999). Analytical issues in nutritional chromium research. Journal of Trace Elements in Experimental Medicine 12: 99–109.

Versieck J, Vanballenberghe L, De Kesel A. (1988). Certification of second-generation biological reference material (freeze-dried human serum) for trace element determinations. Analytica Chimica Acta 204: 63–75.

Verus AP, Samman S. (1994). Urinary zinc as marker of zinc intake: results of a supplementation trial in free-living men. European Journal of Clinical Nutrition 48: 219–221.

Vilter RW, Bozian RC, Hess EV, Zellner DC, Petering HG. (1974). Manifestations of copper deficiency in a patient with systemic sclerosis on intravenous hyperalimentation. New England Journal of Medicine 291: 188–191.

Vincent JB. (2000). The biochemistry of chromium. Journal of Nutrition 130: 715–718.

Vincent JB. (2004). Recent advances in the nutritional biochemistry of trivalent chromium. Proceedings of the Nutrition Society 63: 41–47.

Vitoux D, Arnaud J, Chappuis P. (1999). Are copper, zinc and selenium in erythrocytes valuable biological indexes of nutrition and pathology? Journal of Trace Elements in Medicine and Biology 13: 113–128.

Wada L, Turnlund JR, King JC. (1985). Zinc utilization in young men fed adequate and low zinc intakes. Journal of Nutrition 115: 1345–1354.

Walker BE, Bone I, Mascie-Taylor BH, Kelleher J. (1979). Is plasma zinc a useful investigation? International Journal of Vitamin and Nutrition Research 49: 413–418.

Wallach S, Verch RL. (1984). Placental transport of chromium. Journal of the American College of Nutrition 3: 69–74.

Walravens PA, Hambidge KM. (1976). Growth of infants fed a zinc supplemented formula. American Journal of Clinical Nutrition 29: 1114–1121.

Walravens PA, Krebs NF, Hambidge KM. (1983). Linear growth of low-income preschool children receiving a zinc supplement. American Journal of Clinical Nutrition 38: 195–201.

Wang ST, Demshar HP. (1993). Rapid Zeeman atomic absorption determination of copper in serum and urine. Clinical Chemistry 39: 1907–1910.

Warren DC, Lane HW, Mares M. (1981). Variability of zinc concentrations in human stimulated parotid saliva. Biological Trace Element Research 3: 99–107.

Wastney ME, Aamodt RL, Rumble WF, Henkin RI. (1986). Kinetic analysis of zinc metabolism and its regulation in normal humans. American Journal of Physiology 251: R398–R408.

Watson AR, Stuart A, Wells FE, Houston IB, Addison GM. (1983). Zinc supplementation and its effect on taste acuity in children with chronic renal failure. Human Nutrition: Clinical Nutrition 37: 219–225.

Watson WS. (1988). Plasma zinc uptake and taste acuity. American Journal of Clinical Nutrition 47: 336–337.

Weismann K, Høyer H. (1978). Serum alkaline phosphatase activity in acrodermatitis enteropathica: an index of serum zinc level. Acta Dermato Venereologica 59: 89–90.

Weismann K, Høyer H. (1985). Serum alkaline phosphatase and serum zinc levels in the diagnosis and exclusion of zinc deficiency in man. American Journal of Clinical Nutrition 41: 1214–1219.

Werman MJ, Bhathena SJ (1992). A sensitive and convenient colorimetric assay for measuring lysyl oxidase activity in tissues. Clinical Chemistry and Enzymology Communications 4: 271–277.

Werman MJ, Bhathena SJ, Turnlund JR. (1997). Dietary copper intake influences skin lysyl oxidase in young men. Nutritional Biochemistry 8: 201–204.

White CL, Pschorr J, Jacob ICM, von Lutterotti N, Dahlheim H. (1984). Reduced plasma angiotensin I-converting enzyme and kininase activities in the plasma of zinc deficient rats. In: Mills CF, Bremner I, Chesters JK (eds.) Trace Elements in Man and Animals 5. Commonwealth Agricultural Bureaux, Slough, U.K. pp. 65–70.

Whitehouse RC, Prasad AS, Rabbani PI, Cossack ZT. (1982). Zinc in plasma, neutrophils, lymphocytes, and erythrocytes as determined by flameless atomic absorption spectrophotometry. Clinical Chemistry 28: 475–480.

Whittaker P. (1998). Iron and zinc interactions in humans. American Journal of Clinical Nutrition 68: 442S–446S.

WHO (World Health Organization). (1997). WHO Global Database on Child Growth and Malnutrition. World Health Organization, Geneva.

Wiegand HJ, Ottenwalder H, Bolt HM. (1985). Die Chrombestimmung in Human Erythrozyten. Arbeitsmedizin Sozialmedizin Praventivmedizin 20: 1-4.

Winterbourne CC, Hawkins RE, Brian M, Carrell RW. (1975). The estimation of red cell superoxide dismutase activity. Journal of Laboratory Clinical Medicine 85: 337–342.

Wirth PL, Linder MC. (1985). Distribution of copper among components of human serum. Journal of the National Cancer Institute 75: 277–284.

Wolvekamp MC, de Bruin RW. (1994). Diamine oxidase: an overview of historical, biochemical and functional aspects. Digestive Diseases 12: 2–14.

Wood RJ, Zheng JJ. (1997). High dietary calcium reduces zinc absorption and balance in humans. American Journal of Clinical Nutrition 65: 1803–1809.

Wright AL, King JC, Baer MT, Citron LJ. (1981). Experimental zinc depletion and altered taste perception for NaCl in young adult males. American Journal of Clinical Nutrition 34: 848–852.

Yadrick MK, Kenney MA, Winterfeldt EA. (1989). Iron, copper, and zinc status: response to sup-plementation with zinc or zinc and iron in adult females. American Journal of Clinical Nutrition 49: 145–150.

Zelkowitz M, Verghese JP, Antel J. (1980). Copper and zinc in the nervous system. In: Karcioğlu ZA, Sarper RM (ed.) Zinc and Copper in Medicine. Charles C. Thomas, Springfield, IL, pp. 418–463.

Zhou JR, Canar MM, Erdman JW Jr. (1993). Bone zinc is poorly released in young growing rats fed a marginally zinc-restricted diet. Journal of Nutrition 123: 1383–1388.

Zinc Investigators' Collaborative Group. (1999). Prevention of diarrhea and pneumonia by zinc supplementation in children in developing countries: pooled analysis of randomized controlled trials. Journal of Pediatrics 135: 689–697.

Zober A, Kick K, Schaller KH, Schellmann B, Valentin H. (1984). Normal values of chromium and nickel in human lung, kidney, blood and urine samples. Zentralblatt für Bakteriologie, Mikrobiologie und Hygiene 179: 80–95.

25

Assessment of iodine and selenium status

Iodine and selenium are considered together in this chapter because of their recognized interactions. Deficiencies of the two elements occur in both low-income and more affluent countries, induced primarily by low soil concentrations which are often exacerbated by leaching. Both elements are essential for thyroid hormone metabolism and are required for optimal growth and development. In addition, they have a role in normal reproduction, gene expression, and synthesis of xenobiotic-metabolizing enzymes in the liver (Arthur, 1999). Deficiencies of both elements are associated with serious debilitating clinical effects, some of which are irreversible.

The diverse effects of iodine deficiency on growth and development are well recognized and result from a decrease in the production of the thyroid hormones. The most obvious consequence of iodine deficiency at all ages is goiter, characterized by an enlarged thyroid. Several other adverse effects also occur, and are collectively termed "iodine deficiency disorders" (IDD).

In contrast, there are only two well-characterized diseases linked to selenium deficiency in humans. These are Keshan disease and Kaschin-Beck disease, both of which occur in China and Tibet. There is some evidence that iodine deficiency may additionally be involved in the etiology of Kaschin-Beck disease (Moreno-Reyes et al., 1998). More recently, low selenium status has been implicated in impaired immune function and increased risk of coronary heart disease and cancer.

Selenium is now known to have an essential role in two aspects of thyroid hormone metabolism. Three Se-containing iodothyronine deiodinases (EC 3.8.1.4) control the synthesis and degradation of the biologically active thyroid hormone, $3,5,3'$-triiodothyronine (T_3), in the liver, kidney, and muscle. This regulation of tissue T_3 levels by selenoproteins accounts for the earlier observation that selenium deficiency blocks the thyroid feedback-control system.

In addition, at least five Se-containing glutathione peroxidases (EC 1.11.1.9), and several Se-containing enzymes — thioredoxin reductases (EC 1.6.4.5) — protect the thyroid from lipid peroxides and hydrogen peroxide produced during the synthesis of thyroid hormones (Behne and Kyriakopoulos, 2001). Hence, selenium deficiency also affects the function of the thyroid gland itself (Arthur et al., 1999). Thus selenium deficiency may have an important role in exacerbating hypothyroidism arising from iodine deficiency. It may also be involved in the etiology of myxedematous cretinism (Vanderpas et al., 1993). This is of significance in human nutrition because in some endemically iodine-deficient areas (e.g., Zaire), selenium deficiency also occurs.

There is some evidence that in populations with a relatively low selenium status, treatment of IDD with selenium alone may aggravate hypothyroidism. The effect arises from the stimulation of thyroxine metabolism by the selenoenzyme type I iodothyronine $5'$-deiodinase. Hence, treatment with sel-

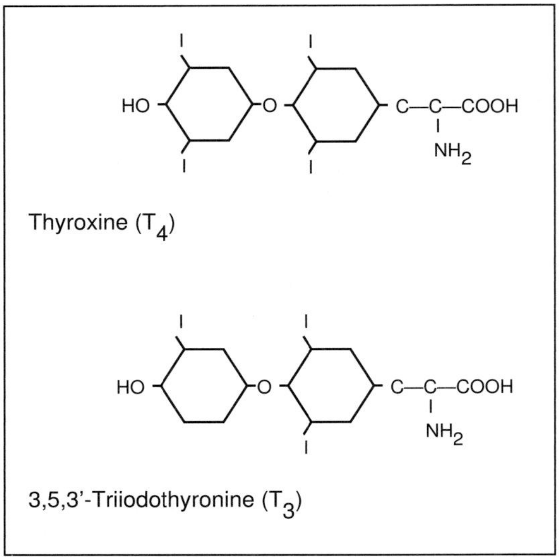

Figure 25.1: Structure of the two thyroid hormones, thyroxine (T_4) and 3,5,3'-triiodothyronine (T_3).

enium should not be given without iodine or thyroid hormone supplementation when deficiencies of both iodine and selenium coexist (Vanderpas et al., 1993).

In contrast to these adverse effects, the existence of concurrent selenium deficiency may also have some beneficial effects in individuals with iodine deficiency. Decreases in the supply of selenium may result in changes in the activities of Se-containing deiodinases that protect the brain from low T_3 concentrations in iodine deficiency. Such effects may help prevent some neurological damage (Arthur et al., 1999). Whether iodine deficiency protects against selenium deficiency warrants further investigation.

25.1 Iodine

The normal adult human body contains about 15–20 mg of iodine, of which 70%–80% is concentrated in the thyroid gland. In the presence of goiter and a low iodine intake, the amount of iodine in the gland can be as little as 1 mg. Iodine occurs in the tissues mainly as organically bound iodine; inorganic iodide is present in very low concentrations.

Functions of iodine

Iodine functions almost exclusively as a component of the thyroid hormones, thyroxine (T_4) and 3,5,3'-triiodothyronine (T_3); their structure is shown in Figure 25.1. These hormones are required for the normal growth and development of tissues such as the central nervous system and for maturation of the whole body. The hormones also regulate the basal metabolic rate and macronutrient metabolism. Although some reports have suggested that iodine may have additional functions such as in the immune response, more research is needed to confirm this suggestion.

Absorption and metabolism of iodine

The amount of iodine absorbed from the diet is largely dependent on the level of dietary iodine, rather than on its chemical form or the composition of the diet. Iodine is ingested in several different forms. Before absorption, iodate is reduced to iodide in the gut. Then, absorption of iodide takes place rapidly, mainly from the upper small intestine and stomach, after which it is taken up immediately by the thyroid gland. Once in the thyroid gland, the iodide participates in a complex series of reactions to produce thyroid hormones.

The thyroid hormones are synthesized in the thyroid gland from thyroglobulin, an iodinated glycoprotein contained in the colloid of the thyroid follicles. Once iodinated, the thyroglobulin is exposed to proteolytic enzymes in the thyroid gland which break it down to release mainly T_4 and some T_3 into the blood.

Production of T_3 and T_4 in the thyroid is controlled by the level of thyroid-stimulating hormone (TSH) — also known as "thyrotropin" — in the circulation. When the circulating levels of T_3 and T_4 are adequate, there is a feedback on the pituitary, which regulates the production of TSH. If the level of circulating T_4 in the blood falls because of mild iodine deficiency, then the secretion of TSH is increased, which, in turn, promotes iodine uptake by the thyroid and enhances the output of T_4 into the circulation. In moderate iodine deficiency, however, the level of circulating T_4 will fall, but TSH levels remain elevated. In conditions of very severe iodine deficiency, the level of T_3 may also decline. Hence, levels of both T_4 and TSH can be used to diagnose hypothyroidism due to iodine deficiency (Clugston and Hetzel, 1994).

Once in the circulation, T_4 and T_3 are rapidly attached to several binding proteins, specifically transthyretin, thyroxine-binding globulin, and albumin. The bound hormone then migrates to target tissues where T_4 is deiodinated to T_3, the metabolically active form. The iodine that is released returns to the serum iodine pool or is excreted in the urine.

Deiodination is controlled by the iodothyronine deiodinases (EC 3.8.1.4), enzymes which require selenocysteine at the active site to function (Arthur, 1999). Hence, as noted earlier, selenium deficiency may impair conversion of T_4 to biologically active T_3 and thus hormone action.

Iodine deficiency in humans

The diverse effects of iodine deficiency on growth and development are termed "iodine deficiency disorders" (IDD) and are itemized in Table 25.1. They include mental retardation, hypothyroidism, goiter, cretinism, and varying degrees of other growth and developmental abnormalities. At all ages, the most common and obvious IDD is goiter, thyroid enlargement. However, thyroid hormone is particularly important for myelination of the central nervous system, which is most active in the perinatal period and during fetal and early postnatal development. Hence, it is not surprising that an inadequate supply of iodine during these critical periods of brain development has a major effect on the neuro-intellectual development of infants and children (Hetzel, 2000). Indeed, the latter has been confirmed by a meta-analysis of 18 studies. Iodine deficiency alone decreased mean IQ scores by 13.5 points in the iodine-deficient compared to noniodine-deficient groups (Bleichrodt and Born, 1994).

Age	Disorder
Fetus	Abortions
	Stillbirth
	Congenital anomalies
	Increased perinatal mortality
	Increased infant mortality
	Neurological cretinism
	Mental deficiency
	Deaf-mutism
	Spastic diplegia
	Squint
	Myxedematous cretinism
	Dwarfism
	Mental deficiency
Neonate	Neonatal goiter
	Neonatal hypothyroidism
Child and adolescent	Goiter
	Juvenile hypothyroidism
	Impaired mental function
	Retarded physical development
Adult	Goiter with its complications
	Hypothyroidism
	Impaired mental function
	Iodine-induced hyperthyroidism

Table 25.1: Iodine deficiency disorders. After Lamberg, European Journal of Clinical Nutrition 47: 1–8, 1993, with permission of the Nature Publishing Group.

Goiter is the major consequence of chronic iodine deficiency and is still very common worldwide. It usually occurs when dietary iodine intakes are $< 50\,\mu g/d$. WHO has established criteria to estimate thyroid gland size in order to standardize results among surveys; details are given in Section 25.1.2.

In areas where endemic goiter exists and iodine deficiency is severe, endemic cretinism may occur. Geographical differences in the clinical manifestations of endemic cretinism are found. The clinical features always include mental deficiency and either a neurological syndrome consisting of hearing and speech defects and characteristic disorders of stance and gait, or predominant hypothyroidism and stunted growth (i.e., the myxedematous form). The former syndrome, known as nervous or neurological cretinism, is more common and appears to result from iodine deficiency of the mother during fetal development. In some areas (e.g., the Himalayas), a mixture of both syndromes occurs (Lamberg, 1993). There is some evidence that the etiology of both neurological and myxedematous cretinism may be influenced by the coexistence of iodine and selenium deficiency in some areas (Vanderpas et al., 1990).

Cases of mild to moderate iodine deficiency, characterized by an impairment of thyroid function, have been detected in some newborn preterm infants in Europe and in neonates elsewhere (Kochupillai et al., 1986). Such transient impairment of thyroid function may be associated, in part, with the neuro-intellectual deficiencies often observed in preterm infants during their subsequent development (Delange, 1985).

Young children (especially those < 5 y), preadolescents, and premenopausal women also appear to be at risk for mild to moderate iodine deficiency, even in some more affluent countries such as Switzerland, Australia, and New Zealand (Burgi et al., 1999; Eastman, 1999; Guttikonda et al., 2002; Skeaff et al., 2002).

The most common cause of iodine deficiency is inadequate dietary intake of iodine. Indeed, a fall in iodine intakes has been linked with the reemergence of mild iodine deficiency in both Australia and New Zealand. This fall has been attributed to a reduction in the use of iodophors in the dairy industry and decreasing consumption of iodized salt (Eastman, 1999; Skeaff et al., 2002).

Secondary dietary factors associated with the development of iodine deficiency include goitrogens, or substances in foods that can block the absorption or utilization of iodine and thus reduce its uptake into the thyroid gland. Vegetables of the Brassicaceae family, especially cabbage, turnips, and rutabagas, contain an active antithyroid agent in a combined form (progoitrin). In general, goitrogens impair the covalent binding of iodine to thyroglobulin and prevent the oxidation of iodine by thyroid iodine peroxidase (Gaitan, 1990). Other goitrogens are linamarin, a cyanoglucoside found in cassava, disulfides of saturated and unsaturated hydrocarbons

from organic sediments in drinking water, soybeans, and bacterial products of *Escherichia coli* in drinking water.

Neonates, and to a lesser extent pregnant women, are more sensitive to the antithyroid action of dietary goitrogens than are infants and children (Delange et al., 1982).

Other dietary factors that are important in relation to iodine include deficiencies of selenium, iron, or vitamin A, each of which exacerbates the effects of iodine deficiency (Vanderpas et al., 1993; Wolde-Gebriel et al., 1993a; Zimmermann et al., 2000a). The role of selenium in iodine metabolism is discussed more fully in Section 25.2.

Certain key steps in iodine metabolism are now known to depend on iron (Beard et al., 1998). In subjects with iron-deficiency anemia, levels of T_4 and T_3 are lower, the conversion of T_4 to T_3 is slowed, and the concentrations of TSH are elevated (Dillman et al., 1980; Beard et al., 1990). Hence, goitrous children with iron-deficiency anemia exhibit a lower response to iodized oil than do iron-replete children (Zimmermann et al., 2000a). In a study of children in Morocco treated with microencapsulated iron and/or iodized salt, there was a greater reduction in the prevalence of hypothyroidism and goiter in the dual fortified salt group compared with those receiving iodized salt alone (Zimmermann et al., 2003a).

Current evidence suggests that the interaction between vitamin A and thyroid metabolism may involve both inhibition of TSH secretion by the pituitary and thyroid hormone transport, mediated in part through two transport proteins, retinol-binding protein and transthyretin. A detailed review is available in Hurrell and Hess (2004). Several studies have reported elevated serum retinol levels in subjects with visible goiters (Wolde-Gebriel et al., 1993a, 1993b; Florentino et al., 1996). So far, few studies have investigated the effect of vitamin A supplementation on thyroid metabolism.

Secondary iodine deficiency may develop in the presence of a number of diseases of the thyroid gland, or pituitary or hypothalamic failure. Under certain conditions, iodide in large doses may block the synthesis of thyroid hormone, usually temporarily, after which hormone synthesis resumes. This phenomenon is known as the Wolff-Chaikoff effect (Wolff and Chaikoff, 1948). Sometimes, in 3%–4% of otherwise healthy individuals, the block persists and a goiter may develop.

Food sources and dietary intakes

Iodine is present in foods largely as inorganic iodide. Foods of marine origin — sea fish, shell fish, and seaweeds — are excellent food sources of iodine but are eaten in small amounts in many countries. Instead dairy products are the major food sources of iodine in most affluent countries (Wilson et al., 1999); cereals comprise the secondary food source, especially in countries where iodized salt or iodates are used in the manufacture of bread. The iodine content of meat, milk, and eggs varies markedly with region, season, and the amount of iodine in the animal feed (Hemken, 1979). Vegetable and fruit products are generally low in iodine (Fisher and Carr, 1974).

Losses of iodine during cooking occur, the extent depending on the temperature, nature of the food, and length of the cooking time (Wang et al., 1999). Freezing and freeze drying can also reduce the iodine content of foods by up to 20%–25% (Lee et al., 1994).

Adventitious sources of iodine may contribute to the iodine content of foods. These include iodates used as dough conditioners as noted above, iodoform used in water as a disinfectant, iodine-containing food colors (e.g., erythrosine and rose bengal), and iodophors used in the dairy industry (Vought et al., 1972; Dunsmore and Wheeler, 1977; Delange, 1985). However, use of iodophors has decreased in some regions, for example, New Zealand and Australia, which has led to a reduction in the iodine levels in milk in these countries (Knowles et al., 1997; Eastman, 1999) and, in turn, to lower iodine intakes and lower urinary iodide excretion (Eastman, 1999; Thomson et al., 2001).

The recommended method for preventing iodine deficiency is to introduce the use of iodized salt, using potassium iodide or potassium iodate as the fortificant. In some countries where the production, distribution, and monitoring of iodized salt is more difficult (e.g., Papua New Guinea, Argentina, Democratic Republic of Congo, China), iodized oil, given either orally or (preferably) intramuscularly, has been used (Delange et al., 2001). Other regions introduced iodized bread (e.g., Tasmania, the Netherlands) (Lamberg 1993), iodized drinking water (e.g., Sicily, China, Malaysia) (Hetzel and Dunn, 1989) or iodized sugar (Eltom et al., 1995). In Finland, iodization of animal feeds has been used (Varo et al., 1982).

Effects of high intakes of iodine

Most individuals with healthy thyroids are very tolerant of habitual excess intakes of iodine from food (Pennington, 1990). In such circumstances, iodine uptake by the thyroid is markedly reduced, but goiter and hypothyroidism are rarely induced. In certain regions of Japan and China, however, where seaweeds rich in iodine are dietary staples (Suzuki et al., 1965; Suzuki and Mashimo, 1973), chronic high intakes of iodine (50,000 to 80,000 μg/d) may produce thyroid enlargement (goiter).

There are also certain subpopulations who respond adversely to sudden excessive intakes of iodine. These include persons living where goiter is endemic and with habitual low intakes of iodine, those sensitive to iodine, and those with preexisting abnormalities of the thyroid gland such as autoimmune thyroid diseases (Delange et al., 1999). Elderly persons, especially females who have had low intakes of iodine throughout their life, tend to be more susceptible to excess iodine intakes (Pennington, 1990). The adverse effects may include hypothyroidism and elevated TSH, goiter, increased incidence of autoimmune thyroid disease, and possibly thyroid papillary cancer (IOM, 2002).

Occasionally, when iodine has been given prophylactically in iodine-deficient areas, a few cases of hyperthyroidism or Jod-Basedow thyrotoxicosis have arisen. These tend to occur in individuals with thyroid nodules that are "autonomous" or "overactive." The hyperthyroidism is generally mild and can be treated readily.

The U.S. Food and Nutrition Board Tolerable Upper Intake Level for the iodine intake of adults >19 y and pregnant and lactating women is $1100 \, \mu g/d$. Levels for children and adolescents are also given in IOM (2002).

Indices of iodine status

The most widely used biochemical method of assessing iodine status is to determine urinary iodine excretion either in 24-h urine samples or casual urine specimens; this method is described below. Measurement of thyroid-stimulating hormone (TSH) in serum is used as a screening test for detecting congenital hypothyroidism in neonates. Whether it can also be used to assess iodine status is less clear. Some investigators claim that serum thyroglobulin concentrations are a sensitive marker of iodine status. Levels of T_3 or T_4 in serum are sometimes also used, although they are relatively insensitive, generally only falling below the normal range when iodine deficiency is very severe.

Methods for assessing the volume of the thyroid gland are also described. Determination of cognitive function in children has sometimes been used as a noninvasive functional measure of iodine status. Several other micronutrients influence cognitive function (e.g., iron, zinc, folate, and vitamin B_{12}), so this test is not very specific and is most useful during double-blind placebo-controlled iodine intervention trials.

25.1.1 Thyroid size by neck palpation

In iodine deficiency, the thyroid gland, which lies in front of the larynx and upper trachea, is enlarged. This thyroid enlargement is known as goiter, and is the most obvious visible clinical consequence of iodine deficiency. Because the thyroid gland may not return to a normal size for months or even years after the correction of iodine deficiency, the preva-

lence of goiter provides a better reflection of past than present iodine status of a population (Delange et al., 2001).

Goiter usually occurs when dietary intakes of iodine are $< 50 \, \mu g/d$, unless it is also associated with goitrogens in the diet. Goitrogens may cause the thyroid to enlarge more than that expected based on iodine intakes alone. Goiter reflects an attempt by the thyroid to compensate for a lack of production of thyroid hormones, induced by iodine deficiency. With the reduced output from the thyroid, the level of T_4 falls, which leads to an increase in TSH secretion by the pituitary. This in turn, increases the uptake of iodide by the thyroid, with increased turnover of iodine associated with hyperplasia of the cells of the thyroid follicles. As a result, the thyroid enlarges.

Initially, the thyroid gland is diffusely and symmetrically enlarged, but as the severity of the iodine deficiency increases and as the subject ages, the gland increases in size and palpable nodules occur. In some circumstances, gross enlargement of the thyroid can cause obstructive symptoms with compression of the trachea or esophagus.

The traditional method of measuring the size of the thyroid is to use neck palpation. Several studies have compared the use of neck palpation with that of ultrasound (Section 25.1.2) for estimating the prevalence of goiter. Results suggest that in areas of mild IDD where the prevalence of visible goiters is low, sensitivity and specificity of palpation are poor, resulting in high rates of misclassification (i.e., 40%) (Vitti et al., 1994; WHO/UNICEF/ICCIDD, 1994). However, in areas of moderate to severe IDD, goiter palpation using the WHO/UNICEF/ICCIDD (1994) criteria (Table 25.2) generally provides a relatively accurate estimate of goiter prevalence, especially for children 6–12 y and pregnant and lactating women.

There is some evidence that thyroid volume varies with sex. Several (Delange et al., 1997; Foo et al., 1999) but not all (Vitti et al., 1994; Xu et al., 1999; Hess and Zimmerman, 2000) reports suggest that girls have larger thyroid volumes than boys.

Interpretive criteria

A simplified classification of goiter based on three grades has been developed by WHO/UNICEF/ICCIDD (1994) and is reproduced in Table 25.2. Neck palpation is especially suitable for children 6–12 y and pregnant and lactating women, but it is not recommended for infants and younger children who have small thyroids. Thyroid volume increases with age, reaching a plateau at about 15 y.

Estimates of grade 1 goiter using neck palpation are not very accurate, as noted earlier. Further, specificity and sensitivity of palpation in grades 0 and 1 are low because of high between-examiner variation. Hence, it is always preferable to confirm low goiter rates by ultrasonography and urinary iodine excretion levels (Section 25.1.3).

Table 25.3 provides epidemiological criteria set by WHO/UNICEF/ICCIDD (1994) for assessing the severity of IDD based on the prevalence of goiter in school-age children. The total goiter rate (TGR) represents the sum of grade 1 and grade 2 goiter rates.

Measurement by neck palpation

Inspection followed by neck palpation is the conventional method for measuring the size of the thyroid. A thyroid gland is considered goitrous when each lateral lobe has a volume greater than the terminal phalanx of

Severity of IDD	Prevalence of goiter (TGR) (%)
Mild	5.0–19.9
Moderate	20.0–29.9
Severe	⩾ 30

Table 25.3: Epidemiological criteria for assessing the severity of IDD based on the prevalence of goiter in school-age children. TGR = total goiter rate. From WHO/UNICEF/ICCIDD (1994), with permission.

the thumb of the subject being examined. In grade 1 goiter, the thyroid lobe is larger than the ends of the thumb and is palpable but not visible when the neck is in the normal position. In grade 2 goiter, the thyroid is enlarged and visible when the neck is in a normal position (WHO/UNICEF/ICCIDD, 1994).

Neck palpation is cheap and easy to perform, requiring only the cost of the examination. Personnel can be trained easily in the technique. In many settings, palpation may be more acceptable and affordable than thyroid ultrasonography, described below (Foo et al., 1999; Zimmermann et al., 2000b).

25.1.2 Thyroid volume by ultrasonography

Ultrasonography measures thyroid volume (T_{vol}) more precisely and objectively than inspection and neck palpation, especially if the visible goiter is small (i.e., grade 1). The method employs sound frequencies in the megahertz range, well above the frequency of audible sound. The impulse is applied to the neck by a small handheld device that both transmits the signal and receives the reflections. The ultrasound penetrates the skin surface and passes through the underlying tissues, with a certain portion of the sound being reflected back. Tissues containing interfaces of different acoustic densities generate dense echoes. Transmission of sound from the transducer to the skin is facilitated by a water-soluble transmission gel, which is applied to the measurement site.

WHO/ICCIDD (1997) suggests using this method with children 8–10 y. The method is

Grade 0	No palpable or visible goiter
Grade 1	A mass in the neck that is consistent with an enlarged thyroid that is *palpable but not visible* when the neck is in a normal position. It moves upward in the neck when the subject swallows. Nodular alteration(s) can occur even when the thyroid is not visibly enlarged.
Grade 2	A swelling in the neck that is *visible* when the neck is in a normal position and is consistent with an enlarged thyroid when the neck is palpated.

Table 25.2: Simplified classification of goiter. From WHO/UNICEF/ICCIDD (1994), with permission.

safe, noninvasive, and feasible even in remote areas because of the availability of portable, rugged, ultrasound equipment. The latter does require electricity but can be operated from a car battery. Well-trained ultrasonographers and care must be used when taking the measurements of thyroid volume, because of the irregular shape of the thyroid gland.

Interpretive criteria

To interpret thyroid ultrasonography correctly for the assessment of the prevalence of goiter, valid reference criteria from iodine-sufficient populations (i.e., where the average iodine intake is >150 µg/d and the median urinary iodine in a casual sample is >100 µg/L) are required.

In 2004, a WHO report from the Nutrition for Health and Development Iodine Deficiency Study Group proposed normative values for thyroid volume in children aged 6–12 y based on the data for 3529 iodine-sufficient children from specific sub-populations in the Americas, central Europe, the eastern Mediterranean, Africa, and the western Pacific. Two examiners performed all ultrasonography using validated techniques.

These reference values for the median and the upper limit of normal (97th percentile) of thyroid volume by age and body surface area (BSA) are given in Table 25.4 (Zimmermann et al., 2004). At ages ≥8 y and BSAs ≥1.0 m², girls had significantly higher median and 97th percentile (*p*.97) values for thyroid volume than boys (*p* < 0.001, ANOVA). The authors noted small but significant differences in the median thyroid volume between the regions but considered these to be modest relative to the population and measurement variability and that a single site-independent set of references was justified. The new reference values should be used in preference to older reference data sets of WHO/ICCIDD (1997) and Zimmermann et al. (2001).

A child is defined as having goiter, when the sex-specific thyroid volume, expressed as a function of age or BSA is >97th percentile value shown in Table 25.4. The thyroid volume data are given as a function

	Boys		Girls	
	Med.	*p*.97	Med.	*p*.97
Age (years)				
6	1.60	2.91	1.57	2.84
7	1.80	3.29	1.81	3.26
8	2.03	3.71	2.08	3.76
9	2.30	4.19	2.40	4.32
10	2.59	4.73	2.76	4.98
11	2.92	5.34	3.17	5.73
12	3.30	6.03	3.65	6.59
BSA (m²)				
0.7	1.47	2.62	1.46	2.56
0.8	1.66	2.95	1.67	2.91
0.9	1.86	3.32	1.90	3.32
1.0	2.10	3.73	2.17	3.79
1.1	2.36	4.20	2.47	4.32
1.2	2.65	4.73	2.82	4.92
1.3	2.99	5.32	3.21	5.61
1.4	3.36	5.98	3.66	6.40
1.5	3.78	6.73	4.17	7.29
1.6	4.25	7.57	4.76	8.32

Table 25.4: WHO reference data for the median and upper limit of normal (*p*.97, 97th percentile) for thyroid volume (mL) by age and body surface area (BSA) measured by ultrasonography in iodine replete children. From Zimmermann et al., American Journal of Clinical Nutrition 79: 231–237, 2004 © Am J Clin Nutr. American Society for Clinical Nutrition.

of BSA because in countries where there is a high prevalence of growth retardation, children weigh less and are shorter than the reference children of a similar age. Such data are also useful when the age of children is uncertain.

Body surface area (BSA) (m²) can be calculated using the following formula:

$$W^{0.425} \times H^{0.725} \times 0.007184$$

where *W* is the weight in kg and *H* is the height in cm.

Currently, no international reference values exist for adults.

Measurement of thyroid volume by ultrasonography

All measurements of thyroid volume by ultrasonography should be performed by well-trained operators who have participated in a calibration exercise with an experienced team, prior to any survey. For the measurement of T_{vol} on small children (i.e., < 6 y), a 7.5 MHz transducer should be used to obtain adequate resolution, whereas for older children a 5.0 MHz transducer is sufficient. The latter results in a resolution of slightly < 1 cm. Measurement of T_{vol} can be taken on children in the supine position with hyperextended neck or when subjects are sitting up in a straight-backed chair with their neck extended (Zimmerman et al., 2004).

An experienced operator can complete up to 200 examinations for thyroid volume per day. Training programs are available internationally. Unfortunately, in practice, the measurement of thyroid volume by ultrasound is often not well standardized, because no standard criteria exist for taking the measurement or the calculation of thyroid volume. As a result, WHO is currently establishing a set of standardized criteria.

A diagram of the thyroid gland showing the two elongate lobes connected across the midline by the isthmus is shown in Figure 25.2. A three-dimensional view is shown for one of the lobes to illustrate that each lobe approximates an ellipsoid. Consequently, lobe volume can be estimated from the measurements of the lengths of the three main axes

(a, b, c) as:

$$V_{lobe} = a \times b \times c \times 0.479$$

Note that the isthmus is not always measured because it can be very small, especially in children. In such cases, its volume is estimated as being 5% of the volume of the two lobes:

$$V_{isthmus} = 0.05 \times (V_{right} + V_{left})$$

To calculate thyroid volume, the volumes are summed:

$$V_{thyroid} = V_{right} + V_{left} + V_{isthmus}$$

Ultrasonography is being increasingly used in large-scale surveys in Europe, South America, and Australia, with the use of a mobile van-based laboratory. Because thyroid volume is not an indicator of current iodine status, neither ultrasonography nor palpation should be used to monitor the efficacy of a salt iodization program: it takes time for the thyroid volume to return to normal after restoration of available iodine levels. Instead, urinary iodine is more suitable and is discussed below.

25.1.3 Urinary iodine excretion

Daily urinary excretion of iodine closely reflects recent iodine intake because only a small fraction is excreted in the feces. Indeed, over 90% of iodine intake is excreted in the urine (Nath et al., 1992). Hence, assuming a median 24-h urine volume of about 0.0009 L/h/kg, and an average bioavailability of iodine in the diet of 92%, daily iodine intake (I_{intake}) in µg can be calculated from urinary iodide as follows:

$$I_{intake} = (0.0009 \times 24 / 0.92) \times Wt \times Ui$$
$$= 0.0235 \times Wt \times Ui$$

where Wt is the body weight (kg) and Ui is the urinary iodine (µg/L). Details are given in IOM (2002).

Other researchers have assumed a 24-h urine volume of 1.5 L and an average iodine bioavailability of 90% (Zimmermann and Delange, 2004).

Urinary iodine has been used as an index

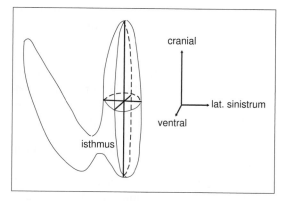

Figure 25.2: Diagram of the thyroid gland, showing a cross-sectional view of the right thyroid lobe. From Szebeni and Beleznay, Journal of Clinical Ultrasound 20: 329–337, 1992 © Wiley & Sons, Inc., with permission.

of iodine nutriture in many large-scale nutrition surveys for the assessment of both deficiency and excess. Twenty-four-hour urine specimens are preferred but are not always practical in field surveys.

Several studies have examined the validity of 24-h urinary iodine excretion as a measure of iodine nutriture at the individual and population levels. Thomson et al. (2001) noted significant correlations between measures of urinary iodine excretion based on two 24-h urine samples per person and thyroid volume and thyroglobulin but not with T_4 or TSH, confirming their use at the individual level in this study of New Zealand adults. Similar results were obtained when subjects ($n = 233$) were ranked into three groups (< 60, 60–90; > 90 μg/d iodine), as shown in Table 25.5.

It is not always practical to collect 24-h urine samples in the field, especially for children. Conscientious and compliant subjects are needed to ensure complete 24-h collections (Section 15.1.12). As an alternative, fasting early morning specimens or casual urine samples are often obtained for population-based estimates. Thomson et al. (1996) reported identical median values for urinary iodine concentrations in adults ($n = 189$) based on fasting urine samples (from part of a 24-h urine), and 24-h urine collection.

	Low $n = 73$	Medium $n = 81$	High $n = 79$
I/creatinine (μg/g Creat.)	34.8 ± 9.5	48.0 ± 14.3	87 ± 43
Urinary iodide (μg/L)	41 ± 19	53 ± 19	83 ± 40
T_{vol} (ml)	16.4 ± 7.0	13.8 ± 6.0	14.1 ± 4.4
Thyroglobin (ng/ml)	8.7 ± 7.7	6.5 ± 4.9	5.9 ± 5.7
TSH (μU/ml)	1.6 ± 0.8	1.7 ± 0.8	1.6 ± 0.7
T_4 (μg/dl)	7.3 ± 1.8	7.6 ± 2.1	7.3 ± 1.5

Table 25.5: Urinary iodide excretion, thyroid hormone levels, and thyroid volume (T_{vol}) of subjects grouped by 24-h urinary iodide excretion (low < 60, medium 60–90, high > 90 μg/d). Data from Thomson et al., European Journal of Clinical Nutrition 55: 387–392, 2001, with permission of the Nature Publishing Group.

	r	p
Fasting iodine (μmol/L)	0.58	0.0001
Fasting iodine (μmol/mol creat.)	0.22	n.s
Body weight (kg)	0.32	0.049

Table 25.6: Correlation coefficients for urinary iodine based on fasting urine samples expressed as μmol/L and as μmol/mol creatinine (creat.) with 24-h urinary iodine excretion (μmol/d). Data from Thomson et al., Journal of Trace Elements in Medicine and Biology 10: 214–222, 1996.

In addition, significant correlations between iodine excretion based on fasting samples (expressed as μmol/L) and 24-h urine samples (expressed as μmol/d) were observed (Table 25.6). Moreover, the proportion of subjects classified as mild, moderate, or severely iodine-deficient was similar, confirming the use of fasting urine samples, at least at the population level in this study. In contrast, Rasmussen et al. (1999) reported that urinary iodine excretion based on a single fasting urine sample was significantly lower than that calculated from the actual 24-h urine concentration.

Some studies have also examined the most appropriate timing for the collection of casual urine samples because urinary iodine excretion exhibits diurnal variation — the lowest values occur in the morning, with peaks occurring 4–5 hours after a meal — and day-to-day (circadian) variation (Als et al., 2000). However, no consensus has been reached and the use of urinary iodine concentrations based on casual samples versus fasting early morning specimens to assess iodine nutriture on a population basis is still hotly debated (Soldin, 2002). Indeed, Soldin (2002) emphasizes that the use of urinary iodine concentrations from casual urine samples may not give a precise estimate of the proportion of the population with a median urinary iodine concentration < 50 μg/L.

Some investigators advocate the additional measurement of creatinine in casual urinary iodine samples, to allow adjustment for factors that may affect the concentrations of iodine (Knudsen et al., 2000), assuming that daily creatinine excretion is constant in a given individual (Section 15.1.12). However, creatinine varies with age and is influenced by several other factors including protein intake, as discussed in Section 16.1.1. Hence, several investigators (Remer and Manz, 1994; Thomson et al., 1996), including WHO/UNICEF/ICCIDD (1994) do not support expressing iodine excretion as an iodine : creatinine ratio, especially for children in developing countries, where urinary creatinine values may be lower because of malnutrition (Furnée et al., 1994; Bourdoux, 1998). As an alternative, ICCIDD/UNICEF/WHO (2001) recommend the measurement of iodine concentration in casual urine samples for assessing iodine status in epidemiological studies.

Nevertheless, in some population surveys in more affluent countries, results for urinary iodine based on casual urine samples have been expressed both as urinary iodine concentrations and as a ratio to creatinine excretion, as shown in Figure 25.3. In the National Health and Nutrition Examination Survey (NHANES) III, the median urinary iodine excretion was nearly 50% lower than the median recorded in NHANES I (145 ± 3 μg/L vs. 320 ± 6 μg/L), based on the same assay, with 11.7% of the population having low urinary iodine concentrations (< 50 μg/L), compared with 2.6% in NHANES I; women of child-bearing age and pregnant women were most at risk. The median urinary iodine concentration in both the NHANES I and III surveys (Figure 25.3) exceeded the level considered to be adequate by WHO/ICCIDD/UNICEF (1994) (Table 25.7).

Interpretive criteria

Urinary iodine values are not usually normally distributed, so the median value should always be reported. Cutoff points for median urinary iodine levels based on casual urine samples have been proposed by WHO/UNICEF/ICCIDD (1994) to assess the severity of IDDs among schoolaged children; they are shown in Table 25.7. The validity of the threshold for urinary iodine levels indicative of iodine sufficiency (e.g., 100–199 μg/L) in Table 25.7 has been confirmed recently using data from 48 populations (Delange et al., 2002).

WHO/UNICEF/ICCIDD (1994) state that no more than 50% of the population should have a urinary iodine concentration below 100 μg/L and no more than 20% of the population should have a urinary iodine concentration below 50 μg/L.

WHO recommends the collection of at least 300 casual urine specimens from any given population to diagnose endemic IDD or to monitor the effectiveness of an interven-

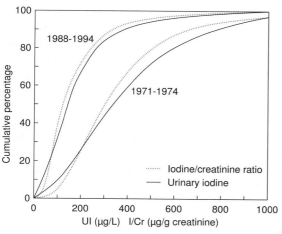

Figure 25.3: Urinary iodine concentrations and iodine/creatinine ratios in the NHANES I and NHANES-III populations. Data from Hollowell et al., Journal of Clinical Endocrinology and Metabolism 83: 3401–3408, 1998.

Median value (μg/L)	Severity of IDD
< 20	Severe IDD
20–49	Moderate IDD
50–99	Mild IDD
100–199	Optimal
200–299	Risk of iodine-induced hyperthyroidism
>300	Risk of adverse health consequences

Table 25.7: Epidemiological criteria for assessing severity of iodine deficiency disorders based on median urinary iodine levels. From ICCIDD/UNICEF/WHO (2001), with permission.

tion. This figure is based on the assumption of a prevalence of abnormal results of 50%, 95% confidence intervals, a design effect of 2, and a relative precision of 16%. Further justification for this sample size is given in WHO/UNICEF/ICCIDD (1994).

Data on the mean, median, and selected percentiles for urinary iodine by age and sex for persons 6 y to >71 y and pregnant and lactating women from NHANES III have been compiled (Appendix A25.1). Median values for the different age groups ranged from 138 to 155 μg/L for men and 110 to 129 μg/L for women, and suggest that dietary intakes of iodine were adequate.

Measurement of urinary iodine

For the measurement of urinary iodine, care must be taken to avoid adventitious sources of contamination. Urine specimens can be collected in special polyethylene tubes, tightly sealed with screw tops. Samples do not require the addition of a preservative or refrigeration during collection and transport to the laboratory. Samples can be stored refrigerated for several months prior to analysis, provided the samples are tightly sealed to avoid evaporation. Frozen urine samples can be kept indefinitely.

Several methods can be used to measure urinary iodine, some of which employ automated equipment allowing the analysis of large numbers of samples (Dunn et al., 1993). Generally, the methods have a low detection limit, and can be used to determine iodine concentrations as low as 5–20 μg/L, with an analytical coefficient of variation (CV) of < 10%.

WHO/UNICEF/ICCIDD (1994) describes a simple method suitable for analyzing urinary iodine in epidemiological surveys, which costs about US$0.50–1.00 per specimen, including labor; 150 specimens can be processed daily using this method.

Many of the methods are based on a chloric acid digestion of organic matter followed by the determination of iodine by the Sandell and Kolthoff reaction. In this reaction, iodine catalyzes the reduction of ceric ammonium sulfate (yellow color) to the cerous form (colorless) using arsenous acid; extinction is measured in a spectrophotometer at 405 nm (Aumont and Tressol, 1986). A certified reference material should be used to control the accuracy of all the analytical methods used. Such materials are available from Seronorm (Sero AS, Asker, Norway).

A new simple, inexpensive, manual urinary iodine acid digestion method has been developed and its performance compared with five other methods in different laboratories. This new method uses a mild chloric acid digestion at a lower temperature and for a shorter period of time to destroy interfering substances, such as thiocyanate and organic matter, eliminating the need for a perchloric acid fume hood. After digestion, the urinary iodine content is again measured via the Sandell-Kolthoff reaction. A high correlation was obtained among the urinary iodine values analyzed by this new, simple method, in all of the participating laboratories, even for the specimens with low urinary iodine values (May et al., 1997).

Qualitative methods that provide information only on iodine deficiency or excess have also been developed for urinary iodine assays. Some are available as commercial kits and require no instrumentation. They produce colored products that can be recognized on a paper strip. These products are summarized in ICCIDD (2000).

Note that measurement of urinary iodine is not appropriate in dietary conditions in which goitrogens prevent the uptake of iodine into the thyroid gland, and subsequent synthesis of thyroid hormones. Urinary iodine does not reflect thyroid function, so in such conditions, urinary iodine excretion may be normal. Instead, the concentration of TSH in the serum or plasma should be used, because it is an excellent indicator of altered thyroid function in individuals.

25.1.4 Thyroid stimulating hormone in serum or whole blood

Levels of TSH in serum or whole blood reflect the availability and adequacy of thyroid hormone and, hence, are an indicator of thyroid function. In chronic severe iodine deficiency, serum TSH concentrations are markedly elevated, as a result of the increased secretion of TSH by the pituitary in an attempt to stimulate thyroid hormone synthesis. However, in mild to moderate iodine deficiency when urinary iodine concentrations are low, serum TSH levels are often within the normal range in adults (Benmiloud et al., 1994; Buchinger et al., 1997; Simsek et al., 2003). Hence, serum TSH levels are not a very sensitive indicator of borderline iodine deficiency in adults (Hetzel et al., 1990). Indeed, WHO/UNICEF/ ICCIDD (1994) do not recommend the use of TSH in serum or whole blood for assessing iodine status in adults or school children.

Because neonates are hypersensitive to iodine deficiency, they exhibit elevated TSH concentrations in serum or whole blood more frequently than adults do. Such elevated levels can be serious because TSH levels directly reflect the adequacy of thyroid hormone in the brain. As a result, testing TSH concentrations in serum, whole blood, or cord blood of newborns is the recommended screening test for congenital hypothyroidism.

Figure 25.4 shows a cumulative distribution of TSH (in 1 mU/L units) measured in dried blood samples taken from neonates, from three developing countries and from two iodine-sufficient areas in Australia and Canada (Sullivan et al., 1997). Note the shift to the right in the cumulative TSH distributions for the neonates from all three developing countries (the Philippines, Malaysia, and Pakistan) when compared with the iodine-sufficient areas (Canada and Australia). In addition, in this study the TSH results were consistent with those of other indicators of IDD (e.g., urinary iodine concentrations) in these areas, although in other studies some discrepancies have been reported (Copeland et al., 2002).

Factors affecting neonatal TSH levels

Maternal iodine deficiency can result in slightly elevated TSH levels in the newborn.

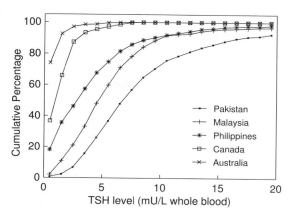

Figure 25.4: A comparison of newborn whole-blood thyroid stimulating hormone (TSH) concentrations in five different countries. From Sullivan et al., Journal of Nutrition 127: 55–58, 1997, with permission of the American Society for Nutritional Sciences.

In Poland, the introduction of iodine supplements during pregnancy and iodized salt in 1997 has led to a decline in the prevalence of elevated neonatal TSH levels (Oltarzewski and Szymborski, 2003).

Stress during the birthing process leads to a surge in TSH during the first few days of life (Copeland et al., 2002).

Time of blood collection may affect neonatal TSH levels, as shown in Table 25.8. In this study both cord blood and heel-prick specimens collected on day one appear to have higher levels than those collected thereafter

Specimen (n)	Median TSH (mU/L)	% with TSH > 5 mU/L (95% CI)
Cord blood (243)	8.3	82.3 (77.1, 86.7)
Heel blood		
day 1 (14)	8.5	85.7 (60.3, 97.5)
day 2 (48)	7.5	79.2 (66.0, 88.9)
day 3[a] (28)	4.7	42.9 (25.7, 61.4)

Table 25.8: Thyroid-stimulating hormone (TSH) results from newborns; comparison of cord blood and whole blood from heel-prick specimens, Crawford Long Hospital, Atlanta, GA, 1996–1997. [a]24 samples were collected on days 3 to 7, and the remainder on days 8 to 34. From Copeland et al., Public Health Nutrition 5: 81–87, 2002, with permission of the authors.

(Copeland et al., 2002). Such trends have not been consistent, however, and the relationship between cord blood TSH and heel-prick collected ⩾ 72 h after birth remains uncertain.

WHO/UNICEF/ICCIDD (1994) have recommended that blood specimens be collected by heel prick after 72 h or from cord blood at the time of birth. Collection by heel prick before 72 h is not recommended, because levels may be elevated as a result of stress during the birthing process. Cord blood TSH may better reflect iodine status at birth than heel-prick TSH levels after 72 h.

Congenital hypothyroidism induces very high TSH levels in affected infants.

Exposure to iodine-containing antiseptics and X-ray contrast media by mothers or neonates can cause increases in TSH levels for 1 mo or longer after birth. Oltarzewski and Szymborski (2003), working in Polish hospitals, reported a positive correlation between the prevalence of elevated TSH levels in neonates and the practice of using iodine-containing antiseptics, and recommended the withdrawal of the latter from all Polish obstetric clinics.

Neonatal exposure to antithyroid medications may elevate TSH levels.

Assay method, manufacturer of the commercial kit, and the type and grade of blood collection paper may all influence the TSH concentrations, and thus comparisons among populations. A microplate ELISA assay that employs monoclonal antibodies is the recommended method because it is more sensitive than the polyclonal test kits and hence can discriminate at low TSH concentrations (i.e., about 2 mU/L) (Sullivan et al., 1997; Copeland et al., 2002).

Interpretive criteria

Cutoff points for whole blood or serum TSH concentrations in neonates have been defined by WHO/UNICEF/ICCIDD (1994). Levels of > 20–25 mU/L whole blood or 40–50 mU/L serum are recommended as cutoffs to screen for congenital hypothyroidism.

Sometimes, TSH testing in newborns is used as an indicator for assessing the prevalence of IDD in epidemiological studies (Figure 25.4). In such cases, TSH levels may be only mildly elevated, and WHO/UNICEF/ICCIDD (1994) suggest a cutoff of > 5 mU/L for whole blood TSH levels in neonates. Based on this cutoff, WHO has defined prevalence estimates for the severity of IDD in neonates, indicative of a mild (3.0%–19.9%), moderate (20.0%–39.9%), or severe (⩾ 40%) public health problem.

Several investigators have noted that the WHO/UNICEF/ICCIDD (1994) criteria must be applied with caution to populations in which iodine solutions are used during prenatal medical procedures (Copeland et al., 2002; Oltarzewski and Szymborski, 2003). Copeland et al. (2002) also note that the appropriateness of the > 5 mU/L cutoff value for different commercial monoclonal TSH kits remains uncertain. There is also some evidence that different cutoffs may be necessary for cord blood versus heel-prick blood samples (Copeland et al., 2002).

Measurement of TSH

Cord blood or heel-prick blood specimens can be collected onto filter paper cards (Grade 903; Schelicher and Schuell) for the assay. Details of the standardized procedures for the collection and storage of heel-prick (and finger-prick) whole blood specimens onto filter paper are summarized in Mei et al. (2001). Note that dried blood spots can be stored at −20°C for many weeks or years, provided these recommended procedures are used. As an alternative, serum from heel-prick samples can be used.

The recommended assay method for TSH is an enzyme-linked immunosorbent assay (ELISA) using monoclonal antibodies. This monoclonal TSH assay does not show the cross-reactions experienced using the earlier polyclonal TSH assays (Sullivan et al., 1997). It also has a high sensitivity (< 2 mU/L), permitting the determination of mild-to-moderate IDD associated with whole blood TSH levels of < 20 mU/L. Further, the reagents have a long shelf life (6 mo) (Miyai et al., 1981). Both internal and external quality-control specimens should be used. The New-born Screening Quality Assurance Program, operated by the U.S. Centers for Disease Control and Prevention (CDC), distributes quality-control materials for TSH (and thy-roxine) assays (Mei et al., 2001).

25.1.5 Serum thyroglobulin

Iodine intake influences the concentrations of both thyroid hormones and thyroglobulin in the blood. Thyroglobulin is the most abundant thyroid protein and is specific to the thyroid, with no known physiological role outside the thyroid. In contrast to urinary iodine, thyroglobulin reflects iodine nutriture over a period of months. When usual iodine intakes are inadequate, thyroid cells proliferate, causing hyperplasia and hypertrophy. In turn, this results in an enhanced turnover of thyroid cells, which release thyroglobulin into the serum. Hence, when habitual intakes of iodine are low, an inverse association between levels of thyroglobulin in serum and iodine intakes is observed.

Rasmussen et al. (2002) suggest that serum thyroglobulin concentration may be a sensitive marker for iodine status, not only when intakes are deficient but also over a broader range of iodine intakes. Further, serum thyroglobulin may be especially useful for detecting short-term changes in thyroid function in response to salt iodization (Zimmerman et al., 2003b).

Missler et al. (1994) examined the response of serum thyroglobulin levels in children in Zimbabwe treated with oral iodized oil at four levels for 1 y (Figure 25.5). The results indicated that serum thyroglobulin was a sensitive indicator of iodine deficiency for children living in an area of severe iodine deficiency. Serum thyroglobulin levels increased before serum TSH became elevated. Indeed, 60% of the children had elevated thyroglobulin levels (i.e., > 20 µg/L) at baseline compared

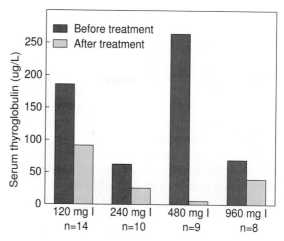

Figure 25.5: Thyroglobulin levels in serum, before and 1 y after single-dose iodine therapy with iodized oil. Comparison of results before and after treatment, using the Wilcoxon signed rank test, showed $p < 0.01$ in all cases. Data from Missler et al., European Journal of Clinical Chemistry and Clinical Biochemistry 32: 137–143, 1994.

with only 9.2% for TSH. Other intervention studies have reported that thyroglobulin is also a more sensitive indicator than thyroxine (T_4) in measuring the response to iodized oil (Benmiloud et al., 1994).

Interpretive criteria

Cutoff points for serum thyroglobulin have not been established, in part because assay methods are not well standardized among laboratories. Further, levels are high at birth, but decline steadily during childhood and adolescence to reach adult concentrations (Penny et al., 1983).

WHO/UNICEF/ICCIDD (1994) currently provide three ranges for median thyroglobulin level (µg/L) in serum for children and adults: 10.0–19.9, 20.0–39.9, and ≥ 40.0 µg/L indicative of IDD of a mild, moderate, or severe public health problem. They also suggest that a median serum thyroglobulin concentration of < 10µg/L at 5 and 12 mo indicates normalization of iodine status. WHO/UNICEF/ICCIDD (1994) caution, however, that different assays may have different normal ranges for both children and adults.

Measurement of thyroglobulin

Thyroglobulin in serum is generally assayed via a sandwich fluoroimmunometric method using microplate technology with commercial kits. A 2-site immunoassay is preferred because it has a low cross-reactivity and improved specificity compared with 1-site assays (Tórrens and Burch, 2001).

Dried blood spot assays are now also available for the assessment of thyroglobulin and use an adaptation of the sandwich fluorescence immunoassay technique (Baumann and Wood, 1985; Zimmermann et al., 2003b). For the assay, blood from a finger, heel, or earlobe puncture can be spotted (3 mm diameter) onto filter paper (grade 903; Schleicher and Schuell), air-dried in a horizontal position for 24 h and then stored at $-20°C$ using the procedures recommended by Mei et al. (2001).

Missler et al. (1994) suggest that the blood spots can be kept at ambient temperature with no decrease of immunoreactivity over a 28-d period, at temperatures between $-5°C$ and $+45°C$, and relative humidities between $< 10\%$ and $> 90\%$. Information on the between- and within-assay precision of this in-house blood spot immunofluorimetric assay is given in Table 25.9 (Missler et al., 1994). This in-house blood spot assay showed better precision than that adapted from a commercial kit by Zimmerman et al. (2003), but a lower correlation with serum thyroglobulin.

More research is required to determine whether it is necessary to measure thyroglobulin antibodies concurrently with thyroglobulin in children from IDD-affected areas to prevent the potential underestimate of thyroglobulin. Likewise, the normal range for thyroglobulin in different age groups using dried whole-blood spot thyroglobulin assays needs to be established (Zimmerman et al. (2003).

In the future, use of the thyroglobulin assay on dried blood spots as an indicator of both thyroid dysfunction and a response to iodine interventions may increase, especially among children. Care must be taken, however, to control the accuracy and precision of these assays by using standardized procedures rec-

Within-assay precision	Median CV(%)
$< 10\,\mu g/L$ ($n = 116$)	9.1
10–$50\,\mu g/L$ ($n = 110$)	8.4
50–$500\,\mu g/L$ ($n = 56$)	7.9
Between-assay precision	Mean CV(%)
$8.9\,\mu g/L$ (low control)	13.9
$66\,\mu g/L$ (medium control)	12.0
$206\,\mu g/L$ (high control)	11.4

Table 25.9: Quality assessment data for an in-house thyroglobulin dry blood spot assay. Data from Missler et al., European Journal of Clinical Chemistry and Clinical Biochemistry 32: 137–143, 1994.

ommended by the Community Bureau of Reference (Spencer 1995). Interassay variability can be large and reproducibility poor between laboratories.

25.1.6 Thyroxine and triiodothyronine in serum

Usually 99.8% of the thyroxine (T_4) and 99.5% of the triiodothyronine (T_3) are bound in serum to thyroxine-binding globulin, transthyretin, and albumin. The levels of these circulating thyroid hormones are used as a measure of thyroid function, although they are not as sensitive as TSH.

Concentrations of both T_4 and T_3 are controlled by the level of TSH. When levels are adequate, there is a feedback on the pituitary which regulates the production of TSH. When supplies of iodine in the diet are moderately limited, stimulation of the thyroid gland by increased serum TSH is often sufficient to maintain circulating T_4 and T_3 concentrations within the normal range. It is only when iodine deficiency becomes more severe that T_4 levels begin to decline, and only in very severe iodine deficiency states (i.e., when median urinary iodine excretion $< 20\,\mu g/L$) that a fall in serum T_3 concentrations occurs. However, even in cases of severe iodine deficiency, levels of T_3 and T_4 often remain within the normal range. Low levels of T_3 are also associated with fasting and malnutrition (Gardner et al., 1988).

As an example, Table 25.10 shows the serum concentrations of T_4, T_3, and TSH, together with the thyroid uptake of ^{131}I in

| Variable | Brussels, Belgium | Ubangi, Zaire | |
		Clinically euthyroid adults	Myxedematous cretins
Serum			
T_4 (μg/dL)	8.1 ± 0.1	4.9 ± 0.2	0.50 ± 0.01
T_3 (ng/dL)	144 ± 3	166 ± 3	46 ± 3
TSH (μU/mL)	1.7 ± 0.1	18.6 ± 2.1	302.7 ± 20
Thyroid uptake of ^{131}I 24 h (% dose)	46.4 ± 1.1	65.2 ± 0.9	28.3 ± 2.6

Table 25.10: Comparison of biochemical indices of iodine status in subjects in Brussels and in the endemic goiter area, Ubangi, Zaire. Results are mean $\pm$ SEM. The differences for each variable between groups are significant ($p < 0.001$). Conversion factors to SI units: T_4 (nmol/L) = $\times$ 12.87; T_3 (nmol/L) = $\times$ 0.01536; TSH (mU/L) = $\times$ 1.00. From Lagasse et al. (1982). Influence of the dietary balance of iodine-thiocyanate and protein on thyroid function in adults and young infants. In: Delange F, Iteke FB, Ermans AM (eds). Nutritional Factors involved in the Goitrogenic Action of Cassava. International Development Research Centre, Ottawa, with permission.

persons living in a severe endemic goiter area in Zaire, compared with Belgian controls. Serum TSH concentrations are higher in those persons living in Zaire, concentrations being particularly high in myxedematous cretins, as a result of the increased secretion of TSH by the pituitary, noted in Section 25.1.4. Also in the clinically euthyroid adults, the values for serum T_3 levels are elevated but those for T_4 in serum are lower than the corresponding values for the Belgian controls. This replacement of T_4 by T_3 represents an iodine sparing effect, because T_3 is a metabolically more active hormone and contains 25% less iodine (Lagasse et al., 1982). It is only in those with very severe iodine deficiency (i.e., myxedematous cretins) that a decline in both T_4 and T_3 levels in serum is apparent when compared with the controls.

Concentrations of T_3 and T_4 are therefore relatively insensitive and unreliable indicators for assessing iodine status. Nevertheless, serum T_4, in particular, is used in clinical medicine to evaluate thyroid function.

Measurement of thyroxine and triiodothyronine

Serum T_4 and T_3 hormones can be accurately and precisely measured (CV 5%–8%) by very sensitive and highly specific competitive radioimmunoassay methods available as commercial kits. However, these methods are expensive and cumbersome, and the assay of serum T_4 and T_3 is not recommended for use in developing countries.

Levels in serum of T_4 and its precursor T_3 can range from 58 to 154 nmol/L and 1.0 to 3.4 nmol/L, respectively (Alexander, 1984).

25.1.7 Radioactive iodine uptake

Measurement of the uptake of radioactive ^{131}I is used as a test of thyroid function in clinical settings. The affinity of the thyroid gland for iodine is estimated by the fraction of an orally administered dose of radioactive iodine that is concentrated in the thyroid (Wayne et al., 1964). In cases of iodine deficiency, the thyroid gland concentrates more radioactive iodine, whereas in conditions of iodine excess, it concentrates less. The uptake of ^{131}I, however, is also affected by other factors. These include hyperthyroidism, hypothyroidism, subacute thyroiditis, and some medications. Variations in renal function also influence radioactive iodine uptake because of variation in the amount of tracer excreted.

Interpretive criteria

In areas where iodine intakes are moderate (i.e., from 100 to 300 μg/d), 20%–50% of the radioactive ^{131}I dose is detected in the thyroid after 24 h. In areas of iodine deficiency, the thyroidal uptake of ^{131}I is much faster and approaches 100% (Dunn, 1978).

Measurement of radioactive iodine uptake

For the test, the radioactive tracer is administered orally, and the thyroid uptake is determined by placing a γ-ray counter over the neck. To account for any nonthyroidal radioactivity in the neck, another area, such as the thigh, is also counted, and any counts obtained are subtracted from those in the neck.

25.1.8 Multiple indices

The choice of the most appropriate indicators to assess iodine status depends on several factors, including their performance, the resources available, the age or lifestage of the subjects, dietary conditions, the iodine status of the study group, and the study objectives (Pardede et al., 1998; Arthur, 1999). WHO/ICCIDD/UNICEF (1994) recommends at least two indicators to reflect the entire spectrum of IDD.

Currently, to assess the prevalence of IDD at the population level, the most practical and widely used indicator is the measurement of urinary iodine excretion in a causal urine specimen. Measurement of serum TSH can be used as a sensitive indicator of IDD in the new born period only (WHO/UNICEF/ICCIDD, 2001). In the future, thyroglobulin in whole blood may be used as an IDD indicator, and to detect short-term changes in thyroid function in response to changes in iodine supply, because urinary iodine does not reflect thyroid function (Van den Briel et al., 2001; Zimmermann et al., 2003b).

In addition, in areas where iodine deficiency is suspected, the prevalence of goiter should be determined on a representative sample of the population, preferably by ultrasonography, as it is a more objective method than palpation. It is noteworthy that the prevalence of IDD determined by these indicators will not necessarily be consistent, because goiter reflects a chronic situation of iodine deficiency, and thyroid size decreases only slowly after iodine repletion, whereas the biochemical markers reflect current iodine nutriture (Pardede et al., 1998).

25.2 Selenium

The selenium content of the human body varies regionally. For adults in the United States it is about 15 mg (Schroeder et al., 1970), whereas in New Zealand, the amount is much lower (Stewart et al., 1978). Skeletal muscle contains the largest fraction of body selenium (Levander, 1985); the liver contains a much smaller proportion.

Functions of selenium

Selenium has an essential role in several important metabolic pathways, including antioxidant defense systems, thyroid hormone metabolism, and redox control of enzymes and proteins. Selenium can influence these metabolic pathways through a number of selenoproteins, all of which contain selenocysteine at the active site; they are itemized in Table 25.11. More recently, its role in the development of the acquired immune system has been emphasized (Kiremidjian-Schumacher and Roy, 1998; Arthur et al., 2003). The precise mechanism whereby selenium maintains optimal immune function is not yet well established, but it is probably related to its function as an antioxidant.

The first selenoprotein identified was cytosolic glutathione peroxidase (GSHPx-1). It is present in all cells. Since then, at least four additional forms of glutathione peroxidase have been characterized: gastrointestinal GSHPx-2, plasma GSHPx-3, phospholipid hydroperoxide GSHPx-4, and sperm nuclei snGPx (Behne and Kyriakopoulos, 2001) (Table 25.11). All forms may function as antioxidants and be involved in eicosanoid metabolism (Roberts and Morrow, 1997). The phospholipid hydroperoxide GSHPx-4 can also metabolize fatty acid hydroperoxides and it may be associated with changes in immune function (Kiremidjian-Schumacher and Roy, 1998; Arthur et al., 2003).

A second major class of selenoproteins are the iodothyronine deiodinases (EC 3.8.1.4); three have been identified and are shown in Table 25.11. These catalyze the conversion of thyroxine (T_4) to biologically active triiodothyronine (T_3), and further inactive thyroid hormone metabolites. As a result, in selenium deficiency there is an increase in levels of plasma T_4 and a decrease in the more active

Enzyme and function
Glutathione peroxidases
Catalyze reduction of hydrogen peroxide and organic hydroperoxides and protect the cells from oxidative damage
GSHPx-1 (cystolic or classical)
GSHPx-2 (gastrointestinal)
GSHPx-3 (extracellular or plasma)
GSHPx-4 (phospholipid hydroperoxide)
snGPx (sperm nuclei) — necessary for sperm maturation and male fertility
Iodothyronine deiodinases
Catalyze activation and inactivation of the thyroid hormones
Type I (liver, kidney, thyroid)
Type II (brain)
Type III (inactivating)
Thioredoxin reductases
Catalyze NADPH-dependent reduction of oxidized thioredoxin
Other enzymes
Selenophosphate synthetase 2 — may be involved in the regulation of selenium homeostasis
Selenoprotein P — may be a transport protein for selenium
Selenoprotein W — may be involved in muscle metabolism

Table 25.11: Functions of some mammalian selenoproteins. NADPH, reduced form of nicotinamide adenine dinucleotide phosphate. From Behne and Kyriakopoulos, reprinted, with permission, from Annual Reviews of Nutrition, 21, 2001 © by Annual Reviews.

T_3. Hence, assessment of the $T_4 : T_3$ ratio in human plasma may provide an indication of the activities of iodothyronine deiodinase in otherwise inaccessible tissues (Olivieri et al., 1995). This selenium–iodine interaction explains why selenium deficiency may exacerbate or ameliorate the effects of coexisting iodine deficiency.

Other selenoproteins include thioredoxin reductases (EC 1.6.4.5). Three forms have been identified; they catalyze the NADPH-dependent reduction of thioredoxin and regenerate ascorbic acid from its oxidized metabolites (May et al., 1998; Sun et al., 1999) (Table 25.11).

Some other selenoproteins have been identified in animal tissues, only some of which have known functions. They include selenophosphate synthetase 2 (EC 2.7.9.3) which may have a role in the regulation of selenium homeostasis (Thomson, 2003), and selenoprotein P which contains 10 Se atoms per molecule. Its metabolic function is unclear, but it may serve as a transport protein for selenium to the brain (Hill et al., 2004) and as an antioxidant (Behne and Kyriakopoulos, 2001; Brown and Arthur, 2001). Selenoprotein W is a selenoprotein that occurs in muscle and other tissues; it may be involved in muscle metabolism (Burk et al., 1997). Several other selenoproteins exist (e.g., a specific selenoprotein in prostate tissue) but their functions have not been identified (Behne and Kyriakopoulos, 2001).

Absorption and metabolism of selenium

Homeostatic regulation of selenium is controlled by selenium excretion in the urine and not by selenium absorption (Levander and Burk, 1994). Hence, subjects with a low selenium status retain selenium through a reduction in urinary excretion (Robinson et al., 1985). As well, the distribution of selenium between organs and tissues is modified to ensure the maintenance of important selenium-dependent functions (Behne, 1988).

Selenium absorption takes place mainly in the duodenum. Absorption from food is generally high, about 80%, although differences in bioavailability of selenium among foods have been described. The main dietary forms of selenium are organic forms — selenocysteine and selenomethionine; their structure is given in Figure 25.6. Selenocysteine is the active form of selenium in selenoproteins, whereas selenomethionine is incorporated nonspecifically into a variety of proteins in place of methionine by a process that is not regulated by selenium status. Selenomethionine contributes to tissue selenium but is not available for synthesis of functional forms until it is catabolized, and converted into selenocysteine. This, together with any ingested selenocysteine and

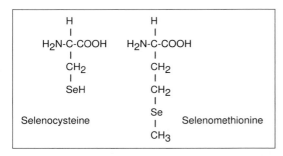

Figure 25.6: The structure of the selenium-containing amino acids, selenocysteine and selenomethionine.

any inorganic selenium from dietary sources (supplements), enters a regulated selenium pool and is incorporated into selenoproteins, as shown in Figure 25.7. Selenomethione is probably better absorbed from supplements than the inorganic forms of selenium (selenite or selenate).

Little is known about either the transport of selenocysteine across the mucosa or the transport of selenium in the body. Selenoprotein P may be a transport protein, but the evidence is weak.

Deficiency of selenium in humans

Decreases in the activities of many of the selenoenzymes and expression of selenoproteins in selenium deficiency have been associated with the onset of disease. In humans, two diseases are linked to severe endemic selenium deficiency: a cardiomyopathy (Keshan disease) and a chondrodystrophy (Kashin-Beck disease). Keshan disease is a naturally occurring selenium-responsive disease that occurs primarily in young children and women of childbearing age living in areas of Northeast China, where the soil is low in selenium (Chen et al., 1980; Xu et al., 1997). Other factors may also trigger this disease, such as environmental toxins, mineral imbalance, or possibly RNA-viruses (Beck, 1997; Levander, 2000; Beck et al., 2003). The suggestion that a virus may be involved is supported by research on the Coxsackie virus B and myocarditis in selenium-deficient mice (Beck and Levander, 2000). Keshan disease is characterized by heart enlargement, gallop rhythm, cardiogenic shock, electrocardiographic changes, and heart failure.

Kashin-Beck disease is an endemic osteoarticular disorder that affects the epiphyseal and articular cartilage and the epiphyseal growth plates of growing bones. It occurs among preadolescents or adolescents and is manifested as enlarged joints; shortened fingers, toes, and extremities; and, in severe cases, dwarfism. This disease is also prevalent in the low-selenium regions of China, but whether selenium deficiency is a primary cause of the disease is uncertain. Other factors such as fulvic acids in drinking water and trichothecene mycotoxins in foods have also been implicated (Peng et al., 1999), as well as low iodine status (Moreno-Reyes et al., 1998).

Selenium-responsive conditions, including cardiomyopathy, muscle pain, and muscular weakness have also been described in some patients receiving long-term total parenteral nutrition (TPN), but no selenium supplements (van Rij et al., 1979; Johnson et al., 1981; Stanley et al., 1982; Vinton et al., 1987; Terada et al., 1996). Once again, other interacting factors may also be involved because not all TPN patients (van Rij et al., 1979) with a low selenium status, or children with inborn errors of metabolism (e.g., phenylketonuria) receiving very low selenium synthetic diets (Jochum et al., 1999), develop clinical symptoms.

It is of note that in an epidemic of optic and peripheral neuropathy in Cuba deficiencies of lycopene, vitamin E, and the B vitamins were all implicated along with selenium. Moreover, in those suffering neuropathological symptoms, a pathogenic strain of Coxsackie virus was isolated. This example together with research on viral isolates from neuropathy patients, supports suggestions that selenium deficiency induces changes in the genetic structure of the Coxsackie virus, increasing its virulence (Beck and Levander, 2000; Beck et al., 2003).

Children with kwashiorkor or marasmus tend to have a low biochemical selenium status (Burk et al., 1967; Squali Houssaini et al., 1997; Ashour et al., 1999). The low

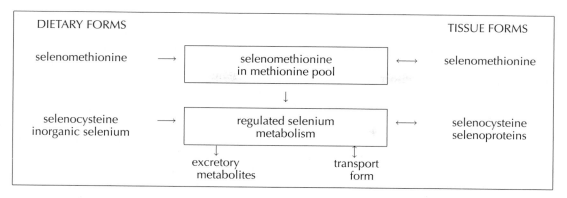

Figure 25.7: Relationships of dietary forms of selenium with tissue forms. Dietary forms of the element are shown on the left, and tissue forms on the right. Excretionary metabolites and the transport form are also present in tissues but only in relatively small quantities. From Levander and Burk (1996). Selenium. In: Ziegler EE, Filer LJ (eds.) Present Knowledge in Nutrition (7th edition), ILSI Press, Washington DC.

biochemical selenium status probably arises from inadequate intakes of protein and selenium, in combination with an increased need for selenium and other antioxidants, induced by malnutrition and infection. Other groups at risk of a low biochemical selenium status include low birth-weight neonates (Darlow et al., 1995), alcoholics, patients with Down's syndrome or acquired immune deficiency disease, and those with malabsorption syndromes such as celiac disease and cystic fibrosis (Navarro-Alarcon and Lopez-Martinez, 2000).

The involvement of selenium in the metabolism of thyroid hormones has led to studies of the selenium status of populations where goiter and myxedematous cretinism occurs. Workers in central Africa have reported a high prevalence of IDD among populations with a relatively low Se status (Vanderpas et al., 1990, 1993; Thilly et al., 1993). In these populations, selenium supplementation may aggravate hypothyroidism by stimulating thyroxine metabolism with selenoenzyme type I iodothyronine 5′-deiodinase. Hence, treatment with selenium should not be given without iodine or thyroid hormone supplementation, when both iodine and selenium deficiencies coexist (Vanderpas et al., 1993).

Suboptimal selenium status arising from low dietary intakes has been documented in persons living in New Zealand (Robinson and Thomson, 1983), parts of Finland (Mutanen, 1984), China (Chen et al., 1980), Scotland (Scott et al., 1997), and areas of the Eastern United States (Snook et al.,1983). So far, however, low selenium intakes appear to have a detrimental effect on health only in China, for reasons which are unclear at the present time.

Attempts have been made to link low selenium status with cancers and coronary heart disease. Animal studies have shown that high intakes of selenium reduce the incidence of cancer (Ip, 1998). In three randomized controlled trials in humans (Blot et al., 1993; Clark et al., 1996; Yoshizawa et al., 1998), the results were inconclusive. However, in the Nutritional Prevention of Cancer (NPC) Trial, supplemental selenium (200 μg/d as Se-enriched yeast) was associated with significant reductions in cancer risks (lung, prostate, colorectal, total cancer) in subjects whose pre-treatment plasma selenium levels were below 1.34–1.54 μmol/L (Clark et al., 1998). In a nested case-control study of Japanese-American men, the lowest risk of prostate cancer was observed in those men with prediagnostic plasma selenium concentrations of above 1.86 μmol/L (Nomura et al., 2000). Combs et al. (2001) suggest that a plasma selenium concentration of about 1.50 μmol/L may be optimal for reducing risk of at least some cancers. More large-scale trials are required to confirm the levels of plasma selenium that are protective.

Selenium may protect against certain cancers through its role as an essential nutrient in antioxidant defense systems and redox-regulatory functions. Relatively high doses of several forms of selenium (supranutritional dose range) may also serve as a source of anti-tumorigenic Se-metabolites, and thus protect the progression of cancer (Combs et al., 2001).

The evidence linking low selenium status and an increased incidence of coronary heart disease is conflicting (Rayman, 2000; Thomson, 2004a). Results of two large studies suggested that subjects with low serum selenium concentrations may be at increased risk of myocardial infarction (Salonen et al., 1982; Suadicani et al., 1992), but this has not been a consistent finding among all studies (Miettinen et al., 1983; Virtamo et al., 1985). Such discrepancies may be due to a threshold in the protective effect of selenium, so that inverse associations would only be apparent in populations with low intakes of selenium (Huttunen, 1997). The protective effect of selenium against cardiovascular disease is most likely to be associated with its antioxidant function (Thomson, 2004a).

Food sources and dietary intakes

Important food sources of selenium are seafoods, organ meats (e.g., liver and kidney), and muscle meats; fruits and vegetables are generally low in selenium. Grain products vary in their selenium content, depending on geographical location. In U.S. diets, five foods (beef, white bread, pork, chicken, and eggs) contribute about 50% of total selenium (Schubert et al., 1987), a trend that has also been reported in the United Kingdom. In New Zealand and Australia, seafood, poultry and eggs, followed by muscle meats, are the main food sources of selenium.

In some industrialized countries, cereals are a major food source of selenium. Hence, any changes in importation of grain can have a marked effect on selenium intakes. Indeed, dietary selenium intakes have fallen in the United Kingdom and other European Union countries, largely because of a decrease in imports of selenium-rich wheat from North America (MacPherson et al.,1997; Zimmerli et al., 1998; Golubkina and Alfthan, 1999). In Britain, for example, the selenium content of diets has declined from 65 to 31 µg/d (Rayman, 1997).

In contrast, selenium intakes increased in Finland from an average of 39 µg/d in 1984 to 92 µg/d in 1986, as a result of the use of selenium-enriched fertilizers (Varo et al., 1994). An increase has also occurred in the North Island of New Zealand, attributed mainly to an increase in the importation of Australian wheat and other products and increased use of supplemental selenium in animal feeds. In the 1997 New Zealand National Nutrition Survey (Wilson et al., 1999), for example, median selenium intakes were 56 and 39 µg/d for male and female adults, respectively, whereas in earlier studies intakes were < 30 µg/d (Robinson and Thomson, 1983).

Effects of high intakes of selenium

The margin between selenium deficiency and toxicity is narrower than for many other trace elements (Olson, 1986). Deleterious effects (nail changes, peripheral neuropathy, and hair loss) have been described in persons taking a selenium supplement — a selenized yeast product containing 182 times more selenium than the stated level (Helzlsouer et al., 1985). Clinical manifestations of selenium toxicity have also been described in certain areas of China (Yang et al., 1983).

The first signs of overexposure to selenium are invariably a garlic odor to the breath, a metallic taste in the mouth, nail changes, and, in severe cases, convulsions and paralysis. Other, more generalized effects, observed in some high-selenium areas such as Venezuela, include pallor, lassitude, irritability, indigestion, and giddiness (Jaffé et al., 1972). Currently, there is no sensitive and specific biochemical test to identify overexposure to selenium.

In the United States, the toxic threshold — defined as an intake above which signs and symptoms of acute or chronic toxicity can be expected — has been set at 800 μg/d (IOM, 2000). The Tolerable Upper Intake Level (UL) for selenium defined by the U.S. Food and Nutrition Board is 400 μg/d for adults. This level is unlikely to be attained through dietary intake alone in most industrialized countries. This UL was also selected for pregnant and lactating women because there are no reports of teratogenicity due to selenosis in infants born to mothers with high but nontoxic intakes of selenium (IOM, 2000). Details for the ULs for children and adolescents are given in IOM (2000).

Indices of selenium status

At present, the potential role of the newer selenoproteins as functional markers of selenium status is unclear. An exception is the Se-dependent iodothyronine deiodinase enzymes, which have an important role in thyroid hormone metabolism. Hence, the total $T_4 : T_3$ ratio may prove to be a useful biochemical functional marker of selenium status in the future. At present, there are no physiological functional tests that can be routinely used. Detection of an impairment of neutrophil function, specifically the inability of the cells to destroy *Candida albicans,* holds promise. However, many other factors can influence neutrophil function, so the test will have to be performed in conjunction with biochemical indicators of selenium status (Arthur, 1999).

When assessing selenium status in relation to disease risk, possible interactions of selenium with other components of the antioxidant defenses of the body (e.g., vitamins A, E, C, β-carotene, and polyunsaturated fat) and heavy metals (e.g., arsenic, cadmium, and lead), may be significant and should also be considered.

As the new biomarkers discussed above are not well established and do not respond equally to changes in selenium status, a series of markers is recommended, the choice depending on which specific function of selenium is under investigation. Some possible choices have been itemized by Arthur (1999)

Plasma or whole blood Se concentrations

Plasma GSHPx-3 activities

Erythrocyte GSHPx-1 activities

Selenoperoxidase activities in blood cells (platelets, lymphocytes, neutrophils)

Plasma selenoprotein P

Thyroid hormone levels.

Box 25.1: Some possible selenium biomarkers. GSH, glutathione. From Arthur, Proceedings of the Nutrition Society 58: 507–512, 1999, with permission of the Nutrition Society.

---

and are shown in Box 25.1 Of these, plasma or serum selenium is most frequently used for international comparisons of selenium status (Thomson, 2004b). The use of each of these markers is discussed in the remainder of this chapter.

25.2.1 Plasma selenium

Plasma selenium is mainly protein-bound and associated with α- and β-globulins and lipoproteins. The selenium content of plasma and serum is comparable, and both respond to short-term changes in dietary selenium intakes (Levander et al., 1981). The response of plasma selenium to changes in dietary selenium intakes is greater for the organic form of selenium (e.g., selenomethionine) than for the inorganic forms used in some dietary supplements. Selenomethionine is incorporated nonspecifically into tissue proteins in place of methionine (Luo et al., 1985a), and is not subject to homeostatic control (Burk and Levander, 1999).

In the past, plasma selenium concentrations of healthy adults in the South Island of New Zealand were frequently < 0.63 μmol/L (Thomson et al., 1982). During the past 10 y, levels have increased (Thomson and Robinson, 1996), due in part to the higher selenium concentrations in meat and poultry arising from selenium supplementation of animal feeds. Changes in food consumption patterns, such as greater intakes of multigrain breads and imported legumes and nuts, have also had a role (Thomson, 2004b). Nevertheless, even in areas in the United States where the soil selenium levels are considered low (Ohio) or only marginally adequate (Maryland), plasma selenium concentrations in healthy adults are still higher than those of adults living in the South Island of New Zealand today (Thomson, 2004b), often ranging from 1.51 and 1.70 µmol/L, respectively (Snook et al., 1983; Levander and Morris, 1984).

Factors affecting plasma selenium

Dietary selenium intake is the major determinant of plasma selenium concentrations (Robberecht and Deelstra, 1994). Plasma and serum selenium concentrations therefore vary widely among countries, reflecting in part variations in soil selenium levels (see above). As a result of these large variations, there are no accepted normal reference ranges for plasma or serum selenium concentrations.

Mode of infant feeding can affect infant plasma or serum selenium concentrations, again probably as a result of differences in selenium intakes. Breast milk has a higher selenium content than most commercial milk formulas. Hence, exclusively breastfed infants have significantly higher serum selenium concentrations than their formula-fed counterparts (Smith et al., 1982, 1995).

Prematurity leads to changes in plasma or serum selenium concentrations: levels fall from the first week of life.

Age-related changes in plasma or serum selenium concentrations during infancy have been noted (Figure 25.8) (Lombeck et al., 1977; McKenzie et al., 1978; van Caillie-Bertrand et al., 1986). Values for German infants were high at birth and then declined to 30%–50% of neonatal values by 5–6 mo. Levels then rose during the remainder of infancy (Lombeck et al., 1978). This trend was ascribed to the low selenium content of the milk formulas used.

During childhood plasma or serum selenium levels gradually increase to adult val-

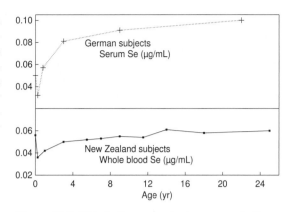

Figure 25.8: Effect of age on selenium concentrations in serum of German subjects and in whole blood of New Zealand subjects. Conversion factor to SI units (µmol/L) = × 12.66. From Thomson and Robinson, *American Journal of Clinical Nutrition* 33: 303–323, 1980 © Am J Clin Nutr. American Society for Clinical Nutrition.

ues, as shown for the German children in Figure 25.8. A similar trend was noted for U.K. children aged 4–18 y, participating in the U.K. Diet and Nutrition Survey (2000). In general, children have lower plasma or serum selenium concentrations than do adults.

During adulthood, plasma serum selenium values appear to be relatively constant (Lane et al., 1983; IOM, 2000), although after 60 y a decline has been noted (Verlinden et al., 1983a, 1983b; Swanson et al., 1990), which has not always been linked with changes in dietary selenium intakes (Olivieri et al., 1994).

Pregnancy and lactation are associated with lower plasma or serum selenium levels (Levander et al., 1987). Concentrations are approximately 20% lower at term compared to the values for nonpregnant women (Behne and Wolters, 1979). The reason for this decline is unknown; it is not related to hemodilution (Levander et al., 1987). Levels in lactating women are unaffected by the stage of lactation (Levander et al., 1987).

Puberty and sex may affect plasma or serum selenium concentrations. Puberty may sometimes lead to lower plasma or serum selenium concentrations in boys than in girls (Marano et al., 1991), although this difference was not observed in U.K. children (Gregory et al., 2000). In younger children (Lombeck et al., 1978; McKenzie et al., 1978; Gregory et al., 2000) and in adults (Kay and Knight, 1979; Lane et al., 1981, 1983), no sex-related differences have been observed.

Race may influence plasma or serum selenium levels, although the differences observed may be diet-related. The mean plasma selenium concentration for African American adult males from Georgia, USA, was slightly lower than in Caucasian males (1.24 μmol/L vs. 1.41 μmol/L) (McAdam et al., 1984).

Smoking impacted negatively on plasma selenium concentrations in the subjects from NHANES III (Kafai and Ganji, 2003). Results for other populations of smokers have been similar (Thomson, 2004). The extent to which the lower plasma selenium levels in smokers is due to an increase in requirements for antioxidants including selenium, or to the effect of an inadequate diet and selenium intake is not clear (Duthie et al., 1993).

Genetic defects such as maple syrup urine disease and phenylketonuria are often associated with below-normal serum selenium concentrations in children, probably arising from the low content of selenium in the synthetic formula diets (Lombeck et al., 1975).

Certain disease states are associated with low plasma or serum selenium concentrations; some are listed in Box 25.2. They include diseases such as HIV (Dworkin, 1994) and chronic renal failure (Marchante-Gayón et al., 1996; Sabé et al., 2002). In cardiovascular disease and cancer, however, the existence of low serum selenium levels has been inconsistent (Salonen et al., 1982; Oster et al., 1983; Auzepy et al., 1987; Suadicani et al., 1992; Rayman, 2000).

Interpretive criteria

Plasma selenium values below 0.1 μmol/L have been observed in several severely de-

---

Disorders of the digestive tract and related organs: short bowel syndrome, Crohn's disease, celiac disease, cystic fibrosis, primary biliary cirrhosis, alcoholic liver cirrhosis, alcoholism, renal failure, hemodialysis, intrahepatic cholestasis of pregnancy.

Muscle disorders: muscular dystrophy, myotonic dystrophy, congestive cardiomyopathy, Keshan disease

Neurological diseases: multiple sclerosis, Down's syndrome, neuronal ceroid lipofuscinosis

Inflammatory diseases: rheumatoid arthritis, AIDS

Chronic renal failure

Cancer

Cardiovascular diseases

Box 25.2: Diseases associated with lower than normal plasma selenium concentrations. From Nève, Journal of Trace Elements and Electrolytes in Health and Disease 5: 1–17, 1991.

---

pleted subjects showing typical clinical features of selenium deficiency; they respond rapidly following selenium repletion (van Rij et al., 1979; Terada et al., 1996).

No universal normal reference values have been established for plasma or serum selenium (Alfthan and Nève, 1996). The values for healthy adults can vary from 0.5 to 2.5 μmol/L, depending on the geographic region. Low plasma selenium values can be interpreted by comparison with those from carefully matched healthy controls who live in the same geographic area (Nève, 1991). Alternatively, the cutoffs for plasma selenium concentrations for assessing the adequacy of selenium status by Thomson (2004a) can be applied. These are shown in Table 25.12.

Data on the mean and selected percentiles for serum selenium for males and females aged ≥ 4 y studied during NHANES III, 1988–1994, are given in Appendix A25.2. Plasma selenium was measured in the U.K. National Diet and Nutrition Survey for young people aged 4–18 y using inductively coupled plasma mass spectrometry (ICP-MS). Mean, median and lower and upper 2.5 percentiles by age and sex are presented (Gregory et al., 2000).

	Se concentration (μmol/L)
Prevention of Keshan disease	> 0.25
Optimal activity of IDIs	> 0.82
Maximization of plasma GSHPx, and selenoprotein P	>1.00–1.20
Protection against some cancers	>1.50

Table 25.12: Proposed cutoff values for plasma selenium indicative of adequate selenium status. IDI, iodothyronine 5'deiodinases; GSHPx, glutathione peroxidase From Thomson, European Journal of Clinical Nutrition 58: 391–402, 2004a.

Measurement of plasma selenium

Plasma and serum selenium levels can now be measured accurately and reliably using hydride generation atomic absorption spectrometry (AAS), or graphite furnace AAS with Zeeman background correction and specially adapted matrix modifiers (McMaster et al., 1990; Nève, 1991). The graphite furnace method, unlike hydride generation AAS, does not require any pretreatment of the samples and was used in NHANES III (IOM, 2000) and the New Zealand Children's Nutrition Survey (McLachlan, 2003).

In the past, fluorometric methods, usually semi-automated (Watkinson, 1979), were adopted for the analysis of plasma or serum selenium, but they required prior sample digestion. Instrumental neutron activation analysis (INAA) (Lombeck et al., 1978; Gibson et al., 1985), and electron capture gas chromatography (McCarthy et al., 1981), are sensitive specialized techniques that have been used, but now inductively coupled plasma mass spectrometry (ICP-MS) is the most frequently adopted technique.

Care must be taken during the collection, preparation, and analysis of samples to avoid adventitious sources of contamination. Several selenium-certified reference materials are available. These include bovine (RM 8419) and human (RM 909) serum from the National Institute of Standards and Technology (Appendix A4.1), as well as human serum (STE 105) from Nycomed, Norway.

25.2.2 Whole blood selenium concentrations

Whole blood selenium concentrations, unlike serum selenium, are an index of long-term selenium status and do not fluctuate from day to day. However, their relationship to selenium intake is complex. In a selenium depletion study of young adult men, for example, whole blood selenium concentrations were not altered after a 6-wk period on a low-selenium diet (19–24 μg/d Se) (Levander et al., 1981), although after a period of months on a low-selenium diet, a response was seen (Thomson and Robinson, 1980). A similar delay in the response was also evident after supplementation with selenium and is due to the long time period required for the incorporation of selenium into erythrocytes.

Table 25.13 shows the relationship between dietary selenium intakes and whole blood (and hair and urine) selenium concentrations in population groups in China with high, normal, and deficient dietary intakes of selenium (Yang et al., 1983).

In the United States, adults have whole blood selenium concentrations ranging from 2.4 to 3.2 μmol/L (Allaway et al., 1968; Burk, 1984). In New Zealand, with lower selenium intakes, whole blood selenium values for adults are lower (0.8 to 0.9 μmol/L) (Griffiths and Thomson, 1974), although they have increased in recent years to levels ranging from

Area	Diet (μg/d)	Blood (μmol/L)	Hair (nmol/g)	Urine (μmol/L)
With Keshan Disease	11	0.27	0.94	0.09
Low-Se area	–	0.34	2.03	–
Se-adequate	116	1.15	4.56	0.33
High-Se area	750	5.57	46.8	1.8
With chronic selenosis	4990	40.5	407.7	33.9

Table 25.13: Mean values of dietary intake, whole blood, hair, and urinary selenium concentrations in different areas of China. Adapted from Yang et al., American Journal of Clinical Nutrition 37: 872–881, 1983 © Am J Clin Nutr. American Society for Clinical Nutrition.

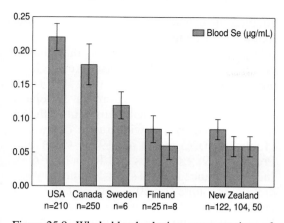

Figure 25.9: Whole blood selenium concentrations of healthy adults in selected countries. From Thomson and Robinson, American Journal of Clinical Nutrition 33: 303–323, 1980 © Am J Clin Nutr. American Society for Clinical Nutrition.

1.1 to 1.4 µmol/L (Thomson and Robinson, 1996; Thomson, 2004b).

In Europe, whole blood selenium concentrations are lower than in North America, but higher than in New Zealand and Finland (Figure 25.9) (Brune et al., 1966; Allaway et al., 1968; Westermarck et al., 1977; Thomson and Robinson, 1980; Oster et al., 1983; Verlinden et al., 1983a; Wąsowicz and Zachara, 1987).

Many of the conditions affecting plasma or serum selenium also influence whole blood selenium concentrations. For instance, low blood selenium concentrations have also been observed in children with kwashiorkor (range 1.1–1.4 µmol/L) (Levine and Olson, 1970), in children with phenylketonuria and maple syrup urine disease on special formula diets low in selenium (range 0.13–0.34 µmol/L) (Lombeck et al., 1978), and in premature infants (Gross, 1976; Amin et al., 1980). Chinese investigators have reported significantly lower whole blood selenium levels in patients with dilated cardiomyopathy than in normal subjects (Nan et al., 1986).

At present, no interpretive criteria have been established for whole blood selenium levels. In a study by Yang et al. (1987), plasma GSHPx-3 plateaued at a whole-blood selenium concentration of 1.13 µmol/L.

Measurement of whole blood selenium

Whole blood selenium concentrations can be measured using the same methods as those described for plasma or serum selenium, although analysis is more difficult. Either venous or capillary blood samples can be used (Van Dael et al., 1994). Reference materials for whole blood available from the International Atomic Energy Authority (IAEA, A-13), and from Nycomed, Norway (STE 904-5-6), are certified for selenium.

25.2.3 Erythrocyte and platelet selenium

A major part of the selenium in erythrocytes is associated with hemoglobin; < 15% of selenium in erythrocytes is actually present in glutathione peroxidase. Erythrocyte selenium concentrations generally reflect long-term selenium status. Positive correlations between selenium concentrations in erythrocytes and plasma, or with dietary intakes have been documented in individuals with a relatively constant parenteral or enteral selenium intake (Lane et al., 1981, 1982). Additionally, consistent correlations between erythrocyte selenium values and signs of chronic toxicity or deficiency have been observed.

Limited data are available on the effects of life-stage group, sex, or race on erythrocyte selenium concentrations, in part because the analysis of erythrocytes is so difficult. Nève (1999) has summarized the influence of disease states on erythrocyte selenium concentrations. In general, levels are low in disease states in which selenium absorption is pathologically decreased (e.g., celiac disease, short bowel syndrome) and in subjects with prolonged inadequate intakes of selenium (e.g., those fed selenium-deficient TPN or with protein-energy malnutrition). Erythrocyte selenium is also altered in some genetic diseases such as sickle cell disease and Down's syndrome.

In selenium supplementation studies, the response of erythrocyte selenium is slower, and the net increase significantly lower, than that of plasma. This difference probably arises, in part, because of the long time period required for the synthesis of erythrocytes, as noted earlier, together with that fact that the major part of erythrocyte selenium is hemoglobin-bound and not readily exchangeable (Nève, 1995). Nevertheless, the changes observed in erythrocytes roughly parallel those of plasma selenium.

Like plasma selenium, the response of erythrocyte selenium concentrations to selenium supplementation depends on the chemical form of the selenium and the selenium status of the subjects. Usually, the inorganic forms (selenite or selenate) only generate an increase in erythrocyte selenium levels after 2–4 wk in severely depleted subjects (i.e., from China), and plateau after 6–10 wk (Luo et al., 1985b; Xia et al., 1992). In subjects who are not so severely depleted, such as those studied in New Zealand, no response was observed after supplementation with inorganic selenium, even after 32 wk (Thomson et al., 1993).

In contrast, when selenomethionine supplements are used or selenium-rich yeast or wheat, most studies have reported increases in erythrocyte selenium (Levander et al., 1983b; Thomson et al., 1985) irrespective of the basal selenium status of the subjects. Moreover, no plateau occurs with selenomethionine because this form of selenium is not subject to homeostatic regulation.

The collection, separation, and analysis of erythrocytes are fraught with problems, and the determination is not recommended (Vitoux et al., 1999).

25.2.4 Urinary selenium

Urine is the main excretory route for selenium, accounting for 50%–60% of selenium losses, with most of the balance being excreted in the feces. Methaneselenol is the major urinary metabolite; trimethylselenonium is a minor metabolite. Losses via the skin, hair, or expired air are small, except when intakes of selenium are toxic.

Homeostasis of selenium is controlled by the regulation of selenium excretion in urine, as noted earlier (Levander and Burk, 1994). Indeed, there is some evidence of a possible adaptation to low selenium status. In New Zealand, for example, excretion of selenium by the kidney appears to be less than that in North America, based on plasma renal clearance of selenium (Robinson et al., 1997).

Daily urinary selenium excretion correlates strongly with plasma selenium and with the dietary intake over a wide range of intakes (Table 25.13) (Yang et al., 1983; Oster and Prellwitz, 1989; Alaejos and Romero, 1993). Indeed, balance studies show that urinary excretion accounts for 50%–60% of the total amount excreted over a wide range of intakes. Hence, dietary intake of selenium may be estimated as twice the daily urinary excretion in subjects with stable and normal intakes (Thomson, 1998). However, when daily intakes fluctuate widely, urinary excretion reflects short-term changes in intake, rather than selenium status (Burk et al., 1972).

Lower urinary excretion of selenium has been noted in females than in males (Tsongas and Ferguson, 1978; Thomson et al., 1996) and in pregnant than in nonpregnant females (Swanson et al., 1983). The effect of age has not been extensively studied, but the elderly appear to excrete lower levels than young adults do (Robberecht and Deelstra, 1984). Both the sex- and age-related trends in selenium excretion may be related to differences in muscle mass (Oster and Prellwitz, 1990). Indeed, Thomson et al. (1996) reported strong correlations between excretion of daily urinary selenium and creatinine, and between 24-h selenium excretion and body weight and body mass index.

Urinary selenium excretion levels are also lower in patients with burns and celiac disease and in alcoholics (Robberecht and Deelstra, 1984). Whether the lowered urinary selenium excretion is a cause or a consequence of the disease or condition is uncertain. In some diseases and conditions, low urinary levels may arise from either reduced intakes or increased retention of selenium.

Interpretive criteria

Interpretive criteria for urinary selenium concentrations have not been established. Urinary selenium concentrations ranging from 0.01 to 490 μmol/L have been reported (Robberecht and Deelstra., 1984), although generally concentrations are < 0.38 μmol/L in nonexposed persons.

Urinary selenium levels have been more frequently used as an index of selenium toxicity and industrial exposure to selenium than as an index of selenium deficiency (Glover, 1967; Hojo, 1981). The proposed maximum allowable urinary selenium concentrations is 1.3 μmol/L (Glover, 1967).

Measurement of urinary selenium

The collection of 24-h urine samples is recommended for measuring urinary selenium (Thomson and Robinson, 1980; Nève and Peretz, 1989), because selenium excretion is affected by dilution, time of day, and the selenium content of the previous meal. However, 24-h urine samples are sometimes impractical. In such circumstances, urinary selenium concentrations (i.e., μmol/L), determined on fasting urine samples (Thomson et al., 1996), can provide a reasonable estimate of total urinary selenium excretion on a population basis, although not for individuals. Results can also be expressed in relation to creatinine excretion (μmol/mol creatinine) (Hojo, 1981; Rodriguez et al., 1995; Mikac-Devic et al., 1993; Thomson et al., 1996). Wąsowicz and Zachara (1987) have reported significant positive correlations of urinary selenium : creatinine ratios and whole blood selenium concentrations in some healthy Polish subjects.

The fluorometric method is normally used for measuring selenium levels in urine (Geahchan and Chambon, 1980). An automated method is also available (Watkinson, 1979). More recently, AAS has also been used. Reference materials for urine certified for selenium are available from NIST (RM 2670) and from Nycomed (STE 108).

25.2.5 Glutathione peroxidase

More specific information on selenium status may be obtained through the measurement of concentrations of individual selenoproteins in blood. There are at least four forms of Se-containing GSH peroxidases (Table 25.11). Erythrocytes and platelets contain the most abundant form — intracellular glutathione peroxidase (GSHPx-1). This enzyme catalyzes the decomposition of hydrogen peroxide and organic hydroperoxides according to the following reaction:

$$ROOH + 2GSH \xrightarrow{GSHPx} ROH + GSSG + H_2O$$

GSHPx-1 activity in erythrocytes

The activity of GSHPx-1 in erythrocytes can only be used to assess the selenium status of individuals with a selenium intake below a "threshold value." Below this threshold level, erythrocyte GSHPx-1 activities correlate significantly with whole blood or erythrocyte selenium concentrations, as shown for the New Zealand subjects in Figure 25.10. In such cases, the activity of GSHPx-1 is dependent on selenium status. However, above the threshold value, the activity of GSHPx-1 reaches a maximum and no correlation is observed. Hence, in such cases, the activity of

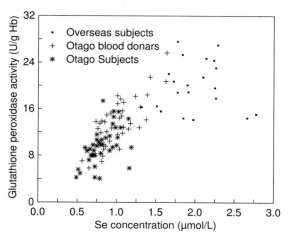

Figure 25.10: Relationship between selenium concentration of erythrocytes and GSHPx activity for subjects from Otago (New Zealand) and overseas. Data from Rea et al., British Journal of Nutrition 42: 201–208, 1979, with permission of the Nutrition Society.

GSHPx-1 can no longer be used to assess selenium status.

Studies have shown that the threshold value corresponds to a whole blood selenium concentration of 1.15 µmol/L (Duffield et al., 1999). The response of erythrocyte GSHPx-1 activity does not appear to be dependent on the chemical form of selenium (Thomson et al., 1993; Nève, 1995).

Whether maximal activity of GSHPx-1 is required for optimal health is not yet known. Moreover, the possible consequences of less than maximal GSHPx activities have not been established.

GSHPx-1 activity in platelets

The activity of GSHPx-1 in platelets has also been investigated, although the separation of the platelets is time consuming and difficult. Platelets contain significantly more selenium than other tissues, have a relatively fast turnover (8–14 d), and contain no hemoglobin (Kasperek et al., 1982). Hence, it is not surprising that GSHPx-1 activity in platelets has been shown to respond quickly to changes in selenium intakes (Thomson and Duncan, 1981; Levander et al., 1983a, 1983b; Thomson et al., 1988; Cohen et al., 1989) and at a faster rate compared with GSHPx-1 activity in erythrocytes, which have a much longer lifespan (120 d) (Nève, 1991).

The validity of platelet GSHPx-1 activity as a sensitive indicator of selenium nutriture in individuals with a low selenium status has been confirmed in several studies. For example, in a selenium supplementation study of Finnish men with low-selenium status, platelet enzyme activity nearly doubled after supplementation for 14 d (Levander et al., 1983b). In New Zealand, after supplementation with selenium for 4 wk, significant positive correlations between platelet GSHPx-1 activity and selenium concentrations in human liver and muscle tissue were observed (Thomson et al., 1988).

Subsequent studies have clearly shown that GSHPx-1 activity in platelets, unlike GSHPx-1 activity in erythrocytes, is sensitive to differences in the chemical form of selenium

administered (Levander et al., 1987; Alfthan et al., 1991; Thomson et al., 1993), although the reason for these differences remains unclear.

GSHPx-3 activity in plasma

Glutathione peroxidase-3 accounts for 12% of the selenium in plasma (Hill et al., 1996). Measurement of extracellular GSHPx-3 in plasma is now the method of choice because its activity can be determined more accurately than that of GSHPx-1 in erythrocytes. Hemoglobin interferes with the GSHPx-1 assay in erythrocytes (Cohen et al., 1985; Xia et al., 1989; Hill et al., 1996).

Several studies have examined relationships between plasma GSHPx-3 and plasma or whole blood selenium concentrations. Figure 25.11 shows a strong association between selenium and glutathione peroxidase activities in plasma of healthy male Chinese adults living in low- and high-selenium areas in China, but, like erythrocyte GSHPx-1 activity, only up to a threshold of 1.0 – 1.2 µmol/L (Duffield et al., 1999; Thomson, 2004a). In the low-selenium area, Keshan disease was endemic, whereas in the control area the

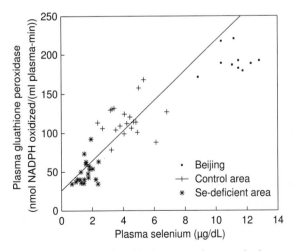

Figure 25.11: Relationship between plasma selenium concentration and plasma GSHPx-3 activity in three groups of Chinese men. The regression line was drawn without inclusion of the Beijing subjects. Data from Xia et al., Journal of Nutrition 119: 1318–1326, 1989, with permission of the American Society for Nutritional Sciences.

	Plasma selenium (μmol/L)	Plasma glutathione peroxidase (U/L)	Plasma seleno-protein P (U/L)
Boys (aged 8–12)			
Low-selenium area	16.5 ± 6.3	29 ± 15	0.10 ± 0.04
Supplemented area	79.8 ± 19.0	111 ± 21	0.76 ± 0.27
Low-selenium/supplemented, %	265.9	26	13
Men (aged 17 and over)			
Low-selenium area	20.26 ± 5.1	51 ± 15	0.13 ± 0.04
Supplemented area	86.1 ± 12.7	137 ± 15	0.57 ± 0.13
Low-selenium/supplemented, %	304	37	23

Table 25.14: Biomarkers of selenium in plasma in boys and men in two areas of China: a selenium-deficient area where Keshan Disease was endemic; and an area supplemented with inorganic selenium. Data in IOM (2000), extracted from Xia et al. (1989) and Hill et al. (1996).

incidence had fallen markedly in part because of selenium supplementation in salt. Results suggest that both plasma GSHPx-3 and plasma selenium measurements are good measures of selenium status. Values are also shown for 10 men from Beijing for comparison purposes; more details are given in Xia et al. (1989).

In Table 25.14, the mean values for plasma selenium, plasma GSHPx-3, and plasma selenoprotein P (Section 25.2.6) are compared from both boys and adult males living in the low- and high-selenium areas. In the low-selenium area, where Keshan disease was endemic, the GSHPx-3 activities in plasma for the boys and men were 26% and 37% of the respective activities for the boys and men from the unaffected supplemented areas. The relative differences parallel those for plasma selenium (Xia et al., 1989).

An increase in plasma GSHPx-3 following selenium supplementation was also reported in a study of 52 New Zealand adults, with a selenium intake of 28 μg/d (Duffield et al., 1999). Fortunately, the response of plasma GSHPx-3 levels to selenium supplementation, unlike that of plasma and erythrocyte selenium concentrations or platelet GSHPx-1 activity, is not dependent on the chemical form of the selenium supplement.

The GSHPx-3 activity in plasma can only be used to assess selenium status in populations with a relatively low selenium status, as noted earlier for the GSHPx-1 activity in erythrocytes and platelets. Thomson (2004a) has concluded that the concentration of selenium in plasma under conditions of maximal expression of plasma GSHPx-3 approximates $1.00 - 1.20$ μmol/L (Table 25.12).

Interpretive criteria

GSHPx activity in erythrocytes, platelets, and probably plasma is affected by many factors other than selenium status. These include age, race, sex, and physical activity; exposure to pro-oxidants, toxicants, or heavy metals; and deficiencies of iron, vitamin B_{12}, or essential fatty acids (Ganther et al., 1976). These factors may have a greater effect when selenium intakes are adequate (Robinson and Thomson, 1983).

Results that can be used to assess GSHPx activity in erythrocytes, platelets, or plasma are limited. Further, they vary with the assay used making comparisons among studies difficult. Data should be compared with a selenium-replete control group living in the same geographic region and for whom the same assay procedure has been used. As an alternative, the change in GSHPx activity values after selenium supplementation can be monitored. GSHPx in erythrocytes was analyzed in the U.K. National Diet and Nutrition Survey on Young People aged 4–18 y. Data for the mean, median, and lower and upper 2.5th percentiles are given (Gregory et al., 2000).

Measurement of GSHPx activity

Measurement of GSHPx activity is useful for the assessment of persons with relatively low selenium status. In general, the assay for GSHPx activity is easier than the analysis of plasma or serum selenium. Of the various forms of GSHPx, the activity of GSHPx-3 in plasma is more stable at −80°C than that of cellular GSHPx-1 in erythrocytes or platelets, and the assay is easier and more accurate.

Commercial enzyme-linked immunoassay kits are available to measure the activity of GSHPx-3 in plasma, provided that heparin is used as the anticoagulant. In the future, a radioimmunoassay may be commercially available to measure glutathione peroxidase protein in plasma or serum. Only 10 µL of plasma or serum is required (Huang and Åkesson, 1993).

Activity of GSHPx-1 is often measured in whole blood rather than in erythrocytes because it is less time consuming. However, there is no standardized method for the assay. A procedure based on the coupled enzyme assay of Paglia and Valentine (1967) is often used. In this assay, GSHPx-1 activity is measured by the oxidation of NADPH with cumene peroxide via glutathione reductase.

An automated enzyme assay for the blood GSHPx activity suitable for large-scale surveys has now been developed (McMaster et al., 1990). GSHPx activities in both whole blood and plasma can be performed using this assay. No standardized reference material is available for assay of GSHPx activity.

25.2.6 Selenoprotein P

Approximately 60%–80% of the selenium in plasma is present as selenoprotein P. This selenoprotein contains 10 selenium atoms per molecule as selenocysteine and has been used as a biomarker of selenium status (Persson-Modchos et al., 1995). It is present in a wide range of tissues and is secreted into the plasma by the liver and into the interstitial space by cells in other tissues (Burk, 1999).

Very few studies have measured plasma selenoprotein P. Table 25.14 presents the data for selenoprotein P levels in stored plasma from the Chinese males discussed earlier, analyzed by Hill et al. (1996). Selenoprotein P concentrations in boys and men in the low-selenium area were 13% and 23%, respectively, of those in the selenium-supplemented area. Corresponding GSHPx-3 activities in plasma were 26% and 37%, respectively. These findings suggest that selenoprotein P concentrations in serum are more sensitive to selenium deficiency than plasma GSHPx-3 activity (Xia et al., 1989).

A similar finding was observed in a study in New Zealand. Again, the response of plasma selenoprotein P concentrations to a selenium supplement, at every dose, was greater than for plasma GSHPx-3 (Duffield et al., 1999). Moreover, in this New Zealand study, maximal expression of plasma selenoprotein P was reached at levels of supplemental selenium that were a little lower than for plasma GSHPx-3. These results again suggest that plasma selenoplasma P may be potentially more sensitive as an index of selenium status than plasma GSHPx-3.

Selenoprotein P and plasma selenium concentrations appear to be positively correlated in subjects with differing selenium status. Figure 25.12 shows the correlation between

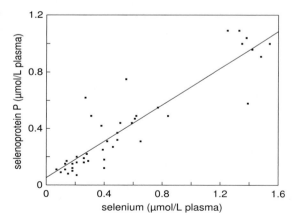

Figure 25.12: Selenoprotein P concentrations versus total selenium in plasma in Chinese male subjects ⩾ 17 y from three different regions. The line is for linear regression (r = 0.91). Redrawn from Hill et al., Journal of Nutrition 126: 138–145, 1996, with permission of the American Society for Nutritional Sciences.

the initial selenoprotein P versus plasma selenium concentrations in Chinese males aged ≥17 y from both the low-selenium and selenium-supplemented areas studied in 1987 by Xia et al. (1989), as well as from 10 men from Beijing. Correlations of plasma selenoprotein P with plasma GSHPx-3 and erythrocyte GSHPx-1 have also been noted (Huang et al., 1995; Åkesson et al., 1997).

Marchaluk et al. (1995) examined serum selenoprotein P in relation to total serum selenium concentrations in adults residing in nine European countries (Figure 25.13). Differences existed in both the level of selenoprotein P in the serum and its proportion in relation to total serum selenium concentrations among countries. Subjects from Spain had the highest serum selenoprotein P levels, as shown in Figure 25.13. Nevertheless, in general, levels of selenoprotein P and total selenium in serum were again significantly correlated.

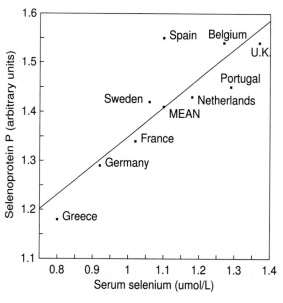

Figure 25.13: Graph showing the mean selenoprotein P and serum selenium concentrations in European countries. Data are for 414 samples from adults aged 37–70 y, from 17 regions in nine countries. Data from Marchaluk et al., European Journal of Clinical Nutrition 49: 42–48, 1995, with permission of the Nature Publishing Group.

Interpretive criteria and measurement of plasma selenoprotein P

At present, an optimal level for plasma selenoprotein P has not been defined. Further, the physiological consequences and implications on health of the reported regional differences in plasma selenoprotein P concentrations that are shown in Figure 25.13 are unknown.

More studies are needed to identify the effects of diet, lifestyle, and disease on plasma selenoprotein P concentrations. At present, the potential role of plasma selenoprotein P and the other newer selenoproteins as functional markers of selenium status is uncertain.

Hill et al. (1996) have developed a competitive radioimmunoassay using ^{75}Se-labeled human selenoprotein P to measure plasma selenoprotein P, but it is not yet commercially available.

25.2.7 Hair selenium

The clinical significance of hair selenium concentrations in human nutrition was first noted by Chinese workers studying Keshan disease. They described a close relationship between hair and whole blood selenium concentrations (Chen et al., 1980). In the Chinese study of population groups with dietary intakes of selenium that were deficient, low, and adequate, average hair selenium concentration in areas where Keshan disease was endemic was 0.94 nmol/g, compared to mean levels of 2.03 nmol/g in low-selenium areas without Keshan disease, and 4.56 nmol/g in selenium-adequate areas (Table 25.13). Low hair selenium levels have also been reported in children with inborn errors of metabolism, treated with semisynthetic diets low in selenium (Lombeck et al., 1978), although none of the classical clinical features of Keshan disease were observed in any of these children.

Hair selenium concentrations also show a positive response to selenium supplementation. For example, increases in hair selenium levels have been observed in subjects after treatment with either selenium-enriched yeast (100 µg/d Se) (Gallagher et al., 1984) or selenium-rich wheat (Djujic et al., 2000).

Hair selenium concentrations can also be used as indices of overexposure to selenium in epidemiological studies, although they are not very sensitive. Elevated hair selenium concentrations were observed in persons living in seleniferous areas of China (Yang et al., 1983) (Table 25.13) and in a child with acute selenium poisoning (Lombeck et al., 1987). Selenium intakes associated with these effects, however, are well above acceptable exposure levels.

The use of selenium-containing antidandruff shampoos in more affluent countries may confound the interpretation of hair selenium levels, because the selenium from the shampoo is not removed during standardized hair washing procedures (Davies, 1982; LeBlanc et al., 1999). The effect of hair color on human hair selenium concentrations has not been firmly established, but selenium concentrations in dyed hair may be lower than that of undyed hair (Borella et al., 1997).

Interpretive criteria

As the type of shampoo and chemical form of selenium in the diet influence hair selenium concentration, universal cutoff points, indicative of selenium deficiency or overexposure, cannot be used for comparisons across populations. Instead, clinical and epidemiological studies should always include carefully selected age- and sex-matched healthy controls living in the same geographic region as the study group.

Measurement of hair selenium

Care must be taken during the collection, preparation, and analyses of hair samples for selenium to avoid adventitious sources of contamination. Hair samples must be carefully sampled and then washed using a standardized procedure (Section 15.1.9).

Concentrations of selenium in hair can be determined using hydride generation AAS or graphite furnace AAS with a Zeeman background correction (Section 25.2.1). For both these methods, the hair samples must first be washed and then digested to remove the organic materials.

Alternatively, INAA can be used (Lombeck et al., 1978; Gibson et al., 1985). The method is especially suitable for the analysis of small hair samples because of its high sensitivity. Sample digestion is not required for INAA. A certified reference material for human hair is available (CRM #397; Institute for Reference Materials and Measurements, Retieseweg, B-2440 Geel, Belgium) and must be used to assess the accuracy of the analytical method.

25.2.8 Toenail selenium

The concentration of selenium in toenails may be a useful indicator of very long-term, retrospective, selenium status because selenium is incorporated into toenails as they grow. Toenail clippings probably reflect selenium status 6–9 mo prior to collection, depending on the nail length and growth rate. Hence, they have the potential to assess prediagnostic intakes in case-control studies of diseases.

The collection of toenails, like hair, is noninvasive and simple, and selenium concentrations are relatively high (Hadjimarkos and Shearer, 1973). Age, gender, cigarette smoking, and alcohol intake have sometimes been reported to influence selenium concentrations in toenails, but may be attributed in part to differences in selenium intakes (Hunter et al., 1990; Swanson et al., 1990). The form of selenium and the content of methionine in the diet also affect toenail selenium concentrations (Salbe and Levander, 1990).

Several investigators have examined toenail selenium concentrations. Morris et al. (1983) reported that toenail selenium concentrations from a high-selenium area (South Dakota) were significantly higher than those from a low-selenium area (New Zealand). Higher toenail selenium concentrations were also noted among U.S. women consuming selenium supplements than in nonsupplement users (11.47 vs. 10.14 nmol/g; $p = 0.02$); the dose response was also significant ($r = 0.50$;

$p = 0.03$) (Hunter et al., 1990). In addition, in this study, the geographic variation in toenail selenium concentrations was consistent with the geographic distribution of selenium in forage crops, as shown in Table 25.15. These findings suggest that toenail selenium concentrations were sufficiently sensitive to delineate relatively small, regional differences in selenium intake.

In some circumstances, a significant association between selenium concentrations in toenails and habitual dietary intakes of selenium at the individual level has been observed. Such a relationship is more likely to occur for analyzed duplicate diet composites that are representative of usual intakes from subjects consuming a relatively wide range of selenium intakes (Swanson et al., 1990; Longnecker et al., 1991). Indeed, in a study by Swanson et al. (1990), the correlations observed between usual selenium intake, based on analyzed duplicate diets, and corresponding selenium concentrations in serum, whole blood, and toenails were very comparable (Table 25.16).

As a result of these findings, toenail selenium concentration has been used as a biomarker in several cohort studies (Van Noord et al., 1987; Hunter et al., 1990; Yoshizawa et al., 1998). For example, in a randomized trial involving the participants in the Health

	Se intake (μg/kg body weight)
Serum (μmol/L)	0.63
Blood (μmol/L)	0.62
Toenails (nmol/g)	0.59
Urine (μmol/d)	0.82

Table 25.16: Pearsons correlation coefficients for the relationship of usual selenium intake to selenium in serum, whole blood, toenails, and urine. All associations are statistically significant ($p < 0.001$). Data from Swanson et al., American Journal of Clinical Nutrition 52: 858–862, 1990 © Am J Clin Nutr. American Society for Clinical Nutrition.

Professional Follow-up Study, an inverse association was seen between the selenium concentration of toenail clippings and the risk of advanced prostate cancer (Yoshizawa et al., 1998), as shown in Table 25.17. These findings were consistent with those of Clark et al. (1998).

Interpretive criteria for toenail selenium

No universal cutoffs for toenail selenium concentrations indicative of selenium deficiency or overexposure can be applied across populations, as noted for hair selenium. Indeed, the approach described for hair should also be adopted for toenail selenium concentrations.

Measurement of toenail selenium

Bank et al. (1981) recommend cleaning nails before clipping with a scrubbing brush and a mild detergent, followed by mechanical scraping to remove any remaining soft tissue. Nails should then be washed in an aqueous nonionic detergent and dried under vacuum prior to analysis. Selenium concentrations in toenails can be determined by the same methods as described for hair.

25.2.9 Multiple indices

At present, the preferred combination of biomarkers for assessing selenium status for those individuals with relatively low selenium status is the measurement of total selenium and GSHPx-3 activity in plasma. For indi-

State (*n*)	Mean toenail Se ± SE (nmol/g)	Level of Se in forage crops
Texas (3)	11.10 ± 0.34	High
California (85)	10.86 ± 0.20	Medium
Michigan (58)	10.70 ± 0.24	Low
Massachusetts (46)	10.42 ± 0.28	Low
Pennsylvania (142)	10.31 ± 0.16	Low
New Jersey (53)	10.18 ± 0.25	Low
New York (110)	10.13 ± 0.18	Low
Ohio (89)	10.08 ± 0.20	Low
Connecticut (31)	10.05 ± 0.33	Low
Florida (8)	9.75 ± 0.66	Very low
Maryland (25)	9.12 ± 0.37	Low

Table 25.15: Mean toenail selenium concentration among 677 U.S. women aged 37–62 y by state of residence. Data from Hunter et al., American Journal of Epidemiology 132: 114–122, 1990, with permission of the Society for Epidemiologic Research.

| | Quintile of Se level | | | | | p for trend |
	1	2	3	4	5	
Se level in toenail – Median	0.66	0.76	0.82	0.88	1.44	
Range (µg/g)	0.53–0.73	0.73–0.79	0.79–0.85	0.85–0.94	0.94–7.09	
Case subjects ($n = 181$)	54	34	29	36	28	
Control subjects ($n = 181$)	35	37	37	35	37	
Odds ratio	1.00	0.57	0.53	0.67	0.49	0.11
95% confidence interval		0.29–1.12	0.28–1.01	0.34–1.32	0.25–0.96	
Multivariate odds ratio	1.00	0.59	0.35	0.76	0.35	0.03
95% confidence interval		0.27–1.30	0.16–0.78	0.34–1.73	0.16–0.78	

Table 25.17: Odds ratio for advanced prostate cancer during a 7-y follow-up according to quintile level of toenail selenium. The significance values are two-sided p values for the trend across quintiles. The multivariate odds ratio is adjusted for quintiles of lycopene, saturated fat, and calcium; for family history of prostate cancer (binary), for body mass index (quintiles); for vasectomy (binary); and for Se content of soil in the region (terciles). From Yoshizawa et al., Journal of the National Cancer Institute 90: 1219–1224, 1998.

viduals with adequate selenium status, total selenium in plasma, as an acute marker, and in erythrocytes for longer-term status, are recommended. For large epidemiological studies within a country, toenail selenium concentrations may be more practical.

Further, when studying selenium status in relation to risk of disease, the interactions of selenium with other components of the antioxidant defenses of the body (e.g. vitamin E, vitamin A, vitamin C, β-carotene, polyunsaturated fat), heavy metals and iodine must also be taken into account.

In the future, measurement of some of the other selenoproteins may be possible, the choice depending on the specific biological function of selenium under investigation, as well as the magnitude of the selenium deficiency state. Measurement of individual selenoproteins are more appropriate than that of total selenium alone. At present, however, the functions of many of these selenoproteins are still uncertain.

Currently, there are no physiological functional tests that can be used routinely for assessing selenium status. Biomarkers of lipid peroxidation or oxidative DNA damage might suggest inadequate antioxidant defense associated with low selenium status, but they are not specific for selenium status. Promising new biomarkers include F 2-isoprostanes (Halliwell, 1999).

Summary

Iodine

Iodine functions exclusively as a component of the thyroid hormones, thyroxine (T_4) and 3,5,3′-triiodothyronine (T_3), which are required for normal growth and development and for maintenance of normal metabolism. Goiter (thyroid enlargement) is the major consequence of chronic iodine deficiency; it generally arises from prolonged inadequate intakes of iodine or exposure to goitrogens in foods. In areas where endemic goiter exists and iodine deficiency is severe, endemic cretinism may occur. However, there are many other adverse effects of iodine deficiency on growth and development. All these diverse effects are collectively termed "iodine deficiency disorders" (IDD). Prolonged excessive intake of iodine in normal persons markedly reduces iodine uptake by the thyroid. Goiter and hypothyroidism are rarely induced, although endemic goiter has been described in certain regions of Japan where seaweeds, rich in iodine, are dietary staples.

Neck palpitation is traditionally used to measure thyroid size. However, in areas of mild IDD, use of thyroid ultrasonography is the preferred method to estimate goiter prevalence. The most commonly used biochemical marker of iodine status is urinary iodine excretion: it closely reflects iodine intake. Measurement of urinary iodine excretion in 24-h urine specimens (μg/d) is generally preferred, although for population studies ICCIDD/UNICEF/WHO recommend the measurement of iodine concentration in casual urine samples. Expression of urinary iodine as a ratio to creatinine excretion is not recommended, especially for children in developing countries.

Concentrations of TSH in serum, whole blood, or cord blood are routinely assayed in neonates in Western countries to detect congenital hypothyroidism, using radioimmuno-assay methods available as commercial kits. With the advent of more sensitive ELISA methods using dried blood spots, TSH assays are now also used in low-income countries. In the future, when assay methods are better standardized, thyroglobulin in serum or dried blood spots may be used as a biomarker of thyroid function in children. Assay methods for T_4 and T_3 in serum are expensive and cumbersome. Further, concentrations are relatively insensitive and unreliable indicators of iodine nutriture and, hence, are rarely used. Uptake of radioactive ^{131}I can be used as a test of thyroid function in clinical settings.

Selenium

Selenium is an essential component of important metabolic pathways, including antioxidant defense systems, thyroid hormone metabolism, and immune function. It exerts these biological effects via its role in a number of selenoproteins. These include at least five Se-containing glutathione peroxidases, all of which function as antioxidants, and possibly in eicosanoid metabolism. Three Se-containing iodothyronine deiodinases also exist. They regulate both the synthesis and the degradation of T_3. Other selenoproteins include selenoprotein P, which may serve as a transport protein for selenium to brain, selenoprotein W, some thioredoxin reductases (EC 1.6.4.5) that catalyze the NADPH-dependent reduction of thioredoxin, and selenophosphate synthetase 2. The latter may

have a role in the regulation of selenium homeostasis.

Selenium-responsive conditions have occurred in patients on long-term TPN and in young children and women of child-bearing age with Keshan's disease. Other factors may trigger this disease. Kashin-Beck disease is also prevalent in low-selenium regions of China, but whether selenium deficiency is the primary cause of this disease is uncertain. Dietary-induced sub-optimal biochemical selenium status has been reported in New Zealand and Finland, but no obvious detrimental health effects are evident. The margin between selenium deficiency and toxicity is relatively narrow, and naturally occurring selenium toxicity occurs in China and Venezuela.

A combination of biomarkers is recommended for assessing selenium status, the choice depending on the expected selenium status of the study group, and the specific biological function under investigation. For those with low-selenium status, the preferred combination is now plasma selenium concentration and plasma GSHPx-3 activity. The latter is used because it is more stable than GSHPx-1 activity in erythrocytes; the assay is easier and more accurate; and an automated method is available. For those with adequate selenium status, plasma GSHPx-3 activity cannot be used because values plateau when intakes reach and exceed an optimal level. Hence, in these circumstances, either plasma selenium for acute status or erythrocyte selenium as a measure of more longer-term status can be used. When blood collection is impractical, toenail selenium concentrations are useful as a measure of long-term selenium exposure, especially for epidemiological studies. Hair selenium, although promising, cannot be used in countries where selenium-containing antidandruff shampoos are used.

Urine is the main excretory route for selenium. Urinary selenium concentrations (in 24-h urine samples) have been used as a measure of toxicity and industrial exposure to selenium, rather than deficiency. Cutoff points for urinary selenium levels to identify deficiency or toxicity are not yet clearly defined.

In the future, plasma selenoprotein P may be used as it is more sensitive than plasma GSHPx-3 to selenium deficiency. Measurement of other selenoproteins may also be possible, the choice depending on which biological function of selenium is under study. Currently, no physiological functional tests for selenium exist, although F 2- isoprostanes hold promise.

References

Åkesson B, Huang W, Persson-Moschos M, Marchaluk E, Jacobsson L, Lingarde F. (1997). Glutathione peroxidase, selenoprotein P and selenium in serum of elderly subjects in relation to other biomarkers of nutritional status and food intake. Journal of Nutritional Biochemistry 8: 508–517.

Alaejos SM, Romero CD. (1993) Urinary selenium concentrations. Clinical Chemistry 39: 2040–2052.

Alexander NM. (1984). Iodine. In: Frieden E (ed.) Biochemistry of the Essential Ultratrace Elements. Plenum Press, New York, pp. 33–53.

Alfthan G, Nève J. (1996). Reference values for serum selenium in various areas, evaluated according to the TRACY protocol. Journal of Trace Elements in Medicine and Biology 10: 77–87.

Alfthan G, Aro A, Arvilomni H, Huttunen JK. (1991). Selenium metabolism and platelet glutathione peroxidase activity in healthy Finnish men: effects of selenium yeast, selenite and selenate. American Journal of Clinical Nutrition 53: 120–25.

Allaway WH, Kubota J, Losée F, Roth M. (1968). Selenium, molybdenum, and vanadium in human blood. Archives of Environmental Health 16: 342–348.

Als C, Helbling A, Peter K, Halidmann M, Zimmerli B, Gerber H. (2000). Urinary iodine concentration follows a circadian rhythm: a study with 3023 spot urine samples in adults and children. Journal of Clinical Endocrinology and Metabolism 85: 1367–1369.

Amin S, Chen SY, Collipp PJ, Castro-Magana M, Maddaiah VT, Klein SW. (1980). Selenium in premature infants. Nutrition and Metabolism 24: 331–340.

Arthur JR. (1999). Functional indicators of iodine and selenium status. Proceedings of the Nutrition Society 58: 507–512.

Arthur JR, Beckett GJ, Mitchell JH. (1999). The interactions between selenium and iodine deficiencies in man and animals. Nutrition Research Reviews 12: 55–73.

Arthur JR, McKenzie RC, Beckett GJ. (2003). Selenium in the immune system. Journal of Nutrition 133: 1457S–1459S.

Ashour MN, Salem SI, El-Gadban HM, Elwan NM, Basu TK. (1999). Antioxidant status in children with protein-calorie malnutrition (PEM) living in Cairo, Egypt. European Journal of Clinical Nutrition 53: 669–673.

Aumont G, Tressol JC. (1986). Improved routine method for the determination of total iodine in urine and milk. Analyst 111: 841–843.

Auzepy PH, Blondeau M, Richard CH, Pradeau D, Therond P, Thuong T. (1987). Serum selenium deficiency in myocardial infarction and congestive cardiomyopathy. Acta Cardiologica 42: 161–166.

Bank HL, Robson J, Bigelow JB, Morrison J, Spell LH, Kantor R. (1981). Preparation of fingernails for trace element analysis. Clinica Chimica Acta 116: 179–190.

Baumann P, Wood WG. (1985). Serum thyroglobulin concentration in the first weeks of life as measured with an immunoluminometric assay. Journal of Clinical Chemistry and Clinical Biochemistry 23: 753–758.

Beard JL, Borel MJ, Derr J. (1990). Impaired thermoregulation and thyroid function in iron-deficiency anemia. American Journal of Clinical Nutrition 52: 813–819.

Beard JL, Brigham DE, Kelley SK, Green MH. (1998). Plasma thyroid hormone kinetics are altered in iron-deficient rats. Journal of Nutrition 128: 1401–1408.

Beck MA (1997). Increased virulence of Coxsackievirus B3 in mice due to vitamin A or selenium deficiency. Journal of Nutrition 127: 966S–970S.

Beck MA, Levander OA. (2000). Host nutritional status and its effect on a viral pathogen. Journal of Infectious Diseases 182: S93–S96.

Beck MA, Levander OA, Handy J. (2003). Selenium deficiency and viral infection. Journal of Nutrition 133: 1463S–1467S.

Behne D. (1988). Selenium homeostasis. In: Nève J, Favier A (eds.) Selenium in Medicine and Biology. Walter de Gruyter, New York, pp. 83–91.

Behne D, Kyriakopoulos A. (2001). Mammalian selenium-containing proteins. Annual Reviews of Nutrition 21: 453–473.

Behne D, Wolters W. (1979). Selenium content and glutathione peroxidase activity in the plasma and erythrocytes of non-pregnant and pregnant women. Journal of Clinical Chemistry and Clinical Biochemistry 17: 133–135.

Benmiloud M, Chaouki M, Gutekunst R, Teichert H-M, Wood WG, Dunn JT. (1994). Oral iodized oil for correcting iodine deficiency: optimal dosing and outcome indicator selection. Journal of Clinical Endocrinology and Metabolism 79: 20–24.

Berr C, Nicole A, Godin J, Ceballos-Picot I, Thevenin M, Dartigues JF, Alperovitch A. (1993). Selenium and oxygen-metabolizing enzymes in elderly community residents: a pilot epidemiological study. Journal of the American Geriatrics Society 41: 143–148.

Bleichrodt N, Born MP. (1994). A metaanalysis of research on iodine and its relationship to cognitive development. In: Stanbury JB (ed.) The Damaged Brain of Iodine Deficiency. Cognizant Communication Corporation, New York, pp. 195–200.

Blot WJ, Li JY, Taylor PR, Guo W, Dawsey S, Wang G, Yang CS, Zheng SF, Gail M, Li GY, Liu BQ, Tangrea J, Sun YH, Liu F, Fraumeni F Jr, Zhang YH, Li B. (1993). Nutrition intervention trials in Linxian, China: supplementation with specific vitamin/mineral combinations, cancer incidence, and disease-specific mortality in the general population. Journal of the National Cancer Institute 85: 1483–1490.

Borella P, Bargellini A, Caselgrandi E, Piccinini L. (1997). Observations of the use of plasma, hair and tissue to evaluate trace element status in cancer. Journal of Trace Elements in Medicine and Biology 11: 162–165.

Bourdoux P. (1998). Evaluation of the iodine intake: problems of the iodine/creatinine ratio—comparison with iodine excretion and daily fluctuations of iodine concentration. Experimental and Clinical Endocrinology 106(suppl.): S17–S20.

Brown KM, Arthur JR. (2001). Selenium, selenoproteins and human health: a review. Public Health Nutrition 4: 593–599.

Brune D, Samsahl K, Wester P. (1966). A comparison between the amounts of As, Au, Br, Cu, Fe, Mo, Se and Zn in normal and uraemic human whole blood by means of neutron activation analysis. Clinica Chimica Acta 13: 285–291.

Buchinger W, Lorenz-Wawschinek O, Semlitsch G, Langsteger W, Binter G, Bonelli RM, Eber O.(1997). Thyrotropin and thyroglobulin as an index of optimal iodine intake: correlation with iodine excretion of 39,913 euthyroid patients. Thyroid 7: 593–597.

Burgi H, Portmann L, Podoba J, Vertongen F, Srbecky M. (1999). Thyroid volumes and urinary iodine in Swiss school children. European Journal of Endocrinology 140: 104–106.

Burk RF. (1984). Selenium. In: Present Knowledge in Nutrition. 5th ed. The Nutrition Foundation, Washington, DC, pp. 519–527.

Burk RF, Hill KE. (1999). Orphan selenoproteins. Bioessays 21: 231–237.

Burk RF, Levander OA. (1999). Selenium. In: Shils ME, Olson JA, Shike M, Ross AC (eds.) Modern Nutrition in Health and Disease. 9th ed. Williams & Wilkins, Baltimore, pp. 265–276.

Burk RF Jr, Pearson WN, Wood RP, Viteri F. (1967). Blood-selenium levels and in vitro red blood cell uptake of 75-Se in kwashiorkor. American Journal of Clinical Nutrition 20: 723–733.

Burk RF, Hill KE, Boeglin ME, Ebner FF, Chittum HS. (1997). Selenoprotein P associates with endothelial cells in rat tissues. Histochemistry and Cell Biology 108: 11–15.

Burk RF, Brown DG, Seely RJ, Scaief CC III. (1972). Influence of dietary and injected selenium on the whole-body retention, route of excretion, and tissue retention of $^{75}SeO_3^{2-}$ in the rat. Journal of Nutrition 102: 1049–1055.

Butler JA, Whanger PD, Tripp MJ. (1982). Blood selenium and glutathione peroxidase activity in pregnant women: comparative assays in primates and other animals. American Journal of Clinical Nutrition 36: 15–23.

Chen XS, Yang GL, Chen JO, Chen XC, Wen ZM, Ge KY. (1980). On the relations of selenium and Keshan disease. Biological Trace Element Research 2: 91–107.

Clark LC, Combs GF Jr, Turnbull BW, Slate EH, Chalker D, Chow J, Curtis D, Davis LS, Glover RA, Graham GF, Gross EG, Krongrad A, Lesher JL Jr, Park HK, Sanders BB Jr, Smith CL, Taylor JR. (1996). Effects of selenium supplementation for cancer prevention in patients with carcinoma of the skin: a randomized controlled trial. Journal of the American Medical Association 276: 1957–1963.

Clark LC, Dalkin B, Krongrad A, Combs GF Jr, Turnbull BW, Slate EH, Witherington R, Herlong JH, Janosko E, Carpenter D, Borosso C, Falk S, Rounder J. (1998). Decreased incidence of prostate cancer with selenium supplementation: results of a double-blind cancer prevention trial. British Journal of Urology 81: 730–734.

Clugston GA, Hetzel BS. (1994). Iodine. In: Shils ME, Olson JA, Shike M (eds.) Modern Nutrition in Health and Disease. 8th ed. Vol 1. Lea & Febiger, Philadelphia, pp. 252–263.

Cohen HJ, Chovaniec ME, Mistretta D, Baker SS. (1985). Selenium repletion and glutathione peroxidase: differential effects on plasma and red blood cell enzyme activity. American Journal of Clinical Nutrition 41: 735–747.

Cohen HJ, Brown MR, Hamilton D, Lyons-Patterson J, Avissar N, Liegey P. (1989). Glutathione peroxidase and selenium deficiency in patients receiving home parenteral nutrition: time course for development of deficiency and repletion of enzyme activity in plasma and red blood cells. American Journal of Clinical Nutrition 49: 132–139.

Combs GF, Clark LC, Turnbull BW. (2001). An analysis of cancer prevention by selenium. BioFactors 14: 153–159.

Copeland DL, Sullivan KM, Houston R, May W, Mendoza I, Salamatullah Q, Solomons N, Nordenberg D, Maberly GF. (2002). Comparison of neonatal thyroid-stimulating hormone levels and indicators of iodine deficiency in school children. Public Health Nutrition 5: 81–87.

Darlow BA, Inder TE, Graham PJ, Sluis KB, Malpas TJ, Taylor BJ, Winterborn CC. (1995). The relationship of selenium status to respiratory outcome in the very low birth weight infant. Pediatrics 96: 314–319.

Davies TS. (1982). Hair analysis and selenium shampoos. Lancet 2(8304): 935.

Delange F. (1985). Physiopathology of iodine nutrition. In: Chandra RK (ed.) Trace Elements in Nutrition of Children. Nestlé Nutrition Workshop Series, Vol. 8. Raven Press, New York, pp. 291–299.

Delange F, Iteke FB, Ermans AM. (1982). Nutritional

factors involved in the goitrogenic action of cassava. International Development Research Centre, Ottawa, pp. 1–100.

Delange F, Benker G, Caron P, Eber O, Ott W, Peter F, Podoba J, Simescu M, Szybinsky Z, Vertongen F, Vitti P, Wiersinga W, Zamrazil V. (1997). Thyroid volume and urinary iodine in European school children: standardization of values for assessment of iodine deficiency. European Journal of Endocrinology 136: 180–187.

Delange F, de Benoist B, Alnwick D. (1999). Risks of iodine-induced hyperthyroidism after correction of iodine deficiency by iodized salt. Thyroid 9: 545–556.

Delange F, de Benoist B, Pretell E, Dunn JT. (2001). Iodine deficiency in the world: where do we stand at the turn of the century? Thyroid 11: 437–447.

Delange F, de Benoist B, Bürgi H, ICCIDD Working Group. (2002). Determining median urinary iodine concentration that indicates adequate iodine intake at population level. Bulletin of the World Health Organization 80: 633–636.

Dillman E, Gale C, Green W, Johnson DG, Mackler B, Finch C. (1980). Hypothermia in iron deficiency due to altered triiodothyronine metabolism. American Journal of Physiology 239: R377–R381.

Djujic IS, Jozanov-Stankov ON, Milovac M, Jankovic V, Djemanovic V. (2000). Bioavailability and possible benefits of wheat intake naturally enriched with selenium and its products. Biological Trace Element Research 77: 273–285.

Duffield AJ, Thomson CD, Hill KE, Williams S. (1999). An estimation of selenium requirements for New Zealanders. American Journal of Clinical Nutrition 70: 896–903.

Dunn JT. (1978). Iodine deficiency in man. In: Rechcigl M (ed.) Section E. Nutritional Disorders. Volume III: Effect of Nutrient Deficiencies in Man. CRC Handbook Series in Nutrition and Food. CRC Press, Boca Raton, FL, pp. 237–257.

Dunn JT, Crutchfield HE, Gutekunst R, Dunn AD. (1993). Two simple methods for measuring iodine in urine. Thyroid 3: 119–123.

Dunsmore DG, Wheeler SM. (1977). Iodophors and iodine in dairy products. 8: The total industry situation. Australian Journal of Dairy Technology 32: 166–171.

Duthie GG, Arthur JR, Beattie JA, Brown KM, Morrice PC, Robertson JD, Shortt CT, Walker KA, James WPT. (1993). Cigarette smoking, antioxidants, lipid peroxidation, and coronary heart disease. Annals New York Academy of Sciences 686: 120–129.

Dworkin BM. (1994). Selenium deficiency in HIV infection and the acquired immunodeficiency syndrome (AIDS). Chemico-Biological Interactions 91: 181–186.

Eastman CJ. (1999). Where has all our iodine gone? Medical Journal of Australia 171: 455–456.

Eltom M, Elnagar B, Sulieman EA, Karlsson FA, Van Thi HV, Bourdoux P, Gebre-Medhin M. (1995). The use of sugar as a vehicle for iodine fortification in endemic iodine deficiency. International Journal of Food Science and Nutrition 46: 281–289.

Fisher KD, Carr CJ. (1974). Iodide in Foods: Chemical Methodology and Sources of Iodine in the Human Diet. Life Sciences Research Office, Federation of American Societies for Experimental Biology, Washington, DC.

Florentino RF, Tanchoco CC, Rodriguez MP, Cruz AJ, Molano WL. (1996). Interactions among micronutrient deficiencies and undernutrition in the Philippines. Biomedical and Environmental Sciences 9: 348–357.

Foo LC, Zulfiqar A, Nafikudin M, Fadzil M, Asmah A. (1999). Local versus WHO/ICCIDD-recommended thyroid volume reference in the assessment of iodine deficiency disorders. European Journal of Endocrinology 140: 491–497.

Furnée CA, van der Haar F, West CE, Hautvast JG. (1994). A critical appraisal of goiter assessment and the ratio of urinary iodine to creatinine for evaluating iodine status. American Journal of Clinical Nutrition 59: 1415–1417.

Gaitan E. (1990). Goitrogens in food and water. Annual Review of Nutrition 10: 21–39.

Gallagher ML, Webb P, Crounse R, Bray J, Webb A, Settle EA. (1984). Selenium levels in new growth hair and in whole blood during ingestion of a selenium supplement for six weeks. Nutrition Research 4: 577–582.

Ganther HE, Hafeman DG, Lawrence RA, Serfass RE, Hoekstra WG. (1976). Selenium and glutathione peroxidase in health and disease: a review. In: Prasad AS, Oberleas D (eds.) Trace Elements in Human Health and Disease. Volume 2: Essential and Toxic Elements. Academic Press, New York, pp. 165–234.

Gardner DF, Centor RM, Utiger RD. (1988). Effects of low dose oral iodide supplementation on thyroid function in normal men. Clinical Endocrinology 28: 283–288.

Geahchan A, Chambon P. (1980). Fluorometry of selenium in urine. Clinical Chemistry 26: 1272–1274.

Gibson RS, Martinez OB, MacDonald AC (1985). The zinc, copper, and selenium status of a selected sample of Canadian elderly women. Journal of Gerontology 40: 296–302.

Glover JR. (1967). Selenium in human urine: a tentative maximum allowable concentration for industrial and rural populations. Annals of Occupational Hygiene 10: 3–14.

Golubkina NA, Alfthan GV. (1999). The human selenium status in 27 regions of Russia. Journal of Trace Elements in Medicine and Biology 13: 15–20.

Gregory J, Lowe S, Bates CJ, Prentice A, Jackson LV, Smithers G, Wenlock R, Farron M. (2000). National Diet and Nutrition Survey: Young People Aged 4 to 18 Years. Volume 1: Report of the Diet and Nutrition Survey. The Stationery Office, London.

Griffiths NM, Thomson CD. (1974). Selenium in whole

blood of New Zealand residents. New Zealand Medical Journal 80: 199–202.

Gross S. (1976). Hemolytic anemia in premature infants: relationship to vitamin E, selenium, glutathione peroxidase and erythrocyte lipids. Seminars in Hematology 13: 187–199.

Guttikonda K, Burgess J, Hynes K, Boyages S, Byth K, Parameswaran V. (2002). Recurrent iodine deficiency in Tasmania, Australia: a salutary lesson in sustainable iodine prophylaxis and its monitoring. Journal of Clinical Endocrinology and Metabolism 87: 2809–2815.

Hadjimarkos DM, Shearer TR. (1973). Selenium content of human nails: a new index for epidemiologic studies of dental caries. Journal of Dental Research 52: 389.

Halliwell B. (1999). Establishing the significance and optimal intake of dietary antioxidants: the biomarker concept. Nutrition Reviews 57: 104–113.

Helzlsouer K, Jacobs R, Morris S. (1985) Acute selenium intoxication in the United States. Federation Proceedings 44: 1670.

Hemken RW. (1979). Factors that influence the iodine content of milk and meat: a review. Journal of Animal Science 48: 981–985.

Hess SY, Zimmermann MB. (2000). Thyroid volumes in a national sample of iodine-sufficient Swiss school children: comparison with the World Health Organization/International Council for the control of iodine deficiency disorders normative thyroid volume criteria. European Journal of Endocrinology 142: 599–603.

Hetzel BS. (2000). Iodine and neuropsychological development. Journal of Nutrition 130: 493–495.

Hetzel BS, Dunn JT. (1989). The iodine deficiency disorders: their nature and prevention. Annual Review of Nutrition 9: 21–38.

Hetzel BS, Potter BJ, Dulberg EM. (1990). The iodine deficiency disorders: nature, pathogenesis and epidemiology. World Review of Nutrition and Dietetics 62: 59–119.

Hill KE, Xia Y, Åkesson B, Boelin ME, Burk RF. (1996). Selenoprotein-P concentration in plasma is an index of selenium status in selenium-deficient and selenium-supplemented Chinese subjects. Journal of Nutrition 126: 138–145.

Hill KE, Zhou J, McMahan WJ, Motley AJ, Burk RF. (2004). Neurological dysfunction occurs in mice with targeted deletion of the selenoprotein P gene. Journal of Nutrition 134: 157–161.

Hojo Y. (1981). Evaluation of the expression of urinary selenium level as ng Se/mg creatinine and the use of single-void urine as a sample for urinary selenium determinations. Bulletin of Environmental Contamination and Toxicology 27: 213–220.

Hollowell JG, Staehling NW, Hannon WH, Flanders DW, Gunter EW, Maberly GF, Braverman LE, Pino S, Miller DT, Garbe PL, DeLozier DM, Jackson RJ. (1998). Iodine nutrition in the United States. Trends and public health implications: iodine excretion data from National Health and Nutrition Examination Surveys I and III (1971–1974 and 1988–1994). Journal of Clinical Endocrinology and Metabolism 83: 3401–3408.

Huang W, Åkesson B. (1993). Radioimmunoassay of glutathione peroxidase in human serum. Clinica Chimica Acta 219: 139–148.

Huang W, Åkesson B, Svensson B, Schutz A, Burk RF, Skerfving S. (1995). Selenoprotein P and glutathione peroxidase (EC 1.11.1.9) in plasma as indices of selenium status in relation to the intake of fish. British Journal of Nutrition 73: 455–461.

Hunter DJ, Morris JS, Chute CG, Kushner E, Colditz G, Stampfer MJ, Speizer FE, Willet WC. (1990). Predictors of selenium concentration in human toenails. American Journal of Epidemiology 132: 114–122.

Hurrell RF, Hess S. (2004). Role for micronutrient interactions in the epidemiology of micronutrient deficiencies: interactions of iron, iodine, and vitamin A. In: Pettifor JM, Zlotkin S (eds.) Micronutrient Deficiencies during the Weaning Period and the First Years of Life. Nestlé Nutrition Workshop Series Pediatric Program, vol. 54, Nestec Ltd, Vevey/S. Karger AG, Basel, pp. 1–19.

Huttunen JK. (1997). Selenium and cardiovascular disease – an update. Biomedical and Environmental Sciences 10; 220–226.

ICCIDD (International Council for the Control of Iodine Deficiency Disorders). (2000). Standardization of ultrasound and urinary iodine determination for assessing iodine status: report of a technical consultation. IDD Newsletter, Vol.16, pp. 19–23.

ICCIDD/UNICEF/WHO (International Council for the Control of Iodine Deficiency Disorders / United Nations Children's Fund / World Health Organization). (2001). Assessment of Iodine Deficiency Disorders and Monitoring their Elimination. 2nd ed. World Health Organization, Geneva.

IOM (Institute of Medicine). (2000). Dietary Reference Intakes for Vitamin C, Vitamin E, Selenium and Carotenoids. National Academy Press, Washington, DC.

IOM (Institute of Medicine). (2002). Dietary Reference Intakes for Vitamin A, Vitamin K, Arsenic, Boron, Chromium, Copper, Iodine, Iron, Manganese, Molybdenum, Nickel, Silicon, Vanadium, and Zinc. National Academy Press, Washington, DC.

Ip C. (1998). Lessons from basic research in selenium and cancer prevention. Journal of Nutrition 128: 1845–1854.

Jaffé WG, Ruphael MD, Mondragon MC, Cuevas MA. (1972). Clinical and biochemical study in school children of a seleniferous zone. Archivos Latinoamericanos de Nutrición 22: 595–611.

Jochum F, Terwolbeck K, Meinhold H, Behne D, Menzel H, Lombeck I. (1999). Is there any health risk of low dietary selenium supply in PKU-children? Nutrition Research 19: 349–360.

Johnson RA, Baker SS, Fallon JT, Maynard EP 3rd, Ruskin JN, Wen Z, Ge K, Cohen HJ. (1981). An occidental case of cardiomyopathy and selenium deficiency. New England Journal of Medicine 304: 1210–1212.

Kafai MR, Ganji V. (2003). Sex, age, geographical location, smoking, and alcohol consumption influence serum selenium concentrations in the USA: Third National Health and Nutrition Examination Survey, 1988–1994. Journal of Trace Elements in Medicine and Biology 17: 13–18.

Kasperek K, Lombeck I, Kiem J, Iyengar GV, Wang Y, Feinendegen LE, Bremer HJ. (1982). Platelet selenium in children with normal and low selenium intake. Biological Trace Element Research 4: 29–34.

Kay RG, Knight GS. (1979). Blood selenium values in an adult Auckland population group. New Zealand Medical Journal 90: 11–13.

Kilinc Y. (1993). Plasma, erythrocyte and urinary selenium levels in sickle cell homozygotes and traits. Turkish Journal of Pediatrics 35: 105–109.

Kiremidjian-Schumacher L, Roy M. (1998). Selenium and immune function. Zeitscruft für Ernahrungswissenschaft 37(Supp.1): 50–56.

Knowles SO, Lee J, Grace ND. (1997). Metabolism of trace elements in lactating cows: perspectives of selenium and iodine in animal health and human nutrition. Proceedings of the Nutrition Society of New Zealand 22: 174–183.

Knudsen N, Christiansen E, Brandt-Christensen M, Nygaard B, Perrild H. (2000). Age- and sex-adjusted iodine/creatinine ratio. A new standard in epidemiological surveys? Evaluation of three different estimates of iodine excretion based on casual urine samples and comparison to 24h values. European Journal of Clinical Nutrition 54: 361–363.

Kochupillai N, Pandav CS, Godbole MM, Mehta M, Ahuja MM. (1986). Iodine deficiency and neonatal hypothyroidism. Bulletin of the World Health Organization 64: 547–551.

Lagasse R, Bourdoux P, Courtois P, Hennart P, Putzeys G, Thilly C, Mafuta M, Yunga Y, Ermans AM, Delange F. (1982). Influence of the dietary balance of iodine-thiocyanate and protein on thyroid function in adults and young infants. In: Delange F, Iteke FB, Ermans AM (eds.) Nutritional Factors Involved in the Goitrogenic Action of Cassava. International Development Research Centre, Ottawa, pp. 84–86.

Lamberg B. (1993). Iodine deficiency disorders and endemic goitre. European Journal of Clinical Nutrition 47: 1–8.

Lane HW, Dudrick S, Warren DC. (1981). Blood selenium levels and glutathione-peroxidase activities in university and chronic intravenous hyperalimentation subjects. Proceedings of the Society of Experimental Biology and Medicine 167: 383–390.

Lane HW, Barroso AO, Englert D, Dudrick SJ, MacFadyen BS. (1982). Selenium status of seven chronic intravenous hyperalimentation patients. Journal of Parenteral and Enteral Nutrition 6: 426–431.

Lane HW, Warren DC, Taylor BJ, Stool E. (1983). Blood selenium and glutathione peroxidase levels and dietary selenium of free-living and institutional-

ized elderly subjects. Proceedings of the Society for Experimental Biology and Medicine 173: 87–95.

LeBlanc A, Dumas P, Lefebvre L. (1999). Trace element content of commercial shampoos: impact on trace element levels in hair. Science of the Total Environment 229: 121–124.

Lee SM, Lewis J, Buss DH, Holcombe GD, Lawrance P. (1994). Iodine in British food and diet. British Journal of Nutrition 72: 435–446.

Levander OA. (1985). Considerations on the assessment of selenium status. Federation Proceedings 44: 2579–2583.

Levander OA. (2000). Coxsackievirus as a model of viral evolution driven by dietary oxidative stress. Nutrition Reviews 58: S17–S24.

Levander OA, Burk RF. (1994). Selenium. In: Shils M, Olson J, Shike M (eds.) Modern Nutrition in Health and Disease. 8th edition. Lea & Febiger, Philadelphia, pp. 242–251.

Levander OA, Burk RF. (1996). Selenium. In: Ziegler E, File LJ (eds.) Present Knowledge in Nutrition. International Life Sciences Institute Press, Washington, DC, pp. 320–328.

Levander OA, Morris VC. (1984). Dietary selenium levels needed to maintain balance in North American adults consuming self-selected diets. American Journal of Clinical Nutrition 39: 809–815.

Levander OA, Sutherland B, Morris VC, King JC. (1981). Selenium balance in young men during selenium depletion and repletion. American Journal of Clinical Nutrition 34: 2662–2669.

Levander OA, DeLoach DP, Morris VC, Moser PB. (1983a). Platelet glutathione peroxidase activity as an index of selenium status in rats. Journal of Nutrition 113: 55–63.

Levander OA, Alfthan G, Arvilommi H, Gref CG, Huttunen J, Kataja M, Koivistoinen P, Pikkarainen J. (1983b). Bioavailability of selenium to Finnish men as assessed by platelet glutathione peroxidase activity and other blood parameters. American Journal of Clinical Nutrition 37: 887–897.

Levander OA, Moser PB, Morris VC. (1987). Dietary selenium intake and selenium concentrations of plasma, erythrocytes and breast milk in pregnant and postpartum lactating and nonlactating women. American Journal of Clinical Nutrition 46: 694–698.

Levine RJ, Olson RE. (1970). Blood selenium in Thai children with protein-calorie malnutrition. Proceedings of the Society for Experimental Biology and Medicine 134: 1030–1034.

Lombeck I, Kasperek K, Feinendegen LE, Bremer HJ. (1975). Serum selenium concentrations in patients with maple-syrup-urine disease and phenylketonuria under dieto-therapy. Clinica Chimica Acta 64: 57–61.

Lombeck I, Kasperek K, Harbish HD, Feinendegen LE, Brewer HJ. (1977). The selenium state of healthy children. I: Serum selenium concentration at different ages; activity of glutathione peroxidase of erythrocytes at different ages; selenium content of food of infants. European Journal of Pediatrics 125: 81–88.

Lombeck I, Kasperek K, Harbisch HD, Becker K, Schumann E, Schröter W, Feinendegen LE, Bremer HJ. (1978). The selenium state of children. II: Selenium content of serum, whole blood, hair and the activity of erythrocyte glutathione peroxidase in dietetically treated patients with phenylketonuria and maple-syrup-urine disease. European Journal of Pediatrics 128: 213–223.

Lombeck I, Menzel H, Frosch D. (1987). Acute selenium poisoning of a 2-year-old child. European Journal of Pediatrics 146: 308–312.

Longenecker MP, Taylor PR, Levander OA, Howe M, Veillon C, McAdam PA, Patterson KY, Holden JM, Stampfer MJ, Morris JS. (1991). Selenium in diet, blood and toenails in relation to human health in a seleniferous area. American Journal of Clinical Nutrition 53: 1288–1294.

Luo XM, Wei HJ, Yang CL, Xing J, Liu X, Qiao CH, Feng YM, Liu J, Liu YX, Wu Z, Liu X, Guo JS, Stoecker BJ, Spallholz JE, Yang SP. (1985a). Bioavailability of selenium to residents in a low-selenium area of China. American Journal of Clinical Nutrition 42: 439–448.

Luo XM, Wei HJ, Yang CL, Xing J, Qiao CH, Feng Y, Liu J, Liu YX, Wu Q, Liu X, Stoecker BJ, Spallholz JE, Yang SP. (1985b). Selenium intake and metabolic balance of 10 men from a low selenium area of China. American Journal of Clinical Nutrition 42: 31–37.

MacPherson A, Barclay MNI, Scott R, Yates RWS. (1997). Loss of Canadian wheat imports lowers selenium intake and status of the Scottish population. In: Fischer PWF, L'Abbé, Cockell KA, Gibson RS (eds.) Trace Elements in Man and Animals 9. National Research Council Press: Ottawa, pp. 203–205.

Marano G, Spagnolo A, Morisi G, Menotti A. (1991). Changes in serum selenium and serum cholesterol in children during sexual maturation. Journal of Trace Elements and Electrolytes in Health and Disease 5: 59–61.

Marchaluk E, Persson-Moschos M, Thorling EB, Åkesson B. (1995). Variation in selenoprotein P concentration in serum from different European regions. European Journal of Clinical Nutrition 49: 42–48.

Marchante-Gayón JM, Sánchez-Uría J, Sanz-Medel A. (1996). Serum and tissue selenium contents related to renal disease and colon cancer as determined by electrothermal atomic absorption spectrometry. Journal of Trace Elements in Medicine and Biology 10: 229–236.

May JM, Cobb CE, Mendiratta S, Hill KE, Burk RF. (1998). Reduction of the ascorbyl free radical to ascorbate by thioredoxin reductase. Journal of Biological Chemistry 273: 23039–23045.

May SL, May WA, Bourdoux PP, Pino S, Sullivan KM, Maberly GF. (1997). Validation of a simple, manual urinary iodine method for estimating the prevalence of iodine-deficiency disorders, and interlaboratory comparison with other methods. American Journal of Clinical Nutrition 65: 1441–1445.

McAdam PA, Smith DK, Felman EB, Hames C. (1984). Effect of age, sex, and race on selenium status of healthy residents of Augusta, Georgia. Biological Trace Element Research 6: 3–9.

McCarthy TP, Brodie B, Milner JA, Bevill RF. (1981). Improved method for selenium determination in biological samples by gas chromatography. Journal of Chromatography 225: 9–16.

McGuire MK, Burgert SL, Milner JA, Glass L, Kummer R, Deering R, Boucek R, Picciano MF. (1993). Selenium status of infants is influenced by supplementation of formula or maternal diets. American Journal of Clinical Nutrition 58: 643–648.

McKenzie HM, Rea HM, Thomson CD, Robinson MF. (1978). Selenium concentration and glutathione peroxidase activity in blood of New Zealand infants and children. American Journal of Clinical Nutrition 31: 1413–1418.

McLachlan SK. (2003). Selenium status of New Zealanders. MSc Thesis, University of Otago, Dunedin, New Zealand.

McMaster D, Bell N, Anderson P, Love AH. (1990). Automated measurement of two indicators of human selenium status, and applicability to population studies. Clinical Chemistry 36: 211–216.

Mei JV, Alexander JR, Adam BW, Hannon WH. (2001). Use of filter paper for the collection and analysis of human whole blood specimens. Journal of Nutrition 131: 1631S–1636S.

Miettinen TA, Alfthan G, Huttunen JK, Pikkarainen J, Naukkarinen V, Mattila S, Kumlin T. (1983). Serum selenium concentration related to myocardial infarction and fatty acid content of serum lipids. British Medical Journal 287: 517–519.

Mikac-Devic D, Vukelic N, Kljaic K. (1993). Urine selenium level in healthy adult populations. Biological Trace Element Research 36: 283–290.

Missler U, Gutekunst R, Wood WG. (1994). Thyroglobulin is a more sensitive indicator of iodine deficiency than thyrotropin: development and evaluation of dry blood spot assays for thyrotropin and thyroglobulin in iodine-deficient geographical areas. European Journal of Clinical Chemistry and Clinical Biochemistry 32: 137–143.

Miyai K, Ishibashi K, Kawashima M. (1981). Two-site immunoenzymometric assay for thyrotropin in dried blood samples on filter paper. Clinical Chemistry 27: 1421–1423.

Moreno-Reyes R, Suetens C, Mathieu F, Begaux F, Zhu D, Rivera MT, Boelaert M, Neve J, Perlmutter N, Vanderpas J. (1998). Kashin-Beck osteoarthropathy in rural Tibet in relation to selenium and iodine status. New England Journal of Medicine 339: 1112–1120.

Morris JS, Stampfer MJ, Willett W. (1983). Dietary selenium in humans: toenails as an indicator. Biological Trace Element Research 5: 529–537.

Mutanen M. (1984). Dietary intake and sources of selenium in young Finnish women. Human Nutrition: Applied Nutrition 38: 265–269.

Nan BS, Li CS, Chen LH. (1986). Significance of low levels of blood and hair selenium in dilated cardiomyopathy. Chinese Medical Journal 99:948–949.

Nath SK, Moinier B, Thuillier F, Rongier M, Desjeux JF. (1992). Urinary excretion of iodine and fluoride from supplemented food grade salt. International Journal of Vitamin Nutrition Research 62: 66–72.

Navarro-Alarcon M, Lopez-Martinez MC. (2000). Essentiality of selenium in the human body: relationship with different diseases. Science of the Total Environment 249: 347–371.

Nève J. (1991). Methods in determination of selenium states. Journal of Trace Elements and Electrolytes in Health and Disease 5: 1–17.

Nève J. (1995). Human selenium supplementation as assessed by changes in blood selenium concentration and glutathione peroxidase activity. Journal of Trace Elements in Medicine and Biology 9: 65–73.

Nève J. (1999). Are copper, zinc and selenium in erythrocytes valuable biological indexes of nutrition and pathology? Journal of Trace Elements in Medicine and Biology 13: 113–128.

Nève J, Peretz A. (1989). Expression of urinary selenium levels in humans. In: Nève J, Favier A (eds.) Selenium in Medicine and Biology. Walter de Gruyter, New York, pp. 189–192.

Nève J, Sinet PM, Molle L, Nicole A. (1983a). Selenium, zinc and copper in Down's syndrome (trisomy 21): blood levels and relations with glutathione peroxidase and superoxide dismutase. Clinica Chimica Acta 133: 209–214.

Nève J, van Geffel R, Hanocq M, Molle L. (1983b). Plasma and erythrocyte zinc, copper, and selenium in cystic fibrosis. Acta Paediatrica Scandinavica 72: 437–440.

Nomura AMY, Lee J, Stemmermann GN, Combs GF Jr (2000). Serum selenium and subsequent risk of prostate cancer. Cancer Epidemiology. Biomarkers & Prevention 9: 883–887.

Olivieri O, Stanzial AM, Girelli D, Trevisan MT, Guarini P, Terzi M, Caffi S, Fontana F, Casaril M, Ferrari S, Corrocher R. (1994). Selenium status, fatty acids, vitamins A and E, and aging: the Nove Study. American Journal of Clinical Nutrition 60: 510–517.

Olivieri O, Girelli D, Azzini M, Stanzial AM, Russo C, Ferroni M, Corrocher R. (1995). Low selenium status in the elderly influences thyroid hormones. Clinical Science 89: 637–642.

Olson OE. (1986). Selenium toxicity in animals with emphasis on man. Journal of the American College of Toxicology 5: 45–70.

Oltarzewski M, Szymborski J. (2003). Neonatal hypothyroid screening in monitoring of iodine deficiency and iodine supplementation in Poland. Journal of Clinical Investigation 26: 27–31.

Oster O, Prellwitz W. (1989). The daily dietary selenium intake of West German adults. Biological Trace Element Research 20: 1–14.

Oster O, Prellwitz W. (1990). The renal excretion of selenium. Biological Trace Element Research 24: 119–146.

Oster O, Prellwitz W, Kasper W, Meinertz T. (1983). Congestive cardiomyopathy and the selenium content of serum. Clinica Chimica Acta 128: 125–132.

Paglia DE, Valentine WN. (1967). Studies on the quantitative and qualitative characterization of erythrocyte glutathione peroxidase. Journal of Laboratory and Clinical Medicine 70: 158–169.

Pardede LVH, Hardjowasito W, Gross R, Dillon DHS, Totoprajogo OS, Yosoprawoto M, Waskito L, Untoro J. (1998). Urinary iodine excretion is the most appropriate outcome indicator for iodine deficiency at field conditions at district level. Journal of Nutrition 128: 1122–1126.

Peng A, Wang WH, Wang CX, Wang ZJ, Rui HF, Wang WZ, Yang ZW. (1999). The role of humic substances in drinking water in Kashin-Beck disease in China. Environmental Health Perspectives 107: 293–296.

Pennington JAT. (1990). A review of iodine toxicity reports. Journal of the American Dietetic Association 90: 1571–1581.

Penny R, Spencer CA, Frasier SD, Nicoloff JT. (1983). Thyroid-stimulating hormone and thyroglobulin levels decrease with chronological age in children and adolescents. Journal of Clinical Endocrinology and Metabolism 56: 177–180.

Persson-Modchos M, Huang W, Srikumar TS, Åkesson B, Lindeberg S. (1995). Selenoprotein P in serum as a biochemical marker of selenium status. Analyst 120: 833–836.

Rasmussen LB, Ovesen L, Christiansen E. (1999). Day-to-day and within-day variation in urinary iodine excretion. European Journal of Clinical Nutrition 53: 401–407.

Rasmussen LB, Ovesen L, Bulow I, Jorgensen T, Knudson N, Laurberg P, Perrild H. (2002). Relations between various measures of iodine intake and thyroid volume, thyroid nodularity, and serum thyroglobulin. American Journal of Clinical Nutrition 76: 1069–1076.

Rayman MP. (1997). Dietary selenium: time to act. British Medical Journal 314: 387–388.

Rayman MP. (2000). The importance of selenium to human health. Lancet 356: 233–241.

Rea HM, Thomson CD, Campbell DR, Robinson MF. (1979). Relation between erythrocyte selenium concentrations and glutathione peroxidase (EC 1.11.1.9) activities of New Zealand residents and visitors to New Zealand. British Journal of Nutrition 42: 201–208.

Remer T, Manz F. (1994). The inadequacy of the urinary iodine-creatinine ratio for the assessment of iodine status during infancy, childhood and adolescence. Journal of Trace Elements and Electrolytes in Health and Disease. 8: 217–219.

Robberecht HJ, Deelstra HA. (1984). Selenium in human urine: concentration levels and medical implications. Clinica Chimica Acta 136: 107–120.

Robberecht HJ, Deelstra HA. (1994). Factors influencing blood selenium concentrations: a literature review. Journal of Trace Elements and Electroytes in Health and Disease 8: 129–143.

Roberts LJ 2nd, Morrow JD. (1997). The generation and actions of isoprostanes. Biochimica et Biophysica Acta 1345: 121–135.

Robinson JR, Robinson MF, Levander OA, Thomson CD. (1985). Urinary excretion of selenium by New Zealand and North American human subjects on differing intakes. American Journal of Clinical Nutrition 41: 1023–1031.

Robinson MF, Thomson CD. (1983). The role of selenium in the diet. Nutrition Abstracts and Reviews Series A. 53: 3–26.

Robinson MF, Thomson CD, Jenkinson CP, Luzhen G, Whanger PD. (1997). Long-term supplementation with selenate and selenomethionine: urinary excretion by New Zealand women. British Journal of Nutrition 77: 551–563.

Rodriguez EMR, Alaejos MTS, Romero CD. (1995). Urinary selenium status of healthy people. European Journal of Clinical Chemistry and Clinical Biochemistry 33: 127–133.

Rudolph N, Wong SL. (1978). Selenium and glutathione peroxidase activity in maternal and cord plasma and red cells. Pediatric Research 12: 789–792.

Sabé R, Rubio R, Garcia-Beltrán L. (2002). Reference values of selenium in plasma in population from Barcelona: comparison with several pathologies. Journal of Trace Elements in Medicine and Biology 16: 231–237.

Salbe AD, Levander OA. (1990). Effect of various dietary factors on the deposition of selenium in the hair and nails of rats. Journal of Nutrition 120: 200–206.

Salonen JH, Alfthan G, Huttunen JK, Pikkarainen J, Puska P. (1982). Association between cardiovascular death and myocardial infarction and serum selenium in matched-pair longitudinal study. Lancet 2(8291): 175–179.

Schroeder HA, Frost DV, Balassa JJ. (1970). Essential trace metals in man: selenium. Journal of Chronic Diseases 23: 227–243.

Schubert A, Holden JM, Wolf WR. (1987). Selenium content of a core group of foods based on a critical evaluation of published analytical data. Journal of the American Dietetic Association 87: 285–299.

Scott R, MacPherson A, Yates RWS. (1997). Selenium supplementation in sub-fertile human males. In: Fischer PWF, L'Abbé MR, Cockell KA, Gibson RS (eds.) Trace Elements in Man and Animals 9, National Research Council Research Press, Ottawa, pp. 458–459.

Simsek E, Safak A,. Yavuz O, Aras S, Dogan S, Kocabay K. (2003). Sensitivity of iodine deficiency indicators and iodine status in Turkey. Journal of Pediatric Endocrinology and Metabolism 16: 197–202.

Skeaff SA, Thomson CD, Gibson RS. (2002). Mild iodine deficiency in a sample of New Zealand school children. European Journal of Clinical Nutrition 56: 1169–1175.

Sluis KB, Darlow BA, George PM, Mogridge N, Dolamore BA, Winterbourn CC. (1992). Selenium and glutathione peroxidase levels in premature infants in a low selenium community (Christchurch, New Zealand). Pediatric Research 32: 189–194.

Smith AM, Picciano MF, Milne RJA. (1982). Selenium intakes and status of human milk and formula fed infants. American Journal of Clinical Nutrition 35: 521–526.

Smith AM, Chen LW, Thomas MR. (1995). Selenate fortification improves selenium status of term infants fed soy formula. American Journal of Clinical Nutrition 61: 44–47.

Snook JT, Palmquist DL, Moxon AL, Cantor AH, Vivian VM. (1983). Selenium status of a rural (predominantly Amish) community living in a low-selenium area. American Journal of Clinical Nutrition 38: 620–630.

Soldin OP. (2002). Controversies in urinary iodine determinations. Clinical Biochemistry 35: 575–579.

Spencer CA. (1995). Thyroglobulin measurement techniques, clinical benefits, and pitfalls. Endocrinology and Metabolism. Clinics of North America 24: 841–863.

Squali Houssaini FZ, Arnaud J, Richard MJ, Renversez JC, Favier A. (1997). Evaluation of oxidative stress and antioxidant defenses in malnourished Morrocan children. Annals of Nutrition and Metabolism 41: 149–159.

Stanley JC, Alexander JP, Nesbitt GA. (1982). Selenium deficiency during total parenteral nutrition: a case report. The Ulster Medical Journal 51:130–132.

Stewart RDH, Griffiths NM, Thomson CD, Robinson MF. (1978). Quantitative selenium metabolism in normal New Zealand women. British Journal of Nutrition 40: 45–54.

Suadicani P, Hein HO, Gyntelberg F. (1992). Serum selenium concentration and risk of ischaemic heart disease in a prospective cohort study of 3000 males. Atherosclerosis 96: 33–42.

Sullivan KM, May W, Nordenberg D, Houston R, Maberly GF. (1997). Use of thyroid stimulating hormone testing in newborns to identify iodine deficiency. Journal of Nutrition 127: 55–58.

Sun QA, Wu Y, Zappacosta F, Jeang KT, Lee BJ, Hatfield DL, Gladyshev VN. (1999). Redox regulation of cell signaling by selenocysteine in mammalian thioredoxin reductases. Journal of Biological Chemistry 274: 24522–24530.

Suzuki H, Mashimo K. (1973). Further studies of "endemic goiter" in Hokkaido, Japan. In: Mashimo K, Suzuki H (eds). Iodine Metabolism and Thyroid Function. Hokkaido University School of Medicine, Sapporo, Japan. p. 143.

Suzuki H, Higuchi T, Sawa K, Ohtaki S, Horiuchi Y. (1965). "Endemic coast goitre" in Hokkaido, Japan. Acta Endocrinologica 50: 161–176.

Swanson CA, Reamer DC, Veillon C, King JC, Levander OA. (1983). Quantitative and qualitative aspects of selenium utilization in pregnant and nonpregnant women: an application of stable isotope methodology. American Journal of Clinical Nutrition 38: 169–180.

Swanson CA, Longnecker MP, Veillon C, Howe M, Levander OA, Taylor PR, McAdam PA, Brown CC, Stampfer MJ, Willet WC. (1990). Selenium intake, age, gender, and smoking in relation to indices of selenium status of adults residing in a seleniferous area. American Journal of Clinical Nutrition 52: 858–862.

Szebeni A, Beleznay E. (1992). New simple method for thyroid volume determination by ultrasonography. Journal of Clinical Ultrasound 20: 329–337.

Terada A, Nakada M, Nakada K, Yamate N, Tanaka Y, Yoshida M, Yoshida K. (1996). Selenium administration to a ten-year-old patient receiving long-term total parenteral nutrition (TPN): changes in selenium concentration in the blood and hair. Journal of Trace Elements in Medicine and Biology 10: 1–5.

Thilly CH, Swennen B, Bourdoux P, Ntambue K, Moreno-Reyes R, Gillies J, Vanderpas JB. (1993). The epidemiology of iodine-deficiency disorders in relation to goitrogenic factors and thyroid-stimulating hormone regulation. American Journal of Clinical Nutrition 57: 267S–270S.

Thomson CD. (1998). Selenium speciation in human body fluids. Analyst 123: 827–831.

Thomson CD. (2003). Selenium: Physiology. In: Caballero B, Trugo LC, Finglas PM (eds.). Encyclopaedia of Food Science, Food Technology and Nutrition. Academic Press, London, pp. 5117–5124.

Thomson CD. (2004a). Assessment of requirements for selenium and adequacy of selenium status: a review. European Journal of Clinical Nutrition 58: 391–402.

Thomson CD. (2004b). Selenium and iodine intakes and status in New Zealand and Australia. British Journal of Nutrition 91: 661–672.

Thomson CD, Duncan A. (1981). Glutathione peroxidase and selenium status. In: Howell JMC, Gawthorne JM, White CL (eds.) Trace Element Metabolism in Man and Animals (TEMA-4). Griffin Press, Netly, South Australia, pp. 22–25.

Thomson CD, Robinson MF. (1980). Selenium in human health and disease with emphasis on those aspects peculiar to New Zealand. American Journal of Clinical Nutrition 33: 303–323.

Thomson CD, Robinson MF. (1996). The changing selenium status of New Zealand residents. European Journal of Clinical Nutrition 50: 107–114.

Thomson CD, Rea HM, Doesburg VM, Robinson MF. (1977). Selenium concentrations and glutathione peroxidase activities in whole blood of New Zealand residents. British Journal of Nutrition 37: 457–460.

Thomson CD, Robinson MF, Campbell DR, Rea HM. (1982). Effect of prolonged supplementation with daily supplements of selenomethionine and sodium selenite on glutathione peroxidase activity in blood of New Zealand residents. American Journal of Clinical Nutrition 36: 24–31.

Thomson CD, Ong LK, Robinson MF. (1985). Ef-

fects of supplementation with high-selenium wheat bread on selenium, glutathione peroxidase and related enzymes in blood components of New Zealand residents. American Journal of Clinical Nutrition 41: 1015–1022.

Thomson CD, Steven SM, van Rij AM, Wade CR, Robinson MF. (1988). Selenium and vitamin E supplementation: activities of glutathione peroxidase in human tissues. American Journal of Clinical Nutrition 48: 316–323.

Thomson CD, Robinson MF, Butler J, Whanger PD. (1993). Long-term supplementation with selenate and selenomethionine: selenium and glutathione peroxidase (EC 1.11.1.9) in blood components of New Zealand women. British Journal of Nutrition 69: 577–588.

Thomson CD, Smith TE, Butler KA, Packer MA. (1996). An evaluation of urinary measures of iodine and selenium status. Journal of Trace Elements in Medicine and Biology 10: 214–222.

Thomson CD, Woodruffe S, Colls A, Joseph J, Doyle T. (2001). Urinary iodine and thyroid status of New Zealand residents. European Journal of Clinical Nutrition 55: 387–392.

Tórrens JL, Burch HB. (2001). Serum thyroglobulin measurement. Endocrinology and Metabolism. Clinics of North America 30: 429–467.

Tsongas TA, Ferguson SW. (1978). Selenium concentration in human urine and drinking water. In: Kirchgessner M (ed.) Trace Element Metabolism in Man and Animals (TEMA-3). Institut für Ernährungs Physiologie Technische Universität München, Freising-Weihenstephan, pp. 320–321.

van Caillie-Bertrand M, Degenhart HJ, Fernandes J. (1986). Influence of age on the selenium status in Belgium and The Netherlands. Pediatric Research 20: 574–576.

Van Dael P, Deschuytere A, Robberecht H, van Caillie-Bertrand M, Lamand M, Deelstra H. (1994). Capillary whole blood selenium determination in assessing selenium status of children. Journal of Trace Elements, Electrolytes, Health and Disease 8: 225–228.

Van den Briel T, West CE, Hautvast JGAJ, Vulsma T, de Vijlder JJM, Ategbo EA. (2001). Serum thyroglobulin and urinary iodine concentration are the most appropriate indicators of iodine status and thyroid function under conditions of increasing iodine supply in school children in Benin. Journal of Nutrition 131: 2701–2706.

Vanderpas JB, Contempre B, Duale N, Goossens W, Bebe N, Thorpe R, Ntambue K, Dumont J, Thilly C, Diplock AT. (1990). Iodine and selenium deficiency associated with cretinism in northern Zaire. American Journal of Clinical Nutrition 52: 1087–1093.

Vanderpas JB, Contempre B, Duale NL, Deckx H, Bebe N, Longombe AO, Thilly CH, Diplock AT, Dumont JE. (1993). Selenium deficiency mitigates hypothyroxinemia in iodine-deficient subjects. American Journal of Clinical Nutrition 57: 271S–275S.

van Noord PA, Collette HJ, Maas MJ, de Waard F. (1987). Selenium levels in nails of premenopausal breast cancer patients assessed prediagnostically in a cohort-nested case-referent study among women screened in the DOM project. International Journal of Epidemiology 16: 318–322.

van Rij AM, Thomson CD, McKenzie JM, Robinson MF. (1979). Selenium deficiency in total parenteral nutrition. American Journal of Clinical Nutrition 32: 2076–2085.

Varo P, Saari E, Paaso A, Koivistoinen P. (1982). Iodine in Finnish foods. International Journal for Vitamin and Nutrition Research 52: 80–89.

Varo P, Alfthan G, Huttunen JK, Aro A. (1994). National selenium supplementation in Finland: effects on diet, blood and tissue levels, and health. In: Burk R (ed.) Selenium in Biology and Human Health. Springer, New York, pp. 197–218.

Verlinden M, Van Sprundel M, Van der Auwera JC, Eylenbosch WJ. (1983a). The selenium status of Belgian population groups. I: Healthy adults. Biological Trace Element Research 5: 91–102.

Verlinden M, Van Sprundel M, Van der Auwera JC, Eylenbosch WJ. (1983b). The selenium status of Belgian population groups. II: Newborns, children, and the aged. Biological Trace Element Research 5: 103–113.

Vinton NE, Dahlstrom KA, Strobel CT, Ament ME. (1987). Macrocytosis and pseudoalbinism: manifestations of selenium deficiency. Journal of Pediatrics 111: 711–717.

Virtamo J, Valkeila E, Alfthan G, Punsar S, Huttunen J, Karvonen MJ. (1985). Serum selenium and the risk of coronary heart disease and stroke. American Journal of Epidemiology 122: 276–282.

Vitoux D, Arnaud J, Chappuis P. (1999). Are copper, zinc and selenium in erythrocytes valuable biological indexes of nutrition and pathology? Journal of Trace Elements in Medicine and Biology 13: 113–128.

Vitti P, Martino E, Aghini-Lombardi F, Rago T, Antonangeli L, Maccherini D, Nasnni P, Loviselloi A, Balestrieri A, Araneo G, et al. (1994). Thyroid volume measurement by ultrasound in children as a tool for the assessment of mild iodine deficiency. Journal of Clinical Endocrinology and Metabolism 79: 600–603.

Vought RL, Brown FA, Wolff J. (1972). Erythrosine: an adventitious source of iodide. Journal of Clinical Endocrinology and Metabolism 34: 747–752.

Wang GY, Zhou RH, Wang Z, Shi L, Sun M. (1999). Effects of storage and cooking on the iodine content in iodized salt and study on monitoring iodine content in iodized salt. Biomedical Environmental Sciences 12: 1–9.

Wąsowicz W, Zachara BA. (1987). Selenium concentrations in the blood and urine of a healthy Polish subpopulation. Journal of Clinical Chemistry and Clinical Biochemistry 25: 409–412.

Watkinson JH. (1979). The semi-automated fluorometric determination of nanogram quantities of selenium in biological material. Analytica Chimica Acta 105: 319–325.

Wayne EJ, Koutras DA, Alexander WD. (1964). Clinical Aspects of Iodine Metabolism. Blackwell Scientific, Oxford.

Westermarck T, Raunu P, Kirjarinta M, Lappalainen L. (1977). Selenium content of blood and serum in adults and children of different ages from different parts of Finland. Acta Pharmacologica et Toxicologica 40: 465–475.

WHO/ICCIDD (World Health Organization / International Council for the Control of Iodine Deficiency Disorders). (1997). Recommended normative values for thyroid volume in children aged 6–15 years. Bulletin of the World Health Organization 75: 95–97.

WHO/UNICEF/ICCIDD. (World Health Organization / United Nations Children's Fund / International Council for the Control of Iodine deficiency Disorders). (1994). Indicators for Assessing Iodine Deficiency Disorders and Their Control through Salt Iodization. World Health Organization, Geneva.

Wilson D, Parnell W, Wilson N, Faed J, Ferguson EL, Herbison P, Horwath C, Nye T, Reid P, Walker R, Wilson B, Tukuitonga C. (1999). NZ Food: NZ People. Key Results of the 1997 National Nutrition Survey, Ministry of Health, Wellington, New Zealand.

Wolde-Gabriel Z, West CE, Gebru H, Tadesse AS, Fisseha T, Gabre P, Aboye C, Ayana G, Hautvast JG. (1993a). Interrelationship between vitamin A, iodine and iron status in school children in Shoa region, central Ethiopia. British Journal of Nutrition 70: 593–607.

Wolde-Gabriel Z, Gebru H, Fisseha T, West C. (1993b). Severe vitamin A deficiency in a rural village in the Harare region of Ethiopia. European Journal of Clinical Nutrition 47: 104–114.

Wolff J, Chaikoff IL. (1948). Plasma inorganic iodide as homeostatic regulator of thyroid function. Journal of Biological Chemistry 174: 555–564.

Xia YM, Hill KE, Burk RF. (1989). Biochemical studies of a selenium-deficient population in China: measurement of selenium, glutathione peroxidase and other oxidant defense indices in blood. Journal of Nutrition 119: 1318–1326.

Xia Y, Zhao X, Zhu L, Whanger PD. (1992). Metabolism of selenate and selenomethionine by a selenium-deficient population of men in China. Journal of Nutritional Biochemistry 3: 202–210.

Xu F, Sullivan K, Houston R, Zhao J, May W, Maberly G. (1999). Thyroid volumes in U.S. and Bangladeshi school children: comparison with European school children. European Journal of Endocrinology 140: 498–504.

Xu GL, Wang SC, Gu BQ, Yang YX, Song HB, Xue HL, Liang WS, Zhang P. (1997). Further investigation on the role of selenium deficiency in the aetiology and pathogenesis of Keshan disease. Biomedical and Environmental Science 10: 316–326.

Yang GQ, Wang SZ, Zhou RH, Sun SZ. (1983). Endemic selenium intoxication of humans in China. American Journal of Clinical Nutrition 37: 872–881.

Yang GQ, Chen JS, Wen ZM, Ge KY, Zhu LZ, Chen XC, Chen XS. (1984). The role of selenium in Keshan Disease. Advances in Nutritional Research 6: 203–231.

Yang GQ, Zhu IZ, Liu LZ, Gu LZ, Qian PC, Huang JH, Lu MD. (1987). Human selenium requirements in China. In: Combs GF, Spallholtz JE, Levander OA, Oldfield JE (eds.). Selenium in Biology and Medicine. Nostrand Reinhold, New York, NY, pp. 589–607.

Yoshizawa K, Willett WC, Morris SJ, Stampfer MJ, Spiegelman D, Rimm EB, Giovannucci E. (1998). Study of prediagnostic selenium level in toenails and the risk of advanced prostate cancer. Journal of the National Cancer Institute 90: 1219–1224.

Zimmerli B, Haldimann M, Sieber R. (1998). Selenium status of the Swiss population. Part 3: Changes and its causes. Mitteilungen aus dem Gebiete der Lebensmitteluntersuchung und Hygiene 89: 257–293.

Zimmermann MB, Delange F. (2004). Iodine supplementation of pregnant women in Europe: a review and recommendations. European Journal of Clinical Nutrition 58: 979–984.

Zimmermann MB, Adou P, Zeder C, Torresani T, Hurrell RF. (2000a). Persistence of goiter despite oral iodine supplementation in goitrous children with iron-deficiency anemia in the Côte d'Ivoire. American Journal of Clinical Nutrition 71: 88–93.

Zimmermann MB, Saad A, Hess S, Torresani T, Chaouki N. (2000b). Thyroid ultrasound compared with World Health Organization 1960 and 1994 palpation criteria for determination of goiter prevalence in regions of mild and severe iodine deficiency. European Journal of Endocrinology 143: 727–731.

Zimmermann MB, Molinari L, Spehl M, Weidinger-Toth J, Podoba J, Hess S, Delange F. (2001). Toward a consensus on reference values for thyroid volume in iodine-replete school children: results of a workshop on inter-observer and inter-equipment variation in sonographic measurement of thyroid volume. European Journal of Endocriniology 144: 2213–2220.

Zimmermann MB, Zeder C, Chaouki N, Torresani T, Saad A, Hurrell RF. (2003a). Addition of microencapsulated iron to iodized salt improves the efficacy of iodine in goitrous, iron deficient children: a randomized, double-blind, controlled trial. European Journal of Endocrinology 147: 747–753.

Zimmermann MB, Moretti D, Chaouki N, Torresani T. (2003b). Development of a dried whole-blood spot thyroglobulin assay and its evaluation as an indicator of thyroid status in goitrous children receiving iodized salt. American Journal of Clinical Nutrition 77: 1453–1458.

Zimmermann MB, Hess SY, Molinari L, De Benoist B, Delange F, Braverman LE, Fujieda K, Ito Y, Jooste PL, Moosa K, Pearce EN, Pretell EA, Shishiba Y. (2004). New reference values for thyroid volume by ultrasound in iodine- sufficient school children: a World Health Organization/Nutrition for Health and Development Iodine Deficiency Study Group Report. American Journal of Clinical Nutrition 79: 231–237.

26

Clinical assessment

Conventionally, clinical assessment consisted of a routine medical history followed by a physical examination to detect and record symptoms (manifestations reported by the patient) and physical signs (observations made by a qualified examiner) associated with malnutrition. These assessment procedures are most useful during advanced nutritional depletion, when overt disease is present.

Some specific nutrient deficiencies, along with protein-energy malnutrition, are known to be associated with loss of immune function, muscle weakness, impaired strength, mobility, and cognitive dysfunction (Jeejeebhoy 1998; Windsor and Hill, 1988). Increasingly, therefore, in hospitalized patients and in institutionalized and independently living elderly tests designed to assess deficits in physiological and cognitive function are included as additional components of clinical assessment. These assessment procedures are used both in clinical and community studies.

Protein-energy undernutrition still occurs among medical and surgical hospitalized patients (Coats et al., 1993; McWhirter and Pennington, 1994; Wyszynski et al., 1998; Sullivan et al., 1999; Edington et al., 2000) and among institutionalized elderly in several industrialized countries (Keller, 1993; Ham, 1994; Morley, 1998; Azad et al., 1999). Micronutrient deficiencies also develop among hospital patients with multiple disease states but are less common. Increasingly, obesity and cases of micronutrient toxicity induced by excessive use of dietary supplements are gaining importance in clinical assessment.

Improvements in nutritional status in hospital patients following appropriate intervention are now well recognized (Keele et al., 1997; Doshi et al., 1998; Potter et al., 1998) and emphasize the need for routine nutritional assessment.

This chapter describes the two major components of clinical assessment included in this definition: the medical history and the physical examination. In addition, a brief discussion of some of the newer functional tests designed to assess strength, mobility, and function is given. Earlier chapters have described the dietary, anthropometric, and laboratory components of nutritional assessment that are also needed, in view of the nonspecific nature of many critical signs and symptoms. So far, few clinical studies have systematically evaluated the ability of clinical assessment alone to reliably identify patients at increased risk for medical complications (Klein et al., 1997).

26.1 Medical history

In clinical medicine, the nutritional and medical history can be obtained by an interview with the patient or from medical records, or both. Source-oriented medical records (SOMRs) have an organizational structure that is based on the source of the information obtained during the course of the health care. The SOMR consists of patient identification data, admission notes, physician's orders, laboratory reports, medication records, consents, consultations, operating room records, progress notes, and flow sheets (Mason et al., 1982).

In many health care settings, the SOMR has been replaced by the problem-oriented medical record (POMR) (Weed, 1971; Ho et al., 1999). Unlike the SOMR, the POMR is organized around a series of problems identified during the data collection process. The POMR consists of a defined database, a complete problem list, the initial care plan, and progress notes, as well as flow sheets and a discharge summary (Fowler and Longabaugh, 1975). Use of either of these types of medical records ensures that all aspects of the care of the patient are noted in one place, as part of the total medical record. In recent years such POMR systems have become computer-based (Ho et al., 1999).

The medical history generally includes a description of the patient and relevant environmental, social, and family factors. For elderly patients especially, reliable information on these factors can be sought discreetly, from other family members or from caregivers such as home care workers, nurses, meals on wheels volunteers, and others who may have visited the home (Ham, 1994). In addition, data on the medical history of the patient and his or her family must be obtained. Such data are obtained by a variety of questions related to weight loss or gain, edema, anorexia, vomiting, diarrhea, and information on decreased or unusual food intake. Again, some of this information may be obtained from the patient or from family members and other caregivers.

Several new tools are now available to enable physicians to rapidly and accurately assess patient's diets and, in some cases, exercise habits. These include a short nutrition history form designed specifically for taking a nutrition history (Hark and Deen, 1999) and two tools, WAVE and REAP, developed by the U.S. Nutrition Academic Award to assist physicians and other health care providers to conduct nutrition assessment and counseling with their patients. WAVE is an acronym for a tool emphasizing the patient's current status in relation to Weight, Activity, Va-

riety and Excess; REAP is a tool for the Rapid Eating and Activity Assessment of Patients. The latter is based on a brief validated questionnaire that focuses on diet and physical activity (Gans et al., 2003).

Other information recorded in a medical history includes previous history of anemia or major surgery, presence of chronic illness, pica (ingestion of clay, starch, paint, etc.), presence of congenital conditions and inborn errors of metabolism, and the use of dietary supplements and medications both prior to and during hospitalization.

Details of both prescription and over-the-counter medications should be obtained as these may interfere with nutritional status in a variety of ways, inducing, for example, changes in appetite, taste, thirst, bowel function, and alterations in absorption, metabolism, or excretion of nutrients. Table 26.1 summarizes the potential effects of some common medications on nutritional status. Details of food allergies and food intolerances should also be obtained. An example of data obtained in a medical history is given in Table 26.2.

Helpful information designed specifically for screening elderly patients can be obtained from the U.S. Nutrition Screening Initiative (NSI). A CD-ROM of a monograph entitled *A Physician's Guide to Nutrition in Chronic Disease Management for Older Adults* is now available from <nsi@gmmb.com>.

The overall objective of nutritional screening is to establish whether a nutrient deficiency is primary, arising from inadequate dietary intake, or secondary in origin. In a secondary deficiency, the diet is potentially adequate, but conditioning factors such as drugs, dietary components, and disease states interfere with the ingestion, absorption, transport, metabolism, utilization, and excretion of the nutrient(s). Examples of disease states associated with increased nutrient metabolism include diabetes mellitus and hyperthyroidism, whereas excessive loss of nutrients is linked with enterocutaneous fistulas (Corish and Kennedy, 2000). Digestive diseases are also major causes of malnutrition, sometimes causing dysphagia (i.e., difficulty or pain on swallowing) or recurrent vomiting,

Class (specific example)	Effect
Amphetamines	↓ Appetite/weight
Anorexiants	↓ Appetite/weight
Antibiotics (*N*-methylthiotetrazole sidechains)	↓ Vitamin K function
Anticonvulsants (phenytoin, phenobarbitol)	↓ Calcium absorption ↓ vitamin D, bone loss, ↓ folate levels
Antipsychotics (clozapine)	↑ Appetite/weight
Bile acid sequestrants	↓ Vitamin A, D, E, K absorption
Corticosteroids	↑ Appetite/fat mass/weight, hyperglycemia, ↓ lean mass ↓ vitamin D, ↓ calcium, bone loss, ↓ vitamin B_6 levels (significance unclear)
Diuretics	↓ Potassium, ↓ magnesium, ↓ thiamin, ↓ sodium, ↑ calcium (thiazides)
Ethanol abuse	↓ Thiamin, ↓ folate, ↓ riboflavin, ↓ vitamin B_6, ↓ vitamin D, ↓ vitamin A
Insulin	↑ Appetite/weight
Isoniazid	↓ Vitamin B_6, ↓ niacin, ↓ vitamin D (significance unclear
Lithium	↑ Appetite/weight
Methotrexate	↓ Folate
Orlistat	↓ Vitamins A, D, E, K absorption
Proton pump inhibitors	↓ Vitamin B_{12}
Selective serotonin reuptake inhibitors	↓ or ↑ Appetite/weight
Sulfasalazine	↓ Folate
Sulfonylureas	↑ Appetite/weight
Theophylline	↓ Appetite/weight
Tricyclic antidepressants	↑ Appetite/weight

Table 26.1: Common medications and potential effects on nutrient status. From Saltzman and Mogensen (2001). Physical assessment. In: Coulston AM, Rock CL, Monsen ER (eds.) Nutrition in the Prevention and Treatment of Disease. © with permission from Elsevier.

chronic diarrhea, intestinal mucosal malabsorption, or recurrent abdominal pain. In hospitalized patients, conditions associated with primary and secondary nutrient deficiencies often coexist, making it difficult to separate their effects on patient outcome (Weinsier and Heimburger, 1997).

Respondent bias may occur during the conduct of the medical history. In general, voluntary information given by the patient tends to be less biased than answers to specific questions on past nutritional and medical history. Consequently, it is preferable to use open-ended questions to elicit such information.

In community surveys, the medical history is obtained by administering a questionnaire in a household (e.g., in U.K. Diet and Nutrition Surveys) or site interview (e.g., in the most recent National Health and Nutrition Examination Survey (NHANES III). Several questions on dietary practices may also be included in this questionnaire to provide information that cannot always be readily obtained from the dietary assessment protocol. These questions may concern slimming diets; smoking behavior; use of alcohol, tea, or coffee; use of medications; and food supplements. The U.K. Diet and Nutrition Survey (Henderson et al., 2002) and NHANES III (NCHS, 1994) asked many of these questions.

Nutrient intake
• Anorexia
• Actual intake
• Gastrointestinal tract malfunction affecting intake, digestion, or absorption

Underlying pathology with nutritional effects
• Chronic infections or inflammatory states
• Neoplasia
• Endocrine disorders
• Chronic illnesses: pulmonary disease, cirrhosis, or renal failure

End-organ effects
• Edema/ascites
• Weight changes
• Obesity
• Muscle mass relative to exercise status

Miscellaneous
• Catabolic medications or therapies: steroids, immunosuppressive agents, radiation, or chemotherapy
• Genetic background: body habitus of parents, siblings, and family
• Other medications: diuretics, laxatives
• Food allergies: food intolerances

Table 26.2: Example of information obtained from a medical history. From Cerra, (1984). Assessment of nutritional and metabolic status. In: Pocket Manual of Surgical Nutrition. ⓒ C.V. Mosby Co., with permission.

Information on medications and dietary supplements is best collected directly from the container labels, by asking the subjects to show the interviewer all drugs (prescription and over-the-counter) and supplements. In this way accurate data on type and dose may be obtained to aid in the interpretation of biochemical indices (Bates et al., 1998; Bates 2000).

In some national nutrition surveys, an oral or dental health component has been included (Henderson et al., 2002; Parnell et al., 2003). Assessment of dental health is especially important in the elderly. There are several reports of a relationship between the degree of edentulousness and indices of nutritional status in this age group (Papas et al., 1998).

Parents can be asked to supply additional information about their children, such as infant feeding history (e.g., breast vs. formula feeding; age of introduction of solid foods), histories of contagious diseases, immunization details, presence of parasites, weight, length, and gestational age of child at birth. For female subjects, questions related to age at first menses, history of pregnancies and miscarriages, oral contraceptive use, and use of noncontraceptive estrogens are also frequently included. In the NHANES III survey, information on the occurrence of fractures was also elicited.

Increasingly, questions on the type and level of habitual physical activity or exercise are being incorporated in national nutrition surveys (e.g., NZ Children's Nutrition Survey (Parnell et al., 2003), and the U.K. National Diet & Nutrition Survey (Ruston et al., 2004)). Details of several physical activity questionnaires have been summarized by Kriska and Caspersen (1997); their validity should always be established prior to use.

26.2 Physical examination

The physical examination corroborates and adds to the findings obtained by the medical history. Serial observations of signs and symptoms are especially useful for assessing the rate of decline in nutritional status or the speed of improvement after nutrition interventions have been initiated. The physical examination may also reveal information on factors that contribute to the etiology of malnutrition.

The physical examination, as defined by Jelliffe (1966), examines "those changes, believed to be related to inadequate nutrition, that can be seen or felt in superficial epithelial tissue, especially the skin, eyes, hair, and buccal mucosa, or in organs near the surface of the body (e.g., parotid and thyroid glands)."

A detailed description and photographs of the physical signs recommended by the WHO Expert Committee on Medical Assessment of Nutritional Status (WHO, 1963) can be found in the Assessment of the Nutritional Status of the Community (Jelliffe, 1966). Additional sources include Pressman and Adams (1990)

System	Nutrient or condition	Sign
Mouth	Deficiencies of riboflavin, niacin, biotin, vitamin B_6, vitamin B_{12}, folate, iron, and zinc	Glossitis
	Deficiencies of riboflavin, niacin, biotin, vitamin B_6, iron	Angular stomatis, cheilosis
	Vitamin C deficiency	Gingivitis and gingival bleeding
	Bulimia nervosa	Parotid hyperplasia, dental erosions
Eyes	Deficiency of vitamin A	Xeropthalmia: night blindness, photophobia, xerosis, Bitot's spots, corneal ulceration, scarring
	Toxicity of vitamin A	Diplopia
	Thiamin deficiency	Nystagmus, deficit of lateral gaze
	Vitamin B_{12} deficiency	Optic nerve atrophy, blindness
	Vitamin E deficiency	Retinitis pigmentosa, visual deficits
	Copper toxicity	Kayser-Fleischer ring, sunflower cataract
Skin	Deficiencies of vitamin B_6, zinc	Seborrheic-like dermatitis
	Deficiencies of vitamin C, zinc	Impaired wound healing
	Niacin deficiency	Erythematous or scaly rash, sun exposed areas arms, legs, neck (Casal's necklace)
	Vitamin C deficiency	Perifollicular petichiae, hemhorrhage
	Vitamin K deficiency	Easy bruising
	Essential fatty acid deficiency	Dry flaky skin
	Protein-energy malnutrition	Depigmentation
	Carotinoid excess	Yellow or orange discoloration
	Deficiencies of iron, vitamin B_{12}, folate	Pallor (due to anemia)
Nails	Iron deficiency	Koilonychia (spoon-shaped nails)
	Selenium toxicity	Discolored or thickened nails
Hair	Vitamin C deficiency	Swan-neck deformity
	Protein-energy malnutrition	Discoloration, dullness, easy pluckability
	Biotin deficiency	Alopecia
	Vitamin A toxicity	Alopecia
Cardio-vascular	Thiamin deficiency	Congestive heart failure, rapid heart rate
	Selenium deficiency	Cardiomyopathy, heart failure
Gastro-intestinal	Niacin deficiency	Stomatitis, proctitis, esophagitis
Musculo-skeletal	Vitamin D deficiency	Generalized or proximal weakness, bone tenderness, fracture
	Hypophosphatemia, hypokalemia, protein-energy malnutrition, hypomagnasemia	Weakness
	Protein-energy malnutrition	Muscle wasting
	Hypocalcemia	Caropedal spasm
Neurologic	Deficiencies of vitamin B_6, E, thiamin; excess vitamin B_6	Peripheral neuropathy
	Vitamin B_{12} deficiency	Sensory neuropathy
	Deficiencies of thiamin vitamin B_6, B_{12}, niacin, biotin, hypophosphatemia, hypermagnasemia	Mental state changes, delerium
	Deficiencies of B_{12}, thiamin, niacin	Dementia

Table 26.3: Signs of nutrient deficiency and excess. From Saltzman and Mogensen (2001). Physical assessment. In: Coulston AM, Rock CL, Monsen ER (eds.) Nutrition in the Prevention and Treatment of Disease. © with permission from Elsevier.

and Lommel and Jackson (1997); only a brief summary is given below.

26.2.1 Limitations of the physical examination

The classical physical signs (Table 26.3) are detected in the general population in industrialized countries less frequently than in populations living in low-income countries. They are also found in patients who enter the hospital for surgery and in those with certain disease states or conditions that result in secondary malnutrition. In clinical medicine, the physical examination is conducted by a clinician; in community surveys, the physical examination can be undertaken by relatively junior personnel, provided that careful training in recognizing the critical signs, and ongoing supervision, is given. The physical examination as a technique for nutritional assessment has several limitations; these are discussed in the following sections.

Nonspecificity of the physical signs is a major limitation, especially in mild or moderate deficiency states. Some physical signs may be produced by more than one nutrient deficiency, as shown in Table 26.3. Examples include nasolabial seborrhea from deficiency of pyridoxine, riboflavin, or niacin; cheilosis and angular stomatitis as a result of deficiencies of riboflavin, niacin, biotin, vitamin B_6, iron; and glossitis of the tongue in deficiencies of riboflavin, niacin, folic acid, or vitamin B_{12}. Other physical signs may be caused by non-nutritional factors, such as eczema and some other allergic manifestations (e.g., follicular hyperkeratosis) and the weather (e.g., Bitot's spots), or may be, in some cases, hereditary.

Multiple physical signs may be exhibited by subjects with coexisting nutrient deficiencies confusing the diagnosis. Such coexisting nutrient deficiencies may be dietary-induced (e.g., nutritional iron and zinc deficiencies) or arise because deficiency of several nutrients may cause disturbances in the metabolic pathways of many enzyme systems, in addition to those directly requiring the nutrient as a coenzyme. Examples include folate deficiency induced by a deficiency of vitamin B_{12} as a result of a reduction in the activity of methionine synthetase (EC 2.1.1.13), an enzyme that uses methylcobalamin as a prosthetic group and is involved in the methylation cycle (Section 22.1). Likewise, severe riboflavin deficiency is often accompanied by other nutrient deficiencies. Severe deficiency may impair the metabolism of vitamin B_6 by limiting the amount of flavin mononucleotide (FMN) required by pyridoxine-5'-phosphate, and the conversion of tryptophan to functional forms of niacin (Section 20.2) (McCormick, 1989).

Signs may be two-directional — occurring during the development of a deficiency or the recovery. For example, an enlarged liver (hepatomegaly) occurs in protein-energy malnutrition and during its treatment.

Examiner inconsistencies may happen during the recording of certain lesions. For example, examiners with very limited experience may record lesions in subjects with mild or borderline evidence of the lesions. Other, more experienced, examiners may record the severe forms only. Such discrepancies have been highlighted by Detsky et al. (1994) during the performance of the physical assessment component of the Subjective Global Assessment (Section 27.2.3).

Table 26.4 presents data for the prevalence

	Examiner		
No. of Examinations	1 (1123)	2 (1127)	3 (589)
Filiform papillary atrophy	4.1	1.1	11.2
Follicular hyperkeratosis	4.0	0.6	6.8
Swollen red gums	2.8	3.7	4.1
Angular lesions	0.4	0.4	1.2
Glossitis	0.6	0.4	0.5
Goiter	3.6	6.6	3.6

Table 26.4: The prevalence, as a percentage, of selected physical signs by three examiners, Texas Nutrition Survey, 1968-1969. From McGanity (1974), with permission.

(as a percentage) of some physical signs recorded by three examiners participating in the 1968 Texas Nutrition Survey (McGanity, 1974). In this cross-sectional survey, the presence of filiform papillary atrophy ranged from 1.1% to 11.2%, according to the examiner. Generally, such inconsistencies are less when the physical signs are severe.

Examiner bias can be minimized by standardizing the criteria used to define the physical signs and by training the examiners. The U.S. Interdepartmental Committee on Nutrition for National Defense (ICNND, 1963) held standardization sessions both before and at intervals during their surveys. In these sessions, each examiner recorded, independently, their clinical findings on 100 persons. Results were compared and any inconsistencies identified. Such standardization sessions will reduce inconsistencies in observations recorded by two or more examiners or by the same examiner on different occasions.

Detsky et al. (1994) recommend that clinicians also undergo a training period involving standardization sessions on a series of patients before using the subjective global assessment tool. Subjective global assessment is designed to assess the nutritional status of hospital patients and is based exclusively on a medical history and physical examination; details are given in Section 27.2.3.

Inconsistencies also arise if the physical lesions are graded during the physical examination. For most lesions, no attempt should be made to grade the severity of the physical signs, especially in the field. Instead, signs should simply be recorded as positive or negative, except in cases where objective measurements using instruments can be used (e.g., tendon jerks or hand grip strength) (Jelliffe, 1966).

Variations in the pattern of physical signs may arise because of genetic factors, activity level, environment, dietary patterns, age, and the degree, duration, and speed of onset of malnutrition. There is no universal set of signs and symptoms suitable for all ages and all countries. Examples of the variations in the prevalence of physical signs of

Deficiency Clinical Signs	Age (Years)		
	0–6	6–16	16+
Protein-energy			
Abnormal hair (color, texture)	2.1	0.6	0.3
Iron or B vitamins			
Filiform papillary atrophy	3.3	4.4	6.2
Vitamin A			
Follicular hyperkeratosis	3.1	4.9	3.9
Vitamin D			
Enlarged wrists	2.8	—	—
Vitamin C			
Swollen, red gums	0.6	5.9	8.5
Riboflavin			
Angular lesions of tongue	1.4	0.9	0.6
Glossitis of tongue	0.4	2.0	8.3
Iodine			
Visible enlargement of thyroid	1.1	5.4	5.5

Table 26.5: Variations in the percentage prevalence of clinical signs associated with nutritional deficiencies with age. From McGanity (1974), with permission.

nutritional deficiencies with age are shown in Table 26.5. Other well known examples include the age-related clinical signs associated with vitamin D deficiency. In children, rickets (Table 26.6) occurs as a result of undermineralization of the growing skeleton, whereas in adults, osteomalacia, induced by demineralization of the adult skeleton, is evident (Zittermann, 2003).

All these limitations of the physical examination confound the diagnosis, making it essential to include laboratory tests to confirm the existence of specific nutrient deficiencies.

26.2.2 Classification and interpretation of physical signs

The World Health Organization has classified the most common physical signs into three groups: (*1*) signs indicating a probable deficiency of one or more nutrients, (*2*) signs indicating probable long-term malnutrition in combination with other factors, and (*3*) signs not related to nutritional status. Generally, in community surveys, only those signs in group 1 should be sought in the physical examination.

To assist in the interpretation, the physical signs (and symptoms) are often com-

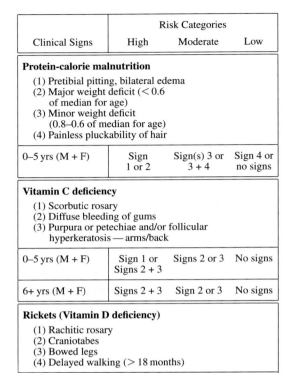

Clinical Signs	Risk Categories		
	High	Moderate	Low
Protein-calorie malnutrition			
(1) Pretibial pitting, bilateral edema			
(2) Major weight deficit (<0.6 of median for age)			
(3) Minor weight deficit (0.8–0.6 of median for age)			
(4) Painless pluckability of hair			
0–5 yrs (M + F)	Sign 1 or 2	Sign(s) 3 or 3 + 4	Sign 4 or no signs
Vitamin C deficiency			
(1) Scorbutic rosary			
(2) Diffuse bleeding of gums			
(3) Purpura or petechiae and/or follicular hyperkeratosis — arms/back			
0–5 yrs (M + F)	Sign 1 or Signs 2 + 3	Signs 2 or 3	No signs
6+ yrs (M + F)	Signs 2 + 3	Sign 2 or 3	No signs
Rickets (Vitamin D deficiency)			
(1) Rachitic rosary			
(2) Craniotabes			
(3) Bowed legs			
(4) Delayed walking (> 18 months)			
0–1 yr (M + F)	Combs. that include Signs 1 + 2	Other combs. with signs 1 + 4	All other combs.
2–5 yrs (M + F)	Signs 1 + 3	Signs 1 + 4	All other combs.

Table 26.6: Examples of the use of combinations of clinical signs in the identification of nutrient deficiencies. From Health and Welfare Canada (1973). Reproduced with permission of the Minister of Supply and Services Canada.

bined into groups associated with a particular nutrient deficiency state. Generally, for any one subject, the greater the number of signs present within a specific group, the greater the probability that the subject has a specific nutrient deficiency. The major physical signs of specific nutrient deficiencies are well established, although their sensitivity and specificity varies. In the NHANES I survey, the major physical signs characteristic of a specific nutrient deficiency were assigned to one of three risk categories (high, moderate, and low), based on their specificity. Individuals with *one* of the physical signs in the high-risk category would be considered at high risk of

developing or having a specific nutrient deficiency. A similar approach was used for the Nutrition Canada National Survey (Health and Welfare Canada, 1973), although in the latter, the risk categories were designated according to specified combinations of physical signs rather than a single sign characteristic of a specified nutrient deficiency. Examples of the combinations of the clinical signs for protein-energy malnutrition and deficiencies of vitamins C, D, and thiamin used in the Nutrition Canada National Survey are shown in Table 26.6.

26.2.3 Functional assessment

Protein-energy malnutrition and other forms of malnutrition are known to be associated with loss of immune function, muscle weakness, fatigue, impaired mobility, and cognitive dysfunction (Jeejeebhoy 1998; Windsor and Hill, 1988). Hence, increasingly, in both hospitalized patients and the institutionalized elderly, methods designed to assess such deficits in physiological, physical, and cognitive function are included as additional components of clinical assessment. Some of these tests have been described in detail in some of the earlier chapters. Examples include immune function (Section 16.5), muscle weakness assessed by voluntary hand-grip strength (Section 16.4.2), and electrical stimulation of the adductor pollicis muscle (Section 16.4.1). Respiratory muscle strength has also been used (Congleton, 1999), but studies of its relationship with malnutrition have been inconsistent (Sauleda et al., 1998; Schols et al., 1998).

In some studies, muscle function tests have been shown to be better than weight loss as a predictor of postoperative complications (Windsor and Hill, 1988). Nevertheless, their use in critically ill patients may be limited by concomitant neuromuscular blockade and illness-associated heightened sensitivity to discomfort associated with the testing, as well as the effects of medication (e.g., opiates, sedatives) (Finn et al., 1996; Corish and Kennedy, 2000). Further, the within-subject variability of these tests can be large (Brooks

Bathing Independent: Bathes self completely or requires help with hard to reach part (i.e., back). Dependent: Does not bathe self, requires assistance with more than one body party, requires assistance with getting into or out of bath or shower.

Dressing Independent: Dresses self, including getting clothes from closet or drawers and manages fastenings. Dependent: Does not dress self.

Toileting Independent: Manages toileting and hygienic activities by self. Dependent: Needs assistance getting to and using toilet or uses commode or bedpan.

Transferring Independent: Gets in and out of bed and chair without assistance. Dependent: Needs assistance getting in and out of bed and chair.

Continence Independent: Self-controlled. Dependent: Partial or total control.

Feeding Independent: Gets food from plate to mouth. Dependent: Needs assistance eating or is dependent on tube or parenteral feeding.

Box 26.1: Activities of daily living. From Chernoff, Nutrition Reviews 52: 132–136, 1994, with permission of the International Life Sciences Institute.

Use of telephone range: Uses telephone, looks up and dials numbers → Does not use telephone at all.

Shopping range: Manages shopping for all needs → Inability to shop.

Food preparation range: Plans, prepares, and serves meals → Requires meals prepared and served by someone else.

Housekeeping range: Can maintain living quarters alone → Does not perform housekeeping tasks.

Laundry range: Does own laundry → Needs laundry done by others.

Transportation range: Travels independently by public transportation or car → Does not travel at all.

Medications range: Manages dose and time of medications → Cannot manage medications.

Finances range: Manages all financial matters → Cannot handle money.

Box 26.2: Instrumental activities of daily living. From Chernoff, Nutrition Reviews, 52, 132–136, 1994, with permission of the International Life Sciences Institute.

et al., 1998). Additional concerns that hamper the use of muscle function tests such as hand grip strength specifically relate to factors such as arthritis or neuromuscular disease, and the reference data used. Age- and sex-specific reference data derived from healthy members of the population under study should be used but are seldom available. Therefore, it is not surprising that it is not yet established whether restoring muscle function with nutritional therapy improves clinical outcome (Christie and Hill, 1990; Keele et al., 1997; Klein et al., 1997).

Other functional methods involve the use of a visual analogue scale as a self-assessment measure of fatigue (Keele et al., 1997; Watters et al., 1997) or a modified version of the Norton scale (Ek and Bjurulf, 1987) to evaluate the effects of postoperative nutrition interventions on clinical outcome. The Norton scale consists of seven subscales: mental condition, activity, mobility, food intake, fluid intake, incontinence, and general physical condition.

Functional status is also of special concern among frail elderly, because of its strong correlation with nutritional status (Sullivan et al., 1993). Hence, in institutionalized elderly, self-care skills are often appraised by a questionnaire on activities of daily living, such as dressing, eating, walking, toileting and bathing (Box 26.1) (Chernoff, 1994). For independently living elderly, functional status can be assessed by a questionnaire regarding instrumental activities of daily living (Box 26.2) (Dywer et al., 1991; Chernoff, 1994). Quality of life measures can also be included, using, for example, questions from the Behavioral Risk Factor Surveillance System (BRFSS) (Keller et al., 2004). Interventions can then be designed to improve the relevant skills and quality of life or provide the necessary assistance and services.

26.3 Summary

In the past, clinical assessment consisted of a routine medical history and a physical examination, but now functional tests of immune function, muscle strength, fatigue, mobility, and cognitive function are often included. Information for the medical history can be obtained by administering a questionnaire, or from medical records, and is used in the study of the etiology of the nutrient deficiency. In the physical examination, physical signs and symptoms related to inadequate and excessive nutrition are investigated. In industrialized countries, mild or moderate (but rarely severe) nutrient deficiencies generally occur, often concomitantly with certain disease states.

Signs associated with such nutrient deficiencies are frequently not very specific and may be two-directional, occurring during both deficiency and recovery, or multiple, co-existing with other nutrient deficiencies. Examiner inconsistencies may also be a source of error, but can be minimized by training examiners and standardizing the criteria used to define the signs. In most cases, signs should be recorded as positive or negative and not in terms of grades of severity. To assist in identifying specific nutrient deficiencies, signs (and symptoms) are grouped with the combinations varying by age, race, country, and so on. Generally, the greater the number of signs present within a specific group, the larger the probability that the individual has a specific nutrient deficiency. The signs within a group are often classified into three risk categories, designated as high, moderate, and low.

Functional status is also of special concern among the frail elderly, because of its strong correlation with nutritional status. Hence, in institutionalized elderly, self-care skills are often appraised by a questionnaire on activities of daily living, such as dressing, eating, walking, toileting, and bathing. For independently living elderly, functional status can be assessed by a questionnaire regarding instrumental activities of daily living (IADLs).

References

ASPEN (American Society for Parenteral and Enteral Nutrition). (1995). Standards for nutrition support:

hospitalized patients. Nutrition in Clinical Practice 10: 208–216.

Azad N, Murphy J, Amos SS, Toppan J. (1999). Nutrition survey in a elderly population following admission to a tertiary care hospital. Canadian Medical Association 161: 511–515.

Bates CJ. (2000). Dietary supplement use at the population level: recent experience from the 1994–5 British National Diet and Nutrition Survey: people aged 65 years and over. Journal of Nutrition, Health, and Aging 4: 51–53.

Bates CJ, Prentice A, van der Pols JC, Walmsley C, Pentieva KD, Finch S, Smithers G, Clarke PC. (1998). Estimation of the use of dietary supplements in the National Diet and Nutrition Survey: people aged 65 years and over – an observed paradox and a recommendation. European Journal of Clinical Nutrition 52: 917–923.

Brooks SD, Gerstman BB, Sucher KP, Kearns PJ. (1998). The reliability of muscle function analysis using different methods of stimulation. Journal of Parenteral and Enteral Nutrition 22: 331–334.

Cerra FB. (1984). Assessment of nutritional and metabolic status. In: Pocket Manual of Surgical Nutrition. The C.V. Mosby, St Louis, pp. 24–48.

Chernoff R. (1994). Meeting the nutritional needs of the elderly in the institutional setting. Nutrition Reviews 52: 132–136.

Christie PM, Hill GL. (1990). Effect of intravenous nutrition on nutrition and function in acute attacks of inflammatory bowel disease. Gastroenterology 99: 730–736.

Coats KG, Morgan SL, Bartolucci AA, Weinsier RL. (1993). Hospital-associated malnutrition: a reevaluation 12 years later. Journal of the American Dietetic Association 93: 27–33.

Congleton J. (1999). The pulmonary cachexia syndrome: aspects of energy balance. Proceedings of the Nutrition Society 58: 321–328.

Corish CA, Kennedy NP. (2000). Protein-energy undernutrition in hospital in-patients. British Journal of Nutrition 83: 575–591.

Detsky AS, Smalley PS, Chang J. (1994). The rational clinical examination. Is this patient malnourished? Journal of the American Medical Association 271: 54–58.

Doshi MK, Lawson R, Ingoe LE, Colligan JM, Barton JR, Cobden I. (1998). Effect of nutritional supplementation on clinical outcome in postoperative orthopedic patients. Clinical Nutrition 17: 19–20.

Dwyer JT, Coletti J, Campbell D. (1991). Maximizing nutrition in the second fifty. Clinical Applied Nutrition 1: 19–31.

Edington J, Boorman J, Durrant ER, Perkins A, Giffin CV, James R, Thomson J, Oldroyd JC, Smith JC, Torrance A, Blackshaw V, Green S, Hill C, Berry C, McKenzie C, Vicca N, Ward JE, Coles SJ, (The Malnutrition Prevalence Group). (2000). Prevalence of malnutrition on admission to four hospitals in England. Clinical Nutrition 19: 191–195.

Ek AC, Bjurulf P (1987). Interrater variability in

a modified Norton scale. Scandinavian Journal of Caring Sciences 11: 99–102.

Finn PJ, Plank LD, Clark MA, Connolly AB, Hill GL. (1996). Assessment of involuntary muscle function in patients after critical injury or severe sepsis. Journal of Parenteral and Enteral Nutrition 20: 332–337.

Fowler DR, Longabaugh R. (1975). The problem-oriented record. Problem definition. Archives of General Psychiatry 32: 831–834.

Gans KM, Ross E, Barner CW, Wylie-Rosett J, McMurray J, Eaton C. (2003). REAP and WAVE: new tools to rapidly assess/discuss nutrition with patients. Journal of Nutrition 133: 556S–562S.

Gregory J, Foster K, Tyler H, Woseman M. (1990). The Dietary and Nutritional Survey of British Adults. The Stationery Office, London.

Ham RJ. (1994). The signs and symptoms of poor nutritional status. Primary Care 21: 33–54.

Hark L, Deen D Jr. (1999). Taking a nutrition history: a practical approach for family physicians. American Family Physicians 59: 1521–1528; 1531–1532.

Health and Welfare Canada. (1973). Nutrition Canada National Survey. Health and Welfare, Ottawa.

Henderson L, Gregory J, Swan G. (2002). National Diet and Nutrition Survey: Adults aged 19 to 64. Volume 1: Types and Quantities of Foods Consumed. The Stationery Office, London.

Ho LM, McGhee SM, Hedley AJ, Leong JC. (1999). The application of a computerized problem-oriented medical record system and its impact on patient care. International Journal of Medical Informatics 55: 47–59.

ICNND (Interdepartmental Committee on Nutrition for National Defense). (1963). Manual for Nutrition Surveys. 2nd ed. Superintendent of Documents, U.S. Government Printing Office, Washington, DC.

Jeejeebhoy KN. (1998). Nutritional assessment. Gastroenterology Clinics of North America 27:347–369.

Jelliffe DB. (1966). The Assessment of the Nutritional Status of the Community. WHO Monograph No. 53. World Health Organization, Geneva.

Keele AM, Bray MJ, Emery PW, Duncan HD, Silk DB. (1997). Two phase randomised controlled clinical trial of postoperative oral dietary supplements in surgical patients. Gut 40: 393–399.

Keller HH. (1993). Malnutrition in institutionalized elderly: how and why? Journal of American Geriatrics Society 41: 1212–1218.

Keller HH, Ostbye T, Goy R. (2004). Nutritional risk predicts quality of life in elderly community-living Canadians. The Journals of Gerontology. Series A. Biological and Medical Sciences 59: 68–74.

Klein S, Kinney J, Jeejeebhoy K, Alpers D, Hellerstein M, Murray M, Twomey P. (1997). Nutrition support in clinical practice: review of published data and recommendations for future research directions. American Journal of Clinical Nutrition 66: 683–706.

Kriska AM, Caspersen CJ (eds.). (1997). A collection of physical activity questionnaires for health-related research. Medicine and Science in Sports and Exercise 29: S1–S205.

Lommel LL, Jackson PL. (1997). Assessing and managing common signs and symptoms: a decision-making approach for health care providers. University of California, San Francisco.

Mason M, Welsh PK, Wenberg BG. (1982). The Dynamics of Clinical Dietetics. 2nd ed. John Wiley and Sons, New York, pp. 66–77.

McCormick DB. (1989). Two interconnected B vitamins: riboflavin and pyridoxine. Physiology Reviews 69: 1170–1198.

McGanity WJ. (1974). The clinical assessment of nutritional status. In: Hawkins WW (ed.) Assessment of Nutritional Status. Miles Symposium II. Miles Laboratories, Rexdale, Ontario, pp. 47–64.

McWhirter JP, Pennington CR. (1994). Incidence and recognition of malnutrition in hospital. British Medical Journal 308: 945–948.

Morley JE. (1998). Protein-energy malnutrition in older subjects. Proceedings of the Nutrition Society 57: 587–592.

NCHS (National Center for Health Statistics). (1994). Plan and Operation of the Third National Health and Nutrition Examination Survey, 1988–94: Vital and Health Statistics 1(32).

Papas AS, Palmer CA, Rounds MC, Russell RM. (1998) The effects of denture status on nutrition. Special Care in Dentistry 18: 17–25.

Parnell W, Scragg R, Wilson N, Schaaf D, Fitzgerald E. (2003). NZ Food NZ Children: Key Results of the 2002 National Children's Nutrition Survey. Ministry of Health, Wellington.

Potter JM, Langhorne P, Roberts M. (1998). Routine protein-energy supplementation in adults: systematic review. British Medical Journal 317: 495–501.

Pressman A, Adams A. (1990). Clinical Assessment of Nutritional Status: A Working Manual. 2nd ed. Lippincott, Williams & Wilkins.

Ruston D, Hoare J, Henderson L, Gregory J. (2004). National Diet and Nutrition Survey: Adults Aged 19 to 64. Volume 4: Nutritional Status (Anthropometry and Blood Analytes), Blood Pressure, and Physical Activity. The Stationery Office, London.

Saltzman E, Mogensen KM. (2001). Physical assessment. In: Coulston AM, Rock CL, Monsen ER (eds.) Nutrition in the Prevention and Treatment of Disease. Academic Press, San Diego, CA, pp. 43–58.

Sauleda J, Gea J, Orozco-Levi M, Corominas J, Minguella J, Aguar C, Broquetas J, Agusti AG. (1998). Structure and function relationships of the respiratory muscle. European Respiratory Journal 11: 906–911.

Schols AM, Mostert R, Soeters PB, Wouters EFM. (1998). Body composition and exercise performance in patients with chronic obstructive pulmonary disease. Thorax 46: 695–699.

Sullivan DH, Martin WE, Flaxman N, Hagen JE. (1993) Oral health problems and involuntary weight loss in a population of frail elderly. Journal of the American Geriatric Society 41: 725–731.

Sullivan DH, Sun S, Walls RC. (1999). Protein-energy undernutrition among elderly hospitalized patients: a prospective study. Journal of American Medical Association 281: 2013–2019.

Watters JM, Kirkpatrick SM, Norris SB, Shamji FM, Wells GA. (1997). Immediate postoperative enteral feeding results in impaired respiratory mechanics and decreased mobility. Annals of Surgery 226: 369–380.

Weed LJ. (1971). The problem oriented record as a basic tool in medical education, patient care and clinical research. Annals of Clinical Research 3: 131–134.

Weinsier RL, Heimburger DC. (1997). Distinguishing malnutrition from disease: the search goes on. American Journal of Clinical Nutrition 66: 1063–1064.

WHO (World Health Organization). (1963). WHO Expert Committee on Medical Assessment of Nutritional Status. WHO Technical Report Series No. 258. World Health Organization, Geneva.

Windsor JA, Hill GL. (1988). Weight loss with physiologic impairment: a basic indicator of surgical risk. Annals of Surgery 207: 290–296.

Wyszynski DF, Crivelli A, Ezquerro S, Rodriguez A. (1998). Assessment of nutritional status in a population of recently hospitalized patients. Medicina 58: 51–57.

Zittermann A. (2003). Vitamin D in preventive medicine: are we ignoring the evidence? British Journal of Nutrition 89: 552–572.

27

Nutritional assessment of hospital patients

Hospital nutritional assessment aims to precisely define the nutritional status of patients, characterize any clinically relevant malnutrition, and monitor any changes in nutritional status during nutritional support (Bozzetti, 1987). Clinically relevant malnutrition has been defined as "the state of altered nutritional status that is associated with an increased risk of adverse clinical events such as complications or death" (Dempsey and Mullen, 1987).

Nutritional assessment was introduced in clinical medicine during the 1970s, when protein and energy malnutrition of hospital patients in North America was first recognized (Blackburn et al., 1977). Even today, protein-energy malnutrition occurs in hospital patients (McWhirter and Pennington, 1994; Edington et al., 2000), notably among the elderly (Sullivan et al., 1999). However, its occurrence is less frequent than in the 1970s (Coats et al., 1993). Indeed, the prevalence of malnutrition during the course of hospitalization may have decreased (Naber et al., 1997). Such a trend is encouraging and may be associated with use by clinicians of improved technologies to provide nutritional support (Weinsier and Heimburger, 1997). Interventions now range from diet modification and counseling to specialized nutrition therapies such as enteral or parenteral nutrition (American Dietetic Association, 1995).

In the early nutritional assessment systems used in the hospital setting, the precision, sensitivity, specificity, and predictive value of the measurements included were rarely considered (Section 1.4). Today, more attention is given to these criteria when selecting the tests for nutritional assessment of hospital patients. Nonetheless, more emphasis on both the design and statistical procedures used in the development of these nutritional assessment tools is still needed (Jones, 2002).

Most of the tests assess protein-energy malnutrition because this is the type of malnutrition most prevalent in hospital patients at the present time (Corish and Kennedy, 2000). Table 27.1 presents a comprehensive list of those tests most frequently used for hospital patients. Tests may include dietary, anthropometric, static biochemical, and functional indices of nutritional status, all of which have been discussed in earlier chapters. The identification of hospital patients at risk for protein-energy malnutrition is especially difficult because many of the parameters measured in the laboratory and listed in Table 27.1 are modified by the underlying disease, making their use to identify malnutrition difficult (Weinsier and Heimburger, 1997).

In many hospitals, nutrition screening is now often routinely applied to high-risk patients, and to identify those who are at risk of becoming malnourished or who are malnourished (Dougherty et al., 1995). Indeed, studies have identified certain disease states and medical conditions associated with a high risk of secondary protein-energy and other nutrient deficiencies; these are outlined in Table 27.2.

Anthropometric measurements		
Height (cm)	Ht:	....
Weight (kg)	Wt:	....
Usual weight (kg)	US-Wt:	....
Body mass index (kg/m^2)	Wt/Ht^2	....
Sex (m/f)	SEX:	....
Ideal body weight (kg)	IBW:	....
Weight as a percentage of IBW (%)	%IBW:	....
Weight as a percentage of usual weight (%)	%US-WT:	....
Triceps skinfold (mm)	TSF:	....
Arm circumference (cm)	AC:	....
Arm muscle circumference (cm)	AMC:	....
Triceps skinfold as % of standard	%TSF:	....
Arm muscle circumference as % of standard	%AMC:	....
Biochemical determinations		
Serum albumin (g/dL)	ALB:	....
Total iron binding capacity (μg/dL)	TIBC:	....
Serum transferrin (mg/dL)	TRANS:	....
Lymphocyte count (%)	LYMPH:	....
White blood cell count (No./mm^3)	WBC:	....
Total lymphocyte count (No./mm^3)	TLC:	....
24-hour urinary urea nitrogen (g)	UUN:	....
24-hour urinary creatinine (mg)	UCR:	....
Creatinine height index as % of standard (%)	CHI:	....
Diet and nutrition status		
Protein intake (g)	PRO:	....
Caloric intake (kJ)	CAL:	....
Nitrogen balance (g)	N-BAL:	....
Obligatory nitrogen loss (g)	N-OBG:	....
Net protein utilization (apparent)	NPU:	....
Basal energy expenditure (kJ/day)	BEE:	....
Caloric intake as % of BEE (%)	%BEE:	....
Skin test results (mm)	ST:	....

Table 27.1: Nutritional and metabolic parameters commonly measured in a full nutritional assessment. Adapted from Blackburn et al., Journal of Parenteral and Enteral Nutrition 1: 11–22, 1977 © American Society for Parenteral and Enteral Nutrition, with permission.

With advance warning, appropriate nutritional support can be implemented to improve the nutritional status of patients at risk. This practice is important because there is consistent evidence that malnutrition among both medical and surgical patients is an important determinant of postoperative morbidity and mortality (Gallagher-Allred et al., 1996).

Numerous protocols have been developed for screening patients for nutritional risk, as well as for conducting a full nutritional assessment. Ideally, the screening protocols used should be simple and inexpensive and be completed by existing staff, preferably on admission of the patient to hospital. To be successful, a nutrition- screening protocol should not only identify malnutrition but also have the ability to anticipate nutritional depletion, so that its onset can be rectified or prevented before the malnutrition becomes clinically significant (Blackburn, 1995).

Some of the screening protocols are based on single anthropometric, biochemical, or functional parameters. In other protocols, the measurements have been aggregated to form multiparameter scoring systems; alternatively they are based exclusively on clinical assessment (Schneider and Hebuterne, 2000). Keller et al. (2000) provide useful guidelines for the development of a protocol for screen-

Body weight aberrations: 20% over ideal body weight; 10% under ideal body weight; more than 10% change in usual body weight in last 6 mo; inappropriate weight for height in children; deviation from normal weight gain in pregnancy

Increased metabolic needs: Fever; infection; hyperthyroidism; burns; recent surgery or soft tissue trauma; skeletal trauma; growth; corticosteroid therapy

Increased nutrient losses: Draining fistulas; open wounds; draining abscesses; effusions; chronic blood losses; chronic renal dialysis; exudative enteropathies; burns

General chronic diseases: Diabetes mellitus; hypertension; hyperlipidemia; coronary artery disease; chronic lung disease; chronic renal disease; chronic liver disease; circulatory problems or heart failure; carcinoma; mental retardation; psychosis; epilepsy; rheumatoid arthritis; peptic ulcer; prolonged comatose state

Diseases or surgery of the gastrointestinal tract: Congenital malformations; pancreatic insufficiency; malabsorption states; blind loop syndrome; severe diarrhea; gastrointestinal fistula; resection of stomach or small bowel; intestinal bypass

Medications: Insulin or other hypoglycemic agents; vitamin-mineral supplements; corticosteroids; anticoagulants; monamine oxidase inhibitors; diuretics; antacids; ethanol; oral contraceptive agents; tricyclic antidepressants; phenylhydantoin

Table 27.2: Conditions associated with an increased risk of protein-energy malnutrition. From Hooley (1986). The nutrition history and physical assessment. In: Krey SH, Murray RL (eds.) Dymanics of Nutrition Support, Assessment, Implementation, Evaluation. © Appleton-Century-Crofts, with permission.

ing nutritional risk in seniors. Examples of several screening protocols are discussed in the following sections.

Details of the parameters that are most commonly included in full nutritional assessment and listed in Table 27.1, have been outlined in earlier chapters, and hence are not discussed below. Some additional functional tests of respiratory muscle strength, wound healing, thermoregulation, fatigue, and so on may also be performed. At present, there is still no consensus on the optimal method of assessing nutritional status in hospital pa-

tients. Regardless of the parameters selected, however, some system for scoring the severity of the malnutrition should be included in the screening protocol, where possible (Dionigi et al., 1986).

27.1 Screening using a single index

Some of the parameters listed in Table 27.1 have been used as single "nutritional assessment" indices. However, their relative value and clinical importance when used individually are uncertain. Some are relatively insensitive (Section 1.4.10); for example, serum albumin and transferrin have relatively long half-lives and, hence, they respond slowly to nutritional depletion and repletion (Shetty et al., 1979). Furthermore, the measurements may be affected by non-nutritional factors that limit their sensitivity and specificity (Section 1.4.11); for example, patients with hepatic disease and nephrosis may also have reduced serum albumin and transferrin levels. Similarly, infection, trauma, immune suppression, and zinc deficiency interfere with the interpretation of delayed hypersensitivity reactivity (Golden et al., 1978). As well, these measurements often have wide confidence limits, restricting their use for individual patients (Collins et al., 1979).

For some nutritional indices, investigators have tried to quantify their clinical relevance by correlating a single measurement of the nutritional status with outcomes such as postoperative complications, morbidity, longer duration in hospital, and increased postoperative mortality. Biochemical or anthropometric measurements and sometimes functional tests are most often used for screening based on a single index; their use is discussed below.

27.1.1 Screening with a single biochemical index

Kaminski et al. (1977) were among the first investigators to demonstrate a relationship between serum transferrin and hospital mortality. Today, serum albumin is probably the most widely used single screening index of nutritional status and predictor of outcome in sick hospital patients. It performs better than most other serum proteins for identifying those patients who fail to respond to nutritional support (Dempsey et al., 1988) or who might benefit from nutritional support (Klein et al., 1997; Vanek, 1998). In a more recent study of medical and surgical Irish patients ($n = 385$), for example, a lower serum albumin value was associated ($p < 0.01$) with a longer hospital stay, reduced ability to return to home, and increased mortality (Corish, 1999). Increasingly, however, serum transthyretin, although more expensive, is also being used to predict the adequacy of nutritional support because it responds more rapidly than serum albumin (Spiekerman, 1993).

27.1.2 Screening using anthropometry

The interpretation of serum protein levels in sick hospital patients is often confounded by the underlying disease state, as noted earlier. This makes it difficult to identify patients with protein-energy malnutrition. As a result, serum protein levels are often replaced by anthropometry for nutrition screening; it is simple, cheap, and noninvasive (McWhirter and Pennington, 1994).

Preadmission and preoperative weight loss are both known to be associated with increases in postoperative complications (Klidjian et al., 1980; Windsor and Hill, 1988; Von Meyenfeldt et al., 1992), duration of hospital stay (Shaw-Stiffel et al., 1993), and postoperative mortality (Busby et al., 1980; Giner et al., 1996). Details of weight loss judged to be clinically significant in the absence of edema or ascites are given in Section 10.2.6. Alternatively, the body mass index (BMI) can be measured. In the past, a BMI of < 20 kg/m^2 has often been used as indicative of under-nutrition in clinical practice (McWhirter and Pennington, 1994), although this cutoff may be too low, especially for the elderly or overweight patients (Corish et al., 2000). Many patients with weight loss or other clinical or nutritional problems will

not be detected if a BMI < 20 kg/m^2 is the sole criterion used to determine whether patients require nutritional support (Corish and Kennedy, 2000).

27.1.3 Screening using other functional indices

The significance of relationships between the functional effects of nutritional depletion and clinical outcomes is increasingly recognized. Examples of such functional effects include muscle weakness, especially of respiratory muscle, poor wound healing, impaired thermoregulation, depression, irritability and fatigue. Physiological functional impairment is likely to occur when $< 20\%$ of body protein is lost (Hill, 1992).

Of the functional tests (Section 15.3) that are available, muscle function as measured by hand-grip strength (Section 16.4.2) appears promising as an index of nutritional status and postoperative risk (Klidjian et al., 1980; Keele et al., 1997), but requires more investigation. In patients with chronic obstructive pulmonary disease, the strength of intercostal muscles has sometimes been measured, although reported relationships with malnutrition have been conflicting (Congleton, 1999). Subjective methods involving, for example, a visual analogue scale for self-assessment of patient fatigue (Christensen et al., 1982) have sometimes been employed to assess the effects of postoperative nutrition interventions (Jensen and Hessov, 1997; Keele et al., 1997).

27.1.4 Characteristics of single-index screening protocols

Very few studies of the clinical importance of nutrition screening using a single index have analyzed the data in terms of sensitivity, specificity, predictive value, and outcome. The sensitivity and specificity of any index can be affected by the cutoff point used, as noted earlier (Section 1.4.11). For example, when the cutoff point is raised (e.g., from < 2.0 g/dL to < 3.5 g/dL for serum albumin), the sensitivity in predicting mortality changes from 20% to 82%, but specificity falls

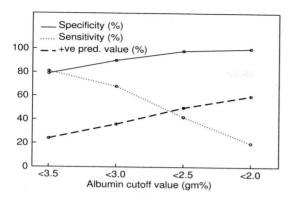

Figure 27.1: The effect of changing the cutoff point for serum albumin on the sensitivity, specificity, and predictive value of albumin as a test for predicting postoperative mortality. From Dempsey and Mullen, Journal of Parenteral and Enteral Nutrition 11: 109S–114S, 1987 © American Society for Parenteral and Enteral Nutrition, with permission.

Parameter	n	SE	SP	PV
Weight loss	46	0.86	0.69	0.72
Serum albumin	3019	0.69	0.82	0.81
Serum transferrin	229	0.77	0.39	0.48
Anergy	1738	0.52	0.86	0.82
Total lymphocyte count	857	0.76	0.62	0.63
Creatinine height index	225	0.65	0.58	0.60

Table 27.3: Single nutritional assessment parameters as predictors of mortality. Abbreviations: *n*, number of subjects; SE, sensitivity; SP, specificity; PV, predictive value. From Dempsey and Mullen, Journal of Parenteral and Enteral Nutrition 11: 109S–114S, 1987 © American Society for Parenteral and Enteral Nutrition, with permission.

from 99% to 80%. This effect is shown in Figure 27.1. The ideal index has a high specificity and a high sensitivity. Hence, to identify the best indices, sensitivity and specificity for predicting the clinical outcome of interest should always be determined.

Further, the predictive value of any index also depends on the sensitivity, specificity, and prevalence of malnutrition, as discussed in Section 1.4.13. Predictive value is the best measure of the clinical usefulness of any index of nutritional status. It can measure the ability of an index to correctly predict the presence or absence of nutrition-associated complications such as postoperative infection, septicemia, and death, or other health and nutrition outcomes such as repeated hospital admissions, duration of hospital stay, and response to a nutritional intervention.

Baker et al. (1982b) compared the ability of three single nutritional indices (serum albumin above or below 30 g/L, serum transferrin above or below 2 g/L, and delayed hypersensitivity reactivity — present or absent) to predict infection in 59 surgical patients. Their results suggested that none of these individual nutritional parameters unambiguously distinguished patients who were at high risk for infection from those who were at low risk.

Dempsey and Mullen (1987) reviewed data on the use of single nutritional assessment parameters, using mortality as the outcome measure. They calculated sensitivity, specificity, and predictive value from these data (Table 27.3) and concluded that mortality was correctly predicted by serum albumin in 81% of individuals in similar populations, whereas for serum transferrin the predictive value was only 48%.

Abnormal values for more than one parameter frequently occur in hospital patients, and no single index is completely satisfactory with regard to sensitivity and specificity. Indeed, there is still no consensus as to which index can best be applied to determine nutritional status and risk of malnutrition (Th et al., 2003). Moreover, comparisons among studies must be made with caution, because of differences in research design, study populations, and disease prevalence. In general, it appears that the predictive value of a single index for nutrition screening is uncertain.

27.2 Multiparameter screening

Recent studies have investigated the use of multiparameter indices of nutritional status in an effort to increase sensitivity and specificity and, hence, predictive value. To be effective, these multiparameter indices, often termed "scoring systems," must be easy to use; cost-effective; and tested for reproducibility, validity, sensitivity, and specificity (Keller et al., 2000; Jones, 2002). Unfortunately, the statistical procedures used to establish the reproducibility and validity of these multi-parameter indices have not always been appropriate. Further, the performance of the indices has not always been tested by health professionals (e.g., physicians, dietitians, or nurses) who were the intended administrators of the tests (Jones, 2002).

Currently, there is no universally accepted multiparameter scoring system of nutritional status. Some systems have been developed to help clinicians decide when specialized nutrition therapy is required (e.g., Prognostic Nutritional Index and Nutritional Risk Index); others predict patients at high risk of developing complications (e.g., Subjective Global Assessment). In some cases, multiparameter scoring systems have been developed specifically to detect malnutrition in elderly patients (e.g., Mini Nutritional Assessment), because some of the other tests are unsuitable (Naber et al., 1997). Examples of multiparameter scoring systems used for nutritional assessment in hospitalized patients are given in Table 27.4; they are discussed in more detail in the following sections.

27.2.1 Prognostic Nutritional Index

The Prognostic Nutritional Index (PNI) was developed by Mullen et al. (1979) to identify those nutritional indices most highly correlated with clinically relevant malnutrition. Researchers examined a series of nutritional assessment parameters, measured on admission in a group of non-emergency surgical patients ($n = 161$). The parameters measured included weight, percentage of weight loss, serum albumin, serum transferrin, total protein, mid-upper-arm muscle circumference, triceps skinfold, total lymphocyte count, delayed hypersensitivity reactivity (assessed using mumps, *Candida*, and streptokinase-streptodornase antigens), selected demographic data (e.g., age, sex, race), and diagnosis. After nutritional assessment, all patients underwent a major surgical procedure, and their clinical course was monitored for objective complications until discharge or death.

Discriminant function analysis and stepwise multiple regression were used to se-

lect those parameters most highly correlated with surgical outcome. The four parameters included in the PNI were serum albumin, serum transferrin, triceps skinfold and delayed hypersensitivity reactivity (DHR). The PNI indicates the risk, expressed as a percentage, of postoperative morbidity and mortality in an individual patient:

$$PNI(\%) = 158 - (16.6 \times ALB) - (0.78 \times TSF) \\ - (0.2 \times TFN) - (5.8 \times DHR)$$

where ALB = serum albumin concentrations (g/dL), TSF = triceps skinfold (in mm), TFN = transferrin (g/dL), and DCH = delayed hypersensitivity (grade of reactivity to any of the three antigens: mumps, streptokinase-streptodornase, *Candida*, all graded 0: nonreactive; 1: < 5 mm induration; 2: > 5 mm induration).

The validity of this model was then tested prospectively on a heterogeneous group of patients undergoing non-emergency gastrointestinal surgery ($n = 100$) (Busby et al., 1980). In these studies, the PNI was calculated before surgery, and patients were classified according to the risk of complications (low-risk PNI, < 40%; intermediate-risk PNI, 40% to 50%; high-risk PNI, > 50%). Patients were then followed until discharge or death, and monitored for postsurgical complications by an observer not involved in the patient care and with no knowledge of the predicted outcome. The accuracy of the PNI model for predicting the occurrence of complications was assessed by comparing the predicted risk of complications with the actual occurrences. The results, shown in Figure 27.2, demonstrate that the incidence of complications and death generally increased with an increase in PNI; those patients identified as high risk by the PNI did indeed have a significantly increased risk of complications, sepsis, and mortality, compared with those identified as low risk.

In terms of sensitivity, specificity, and predictive value, when the cutoff point for an abnormal PNI was taken as > 50%, the index predicted mortality with a sensitivity of 86%, a specificity of 69%, and a predictive value of 72%. Changing the cutoff point of the PNI from > 50% to > 40%, increased the sensi-

System and variables measured	Comment
Prognostic Nutritional Index (Busby et al., 1980): Serum albumin, transferrin, triceps skinfold, delayed hypersensitivity reactivity	Impractical and expensive for routine preoperative assessment; designed for surgical patients.
Nutrition Risk Index (Veterans Affairs Total Parenteral Nutrition Cooperative Study Group, 1991): Percentage weight loss from normal; current serum albumin	The factors that affect the components of this score affect the score result; designed for surgical patients.
Mini Nutritional Assessment: Original consisted of 18 items grouped into four components: anthropometric, general, dietary, subjective assessment (Guigoz et al., 1994). New two-step version for low-risk populations (Rubenstein, 1998). Step I (screening): 6 items — 3 min to complete. If initial screening score is ≤ 11, then proceed to Step II (assessment) with 12 items. Add score for I and II: total score 17–23.4: risk of malnutrition; < 17, malnutrition.	Developed specifically for detecting malnutrition in elderly patients.
Subjective Global Assessment (Detsky et al., 1987): Percentage weight loss from normal; duration and degree of abnormal dietary intake (starvation, hypocaloric fluids; liquid diet, suboptimal solid diet), gastrointestinal symptoms (anorexia, vomiting, diarrhea, nausea); functional capacity (bedridden to full capacity); disease state, physical examination (loss of fat and muscle, presence of edema or ascites).	Large subjective element to assessment; need specialized training; technique more suitable for medical staff; designed for surgical patients.

Table 27.4: Multiparameter scoring systems used for nutritional assessment in hospitalized patients.

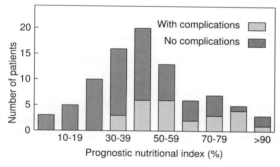

Figure 27.2: Distribution of gastrointestinal surgical patients with and without complications as a function of the prognostic nutritional index (PNI). From Mullen (1981). Reproduced with permission from Clinical Consultations in Nutritional Support, Vol. 1, No. 1, 1981, Medical Directions, Inc., Chicago, IL.

tivity to 93%, but, as expected, decreased the specificity to 44% and lowered the predictive value for mortality to 51%.

The use of the PNI model for the prospective identification of patients who would benefit from preoperative support has also been tested using both prospective nonrandomized and randomized intervention studies in adult surgical patients (Mullen et al., 1980) and patients with gastrointestinal cancer (Muller et al., 1982), respectively. In both studies, those patients classified as high risk on the basis of a PNI $> 50\%$ benefited from preoperative support, as indicated by a significant reduction in mortality when compared with those patients with a PNI $< 50\%$.

Nevertheless, several limitations of the PNI have been identified. Subsequent studies have failed to show that the PNI predicts the outcome of patients with acute abdominal trauma (Jones et al., 1983). In addition, it may not be appropriate for predicting survival in patients who do not undergo surgery. Furthermore, the PNI does not give information about the type of nutritional abnormalities.

The indices selected for inclusion in the PNI have also been criticized because serum albumin and transferrin are not independent of one another, an assumption of stepwise multiple regression procedures. Moreover, the indices selected may be affected by nonnutritional factors, as noted in Section 27.1. Hence, it becomes very difficult to separate the effects of an actual nutrient deficiency from those of the disease process on the basis of the measurements (Baker et al., 1982b). Indeed, Pettigrew and Hill (1986) suggested that the PNI offers no advantage over simple measurements of plasma protein levels in predicting risk of postoperative complications.

27.2.2 Nutritional Risk Index

The Nutritional Risk Index (NRI) was developed by the Veterans Affairs Total Parenteral Nutrition Cooperative Study Group (1991) for use in their clinical trial evaluating the efficacy of perioperative total parenteral nutrition in malnourished patients undergoing major abdominal or thoracic surgery. It uses serum albumin and present weight compared with usual weight:

$$NRI = (1.519 \times ALB)$$
$$+ (41.7 \times (present\ weight\ /\ usual\ weight))$$

where: ALB = serum albumin (g/L). An NRI > 100, no malnutrition; NRI = 97.5–100, mild malnutrition; NRI = 83.5 –97.5, moderate malnutrition; NRI < 83.5, severe malnutrition. Usual weight is generally defined as the stable weight > 6 mo before admission.

The NRI has been used to define nutritional risk in several studies. For example, the NRI was reported to be sensitive and specific and a positive predictor for identifying patients at risk for complications in a study of malnourished patients ($n = 396$) who required laparotomy or noncardiac thoracotomy. When compared with Subjective Global Assessment (SGA) (Section 27.2.3), the performance of NRI for detecting those severely malnourished patients who should receive perioperative total parenteral nutrition, was better, as shown in Figure 27.3.

Nevertheless, one of the limitations of the NRI as a screening tool is that it relies on current and previous body weight. These measurements are affected by a relative increase in total body water in patients with hepatic, renal, or cardiac disease (Corish, 1999). In addition, caution is needed when self-reported weight is used as the basis of current and usual weight for the NRI. There have been several reports of failures to report current weights accurately, especially among undernourished and obese patients (Doyle et al., 1998). As well, the confounding effect

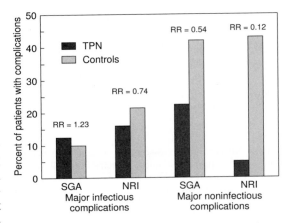

Figure 27.3: Effect of perioperative total parenteral nutrition in severely malnourished patients as assessed by Subjective Global Assessment (SGA) versus Nutrient Risk Index (NRI). RR, relative risk. Data from the Veterans Affairs Total Parenteral Nutrition Cooperative Study Group (1991).

of stress on serum albumin concentrations is also a recognized limiting factor (Klein, 1990).

27.2.3 Subjective Global Assessment

The usefulness of performing objective measurements of nutritional assessment in hospital patients has been questioned in view of the confounding effects of the disease process on many of the measurements, as noted earlier. The Subjective Global Assessment (SGA) method (Table 27.5) is an alternative method of nutritional assessment based exclusively on a carefully performed medical history and physical examination. No anthropometric or laboratory indices are included.

Five features are emphasized in the medical history component: (*1*) weight change, (*2*) changes in dietary intake, (*3*) presence of gastrointestinal symptoms, (*4*) functional capacity or energy level (bedridden to full capacity), and (*5*) the metabolic demands of the patient's underlying disease state. Both the extent of the weight loss and the rate and pattern of weight loss are considered. Dietary intake is classified as normal or abnormal, with the duration and degree of abnormal intake being recorded. The presence of gastrointestinal symptoms, classified as

HISTORY: Weight loss in past 6 months:		......kg	% loss ......
Change in past 2 weeks:	increase ☐	no change ☐	decrease ☐

Dietary changes: no changes ☐   changes ☐   duration...wk
If changes indicate type:
suboptimal solid diet ☐   full liquid diet ☐
hypocaloric liquids ☐   starvation ☐

Gastrointestinal symptoms (persisting for more than 2 weeks)   none ☐
     nausea ☐   vomiting ☐   diarrhea ☐   anorexia ☐

Functional capacity   none ☐   dysfunction ☐   duration ...
     working suboptimally ☐   ambulatory ☐   bedridden ☐

Disease and its relation to nutritional requirements
Primary diagnosis ....
....
Metabolic demand:
     no stress ☐   low stress ☐   modest stress ☐   high stress ☐

PHYSICAL: For each trait specify: 0 = normal, 1 = mild, 2 = moderate, 3 = severe
loss of subcutaneous fat (triceps,chest) ...   ankle edema...
muscle wasting (quadriceps, deltoids) ...   sacral edema ...   ascites ...

SGA rating (select one)	well nourished ☐	moderately nourished ☐	severely malnourished ☐

Table 27.5: Components of subjective global assessment. From Detsky et al., Journal of Parenteral and Enteral Nutrition 11: 8–13, 1987 © American Society for Parenteral and Enteral Nutrition, with permission.

anorexia, nausea, vomiting, and diarrhea, is also noted if they persist on a daily basis for more than 2 wk. Intermittent diarrhea or vomiting is not included, although vomiting that occurs secondary to obstruction, once or twice daily, is recorded. The fourth feature of the medical history concerns the functional capacity or energy level of the patient, noted in relation to both degree of dysfunction (i.e., bedridden to full capacity) and duration. The final feature of the history considers the metabolic demands or stress associated with the underlying disease state of the patient and categorizes the degree of stress as high, moderate, or low.

The physical examination of the SGA also emphasizes five features: (*1*) loss of subcutaneous fat, (*2*) muscle wasting, (*3*) presence of edema in the ankles, (*4*) presence of edema in the sacral region, and (*5*) presence of ascites. Each of these features is classified as normal (0), mild (1+), moderate (2+), or severe (3+). The presence of coexisting disease states such as congestive heart failure and neurological deficits is also taken into consideration when grading edema and muscle wasting, respectively.

Physicians assign an SGA rank for each patient's nutritional status, based on the features emphasized in the history and physical examination. The SGA rank is assigned on the basis of subjective weighting, using particularly the variables weight loss, poor dietary intake, loss of subcutaneous tissue, and muscle wasting. A rigid scoring system based on a numerical weighting is not used.

The SGA rank can be one of three categories: (*1*) well nourished, (*2*) moderate or suspected malnutrition, and (*3*) severe malnutrition; the rank is used to predict a patient's risk for medical complications. A more detailed description of the method of rating can be found in Detsky et al. (1987). Note that nursing staff are unlikely to be able to carry out the physical examination included in the SGA, without additional training.

The validity of the SGA has been established by (a) the presence of significant correlations of objective nutritional assessment (both anthropometric and laboratory measurements) and three measures of hospital morbidity (the incidence of infection, the use of antibiotics, and the length of hospital stay) (Baker et al., 1982a); (b) the absence of any significant differences between the number of patients classified as malnourished on the basis of SGA compared with objective assessment techniques (Detsky et al., 1984); and (c) the ability of SGA to predict the tendency to develop an infection in general surgical patients (Baker et al., 1982b).

Subjective Global Assessment also appears to be a good predictor of complications in several prospective studies on a wide variety of other hospital patients. These have included those receiving dialysis (Enia et al., 1993) and liver transplants (Pikul et al., 1994). As well, in a study of HIV-infected adults, SGA was reported to detect a worsening of nutritional status and serve as a basis for prescribing parenteral nutrition (Niyongabo et al., 1999).

Nonetheless, other investigators have suggested that inclusion of some objective indices with the SGA may be advisable (Pettigrew et al., 1984), especially for detecting less advanced cases of protein-energy malnutrition. For example, inclusion of serum albumin, delayed hypersensitivity reactivity, and creatinine-height index with SGA increased the ability to identify patients who developed complications from 82% to 90%, although the proportion of patients identified as "malnourished" but who did not develop a postoperative complication was also increased (from 25% to 30%) (Detsky et al., 1984). Kalantar-Zadeh et al. (1999), in a study of hemodialysis patients, concluded that a modified SGA which included three laboratory parameters (total iron-binding capacity, serum albumin, and total serum protein) was needed to assess their nutritional status more reliably.

Finally, one of the major limitations of the SGA is that it is subjective, and its reproducibility depends on the training and experience of the examiners. In a study of general surgical patients ($n = 59$), two experienced examiners agreed on the nutritional status, as indicated by a SGA rating, in 81% of the cases (Baker et al., 1982a); with the gastrointestinal surgical patients, the percentage agreement was 91% (Detsky et al., 1987). However, in a study of newly admitted geriatric patients ($n = 90$), the between-observer reproducibility of the SGA ratings was poor. Of these geriatric patients, 30% were judged to be malnourished upon admission based on objective criteria. When using SGA, however, the clinician judged 6.7% and 45.5% of the patients to be severely and moderately malnourished, compared with 21.1% and 26.7%, respectively, by the researcher (Ek et al., 1996). It appears, therefore, that SGA is probably most suited for use by clinicians; nursing staff would probably require considerable training before they could carry out the physical examination required. Therefore, implementing SGA as a routine nutritional screening tool in a large hospital may be impractical (Reilly, 1996).

27.2.4 Mini Nutritional Assessment

The Mini Nutritional Assessment (MNA) was developed specifically for detecting malnutrition in elderly patients (Guigoz et al., 1994), because of the poor performance of many of the other multiparameter indices in this age group (Naber et al., 1997). Barone et al. (2003), for example, concluded that the MNA was better able than the SGA to identify severely malnourished patients over 65 y, and can be used for detecting malnutrition among the elderly in hospitals, in general practice, in nursing home admissions, and home-care patients (Soini et al., 2004).

The original form used for the MNA consisted of 18 items grouped into four components: anthropometric assessment (weight, height, and weight loss); general assessment (lifestyle, medication, and mobility); dietary assessment (number of meals, food and fluid intake, and autonomy of feeding); and subjective assessment (self perception of health and nutrition). It could be used by relatively untrained personnel, and took < 20 min to

Mini Nutritional Assessment — I. Screening	**N Mode of feeding.** 0 = unable to eat without assistance; 1 = self-fed with some difficulty; 2 = self-fed without any problem ☐

Mini Nutritional Assessment — I. Screening

Name _____ Sex ___ Date_____
Age _____ Weight (kg) _____ Height (cm) _____

A **Has food intake declined** over the past three months due to loss of appetite, digestive problems, chewing or swallowing difficulties? 0 = severe loss of appetite, 1 = moderate loss of appetite, 2 = no loss of appetite ☐

B **Weight loss** over past three months? 0 = weight loss > 3 kg; 1 = does not know; 2 = weight loss of 1–3 kg; 3 = no weight loss ☐

C **Mobility** 0 = bed or chair bound; 1 = able to get out of bed/chair but does not go out; 2 = goes out ☐

D **Psychological stress or acute disease** suffered in the past three months. 0 = yes; 2 = no ☐

E **Neuropsychological problems** 0 = severe dementia or depression; 1 = mild dementia; 2 = no psychological problems ☐

F **Body Mass Index (BMI)** 0 = BMI < 19; 1 = BMI 19 to < 21; 2 = BMI 21 to < 23; 3 = BMI $\geqslant$ 23 ☐

Total Screening Score (Max. = 14 points) $\geqslant$ 12 points = normal, not at risk, no need to continue assessment; $\leqslant$ 11 points = possible malnutrition. Continue below with II: Assessment. ☐

Mini Nutritional Assessment — II. Assessment

G **Lives independently.** (Not in nursing home or hospital). 0 = no; 1 = yes ☐

H **Prescription drugs** taken (More than three drugs per day?). 0 = yes; 1 = no ☐

I **Pressures sores or skin ulcers.** 0 = yes; 1 = no ☐

J **Full meals.** How many per day? 0 = 1 meal; 1 = 2 meals; 2 = 3 meals ☐

K **Protein intake.** (a) At least one serving of dairy products (milk, cheese, yogurt per day (Yes/No)? (b) Two or more servings of legumes or eggs per week (Yes/No). (c) Meat, fish, or poultry every day (Yes/No). 0.0 = if 0 or 1 yes; 0.5 = if 2 yes; 1.0 = if 3 yes ☐

L **Fruits or Vegetables** Consumes two or more servings per day? 0 = no; 1 = yes ☐

M **Fluids.** Consumption of water, juice, coffee, tea, or milk per day 0.0 = < 3 cups; 0.5 = 3–5 cups; 1.0 > 5 cups ☐

N **Mode of feeding.** 0 = unable to eat without assistance; 1 = self-fed with some difficulty; 2 = self-fed without any problem ☐

O **Self view of nutritional status.** 0 = views self as being malnourished; 1 = is uncertain of nutritional state; 2 = views self as having no nutritional problems ☐

P **Health status.** In comparison with others in the same age group, how do they view their health? 0 = not as good; 0.5 = does not know; 1.0 = as good; 2.0 = better ☐

Q **Mid-upper-arm circumference.** (MUAC) in cm 0 = MUAC < 21; 0.5 = MUAC 21–22; 1 = MUAC $\geqslant$ 22 ☐

R **Calf circumference.** (CC) in cm 0 = CC < 31; 1 = CC $\geqslant$ 31 ☐

I. Screening Score ☐

II. Assessment Score ☐

Total Malnutrition Indicator Score (max 30 points)
17–23.5 points— at risk of malnutrition
Less than 17 points — malnourished ☐

Table 27.6: Mini Nutritional Assessment. I Screening and II Assessment. Adapted from Murphy et al., European Journal of Clinical Nutrition 54: 555–562, 2000 © with permission of the Nature Publishing Group.

complete. The final total score was used to classify patients as normal, at risk of malnutrition, or undernourished. This original 18-item version is best used with at-risk or ill elderly with a high likelihood of malnutrition.

The original MNA gave a maximum score of 30 and was extensively validated in studies on more than 600 elderly from Toulouse, France and New Mexico, USA varying from frail to healthy elderly (Garry et al., 1982; Guigoz et al., 1994,1996; Vellas et al., 2000).

A new two-step version of the MNA is also available: it is shown in Table 27.6. This version consists of an initial section (Step I: Screening) comprised of six items, followed by a more detailed nutritional assessment of subjects who score $\leqslant$ 11 on the initial screen (Step II: Assessment). Subjects are classified as malnourished with a final total malnutrition indicator score of < 17 and at risk of malnutrition with a score 17–23.5. This new two-step version of the MNA is especially useful in low-risk populations, and the screening section takes only 3 min to administer (Rubenstein, 1998).

Murphy et al. (2000) evaluated the use of the new two-step version of MNA on 49 elderly U.K. hospitalized orthopedic female patients and confirmed its use as a diagnostic tool for identifying elderly patients at risk from malnutrition and those who are already malnourished. Guigoz et al. (2002) also evaluated this version in community-dwelling elderly, and concluded that MNA detects risk of malnutrition and lifestyle characteristics associated with nutritional risk, even when serum albumin and BMI are within the normal range. In a Swiss study of patients $\geqslant 70\,$y ($n = 166$) admitted to a geriatric department, an MNA score of < 17 was associated with higher costs of care and a longer hospital stay (Quadri et al., 1999).

Nevertheless, further studies are needed to establish whether the two-step version of the MNA is an effective tool for monitoring response to treatment, as well as the relationship between the MNA score and clinical outcome of elderly medical or surgical patients.

27.2.5 Nutritional scores for use by nurses

Several tools that can be used by nursing staff or registered dietitians to screen large numbers of patients on admission who are potentially at nutritional risk for malnutrition have been developed. They include the Registered Nurses Nutritional Risk Classification (RNNRC), and the Nursing Nutritional Screening Form (NNSF).

The RNNRC was developed by Kovacevich et al. (1997) and is shown in Table 27.7. The RNNRC is based on the U.S. nursing admission assessment form, modified to include questions about weight loss history, percentage of ideal body weight, and alterations in dietary intake and gastrointestinal functions. The items listed must be completed in a fixed order within 48 h of a patient's admission, then scored by both nurses and a

---

A. Diagnosis *If the patient has one or more of the following, circle and proceed to section E to assess the patient's nutritional risk.*
Anorexia nervosa, bulimia nervosa; malabsorption (celiac sprue, ulcerative colitis, Crohn's disease, short bowel syndrome); Multiple trauma (closed head injury, penetrating trauma, multiple fractures); Decibitus ulcers; Major gastrointestinal surgery within the past year; Cachexia (temporal wasting, muscle wasting, cancer, cardiac disease); Coma; Diabetes; end-stage liver disease; end-stage renal disease; nonhealing wounds.

B. Nutrition History *If the patient has one or more of the following, circle and proceed to section E to assess the patient's nutritional risk.*
Diarrhea ($>500\,$ml $\times 2\,$days; Vomiting ($>5\,$d). Reduced intake ($<$ one-half normal intake for $>5\,$d.)

C. Ideal Body Weight Standards *Compare the patient's current weight for height to the ideal body weight for the appropriate height and sex. If $\leqslant 80\%$ of ideal body weight, proceed to section E to consider the patient at nutritional risk and stop here.*

D. Weight History
Any recent unplanned weight loss (No/Yes) ___ Amount (kg) ___ If yes, within the past ___ weeks or ___ months. Current weight (kg) ___ Usual weight (kg) ___ Height (cm) ___. Percentage weight loss (%) ___. Weight loss is significant if, over the indicated period, it is within the limits specified, and severe if it exceeds these limits. 1 week (1%–2% loss); 2–3 weeks (2%–3% loss); 1 month (4%–5% loss); 3 months (7%–8% loss); 5+ months (10% loss). *If the patient has experienced significant or severe weight loss, proceed to section E to assess the patient's nutritional risk.*

E. Nurse Assessment. Using the above criteria, what is the patients nutritional risk? (circle one) Low nutrition risk OR At nutritional risk.

Table 27.7: Registered Nurses Nutritional Risk Classification. From Schneider and Hebuterne, Nutrition Reviews, 58, 31–38, 2000.

dietitian. After completion of the screening tool, nurses classify patients as at nutritional risk or low nutritional risk.

The reproducibility of the RNNRC was established in a prospective study in which the classification of 186 consecutive adult admissions by staff registered nurses and a

	A	B	C	Score
Weight change	< 10%	10%–20%	> 20%	
Clinical appearance	Good	Moderate	Poor	
Appetite[a]	Good	Moderate	Poor	
Food intake: restrictions	None	Support needed	Starvation	
Diarrhea, nausea, vomiting	Little	Regular	Continuous	
Seriousness of illness, treatment, intervention	Mild	Moderate	Severe	

Table 27.8: Nursing Nutritional Screening Form for the classification of the risk of malnutrition or actual malnutrition. Each item is separately scored as normal (A), moderate (B), or severe (C). If all items are answered with an A, the patient is considered not to be at risk of malnutrition. If a B or C is entered more than once, the patient is potentially at risk of malnutrition. [a]Scored as A during complete enteral or parenteral feeding. From Th et al., British Journal of Nutrition 90: 829–836, 2003, with permission of the authors.

nutritionist was compared (Kovacevich et al., 1997). The agreement was reported to be 97.3%, and the sensitivity was 84.6%. These measures of agreement were, however, based on a test of proportions (i.e., the chi-square goodness-of-fit test), and not the kappa statistic or intraclass correlation recommended earlier (Section 6.3.5) (Jones, 2002). Validity of the RNNRC was assessed by calculating sensitivity and specificity, using serum transthyretin levels (low or normal) as the "gold standard." Serum transthyretin is itself influenced by the presence and severity of illness, thus limiting the interpretation of these results.

A second method developed to allow nursing staff to detect malnourished patients or patients at risk of malnutrition at an early stage of their hospitalization is the Nursing Nutritional Screening Form (NNSF) (Th et al., 2003). The NNSF was developed by a panel of experts, nurses, dietitians, and clinicians and consists of five clinical variables shown in Table 27.8, each of which can be scored as normal–mild (A), moderate (B), or severe (C). A patient is considered potentially at risk of malnutrition if the dietitian agrees with a B or C score based on the assessment of the nurses. Patients are classified as actually malnourished if a weight loss of > 10% and an energy intake of < 75% of that required is established. Nurses require no special training to score the items on the NNSF.

The reproducibility of the NNSF was assessed in two phases: first on 69 patients by pairs of nurses, dietitians, and clinicians and then, after some modification to certain items, again on 40 patients. The extent of agreement was tested by Cohen's kappa statistic. The validity of the NNSF was also evaluated by applying the opinion of the dietitian as the "gold standard," although such an assessment is not appropriate as a criterion validation (Keller et al., 2002).

27.3 The prognostic value of multi-parameter scoring systems

All of the considerations discussed in relation to the design of nutritional assessment systems in Section 1.3 are also applicable when selecting and evaluating hospital multiparameter scoring systems. Such considerations include study objectives, sampling protocols, validity, reproducibility, random and systematic measurement errors, accuracy, sensitivity, specificity, and predictive value. The ideal multiparameter scoring systems are those that are accurate markers of nutritional status, accurate predictors of outcome, and easily monitored during nutritional repletion (Bozzetti, 1987). Care must be taken to ensure that the reproducibility and validity of the multiparameter scoring systems are established prior to use with procedures based on appropriate sample sizes, designs, and statistical analysis (Jones, 2002). Where possible, validity should be assessed by comparison with a gold standard or criterion method, although in practice such a method is not

Patient group (Reference)	n	Method of assessment	Critical outcome in high-risk group
Elective gastrointestinal surgery (Busby et al., 1980)	100	Prognostic nutritional index	Increased postoperative complications, major sepsis, and mortality
General surgery (Haydock and Hill, 1986)	68	Percentage weight loss from normal, BMI, MAC, TSF, serum albumin, transferrin, transthyretin	Impaired wound healing response
Gastrointestinal surgery (Detsky et al., 1987)	202	Subjective global assessment	67% suffered major postoperative complications vs. 10% overall
Cardiac valve replacement (Sagar and MacFie, 1994)	936	BMI	Increased risk of major and septic complications
Elderly (Potter et al., 1995)	69	BMI, MAMA	Increased mortality and rate of discharge to residential care, decreased ability to go home.
Elderly (Muhlethaler et al., 1995)	219	Weight, MAMA	Decreased overall survival and ability to live at home.
Fractured femur (Lumbers et al., 1996)	60	Weight, TSF, MAMC, serum albumin, hemoglobin	Increased length of convalescence and dependence on walking frames
Intensive care (Giner et al., 1996)	129	Serum albumin, weight:height ratio	Increased complication rate, length of stay and "not discharged"

Table 27.9: Effects of poor nutritional status on clinical outcome in hospitalized patients. BMI, body mass index; MAC, mid-arm circumference; TSF, triceps skinfold thickness; MAMA, mid-arm muscle area; MAMC, mid-arm muscle circumference. From Corish and Kennedy, British Journal of Nutrition 83: 575–591, 2000, with permission of the Nutrition Society.

always available, and surrogate measures are often used (Keller et al., 2000).

For the adequate evaluation of any multiparameter screening protocol, the performance of the protocol must be evaluated in relation to its intended purpose, by health professionals who are similar to the intended administrators of the test. All too often, a screening tool may be used in a capacity that far exceeds that for which it was originally intended (Jensen et al., 2001). In addition, the screening protocols should be conducted on well-nourished subjects and on patients (well-nourished and malnourished) with other diseases, to try to establish the effects of nutritional and non-nutritional factors on the test result (Dempsey and Mullen, 1987). Moreover, as well as correlating the test measurements with clinical outcomes, including postoperative morbidity and mortality, their ability to predict other important health and nutrition outcomes should also be tested. Examples include prediction of

future hospital admissions, response to nutrition therapy, and other outcomes listed in Table 27.9.

There is an urgent need to ensure that protocols for nutritional screening based on single and multiparameter indices, as well as on nutritional assessment of hospital patients, are developed and evaluated using procedures based on good design and statistical practice (Keller et al., 2000; Jones, 2002).

27.4 Summary

The objectives of nutritional assessment of hospital patients are to accurately define the nutritional status of the patient, to define clinically relevant malnutrition, and to monitor any changes in nutritional status during nutritional support. Generally, nutritional assessment is routinely applied to high-risk patients using single or multiparameter scoring systems. A single static biochemical, anthropometric, or functional index can be used. The sensitivity, specificity, and predictive value of a single index such as serum transferrin, serum albumin, or delayed hypersensitivity reactivity is low because of the confounding effects of non-nutritional factors. To increase their predictive value, multiparameter scoring systems have been developed. Some of these are designed to be prognostic of health outcomes and thus provide information that can help clinicians decide when specialized nutrition therapy is needed. Examples include the prognostic nutritional index (PNI), the Nutrition Risk Index, and the Mini Nutritional Assessment (MNA) tool, developed specifically to determine malnutrition in elderly patients. Several tools have also been developed for use by registered nurses to assess hospitalized patients within 48 h of their admission. Examples include the Registered Nurses Nutritional Risk Classification and the Nursing Nutritional Screening Form (NNSF).

Because the interpretation of many of the laboratory indices is confounded by the effects of the disease process, an approach based exclusively on a medical history and physical examination has been developed. This technique, the Subjective Global Assessment, is able to provide a valid and reproducible prediction of morbidity in surgical patients, but it must be performed by a physician because of its subjective nature. All of the multiparameter scoring systems must be tested in well-nourished subjects and in well-nourished and malnourished patients with other diseases before their sensitivity, specificity, and predictive value can be firmly established. Such tests must be undertaken by the intended administrator of the scoring system. There is an urgent need to ensure that protocols for both nutritional screening and nutritional assessment of hospital patients are developed and evaluated using procedures based on good design and statistical practice.

References

American Dietetic Association. (1995). Position of the American Dietetic Association: cost-effectiveness of medical nutrition therapy. Journal of the American Dietetic Association 95: 88–91.

Baker JP, Detsky AS, Wesson DE, Wolman SL, Stewart S, Whitewell J, Langer B, Jeejeebhoy K. (1982a). Nutritional assessment: a comparison of clinical judgment and objective measurements. New England Journal of Medicine 306: 969–972.

Baker JP, Detsky AS, Whitewell J, Langer B, Jeejeebhoy KN. (1982b). A comparison of the predictive value of nutritional assessment techniques. Human Nutrition: Clinical Nutrition 36C: 233–241.

Barone L, Milosavljevic M, Gazibarich B. (2003). Assessing the older person: is the MNA a more appropriate nutritional assessment tool than the SGA? Journal of Nutrition, Health and Aging 7: 13–17.

Blackburn GL. (1995). Skeleton in the hospital closet: then and now. Nutrition 11(Suppl): 193–195.

Blackburn GL, Bistrian BR, Maini BS, Schlamm HT, Smith MF. (1977). Nutritional and metabolic assessment of the hospitalized patient. Journal of Parenteral and Enteral Nutrition 1: 11–22.

Bozzetti F. (1987). Nutritional assessment from the perspective of a clinician. Journal of Parenteral and Enteral Nutrition 11: 115S–121S.

Busby GP, Mullen JL, Matthews DC, Hobbs CL, Rosato EF. (1980). Prognostic nutritional index in gastrointestinal surgery. American Journal of Surgeons 139: 160–167.

Christensen T, Bendix T, Kehlet H. (1982). Fatigue and cardio-respiratory function following abdominal surgery. British Journal of Surgery 69: 417–419.

Coats KG, Morgan SL, Bartolucci AA, Weinsier RL. (1993). Hospital-associated malnutrition: a reevaluation 12 years later. Journal of the American Dietetic Association 93: 27–33.

Collins JP, McCarthy ID, Hill GL. (1979). Assessment of protein nutriture in surgical patients: the value of anthropometrics. American Journal of Clinical Nutrition 32: 1527–1530.

Congleton J. (1999). The pulmonary cachexia syndrome: aspects of energy balance. Proceedings of the Nutrition Society 58: 321–328.

Corish CA. (1999). Pre-operative nutritional assessment. Proceedings of the Nutrition Society 58: 821–829.

Corish CA, Kennedy NP. (2000). Protein-energy undernutrition in hospital inpatients. British Journal of Nutrition 83: 575–591.

Corish CA, Flood P, Mulligan S, Kennedy NP. (2000). Apparent low frequency of undernutrition in Dublin hospital in-patients: should we review the anthropometric thresholds for clinical practice. Proceedings of the Nutrition Society 84: 325–335.

Dempsey DT, Mullen JL. (1987). Prognostic value of nutritional indices. Journal of Parenteral and Enteral Nutrition 11: 109S–114S.

Dempsey DT, Mullen JL, Busby GP. (1988). The link between nutritional status and clinical outcome: can nutritional intervention modify it? American Journal of Clinical Nutrition 47: 352–356.

Detsky AS, Baker JP, Mendelson R, Wolman SL, Wesson DE, Jeejeebhoy KN. (1984). Evaluating the accuracy of nutritional assessment techniques applied to hospitalized patients: methodology and comparisons. Journal of Parenteral and Enteral Nutrition 8: 53–159.

Detsky AS, McLaughlin JR, Baker JP, Johnson N, Whittaker S, Mendelson R, Jeejeebhoy KN. (1987). What is subjective global assessment of nutritional status? Journal of Parenteral and Enteral Nutrition 11: 8–13.

Dionigi R, Cremaschi RE, Jemos V, Dominioni L, Monico R. (1986). Nutritional assessment and severity of illness classification systems: a critical review on their clinical relevance. World Journal of Surgery 10: 2–11.

Dougherty D, Bankhead R, Kushner R, Mirtallo J, Winkler M. (1995). Nutrition care given new importance in JCAHO standards. Nutrition in Clinical Practice 10: 26–31.

Doyle M, Corish C, Flood P, Kennedy NP. (1998). Can patients' knowledge of their own weight and height be used to replace measured weight and height in the calculation of BMI. Proceedings of the Nutrition Society 57: 165A.

Edington J, Boorman J, Durrant ER, Perkins A, Giffin CV, James R, Thomson JM, Oldroyd JC, Smith JC, Torrance AD, Blackshaw V, Green S, Hill CJ, Berry C, McKenzie C, Vicca N, Ward JE, Coles, SJ. (2000). Prevalence of malnutrition on admission to four hospitals in England. Clinical Nutrition 19: 191–195.

Ek A, Unosson M, Larsson J, Bjurulf P. (1996). Interrater variability in subjective global assessment of elderly patients. Scandinavian Journal of Caring Sciences 10: 163–168.

Enia G, Sicuso C, Alati G, Zoccali C. (1993). Subjective global assessment of nutrition in dialysis patients. Nephrology, Dialysis, Transplantation 8: 1094–1098.

Gallagher-Allred CR, Voss AC, Finn SC, McCamish MA. (1996). Malnutrition and clinical outcomes: the case for medical nutrition therapy. Journal of the American Dietetic Association 96: 361–369.

Garry PJ, Goodwin JS, Hunt WC, Hooper EM. (1982). Nutritional status in a healthy elderly population: dietary and supplemental intake. American Journal of Clinical Nutrition 36: 319–331.

Giner M, Laviano A, Meguid MM, Gleason JR. (1996). In 1995 a correlation between malnutrition and poor outcome in critically ill patients still exists. Nutrition 12: 23–29.

Golden MH, Harland PS, Golden BE, Jackson AA. (1978). Zinc and immunocompetence in protein-energy malnutrition. Lancet 1(8076): 1226–1228.

Guigoz Y, Vellas BJ, Garry PJ. (1994). Mini Nutritional Assessment: a practical assessment tool for grading the nutritional state of elderly patients. Facts and Research in Gerontology 4 (suppl. 2): 15–59.

Guigoz Y, Vellas BJ, Garry PJ. (1996). Assessing the nutritional status of the elderly: the Mini Nutritional Assessment as part of the geriatric evaluation. Nutrition Reviews 54: S59–S65.

Guigoz Y, Lauque S, Vellas BJ. (2002). Identifying the elderly at risk for malnutrition: the Mini Nutritional Assessment. Clinics in Geriatric Medicine 18: 737–757.

Haydock DA, Hill GL. (1986). Impaired wound healing in surgical patients with varying degrees of malnutrition. Journal of Parenteral and Enteral Nutrition 10: 550–554.

Hill GL. (1992). Body composition research: implications for the practice of clinical nutrition. Journal of Parenteral and Enteral Nutrition 16: 197–218.

Hooley R. (1986). The nutrition history and physical assessment. In: Krey SH, Murray RL (eds.) Dynamics of Nutrition Support: Assessment, Implementation, Evaluation. Appleton-Century-Crofts, Norwalk, CT, pp. 53–81.

Jensen GL, Friedman JM, Coleman CD, Smiciklas-Wright H. (2001). Screening for hospitalization and nutritional risk among community dwelling older persons. American Journal of Clinical Nutrition 74: 201–205.

Jensen MB, Hessov I. (1997). Randomization to nutritional intervention at home did not improve postoperative function, fatigue or well-being. British Journal of Surgery 84: 113–118.

Jones JM. (2002). The methodology of nutritional screening and assessment methods. Journal of Human Nutrition and Dietetics 15: 59–71.

Jones TN, Moore EE, Van Way CW. (1983). Factors influencing nutritional assessment in abdominal trauma patients. Journal of Parenteral and Enteral Nutrition 7: 115–116.

Kalantar-Zadeh K, Kleiner M, Dunne E, Lee GH, Luft FC. (1999). A modified quantitative subjective global assessment of nutrition for dialysis patients. Nephrology, Dialysis, Transplantation 14: 1732–1738.

Kaminski MV Jr, Fitzgerald MJ, Murphy RJ, Pagast P, Hoppe MC, Winborn AL, Pluta J. (1977). Correlation of mortality with serum transferrin and anergy. (Abstract). Journal of Parenteral and Enteral Nutrition 1: 27 (Abstract).

Keele AM, Bray MJ, Emery PW, Duncan HD, Silk DB. (1997). Two phase randomised controlled clinical trial of postoperative oral dietary supplements in surgical patients. Gut 40: 393–399.

Keller HH, Hedley MR, Wong Brownlea S. (2000). The Development of Seniors in the Community: Risk Evaluation for Eating and Nutrition (SCREEN). Canadian Journal of Dietetic Practice Research 61: 67–72.

Klein S. (1990). The myth of serum albumin as a measure of nutritional status. Gastroenterology 99: 1845–1851.

Klein S, Kinney J, Jeejeeebhoy K, Alpers D, Hellerstein M, Murray M, Twomey P. (1997). Nutrition support in clinical practice: review of published data and recommendations for future research directions: summary of a conference sponsored by the National Institute of Health, American Society for Parenteral and Enteral Nutrition, and American Society for Clinical Nutrition. American Journal of Clinical Nutrition 66: 683–706.

Klidjian AM, Foster KJ, Kammerling RM, Cooper A, Karran SJ. (1980). Relation of anthropometric and dynamometric variables to serious postoperative complications. British Medical Journal 281: 899–901.

Kovacevich DS, Boney AR, Braunschweig C, Perez A, Stevens M. (1997). Nutrition Risk Classification: a reproducible and valid tool for nurses. Nutrition in Clinical Practice 12: 20–25.

Lumbers M, Driver LT, Howland RJ, Older MWJ, Williams CM. (1996). Nutritional status and clinical outcome in elderly female surgical orthopedic patients. Clinical Nutrition 15, 101–107.

McWhirter JP, Pennington CR. (1994). Incidence and recognition of malnutrition in hospital. British Medical Journal 308: 945–948.

Muhlethaler R, Stuck AE, Minder CE, Frey B. (1995). The prognostic significance of protein-energy malnutrition in geriatric patients. Age and Ageing 24: 193–197.

Mullen JL. (1981). Nutritional assessment: its role in nutritional and metabolic support. Clinical Consultations in Nutritional Support 1: 3–9.

Mullen JL, Buzby GP, Waldman MT, Gertner MH, Hobbs CL, Rosato EF. (1979). Prediction of operative morbidity and mortality by preoperative nutritional assessment. Surgical Forum 30: 80–82.

Mullen JL, Buzby GP, Matthews DC, Smale BF, Rosato EF. (1980). Reduction of operative morbidity and mortality by combined preoperative and postoperative nutritional support. Annals of Surgery 192: 604–613.

Muller JM, Brenner U, Dienst C, Brenner U, Pichlmaier H. (1982). Preoperative parenteral feeding in patients with gastrointestinal carcinoma. Lancet 1(8263): 68–71.

Murphy MC, Brooks CN, New SA, Lumbers ML. (2000). The use of the Mini-Nutritional Assessment (MNA) tool in elderly orthopaedic patients. European Journal of Clinical Nutrition 54: 555–562.

Naber HJ, de Bree A, Schermer TRJ, Bakkeren J, Bar B, de Wild G, Katan MB. (1997). Specificity of indexes of malnutrition when applied to apparently healthy people: the effect of age. American Journal of Clinical Nutrition 65: 1721–1725.

Niyongabo T, Melchior JC, Henzel D, Bouchard O, Larouze B. (1999). Comparison of methods for assessing nutritional status in HIV-infected adults. Nutrition 15: 740–743.

Pettigrew RA, Hill GL. (1986). Indicators of surgical risk and clinical judgment. British Journal of Surgery 73: 47–51.

Pettigrew RA, Charlesworth PM, Farmilo RW, Hill GL. (1984). Assessment of nutritional depletion and immune competence: a comparison of clinical examination and objective measurements. Journal of Parenteral and Enteral Nutrition 8: 21–24.

Pikul J, Sharpe MD, Lowndes R, Ghent CN. (1994). Degree of preoperative malnutrition is predictive of postoperative morbidity and mortality in liver transplant recipients. Transplantation 57: 469–472.

Potter J, Klipstein K, Reilly JJ, Roberts M. (1995). The nutritional status and clinical course of acute admissions to a geriatric unit. Age and Ageing 24: 131–136.

Quadri P, Fragiacomo C, Pertoldi W, Quigoz Y, Herrmann F, Rapin ChH. (1999). MNA and Cost of Care. Mini Nutritional Assessment (MNA): Research and Practice in the Elderly. Nestlé Nutrition Workshop Series Clinical and Performance Programme. Vevey/S. Karger AG, Basel, vol. 1, pp. 141–148.

Reilly HM. (1996). Screening for nutritional risk. Proceedings of the Nutrition Society 55: 841–853.

Rubenstein LZ. (1998). Development of a short version of the Mini Nutritional Assessment. In: Mini Nutritional Assessment (MNA): Research and Practice in the Elderly. Nestlé Nutrition Workshop Series Clinical and Performance Programme. Vevey/S. Karger AG, Basel, vol. 1, pp. 101–116.

Sager PM, MacFie J. (1994). Effect of preoperative nutritional status on the outcome of cardiac valve replacement. Nutrition 10: 490A.

Schneider SM, Hebuterne X. (2000). Use of nutritional scores to predict clinical outcomes in chronic disease. Nutrition Reviews 58: 31–38.

Shaw-Stiffel TA, Zarny LA, Pleban WE, Rosman DD, Rudolf RA, Bernstein LH. (1993). Effect of nutrition status and other factors on length of hospital stay after major gastrointestinal surgery. Nutrition 9: 140–145.

Shetty PS, Watrasiewicz KE, Jung RT, James WP. (1979). Rapid-turnover transport proteins: an index of subclinical protein-energy malnutrition. Lancet 2(8136): 230–232.

Soini H, Routasalo P, Lagström H. (2004). Characteristics of the Mini-Nutritional Assessment of elderly home-care patients. European Journal of Clinical Nutrition 58: 64–70.

Spiekerman AM. (1993). Proteins used in nutritional assessment. Clinical Laboratory Medicine 13: 353–369.

Sullivan DH, Sun S, Walls RC. (1999). Protein-energy undernutrition among elderly hospitalized patients. Journal of the American Medical Association 281: 2013–2019.

Th J, de kruif CM, Vos A. (2003). An algorithm for the clinical assessment of nutritional status in hospitalized patients. British Journal of Nutrition 90: 829–836.

Vanek VW. (1998). The use of serum albumin as a prognostic or nutritional marker and the pros and cons of IV albumin therapy. Nutrition in Clinical Practice 13: 110–122.

Vellas B, Guigoz Y, Baumgartner M, Garry PJ, Lauque S, Albarede J-L. (2000). Relationships between nutritional markers and the Mini-Nutritional Assessment in 155 older persons. Journal of American Geriatrics Society 48: 1300–1309.

Veterans Affairs Total Parenteral Nutrition Cooperative Study Group. (1991). Perioperative total parenteral nutrition in surgical patients. New England Journal of Medicine 325: 525–532.

Von Meyenfeldt MF, Meijerink WJHJ, Rouflart MMJ, Buil-Massen MTHJ, Soeters PB. (1992). Perioper-ative nutritional support: a randomised clinical trial. Clinical Nutrition 11: 180–186.

Weinsier RL, Heimburger DC. (1997). Distinguishing malnutrition from disease: the search goes on. American Journal of Clinical Nutrition 66: 1063–1064.

Windsor JA, Hill GL. (1988). Weight loss with physiologic impairment: a basic indicator of surgical risk. Annals of Surgery 207: 290–296.

Appendix A

Dietary recommendations and other miscellaneous data

United States CDC Growth Charts

Anthropometric data from NHANES III

Biochemical data from NHANES III (1988–1994)

Country: Guatemala Year: 2001 Population 11,687,000	Domestic Supply					Domestic Utilisation						Per caput supply			
	Production	imports	Stock changes	Exports	Total	Feed	Seed	Processing	Waste	Other uses	Food	kg/y	Calories	Per day Protein (g)	Fat (g)
	1000 metric tons					1000 metric tons									
Grand Total													2194	55.6	49.4
Vegetable products													1993	41.4	36.0
Animal products													201	14.1	13.3
Cereals — Excluding Beer	1184	1081	-97	115	2053	436	22	22	46	17	154	129.1	1135	30.8	10.9
Wheat	10	442	4	54	402		2	0	3	0	397	33.8	244	7.9	0.8
Rice (milled equivalent)	30	50	0	20	60		1	0	2	0	55	4.7	44	0.9	0.1
Barley (excluding beer)	2	22	0	0	23	1		22			0.0	0.1	0.0	0.1	
Maize	1091	540	-100	31	1501	389	19	0	40	10	1043	89.0	836	21.8	10.0
Rye	0	0	0	0	0	0					0	0.0	0	0.0	0.0
Oats		2	0	6	-4	1					0	0.0	0	0.0	0.0
Millet		1	0	0	1	1									
Sorghum	51	0	-1	0	49	43	0		1		5	0.4	4	0.1	0.0
Cereals, other		24	0	4	21	1					14	1.7	7	0.2	0.0
Starchy Roots	243	16	0	79	179		5		6	101	67	5.7	12	0.2	0.0
Cassava	16	0	0	0	16				2		14	1.2	3	0.0	0.0
Potatoes	227	16	0	79	164		5		5	101	53	4.5	9	0.2	0.0
Sweet potatoes				0	0										
Roots, other		0		0	0						0	0.0	0		
Sugar Crops	16935	0	0	0	16935	30		16700	169	36	0	0.0	0		
Sugar cane	16935	0	0	0	16935	30		16700	169	36					
Sugar beet etc.				0	0										

Appendix A2.1: The uppermost portion of the FAO food balance sheet for Guatemala for the year 2001. Other major food categories included in the complete sheet are: pulses, treenuts, oilcrops, vegetable oils, fruit, stimulants, spices, alcoholic beverages, meat, offal, animal fats, milk, eggs, fish & seafood, and miscellaneous. The complete table, and similar data for other years and countries is available from http://www.fao.org/

American Association of Cereal Chemists
  3340 Pilot Knob Road, St. Paul, MN, 55121-2097 USA
  Tel: +1 651 454 7250   Fax: +1 651 454 0766
  http://www.aaccnet.org/ApprovedMethods/top.htm

Analytical Quality Control Services, Laboratories Seibersdorf
  International Atomic Energy Agency
  PO Box 100, A-1400 Vienna, Austria
  Tel: +43 1 2600 28226   Fax: +43 1 2600 28222
  E-mail: AQCS@IAEA.org

Association of Official Analytical Chemists, Method validation programs
  AOAC INTERNATIONAL.
  481 North Frederick Avenue Suite 500
  Gaithersburg, Maryland 20877 USA
  E-mail: webmaster@aoac.org

European Commission - Joint Research Centre, Institute for Reference Materials and Measurements
  Reference Materials Unit
  Retieseweg 111, B-2440 Geel, Belgium
  Tel: +32 14 571 705   Fax: +32 14 590 406
  E-mail: jrc-irmm-rm-sales@cec.eu.int

Federal Institute for Materials Research and Testing (BAM)
  Unter den Eichen 87
  12205 Berlin, Germany
  Tel: +49 30 8104-0   Fax: +49 30 8112029
  E-mail: info@bam.de

Laboratory of the Government Chemist (LGC), Queens Road, Teddington
  Middlesex, TW11 0LY, UK
  Tel: +44 (0)20 8943 7000   Fax: +44 (0)20 8943 2767
  E-mail: info@lgc.co.uk

National Institute of Standards and Technology (NIST), Standard Reference Materials Program
  100 Bureau Drive, Stop 2322
  Bldg. 202, Room 204
  Gaithersburg, MD 20899-2322, USA
  E-mail: srminfo@nist.gov
  http://ts.nist.gov/srm/

Netherlands Meetinstituut (NMi), Netherland Bureau of Reference Materials
  P.O. Box 654, NL-2600 AR Delft
  The Netherlands
  Tel: +31 152 691 500   Fax: +31 152 612 971
  E-mail: NMi@NMi.nl

Appendix A4.1: Some suppliers of certified reference materials and/or certified analytical methods or procedures. This information is provided for the use of readers. Many such suppliers exist. No significance should be attached to the presence/absence from this list of any particular company or organization.

σ_w^2/σ_b^2	Number of Measurements per Subject										
	1	2	3	4	5	6	7	8	10	12	14
0.00	1.00	1.00	1.00	1.00	1.00	1.00	1.00	1.00	1.00	1.00	1.00
0.25	0.89	0.94	0.96	0.97	0.98	0.98	0.98	0.98	0.99	0.99	0.99
0.50	0.82	0.89	0.93	0.94	0.95	0.96	0.97	0.97	0.98	0.98	0.98
1.00	0.71	0.82	0.87	0.89	0.91	0.93	0.94	0.94	0.95	0.96	0.97
1.50	0.63	0.76	0.82	0.85	0.88	0.89	0.91	0.92	0.93	0.94	0.95
2.00	0.58	0.71	0.77	0.82	0.85	0.87	0.88	0.89	0.91	0.93	0.94
2.50	0.53	0.67	0.74	0.78	0.82	0.84	0.86	0.87	0.89	0.91	0.92
3.00	0.50	0.63	0.71	0.76	0.79	0.82	0.84	0.85	0.88	0.89	0.91
3.50	0.47	0.60	0.68	0.73	0.77	0.79	0.82	0.83	0.86	0.88	0.89
4.00	0.45	0.58	0.65	0.71	0.75	0.77	0.80	0.82	0.85	0.87	0.88
4.50	0.43	0.55	0.63	0.69	0.73	0.76	0.78	0.80	0.83	0.85	0.87
5.00	0.41	0.53	0.61	0.67	0.71	0.74	0.76	0.78	0.82	0.84	0.86

Appendix A6.1: Attenuation factors for simple correlation coefficients. (σ_w^2 = within-subject variation, σ_b^2 = between-subject variation). For example, if the ratio of within- to between-subject variances for a given nutrient is 2.5, and three 24-h recalls are used to estimate the intake, the observed correlation coefficient between the estimated intake and a biochemical measurement is 74% of the true correlation. From Anderson (1986). Guidelines for Use of Dietary Data. Life Sciences Research Office, Federation of American Societies for Experimental Biology.

σ_w^2/σ_b^2	Number of Measurements per Subject										
	1	2	3	4	5	6	7	8	10	12	14
0.00	1.00	1.00	1.00	1.00	1.00	1.00	1.00	1.00	1.00	1.00	1.00
0.25	0.80	0.89	0.92	0.94	0.95	0.96	0.97	0.97	0.98	0.98	0.98
0.50	0.67	0.80	0.86	0.89	0.91	0.92	0.93	0.94	0.95	0.96	0.97
1.00	0.50	0.67	0.75	0.80	0.83	0.86	0.88	0.89	0.91	0.92	0.93
1.50	0.40	0.57	0.67	0.73	0.77	0.80	0.82	0.84	0.87	0.89	0.90
2.00	0.33	0.50	0.60	0.67	0.71	0.75	0.78	0.80	0.83	0.86	0.88
2.50	0.29	0.44	0.55	0.62	0.67	0.71	0.74	0.76	0.80	0.83	0.85
3.00	0.25	0.40	0.50	0.57	0.63	0.67	0.70	0.73	0.77	0.80	0.82
3.50	0.22	0.36	0.46	0.53	0.59	0.63	0.67	0.70	0.74	0.77	0.80
4.00	0.20	0.33	0.43	0.50	0.56	0.60	0.64	0.67	0.71	0.75	0.78
4.50	0.18	0.31	0.40	0.47	0.53	0.57	0.61	0.64	0.69	0.73	0.76
5.00	0.17	0.29	0.38	0.44	0.50	0.55	0.58	0.62	0.67	0.71	0.74

Appendix A6.2: Attenuation factors for simple linear regression coefficients (σ_w^2 = within-subject variation, σ_b^2 = between-subject variation). For example, if the ratio of the within- to between-subject variance is equal to 2.0, and three measurements are taken of the dietary intake, then the regression coefficient of a biological variable on the estimated value of the dietary factor is 60% of the true coefficient. From Anderson (1986). Guidelines for Use of Dietary Data. Life Sciences Research Office, Federation of American Societies for Experimental Biology.

Age	Ca (mg/d)	P ^{a} (mg/d)	K (mg/d)	Fe (mg/d)	Zn (mg/d)	Cu (mg/d)	Se (μg/d)	I (μg/d)
0–3 mo	525	400	800	1.7	4.0	0.3	10	50
4–6 mo	525	400	850	4.3	4.0	0.3	13	60
7–9 mo	525	400	700	7.8	5.0	0.3	10	60
10–12 mo	525	400	700	7.8	5.0	0.3	10	60
1–3 y	350	270	800	6.9	5.0	0.4	15	70
4–6 y	450	350	1100	6.1	6.5	0.6	20	100
7–10 y	550	450	2000	8.7	7.0	0.7	30	110
Males 11–14 y	1000	775	3100	11.3	9.0	0.8	45	130
15–18 y	1000	775	3500	11.3	9.5	1.0	70	140
19–50 y	700	550	3500	8.7	9.5	1.2	75	140
50+ y	700	550	3500	8.7	9.5	1.2	75	140
Females 11–14 y	800	625	3100	14.8 ^{b}	9.0	0.8	45	130
15–18 y	800	625	3500	14.8 ^{b}	7.0	1.0	60	140
19–50 y	700	550	3500	14.8 ^{b}	7.0	1.2	60	140
50+ y	700	550	3500	8.7	7.0	1.2	60	140
Pregnancy	*	*	*	*	*	*	*	*
Lactation 0-4 mo	+550	+440	*	*	+6.0	+0.3	*	*
4+ mo	+550	+440	*	*	+2.5	+0.3	*	*

Appendix A8.1: United Kingdom Reference Nutrient Intakes for minerals. * No increment. ^{a} Phosphorus RNI is set equal to calcium in molar terms. ^{b} Insufficient for women with high menstrual losses where the most practical way of meeting iron requirements is to take iron supplement. Abstracted from COMA (1991). Crown copyright material is reproduced with the permission of the Controller of HMSO and the Queen's Printer for Scotland.

Age (yr)	Fat-soluble Vitamins		Water-soluble Vitamins						
	Vit. A (RE) (μg/d)	Vit. D (μg/d)	Vit. C (mg/d)	Thia-min (mg/d)	Ribo flavin (mg/d)	Niacin (NE) (mg/d)	Vit. B$_6$ (mg/d †)	Fol-ate (μg/d)	Vit. B$_{12}$ (μg/d)
0–3 mo	350	8.5	25	0.2	0.4	3	0.2	50	0.3
4–6 mo	350	8.5	25	0.2	0.4	3	0.2	50	0.3
7–9 mo	350	7	25	0.2	0.4	4	0.3	50	0.4
10–12 mo	350	7	25	0.3	0.4	5	0.4	50	0.4
1–3 y	400	7	30	0.5	0.6	8	0.7	70	0.5
4–6 y	500	–	30	0.7	0.8	11	0.9	100	0.8
7–10 y	500	–	30	0.7	1.0	12	1.0	150	1.0
Males 11–14 y	600	–	35	0.9	1.2	15	1.2	200	1.2
15–18 y	700	–	40	1.1	1.3	18	1.5	200	1.5
19–50 y	700	–	40	1.0	1.3	17	1.4	200	1.5
50+ y	700	**	40	0.9	1.3	16	1.4	200	1.5
Females 11–14 y	600	–	35	0.7	1.1	12	1.0	200	1.2
15–18 y	600	–	40	0.8	1.1	14	1.2	200	1.5
19–50 y	600	–	40	0.8	1.1	13	1.2	200	1.5
50+ y	600	**	40	0.8	1.1	12	1.2	200	1.5
Pregnancy	+100	10	+10	+0.1***	+0.3	*	*	+100	*
Lactation 0–4 mo	+350	10	+30	+0.2	+0.5	+2	*	+60	+0.5
4+ mo	+350	10	+30	+0.2	+0.5	+2	*	+60	+0.5

Appendix A8.2: United Kingdom Reference Nutrient Intakes for vitamins. * No increment. ** After age 65 the RNI is 10 μg/d for men and women. *** For last trimester only. † Based on protein providing 14.7% of EAR for energy. From COMA (1991). Crown copyright material is reproduced with the permission of the Controller of HMSO and the Queen's Printer for Scotland.

Group	Age (yr)	Macronutrients			Elements					
		Carbo-hydrate (g/d)	fat (g/d)	Pro-tein (g/d)	Ca (mg/d)	P (mg/d)	Mg (mg/d)	Fe [a] (mg/d)	Zn [b] (mg/d)	Iodine (μg/d)
Infants	0–0.5	60*	ND	9.1*	210*	100*	30*	0.27*	2*	110*
	0.5–1.0	95*	ND	13.5	270*	275*	75*	11	3	130*
Children	1–3	130	19*	13	500*	460	80	7	3	90
	4–8	130	25*	19	800*	500	130	10	5	90
Males	9–13	130	31*	34	1300*	1250	240	8	8	120
	14–18	130	38*	52	1300*	1250	410	11	11	150
	19–30	130	38*	56	1000*	700	400	8	11	150
	31–50	130	38*	56	1000*	700	420	8	11	150
	50–70	130	30*	56	1200*	700	420	8	11	150
	>70	130	30*	56	1200*	700	420	8	11	150
Females	9–13	130	26*	34	1300*	1250	240	8	8	120
	14–18	130	26*	46	1300*	1250	360	15	9	150
	19–30	130	25*	46	1000*	700	310	18	8	150
	31–50	130	25*	46	1000*	700	320	18	8	150
	50–70	130	21*	46	1200*	700	320	8	8	150
	>70	130	21*	46	1200*	700	320	8	8	150
Pregnancy	≤18	175	28*	71	1300*	1250	400	27	13	220
	19–30	175	28*	71	1000*	700	350	27	11	220
	31–50	175	28*	71	1000*	700	360	27	11	220
Lactation	≤18	210	29*	71	1300*	1250	360	10	14	290
	19–30	210	29*	71	1000*	700	310	9	12	290
	1–50	210	29*	71	1000*	700	320	9	12	290

Appendix A8.3: United States Recommended Dietary Allowances (RDAs): selected macronutrients and elements. Where not available, the Adequate Intake (AI) is shown and followed by an asterisk (*). RDAs and AIs may both be used as goals for average daily individual intake. Sources: IOM (1997, 1998, 2000, 2001). These reports may be accessed via http://www.nap.edu/ and are copyright 2001 by The National Academies. All rights reserved.

[a] Non-heme iron absorption is lower for those consuming vegetarian diets than for those eating nonvegetarian diets. Therefore, it has been suggested that the iron requirement for those consuming a vegetarian diet is approximately twofold greater than for those consuming a nonvegetarian diet. Recommended intake assumes 75% of iron is from heme iron sources.

[b] Zinc absorption is lower for those consuming vegetarian diets than for those eating nonvegetarian diets. Therefore, it has been suggested that the zinc requirement for those consuming a vegetarian diet is approximately twofold greater than for those consuming a nonvegetarian diet.

Group	Age (yr)	Fat-soluble Vitamins			Water-soluble Vitamins						
		Vit.A RAE[a] (µg/d)	Vit. D[b] (µg/d)	Vit. E[c] (mg/d)	Vit. C[d] (mg/d)	Thia-min[e] (mg/d)	Ribo-flavin[f] (mg/d)	Nia-cin[g] (NE/d)	Vit. B6[h] (mg/d)	Fol-ate[i] (µg/d)	Vit. B12[j] (µg/d)
Infants	0–0.5	400*	5*	4*	40*	0.2*	0.3*	2*	0.1*	65*	0.4*
	0.5–1.0	500*	5*	5*	50*	0.3*	0.4*	4*	0.3*	80*	0.5*
Children	1–3	300	5*	6	15	0.5	0.5	6	0.5	150	0.9
	4–8	400	5*	7	25	0.6	0.6	8	0.6	200	1.2
Males	9–13	600	5*	11	45	0.9	0.9	12	1.0	300	1.8
	14–18	900	5*	15	75	1.2	1.3	16	1.3	400	2.4
	19–30	900	5*	15	90	1.2	1.3	16	1.3	400	2.4
	31–50	900	5*	15	90	1.2	1.3	16	1.3	400	2.4
	50–70	900	10*	15	90	1.2	1.3	16	1.7	400	2.4
	>70	900	15*	15	90	1.2	1.3	16	1.7	400	2.4
Females	9–13	600	5*	11	45	0.9	0.9	12	1.0	300	1.8
	14–18	700	5*	15	65	1.0	1.0	14	1.2	400	2.4
	19–30	700	5*	15	75	1.1	1.1	14	1.3	400	2.4
	31–50	700	5*	15	75	1.1	1.1	14	1.3	400	2.4
	50–70	700	10*	15	75	1.1	1.1	14	1.5	400	2.4
	>70	700	15*	15	75	1.1	1.1	14	1.5	400	2.4
Pregnancy	≤18	750	5*	15	80	1.4	1.4	18	1.9	600	2.6
	19–30	770	5*	15	85	1.4	1.4	18	1.9	600	2.6
	31–50	770	5*	15	85	1.4	1.4	18	1.9	600	2.6
Lactation	≤18	1200	5*	19	115	1.4	1.6	17	2.0	500	2.8
	19–30	1300	5*	19	120	1.4	1.6	17	2.0	500	2.8
	31–50	1300	5*	19	120	1.4	1.6	17	2.0	500	2.8

Appendix A8.4: United States Recommended Dietary Allowances (RDAs): selected vitamins. Where not available, the Adequate Intake (AI) is shown and followed by an asterisk (*). RDAs and AIs may both be used as goals for average daily individual intake. Sources: IOM (1997; 1998; 2000; 2001). These reports may be accessed via http://www.nap.edu/ and are copyright 2001 by The National Academies. All rights reserved.

[a] Vitamin A. Includes provitamin A carotenoids that are dietary precursors of retinol. Note: given as retinol activity equivalents (RAEs). 1 RAE = 1 µg retinol, 12 µg β-carotene, 24 µg α-carotene, or 24 µg β-cryptoxanthin.

[b] Vitamin D. Also known as calciferol. Note: 1 g calciferol = 40 IU vitamin D. The DRI values are based on the absence of adequate exposure to sunlight.

[c] Vitamin E. Also known as α-tocopherol. Note: given as α-tocopherol, which includes RRR-α-tocopherol, the only form of α-tocopherol that occurs naturally in foods, and the 2R-stereoisomeric forms of α-tocopherol (RRR-, RSR-, RRS-, and RSS-α-tocopherol) that occur in fortified foods and supplements. It does not include the 2S-stereoisomeric forms of α-tocopherol (SRR-, SSR-, SRS-, and SSS-α-tocopherol), also found in fortified foods and supplements.

[d] Vitamin C. Also known as ascorbic acid or dehydroascorbic acid (DHA).

[e] Thiamin. Also known as Vitamin B_1.

[f] Riboflavin. Also known as Vitamin B_2.

[g] Niacin. Includes nicotinic acid amide, nicotinic acid (pyridine-3-carboxylic acid), and derivatives that exhibit the biological activity of nicotinamide. Note: given as mg/d of niacin equivalents (NE).

[h] Vitamin B_6 comprises a group of six related compounds: pyridoxal, pyridoxine, pyridoxamine, and 5-phosphates (PLP, PNP, PMP).

[i] Folate. Also known as folic acid and folacin pteroylpolyglutamates. Note: given as dietary folate equivalents (DFE).

[j] Vitamin B_{12}. Also known as cobalamin.

	Ca μg/d	P mg/d	K mg/d	Fe mg/d	Zn mg/d	Cu mg/d	Se μg/d	I μg/d
Infants 6–11 mo	400	300	800	6	4	0.3	8	50
Children 1–3 y	400	300	800	4	4	0.4	10	20
4–6 y	450	350	1100	4	6	0.6	15	50
7–10 y	550	450	2000	6	7	0.7	25	100
Males 11–14 y	1000	775	3100	10	9	0.8	35	120
15–17 y	1000	775	3100	13	9	1.0	45	130
18+ y	700	350	3100	9	9.5	1.1	55	130
Females 11–14 y	800	625	3100	22* 18**	9	0.8	35	120
15–17 y	800	625	3100	21* 17**	7	1.0	45	130
18+ y	700	550	3100	20* 16**	7	1.1	55	130
postmenopausal				8				
Pregnancy	700	550	3100	***	7	1.1	55	130
Lactation	1200	900	3100	10	12	1.4	70	160

Appendix A8.5: European population reference intakes — minerals. *To cover 95% of population. **To cover 90% of the population. ***Supplements necessary. From: European Communities — Commission (1993) Reports of the Scientific Committee for food (thirty-first series). Office for Official Publications of the European Communities, Luxembourg.

	Protein g/kg body wt.	Vit. A μg	Thia-min μg/MJ	Ribo-Flavin mg	Niacin mg/MJ	Vit.B-6 μg/g protein	Folate μg	Vit. B-12 μg	Vit. C mg
Infants 6–11 mo	1.6	350	100	0.4	1.6	15	50	0.5	20
Children 1–3 y	1.1	400	100	0.8	1.6	15	100	0.7	25
4–6 y	1.0	400	100	1.0	1.6	15	130	0.9	25
7–10 y	1.0	500	100	1.2	1.6	15	150	1.0	30
Males 11–14 y	1.0	600	100	1.4	1.6	15	180	1.3	35
15–17 y	0.9	700	100	1.6	1.6	15	200	1.4	40
18+ y	0.75	700	100	1.6	1.6	15	200	1.4	45
Females 11–14 y	0.95	600	100	1.2	1.6	15	180	1.3	35
15–17 y	0.85	600	100	1.3	1.6	15	200	1.4	40
18+ y	0.75	600	100	1.3	1.6	15	200(a)	1.4	45
Pregnancy	0.75 (+10 g/d)	700	100	1.6	1.6	15	400	1.6	55
Lactation	0.75 (+16 g/d)	950	100	1.7	1.6 (+2mg/d)	15	350	1.9	70

Appendix A8.6: European population reference intakes — protein, polyunstaturated fatty acids (PUFA), and vitamins. The population reference intakes for n-6 PUFA, expressed as percentage of dietary energy, 4.5% for infants, 3% for children 1–3 y, and 2% for all other subjects. The population reference intakes for n-3 PUFA are 0.5% for all subjects. (a) Neural tube defects have been shown to be prevented in offspring by periconceptual ingestion of 400 μg folic acid in the form of supplements. From: European Communities — Commission (1993) Reports of the Scientific Committee for food (thirty-first series). Office for Official Publications of the European Communities, Luxembourg.

	Ca (c) mg/d	Mg mg/d	Se µg/d	Zn Bioavailability High Mod. Low mg/d			Fe Bioavailability (i) 15% 12% 10% 5% mg/d				Iodine (o) µg/d
Infants Premature											30 µg/kg(p)
0–6 mo	300 (a) 400 (b)	26 (a) 36 (b)	6	1.1 (e)	2.8 (f)	6.6 (g)	(k)	(k)	(k)	(k)	15 µg/kg
7–11 mo	400	53	10	0.8 (e) 2.5 (h)	4.1 (h)	8.3 (h)	6 (l)	8 (l)	9 (l)	19 (l)	135
Children 1–3 y	500	60	17	2.4	4.1	8.4	4	5	6	13	75
4–6 y	600	73	21	3.1	5.1	10.3	4	5	6	13	110
7–9 y	700	100	21	3.3	5.6	11.3	6	7	9	18	100
Adolescents											
Males 10–18 y	1300 (d)	250	34	5.7	9.7	19.2	10	12 (10–14 y)	15	29	135 (10–11 y)
							12	16 (15–18 y)	19	38	110 (12 + y)
Females 10–18 y	1300 (d)	230	26	4.6	7.8	15.5	9	12 (10–14 y) (m)	14	28	140 (10–11 y)
							22	28 (10–14 y)	33	65	100 (12 + y)
							21	26 (15–18 y)	31	62	
Adults											
Males 19–65 y	1000	260	34	4.2	7.0	14.0	9	11	14	27	130
Females											
19–50 y (pre-meno.)	1000	220	26	3.0	4.9	9.8	20	24	29	59	110
51–65 y (meno.)	1300	220	26	3.0	4.9	9.8	8	9	11	23	110
Males (65+ y)	1300	230	34	4.2	7.0	14.0	9	11	14	27	130
Females (65+ y)	1300	190	26	3.0	4.9	9.8	8	9	11	23	110
Pregnancy 1st trim.		220		3.4	5.5	11.0	(n)	(n)	(n)	(n)	200
2nd trim.		220	28	4.2	7.0	14.0	(n)	(n)	(n)	(n)	200
3rd trim.	1200	220	30	6.0	10.0	20.0	(n)	(n)	(n)	(n)	200
Lactation 0–3 mo	1000	270	35	5.8	9.5	19.0	32	40	48	95	200
4–6 mo	1000	270	35	5.3	8.8	17.5	32	40	48	95	200
7–12 mo	1000	270	42	4.3	7.2	14.4	32	40	48	95	200

Appendix A8.7: FAO/WHO Recommended nutrient intakes — minerals (a) Human breast milk. (b) Infant formula. (c) The data used in developing calcium RNIs originate from developed countries, and there is controversy as to their appropriateness for developing countries. This notion also holds true for most nutrients, but based on current knowledge, the impact appears to be most marked for calcium. (d) Particularly during the growth spurt. (e) Human-milk fed infants only. (f) Formula-fed infants, moderate zinc bio-availability. (g) Formula-fed infants, low zinc bio-availability due to infant consumption of phytate rich cereals and vegetable protein based formula. (h) Not applicable to infants consuming human milk only. (i) There is evidence that iron absorption can be significantly enhanced when each meal contains a minimum of 25 mg of Vitamin C, assuming three meals per day. This is especially true if there are iron absorption inhibitors in the diet such as phytate or tannins. (k) Neonatal iron stores are sufficient to meet the iron requirement for the first 6 mo in full-term infants. Premature infants and low birth weight infants require additional iron. (l) Bio-availability of dietary iron during this period varies greatly. (m) Non-menstruating adolescents. (n) It is recommended that iron supplements in tablet form be given to all pregnant women because of the difficulties in correctly evaluating iron status in pregnancy. In the non-anaemic pregnant woman, daily supplements of 100 mg of iron (e.g., as ferrous sulphate) given during the second half of pregnancy are adequate. In anaemic women higher doses are usually required. (o) Data expressed on a per kg body weight basis is sometimes preferred, and this data is as follows: children 1–6 y = 6 µg/kg/day, children 7–11 y = 4 µg/kg/day, adolescents and adults 12+ y = 2 µg/kg/day, pregnancy and lactation = 3.5 µg/kg/day. (p) In view of the high variability in body weights at these ages the RNIs are expressed as g/kg body weight/day.

	Thia-min mg/d	Ribo-flavin mg/d	Niacin NE(a) mg/d	Vit. B6 mg/d	Panto-thenate mg/d	Bio-tin μg	Folate DFE(c) μg/d	Vit. B12 μg/d	Vit. C(d) mg/d	Vit. A RE(f)(g) μg/d	Vit. D μg/d	Vit. E a-TE mg/d	Vit. K μg/d
Infants													
0–6 mo	0.2	0.3	2 (b)	0.1	1.7	5	80	0.4	25	375	5	2.7 (i)	5 (m)
7–11 mo	0.3	0.4	4	0.3	1.8	6	80	0.5	30	400	5	2.7 (i)	10
Children													
1–3 y	0.5	0.5	6	0.5	2	8	160	0.9	30	400	5	5 (k)	15
4–6 y	0.6	0.6	8	0.6	3	12	200	1.2	30	450	5	5 (k)	20
7–9 y	0.9	0.9	12	1.0	4	20	300	1.8	35	500	5	7 (k)	25
Adolescents													
Males													
10–18 y	1.2	1.3	16	1.3	5	25	400	2.4	40	600	5	10	35-65
Females													
10–18 y	1.1	1.0	16	1.2	5	25	400	2.4	40	600	5	7. 5	35-55
Adults													
Males													
19–65 y	1.2	1.3	16		5	30	400	2.4	45	600		10	65
19–50 y				1.3							5		
50+ y				1.7							10		
Females													
19–50 y (pre-meno.)	1.1	1.1	14	1.3	5	30	400	2.4	45	500	5	7.5	55
51–65 y (meno.)	1.1	1.1	14	1.5	5	30	400	2.4	45	500	10	7.5	55
Adults 65+ y													
Males	1.2	1.3	16	1.7	5		400	2.4	45	600	15	10	65
Females	1.1	1.1	14	1.5	5		400	2.4	45	600	15	7.5	55
Pregnancy	1.4	1.4	18	1.9	6	30	600	2.6	55	800	5	(i)	55
Lactation	1.5	1.6	17	2.0	7	35	500	2.8	70 (e)	850	5	(i)	55

Appendix A8.8: FAO/WHO Recommended nutrient intakes — vitamins. (a) NE = niacin equivalents, 60-to-1 conversion factor for tryptophan to niacin. (b) Preformed niacin. (c) DFE = dietary folate equivalents; mg of DFE provided = [mg of food folate + (1.7 x mg of synthetic folic acid)]. (d) An RNI of 45 mg was calculated for adult men and women and 55 mg recommended during pregnancy. It is recognized however that larger amounts would promote greater iron absorption if this can be achieved. (e) An additional 25 mg is needed for lactation. (f) Vitamin A values are "recommended safe intakes" instead of RNIs. This level of intake is set to prevent clinical signs of deficiency, allow normal growth, but does not allow for prolonged periods of infections or other stresses. (g) Recommended safe intakes as g RE/day; 1 μg retinol = 1 μg RE; 1 μg β-carotene = 0.167 μg RE; 1 μg other provitamin A carotenoids = 0.084 μg RE. (h) Data were considered insufficient to formulate recommendations for this vitamin so that "acceptable intakes" are listed instead. This represents the best estimate of requirements, based on the currently acceptable intakes that support the known function of this vitamin. (i) For pregnancy and lactation there is no evidence of requirements for vitamin E that are any different from those of older adults. Increased energy intake during pregnancy and lactation is expected to compensate for increased need for infant growth and milk synthesis. Breast milk substitutes should not contain less than 0.3 mg a-tocopherol equivalents (TE)/100 ml of reconstituted product, and not less than 0.4 mg TE/g PUFA. Human breast milk vitamin E is fairly constant at 2.7 mg for 850 ml of milk. (k) Values based on a proportion of the adult acceptable intakes. (l) The RNI for each age group is based on a daily intake of 1 g/kg/day of phylloquinone, the latter being the major dietary source of vitamin K. (m) This intake cannot be met by infants who are exclusively breastfed. To prevent bleeding due to vitamin K deficiency, all breastfed babies should receive vitamin K supplementation at birth according to nationally approved guidelines.

Disclaimer: The information below should not be taken as an endorsement by the author or publisher of the listed products, manufacturers, or suppliers. No significance should be attached to the absence from this list of any product, manufacturer, or supplier.

Lightweight Infantometer (Length Measuring Board)
> Description: Lightweight and portable. Measuring range 100 cm.
> Supplier: Perspective Enterprises; 7829 Sprinkle Road; Portage, MI 49002, USA
> Tel: +1-269-327-0869   Fax: +1-269-327-0837   E-mail: pepdc@perspectiveent.com

Length Measuring Mat
> Description: Flexible mat of non-stretch, non-shrink closed-cell plastic foam with rigid plastic head-board. For measuring length, from birth to approximately 3 y of age. Measuring range 100 cm, accuracy 1–3 mm. Supplied with plastic draw-string bag for storage/transport. Estimated weight: 1.6 kg
> Supplier: Supply Division, UNICEF Plads, Freeport, DK-2100, Copenhagen, Denmark
> Tel: +45 35 27 35 27;   Fax: +45 35 26 94 21;   E-mail: supply@unicef.org

The Portable Adult/Infant Length/Stature Measuring Board
> Description: Single versatile portable unit, usable as an infantometer and child/adult stadiometer. Use in transient programs or when wall space is unavailable.
> Supplier: Perspective Enterprises, 7829 Sprinkle Road, Portage, MI 49002, USA
> Tel: +1-269-327-0869   Fax: +1-269-327-0837   E-mail: pepdc@perspectiveent.com

Digital Office Infantometer
> Description: Electronic length board with measurements to 0.01cm. Battery operated.
> Supplier: QuickMedical, P.O. Box 1052, Snoqualmie, WA 98065, USA
> Tel: +1-425-831-5963   Fax: +1-425-831-6032
> E-mail: CustomerService@quickmedical.com.

Harpenden Portable Stadiometer
> Description: This instrument is a portable form of the "Harpenden" standard Stadiometer. Measuring range: 850–2060 mm. Easy to erect, free-standing unit. Measures to the nearest millimeter. Dimensions: Base 120 cm x 36 cm x 7.5 cm. Weight (including base): 20.5 kg.
> Supplier: Seritex, Inc., One Madison Street, East Rutherford, NJ 07073, USA
> Tel: +1-973-472-4200   Fax: +1-973-472-0222   http://www.seritex.com/

Wall-mounted Stadiometer SECA 216
> Description: Stadiometer with built-in leveling bubble. The headpiece has a lock knob for measurement accuracy. Readings can be taken in feet and inches or in centimeters. Measuring range: 61–212 cm / 24–83 in. Dimensions $4 \times 60 \times 9$ in.
> Supplier: Seca Ltd. Medical Scales and Measuring Systems, 40 Barn Street, Birmingham B5 5QB, UK Tel: +44-121-643-9349   Fax: +44-121-633-3403   E-mail: uk@seca.com

Electronic Wall-mounted Rod Stadiometer
> Description: Electronic unit transmits the determined height by radio from the measuring slide to a separate display. The large-area head slide and the foot positioner help ensure that the measurements are made correctly. Measuring range 62–210 cm / 25–82.5 in. Graduations 1 mm / 0.05 in Dimensions 300 x 2200 x 250 mm. Power supply: batteries
> Supplier: Seca Ltd. Medical Scales and Measuring Systems, 40 Barn Street, Birmingham B5 5QB, UK Tel: +44-121-643-9349   Fax: +44-121-633-3403   E-mail: uk@seca.com

Handi-Stat Measuring Device Kit
> Description: Right angle head-piece with measuring tape. Graduations: 1/16th inch and millimeters. Suitable for those wishing to manufacture their own measuring equipment.
> Supplier: Perspective Enterprises, 7829 Sprinkle Road, Portage, MI 49002, USA
> Tel: +1-269-327-0869   Fax: +1-269-327-0837   E-mail: pepdc@perspectiveent.com

Microtoise Modified Tape Measure
> Supplier: CMS Weighing Equipment Ltd., 18 Camden High St., London, NW1 OJH, UK
> Tel (+44) 020 7383 7030

Appendix A10.1: Some suppliers of anthropometric equipment for measuring length and height.

Disclaimer: The information below should not be taken as an endorsement by the author or publisher of the listed products, manufacturers, or suppliers. No significance should be attached to the absence from this list of any product, manufacturer, or supplier.

Siltec Digital Baby Scale
Digital scale for office, clinic, or hospital use. Capacity: 0–20 lb × 0.5 oz and 20–44 lb × 1 oz (0–10 kg × 10 g, and 10–20 kg × 20 g). Automatic hold. Powered by AC adapter or 9 v battery. One button tare function. Large platform. Large 4-digit display. Removal of weighing tray allows scale to be used for weighing children. Dimensions: 10" × 10 × 2"
Supplier: Precision Weighing Balances, 10 Peabody St., Bradford, MA 01835-7614, USA
Tel: +1-978-521-7095   Fax: 978-374-5568   E-mail: sales@balances.com

Suspended Infant Weighing Pack
Dial scale made of durable plastic with an easy to read face. Capacity 0–25 kg × 100 g. The 1-kg pack includes a sling, weighing trousers, a detachable handle for weighing larger children, and a vinyl shoulder bag. Extra slings and trousers are available.
Supplier: Perspective Enterprises, 7829 Sprinkle Road, Portage, MI 49002, USA
Tel: +1-269-327-0869   Fax: +1-269-327-0837   E-mail: pepdc@perspectiveent.com

Salter Lightweight Scale Model 235-6S
Lightweight scale in a non-rust metal case with plastic face. Capacity 25 kg × 100 g.
Supplier: Salter Industrial Measurement,Ltd., George Street, West Bromwich, West Midlands, B70 6AD, UK   Tel:+44-121-553-1855.

Seca 881 Digital Medical Floor Scale
Large LCD display and tare function. 400 lb / 180 kg capacity with 2 oz / 50 g readability.
Supplier: Seca Ltd. Medical Scales and Measuring Systems, 40 Barn Street, Birmingham, B5 5QB, UK.   Tel: +44-121-643-9349   Fax +44-121-633-3403   E-mail: uk@seca.com

Standard Weights for Calibration
Precision weights, including all ASTM, OIML, and NBS classes, for balances and scales.
Supplier: Rice Lake Weighing Systems, 230 W. Coleman St, Rice Lake, WI 54868, USA
Tel: +1-715-234-9171   Fax: +1-715-234-6967   E-mail: prodinfo@rlws.com

Harpenden Skinfold Caliper
Supplier: Hemco Corporation, 455 Douglas Avenue, Holland, Michigan 49424, USA
Tel: +1-616-396-4604   Fax: +1-616-396-0413   E-mail: mhop@hemcogages.com

Lange Skinfold Caliper
Supplier: QuickMedical, P.O. Box 1052, Snoqualmie, WA 98065, USA
Tel: +1-425-831-5963 Fax: +1-425-831-6032 E-mail: CustomerService@quickmedical.com

Holtain Skinfold Caliper
Supplier: Holtain Ltd., Crosswell, Crymych, Dyfed SA41 3UF, UK
Tel: +44-1239-891656   Fax: +44-1239-891453

Skyndex I Digital Skinfold Caliper
Supplier: Creative Health Products, Inc., 5148 Saddle Ridge Rd., Plymouth, MI 48170, USA
Tel: +1-734-996-5900   FAX: +1-734-996-4650   E-mail: sales@chponline.com

Elbow Breadth Sliding Caliper (Martin Type)
0–20 cm. GPM Anthropological Instruments. http://www.siberhegner.com/

Knee Height Caliper
Suppliers: Seritex, Inc., One Madison Street, East Rutherford, NJ 07073, USA
Tel: +1-973-472-4200   Fax: +1-973-472-0222   http://www.seritex.com/   OR
Shorr Productions, 17802 Shotley Bridge Place, Olney, Maryland 20832, USA
Tel: +1-301-774-9006;   Fax: +1-301-774-0436;   E-mail: ijshorr@shorrproductions.com

Insertion Circumference Tapes
For arm and head circumference. TALC, PO Box 49, St Albans, Herts, AL1 5TX, UK
Tel: +44-1727-853869   Fax: +44-1727-846852   E-mail: info@talcuk.org

Appendix A10.2: Some suppliers of weighing scales and anthropometric calipers and tapes.

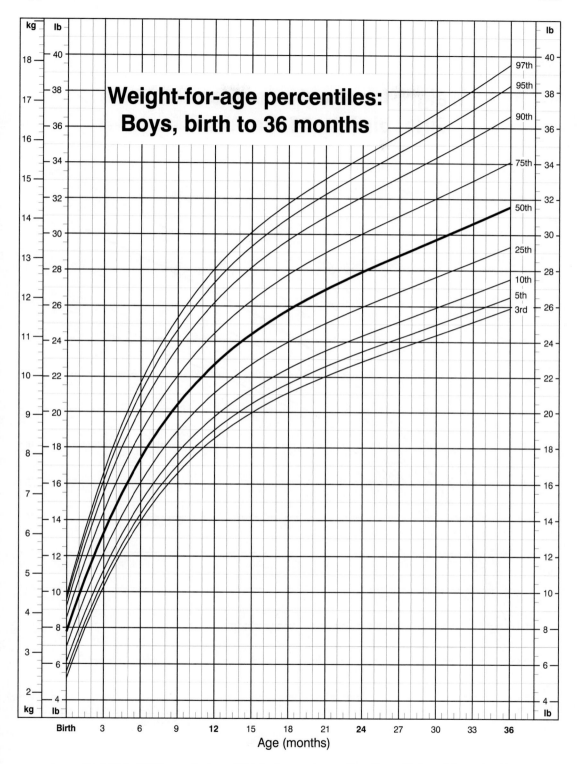

Appendix A12.1: CDC growth chart. Weight-for-age percentiles: Boys, birth to 36 months. From Kuczmarski et al. (2000).

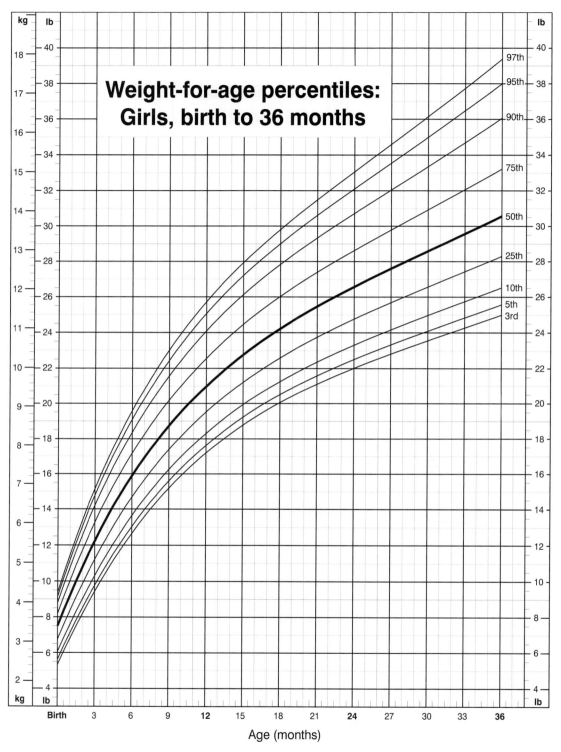

Appendix A12.2: CDC growth chart. Weight-for-age percentiles: Girls, birth to 36 months. From Kuczmarski et al. (2000).

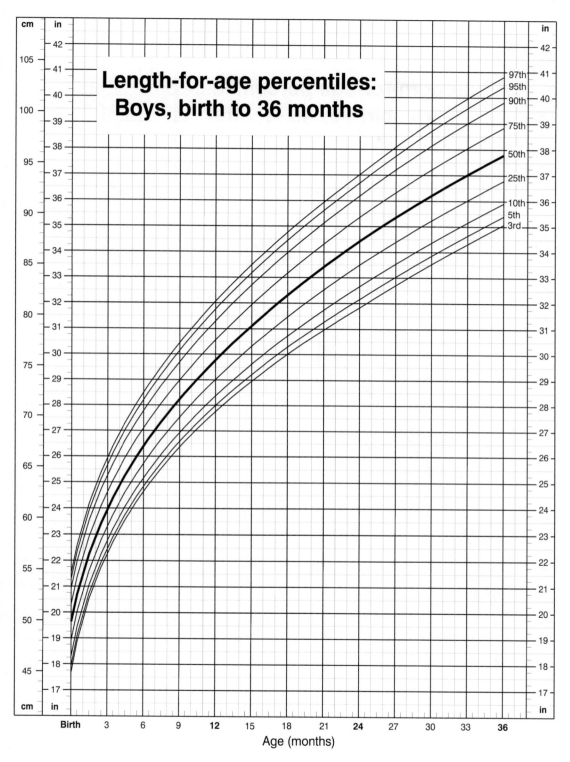

Appendix A12.3: CDC growth chart. Length-for-age percentiles: Boys, birth to 36 months. From Kuczmarski et al. (2000).

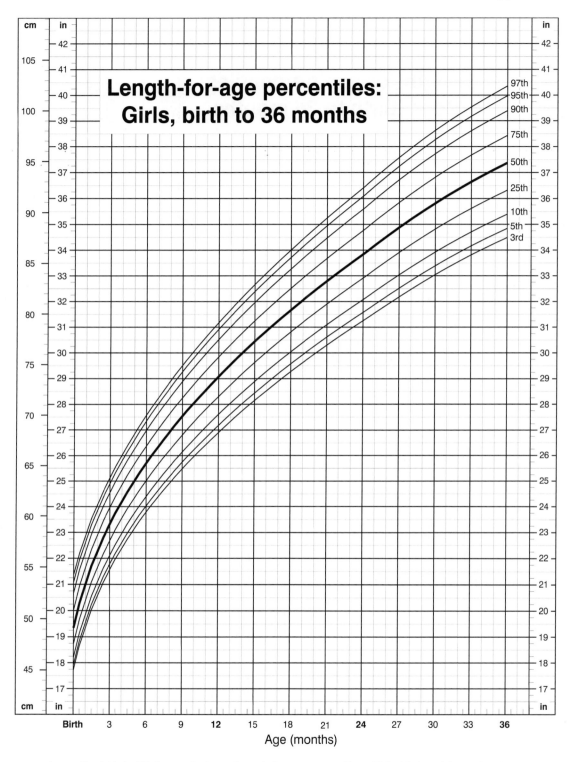

**Length-for-age percentiles:
Girls, birth to 36 months**

Appendix A12.4: CDC growth chart. Length-for-age percentiles: Girls, birth to 36 months. From Kuczmarski et al. (2000).

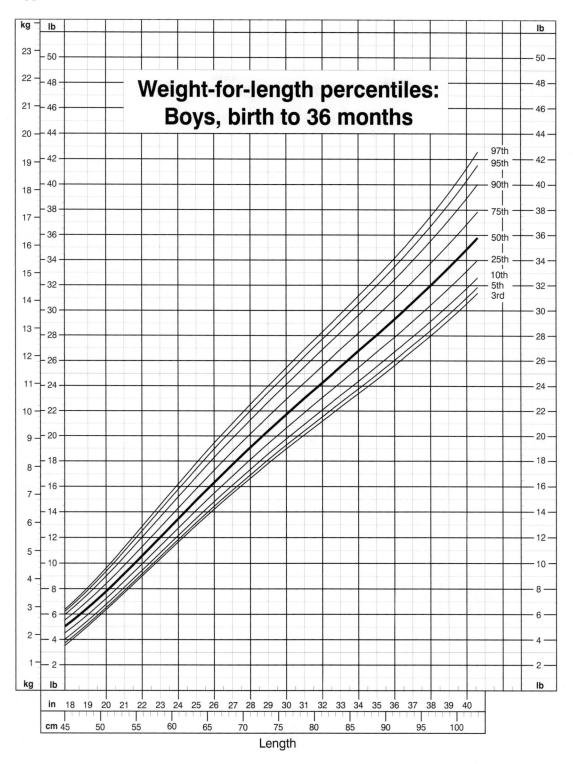

Appendix A12.5: CDC growth chart. Weight-for-Length percentiles: Boys, birth to 36 months. From Kuczmarski et al. (2000).

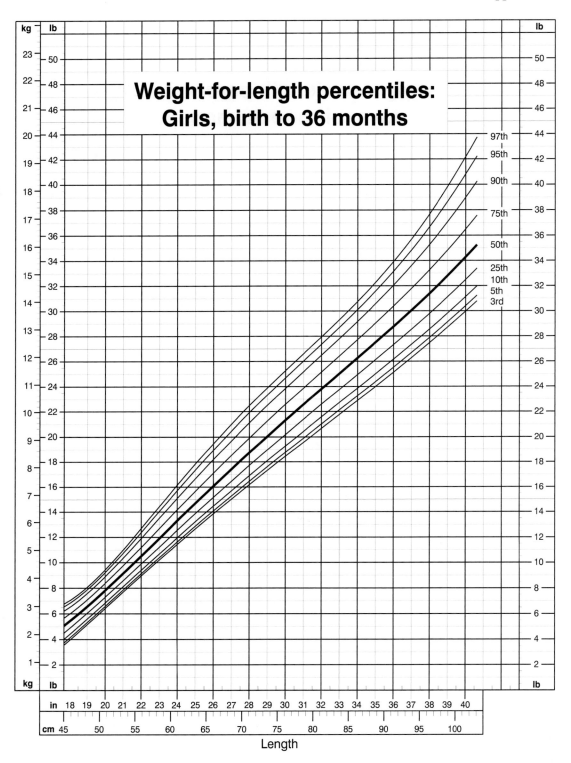

Appendix A12.6: CDC growth chart. Weight-for-Length percentiles: Girls, birth to 36 months. From Kuczmarski et al. (2000).

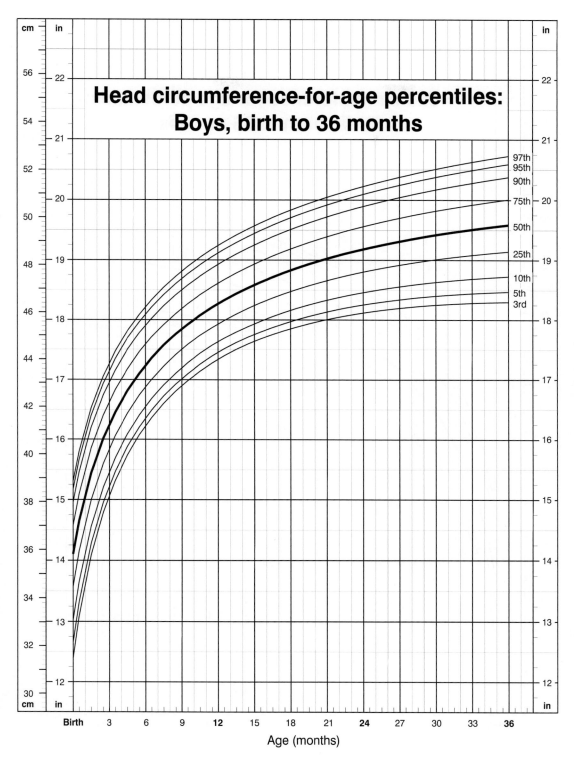

Head circumference-for-age percentiles: Boys, birth to 36 months

Appendix A12.7: CDC growth chart. Head circumference-for-age percentiles: Boys, birth to 36 months. From Kuczmarski et al. (2000).

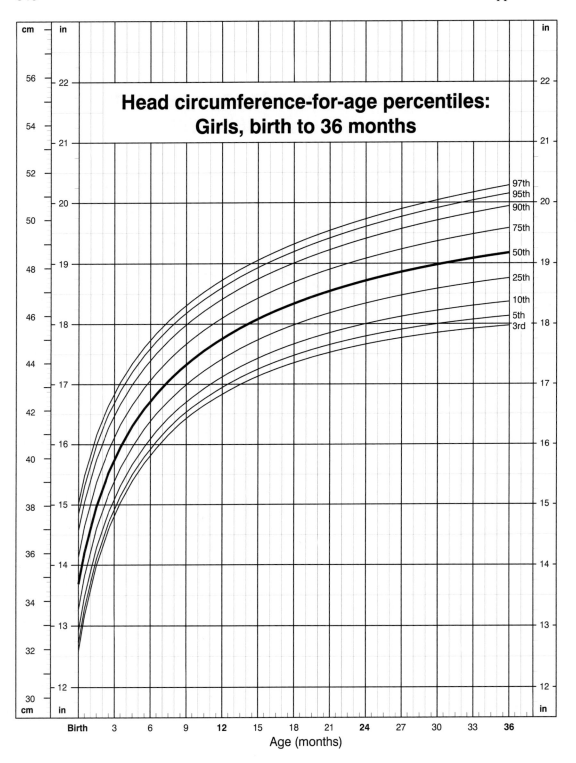

Appendix A12.8: CDC growth chart. Head circumference-for-age percentiles: Girls, birth to 36 months. From Kuczmarski et al. (2000).

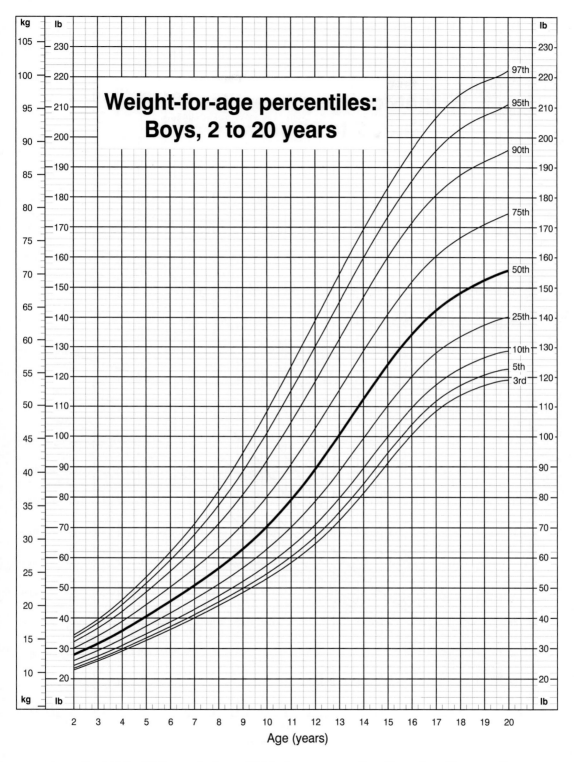

Appendix A12.9: CDC growth chart. Weight-for-age percentiles: Boys, 2 to 20 years. From Kuczmarski et al. (2000).

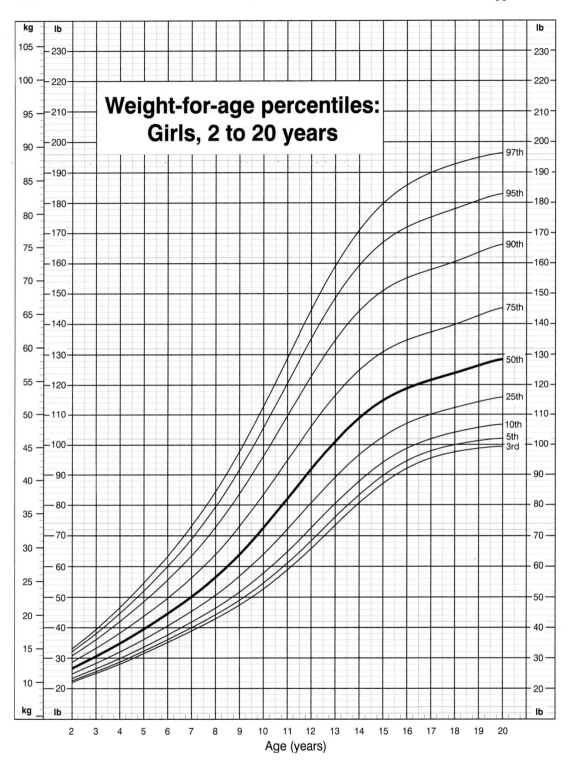

Appendix A12.10: CDC growth chart. Weight-for-age percentiles: Girls, 2 to 20 years. From Kuczmarski et al. (2000).

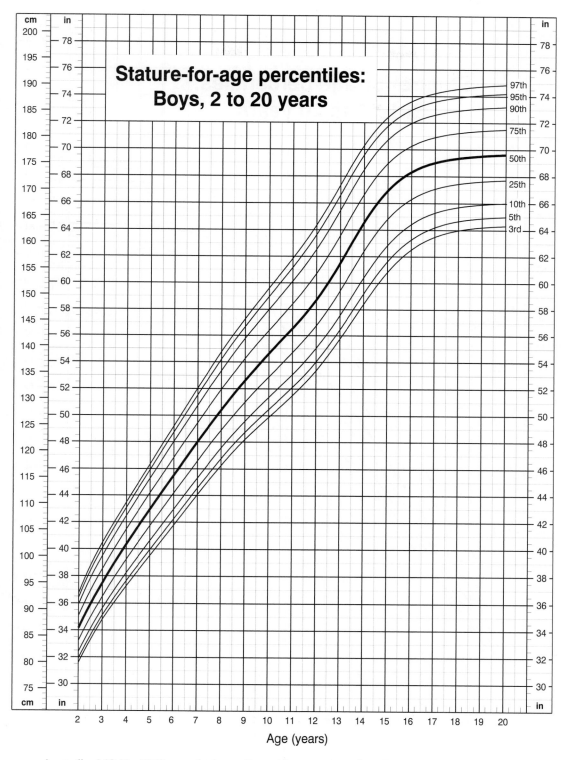

Appendix A12.11: CDC growth chart. Stature-for-age percentiles: Boys, 2 to 20 years. From Kuczmarski et al. (2000).

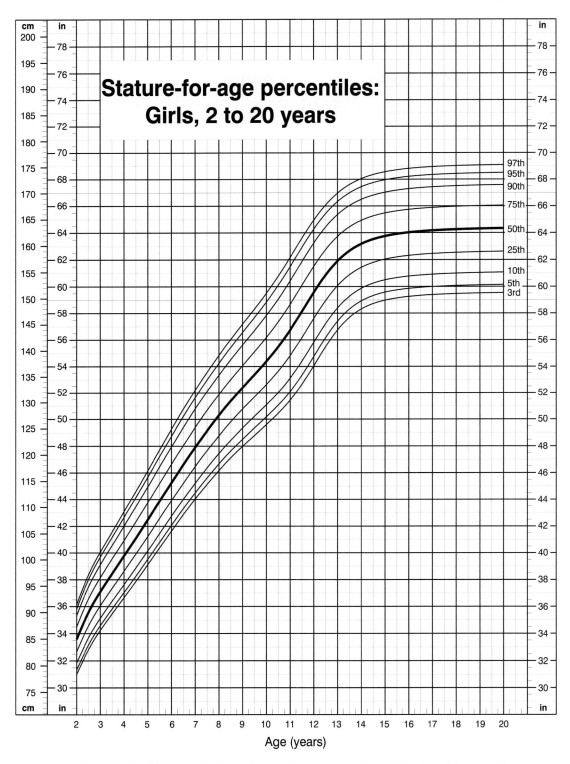

Appendix A12.12: CDC growth chart. Stature-for-age percentiles: Girls, 2 to 20 years. From Kuczmarski et al. (2000).

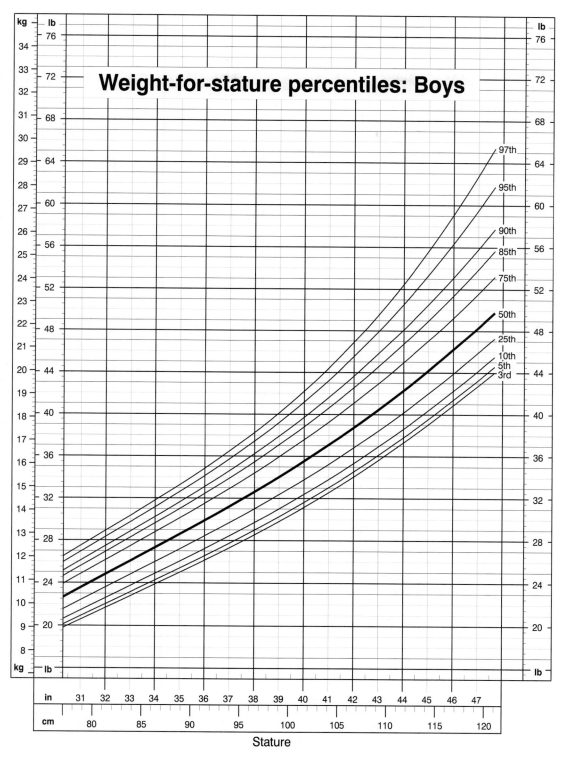

Appendix A12.13: CDC growth chart. Weight-for-stature percentiles: Boys, 2 to 20 years. From Kuczmarski et al. (2000).

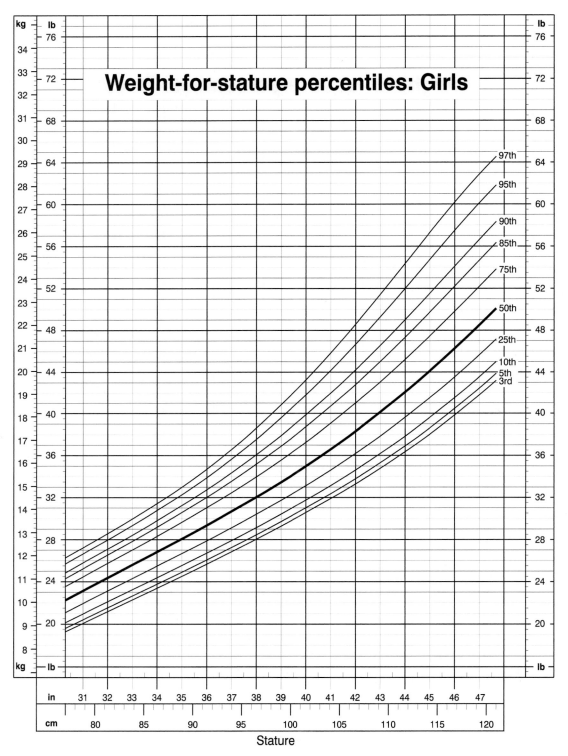

Appendix A12.14: CDC growth chart. Weight-for-stature percentiles: Girls, 2 to 20 years. From Kuczmarski et al. (2000).

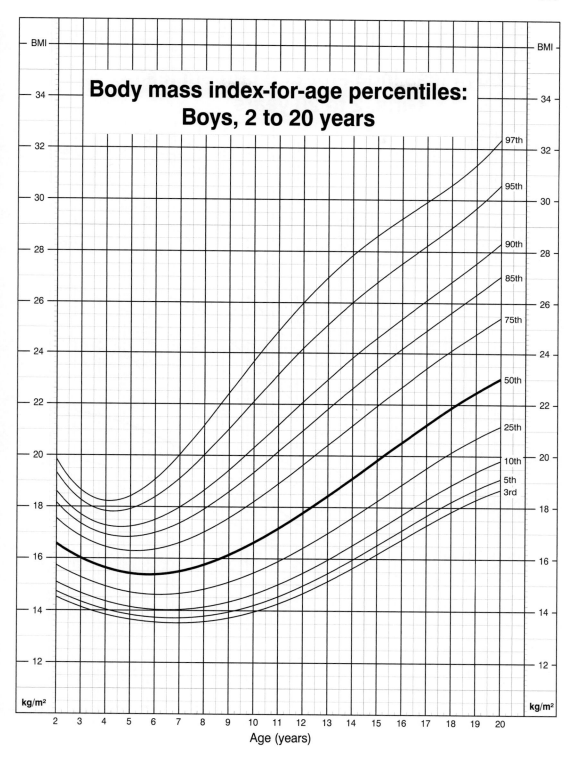

Appendix A12.15: CDC growth chart. Body mass index-for-age percentiles: Boys, 2 to 20 years. From Kuczmarski et al. (2000).

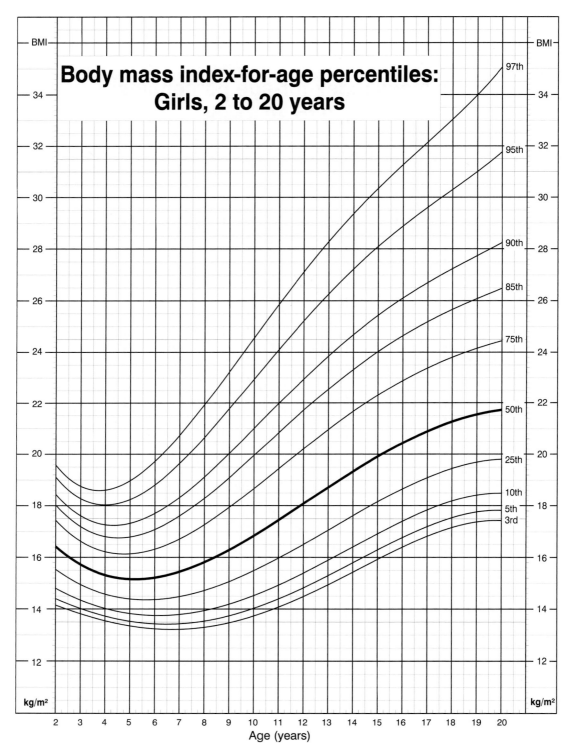

Appendix A12.16: CDC growth chart. Body mass index-for-age percentiles: Girls, 2 to 20 years. From Kuczmarski et al. (2000).

Age group	n	Mean	SEM	5th	10th	15th	25th	50th	75th	85th	90th	95th
Caucasian												
20–29 y	393	177.4	0.34	167.1	169.1	170.8	172.7	177.2	182.1	185.1	186.2	188.2
30–39 y	454	177.9	0.33	167.6	169.5	170.6	173.1	177.5	182.3	185.6	187.6	189.3
40–49 y	428	177.2	0.34	166.0	168.3	169.9	173.1	177.0	181.8	183.9	185.7	188.2
50–59 y	418	176.7	0.31	166.7	168.5	170.1	172.3	176.8	180.7	183.2	184.5	187.3
60–69 y	510	175.0	0.29	165.0	167.2	168.5	170.6	174.7	179.4	181.6	183.4	185.8
70–79 y	524	172.2	0.29	161.8	163.5	164.9	167.4	172.2	176.7	179.2	180.5	183.6
⩾ 80 y	559	169.8	0.30	158.3	160.9	162.9	165.1	169.7	174.3	177.2	178.9	180.7
African American												
20–29 y	488	177.0	0.35	165.6	167.9	169.7	172.4	176.5	182.0	184.9	187.1	188.9
30–39 y	497	177.2	0.32	165.9	168.6	170.7	173.1	177.0	181.2	184.0	186.1	188.9
40–49 y	370	176.7	0.40	165.0	167.1	168.5	171.6	176.6	181.8	185.1	186.6	188.6
50–59 y	217	175.4	0.48	164.6	167.7	168.5	170.6	175.7	179.6	182.7	183.8	185.2
60–69 y	295	173.5	0.42	162.2	164.7	166.0	168.7	173.3	178.3	180.4	182.9	184.7
70–79 y	187	172.4	0.54	*	163.8	164.6	167.8	172.7	177.9	179.7	181.5	*
⩾ 80 y	59	168.8	1.22	*	*	*	165.2	170.2	174.4	*	*	*
Mexican American												
20–29 y	675	169.8	0.30	159.3	161.4	163.4	165.5	169.7	174.0	176.6	178.2	180.6
30–39 y	474	170.6	0.38	159.7	162.0	163.4	166.6	170.3	174.9	177.7	179.3	182.6
40–49 y	381	169.8	0.39	160.3	161.9	163.6	165.5	169.3	173.9	176.6	178.2	181.7
50–59 y	178	169.3	0.53	*	161.8	163.0	165.0	169.4	173.0	175.2	177.3	*
60–69 y	338	168.4	0.39	158.0	160.7	162.1	164.1	168.4	172.7	175.2	176.2	178.1
70–79 y	149	165.7	0.56	*	158.5	159.9	162.4	165.1	169.2	172.6	173.5	*
⩾ 80 y	63	162.6	0.90	*	*	*	157.6	163.2	165.9	*	*	*

Appendix A12.17: Height in centimeters for males 20 years and over, number of examined persons (n), mean, standard error of the mean (SEM), and selected percentiles, by race/ethnicity and age. NHANES III, 1988–1994. *Figure does not meet standard of reliability or precision. Data from http://www.cdc.gov/nchs/nhanes.htm

Age group	n	Mean	SEM	5th	10th	15th	25th	50th	75th	85th	90th	95th
Caucasian												
20 – 29 y	499	163.6	0.40	152.7	155.5	156.7	159.3	163.2	168.1	170.9	172.3	175.1
30 – 39 y	600	164.5	0.35	153.9	156.3	157.8	160.0	164.5	168.7	171.0	172.7	175.4
40 – 49 y	478	163.5	0.37	153.8	156.3	157.5	159.7	163.3	167.7	170.0	171.0	173.2
50 – 59 y	485	162.4	0.36	152.8	155.2	156.5	158.1	162.6	166.6	168.8	170.7	172.6
60 – 69 y	501	160.7	0.36	150.7	153.2	154.7	156.7	160.6	165.0	166.7	168.7	171.4
70 – 79 y	644	158.1	0.35	147.3	150.1	152.4	154.3	158.4	162.7	164.8	166.1	168.0
⩾ 80 y	624	155.0	0.36	143.9	147.0	148.5	151.1	155.1	159.5	161.9	163.5	165.8
African American												
20 – 29 y	624	163.7	0.29	153.4	155.9	157.1	159.6	163.9	167.9	169.9	171.7	173.5
30 – 39 y	654	163.6	0.31	153.0	155.5	156.8	158.6	163.9	168.1	170.9	172.5	175.0
40 – 49 y	457	164.1	0.33	154.3	156.3	157.6	159.7	163.9	168.3	170.2	171.9	174.5
50 – 59 y	275	162.8	0.42	153.0	155.1	156.8	158.6	162.8	167.1	169.5	170.2	172.2
60 – 69 y	301	161.3	0.42	150.5	153.3	154.8	157.0	161.1	165.4	167.7	169.7	172.1
70 – 79 y	182	159.8	0.51	*	152.0	153.4	155.7	160.2	164.2	166.3	167.5	*
⩾ 80 y	92	156.1	0.77	*	*	150.1	152.7	156.3	160.3	162.9	*	*
Mexican American												
20 – 29 y	663	157.4	0.29	147.9	149.9	151.2	153.2	157.6	161.1	163.7	165.4	167.9
30 – 39 y	530	157.1	0.35	147.4	149.1	150.8	153.1	156.9	161.1	163.0	164.7	168.6
40 – 49 y	368	157.4	0.36	148.7	150.7	151.8	153.5	157.1	161.1	162.9	164.7	167.2
50 – 59 y	195	155.7	0.50	*	148.7	150.2	151.8	155.5	159.6	162.1	162.9	*
60 – 69 y	325	154.2	0.40	144.7	146.8	148.4	150.1	154.3	158.0	160.2	161.4	163.3
70 – 79 y	127	152.6	0.75	*	*	147.0	149.0	153.1	157.1	158.8	*	*
⩾ 80 y	59	146.3	1.04	*	*	*	143.2	145.7	150.5	*	*	*

Appendix A12.18: Height in centimeters for females 20 years and over, number of examined persons (n), mean, standard error of the mean (SEM), and selected percentiles, by race/ethnicity and age. NHANES III, 1988–1994. *Figure does not meet standard of reliability or precision. Data from http://www.cdc.gov/nchs/nhanes.htm

Age group	n	Mean	SEM	5th	10th	15th	25th	50th	75th	85th	90th	95th
Caucasian												
20 – 29 y	393	79.0	0.90	59.4	62.4	65.0	68.0	75.6	85.6	93.7	99.7	106.7
30 – 39 y	454	84.4	0.89	63.0	66.0	69.2	73.7	81.6	93.0	100.2	103.1	114.1
40 – 49 y	428	86.2	0.93	63.6	67.5	70.5	75.6	82.7	94.1	102.0	106.0	117.8
50 – 59 y	418	87.1	0.82	66.0	70.5	73.6	77.0	85.1	95.3	102.1	105.9	114.9
60 – 69 y	510	84.3	0.71	62.6	65.3	69.0	74.4	83.6	93.3	98.8	102.6	107.6
70 – 79 y	524	79.6	0.66	60.1	63.2	65.5	69.8	78.5	87.6	93.6	96.2	103.3
⩾ 80 y	560	72.3	0.59	52.1	56.6	59.8	64.1	71.5	79.0	84.5	88.0	93.3
African American												
20 – 29 y	488	82.6	0.97	59.2	61.9	64.0	69.1	79.1	89.7	99.8	108.5	122.3
30 – 39 y	497	82.9	0.91	59.9	64.2	66.6	69.6	80.3	90.6	98.1	104.5	119.0
40 – 49 y	370	84.3	0.96	59.8	63.6	66.2	71.0	81.4	94.4	101.1	106.7	115.5
50 – 59 y	217	84.6	1.41	58.6	61.4	65.8	72.1	82.9	94.5	101.6	105.6	121.0
60 – 69 y	295	80.4	1.02	56.5	60.7	64.3	69.4	78.3	90.5	98.3	102.8	109.5
70 – 79 y	187	77.2	1.19	*	59.2	60.0	65.5	76.2	86.6	91.9	96.8	*
⩾ 80 y	59	70.7	2.04	*	*	*	60.5	71.8	78.8	*	*	*
Mexican American												
20 – 29 y	674	73.8	0.66	56.1	58.7	61.3	64.5	71.6	80.0	87.1	91.4	100.0
30 – 39 y	474	78.7	0.83	57.7	62.1	65.0	69.6	77.0	86.3	92.8	95.6	106.6
40 – 49 y	381	82.5	0.97	63.3	65.6	68.1	72.8	79.6	92.0	97.4	101.5	109.5
50 – 59 y	178	82.8	1.40	*	65.8	68.2	72.0	81.5	90.6	97.1	100.6	*
60 – 69 y	337	78.3	0.87	61.3	63.3	64.6	68.3	77.3	87.1	92.0	96.9	101.6
70 – 79 y	149	73.1	1.31	*	57.7	59.9	63.6	74.7	81.2	84.9	88.0	*
⩾ 80 y	63	66.3	1.62	*	*	*	58.9	66.8	70.2	*	*	*

Appendix A12.19: Weight in kilograms for males 20 years and over, number of examined persons (n), mean, standard error of the mean (SEM), and selected percentiles, by race/ethnicity and age. NHANES III, 1988–1994. *Figure does not meet standard of reliability or precision. Data from http://www.cdc.gov/nchs/nhanes.htm

Age group	n	Mean	SEM	5th	10th	15th	25th	50th	75th	85th	90th	95th
Caucasian												
20–29 y	452	63.7	0.87	46.8	49.4	50.6	53.7	59.3	69.5	77.8	84.4	99.5
30–39 y	579	68.9	0.94	47.9	50.9	53.0	56.2	64.3	77.2	87.6	94.4	103.6
40–49 y	477	70.5	0.96	49.9	53.3	55.8	58.7	67.1	78.3	87.2	92.1	103.3
50–59 y	484	74.3	0.99	52.3	54.8	57.2	61.5	71.4	84.3	91.1	96.1	109.0
60–69 y	501	70.7	0.87	50.0	52.7	55.5	59.5	68.9	78.6	86.8	91.5	99.8
70–79 y	644	66.8	0.74	45.8	50.5	52.9	56.6	64.4	74.8	81.1	85.2	93.7
⩾ 80 y	621	60.4	0.63	41.8	45.5	47.9	51.9	59.7	67.8	72.2	76.1	84.6
African American												
20–29 y	563	70.8	0.83	48.6	51.0	53.7	58.2	66.8	80.7	87.8	94.5	101.9
30–39 y	626	76.8	0.92	52.2	54.9	57.8	62.2	72.7	87.3	97.8	104.9	114.3
40–49 y	456	81.9	1.15	53.0	56.4	61.1	66.5	78.1	93.1	103.5	111.6	125.7
50–59 y	275	80.8	1.34	51.2	56.3	62.5	67.4	79.3	92.6	100.1	107.4	113.7
60–69 y	300	78.8	1.29	51.9	57.1	61.5	66.0	76.4	87.9	95.1	100.1	115.1
70–79 y	182	75.5	1.57	*	56.4	58.0	62.8	72.6	84.2	93.3	103.9	*
⩾ 80 y	93	63.1	1.66	*	*	50.4	53.2	61.8	68.6	80.2	*	*
Mexican American												
20–29 y	575	64.8	0.76	46.1	48.1	50.2	54.1	62.2	71.5	80.7	85.5	93.6
30–39 y	493	70.3	0.93	48.7	52.1	54.6	59.0	66.2	79.2	87.0	94.5	104.4
40–49 y	367	74.1	0.97	53.2	57.0	59.5	63.5	71.8	81.8	88.1	93.0	102.7
50–59 y	193	70.9	1.20	*	55.2	56.1	61.3	70.0	80.0	83.1	87.3	*
60–69 y	321	70.2	0.99	52.1	53.9	56.8	60.6	67.5	77.8	82.3	87.9	97.5
70–79 y	127	63.7	1.38	*	*	51.7	55.3	61.6	69.6	74.5	*	*
⩾ 80 y	59	53.8	1.74	*	*	*	44.0	52.7	61.4	*	*	*

Appendix A12.20: Weight in kilograms for females 20 years and over, number of examined persons (*n*), mean, standard error of the mean (SEM), and selected percentiles, by race/ethnicity and age. NHANES III, 1988–1994. * Figure does not meet standard of reliability or precision. Note: pregnant women are excluded. Data from http://www.cdc.gov/nchs/nhanes.htm

Age group	n	Mean	SEM	5th	10th	15th	25th	50th	75th	85th	90th	95th
Caucasian												
20 – 29 y	393	25.0	0.27	19.4	20.4	20.9	21.9	24.2	27.0	29.1	30.6	33.6
30 – 39 y	454	26.6	0.25	20.7	21.6	22.5	23.6	26.0	28.4	30.6	32.1	35.1
40 – 49 y	428	27.4	0.28	21.5	22.4	22.7	24.2	26.4	29.5	32.0	33.3	36.5
50 – 59 y	418	27.9	0.25	21.6	22.6	23.6	24.7	27.1	30.8	32.3	33.7	36.7
60 – 69 y	510	27.5	0.21	20.7	21.9	23.3	24.7	27.3	30.0	31.7	32.7	33.9
70 – 79 y	524	26.8	0.20	20.6	21.7	22.6	24.0	26.2	29.3	30.7	32.0	35.0
⩾ 80 y	559	25.0	0.18	18.6	19.9	21.1	22.7	25.1	27.1	28.7	29.5	31.7
African American												
20 – 29 y	488	26.2	0.28	19.7	20.6	21.3	22.4	25.0	28.8	30.9	33.0	37.0
30 – 39 y	497	26.4	0.27	19.4	20.5	21.5	22.7	25.4	28.8	31.2	33.3	36.7
40 – 49 y	370	26.9	0.27	19.7	21.0	22.0	23.7	26.4	29.7	31.5	33.4	35.3
50 – 59 y	217	27.4	0.42	19.3	20.6	21.8	23.9	27.1	29.7	31.5	33.5	38.3
60 – 69 y	295	26.7	0.31	18.5	20.4	22.0	23.2	26.4	30.0	31.8	33.1	35.2
70 – 79 y	187	25.9	0.38	*	20.0	20.9	22.4	25.4	28.8	31.1	31.5	*
⩾ 80 y	59	24.9	0.78	*	*	*	21.5	24.7	27.7	*	*	*
Mexican American												
20 – 29 y	674	25.5	0.20	20.1	20.8	21.6	22.6	24.9	27.7	29.6	30.5	33.1
30 – 39 y	474	27.0	0.25	20.6	21.8	22.8	24.3	26.7	28.9	30.6	32.1	35.3
40 – 49 y	381	28.5	0.28	22.6	23.9	24.3	25.3	27.8	31.5	33.3	34.2	36.3
50 – 59 y	178	28.8	0.41	*	23.6	24.1	25.7	28.5	31.1	33.5	34.1	*
60 – 69 y	337	27.6	0.27	21.7	22.7	23.3	24.7	27.4	30.1	32.2	32.9	34.1
70 – 79 y	149	26.5	0.40	*	20.9	22.9	23.8	26.6	29.4	30.3	31.9	*
⩾ 80 y	63	25.0	0.51	*	*	*	23.9	25.2	26.5	*	*	*

Appendix A12.21: Body mass index for males 20 years and over, number of examined persons (*n*), mean, standard error of the mean (SEM), and selected percentiles, by race/ethnicity and age. NHANES III, 1988–1994. *Figure does not meet standard of reliability or precision. Data from http://www.cdc.gov/nchs/nhanes.htm

Age group	n	Mean	SEM	5th	10th	15th	25th	50th	75th	85th	90th	95th
Caucasian												
20–29 y	452	23.8	0.30	18.4	19.0	19.4	20.2	22.2	25.6	28.3	31.5	35.5
30–39 y	579	25.5	0.33	18.5	19.2	19.6	20.6	23.5	28.7	32.0	34.9	38.7
40–49 y	477	26.4	0.36	19.2	20.4	21.0	22.1	24.8	29.3	32.4	34.4	39.4
50–59 y	484	28.2	0.36	19.9	21.0	22.0	23.3	26.9	31.8	35.0	37.0	40.6
60–69 y	501	27.3	0.32	19.5	20.7	21.7	23.4	26.4	30.4	33.3	35.5	38.3
70–79 y	643	26.7	0.28	19.5	20.9	21.4	22.6	25.8	29.7	31.7	33.4	37.3
≥ 80 y	621	25.1	0.24	17.7	19.2	20.3	21.7	24.9	28.2	29.9	31.0	33.5
African American												
20–29 y	563	26.3	0.30	18.7	19.5	20.6	22.0	24.9	29.5	32.9	35.3	38.3
30–39 y	626	28.7	0.34	19.6	20.5	21.5	23.2	27.3	32.8	36.1	38.2	42.5
40–49 y	456	30.4	0.42	20.4	21.5	22.7	25.0	28.9	34.7	38.6	40.8	46.2
50–59 y	275	30.5	0.50	19.9	21.7	23.0	25.6	29.9	34.6	38.3	40.0	42.4
60–69 y	300	30.3	0.49	20.4	22.1	24.0	25.5	29.5	33.7	36.4	38.6	43.9
70–79 y	181	29.4	0.59	*	21.9	22.9	25.0	28.3	32.9	36.0	39.2	*
≥ 80 y	92	25.9	0.66	*	*	20.4	22.1	25.2	29.1	31.3	*	*
Mexican American												
20–29 y	575	26.1	0.30	18.7	19.7	20.5	22.0	25.2	29.2	31.5	33.0	36.7
30–39 y	493	28.5	0.36	20.1	20.9	22.2	23.8	27.3	32.1	35.0	37.1	40.8
40–49 y	366	29.9	0.41	22.1	23.3	24.1	25.3	29.3	33.2	35.7	37.4	42.3
50–59 y	193	29.2	0.49	*	22.6	23.6	25.2	29.1	32.6	34.1	35.7	*
60–69 y	321	29.5	0.42	21.7	22.5	23.6	25.2	28.7	32.3	35.9	37.8	41.4
70–79 y	126	27.4	0.60	*	*	21.9	23.3	26.8	29.9	33.6	*	*
≥ 80 y	58	25.1	0.72	*	*	*	21.3	25.0	28.3	*	*	*

Appendix A12.22: Body mass index for females 20 years and over, number of examined persons (*n*), mean, standard error of the mean (SEM), and selected percentiles, by race/ethnicity and age. NHANES III, 1988–1994. *Figure does not meet standard of reliability or precision. Note: pregnant women are excluded. Data from http://www.cdc.gov/nchs/nhanes.htm

Age group	n	Mean	SEM	5th	10th	15th	25th	50th	75th	85th	90th	95th
Male												
2 y	524	47.9	0.20	43.5	44.4	45.0	46.0	47.7	49.5	50.8	51.8	53.1
3 y	485	49.8	0.31	45.1	46.0	46.6	47.5	49.3	51.2	52.5	53.2	55.5
4 y	542	51.4	0.25	46.4	47.2	47.8	48.9	51.4	52.9	54.4	55.3	57.2
5 y	492	53.0	0.31	47.6	48.4	48.8	50.1	52.5	54.9	56.0	57.3	61.2
6 y	279	55.7	0.64	*	49.6	50.5	51.5	54.1	57.8	59.7	66.5	*
7 y	268	57.4	0.63	*	51.4	52.1	53.0	55.7	59.4	62.7	64.2	*
8 y	262	60.0	0.72	*	52.7	53.6	54.6	58.0	63.7	67.2	72.0	*
9 y	273	63.3	0.91	*	54.1	55.0	56.7	59.6	68.8	75.0	78.1	*
10 y	293	65.1	0.83	*	55.1	56.1	57.9	62.9	69.5	76.7	77.5	*
11 y	281	68.7	1.02	*	58.2	59.0	61.0	65.1	74.1	81.1	84.4	*
12 y	202	72.2	1.20	*	*	61.1	64.5	69.1	80.2	84.5	*	*
13 y	181	73.0	1.35	*	*	61.7	65.0	69.6	80.4	85.5	*	*
14 y	185	77.4	1.91	*	*	66.6	67.5	73.1	79.5	85.5	*	*
15 y	182	78.7	1.54	*	*	66.8	69.6	75.4	85.4	92.1	*	*
16 y	191	78.3	1.25	*	*	70.1	71.4	75.0	82.0	85.8	*	*
17 y	190	81.0	1.26	*	*	70.9	73.0	77.6	84.5	94.7	*	*
18 y	169	80.2	1.35	*	*	71.0	71.9	77.0	84.9	91.0	*	*
19 y	162	82.1	1.33	*	*	73.1	75.1	79.2	86.2	94.6	*	*
Female												
2 y	507	48.0	0.28	*	44.2	44.8	45.9	48.0	49.8	50.8	52.0	*
3 y	562	49.8	0.35	43.6	45.5	46.1	47.1	49.3	51.6	53.3	54.5	57.2
4 y	527	52.1	0.46	*	47.2	47.8	49.0	51.1	53.7	55.6	56.8	*
5 y	554	53.3	0.41	*	47.9	48.6	49.6	52.6	55.4	57.4	59.8	*
6 y	273	54.6	0.78	*	*	49.1	50.4	53.0	56.5	60.1	*	*
7 y	268	57.6	0.92	*	*	50.7	52.2	55.4	60.4	64.6	*	*
8 y	244	59.4	0.94	*	*	53.1	54.1	58.2	62.1	65.4	*	*
9 y	273	62.9	1.14	*	*	53.5	55.9	59.8	66.6	73.0	*	*
10 y	254	64.7	1.22	*	*	56.0	57.1	61.3	69.5	76.1	*	*
11 y	266	67.4	1.05	*	*	58.7	60.5	65.8	72.6	77.6	*	*
12 y	233	69.9	1.36	*	*	59.8	61.7	67.8	77.1	79.5	*	*
13 y	216	74.0	1.49	*	*	62.9	66.4	71.6	80.3	85.6	*	*
14 y	217	76.4	1.40	*	*	65.6	69.2	74.0	82.9	89.3	*	*
15 y	188	74.1	1.43	*	*	65.3	68.1	71.6	77.6	81.3	*	*
16 y	204	76.5	1.69	*	*	67.1	68.7	72.2	81.3	86.8	*	*
17 y	191	78.5	1.50	*	*	69.1	70.1	76.5	81.6	91.3	*	*
18 y	169	76.5	1.72	*	*	*	69.0	74.6	81.1	*	*	*
19 y	170	78.6	1.88	*	*	*	69.6	75.2	82.5	*	*	*

Appendix A12.23: Waist circumference in centimeters for persons 2–19 years, number of examined persons (*n*), mean, standard error of the mean (SEM), and selected percentiles, by sex and age: NHANES III, 1988–1994. * Figure does not meet standard of reliability or precision. Note: pregnant women are excluded. Data from http://www.cdc.gov/nchs/nhanes.htm

Age group	n	Mean	SEM	5th	10th	15th	25th	50th	75th	85th	90th	95th
Caucasian												
20–29 y	383	88.1	0.63	73.6	76.0	77.5	79.5	86.1	94.3	100.0	103.7	111.6
30–39 y	445	94.6	0.61	77.7	81.2	83.2	87.0	93.2	100.5	103.6	108.5	117.3
40–49 y	416	98.4	0.66	80.5	84.3	87.1	91.0	97.1	104.6	110.0	112.7	121.6
50–59 y	402	100.9	0.61	84.4	86.4	89.2	92.5	100.1	107.1	113.4	117.9	121.6
60–69 y	479	102.3	0.55	84.1	88.3	91.0	95.3	102.5	109.5	112.5	116.7	121.0
70–79 y	469	100.7	0.52	81.9	88.3	90.0	93.5	100.6	107.5	111.2	114.5	121.0
⩾ 80 y	430	98.2	0.55	80.0	85.4	87.8	91.9	97.9	104.5	108.6	111.3	115.1
African American												
20–29 y	473	87.1	0.72	70.4	72.0	73.4	76.6	84.0	94.7	100.6	104.7	113.9
30–39 y	473	90.3	0.69	71.5	74.2	76.8	80.2	88.5	96.8	103.7	108.9	119.0
40–49 y	341	93.9	0.77	74.2	78.3	79.6	84.0	92.4	102.2	106.3	111.6	118.5
50–59 y	203	97.1	1.08	75.0	79.0	83.3	88.0	96.2	103.1	109.9	114.0	125.6
60–69 y	271	97.7	0.85	75.6	80.2	83.3	88.9	96.8	106.7	111.5	115.1	117.7
70–79 y	162	96.7	1.05	*	80.1	82.6	87.1	97.7	104.5	108.0	110.7	*
⩾ 80 y	46	94.0	1.74	*	*	*	86.1	93.6	102.1	*	*	*
Mexican American												
20–29 y	652	87.8	0.52	73.1	75.5	77.2	80.0	86.8	93.6	98.4	102.2	107.8
30–39 y	456	93.7	0.62	77.8	80.5	83.2	86.6	93.0	99.1	103.6	106.8	112.6
40–49 y	370	99.0	0.75	83.5	86.7	88.3	91.0	97.6	106.0	110.6	113.3	120.2
50–59 y	169	101.9	1.10	*	87.5	89.5	93.5	102.5	108.7	113.0	116.5	*
60–69 y	319	100.9	0.67	84.0	88.6	90.6	95.1	100.1	108.0	111.5	113.3	117.2
70–79 y	130	98.3	1.24	*	83.6	84.3	91.4	99.8	104.5	106.8	111.1	*
⩾ 80 y	48	95.4	1.47	*	*	*	*	95.6	*	*	*	*

Appendix A12.24: Waist circumference in centimeters for males 20 years and over, number of examined persons (*n*), mean, standard error of the mean (SEM), and selected percentiles, by race/ethnicity and age: NHANES III, 1988–1994. *Figure does not meet standard of reliability or precision. Data from http://www.cdc.gov/nchs/nhanes.htm

Age group	n	Mean	SEM	5th	10th	15th	25th	50th	75th	85th	90th	95th
Caucasian												
20–29 y	440	79.4	0.76	65.6	67.1	68.7	70.5	75.2	85.1	92.5	98.7	106.9
30–39 y	558	84.8	0.79	66.8	68.5	70.2	74.1	81.8	91.6	101.9	107.1	114.5
40–49 y	457	88.4	0.85	69.5	72.1	73.8	77.7	85.1	96.9	105.0	108.6	116.0
50–59 y	469	94.0	0.86	72.6	76.4	78.5	82.5	92.0	104.1	109.8	113.1	120.7
60–69 y	466	94.0	0.79	72.1	75.7	78.7	84.3	93.6	101.9	108.2	111.8	119.0
70–79 y	564	93.3	0.70	74.0	76.4	79.2	83.3	92.2	102.1	106.1	108.8	116.8
⩾ 80 y	441	91.8	0.63	74.0	78.1	81.1	85.0	91.1	99.8	103.2	105.5	108.2
African American												
20–29 y	547	84.6	0.71	65.7	68.9	70.2	73.9	81.9	93.7	99.3	103.1	112.2
30–39 y	593	91.4	0.80	69.8	72.4	74.5	79.9	88.2	101.7	109.7	114.9	123.4
40–49 y	424	96.7	0.98	72.5	76.2	79.1	85.0	94.4	106.2	115.2	119.2	125.8
50–59 y	257	99.3	1.12	73.5	79.1	84.3	89.5	98.5	108.6	115.0	118.9	126.8
60–69 y	261	100.6	1.09	78.8	83.3	86.5	89.6	100.0	110.0	114.0	118.9	129.0
70–79 y	151	97.9	1.29	*	80.5	85.0	88.6	96.7	107.2	112.8	117.1	*
⩾ 80 y	63	91.2	1.95	*	*	*	82.7	90.6	102.1	*	*	*
Mexican American												
20–29 y	555	84.7	0.70	67.1	69.5	71.1	74.2	83.5	92.6	97.4	102.5	110.0
30–39 y	479	90.6	0.82	70.4	73.4	75.6	80.1	89.9	99.2	104.6	110.2	116.3
40–49 y	347	95.8	0.85	77.4	80.7	83.0	86.9	95.5	103.1	107.8	112.5	117.6
50–59 y	185	96.3	1.13	*	79.3	83.3	88.2	96.8	104.3	108.0	109.8	*
60–69 y	299	99.2	1.00	78.5	82.8	85.3	88.8	97.6	108.2	113.1	117.4	124.6
70–79 y	110	96.7	1.57	*	*	82.1	88.6	96.5	105.9	111.4	*	*
⩾ 80 y	44	90.3	2.02	*	*	*	*	*	*	*	*	*

Appendix A12.25: Waist circumference in centimeters for females 20 years and over, number of examined persons (*n*), mean, standard error of the mean (SEM), and selected percentiles, by race/ethnicity and age: NHANES III, 1988–1994. *Figure does not meet standard of reliability or precision. Note: pregnant women are excluded. Data from http://www.cdc.gov/nchs/nhanes.htm

Age group	n	Mean	SEM	5th	10th	15th	25th	50th	75th	85th	90th	95th
Male												
3 – 5 mo	290	10.5	0.21	*	7.9	8.4	9.2	10.7	11.7	12.5	13.2	*
6 – 8 mo	320	10.2	0.23	*	7.3	7.9	8.5	9.9	11.6	12.5	13.3	*
9 – 11 mo	275	9.5	0.20	*	7.1	7.4	8.1	9.2	10.7	11.1	11.8	*
1 y	647	9.4	0.15	6.4	6.9	7.2	7.9	9.1	10.7	11.7	12.1	13.1
2 y	555	9.1	0.13	6.4	6.7	7.3	7.9	8.9	10.4	11.1	11.5	12.4
3 y	479	8.9	0.20	*	6.4	6.8	7.3	8.6	10.0	10.8	11.6	*
4 y	538	9.0	0.18	6.0	6.6	6.8	7.3	8.6	10.0	11.4	12.0	12.9
5 y	493	8.7	0.20	6.0	6.3	6.8	7.2	8.1	9.5	10.3	11.3	13.0
6 y	278	9.8	0.46	*	6.0	6.4	7.1	8.5	10.8	12.9	14.9	*
7 y	268	9.7	0.45	*	6.1	6.4	7.1	8.7	10.7	13.3	16.8	*
8 y	262	10.8	0.59	*	6.3	6.4	7.3	8.8	12.3	15.7	20.1	*
9 y	276	12.4	0.69	*	6.6	6.8	7.4	9.7	15.4	21.3	23.9	*
10 y	293	12.5	0.63	*	6.0	6.9	8.2	10.4	15.5	20.8	22.3	*
11 y	282	13.6	0.70	*	6.7	7.2	8.6	11.3	18.2	19.5	22.3	*
12 y	200	13.5	0.77	*	*	7.6	8.6	12.9	17.4	19.2	*	*
13 y	182	12.4	0.89	*	*	6.4	7.1	10.5	15.7	19.7	*	*
14 y	183	11.0	0.82	*	*	6.2	6.7	8.3	13.4	17.0	*	*
15 y	182	12.1	1.00	*	*	6.0	6.7	9.5	13.8	19.2	*	*
16 y	191	11.1	0.86	*	*	6.6	7.1	8.6	13.6	17.0	*	*
17 y	191	11.3	0.82	*	*	5.8	7.2	8.9	12.8	19.2	*	*
18 y	168	10.9	0.90	*	*	5.7	6.3	8.3	12.6	16.8	*	*
19 y	160	12.1	1.05	*	*	6.3	7.5	9.5	12.2	21.9	*	*
Female												
3 – 5 mo	309	10.4	0.21	*	7.9	8.2	8.7	10.3	11.8	12.3	12.6	*
6 – 8 mo	261	9.9	0.28	*	*	7.6	8.2	9.4	11.3	12.2	*	*
9 – 11 mo	316	9.6	0.24	*	7.1	7.4	8.0	9.2	10.9	11.9	12.7	*
1 y	626	9.7	0.16	6.5	7.1	7.4	8.1	9.6	11.0	11.9	12.4	13.5
2 y	545	9.5	0.17	*	7.1	7.4	7.9	9.2	10.9	11.6	12.3	*
3 y	554	9.7	0.21	*	7.1	7.4	8.1	9.1	10.9	11.6	12.4	*
4 y	529	10.3	0.29	*	7.3	7.7	8.4	9.6	11.6	12.8	13.4	*
5 y	554	10.3	0.27	*	7.3	7.6	8.2	9.6	11.4	12.8	14.4	*
6 y	273	10.3	0.48	*	*	7.1	7.5	9.3	11.1	13.6	*	*
7 y	269	11.9	0.59	*	*	7.4	7.9	10.6	14.5	18.0	*	*
8 y	244	12.4	0.64	*	*	7.8	8.5	10.7	14.2	17.6	*	*
9 y	270	14.4	0.84	*	*	8.2	8.9	12.1	16.5	23.9	*	*
10 y	255	15.0	0.81	*	*	8.7	10.1	12.9	18.1	21.7	*	*
11 y	268	15.1	0.78	*	*	8.9	9.9	12.9	19.8	21.2	*	*
12 y	233	15.2	0.90	*	*	8.2	9.6	13.2	19.4	23.4	*	*
13 y	218	17.5	0.89	*	*	10.4	11.7	15.9	22.3	24.4	*	*
14 y	216	18.7	0.90	*	*	11.6	12.4	17.5	22.5	25.4	*	*
15 y	188	17.8	0.98	*	*	11.1	12.4	16.7	20.7	25.7	*	*
16 y	202	18.6	0.89	*	*	12.0	14.0	16.8	21.8	25.4	*	*
17 y	191	20.0	0.98	*	*	12.4	14.2	19.6	24.8	27.3	*	*
18 y	165	19.4	1.07	*	*	*	13.8	14.2	17.9	24.2	*	*
19 y	167	19.6	1.18	*	*	*	14.0	18.5	24.1	*	*	*

Appendix A12.26: Triceps skinfold in millimeters for persons 3 months–19 years, number of examined persons (n), mean, standard error of the mean (SEM), and selected percentiles, by sex and age: NHANES III, 1988–1994. * Figure does not meet standard of reliability or precision. Note: pregnant women are excluded. Data from http://www.cdc.gov/nchs/nhanes.htm

Age group	n	Mean	SEM	5th	10th	15th	25th	50th	75th	85th	90th	95th
Caucasian												
20–29 y	382	12.3	0.35	5.3	5.9	6.5	7.9	10.7	15.4	18.0	20.3	24.2
30–39 y	440	13.3	0.34	5.9	7.1	7.5	9.0	11.8	15.7	18.3	21.0	27.0
40–49 y	410	13.8	0.33	6.3	7.1	8.1	9.8	12.5	16.4	20.2	22.0	25.0
50–59 y	402	13.8	0.33	6.8	7.6	8.3	9.4	12.9	16.2	18.7	21.8	25.1
60–69 y	486	14.6	0.31	7.5	8.1	9.0	10.5	13.1	17.4	21.4	23.3	26.0
70–79 y	500	13.5	0.29	6.4	7.4	8.0	9.3	12.4	16.4	18.8	20.6	24.7
≥ 80 y	515	12.0	0.25	5.4	6.8	7.6	8.8	11.3	13.9	16.2	18.0	22.2
African American												
20–29 y	456	11.8	0.35	4.4	5.1	5.6	6.4	9.8	15.0	18.9	21.7	26.2
30–39 y	471	11.8	0.31	4.4	5.0	5.6	6.9	10.4	14.9	17.9	20.3	25.9
40–49 y	341	12.5	0.39	4.2	5.2	5.9	7.7	10.7	15.4	19.4	22.8	26.2
50–59 y	200	12.5	0.48	5.0	5.9	6.6	7.9	10.9	14.8	18.3	22.5	25.7
60–69 y	279	12.6	0.44	4.8	5.4	6.1	7.5	10.7	15.6	19.3	24.0	29.4
70–79 y	168	12.5	0.54	*	6.1	6.9	7.8	10.7	14.9	19.2	20.7	*
≥ 80 y	50	11.6	0.87	*	*	*	7.6	10.7	13.4	*	*	*
Mexican American												
20–29 y	646	11.7	0.26	5.2	6.0	6.7	7.7	10.8	14.0	16.6	18.7	21.9
30–39 y	455	12.8	0.35	5.4	6.5	7.5	8.8	10.9	15.3	18.2	20.5	25.4
40–49 y	368	12.5	0.35	6.1	7.0	7.6	8.5	11.5	14.7	18.0	20.1	23.8
50–59 y	169	13.6	0.61	*	7.2	8.3	9.3	12.3	16.1	18.6	22.6	*
60–69 y	325	12.2	0.34	6.6	7.1	8.2	9.2	11.4	13.7	15.8	17.9	22.1
70–79 y	143	10.7	0.40	*	6.4	7.1	8.0	10.3	12.9	14.4	15.3	*
≥ 80 y	58	11.2	0.58	*	*	*	8.8	10.3	13.2	*	*	*

Appendix A12.27: Triceps skinfold in millimeters for males 20 years and over, number of examined persons (*n*), mean, standard error of the mean (SEM), and selected percentiles, by race/ethnicity and age: NHANES III, 1988–1994. * Figure does not meet standard of reliability or precision. Data from http://www.cdc.gov/nchs/nhanes.htm

Age group	n	Mean	SEM	5th	10th	15th	25th	50th	75th	85th	90th	95th
Caucasian												
20 – 29 y	438	20.6	0.50	10.1	11.0	12.2	13.9	18.8	25.8	31.6	33.4	37.0
30 – 39 y	549	22.9	0.48	10.2	12.3	13.5	15.6	21.5	30.6	33.9	36.2	38.6
40 – 49 y	445	25.1	0.46	12.0	14.3	16.3	19.4	25.1	30.7	33.8	35.5	38.4
50 – 59 y	460	26.7	0.44	14.5	16.4	18.4	20.6	26.7	32.0	35.1	37.0	39.5
60 – 69 y	473	24.3	0.44	12.5	14.8	16.3	18.3	24.3	29.6	32.8	34.8	37.9
70 – 79 y	601	22.2	0.38	11.2	12.5	14.0	16.4	21.6	27.5	30.2	31.8	35.4
≥ 80 y	561	18.7	0.37	7.6	10.0	11.2	13.4	18.4	23.4	26.3	28.9	31.7
African American												
20 – 29 y	517	21.9	0.46	9.0	10.8	12.3	14.1	20.6	28.6	33.2	35.9	38.1
30 – 39 y	546	25.4	0.48	10.2	11.7	14.4	17.7	25.2	33.9	37.1	38.6	40.6
40 – 49 y	389	27.3	0.53	11.3	14.6	17.7	20.8	28.1	34.4	37.4	39.0	41.1
50 – 59 y	240	27.5	0.67	11.0	13.9	16.6	21.8	29.2	33.6	36.5	37.9	39.9
60 – 69 y	268	26.0	0.61	11.8	13.8	15.9	19.4	26.8	32.9	35.4	36.7	38.6
70 – 79 y	154	23.9	0.80	*	12.6	14.0	18.8	24.1	28.9	33.8	36.5	*
≥ 80 y	77	17.1	0.98	*	*	9.2	11.3	16.2	22.8	26.2	*	*
Mexican American												
20 – 29 y	553	22.8	0.42	10.7	12.8	14.2	16.6	22.2	28.6	32.3	34.3	36.6
30 – 39 y	460	25.5	0.49	12.6	14.6	16.2	18.7	25.0	32.2	36.0	37.8	39.1
40 – 49 y	338	27.5	0.47	15.8	18.1	19.3	22.5	27.7	33.2	35.1	36.4	37.9
50 – 59 y	179	26.1	0.67	*	16.6	18.2	20.8	25.6	30.7	35.0	36.1	*
60 – 69 y	301	24.8	0.49	14.2	16.4	17.5	20.1	24.7	30.0	32.6	33.9	35.6
70 – 79 y	117	21.0	0.87	*	*	14.7	15.6	19.6	26.4	29.5	*	*
≥ 80 y	52	16.1	1.02	*	*	*	11.8	14.4	20.2	*	*	*

Appendix A12.28: Triceps skinfold in millimeters for females 20 years and over, number of examined persons (n), mean, standard error of the mean (SEM), and selected percentiles, by race/ethnicity and age: NHANES III, 1988–1994. *Figure does not meet standard of reliability or precision. Note: Data from http://www.cdc.gov/nchs/nhanes.htm

Age group	n	Mean	SEM	5th	10th	15th	25th	50th	75th	85th	90th	95th
Male												
3 – 5 mo	283	7.8	0.18	*	5.8	6.2	6.5	7.6	8.7	9.4	10.1	*
6 – 8 mo	313	7.6	0.19	*	5.4	5.7	6.2	7.4	8.6	9.6	10.0	*
9 – 11 mo	269	7.2	0.16	*	5.5	5.9	6.2	7.0	8.0	8.6	9.4	*
1 y	644	6.9	0.11	4.6	5.0	5.3	5.7	6.7	7.9	8.7	9.0	9.6
2 y	549	6.4	0.11	4.4	4.8	5.0	5.4	6.2	7.3	8.0	8.6	9.1
3 y	479	6.2	0.22	*	4.5	4.6	5.0	5.7	6.5	7.2	7.9	*
4 y	537	6.0	0.15	4.1	4.4	4.5	5.0	5.6	6.4	7.3	8.0	9.2
5 y	491	5.8	0.18	4.0	4.3	4.4	4.7	5.3	6.0	6.6	7.4	9.3
6 y	278	6.9	0.45	*	4.5	4.7	4.8	5.5	6.5	8.2	13.6	*
7 y	267	6.7	0.52	*	4.3	4.5	4.6	5.4	6.5	7.8	9.6	*
8 y	261	7.6	0.50	*	4.4	4.6	4.8	5.8	8.4	9.5	15.0	*
9 y	271	8.6	0.58	*	4.5	4.7	5.0	6.3	10.0	13.1	18.2	*
10 y	292	9.1	0.53	*	4.7	4.9	5.4	6.4	12.4	14.8	17.2	*
11 y	280	10.5	0.75	*	5.0	5.2	5.7	7.2	11.9	18.6	26.0	*
12 y	199	10.8	0.82	*	*	5.6	6.0	8.3	13.5	18.5	*	*
13 y	180	10.2	0.90	*	*	5.3	5.9	7.2	11.5	16.0	*	*
14 y	182	11.0	1.04	*	*	6.1	6.8	8.1	11.9	14.7	*	*
15 y	181	11.7	0.97	*	*	6.4	6.9	8.5	14.4	21.5	*	*
16 y	187	10.9	0.82	*	*	6.7	7.4	8.4	11.3	15.5	*	*
17 y	190	12.7	0.93	*	*	7.3	8.0	10.1	13.6	17.7	*	*
18 y	168	12.3	0.87	*	*	7.3	8.0	9.8	13.3	17.1	*	*
19 y	159	13.9	0.98	*	*	*	9.2	11.7	15.3	*	*	*
Female												
3 – 5 mo	307	8.1	0.22	*	6.0	6.3	6.8	7.8	9.4	10.0	10.6	*
6 – 8 mo	255	7.9	0.29	*	*	5.7	6.3	7.4	9.0	10.0	*	*
9 – 11 mo	312	7.6	0.19	*	5.7	5.9	6.5	7.5	8.7	9.3	9.7	*
1 y	624	7.1	0.15	4.9	5.3	5.5	5.9	6.8	7.9	8.6	9.5	10.8
2 y	541	6.9	0.17	*	5.2	5.3	5.6	6.6	7.7	8.4	9.0	*
3 y	553	6.9	0.23	*	4.9	5.1	5.5	6.3	7.6	8.3	9.0	*
4 y	526	7.3	0.35	*	5.0	5.2	5.4	6.2	7.7	8.9	9.8	*
5 y	555	7.4	0.36	*	4.8	4.9	5.3	6.3	7.8	9.4	10.5	*
6 y	273	7.6	0.61	*	*	4.9	5.1	6.1	7.6	10.4	*	*
7 y	265	9.1	0.81	*	*	5.0	5.3	6.2	10.3	14.4	*	*
8 y	243	9.0	0.75	*	*	5.0	5.6	6.7	10.7	12.8	*	*
9 y	269	11.0	1.00	*	*	5.5	6.1	7.9	12.0	17.6	*	*
10 y	253	11.5	0.99	*	*	5.8	6.5	8.5	14.9	19.9	*	*
11 y	263	11.9	0.98	*	*	6.2	6.9	8.8	15.0	20.5	*	*
12 y	231	12.6	1.05	*	*	6.1	6.9	9.9	15.0	18.9	*	*
13 y	215	13.9	1.10	*	*	7.2	8.4	10.7	18.0	22.3	*	*
14 y	214	15.3	1.15	*	*	8.4	9.1	13.6	17.8	22.1	*	*
15 y	183	14.9	1.17	*	*	*	9.4	12.3	18.5	*	*	*
16 y	199	16.0	1.10	*	*	10.1	10.5	13.0	18.9	22.7	*	*
17 y	184	17.8	1.14	*	*	*	11.2	16.7	21.5	*	*	*
18 y	160	16.4	1.20	*	*	*	11.0	13.2	22.3	*	*	*
19 y	162	16.3	1.30	*	*	*	10.9	13.8	18.4	*	*	*

Appendix A12.29: Subscapular skinfold in millimeters for persons 3 months–19 years, number of examined persons (*n*), mean, standard error of the mean (SEM), and selected percentiles, by sex and age: NHANES III, 1988–1994. *Figure does not meet standard of reliability or precision. Note: pregnant women are excluded. Data from http://www.cdc.gov/nchs/nhanes.htm

Age group	n	Mean	SEM	5th	10th	15th	25th	50th	75th	85th	90th	95th
Caucasian												
20–29 y	381	15.9	0.44	7.9	8.6	9.0	10.3	13.8	19.3	23.5	26.8	31.9
30–39 y	440	18.9	0.39	8.9	10.2	11.4	13.5	18.3	23.5	26.5	28.9	32.6
40–49 y	400	20.2	0.41	9.6	11.2	12.7	14.8	19.5	24.4	28.2	30.4	33.7
50–59 y	382	20.5	0.44	10.4	11.5	12.8	14.7	19.5	26.0	28.5	30.6	33.6
60–69 y	461	21.3	0.40	10.5	12.0	13.5	15.7	20.7	25.9	29.3	32.1	35.1
70–79 y	462	19.4	0.36	9.1	11.2	12.3	14.2	18.7	24.1	26.3	28.2	31.8
⩾ 80 y	429	16.7	0.33	7.6	8.9	10.2	12.5	16.7	20.1	22.4	23.6	26.9
African American												
20–29 y	450	17.2	0.39	7.6	8.5	9.1	10.5	14.4	22.8	26.6	30.1	33.1
30–39 y	443	18.2	0.42	7.7	8.7	9.4	11.1	16.4	23.6	27.7	31.2	37.0
40–49 y	320	20.1	0.48	8.1	9.6	10.7	13.7	18.9	25.8	30.0	33.1	35.3
50–59 y	187	20.8	0.63	*	9.7	11.9	14.0	20.1	26.3	30.6	33.9	*
60–69 y	257	20.8	0.56	7.5	8.9	10.9	13.5	20.2	27.0	31.1	33.2	37.2
70–79 y	154	20.5	0.66	*	9.7	11.1	13.5	20.2	26.9	29.2	32.1	*
⩾ 80 y	44	17.6	1.03	*	*	*	12.3	16.3	23.0	*	*	*
Mexican American												
20–29 y	639	17.5	0.34	8.4	9.5	10.2	11.8	16.5	21.5	24.8	27.1	31.4
30–39 y	442	20.2	0.42	8.9	10.4	11.8	14.8	19.7	25.2	28.3	30.5	33.0
40–49 y	342	21.5	0.47	10.1	13.4	14.6	16.0	20.2	26.0	29.3	30.7	35.9
50–59 y	159	22.6	0.66	*	14.5	16.1	17.7	21.7	27.4	29.7	32.9	*
60–69 y	313	21.9	0.51	11.5	13.2	14.5	16.8	20.8	26.6	29.5	32.3	36.3
70–79 y	133	18.5	0.63	*	10.9	12.9	14.6	18.3	21.9	24.0	25.6	*
⩾ 80 y	49	16.7	0.86	*	*	*	*	17.4	*	*	*	*

Appendix A12.30: Subscapular skinfold in millimeters for males 20 years and over, number of examined persons (*n*), mean, standard error of the mean (SEM), and selected percentiles, by race/ethnicity and age: NHANES III, 1988–1994. *Figure does not meet standard of reliability or precision. Data from http://www.cdc.gov/nchs/nhanes.htm

Age group	n	Mean	SEM	5th	10th	15th	25th	50th	75th	85th	90th	95th
Caucasian												
20 – 29 y	424	17.4	0.52	8.0	8.7	9.5	11.0	14.2	22.4	28.0	31.5	36.6
30 – 39 y	533	20.0	0.51	7.8	9.2	9.8	11.5	18.1	26.8	31.8	34.6	38.2
40 – 49 y	428	21.9	0.52	8.9	10.8	12.0	14.7	21.1	28.9	32.4	34.1	38.0
50 – 59 y	450	24.1	0.52	10.0	12.2	14.0	17.3	23.4	30.4	35.0	37.0	39.9
60 – 69 y	464	22.1	0.49	8.9	10.2	12.2	15.3	21.4	28.4	32.0	33.8	38.2
70 – 79 y	558	19.3	0.40	8.4	9.5	11.0	12.7	18.9	24.4	28.3	30.4	33.5
⩾ 80 y	445	16.1	0.40	6.6	7.8	8.8	10.7	14.5	21.2	23.8	26.1	29.7
African American												
20 – 29 y	493	21.6	0.47	9.0	10.1	11.5	13.9	19.8	28.8	33.0	35.1	38.1
30 – 39 y	505	25.0	0.51	9.4	12.0	13.4	17.5	23.6	33.2	37.4	39.4	41.9
40 – 49 y	350	27.6	0.55	12.2	14.7	16.2	20.9	28.1	35.2	38.2	39.7	40.7
50 – 59 y	212	27.6	0.74	*	13.6	15.5	21.2	29.4	35.1	37.7	38.7	*
60 – 69 y	239	26.7	0.64	11.7	15.1	16.7	20.4	27.2	32.5	37.1	39.1	40.1
70 – 79 y	143	24.3	0.87	*	11.4	14.4	18.8	24.1	30.3	34.4	37.9	*
⩾ 80 y	62	18.9	1.28	*	*	*	12.9	17.2	24.9	*	*	*
Mexican American												
20 – 29 y	522	22.2	0.45	9.9	11.1	12.8	14.9	21.2	28.5	32.6	35.1	37.9
30 – 39 y	442	25.2	0.51	11.0	13.1	15.0	18.2	25.3	32.9	36.2	37.4	39.4
40 – 49 y	321	27.3	0.47	15.3	18.4	19.7	22.5	27.5	32.2	35.6	37.2	39.0
50 – 59 y	173	25.9	0.68	*	15.8	16.8	20.4	26.9	30.9	33.7	36.2	*
60 – 69 y	282	25.1	0.57	10.8	14.0	16.5	19.5	24.9	31.8	34.0	35.0	38.1
70 – 79 y	108	20.5	0.90	*	*	12.6	15.0	19.3	25.4	29.2	*	*
⩾ 80 y	44	15.2	1.16	*	*	*	*	*	*	*	*	*

Appendix A12.31: Subscapular skinfold in millimeters for females 20 years and over, number of examined persons (*n*), mean, standard error of the mean (SEM), and selected percentiles, by race/ethnicity and age: NHANES III, 1988–1994. * Figure does not meet standard of reliability or precision. Note: pregnant women are excluded. Data from http://www.cdc.gov/nchs/nhanes.htm

Age group	n	Mean	SEM	5th	10th	15th	25th	50th	75th	85th	90th	95th
Male												
3 – 5 mo	289	14.6	0.12	*	13.2	13.5	13.9	14.5	15.4	15.7	16.0	*
6 – 8 mo	319	15.3	0.12	*	13.8	14.0	14.4	15.2	16.1	16.6	17.0	*
9 – 11 mo	275	15.6	0.12	*	14.1	14.5	14.8	15.7	16.4	16.8	17.1	*
1 y	651	16.1	0.08	14.4	14.8	15.0	15.4	16.0	16.9	17.3	17.7	18.3
2 y	574	16.5	0.08	14.8	15.1	15.4	15.6	16.3	17.2	17.8	18.0	18.5
3 y	483	16.9	0.13	15.0	15.4	15.7	15.9	16.8	17.7	18.2	18.6	19.0
4 y	542	17.3	0.11	15.3	15.6	16.0	16.4	17.1	18.0	18.4	19.0	19.5
5 y	495	17.9	0.13	15.5	16.0	16.2	16.8	17.7	18.6	19.3	19.6	20.7
6 y	279	18.9	0.28	*	16.4	16.8	17.1	18.4	19.6	20.5	22.7	*
7 y	268	19.3	0.24	*	17.1	17.6	17.9	18.9	20.3	21.3	21.7	*
8 y	261	20.4	0.31	*	17.5	18.0	18.4	19.6	21.8	23.4	24.7	*
9 y	276	21.7	0.34	*	18.3	18.6	19.2	20.7	24.2	25.3	27.0	*
10 y	294	22.6	0.34	*	18.7	19.2	20.1	22.0	25.0	26.6	27.5	*
11 y	281	23.6	0.38	*	19.7	20.0	21.1	22.7	25.5	27.4	28.1	*
12 y	202	25.2	0.45	*	*	21.6	23.1	24.1	27.3	28.5	*	*
13 y	181	25.7	0.49	*	*	22.0	23.6	24.6	27.8	28.6	*	*
14 y	185	28.1	0.78	*	*	23.9	24.3	27.0	29.8	30.6	*	*
15 y	183	28.5	0.51	*	*	24.9	25.9	27.5	31.1	33.3	*	*
16 y	191	29.2	0.50	*	*	25.6	26.6	28.4	31.2	32.6	*	*
17 y	193	30.7	0.51	*	*	26.7	27.7	30.0	33.1	35.3	*	*
18 y	168	30.1	0.55	*	*	25.9	27.4	29.6	31.8	34.5	*	*
19 y	161	31.5	0.52	*	*	27.8	28.6	30.8	33.7	35.8	*	*
Female												
3 – 5 mo	309	14.0	0.13	*	12.7	12.9	13.3	14.0	14.8	15.2	15.6	*
6 – 8 mo	262	14.8	0.14	*	*	13.6	13.9	14.7	15.4	16.1	*	*
9 – 11 mo	315	15.2	0.12	*	13.8	14.0	14.4	15.2	15.9	16.4	16.7	*
1 y	627	15.9	0.09	14.0	14.4	14.7	15.0	15.9	16.7	17.0	17.5	17.9
2 y	556	16.3	0.09	*	15.0	15.2	15.5	16.2	17.0	17.4	17.9	*
3 y	561	17.0	0.11	15.1	15.5	15.8	16.1	16.8	17.6	18.1	18.5	19.3
4 y	527	17.6	0.17	*	15.6	15.9	16.4	17.3	18.2	19.0	19.6	*
5 y	555	18.1	0.15	*	16.1	16.3	16.8	17.8	19.0	19.7	20.6	*
6 y	273	18.7	0.28	*	*	16.7	17.2	18.1	19.5	21.1	*	*
7 y	270	19.9	0.34	*	*	17.1	17.6	19.3	21.4	23.5	*	*
8 y	245	20.6	0.35	*	*	17.9	18.6	20.0	21.5	23.3	*	*
9 y	272	22.1	0.47	*	*	18.4	19.3	20.9	24.0	26.5	*	*
10 y	255	22.6	0.42	*	*	19.0	19.8	21.8	24.6	26.5	*	*
11 y	268	23.7	0.40	*	*	20.1	21.2	23.5	25.7	27.4	*	*
12 y	233	24.5	0.48	*	*	20.0	21.5	23.8	27.1	28.3	*	*
13 y	217	26.3	0.53	*	*	22.1	23.0	25.4	29.1	31.1	*	*
14 y	218	26.9	0.49	*	*	23.0	24.0	25.9	29.5	31.1	*	*
15 y	189	26.7	0.49	*	*	23.8	24.2	25.9	28.1	30.1	*	*
16 y	204	27.3	0.47	*	*	23.5	24.7	26.4	29.5	31.3	*	*
17 y	195	27.7	0.50	*	*	24.2	25.2	27.0	29.3	31.2	*	*
18 y	170	27.4	0.59	*	*	*	24.4	26.5	29.8	*	*	*
19 y	168	28.2	0.63	*	*	*	25.2	27.2	29.6	*	*	*

Appendix A12.32: Mid-upper arm circumference in centimeters for persons 3 months–19 years, number of examined persons (*n*), mean, standard error of the mean (SEM), and selected percentiles, by sex and age: NHANES III, 1988–1994. * Figure does not meet standard of reliability or precision. Note: pregnant women are excluded. Data from http://www.cdc.gov/nchs/nhanes.htm

Age group	n	Mean	SEM	5th	10th	15th	25th	50th	75th	85th	90th	95th
Caucasian												
20 – 29 y	386	32.5	0.20	27.2	28.2	28.8	29.7	32.6	34.6	36.1	37.1	38.7
30 – 39 y	444	33.6	0.19	27.9	29.1	29.9	31.2	33.5	35.7	37.1	38.2	39.9
40 – 49 y	417	33.9	0.19	29.0	29.8	30.5	31.4	33.3	35.7	37.5	38.2	41.1
50 – 59 y	406	33.7	0.19	27.9	29.4	30.1	31.1	33.7	35.8	37.2	38.0	39.3
60 – 69 y	487	32.9	0.16	27.1	28.6	29.4	30.9	33.0	35.2	36.2	37.0	37.8
70 – 79 y	502	31.6	0.16	26.5	27.5	28.3	29.4	31.3	33.5	35.2	36.1	37.2
≥ 80 y	517	29.5	0.16	23.6	25.5	26.3	27.3	29.5	31.5	32.6	33.2	35.1
African American												
20 – 29 y	473	33.7	0.23	27.5	28.4	29.4	30.4	33.0	36.5	38.3	39.8	41.9
30 – 39 y	480	33.9	0.21	27.9	29.1	29.8	30.8	33.3	36.4	38.1	39.9	42.0
40 – 49 y	344	33.9	0.23	27.2	29.1	30.0	31.2	33.8	36.2	37.6	39.2	40.9
50 – 59 y	207	33.9	0.35	26.5	28.0	29.2	31.0	33.8	36.4	38.0	39.2	41.3
60 – 69 y	282	32.9	0.28	25.9	26.7	28.6	30.2	32.8	35.8	37.8	38.6	39.9
70 – 79 y	172	31.9	0.33	*	26.8	27.9	29.3	31.6	34.2	36.0	36.8	*
≥ 80 y	50	30.0	0.65	*	*	*	27.6	30.0	32.2	*	*	*
Mexican American												
20 – 29 y	655	31.7	0.16	26.7	27.5	28.3	29.4	31.4	33.7	35.1	36.2	38.0
30 – 39 y	457	33.0	0.20	27.3	28.6	29.5	30.6	33.1	35.1	36.5	37.5	39.4
40 – 49 y	371	33.7	0.21	28.7	29.9	30.4	31.3	33.5	36.1	37.1	37.8	39.2
50 – 59 y	169	33.5	0.30	*	29.9	30.0	31.2	33.3	35.1	36.6	37.4	*
60 – 69 y	325	31.9	0.21	27.4	27.7	28.4	29.4	31.9	34.0	35.4	36.4	37.2
70 – 79 y	145	30.3	0.32	*	26.0	27.4	28.0	30.5	32.7	33.9	34.4	*
≥ 80 y	58	28.4	0.43	*	*	*	27.3	28.3	30.0	*	*	*

Appendix A12.33: Mid-upper arm circumference in centimeters for males 20 years and over, number of examined persons (n), mean, standard error of the mean (SEM), and selected percentiles, by race/ethnicity and age: NHANES III, 1988–1994. *Figure does not meet standard of reliability or precision. Data from http://www.cdc.gov/nchs/nhanes.htm

Age group	n	Mean	SEM	5th	10th	15th	25th	50th	75th	85th	90th	95th
Caucasian												
20 – 29 y	442	28.6	0.25	23.4	24.2	24.8	25.6	27.5	30.7	33.3	34.8	37.4
30 – 39 y	561	30.2	0.27	24.0	24.7	25.4	26.6	28.9	33.0	35.8	37.0	39.6
40 – 49 y	459	31.0	0.27	24.8	25.7	26.5	27.9	30.4	33.6	35.4	37.0	39.7
50 – 59 y	472	32.4	0.28	25.5	26.6	27.5	28.6	31.9	35.0	37.3	38.8	42.4
60 – 69 y	485	31.5	0.26	24.3	26.0	26.8	28.3	31.0	34.1	36.0	37.7	40.2
70 – 79 y	608	30.4	0.22	24.1	25.4	26.2	27.4	29.9	32.6	34.9	36.2	38.6
⩾ 80 y	568	28.5	0.23	21.5	23.0	23.9	25.6	28.4	31.5	33.0	34.0	35.7
African American												
20 – 29 y	548	30.3	0.24	23.4	24.5	25.2	26.8	29.5	33.1	35.2	37.3	39.8
30 – 39 y	593	32.4	0.26	24.7	25.8	26.7	28.2	31.6	35.8	38.4	40.1	42.2
40 – 49 y	426	34.0	0.33	26.0	27.1	27.9	29.8	33.1	37.5	39.6	42.1	44.4
50 – 59 y	261	34.1	0.41	25.2	26.3	27.8	30.1	34.2	37.9	40.0	41.1	44.3
60 – 69 y	280	34.0	0.39	25.4	27.5	28.7	30.1	33.6	37.1	39.5	41.0	42.9
70 – 79 y	161	32.8	0.51	*	26.3	27.5	29.4	32.1	36.2	37.8	40.7	*
⩾ 80 y	78	28.9	0.63	*	*	23.5	24.9	29.1	32.9	34.1	*	*
Mexican American												
20 – 29 y	559	29.7	0.24	23.6	24.3	25.2	26.5	29.0	32.4	34.7	35.8	37.9
30 – 39 y	481	31.9	0.27	25.2	26.3	26.9	28.5	31.2	35.1	36.8	38.5	41.4
40 – 49 y	348	33.1	0.29	27.0	27.9	28.9	29.9	32.9	35.5	37.2	38.8	41.3
50 – 59 y	185	32.9	0.41	*	28.0	28.5	30.0	32.5	35.5	36.7	38.3	*
60 – 69 y	309	32.8	0.34	26.2	27.8	28.1	29.4	32.3	35.4	37.0	38.6	43.4
70 – 79 y	115	30.5	0.62	*	*	25.5	26.2	29.9	33.4	37.2	*	*
⩾ 80 y	51	27.2	0.75	*	*	*	23.1	27.2	30.1	*	*	*

Appendix A12.34: Mid-upper arm circumference in centimeters for females 20 years and over, number of examined persons (n), mean, standard error of the mean (SEM), and selected percentiles, by race/ethnicity and age: NHANES III, 1988–1994. *Figure does not meet standard of reliability or precision. Note: pregnant women are excluded. Data from http://www.cdc.gov/nchs/nhanes.htm

Age group	n	Mean	SEM	5th	10th	15th	25th	50th	75th	85th	90th	95th
Caucasian												
20–29 y	485	6.3	0.02	5.6	5.7	5.8	6.0	6.2	6.5	6.7	6.8	7.0
30–39 y	581	6.4	0.03	5.7	5.9	6.0	6.1	6.4	6.7	6.9	7.0	7.3
40–49 y	462	6.5	0.03	5.8	5.9	6.0	6.2	6.5	6.7	7.0	7.1	7.4
50–59 y	472	6.7	0.03	6.0	6.0	6.1	6.3	6.6	7.0	7.2	7.4	7.6
60–69 y	469	6.6	0.03	6.0	6.1	6.1	6.3	6.6	6.9	7.1	7.2	7.5
70–79 y	571	6.6	0.03	5.9	6.0	6.1	6.2	6.6	6.9	7.2	7.3	7.7
≥ 80 y	462	6.5	0.03	5.8	6.0	6.1	6.2	6.5	6.9	7.0	7.1	7.3
African American												
20–29 y	603	6.4	0.02	5.7	5.9	6.0	6.1	6.4	6.7	6.9	7.1	7.3
30–39 y	628	6.5	0.03	5.9	6.0	6.0	6.2	6.5	6.8	7.1	7.3	7.5
40–49 y	432	6.8	0.04	5.9	6.1	6.1	6.3	6.7	7.2	7.4	7.6	7.8
50–59 y	259	6.9	0.05	6.0	6.1	6.2	6.5	6.8	7.2	7.5	7.6	7.9
60–69 y	273	6.9	0.05	6.0	6.2	6.3	6.5	6.9	7.2	7.5	7.7	8.0
70–79 y	160	6.8	0.06	*	6.2	6.3	6.5	6.8	7.2	7.4	7.5	*
≥ 80 y	72	6.7	0.07	*	*	*	6.5	6.7	7.1	*	*	*
Mexican American												
20–29 y	638	6.1	0.02	5.5	5.6	5.7	5.8	6.1	6.4	6.6	6.7	7.0
30–39 y	515	6.4	0.03	5.6	5.8	5.9	6.0	6.3	6.7	6.9	7.0	7.3
40–49 y	351	6.5	0.04	5.7	5.9	6.0	6.2	6.5	6.8	7.0	7.1	7.4
50–59 y	185	6.6	0.05	*	6.0	6.0	6.2	6.6	6.8	7.1	7.2	*
60–69 y	302	6.6	0.04	5.9	6.0	6.1	6.3	6.6	6.9	7.2	7.3	7.6
70–79 y	113	6.5	0.05	*	*	6.0	6.2	6.5	6.8	6.9	*	*
≥ 80 y	49	6.3	0.07	*	*	*	*	6.2	*	*	*	*

Appendix A12.37: Elbow breadth in centimeters for females 20 years and over, number of examined persons (*n*), mean, standard error of the mean (SEM), and selected percentiles, by race/ethnicity and age: NHANES III, 1988–1994. * Figure does not meet standard of reliability or precision. Data from http://www.cdc.gov/nchs/nhanes.htm

Sex/Age	n	Mean	SEM	5th	10th	25th	50th	75th	90th	95th
Both sexes 1–3 y	2389	120.9	0.2	108.0	110.8	115.7	120.4	125.7	130.5	133.3
Both sexes 4–8 y	2910	126.9	0.2	113.5	116.4	121.1	127.2	132.1	136.4	139.2
M 9–13 y	1110	135.2	0.5	120.3	123.2	128.3	134.6	141.2	146.3	150.1
M 14–18 y	830	149.0	0.6	131.6	135.3	141.5	149.4	156.1	161.0	164.2
M 19–30 y	1804	154.0	0.4	138.9	142.1	147.1	153.7	160.1	164.9	168.5
M 31–50 y	2416	152.0	0.4	135.2	139.3	145.6	152.2	158.2	164.5	167.8
M 51–70 y	1874	148.8	0.2	128.7	134.7	141.7	149.1	155.7	162.2	166.6
M 71+ y	1189	143.7	0.6	117.6	125.1	135.8	144.2	152.6	159.7	164.3
F 9–13 y	1090	131.8	0.5	117.9	121.3	126.3	130.6	136.5	143.1	146.2
F 14–18 y	883	132.4	0.5	116.8	120.3	125.9	132.5	138.8	143.8	147.3
F 19–30 y	1809	132.8	0.3	115.8	119.8	126.3	133.0	139.2	144.8	147.7
F 31–50 y	2805	132.2	0.3	112.9	118.3	126.0	132.5	139.1	145.2	149.5
F 51–70 y	1976	135.1	0.3	117.4	121.7	128.3	135.0	141.7	147.8	151.6
F 71+ y	1306	134.1	0.4	113.7	119.5	127.4	134.1	141.3	147.7	152.4
F Pregnant	317	121.0	1.0	*	108.9	114.5	120.7	126.2	136.1	*
F Lactating	96	134.2	2.1	*	*	*	134.4	*	*	*

Appendix A17.1: Mean and percentiles for hemoglobin (g/L), NHANES III (1988–1994). Note: Means, standard errors, and percentiles calculated with WesVar Complex Samples 3.0. Children fed human milk and females who had "blank but applicable" pregnancy and lactating status data or who responded "I don't know" to questions on pregnancy and lactating status were excluded from all analyses. * Figure does not meet standard of reliability or precision. Source: ENVIRON International Corporation, 2000.

Sex/Age	n	Mean	SEM	5th	10th	25th	50th	75th	90th	95th
Both sexes 1–3 y	1935	18.6	0,3	5.6	7.6	11.4	17.6	24.6	29.8	35.3
Both sexes 4–8 y	2865	21.4	0.2	8.9	11.1	15.3	20.5	26.6	31.9	37.4
M 9–13 y	1097	22.5	0.5	9.4	11.8	15.5	20.9	27.9	33.7	39.2
M 14–18 y	836	27.7	0.7	12.4	14.4	19.2	25.1	34.8	44.2	49.7
M 19–30 y	1802	30.4	0.4	13.1	16.2	21.8	29.6	36.8	46.0	52.3
M 31–50 y	2413	29.1	0.3	15.3	17.0	21.5	27.5	34.9	43.0	48.9
M 51–70 y	1879	27.5	0.4	13.0	15.9	20.6	26.5	33.2	39.7	45.1
M 71+ y	1188	27.1	0.4	12.2	14.5	19.6	25.9	33.2	39.9	45.9
F 9–13 y	1087	22.6	0.6	8.8	10.7	16.1	21.3	27.2	34.3	41.2
F 14–18 y	884	23.4	0.5	7.3	10.0	15.9	22.0	29.5	36.0	44.4
F 19–30 y	1795	25.4	0.5	8.5	11.3	16.5	23.5	31.6	40.6	47.7
F 31–50 y	2802	23.4	0.4	7.3	9.9	15.0	21.4	29.8	39.0	45.1
F 51–70 y	1980	23.6	0.3	11.1	13.0	17.0	22.4	28.6	35.2	41.3
F 71+ y	1301	23.9	0.3	11.0	13.2	17.5	22.2	29.2	35.6	40.7
F Pregnant	318	22.8	1.0	*	10.5	14.0	21.4	28.5	38.2	*
F Lactating	93	*	*	*	*	*	*	*	*	*

Appendix A17.2: Mean and percentiles for serum transferrin saturation (%), NHANES III (1988–1994). Note: Means, standard errors, and percentiles calculated with WesVar Complex Samples 3.0. Children fed human milk and females who had "blank but applicable" pregnancy and lactating status data or who responded "I don't know" to questions on pregnancy and lactating status were excluded from all analyses. * Figure does not meet standard of reliability or precision. Source: ENVIRON International Corporation, 2000.

Sex/Age	n	Mean	SEM	5th	10th	25th	50th	75th	90th	95th
Both sexes 1–3 y	2429	27.9	0.7	6.0	9.0	15.0	23.0	34.0	49.0	64.0
Both sexes 4–8 y	2906	34.1	0.5	14.3	17.0	21.8	29.8	41.2	56.6	68.9
M 9–13 y	1098	38.8	1.1	16.2	19.2	25.4	34.8	47.7	65.4	75.2
M 14–18 y	837	56.6	2.1	20.0	24.0	33.0	48.0	70.0	99.0	123.0
M 19–30 y	1801	131.0	2.5	42.0	54.0	80.0	118.0	168.0	224.0	263.0
M 31–50 y	2418	189.4	3.6	41.0	60.0	101.0	157.0	235.0	355.0	455.0
M 51–70 y	1877	204.2	6.8	37.0	53.0	92.0	161.0	267.0	408.0	519.0
M 71+ y	1189	184.8	6.4	28.0	41.0	74.0	136.0	239.0	385.0	506.0
F 9–13 y	1092	36.4	1.1	12.3	16.0	22.5	31.7	44.2	60.7	76.4
F 14–18 y	888	35.8	2.9	9.0	12.0	19.0	29.0	42.0	63.0	86.0
F 19–30 y	1797	47.8	1.5	9.0	13.0	22.0	37.0	60.0	94.0	124.0
F 31–50 y	2808	64.0	3.1	7.0	11.0	21.0	42.0	75.0	133.0	194.0
F 51–70 y	1980	121.0	3.3	19.0	28.0	50.0	91.0	157.0	247.0	321.0
F 71+ y	1300	135.1	5.0	21.0	30.0	53.0	96.0	170.0	281.0	380.0
F Pregnant	320	37.6	3.9	12.0	15.0	22.0	33.0	47.0	65.0	80.0
F Lactating	94	47.3	6.1	18.0	21.0	29.0	41.0	59.0	81.0	98.0

Appendix A17.3: Mean and percentiles for serum ferritin (μg/L) NHANES III (1988–1994). Note: For all groups greater than 3 y, data were adjusted using the Iowa State University Method. Mean, standard errors, and percentiles were obtained using C-Side. Standard errors were estimated via jacknife replication. Infants and children fed human milk and females who had "blank but applicable" pregnancy and lactating status data or who responded "I don't know" to questions on pregnancy and lactating status were excluded from all analyses. The sample sizes for the Pregnant and Lactating categories were very small so their estimates of usual serum ferritin distributions are not reliable. Source: ENVIRON International Corporation, 2000.

Sex/Age	n	Mean	SEM	5th	10th	25th	50th	75th	90th	95th
Both sexes 4–8 y	2704	1.22	0.01	0.84	0.91	1.04	1.20	1.35	1.49	1.58
M 9–13 y	1076	1.43	0.01	0.99	1.06	1.21	1.40	1.57	1.81	1.89
M 14–18 y	8,23	1.76	0.02	1.22	1.31	1.52	1.71	1.95	2.20	2.34
M 19–30 y	1784	2.01	0.02	1.38	1.50	1.69	1.95	2.23	2.54	2.72
M 31–50 y	2397	2.22	0.01	1.43	1.59	1.85	2.16	2.52	2.88	3.11
M 51–70 y	1870	2.27	0.02	1.48	1.65	1.90	2.21	2.58	2.94	3.17
M 71+ y	1174	2.34	0.03	1.42	1.62	1.88	2.19	2.65	3.17	3.47
F 9–13 y	1070	1.40	0.01	1.01	1.09	1.20	1.34	1.54	1.72	1.82
F 14–18 y	877	1.61	0.02	1.07	1.16	1.32	1.55	1.78	2.08	2.34
F 19–30 y	1786	1.87	0.02	1.14	1.26	1.48	1.77	2.16	2.56	2.80
F 31–50 y	2781	1.79	0.02	1.14	1.23	1.44	1.71	2.01	2.36	2.63
F 51–70 y	1965	2.14	0.02	1.32	1.48	1.73	2.06	2.41	2.79	3.10
F 71+ y	1282	2.24	0.02	1.32	1.49	1.81	2.16	2.56	3.00	3.32
F Pregnant	316	1.47	0.04	*	0.99	1.22	1.45	1.67	1.94	*
F Lactating	94	*	*	*	*	*	*	*	*	*

Appendix A18.1: Mean and percentiles for serum vitamin A (retinol) (μmol/L), NHANES III (1988–1994). Note: Means, standard errors, and percentiles calculated with WesVar Complex Samples 3.0. Females who had "blank but applicable" pregnancy and lactating status data or who responded "I don't know" to questions on pregnancy and lactating status were excluded from all analyses. *Figure does not meet standard of reliability or precision. Source: ENVIRON International Corporation, 2000.

Sex/Age	n	Mean	5th	10th	25th	50th	75th	90th	95th
Both sexes 4–8 y	2834	18.7	8.2	9.5	12.4	16.6	22.5	30.1	36.2
Standard error		0.3	0.2	0.3	0.4	0.3	0.9	0.9	1.2
M 9–13 y	1072	16.7	6.3	7.7	10.6	14.7	19.9	27.0	33.5
Standard error		0.6	0.3	0.3	0.4	0.4	0.5	1.5	2.7
M 14–18 y	816	12.4	5.1	5.9	7.7	10.8	15.1	20.0	24.4
Standard error		0.4	0.3	0.3	0.4	0.4	0.5	1.2	2.3
M 19–30 y	1782	12.9	4.0	5.0	6.9	9.8	15.3	24.3	32.2
Standard error		0.5	0.2	0.1	0.3	0.2	0.5	1.3	2.0
M 31–50 y	2388	16.2	4.1	5.3	7.9	12.4	19.5	29.7	39.7
Standard error		0.5	0.2	0.2	0.2	0.3	0.5	1.0	1.8
M 51–70 y	1892	19.5	4.7	6.3	9.6	15.3	24.1	35.9	46.8
Standard error		0.6	0.4	0.3	0.4	0.4	0.8	1.9	3.5
M 71+ y	1193	23.4	5.7	7.6	11.6	18.0	28.1	44.1	59.2
Standard error		0.9	0.2	0.3	0.6	0.6	1.8	2.4	3.7
F 9–13 y	1094	15.7	6.7	7.9	10.4	14.1	19.2	25.5	30.2
Standard error		0.4	0.2	0.2	0.3	0.4	0.5	0.7	0.9
F 14–18 y	937	14.3	5.6	6.4	8.4	11.7	17.2	25.0	31.6
Standard error		0.6	0.2	0.2	0.2	0.3	0.7	1.5	2.4
F 19–30 y	2028	15.0	4.6	5.7	7.9	12.0	18.6	27.0	34.5
Standard error		0.4	0.1	0.1	0.2	0.3	0.5	0.9	1.4
F 31–50 y	2839	21.7	5.7	7.4	11.0	17.2	26.8	39.6	51.4
Standard error		0.5	0.2	0.2	0.3	0.4	0.6	1.1	1.9
F 51–70 y	1955	26.4	6.4	8.5	13.1	20.6	32.3	49.9	65.8
Standard error		0.8	0.3	0.4	0.6	0.6	1.7	1.9	3.4
F 71+ y	1289	31.1	8.4	10.6	15.7	24.5	38.7	58.8	75.8
Standard error		1.0	0.4	0.4	0.5	0.7	1.2	2.4	3.8

Appendix A18.2: Mean and percentiles for serum β-carotene (μg/dL), NHANES III (1988–1994).
Source: Iowa State University Department of Statistics, 1999.

Sex/Age	n	Mean	5th	10th	25th	50th	75th	90th	95th
Both sexes 4–8 y	2835	814	617	648	713	793	890	1004	1089
Standard error		7.3	8.9	7.8	6.6	6.7	9.3	16.2	23.4
M 9–13 y	1072	790	571	609	679	771	880	995	1073
Standard error		7.9	6.1	6.0	7.2	9.0	10.3	12.6	15.6
M 14–18 y	816	739	522	558	624	710	821	956	1058
Standard error		9.1	7.3	7.8	8.9	7.9	13.4	18.7	24.6
M 19–30 y	1782	894	594	648	741	853	996	1185	1335
Standard error		10.3	10.0	7.9	7.9	9.7	15.0	22.5	32.8
M 31–50 y	2391	1128	675	746	885	1062	1269	1551	1815
Standard error		13.9	9.0	9.7	10.2	11.4	18.2	30.2	45.1
M 51–70 y	1895	1294	739	833	985	1117	1465	1878	2232
Standard error		18.2	52.4	30.7	36.0	15.7	44.9	85.3	149.0
M 71+ y	1193	1303	724	796	940	1157	1489	1967	2375
Standard error		30.9	10.7	12.3	16.8	19.0	33.0	64.0	119.0
F 9–13 y	1094	795	563	606	678	765	875	1018	1129
Standard error		11.3	8.0	7.9	8.3	9.5	14.0	22.1	30.8
F 14–18 y	937	810	548	592	678	786	902	1041	1159
Standard error		10.5	15.0	17.8	12.3	25.6	17.0	46.2	43.7
F 19–30 y	2028	932	618	671	765	880	1036	1248	1422
Standard error		9.5	7.9	7.5	6.7	10.0	11.2	29.9	40.4
F 31–50 y	2839	1074	686	745	856	1007	1207	1470	1691
Standard error		10.3	6.4	6.8	7.8	9.7	12.7	20.1	32.7
F 51–70 y	1957	1424	793	890	1058	1279	1597	2078	2534
Standard error		25.7	24.6	14.0	20.7	16.7	28.8	54.0	99.2
F 71+ y	1290	1489	834	946	1138	1373	1696	2156	2543
Standard error		19.2	37.4	20.8	16.0	18.2	23.0	41.5	73.1

Appendix A18.3: Mean and percentiles for serum vitamin E (μg/dL), NHANES III (1988–1994).
Source: Iowa State University Department of Statistics, 1999.

Sex/Age	n	Mean	5th	10th	25th	50th	75th	90th	95th
Both sexes 4–8 y	1216	1.1	0.9	0.9	1.0	1.1	1.2	1.3	1.4
Standard error		0.02	0.12	0.09	0.05	0.02	0.05	0.1	0.13
M 9–13 y	1019	0.9	0.4	0.5	0.7	0.9	1.2	1.4	1.5
Standard error		0.03	0.03	0.03	0.03	0.03	0.03	0.04	0.06
M 14–18 y	789	0.7	0.2	0.3	0.5	0.7	0.9	1.2	1.3
Standard error		0.03	0.04	0.03	0.03	0.04	0.03	0.03	0.04
M 19–30 y	1715	0.7	0.1	0.2	0.4	0.6	0.9	1.1	1.3
Standard error		0.02	0.01	0.01	0.02	0.02	0.02	0.03	0.0'
M 31–50 y	2314	0.6	0.1	0.2	0.3	0.6	0.9	1.1	1.3
Standard error		0.02	0.01	0.01	0.02	0.02	0.02	0.04	0.07
M 51–70 y	1836	0.7	0.1	0.2	0.4	0.7	1.0	1.2	1.4
Standard error		0.02	0.01	0.01	0.02	0.02	0.02	0.04	0.05
M 71+ y	1150	0.8	0.2	0.2	0.5	0.7	1.0	1.3	1.5
Standard error		0.02	0.02	0.02	0.03	0.02	0.03	0.04	0.06
F 9–13 y	1045	1.0	0.4	0.5	0.8	1.0	1.2	1.4	1.5
Standard error		0.03	0.03	0.03	0.03	0.04	0.03	0.05	0.07
F 14–18 y	906	0.9	0.3	0.4	0.6	0.8	1.1	1.3	1.5
Standard error		0.04	0.03	0.03	0.03	0.03	0.04	0.06	0.07
F 19–30 y	1973	0.7	0.2	0.3	0.5	0.7	1.0	1.2	1.3
Standard error		0.02	0.03	0.03	0.03	0.05	0.05	0.05	0.05
F 31–50 y	2778	0.8	0.2	0.3	0.5	0.7	1.0	1.2	1.1
Standard error		0.02	0.01	0.02	0.02	0.01	0.02	0.03	0.04
F 51–70 y	1907	0.9	0.3	0.4	0.6	0.9	1.1	1.4	1.6
Standard error		0.03	0.02	0.02	0.03	0.03	0.03	0.04	0.06
F 71+ y	1251	1.0	0.3	0.5	0.7	1.0	1.3	1.:5	1.7
Standard error		0.02	0.02	0.02	0.03	0.02	0.02	0.03	0.05

Appendix A19.1: Mean and percentiles for serum vitamin C (mg/dL), NHANES III (1988–1994). Source: Iowa State University Department of Statistics, 1999.

Sex/Age	n	Mean	SEM	5th	10th	25th	50th	75th	90th	95th
Both sexes 4–8 y	3,128	11.0	0.3	4.4	5.3	6.9	9.4	12.8	16.9	21.8
M 9–13 y	1129	9.0	0.3	3.4	4.0	5.6	7.7	10.9	15.3	18.1
M 14–18 y	865	6.0	0.4	2.3	2.6	3.4	4.7	7.4	10.5	13.2
M 19–30 y	1856	5.0	0.1	1.8	2.2	2.9	4.0	6.2	8.7	11.1
Males 31–50 y	2493	5.7	0.2	1.9	2.3	3.2	4.6	7.1	10.5	12.8
M 51–70 y	1987	7.4	0.2	2.2	2.7	3.7	5.7	9.3	14.3	17.8
M > 70 y	1370	9.0	0.3	2.3	3.1	4.5	6.9	11.1	17.9	21.7
F 9–13 y	1149	8.2	0.3	3.1	3.8	4.9	6.8	10.3	13.9	17.8
F 14–18 y	936	5.7	0.2	2.1	2.5	3.2	4.9	7.2	9.7	12.1
F 19–30 y	1915	5.8	0.2	1.8	2.3	3.1	4.6	7.2	10.5	13.1
F 31–50 y	2929	6.5	0.2	1.9	2.3	3.3	4.9	8.2	12.4	16.0
F 51–70 y	2087	8.9	0.3	2.4	2.9	4.2	6.6	11.4	17.0	22.2
F > 70 y	1534	10.7	0.4	2.9	3.6	5.1	8.0	13.7	20.6	26.6
Pregnant F 14–55 y	327	10.5	0.8	*	3.4	4.7	8.4	13.9	18.5	*

Appendix A22.1: Mean and selected percentiles for serum folate (ng/mL), NHANES III (1988–1994). NOTE: Values have been adjusted by following recommendations in Life Sciences Research Office/Federation of American Societies for Experimental Biology. 1994. Assessment of the Folate Methodology Used in the Third National Health and Nutrition Examination Survey (NHANES III, 1988–1994). Raiten Di, Fisher KD, eds. Bethesda, MD: LSRO/ FASEB. *Figure does not meet standard of reliability or precision. Source: C.I. Johnson and J.D. Wright, National Center for Health Statistics, Centers for Disease Control and Prevention, 1997.

Sex/Age	n	Mean	SEM	5th	10th	25th	50th	75th	90th	95th
Both sexes, 4–8 y	3,157	222	12.6	123	140	170	212	258	312	359
M 9–13 y	1137	202	4.2	102	116	149	190	242	306	342
M 14–18 y	864	164	4.4	83	94	116	149	197	261	301
M 19–30 y	1853	164	2.8	84	95	119	151	192	244	300
M 31–50 y	2484	182	3.0	86	102	127	166	217	282	335
M 51–70 y	1968	216	4.5	93	108	139	188	269	353	425
M > 70 y	1266	242	7.3	93	113	149	207	305	419	471
F 9–13 y	1145	175	3.4	87	104	129	167	216	260	288
F 14–18 y	934	157	4.0	77	89	115	141	190	240	269
F 19–30 y	1917	168	3.3	77	88	116	149	206	270	315
F 31–50 y	2924	194	3.4	84	97	125	172	239	324	369
F 51–70 y	2059	238	5.5	95	113	149	206	296	408	462
F > 70 y	1374	259	7.3	96	116	160	228	325	432	519
Pregnant F 14–55 y	322	261	12.5	*	123	164	248	344	429	*

Appendix A22.2: Mean and selected percentiles for erythrocyte folate (ng/mL), NHANES III (1988–1994). NOTE: Values have been adjusted by following recommendations in Life Sciences Research Office/Federation of American Societies for Experimental Biology. 1994. Assessment of the Folate Methodology Used in the Third National Health and Nutrition Examination Survey (NHANES III, 1988–1994). Raiten Di, Fisher KD, eds. Bethesda, MD: LSRO/FASEB. * Figure does not meet standard of reliability or precision. Source: C.I. Johnson and J.D. Wright, National Center for Health Statistics, Centers for Disease Control and Prevention, 1997.

Sex/Age	n	Mean	SEM	5th	10th	25th	50th	75th	90th	95th
M 12–13 y	177	6.61	0.20	3.90	4.40	5.30	6.50	7.70	8.61	9.51
M 14–18 y	395	8.39	0.34	4.80	5.40	6.20	7.40	9.01	11.60	15.30
M 19–30 y	816	10.29	0.26	5.70	6.40	7.60	9.20	11.20	13.90	17.53
M 31–50 y	1055	9.93	0.20	6.00	6.40	7.70	9.00	10.89	13.90	16.38
M 51–70 y	821	11.94	0.49	6.40	7.40	8.51	10.20	12.89	15.30	18.38
M > 70 y	502	13.40	0.49	6.80	7.90	9.31	12.11	15.70	19.01	22.70
F 12–13 y	226	6.19	0.22	3.40a	3.70	4.70	5.80	7.20	8.51	9.51
F 14–18 y	448	7.08	0.19	3.50	4.20	5.60	6.50	7.90	9.90	12.10
F 19–30 y	938	8.05	0.15	4.70	5.10	5.90	7.20	9.40	12.20	14.09
F 31–50 y	1446	8.36	0.16	4.50	5.09	6.10	7.50	9.20	12.40	14.30
F 51–70 y	937	9.68	0.19	5.20	5.70	7.40	8.90	11.01	14.10	16.01
F > 70 y	681	11.83	0.36	6.40	7.01	8.40	10.61	13.40	17.30	20.53
Pregnant F 14–55 y	143	5.41	0.36	*	*	3.50	4.90	6.40	*	*

Appendix A22.3: Mean and percentiles for serum homocysteine (μmol/L), NHANES III (1988–1994). * Figure does not meet standard of reliability or precision. Source: C.I. Johnson and J.D. Wright, National Center for Health Statistics, Centers for Disease Control and Prevention, 1997.

Sex/Age	n	Mean	SEM	5th	10th	25th	50th	75th	90th	95th
Both sexes, 4–8 y	1519	781	13.2	409	474	569	720	909	1103	1270
M 9–13 y	550	620	12.7	344	379	470	590	746	868	947
M 14–18 y	458	516	14.0	261	335	395	485	589	767	871
M 19–30 y	891	470	8.1	251	281	355	466	550	666	762
M 31–50 y	1201	473	8.4	236	287	348	436	556	681	803
M 51–70 y	937	460	23.7	190	247	317	414	540	688	884
M > 70 y	614	449	21.0	187	218	298	382	512	719	881
F 9–13 y	595	612	13.6	344	383	453	569	694	880	1060
F 14–18 y	496	509	14.6	276	300	362	460	618	791	871
F 19–30 y	1049	479	42.1	214	250	328	437	580	721	805
F 31–50 y	1639	497	42.8	223	262	332	427	589	729	827
F 51–70 y	1078	504	12.7	224	266	344	465	605	769	919
F > 70 y	824	536	66.1	186	232	315	436	622	795	953
Pregnant F 14–55 y	173	426	53.1	*	246	293	421	501	579	*

Appendix A22.4: Mean and percentiles for serum vitamin B_{12} (pg/mL), NHANES III (1988–1994). * Figure does not meet standard of reliability or precision. Source: C.I. Johnson and J.D. Wright, National Center for Health Statistics, Centers for Disease Control and Prevention, 1997.

Sex/Age	n	Mean	SEM	5th	10th	25th	50th	75th	90th	95th
Both sexes 6–8 y	1369	30.0	1.7	6.0	9.2	15.1	25.5	36.9	53.3	64.0
M 9–13 y	1184	96.1	73.7	7.0	9.0	14.3	23.7	39.6	57.6	70.5
M 14–18 y	876	26.0	1.4	6.0	8.4	12.5	21.0	30.2	44.6	58.9
M 19–30 y	1852	21.3	0.9	3.8	5.7	10.0	15.3	23.9	38.3	52.7
M 31–50 y	2481	18.2	0.7	2.9	4.6	8.3	13.8	21.6	34.4	45.7
M 51–70 y	1896	29.7	6.2	3.6	4.6	8.0	14.1	23.2	37.7	50.0
M 71+ y	1181	33.0	4.1	4.4	5.8	9.5	15.5	27.1	43.8	68.0
F 9–13 y	1146	23.3	1.0	4.6	7.0	11.4	17.9	26.5	42.3	52.2
F 14–18 y	897	26.9	2.8	4.4	6.2	10.5	17.2	27.5	49.0	66.6
F 19–30 y	1860	31.9	13.4	2.9	4.6	7.8	12.9	19.9	29.4	41.2
F 31–50 y	2886	18.8	1.6	2.1	2.9	5.5	11.1	19.0	31.9	41.3
F 51–70 y	2009	23.5	1.8	2.4	3.3	5.8	11.0	19.0	31.2	44.4
F 71+ y	1228	39.7	11.5	3.5	4.4	6.8	12.6	21.4	36.1	50.3
F Pregnant	343	19.6	1.1	*	5.8	9.2	14.0	25.2	39.7	*
F Lactating	95	*	*	*	*	*	*	*	*	*

Appendix A25.1: Mean, standard error of the mean (SEM), and percentiles for urinary iodine (μg/dL) NHANES III. Note: Means, standard errors, and percentiles calculated with WesVar Complex Samples 3.0. Females who had "blank but applicable" pregnancy and lactating status data or who responded "I don't know" to questions on pregnancy and lactating status were excluded from all analyses. * Figure does not meet standard of reliability or precision. Source: ENVIRON International Corporation, 2000.

Index

Appendix entries are marked with a suffix "A"